GI/LIVER
SECRETS

GI/LIVER SECRETS

Third Edition

Peter R. McNally, DO, FACP, FACG
Chief, GI/Hepatology
Evans Army Hospital
Colorado Springs, Colorado
Formerly, Director, GI/Hepatology Fellowship Program
University of Colorado Health Sciences Center
Denver, Colorado

ELSEVIER
MOSBY

ELSEVIER
MOSBY

1600 John F. Kennedy Boulevard, Suite 1800
Philadelphia, PA 19103-2899

GI/Liver Secrets ISBN: 1-56053-618
Third Edition

Notice

Previous editions copyrighted 2001, 1996

Library of Congress Cataloging-in-Publication Data
GI/liver secrets/[edited by] Peter R. McNally.–3rd ed.
     p. ; cm.
  Includes bibliographical references and index.
  ISBN 1-56053-618-7
  1. Digestive organs–Diseases–Examinations, questions, etc. I. McNally, Peter R., 1954
  [DNLM: 1. Digestive System Diseases–Examination Questions. WI 18.2 G428 2006]
RC802.G52 2006
616.3'0076–dc22

20050478

Vice President, Medical Education: Linda Belfus
Developmental Editor: Stan Ward
Senior Project Manager: Cecelia Bayruns
Marketing Manager: Kate Rubin

Printed in China.

Last digit is the print number: 9 8 7 6 5 4 3 2 1

Working together to grow
libraries in developing countries

www.elsevier.com | www.bookaid.org | www.sabre.org

ELSEVIER   BOOK AID International   Sabre Foundation

CONTENTS

op 100 Secrets 1

I. ESOPHAGUS

1. Swallowing Disorders and Dysphagia 11
   Mehnaz A. Shafi, MD, and Gulchin A. Ergun, MD

2. Gastroesophageal Reflux Disease 19
   Peter R. McNally, DO

3. Esophageal Infections 29
   Dirk R. Davis, MD

4. Esophageal Causes of Chest Pain 34
   Brian T. Johnston, MD, and Donald O. Castell, MD

5. Achalasia 43
   Xiaotuan Zhao, MD, PhD, and Pankaj Jay Pasricha, MD

6. Esophageal Cancer 51
   Nimish Vakil, MD

7. Pill-Induced and Corrosive Injury of the Esophagus 56
   Matthew Bachinski, MD

8. Barrett's Esophagus 69
   Richard E. Sampliner, MD

9. Esophageal Anomalies 73
   John H. Meier, MD

II. STOMACH

10. Gastritis 79
    Frank L. Lanza, MD

11. Gastric Cancer 85
    John C. Deutsch, MD

12. Peptic Ulcer Disease and *Helicobacter pylori* 90
    Khalouck M. Abdrabbo, MD, and David A. Peura, MD

13. Gastric Polyps and Thickened Gastric Folds 98
    Gregory G. Ginsberg, MD

14. Gastroparesis 110
     Erik G. Kerekes, MD, and Michael H. Walter, MD

III. LIVER AND BILIARY TRACT DISORDERS

15. Evaluation of Abnormal Liver Tests 119
     Kenneth E. Sherman, MD, PhD

16. Viral Hepatitis 120
     Kenneth E. Sherman, MD, PhD

17. Antiviral Therapy for Hepatitis C Infection 130
     Jorge L. Herrera, MD

18. Antiviral Therapy for Hepatitis B 143
     Jorge L. Herrera, MD

19. Autoimmune Hepatitis: Diagnosis 151
     Albert J. Czaja, MD

20. Autoimmune Hepatitis: Treatment 160
     Albert J. Czaja, MD

21. Primary Biliary Cirrhosis and Primary Sclerosing
     Cholangitis 177
     Jayant A. Talwalkar, MD, MPH, and Nicholas F. LaRusso, MD

22. Hepatitis Vaccines and Immunoprophylaxis 188
     Col. Maria H. Sjögren, MD, and Marcos Amorim, MD

23. Liver Problems in Pregnancy 196
     Anca I. Pop, MD, and Caroline A. Riely, MD

24. Rheumatologic Manifestations of Hepatobiliary Diseases 207
     Sterling G. West, MD

25. Evaluation of Focal Liver Masses 214
     Steven P. Lawrence, MD

26. Drug-Induced Liver Disease 222
     Peter R. McNally, DO

27. Alcoholic Liver Disease 231
     Thomas E. Trouillot, MD

28. Vascular Liver Disease 236
     Augustin R. Attwell, MD, and Marcelo Kugelmas, MD

29. Nonalcoholic Fatty Liver Disease 245
     Steven Zacks, MD, MPH, and Roshan Shrestha, MD

30. Liver Transplantation 254
     Kevin S. Sieja, MD, and James F. Trotter, MD

31. Ascites 268
    Carlos Guarner, MD, and Bruce A. Runyon, MD

32. Liver Abscess 281
    Jorge L. Herrera, MD, and Jason M. Wilkes, MD

33. Inheritable Forms of Liver Disease 287
    Bruce R. Bacon, MD

34. Liver Histopathology 296
    Janet K. Stephens, MD, PhD, and George H. Warren, MD

35. Hepatobiliary Cystic Disease 310
    Randall E. Lee, MD

36. Gallbladder: Stones, Sludge, and Polyps 317
    Cynthia W. Ko, MD, MS, and Sum P. Lee, MD, PhD

37. Sphincter of Oddi Dysfunction 324
    Erik W. Springer, MD, and Raj J. Shah, MD

V. PANCREATIC DISORDERS

38. Acute Pancreatitis 331
    Michael W. Cheng, MD, and Jamie S. Barkin, MD

39. Chronic Pancreatitis 342
    Michael W. Cheng, MD, and Jamie S. Barkin, MD

40. Pancreatic Cancer 352
    Sergey V. Kantsevoy, MD, PhD, and Anthony N. Kalloo, MD

41. Cystic Disease of the Pancreas 356
    Randall E. Lee, MD

V. SMALL AND LARGE BOWEL DISORDERS

42. Celiac Disease, Tropical Sprue, Whipple's Disease,
    Lymphangiectasia, Immunoproliferative Small Intestinal Disease,
    and Nonsteroidal Anti-Inflammatory Drugs 361
    David J. Kaufman, DO, and Ingram M. Roberts, MD

43. Crohn's Disease 368
    Aaron Brzezinski, MD, and Bret A. Lashner, MD

44. Ulcerative Colitis 379
    Ramona O. Rajapakse, MD, and Burton I. Korelitz, MD

45. Eosinophilic Gastroenteritis 388
    Christian Jost, MD, and Michael B. Wallace, MD, MPH

46. Bacterial Overgrowth 397
    Jack A. DiPalma, MD

47. Colorectal Cancer and Colon Cancer Screening 40
Stephen P. Laird, MD, MS, and Neil W. Toribara, MD, PhD

48. Constipation and Fecal Incontinence 41
Peter E. Legnani, MD, and Suzanne Rose, MD, MSEd

49. Diverticulitis 42
Erik J. Pieramici, MD, JD, and Stephen R. Freeman, MD

50. Diseases of the Appendix 43
Jonathan A. Schoen, MD, and Frank H. Chae, MD

51. Colitis: Pseudomembranous, Microscopic, and Radiation 43
Jill M. Watanabe, MD, MPH, and Christina M. Surawicz, MD

52. Upper Gastrointestinal Tract Hemorrhage 44
John S. Goff, MD

53. Lower Gastrointestinal Tract Bleeding 44
Peter R. McNally, DO

54. Occult and Obscure Gastrointestinal Bleeding 45
John S. Goff, MD

55. Evaluation of Acute Abdominal Pain 45
Peter R. McNally, DO, and James E. Cremins, MD

56. Evaluation of Acute Diarrhea 46
Col. Kent C. Holtzmuller, MD

57. Chronic Diarrhea 47
Lawrence R. Schiller, MD

58. AIDS and the Gastrointestinal Tract 49
C. Mel Wilcox, MD

59. Intestinal Ischemia 500
Arvey I. Rogers, MD, and David S. Estores, MD

60. Nutrition and Malnutrition 511
Peter R. McNally, DO, and Jonathan P. Kushner, MD

61. Potpourri: Nausea and Vomiting, Hiccups,
Bulimia/Anorexia, and Rumination 518
Steven S. Shay, MD

62. Foreign Bodies and the Gastrointestinal Tract 527
George Triadafilopoulos, MD

63. Irritable Bowel Syndrome 531
Ashok K. Tuteja, MD, MRCP, MPH

64. Endoscopic Cancer Screening and Surveillance 538
Peter R. McNally, DO, and Scot M. Lewey, DO

VI. MULTISYSTEM MANIFESTATIONS OF GASTROINTESTINAL DISEASE

65. Rheumatologic Manifestations of Gastrointestinal Disease 547
Sterling G. West, MD

66. Dermatologic Manifestations of Gastrointestinal Disease 559
James E. Fitzpatrick, MD

67. Endocrine Disorders and the Gastrointestinal Tract 567
John A. Merenich, MD, and William J. Georgitis, MD

VII. GASTROINTESTINAL RADIOLOGY

68. Radiography and Radiographic/Fluoroscopic Contrast
Examinations 575
Bernard E. Zeligman, MD

69. Interventional Radiology 591
Paul D. Russ, MD, Stephen W. Subber, MD, Dale L. McCarter, MD, and Keith M. Shonnard, MD

70. Interventional Radiology: Fluoroscopic and Angiographic
Procedures 603
Stephen W. Subber, MD, Paul D. Russ, MD, Dale L. McCarter, MD, and Keith M. Shonnard, MD

71. Noninvasive Gastrointestinal Imaging: Ultrasound,
Computed Tomography, Magnetic Resonance Scanning 612
Michael G. Fox, MD, David W. Bean, Jr., MD, Steven H. Peck, MD, and Kevin M. Rak, MD

72. Nuclear Medicine Studies 637
Cyrus W. Partington, MD, and Col. Mike McBiles, II, MD

73. Endoscopic Ultrasound 653
Peter R. McNally, DO

74. Advanced Endoscopic Ultrasound 664
Erik W. Springer, MD, and Mainor Antillon, MD, MBA, MPH

VIII. SURGERY AND THE GASTROINTESTINAL TRACT

75. Surgery of the Esophagus 673
Todd A. Kellogg, MD, Brant K. Oelschlager, MD, and Carlos A. Pellegrini, MD

76. Surgery for Peptic Ulcer Disease 687
Jaimie D. Nathan, MD, and Theodore N. Pappas, MD

77. Surgical Approach to the Acute Abdomen 700
Jonathan A. Schoen, MD, and Frank H. Chae, MD

78. Colorectal Surgery 706
Martin D. McCarter, MD

79. Obesity and Surgical Weight Loss 718
Jonathan A. Schoen, MD, and Frank H. Chae, MD

80. Hepatobiliary Surgery .... 72?

Anthony J. Canfield, MD, John D. Moffat, MD, Michael C. Hotard, MD, and F. Calvin Bigler, MD

81. Laparoscopic Surgery 730

Anthony J. LaPorta, MD, and Brian Barbick, MD

Index 74

CONTRIBUTORS

Khalouck M. Abdrabbo, MD
Assistant Professor of Internal Medicine, Division of Gastroenterology and Hepatology, University of Virginia Health System, Charlottesville, Virginia

Marcos Amorim, MD
Walter Reed Army Medical Center, Washington, District of Columbia

Mainor Antillon, MD, MBA, MPH
Associate Professor of Medicine, Department of Gastroenterology and Hepatology, University of Colorado Health Sciences Center; Anschutz Centers for Advanced Medicine, Aurora, Colorado

Augustin R. Attwell, MD
Department of Gastroenterology and Hepatology, University of Colorado Health Sciences Center, Denver, Colorado

Matthew Bachinski, MD, FACP
Digestive Disease Group, Greenwood, South Carolina

Bruce R. Bacon, MD
James King, MD, Endowed Chair in Gastroenterology; Professor of Medicine; Director of the Division of Gastroenterology, St. Louis University, St. Louis, Missouri

Brian Barbick, MD
Department of Surgery, University of Colorado Health Sciences Center, Denver, Colorado

Jamie S. Barkin, MD, FACP, FACG
Professor of Medicine, Division of Gastroenterology, University of Miami School of Medicine; Chief, Division of Gastroenterology, Mount Sinai Medical Center, Miami, Florida

David W. Bean, Jr., MD
Diagnostic Radiologist, Medical X-Ray Center, PC, Sioux Falls, South Dakota

F. Calvin Bigler, MD, FACS
Southwest Medical Center, Liberal, Kansas

Aaron Brzezinski, MD
Center for Inflammatory Bowel Disease, Department of Gastroenterology, Cleveland Clinic Foundation, Cleveland, Ohio

Anthony J. Canfield, MD, FACS
Southwest Medical Center, Liberal, Kansas

Donald O. Castell, MD
Professor of Medicine, Division of Gastroenterology and Hepatology, Medical University of South Carolina, Charleston, South Carolina

Frank H. Chae, MD, CM, FACS
Head, Bariatric Surgery Fellowship Program; Head, Advanced Laparoscopic Surgery Fellowship Program; Department of Surgery, University of Colorado Health Sciences Center, Denver, Colorado

Michael W. Cheng, MD
Division of Gastroenterology, University of Miami School of Medicine, Miami, Florida

James E. Cremins, MD
Robinwood Medical Center, Hagerstown, Maryland

Albert J. Czaja, MD
Professor of Medicine, Mayo Clinic College of Medicine; Consultant in Gastroenterology and Hepatology, Mayo Clinic, Rochester, Minnesota

Dirk R. Davis, MD, FACG
Northern Utah Gastroenterology, Logan, Utah

John C. Deutsch, MD
Consultant in Gastroenterology, Hepatology, and Oncology, St. Mary's Duluth Clinic Health, Duluth, Minnesota

Jack A. DiPalma, MD
Professor of Medicine, Chief, Division of Gastroenterology, University of South Alabama College of Medicine, Mobile, Alabama

Gulchin A. Ergun, MD
Associate Professor of Medicine, Baylor College of Medicine; Clinical Chief, Digestive Disease Section and Medical Director, Reflux Center, Methodist Hospital, Houston, Texas

David S. Estores, MD
Assistant Professor of Clinical Medicine, University of Miami School of Medicine; Staff Physician, Veterans Affairs Medical Center; Jackson Memorial Hospital, Miami, Florida

James E. Fitzpatrick, MD
Associate Professor, Department of Dermatology, University of Colorado Health Sciences Center, Aurora, Colorado

Michael G. Fox, MD
Radiology Specialists of Denver, PC, Denver, Colorado

Stephen R. Freeman, MD
Associate Professor of Medicine, University of Colorado Health Sciences Center, Aurora, Colorado

William J. Georgitis, MD
Clinical Professor of Medicine, University of Colorado Health Sciences Center, Denver, Colorado

Gregory G. Ginsberg, MD
Associate Professor of Medicine, Division of Gastroenterology, University of Pennsylvania School of Medicine; Director of Endoscopic Services, Hospital of the University of Pennsylvania, Philadelphia, Pennsylvania

John S. Goff, MD, FACG, FACP
Clinical Professor of Medicine, Division of Gastroenterology, University of Colorado Health Sciences Center, Denver, Colorado; Rocky Mountain Clinical Research and Lakewood Endoscopy Center, Lakewood, Colorado

Carlos Guarner, MD
Chief of Liver Section, Gastroenterology Service, Hospital de Saint Pau; Autonomous University of Barcelona, Barcelona, Spain

Jorge L. Herrera, MD
Professor of Medicine, Division of Gastroenterology, University of South Alabama College of Medicine, Mobile, Alabama

Col. Kent C. Holtzmuller, MD
Consultant, Surgeon General's Office; Division of Gastroenterology, Walter Reed Army Medical Center, Washington, District of Columbia

Michael C. Hotard, MD, FACS
Southwest Medical Center, Liberal, Kansas

Brian T. Johnston, MD
Department of Medicine, Royal Victoria Hospital, Belfast, Northern Ireland

Christian Jost, MD
University Hospital Zurich, Zurich, Switzerland

Anthony N. Kalloo, MD
Division of Gastroenterology, Johns Hopkins University School of Medicine, Baltimore, Maryland

Sergey V. Kantsevoy, MD, PhD
Assistant Professor of Medicine, Division of Gastroenterology, Johns Hopkins University School of Medicine, Baltimore, Maryland

David J. Kaufman, DO
Gastroenterology Section, Bridgeport Hospital, Bridgeport, Connecticut

Todd A. Kellogg, MD
Assistant Professor of Surgery, University of Minnesota Medical School, Minneapolis, Minnesota; Regions Hospital, St. Paul, Minnesota

Erik G. Kerekes, MD
Division of Gastroenterology, Loma Linda University Medical Center, Loma Linda, California

Cynthia W. Ko, MD, MS
Division of Gastroenterology, Department of Medicine, University of Washington School of Medicine, Seattle, Washington

Burton I. Korelitz, MD
Clinical Professor of Medicine, Division of Gastroenterology, New York University School of Medicine, New York, New York

Marcelo Kugelmas, MD
Department of Hepatology, University of Colorado Health Sciences Center, Denver, Colorado

Jonathan P. Kushner, MD
Division of Digestive Diseases, University of Cincinnati School of Medicine, Cincinnati, Ohio

Stephen P. Laird, MD, MS
Clinical Instructor, Section of Gastroenterology and Hepatology, Department of Medicine, University of Colorado Health Sciences Center and Denver Health Medical Center, Denver, Colorado

Frank L. Lanza, MD, FACG
Clinical Professor of Medicine, Section of Gastroenterology, Baylor College of Medicine, Houston, Texas

Anthony J. LaPorta, MD, FACS
Clinical Professor of Surgery, University of Colorado Health Sciences Center; Chairman, Department of Surgery, Rose Medical Center, Denver, Colorado

Nicholas F. LaRusso, MD
Professor of Medicine and Biochemistry and Molecular Biology, Division of Hepatology, Mayo Clinic College of Medicine, Rochester, Minnesota

Bret A. Lashner, MD
Director, Center for Inflammatory Bowel Disease, Department of Gastroenterology, Cleveland Clinic Foundation, Cleveland, Ohio

Steven P. Lawrence, MD, FACP, FACG
Arapahoe Gastroenterology, PC, Littleton, Colorado

Randall E. Lee, MD, FACP
Gastroenterologist, Department of Veterans Affairs Northern California Health Care System, Martinez, California; Associate Professor of Medicine, University of California at Davis School of Medicine, Davis, California

Sum P. Lee, MD, PhD
Professor and Head, Division of Gastroenterology, Department of Medicine, University of Washington School of Medicine, Seattle, Washington

Peter E. Legnani, MD
Division of Gastroenterology, Mount Sinai School of Medicine, New York, New York

Scot M. Lewey, DO, FACP
Gastroenterology Associates of Colorado Springs, Colorado Springs, Colorado

Col. Mike McBiles, II, MD
Department of Radiology, University of Texas at San Antonio Health Sciences Center; Brooke Army Medical Center, San Antonio, Texas

Dale L. McCarter, MD
Interventional Radiology, Carmel, Indiana

Martin D. McCarter, MD
Assistant Professor of Surgery, University of Colorado Health Sciences Center, Denver, Colorado

Peter R. McNally, DO, FACP, FACG
Chief, GI/Hepatology, Evans Army Hospital, Colorado Springs, Colorado; Clinical Professor of Medicine, Division of Gastroenterology, University of Colorado Health Sciences Center; Denver, Colorado

John H. Meier, MD
Consultant in Gastroenterology, Gastroenterology Associates, Hickory, North Carolina

John A. Merenich, MD
Clinical Associate Professor of Medicine, University of Colorado Health Sciences Center; Kaiser Permanente Denver, Colorado

John D. Moffat, MD, FACS
Southwest Medical Center, Liberal, Kansas

Jaimie D. Nathan, MD
Department of Surgery, Duke University Medical Center, Durham, North Carolina

Brant K. Oelschlager, MD
Department of Surgery, University of Washington School of Medicine; Eastside Specialty Center, Seattle, Washington

Theodore N. Pappas, MD
Professor, Department of Surgery, Duke University School of Medical; Duke University Medical Center, Durham, North Carolina

Cyrus W. Partington, MD, FACNM, FACR
Department of Radiology, Evans Army Hospital, Fort Carson, Colorado

Pankaj Jay Pasricha, MD
Professor of Internal Medicine; Chief, Division of Gastroenterology and Hepatology, University of Texas Medical Branch, Galveston, Texas

Steven H. Peck, MD
Radiology Specialists of Denver, PC, Denver, Colorado

Carlos A. Pellegrini, MD
Department of Surgery, University of Washington School of Medicine, Seattle, Washington

David A. Peura, MD
Professor of Internal Medicine, Associate Chief of Gastroenterology and Hepatology, Division of Gastroenterology and Hepatology, Department of Internal Medicine, University of Virginia School of Medicine; Digestive Health Center of Excellence, University of Virginia Health System, Charlottesville, Virginia

Erik J. Pieramici, MD, JD
Division of Gastroenterology and Hepatology, Department of Medicine, University of Colorado Health Sciences Center, Denver, Colorado

Anca I. Pop, MD
Division of General Internal Medicine, James H. Quillen Veterans Affair Medical Center, Johnson City, Tennessee

Ramona O. Rajapakse, MD
Division of Gastroenterology, New York University School of Medicine, New York, New York

Kevin M. Rak, MD
Chief, Department of Radiology, Divine Savior Healthcare, Portage, Wisconsin

Caroline A. Riely, MD
Professor of Medicine and Pediatrics, Chief of Hepatology, University of Tennessee School of Medicine, Memphis, Tennessee

Ingram M. Roberts, MD
Associate Clinical Professor of Medicine, Yale University School of Medicine, New Haven, Connecticut; Vice Chair of Medicine, St. Vincent's Hospital, Bridgeport, Connecticut

Arvey I. Rogers, MD, FACP, FACG
Professor Emeritus, Division of Gastroenterology, Department of Medicine, University of Miami School of Medicine, Miami, Florida

Suzanne Rose, MD, MSEd
Associate Professor, Division of Gastroenterology, Department of Medicine; Associate Professor of Medical Education, Mount Sinai School of Medicine, New York, New York

Bruce A. Runyon, MD
Chief, Liver Service, Loma Linda University Medical Center, Loma Linda, California

Paul D. Russ, MD
Professor, Department of Diagnostic Radiology, University of Colorado Health Sciences Center, Denver, Colorado

Richard E. Sampliner, MD
Professor of Medicine, Section of Gastroenterology, University of Arizona College of Medicine; Southern Arizona Veterans Affairs Health Care Center, Tucson, Arizona

Lawrence R. Schiller, MD, FACP, FACG
Program Director, Gastroenterology Fellowship, Baylor University Medical Center, Dallas, Texas

Jonathan A. Schoen, MD
Clinical Instructor in Surgery, University of Colorado Health Sciences Center, Denver, Colorado

Mehnaz A. Shafi, MD
Assistant Professor of Medicine, Gastroenterology Section, Baylor College of Medicine; Methodist Hospital, Houston, Texas

Raj J. Shah, MD
Assistant Professor of Medicine, Department of Gastroenterology and Hepatology, University of Colorado Health Sciences Center; Anschutz Centers for Advanced Medicine, Aurora, Colorado

Steven S. Shay, MD
Department of Gastroenterology, Cleveland Clinic Foundation, Cleveland, Ohio

Kenneth E. Sherman, MD, PhD
Gould Professor of Medicine; Director, Division of Digestive Diseases, University of Cincinnati College of Medicine, Cincinnati, Ohio

Keith M. Shonnard, MD
Interventional Radiology, Carson City, Nevada

Roshan Shrestha, MD
Associate Professor of Medicine, Medical Director of Liver Transplantation, University of North Carolina at Chapel Hill School of Medicine, Chapel Hill, North Carolina

Kevin S. Sieja, MD
Division of Gastroenterology and Hepatology, Department of Medicine, University of Colorado Health Sciences Center, Denver, Colorado

Col. Maria H. Sjögren, MD
Chief, Department of Clinical Investigation, Walter Reed Army Medical Center, Washington, District of Columbia

Erik W. Springer, MD
Department of Gastroenterology and Hepatology, University of Colorado Health Sciences Center, Denver, Colorado

Janet K. Stephens, MD, PhD
Division of Pathology, University of Colorado Health Sciences Center, Denver, Colorado

Stephen W. Subber, MD
Associate Professor, Department of Diagnostic Radiology, University of Colorado Health Sciences Center, Denver, Colorado

Christina M. Surawicz, MD
Professor of Medicine, Division of Gastroenterology, University of Washington School of Medicine; Chief, Division of Gastroenterology, Harborview Medical Center, Seattle, Washington

Jayant A. Talwalkar, MD, MPH
Assistant Professor of Medicine, Division of Hepatology, Mayo Clinic College of Medicine, Rochester, Minnesota

Neil W. Toribara, MD, PhD
Associate Professor of Medicine and Cellular and Structural Biology, University of Colorado Health Sciences Center; Chief, Division of Gastroenterology and Hepatology, Denver Health Medical Center, Denver, Colorado

George Triadafilopoulos, MD
Chief of Gastroenterology, Veterans Affairs Palo Alto Health Care System, Palo Alto, California

Thomas E. Trouillot, MD
Mile High Gastroenterology, PC, Denver, Colorado

James F. Trotter, MD
Assistant Professor of Medicine, University of Colorado Health Sciences Center, Denver, Colorado

Ashok K. Tuteja, MD, MRCP, MPH
Assistant Professor of Medicine, Division of Gastroenterology, University of Utah Health Sciences Center, Salt Lake City, Utah

Nimish Vakil, MD, FACP, FACG
Clinical Professor of Medicine, University of Wisconsin Medical School, Milwaukee, Wisconsin

Michael B. Wallace, MD, MPH
Associate Professor of Gastroenterology, Director of Endoscopic Research, Mayo Clinic, Jacksonville, Florida

Michael H. Walter, MD
Professor of Medicine, Loma Linda University School of Medicine; Chief, Division of Gastroenterology, Loma Linda University Medical Center, Loma Linda, California

George H. Warren, MD
Clinical Associate Professor of Pathology and Medicine, Division of Gastroenterology, University of Colorado Health Sciences Center, Denver, Colorado

Jill M. Watanabe, MD, MPH
Assistant Professor of Medicine, Division of General Internal Division, University of Washington School of Medicine; Harborview Medical Center, Seattle, Washington

Sterling G. West, MD
Professor of Medicine, University of Colorado Health Sciences Center, Denver, Colorado

C. Mel Wilcox, MD
Professor of Medicine and Director, Division of Gastroenterology and Hepatology, University of Alabama School of Medicine, Birmingham, Alabama

Jason M. Wilkes, MD
Division of Gastroenterology, University of South Alabama College of Medicine, Mobile, Alabama

Steven Zacks, MD, MPH
Assistant Professor of Medicine, University of North Carolina at Chapel Hill School of Medicine, Chapel Hill, North Carolina

Bernard E. Zeligman, MD
Associate Professor of Radiology, University of Colorado Health Sciences Center, Denver, Colorado

Xiaotuan Zhao, MD, PhD
Division of Gastroenterology, University of Texas Medical Branch, Galveston, Texas

PREFACE

To practice the art of medicine, one must learn the secrets of physiology, disease, and therapy. In this text you will find the answers to many questions about the hepatic and digestive diseases. We hope that medical students, residents, fellows, and, yes, even attending physicians will find the third edition of *GI/Liver Secrets* instructive and insightful.

As editor, I am most appreciative of all my contributing authors who have shared their invaluable secrets and made this book an enjoyable as well as an educational experience.

Peter R. McNally, DO, FACP, FACG

TOP 100 SECRETS

These secrets are 100 of the top board alerts. They summarize the concepts, principles, and most salient details of gastroenterology and hepatology.

1. Oropharyngeal dysphagia is caused by neuromuscular (80%) or structural disorders (20%). The most common causes are cerebrovascular accident, followed by Parkinson's disease, motor neuron disease, and skeletal myopathy. Think Schatzki's ring in the patient with intermittent solid-food dysphagia.

2. Wait 2 weeks after a stroke-induced oropharyngeal dysphagia before initiation of swallow evaluation or placement of a percutaneous gastrostomy tube.

3. Routine barium swallow radiograph is inadequate to evaluate swallowing disorders. The rapidity of swallowing events requires video imaging to analyze adequately. The anticholinesterase antibody test is 90% sensitive for diagnosis of myasthenia gravis.

4. Nocturnal acid reflux is seen in 54–72% of persons with obstructive sleep apnea. Administration of nighttime continuous positive airway pressure and/or proton pump inhibitor therapy will decrease apnea and acid reflux events. Morbid obesity, body mass index (BMI) >35, is a significant risk factor for antireflux surgery failure.

5. Cytomegalovirus (CMV) is the most common cause of viral esophagitis in an immunocompromised patient; herpes simplex virus (HSV) esophagitis, although rare, is the etiology of viral esophagitis in an immunocompetent patient.

6. Most cases of achalasia are acquired in mid-adult life (ages 30–60) and affect both sexes and all races nearly equally. Rare cases of achalasia may be found as part of a congenital syndrome, such as triple-A syndrome (achalasia, alacrima, and resistance to adrenocorticotropic hormone), also called Allgrove syndrome. Patients with long-standing and untreated achalasia are at a 16-fold increased risk for esophageal cancer. Cancer is often far advanced at the time of presentation.

7. Squamous cell esophageal carcinoma is much more frequent in African Americans than in whites. Obesity has been shown to be an independent risk factor for the development of esophageal cancer.

8. Causes of pill-induced esophagitis include doxycycline, tetracycline, aspirin, quinidine, alendronate sodium (Fosamax), phenytoin, vitamin C, iron, nonsteroidal anti-inflammatory drugs (NSAIDs), and alprenolol. Endoscopy showing deep ulceration with black discoloration after caustic ingestion suggests third-degree chemical burn. Transmural injury with erosions into the mediastinum and/or peritoneal structures is likely.

9. Barrett's esophagus is associated with increased risk for esophageal cancer; the risk appears to be 0.4–0.5% per year. Management of patients with Barrett's esophagus and high-grade dysplasia is controversial. Many experts recommend more frequent surveillance (every 3 months) until cancer is detected, then esophagectomy or referral to a tertiary center for consideration of experimental endoscopic reversal therapy.

10. In patients infected with *Helicobacter pylori* who fail standard treatment, get a culture of the gastric mucosa to determine antibiotic resistance.

11. *H. pylori* is estimated to infect 60% of the world's adult population, possibly making it the most common chronic human bacterial infection. Reasonable indications for the eradication of active *H. pylori* infection include active or past gastric or duodenal ulcer disease, low-grade mucosa-associated lymphoid tissue (MALT) lymphoma, increased risk of gastric cancer (i.e., positive family history or gastric metaplasia on prior biopsies), and initiation of NSAID therapy in older patients.

12. Most gastric polyps are benign; however, curative endoscopic resection is recommended for gastric polyps greater than 5 mm in diameter because forceps biopsy tissue sampling alone may be misleading.

13. Endoscopic ultrasound (EUS) should be used in the evaluation of thickened gastric folds. Routine mucosal biopsy forceps tissue sampling alone will commonly fail to detect infiltrating gastric carcinoma and lymphoma. When thickening or disruption of deeper wall layers is observed on EUS and forceps biopsy is negative, a tunnel of operative full-thickness biopsy should be pursued.

14. Gastrointestinal stromal tumors (GISTs) are the most common subepithelial gastric lesion and have a characteristic appearance on EUS. Older literature commonly misclassified these lesions as leiomyomas. Large (>3 cm) and symptomatic (bleeding, ulceration, abdominal pain) GISTs should be operatively resected. Small, asymptomatic GISTs can be observed with periodic inspection to affirm stability.

15. The number one cause of nausea in women is pregnancy.

16. The hepatitis C virus (HCV) is underdiagnosed in women. Look for risk factors, not abnormal transaminases. Acute HCV may be missed by standard serologic (EIA) testing. Use HCV RNA test methods.

17. The hepatitis D virus (HDV) always occurs with the hepatitis B virus (HBV). Don't waste money on HDV testing, unless the clinical suspicion is high and HBV is present.

18. Hepatitis A and hepatitis B viruses are preventable diseases! Always vaccinate patients at risk.

19. Pegylated interferon, in combination with ribavirin, is the therapy of choice for chronic hepatitis C infection. Sustained viral remission can be achieved with 24 weeks of therapy in 80–85% of patients infected with genotype 2 or 3 and in 45–55% of patients infected with genotype 1. Failure after 12 weeks of antiviral treatment to decrease pretreatment HCV viral load by two log orders is predictive that viral clearance will not occur even with continuation of therapy.

20. Antiviral therapy is indicated for patients with chronic hepatitis B infection, high viral load (>100,000 copies/mL by HBV-DNA PCR assay), and elevated liver enzymes. The goal of antiviral therapy in chronic hepatitis B infection is to normalize serum ALT, achieve e-antigen seroconversion, and improve histology. Most patients remain (HBsAG) HBsAG-positive, despite successful therapy.

21. Hepatitis B virus carriers, defined as HBsAG-positive, have normal liver enzyme levels, negative HBeAg, positive HBeAb, and low levels of circulating virus (<100,000 copies/mL by HBV-DNA PCR assay); they do not require antiviral therapy.

22. Consider autoimmune hepatitis in patients with unexplained acute, or even fulminant, hepatitis. HLA DR3 identifies patients with disease that is more difficult to treat and control. Graft dysfunction after liver transplantation may indicate recurrent or de novo autoimmune hepatitis.

23. Celiac disease may be associated with chronic hepatitis, and immunoglobulin A (IgA) antibodies to endomysium (EMA) and/or tissue transglutaminase (anti-tTG) should be performed in all patients with cryptogenic chronic hepatitis to exclude this diagnosis. Refractoriness to corticosteroids and/or cholestatic features suggest a misdiagnosis of autoimmune hepatitis or an unrecognized variant form of the disease ("overlap syndrome").

24. Up to 80% of patients with primary biliary cirrhosis (PBC) also have coexisting autoimmune diseases. They include sicca (Sjögren's) syndrome; thyroiditis; scleroderma; calcinosis, Raynaud's phenomenon, esophageal dysfunction, sclerodactyly, and telangiectasia (CREST); rheumatoid arthritis, dermatomyositis, systemic lupus erythematosus, renal tubular acidosis, and idiopathic pulmonary fibrosis. The antimitochondrial antibody (AMA) test is positive in 95% of patients with PBC.

25. Most liver-associated enzyme tests should remain within normal ranges during pregnancy, including aspartate aminotransferase, alanine aminotransferase, γ-glutamyl transpeptidase, bilirubin, and prothrombin time. Total alkaline phosphatase (AP) is elevated during pregnancy. The placenta is the major source of AP; levels return to normal within 20 days after delivery.

26. Spider angiomas and palmar erythema appear in about two thirds of pregnant women without liver disease; small esophageal varices are present in approximately 50% of healthy pregnant women without liver disease because of the increased flow in the azygous system. Viral hepatitis is the most common cause of jaundice in pregnancy.

27. All patients with significant liver disease should be screened for osteoporosis and osteomalacia.

28. A serum α-fetoprotein level >500 ng/mL in a patient with cirrhosis and a liver mass is virtually diagnostic of hepatocellular carcinoma. Hepatic adenomas are directly related to the use of oral contraceptive agents or anabolic steroids, and risk directly correlates with duration of use.

29. Simple hepatic cysts, which are the most common incidental liver lesions, need no further evaluation when definitely documented by radiographic study.

30. Metastatic disease is the most common malignancy found on liver imaging, and it almost always presents as multiple lesions.

31. The thiazolidinediones, or the "-glitazone" class of insulin-modulating drugs, is associated with acute hepatitis and liver failure. Elevations of liver enzyme tests during the first year of treatment with rosiglitazone (Avandia) or pioglitazone (Actos) should prompt concern and possible discontinuation of the medication.

32. Drugs that mimic mononucleosis-like hepatitis include diphenylhydantoin, para-amino salicylic acid, sulfonamides, and dapsone. Amoxicillin-clavulanate, chlorpromazine, and erythromycin have been associated with an acute, purulent inflammation of the bile ducts that mimics acute cholecystitis. Nitrofurantoin and minocycline are the most frequent causes of drug-induced chronic hepatitis.

33. Alcohol hepatitis is manifest as jaundice, hepatomegaly, a moderate elevation in the aspartate aminotransferase (AST), and an elevated white blood cell count.

34. Use the discriminant function (DF) formula to help determine whether a patient with alcohol hepatitis will benefit from the use of corticosteroids.

$$DF = [4.6 \times (\text{prothrombin time seconds} - \text{control time})] + \text{serum bilirubin mg/dL}$$

or

$$DF = [4.6 \times (\text{prothrombin time seconds} - \text{control time})] + \text{serum bilirubin mmol/L/17}$$

A DF value >32 is associated with severe alcoholic hepatitis and a high short-term mortality rate (within approximately 1 month). Treatment with corticosteroids is indicated, provided there is no active gastrointestinal hemorrhage or infection.

35. Patients with cirrhotic alcohol liver disease may be candidates for liver transplantation, if they meet proper guidelines for abstinence established by the local transplantation program. Usually a sobriety period of 6 months is mandatory before liver transplant will be considered.

36. The key clinical features of Budd-Chiari syndrome (BCS) include abdominal pain, ascites, and hepatomegaly developing over weeks to months and caudate lobe hypertrophy seen on imaging studies.

37. Up to 40% of patients with nonalcoholic fatty liver disease (NAFLD), exhibiting fibrosis on liver biopsy, will progress to cirrhosis. Liver enzyme tests and radiographic imaging do *not* predict which patients with NAFLD have fibrosis or early cirrhosis. Liver biopsy is the only way to identify steatohepatitis or fibrotic stage. Risk factors for NAFLD include female gender, age >50, morbid obesity, diabetes, hyperlipidemia, and AST/ALT ratio greater than 1. As many as 75% of type 2 diabetics have some form of NAFLD.

38. The Model for Endstage Liver Disease (MELD) score is the basis for prioritizing patients for cadaveric liver transplant:

$$R = (0.957 \times \log_e[\text{creatinine mg/dL}] + 0.378 \times \log_e[\text{total bilirubin mg/dL}] + 1.120 \times \log_e[\text{INR}] + 0.643) \times 10$$

Patients with chronic liver disease should be considered for listing as candidates for transplantation, if they have a MELD score ≥14 or life-threatening complications of end-stage liver disease.

39. The King's College Criteria (arterial blood pH <7.30 or a combination of PT >100 seconds, serum creatinine >3.3 mg/dL, and grade III or IV encephalopathy) are the most widely used criteria to determine which patients with fulminant hepatic failure due to acetaminophen poisoning are most likely to benefit from a liver transplant.

40. All patients with new-onset ascites should undergo abdominal paracentesis. The initial laboratory investigation of ascitic fluid should include an ascitic fluid cell count and differential, ascitic fluid total protein, and serum-ascites albumin gradient (SAAG). If ascitic infection is suspected, ascitic fluid should be cultured at the bedside in blood culture bottles.

41. Cirrhosis is the most common cause of ascites (85%). First-line treatment of patients with cirrhosis and ascites consists of sodium restriction (88 mmol per day [2000 mg per day]) and diuretics (oral spironolactone and furosemide). Patients with ascitic fluid polymorphonuclear (PMN) counts ≥250 cells/mm^3 should receive empiric antibiotic therapy.

42. Amebic liver abscesses are usually solitary, located in the right lobe of the liver, and present with right upper quadrant pain and fever; a history of amebic colitis is often not present. Amebic liver

abscesses are managed with parenteral antibiotics alone and rarely, if ever, require percutaneous drainage.

43. The most common cause of pyogenic liver abscess is biliary tract disease; gram-negative organisms are commonly implicated. Pyogenic liver abscesses should be percutaneously drained.

44. Wilson's disease is an autosomal recessive disorder leading to excessive bodily accumulations of copper that can cause cirrhosis, neurologic defects, psychosis, nephrolithiasis, arthropathy, and hemolytic anemia.

45. Gallbladder sludge and stones are common but often asymptomatic. Ultrasonography should be the initial diagnostic modality in patients suspected of having gallbladder sludge or stones. Magnetic resonance (MR) cholangiopancreatography is useful to diagnose common bile duct stones noninvasively. Laparoscopic cholecystectomy is the definitive therapy for sludge or stones with associated symptoms or complications.

46. The sphincter of Oddi functions primarily to regulate bile and pancreatic juice flow into the duodenum and to prevent reflux of duodenal contents into the ducts. If you suspect that someone with upper abdominal pain has sphincter of Oddi dysfunction, obtain hepatic and pancreatic enzymes during an episode of pain. For diagnosis of sphincter of Oddi dysfunction, endoscopic retrograde cholangiopancreatography (ERCP) with manometry is considered to be the gold standard. Suspected sphincter of Oddi dysfunction alone is an independent risk factor for post-ERCP pancreatitis.

47. Absence of a family history of diabetes mellitus with new-onset diabetes mellitus may help identify persons with new-onset pancreatic carcinoma. Patients with hereditary pancreatitis carry a 50- to 70-fold increased risk of pancreatic carcinoma. Screening should begin at ages 35–40 or a decade younger than the first diagnosed case of familial pancreatic carcinoma.

48. Asymptomatic elevation of liver function tests is a new extra-intestinal manifestation seen in up to 42% of celiac patients. Strict adherence to a gluten-free diet will lead to a reduction in aminotransferase levels in the majority of individuals. Failure of liver function test improvement, despite treatment with a gluten-free diet, should prompt consideration of coexistent forms of autoimmune liver disease, such as autoimmune hepatitis, primary biliary cirrhosis, or primary sclerosing cholangitis.

49. Immunoproliferative small intestinal disease (IPSID) is also known as α-heavy-chain disease. IPSID is a type of lymphoma composed of dense lymphoplasmacytic mucosal infiltrate that secretes an abnormal α-heavy-chain protein. The disease affects usually the small intestine from the second part of the duodenum distally into the jejunum. It presents in young adults and is usually associated with poor socioeconomic conditions in the Mediterranean region and many developing nations.

50. The Crohn's Disease Activity Index (CDAI) is currently the standard measure of disease activity for all clinical trials. CDAI scores <150 indicate a clinical remission, and scores >450 indicate a severely active disease. The so-called "string sign" is the radiographic finding of advanced ileal Crohn's disease, causing separation of bowel loops, a narrowed and ulcerated terminal ileum.

51. Antibody tests for the diagnosis of inflammatory bowel disease include anti-saccharomyces cerevisiae antibody (ASCA), which is seen in over 60% of patients with Crohn's disease and in less than 10% of patients with other gastrointestinal diseases; and perinuclear antineutrophil cytoplasmic antibody (pANCA), a test with a 70% sensitivity for ulcerative colitis.

52. The incidence of inflammatory bowel disease (IBD) in first-degree relatives of patients with IBD is 30–100 times higher than in the general population.

53. Severe ulcerative colitis is defined as more than six stools daily with blood and systemic disturbance as shown by fever, tachycardia, anemia, or erythrocyte sedimentation rate (ESR) >30. *Toxic megacolon* is defined as a severe attack of colitis with total or segmental dilation of the colon (diameter of transverse colon usually >5–6 cm).

54. Peripheral eosinophilia is present in most (80%) but not all patients with eosinophilic gastroenteritis. Eosinophilic esophagitis presents with circumferential rings or feline esophagus. Therapy of eosinophilic gastroenteritis with per oral prednisone 0.5 mg/kg/day for 2 weeks will induce remission in 90% of patients, irrespective of the affected gut layer.

55. The clinical manifestations of bacterial overgrowth may be subtle and appear identical to irritable bowel syndrome (IBS). Patients with a history of prior surgery, especially Roux-en-Y limb or Billroth II anastomosis for ulcer disease, are susceptible to bacterial overgrowth.

56. Small bowel diverticula are more common among patients with connective tissue disorder, and they may present with intestinal complaints due to bacterial overgrowth.

57. Colonic inertia is an uncommon cause of constipation characterized by a loss of propulsive forces of the colon. The disorder requires exclusion of colonic or anorectal obstruction and persistence of radiopaque markers throughout the left and right colon 5–7 days after ingestion. 5-HT$_4$ agonists are a new class of compounds shown to be effective in the treatment of IBS-related constipation.

58. Diverticulosis is a common condition related to age and a low fiber diet and remains asymptomatic in 70–80% of people. Diverticulitis occurs in 15–25% of patients with diverticulosis and is mild and successfully managed medically in 80%.

59. The peak incidence of acute appendicitis is ages 15–19. However, appendicitis should be considered among all age groups with abdominal pain and fever, regardless of pain location.

60. A patient with chronic diarrhea and a grossly negative colonoscopy should undergo biopsy of the normal-appearing colonic mucosa to evaluate for microscopic changes consistent with collagenous colitis or lymphocytic colitis.

61. For patients presenting with upper gastrointestinal (UGI) bleeding, the finding of orthostatic changes in hemodynamic measurements (fall of 10–20 mmHg in systolic BP and a pulse rise of 20 beats/min) suggests a blood loss of >1000 mL. Rectal bleeding without signs of orthostatic BP changes or syncope is unlikely due to a UGI bleeding source.

62. Most lower gastrointestinal (LGI) bleeding will stop spontaneously—about 80%. The most common cause of hemodynamically significant LGI bleeding is diverticulosis—30% of all cases.

63. Acute, continuous abdominal pain lasting ≥6 hours will likely require surgical intervention. The most common cause of acute abdominal pain in elderly patients is biliary tract disease— responsible for 25% of all cases.

64. When the appendix is found to be entirely normal during a laparotomy performed for presumed appendicitis in a gravid woman, the appendix should *not* be removed. Removal of the normal appendix triples the risk of fetal loss.

65. Most cases of diarrhea are self-limited and do not require treatment with antibiotics. The most common causes of acute dysentery in the United States are *Campylobacter, Salmonella, Shigella*, and enterohemorrhagic *Escherichia coli. Clostridium difficile* is the most common cause of hospital-acquired diarrhea. *E. coli* O157:H7 should be considered, if a patient with diarrhea develops hemolytic uremia syndrome following the administration of antibiotics. Patients with iron overload are more susceptible to *Yersinia* infections.

66. The likely causes of osmotic watery diarrhea are osmotic laxatives (Mg^{2+}, PO_4^{-3}, SO_4^{-2}) and carbohydrate malabsorption. Celiac disease is a common cause of chronic fatty diarrhea. Serologic testing for IgA antibodies to tissue transglutaminase is the preferred indirect test, but mucosal biopsy remains the gold standard for diagnosis.

67. Microscopic colitis is a syndrome characterized by chronic secretory diarrhea, a normal gross appearance of the colonic mucosa, and a typical pattern of inflammation in colon biopsy specimens. It occurs frequently in older patients and is often associated with fecal incontinence. Treatment with budesonide, bile-acid-binding resins, or bismuth subsalicylate (Pepto-Bismol) has the best reported response rates.

68. Among HIV-infected patients, cytomegalovirus is the most common colonic cause of chronic unexplained diarrhea, and flexible sigmoidoscopy is often adequate to establish the diagnosis. Cryptosporidia and microsporidia (*Enterocytozoon bieneusi*), parasites for which there is no specific antimicrobial treatment, may be "cured" by highly active antiretroviral therapy.

69. Right upper quadrant pain associated with a dilated bile duct in a patient with AIDS is most likely due to papillary stenosis, which is usually infectious in etiology. Drugs are the most common cause of pancreatitis in patients with AIDS.

70. The three major collateral channels of the visceral circulatory system are the pancreaticoduodenal cascade, marginal artery of Drummond, and arc of Riolan.

71. The three clinical forms of ischemic bowel disease are acute mesenteric ischemia from emboli, arterial or venous thrombi, or vasoconstriction; chronic mesenteric ischemia; and colonic ischemia. Acute mesenteric ischemia should be suspected in patients complaining of severe abdominal pain out of proportion to findings on physical examination and when pain is present for more than 2 hours.

72. Morbid obesity is defined as BMI >40. In 2000, over 30% of American adults were considered obese and over 60% were overweight.

73. Vitamin B_{12} deficiency is seen in 37% of patients after bariatric surgery. Routine B_{12} supplementation is recommended postoperatively.

74. Mallory-Weiss esophageal laceration and Boerhaave's syndrome (transmural tear of the esophagus) are the dreaded severe complications of severe vomiting.

75. Most patients with anorexia nervosa are women, but men account for 5–10% of all cases. After suicide, cardiac arrhythmias are the most common cause of death among patients with anorexia nervosa.

76. Identify the location, size, and nature of an ingested foreign body, and adjust management accordingly. Always consider a hitherto unrecognized anatomic or functional defect that would impair spontaneous passage.

77. Major changes included in New Guidelines on Colorectal Cancer Screening and Surveillance consist of the following:
    - Double contrast barium enema has been downgraded from every 5–10 years to every 5 years because of evidence that its sensitivity is much lower than colonoscopy.
    - Colonoscopy is relied on exclusively for the diagnostic investigation of patients with findings on screening, for postpolypectomy surveillance, and for patients with a family history of non-polyposis colorectal cancer.
    - For people with a family history of colorectal cancer, there is a greater degree of risk stratification.
    - Virtual colonoscopy remains an investigational tool.
    - Most persons with only one or two tubular adenomas <1 cm in size at colonoscopy should have their next colonoscopy at 5 years rather than 3 years.

78. Nighttime back pain with morning stiffness in a patient with inflammatory bowel disease should prompt an evaluation for ankylosing spondylitis.

79. Episodes of peripheral arthritis coincide with flares of colonic inflammation, whereas spinal arthritis occurs independently of bowel disease severity in patients with inflammatory bowel disease.

80. Sister Mary Joseph's nodule is an umbilical metastasis from an underlying visceral malignancy, with the most common sites being stomach, large bowel, ovary, and pancreas. It may be the presenting sign of internal malignancy.

81. Surgical therapy of active pyoderma gangrenosum is contraindicated because of pathergy, the term used for induction and propagation of cutaneous disease in sites of trauma.

82. Children with type 1 diabetes mellitus and malabsorption, growth failure, unstable diabetes, or even subtle gastrointestinal (GI) upset should be screened for celiac disease.

83. In patients being evaluated for hypoglycemia, absence of Whipple's triad makes the diagnosis of insulinoma and other causes of pathologic hypoglycemia very unlikely.

84. Investigating the cause of an acute abdomen with radiography warrants a three-way abdomen series, nothing less.

85. Barium is the contrast medium of choice for diagnostic fluoroscopic-radiographic examinations of the gut, unless contraindicated because of suspected perforation or because barium may accumulate above a mechanical colon obstruction. Findings on barium swallow that help distinguish secondary from primary achalasia include an eccentric, irregular, abruptly marginated "beak," luminal dilatation <4.0 cm above the beak, and a long, narrow segment "beak" (3.5 cm).

86. The single most important indication for enteroclysis is suspected low-grade mechanical obstruction of small bowel.

87. Ultrasound- and computed tomographic (CT)–guided fine needle aspiration (FNA) of suspected neoplasms has 90% sensitivity and 98% specificity. The initial diagnosis of some neoplasms, particularly hepatocellular carcinoma and lymphoma, often requires more tissue obtained from 18-G core biopsy to evaluate histologic architecture and for immunohistochemistry.

88. With some exceptions, most intra-abdominal and retroperitoneal abscesses can be drained successfully with an 8 Fr, self-retaining, locking pigtail, all-purpose catheter, introduced using either the Seldinger or trocar technique.

89. Hepatic transarterial chemoembolization (TACE) is often used in the treatment of hepatocellular carcinoma (HCC). TACE is palliative in the treatment of HCC; emerging data suggest some increase in overall mean survival following TACE.

90. Mesenteric angiography can detect the site of gastrointestinal hemorrhage, if there is active bleeding at the time of the study and if the rate of bleeding exceeds 1.5–2.0 mL/min.

91. By reducing the portosystemic pressure gradient to <12 mmHg, percutaneous placement of a transjugular intrahepatic portosystemic shunt (TIPS) between the portal and hepatic veins significantly reduces the complications caused by portal hypertension.

92. In the evaluation of the pancreatobiliary tree, magnetic resonance cholangiopancreatography (MRCP) is noninvasive and less expensive than endoscopic retrograde cholangiopancreatography (ERCP). In addition, it does not require radiation or sedation, can detect extraductal pathology, better visualizes ducts proximal to an obstruction, and visualizes the ducts in their "native" state.

93. An appendix larger than 6 mm on ultrasonography (US) is abnormal. Acute appendicitis is suspected when it is distended and noncompressible, contains an appendicolith, adjacent fluid collection, peritoneal fluid, and/or a focal mixed echogenic mass representing a phlegmon or abscess. US is 85–90% sensitive in the diagnosis of appendicitis.

94. In pediatric cases of GI bleeding, Tc-99 pertechnetate scanning is particularly useful in detecting Meckel's diverticula containing gastric mucosa.

95. Decreased gallbladder ejection fraction (<40%), as determined by cholescintigraphy and sincalide infusion, is predictive of acalculous cholecystitis and symptom relief with cholecystectomy. Cholescintigraphy is a very sensitive and specific test for identification of bile leak after cholecystectomy.

96. A gallium-67 avid liver lesion is highly suspicious for hepatoma.

97. In 77% of patients with recurrent idiopathic pancreatitis and negative CT, US, or ERCP testing, EUS identified stones in the gallbladder and/or common bile duct. EUS identification of large paraesophageal varices >5 mm is predictive of future variceal hemorrhage.

98. A large hiatal hernia, stricture with persistent dysphagia, and Barrett's esophagus are characteristics of advanced gastroesophageal reflux disease (GERD) and may predict less than ideal results from surgical antireflux procedure.

99. More than 10 polyps found at endoscopy may indicate familial adenomatous polyposis (FAP) or attenuated FAP. For children with FAP, a total proctocolectomy with ileal J-pouch anal anastomosis should be planned during their mid-teenage years to reduce the risk of cancer.

100. The surgical goal for treating Crohn's disease is to preserve as much intestinal length as possible.

SWALLOWING DISORDERS AND DYSPHAGIA

Mehnaz A. Shafi, MD, and Gulchin A. Ergun, MD

1. **What is the most difficult substance to swallow?**

   Water. Swallowing involves several phases. First, a preparatory phase involves chewing, sizing, shaping, and positioning of the bolus on the tongue. Then, during an oral phase, the bolus is propelled from the oral cavity into the pharynx while the airway is protected. Finally, the bolus is transported into the esophagus. Water is the most difficult substance to size, shape, and contain in the oral cavity. This makes it the hardest to control as it is passed from the oral cavity into the pharynx. Thus, viscous foods are used to feed patients with oropharyngeal dysphagia.

2. **What sensory cues elicit swallowing?**

   The sensory cues are not entirely known, but entry of food or fluid into the hypopharynx, specifically the sensory receptive field of the superior laryngeal nerve, is paramount. Swallowing may also be initiated by volitional effort, if food is present in the oral cavity. The required signal for initiation of the swallow response is a mixture of both peripheral sensory input from oropharyngeal afferents and superimposed control from higher nervous system centers. Neither is capable of initiating swallowing independent of the other. Thus, swallowing cannot be initiated during sleep when higher centers are turned off or with deep anesthesia to the oral cavity when peripheral afferents are disconnected.

3. **What is flexible endoscopic evaluation of swallowing with sensory testing (FEESST)?**

   FEESST is an endoscopic test that allows direct visualization of the hypopharynx and larynx during swallowing evaluation. It can directly assess airway protection during a swallow. A thin, flexible endoscope is passed transnasally into the hypopharynx. Pooling of hypopharyngeal secretions is recorded and is used to gauge aspiration risk. Next, swallowing assessment is done with liquids (mixed with food coloring) of varying consistency, given serially to the patient and observed as they traverse the hypopharynx. Any penetration into the larynx (aspiration) is noted. Finally, discrete pulses of air are given, endoscopically, to the mucosa innervated by the superior laryngeal nerve to elicit the protective laryngeal adductor reflex. This results in brief closure of the vocal cords with or without a swallow. An intact reflex supports a low aspiration risk. FEESST is a safe procedure that can be performed at the bedside or office, and it does not require sedation.

4. **What is the difference between globus sensation (globus hystericus) and dysphagia?**

   Globus sensation is the feeling of a lump in the throat. It is present continually and is not related to swallowing. It may even be temporarily alleviated during a swallow. Dysphagia is difficulty in swallowing and is noted by the patient only during swallowing.

5. **What are common causes of globus sensation?**
   - Gastroesophageal reflux disease
   - Anxiety disorder (must exclude organic disease)
   - Early hypopharyngeal cancer
   - Goiter

   Table 1-1 summarizes the causes of oropharyngeal dysphagia.

TABLE 1-1.   CAUSES OF OROPHARYNGEAL DYSPHAGIA

Propulsive	Structural	Iatrogenic
Neurologic	**Benign**	**Drug induced**
Cerebrovascular accident (medulla, large territory cortical)	Cricopharyngeal bars	Steroid myopathy
	Hypopharyngeal diverticula (Zenker's)	Tardive dyskinesia
Parkinson's disease		Mucositis due to chemotherapy
Amyotrophic lateral sclerosis	Cervical vertebral body osteophytes	
Multiple sclerosis		**Radiation induced**
Degenerative diseases (Alzheimer's, Huntington's, Friedreich's ataxia)	**Skin diseases**	Xerostomia
	Epidermolysis bullosa, pemphigoid, graft vs. host disease	Myopathy
Brain neoplasm (brain stem)		**Prosthetics**
Polio and postpolio syndrome	Lymphadenopathy	Neck stabilization hardware
Cerebral palsy	**Caustic injury**	Ill-fitting dental or intra-oral prostheses
Cranial nerve palsies	Lye	
Recurrent laryngeal nerve palsy	Pill-induced	**Surgery**
Muscular	**Infections**	Oropharyngeal resection
Muscular dystrophy (Duchenne, oculopharyngeal)	Abscess	
	Ulceration	
Myositis and dermatomyositis	Pharyngitis	
Myasthenia gravis	**Autoimmune**	
Eaton-Lambert syndrome	Oral ulcers in Crohn's, Behçet's disease	
Metabolic		
Hypothyroidism with myxedema	Dental	
Hyperthyroidism	Dental anomalies	
Inflammatory/autoimmune	**Neoplasms**	
Systemic lupus erythematosus		
Amyloidosis		
Sarcoidosis		
Infectious		
AIDS with CNS involvement		
Syphilis (tabes dorsalis)		
Botulism		
Rabies		
Diphtheria		
Meningitis		
Viral (coxsackie, herpes simplex)		

CNS = central nervous system.

6. Do patients accurately localize the site of dysphagia?

No. Patients with esophageal dysphagia localize the abnormal site correctly only 60–70% of the time. Patients incorrectly localize the site of dysphagia proximal to the actual site in the remainder. Differentiating between proximal and distal lesions may be difficult, based on the patient's perception only. Patients with oropharyngeal dysphagia usually recognize that the swallow dysfunction is in the oropharynx. They may perceive food accumulating in the mouth or an inability to initiate a pharyngeal swallow. They can generally recognize aspiration before, during, or after a swallow. Associated symptoms, such as difficulty with chewing, drooling, coughing or choking after a swallow, are more suggestive of oropharyngeal than esophageal dysphagia.

7. What are the differences between esophageal and oropharyngeal dysphagia?

See Table 1-2.

TABLE 1-2. ESOPHAGEAL VERSUS OROPHARYNGEAL DYSPHAGIA	
Esophageal Dysphagia	**Oropharyngeal Dysphagia**
Associated symptoms: chest pain, water brash, regurgitation	Associated symptoms: weakness, ptosis, nasal voice, pneumonia, cough
Organ-specific diseases (e.g., esophageal cancer, esophageal motor disorder)	Systemic diseases (e.g., myasthenia gravis, Parkinson's disease)
Treatable (e.g., dilation)	Rarely treatable
Expendable organ (one function only)	Nonexpendable organ (functions include speech, respiration, and swallowing)

8. What symptoms can be seen in oropharyngeal dysphagia?

- Inability to initiate a swallow
- Sensation of food getting stuck in the throat
- Coughing or choking (aspiration) during swallowing
- Nasopharyngeal regurgitation
- Changes in speech or voice (nasality)
- Ptosis
- Photophobia or visual changes
- Weakness, especially progressive toward the end of the day

9. What are the causes of oropharyngeal dysphagia?

Oropharyngeal dysphagia can result from propulsive failure or structural abnormalities of either the oropharynx or esophagus. Propulsive abnormalities can result from dysfunction of the central nervous system control mechanisms, intrinsic musculature, or peripheral nerves. Structural abnormalities may result from neoplasm, surgery, trauma, caustic injury, or congenital anomalies. If dysphagia occurs in the absence of radiographic findings, motor abnormalities may be demonstrable by more sensitive methods, such as electromyography or nerve stimulation studies. If all studies are normal, impaired swallowing sensation may be the primary abnormality (see Table 1-1).

10. What causes oropharyngeal dysphagia in the elderly?

- 80% caused by neuromuscular disorders: Leading cause is cerebrovascular accidents (CVAs); others include Parkinson's disease, myasthenia gravis, and dermatomyositis.
- 20% caused by structural disorders: Cancer is the most worrisome cause.

11. **Why is a brain stem stroke more likely to cause severe oropharyngeal dysphagia than a hemispheric stroke?**

The swallowing center is situated bilaterally, in the reticular substance below the nucleus of the solitary tract, in the brain stem. Efferent fibers from the swallow centers travel to the motor neurons controlling the swallow musculature located in the nucleus ambiguus. Therefore, brain stem strokes are more likely to cause the most severe impairment of swallowing with difficulty in initiating a swallow or absence of the swallow response.

12. **When is it appropriate to evaluate stroke-related dysphagia?**

About 25–50% of strokes will result in oropharyngeal dysphagia. Most stroke-related swallowing dysfunction improves spontaneously within the first 2 weeks. Unnecessary diagnostic or therapeutic procedures, such as percutaneous gastrostomy, should be avoided immediately after a cerebrovascular accident. When symptoms persist *beyond* the 2-week period, swallowing function should be evaluated.

13. **Is a barium swallow examination adequate to evaluate oropharyngeal dysphagia?**

No. A barium swallow focuses on the esophagus, is done in a supine position, and takes only a few still images as the barium passes through the oropharynx. Therefore, aspiration may be missed if a conventional barium swallow is ordered.

Oropharyngeal dysphagia is best evaluated with a cineradiographic or videofluoroscopic swallowing study, commonly called the *modified barium swallow.* The oropharyngeal swallow rapid and transpires in less than 1 second, images must be obtained and recorded at a rate of 15–30/sec to capture adequately the motor events. The recorded study can be played back in slow motion for careful evaluation. This study is done with the patient in the upright position and resembles normal eating position more than the conventional barium swallow.

14. **Can childhood polio cause dysphagia to develop years later in adulthood?**

Yes, even if the initial presentation did not include bulbar involvement. The post polio syndrome is a disorder of the medullary motor neuron resulting from new or continuing instability of previously injured motor neurons. Typically, the syndrome consists of new musculoskeletal symptoms, such as weakness and atrophy in previously affected muscles. Patients become symptomatic 25–35 years after the original illness, and even muscular units (limb or bulbar) that appeared untouched in the original infection may develop signs clinical weakness. Bulbar neuron involvement was reported previously in only 15% of patients with the acute infection. Recent studies demonstrate that some bulbar muscle dysfunction can be demonstrated in all patients with post polio syndrome, although few report dysphagia. Swallowing problems are most severe in patients with bulbar involvement at the onset.

15. **What is the characteristic feature of dysphagia in myasthenia gravis?**

Myasthenia gravis is an autoimmune disorder characterized by progressive destruction of acetylcholine receptors at the neuromuscular junction. It affects the striated portion of the esophageal musculature. A distinct feature is increased muscle weakness with repetitive muscle contraction, such that dysphagia worsens with repeated swallows or as the meal progresses. Resting to allow reaccumulation of acetylcholine in nerve endings improves pharyngo-esophageal functions and symptoms simultaneously. Muscles of facial expression, mastication and swallowing are frequently involved, and dysphagia is a prominent symptom in more than one third of cases. *An anticholinesterase antibody test is about 90% sensitive in diagnosing myasthenia gravis.* If clinical suspicion is strong, a therapeutic trial with an acetylcholinesterase inhibitor, such as Tensilon, or a cholinomimetic, such as Mestinon, should be considered even the absence of the anticholinesterase antibody.

. **Why is simultaneous involvement of the oropharynx and esophagus extremely unusual for any disease process other than infection?**
The oropharynx and the esophagus are fundamentally different in respect to musculature, inner-vation, and neural regulation (Table 1-3). Because most disease processes are specific for a par-ticular type of muscle or nervous system element, it is unlikely that they would involve such diverse systems.

TABLE 1-3. BASIC DIFFERENCES BETWEEN THE OROPHARYNX AND ESOPHAGUS	
Oropharynx	**Esophagus**
Striated muscle	Striated muscle (proximal), smooth muscle (middle and distal)
Direct nicotinic innervation	Myenteric plexus within longitudinal and circular smooth muscles
Cholinergic	Cholinergic, nitric oxide, vasoactive intestinal peptide

. **What is a Zenker's diverticulum?**
A diverticulum of the hypopharynx. It is located posteriorly in an area of potential weakness at the intersection of the trans-verse fibers of the cricopharyngeus and the obliquely oriented fibers of the inferior pharyngeal constrictors, also called the *Killian's dehiscence* (see Fig. 1-1).

. **Is a Zenker's diverticulum the result of an obstructive or propulsive defect?**
Obstructive defect. Previously, it was believed that the pathogenesis of the diverticulum was due to abnormally high hypopharyngeal pressures caused by defective coordination of upper esophageal sphincter (UES) relaxation during pharyngeal bolus propulsion. It is now known that Zenker's diverticulum is caused by a constrictive myopathy of the cricopharyngeus (poor sphincter compli-ance). Increased resistance at the cricopharyngeus and increased intrabolus pressures above this relative obstruction cause muscular stress in the hypopharynx with herniation and diverticulum formation. Thus, Zenker's diverticulum is an *obstructive* rather than propulsive disease.

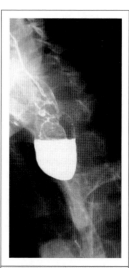

Figure 1-1. Radiograph of Zenker's diverticulum.

. **What are the indications and risks of a cricopharyngeal myotomy?**
See Table 1-4.

. **What is the differential diagnosis of dysphagia in a patient who has had surgery, radiation, and chemotherapy for head and neck cancer?**
- Radiation myositis and/or fibrosis
- Xerostomia (hyposalivation)
- Anatomic defects due to surgery
- Recurrence of malignancy

TABLE 1-4. INDICATIONS AND RISKS OF CRICOPHARYNGEAL MYOTOMY	
Indications	**Risks**
Zenker's diverticulum	Aspiration in patients with gastroesophageal
Cricopharyngeal bar with symptoms	reflux disease
Parkinson's disease with impaired UES relaxation	Worsening of swallow function

UES = upper esophageal sphincter.

KEY POINTS: DYSPHAGIA

1. Water is the most difficult substance to swallow.

2. Critical narrowing of the esophageal lumen for onset of dysphagia is approximately 12 mm.

3. Zenker's diverticulum is caused by relative obstruction by the cricopharyngeus muscle.

21. **What therapies can be used to improve swallowing?**
    The goal of swallow therapy is to help minimize the risk of aspiration and to optimize oral delivery of nutrition.
    - Direct swallow therapies attempt to improve the swallow physiology. Examples include treatment of the primary disease, oral and maxillofacial prosthetics, cricopharyngeal myotomy, and swallow maneuvers, such as the supraglottic swallow.
    - Compensatory techniques help elimiate symptoms but do not change the swallowing dysfunction. They include adjustment of the patient's head and neck, changing food viscosity and optimizing the volume and rate of food delivery.
    - Indirect swallow therapies address the neuromuscular coordination needed for swallowing. Examples include exercise regimens for tongue coordination and chewing.

22. **Which patients are ideal candidates for swallow therapy?**
    Patients who are mentally competent and motivated have the best results with swallow therapy. Therapy is most effective for aspiration (during and after swallow) and unilateral pharyngeal paresis.

23. **What are the etiologies of dysphagia in gastroesophageal reflux disease?**
    - Inflammation: 30% of patients with esophagitis experience dysphagia.
    - Stricture: dysphagia occurs when the lumen diameter is less than 11–13 mm.
    - Peristaltic dysfunction: this is seen with advanced disease.
    - Hiatus hernia: up to 30% of patients with a hiatus hernia may have dysphagia.

24. **What are the common symptoms and causes of xerostomia?**

Symptoms	*Causes*
Dysphagia	Sjögren's syndrome
Dry mouth with viscous saliva	Rheumatoid arthritis
Bad taste in mouth	Drugs (e.g., anticholinergics, antidepressants)
Oral burning	Radiation therapy
Dental decay	
Bad breath	

Why is "cricopharyngeal achalasia" a misnomer? How does it differ from classic achalasia?

The upper esophageal sphincter (UES) is a *striated muscle,* which is dependent on tonic excitation to maintain contractility. If innervation to the cricopharyngeus is lost, the UES relaxes and becomes flaccid. This is in contrast to the lower esophageal sphincter (LES). The LES is a 3–4 cm long segment of tonically contracted *smooth muscle* at the distal end of the esophagus. LES tonic contraction is a property of both the muscle itself and its extrinsic innervation (Table 1-5). Normal resting tone of the LES varies from 10–30 mmHg, being least in the postcibal period and greatest at night. Classic achalasia is caused by loss of the inhibitory myenteric plexus neurons in the distal esophagus, thereby leaving no mechanism to inhibit myogenic contraction.

TABLE 1-5. LOWER VERSUS UPPER ESOPHAGEAL SPHINCTER		
	LES	**UES**
Resting tone	Myogenic	None
Result of denervation	Contraction	Relaxation
Cause of impaired opening	Failure of relaxation	Failure of traction (pulling open)
Source of opening force	Bolus	Suprahyoid and infrahyoid musculature

LES = lower esophageal sphincter; UES = upper esophageal sphincter.

When is botulinum toxin (BTX) used for dysphagia?

BTX has been best studied in dysphagia due to achalasia. Achalasia is caused by selective loss of inhibitory neurons at the LES, resulting in unopposed (tonic) excitation of the LES. BTX injection into the distal esophagus can reduce LES pressure by blocking acetylcholine release from the presynaptic cholinergic nerve terminals in the myenteric plexus. Surgical myotomy is the definitive treatment for achalasia, because repeated BTX therapy is required to maintain efficacy. Ideal candidates for BTX are the elderly and those at high operative risk.

Surgical cricopharyngeal myotomy is the treatment of choice for Zenker's diverticulum. Endoscopic injection of BTX into the diverticular spur, as an alternative to surgery, has shown favorable results in case reports. BTX in Parkinson's disease with dysphagia, due to impaired relaxation of the UES, has also shown marked improvement by videofluoroscopic and electromyographic studies. Potential side effects include persistent stenosis and the risk of local BTX diffusion into the larynx or hypopharynx.

WEBSITES

1. http://www.nlm.nih.gov/medlineplus/dysphagia.html
2. http://www.pentaxmedical.com/products/ENT.asp

BIBLIOGRAPHY

1. Aviv JE, Kaplan ST, Thomson JE, et al: The safety of flexible endoscopic evaluation of swallowing with sensor testing (FEESST): An analysis of 500 consecutive evaluations. Dysphagia 15(1):39–44, 2000.

2. Cook IJ, Gabb M, Panagopoulos V, et al: Pharyngeal (Zenker's) diverticulum is a disorder of upper esophageal sphincter opening. Gastroenterology 103:1229–1235, 1992.

3. Cook IJ, Kahrilas PJ: AGA technical review of management of oropharyngeal dysphagia. Gastroenterology 116:455–478, 1999.

4. Kahrilas PJ, Logemann JA, Lin S, Ergun G: Pharyngeal clearance during swallowing: A combined manometric and videofluoroscopic study. Gastroenterology 103:128–136, 1992.

5. Kolbasnik J, Waterfall WE, Fachnie B: Long term efficacy of botulinum toxin in classical achalasia: A prospective study. Am J Gastroenterol 94:3434–3439, 1999.

6. Ramsey DJ, Smithard DG, Kalra L: Early assessment of dysphagia and aspiration risk in acute stroke patients. Stroke 34(5):1252–1257, 2003.

7. Restivo DA, Palmeri A, Marchese-Ragona R: Botulinum toxin for cricopharyngeal dysfunction in Parkinson's disease. N Engl J Med 346(15):1174–1175, 2002.

8. Sonies BC, Dalakas MC: Dysphagia in patients with the post-polio syndrome. N Engl J Med 324:1162–1167, 1991.

9. Spechler S: American Gastroenterological Association technical review on treatment of patients with dysphagia caused by benign disorders of the distal esophagus. Gastroenterology 117(1):229–233, 1999.

10. Spinelli P, Ballardini G: Botulinum toxin type A (Dysport) for the treatment of Zenker's diverticulum. Surg End 17(4):660, 2003.

GASTROESOPHAGEAL REFLUX DISEASE

Peter R. McNally, DO

CHAPTER 2

What is gastroesophageal reflux disease (GERD)? How common is it?

GERD is a pathologic condition of symptoms and injury to the esophagus caused by percolation of gastric or gastroduodenal contents into the esophagus. GERD is extremely common. One survey of hospital employees showed that 7% experienced heartburn daily, 14% experienced symptoms weekly, and 15% monthly. Other studies have suggested a 3–4% prevalence of GERD among the general population, with a prevalence increase to approximately 5% in people older than age 55. Pregnant women have the highest incidence of daily heartburn at 48–79%. The distribution of GERD between the sexes is equal, but men are more likely to suffer complications of GERD esophagitis (2–3:1) and Barrett's esophagus (10:1).

What are the typical symptoms of GERD?

Heartburn is usually characterized as a midline retrosternal burning sensation that radiates to the throat and, occasionally, to the intrascapular region. Patients often place the open hand over the sternal area and flip the wrist in an up-and-down motion to simulate the nature and location of the heartburn symptoms. Mild symptoms of heartburn are often relieved within 3–5 minutes of ingesting milk or antacids. Other symptoms of GERD include the following:

- *Regurgitation* consists of eructation of gastric juice or stomach contents into the pharynx and is often accompanied by a noxious bitter taste. Regurgitation is most common after a large meal and occurs usually with stooping or assuming a recumbent posture.
- *Dysphagia* (difficulty in swallowing) is usually caused by a benign stricture of the esophagus in patients with long-standing GERD. Solid foods, such as meat and bread, are often precipitants of dysphagia. Dysphagia implies significant narrowing of the esophageal lumen, to usually a luminal diameter <13 mm. Prolonged dysphagia, associated with inability to swallow saliva, requires prompt evaluation and often endoscopic removal (see Chapter 66, Dermatologic Manifestations of Gastrointestinal Disease).
- *Waterbrash* is an uncommon symptom but highly suggestive of GERD. Patients literally foam at the mouth because the salivary glands produce up to 10 mL/min of saliva as an esophago-salivary reflex response to acid reflux.

Is gastrointestinal (GI) hemorrhage a common symptom of GERD?

No. Endoscopic evaluation of patients with upper GI hemorrhage has identified erosive GERD as the cause in only 2–6% of cases.

What is odynophagia? Is it a common symptom of GERD?

Odynophagia is a painful substernal sensation associated with swallowing that should not be confused with dysphagia. Odynophagia rarely results from GERD. Instead, odynophagia is caused by infections (monilia, herpes simplex virus, and cytomegalovirus), ingestion of corrosive agents or pills (tetracycline, vitamin C, iron, quinidine, estrogen, aspirin, alendronate [Fosamax], or nonsteroidal anti-inflammatory drugs), or cancer.

5. **What clues about GERD can be gleaned from the physical exam?**
   - Severe kyphosis is often associated with hiatal hernia and GERD, especially when a body brace is necessary.
   - Tight-fitting corsets or clothing (in men or women) can increase intra-abdominal pressure and may cause stress reflux.
   - Abnormal phonation may suggest high GERD and vocal cord injury. When hoarseness is due to high GERD, the voice is often coarse or gravelly and may be worse in the morning, whereas in other causes of hoarseness, excessive voice use or abuse leads to worsening later in the day.
   - Wheezing or asthma and pulmonary fibrosis have been associated with GERD. Patients often give a history of postprandial or nocturnal regurgitation with episodes of coughing or choking caused by near or partial aspiration.
   - Loss of enamel on the lingual surface of the teeth may be seen in severe GERD, although it is more common in patients with rumination syndrome or bulimia.
   - Esophageal dysfunction may be the predominant component of scleroderma or mixed connective tissue disease. Inquiry about symptoms of Raynaud's syndrome and examination for sclerodactyly, taut skin, and calcinosis are important.
   - Cerebral palsy, Down syndrome, and mental retardation are commonly associated with GERD
   - Children with peculiar head movements during swallowing may have Sandifer's syndrome.
   - Some patients unknowingly swallow air (aerophagia) that triggers a burp, belch, and heartburn cycle.

   The observant clinician may detect this behavior during the interview and physical exam.

6. **Do healthy persons have GERD?**
   Yes. Healthy persons may regurgitate acid or food contents into the esophagus, especially after a large meal late at night. In normal persons, the natural defense mechanisms of the lower esophageal sphincter barrier and esophageal clearance are not overwhelmed, hence symptoms and injury do not occur. Ambulatory esophageal pH studies have shown that healthy persons have acid reflux into the esophagus <2% of the daytime (upright position) and <0.3% of the nighttime (supine position).

7. **How can swallowing and salivary production be associated with GERD?**
   Reflux of gastric contents into the esophagus often stimulates salivary production and increase swallowing. Saliva has a neutral pH, which helps to neutralize the gastric refluxate. Furthermore the swallowed saliva initiates a peristaltic wave that strips the esophagus of refluxed material (clearance). During the awake upright period, persons swallow 70 times/h; this rate increases to 200 times/h during meals. Swallowing is least common during sleep (<10 times/h), and arousa from sleep to swallow during GERD may be reduced by sedatives or alcohol ingestion. Patients with Sjögren's syndrome and smokers have reduced salivary production and prolonged esophageal acid clearance times.

8. **What are the two defective anatomic mechanisms in patients with GERD?**
   Ineffective clearance and defective gastroesophageal barrier.

9. **What clearance defects are associated with GERD?**
   - Esophageal. Normally, reflux of gastric contents into the esophagus stimulates a secondary peristaltic or clearance wave to remove the injurious refluxate from the esophagus. The wors case of ineffective esophageal clearance is seen in patients with scleroderma. The lower esophageal sphincter barrier is nonexistent, and there is no primary or secondary peristalsis of the esophagus (hence, no clearance).
   - Gastric. Gastroparesis may lead to excessive quantities of retained gastroduodenal and food contents. Larger volumes of stagnant gastric contents predispose to esophageal reflux.

How may the gastroesophageal (GE) barrier be compromised?
The normal lower esophageal sphincter (LES) is 3–4 cm long and maintains a resting tone of 10–30 mmHg pressure. The LES acts as a barrier against GERD. When the LES pressure is <6 mmHg, GERD is common; however, the presence of "normal" LES pressure does not predict absence of GERD. In fact, LES pressure <10 mmHg is found in a minority of people with GERD. Recent studies have shown that transient LES relaxations (tLESRs) are important in the pathogenesis of GERD. During tLESR, the sphincter inappropriately relaxes and free gastric reflux occurs.

What foods and medications influence resting LES pressure?
See Table 2-1.

TABLE 2-1. INCREASED VERSUS DECREASED LOWER ESOPHAGEAL SPHINCTER PRESSURE

	Increased LES Pressure	Decreased LES Pressure
Food	Protein	Fat
		Chocolate
		Ethanol
		Peppermint
Medications	Antacids	Calcium channel antagonists
	Metoclopramide	Theophylline
	Cisapride	Diazepam
	Domperidone	Meperidine
		Morphine
		Dopamine
		Barbiturates

What other medical conditions may mimic symptoms of GERD?
The differential diagnosis of GERD includes coronary artery disease, gastritis, gastroparesis, infectious and pill-induced esophagitis, peptic ulcer disease, biliary tract disease, and esophageal motor diseases.

What medical condition clinically presents with dysphagia and is often mistaken for GERD?
Eosinophilic esophagitis. The condition is usually accompanied by atopy, allergies, or asthma. Symptoms of heartburn are usually mild or nonexistent. Endoscopic findings include "coiled rings," vertical linear lines, and a narrowed esophageal lumen (Fig. 2-1). Esophageal biopsy showing >25 eosinophils per high power field is diagnostic.

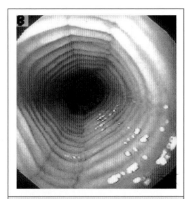

Figure 2-1. Endoscopic photograph showing multiple concentric rings with vertical lines seen in eosinophilic esophagitis.

14. **How can GERD be distinguished from coronary artery disease?**

In the evaluation of patients with retrosternal chest pain, the clinician must always be mindful patients with GERD do not die, but patients with new-onset angina or an acute myocardial infarction with symptoms mimicking GERD can. Clues that a patient's chest pain is cardiac in origin include radiation of the pain to the neck, jaw, or left shoulder/upper extremity; associated shortness of breath and/or diaphoresis; precipitation of pain by exertion; and relief of pain with sublingual nitroglycerin. Physical findings of new murmurs or gallops or abnormal rhythms are also suggestive of a cardiac origin. Although positive findings on an electrocardiogram (ECG) are helpful in the evaluation of patients with chest pain, the absence of ischemic ECG changes sho not discourage the clinician from excluding a cardiac etiology for the patient's symptoms.

15. **How should patients with symptoms of GERD be evaluated?**

Evaluation of patients with GERD may be guided by the severity of symptoms. Patients without symptoms of high GERD (aspiration or hoarseness) or dysphagia may be given careful instruction about lifestyle modification and a diagnostic trial of H_2-blocker therapy and followed clinically. Diagnostic evaluation is warranted when symptoms of GERD are chronic or incompletely responsive to medical therapy. Esophagogastroduodenoscopy (EGD) is the single best test for evaluation of GERD. Up to 50% of patients with GERD do not have macroscopic evidence of esophagitis at the time of endoscopy. In this group, more sensitive GER testing may be necessary or alternative diagnoses considered.

16. **Describe a commonly used endoscopic grading system for GERD.**

Grade 0   Macroscopically normal esophagus; only histologic evidence of GERD
Grade 1   One or more nonconfluent lesions with erythema or exudate above the GE junction
Grade 2   Confluent, noncircumferential, erosive, and exudative lesions
Grade 3   Circumferential, erosive, and exudative lesions
Grade 4   Chronic mucosal lesions (ulceration, stricture, or Barrett's esophagus)

17. **What are the more sophisticated esophageal function tests? How can they be used appropriately in the evaluation of patients with GERD?**

Clinical tests of GERD may be divided into three categories:

1. Acid sensitivity
   - Acid perfusion (Bernstein) test
   - 24- to 48-hour ambulatory esophageal pH monitoring
2. Esophageal barrier and motility
   - Esophageal manometry
   - Gastroesophageal scintiscanning
   - Standard acid reflux (modified Tuttle) test
   - 24- to 48-hour ambulatory esophageal pH monitoring
3. Esophageal acid clearance time
   - Standard acid reflux clearance test (SART)
   - 24- to 48-hour ambulatory esophageal pH monitoring

18. **Do all patients with GERD need esophageal function testing?**

No. Testing should be reserved for patients who fail medical therapy or in whom the correlation of reflux symptoms is in doubt.

19. **What is the utility of multichannel intraluminal impedance and pH (MII-pH) technology in the evaluation of GERD?**

The normal pH of the esophagus ranges between 5.0 and 6.8, making it difficult for conventional intra-esophageal pH measurements to detect *non*-acid reflux events. The MII-pH (impedance) technology is a major advance in esophageal testing that can detect both *acid* and *nonacid* reflux events.

When is ambulatory esophageal pH monitoring helpful?

Ambulatory esophageal pH monitoring is helpful in evaluating patients refractory to standard medical therapy. Acid hypersecretion is often seen in patients with GERD, and esophageal pH monitoring may be helpful in titrating the dose of H_2-blocker or proton pump inhibitor (PPI). Persistence of acid reflux on "adequate" doses of a PPI should raise the possibility of patient noncompliance or Zollinger-Ellison syndrome.

The Bravo capsule (Medtronix, Inc., Minneapolis, MN) is a new wireless technology that permits more physiologic intraesophageal monitoring for acid reflux. The Bravo capsule is the size of a gel cap and placed with or without endoscopic assistance 6 cm above the squamocolumnar junction. The capsule is "stapled" to the esophageal mucosal permitting more physiologic and prolonged intra-esophageal monitoring. Some investigators have begun to "staple" the capsule in the proximal esophagus to evaluate patients with atypical reflux symptoms, such as hoarseness, throat tightness, asthma, and interstitial lung disease.

When are esophageal manometry and scintiscanning helpful?

Esophageal manometry is helpful in evaluating the competency of the LES barrier and the body of the esophagus for motor dysfunction. Severe esophagitis may be the sole manifestation of early scleroderma. When ambulatory pH testing is not available, scintiscanning has been shown to be helpful.

Define the various types of medical therapy for GERD, and give a logical approach to prescription therapy for patients with long-standing GERD.

For patients with mild, uncomplicated symptoms of heartburn, empiric H_2-blocker therapy without costly and sophisticated diagnostic testing is reasonable. For patients recalcitrant to conventional therapy or with complications of high GERD (aspiration, asthma, hoarseness), Barrett's esophagus, or stricture, diagnostic and management decisions become more complicated. Medical or surgical therapy depends on patient preference, health care cost, risk of medical or surgical complications, and other related factors (Table 2-2).

Describe the commonly recommended approach to graded treatment of GERD.

Stage I   Lifestyle modifications:
             Antacids, prokinetics, over-the-counter H_2-blockers, or sucralfate
Stage II H_2-blocker therapy:
             Reinforce need for lifestyle modifications
Stage III   PPIs:
             Reinforce need for lifestyle modifications
Stage IV   Surgical or endoscopic antireflux procedure

The author favors initiation of aggressive lifestyle modification (especially weight reduction and dietary changes) and pharmacologic therapy to achieve endoscopic healing of esophagitis (usually a PPI). When esophagitis is healed, an effective dose of an intermediate-potency H_2 blocker is substituted for the PPI. Then the patient is counseled about the risks, benefits, and alternatives to long-term medical therapy. Surgery is encouraged for the fit patient who requires chronic high doses of pharmacologic therapy to control GERD or who dislikes taking medicines. Endoscopic treatments for GERD are very promising, but controlled long-term comparative trials with proton pump inhibitors and/or surgery are lacking.

Do patients scheduled for surgical antireflux procedures need to undergo sophisticated esophageal function testing before surgery?

There is no absolute correct answer. However, it is prudent to do esophageal motility studies to ensure that esophageal motor disease is not present. Patients with scleroderma may have a paucity of systemic complaints, and the diagnosis may go undetected without esophageal manometry. Generally, surgical antireflux procedures are avoided or modified in such patients. In addition, esophageal motility studies and ambulatory 24-hour pH monitoring may confirm or refute that the patient's symptoms are attributable to GERD before performance of a surgical procedure.

TABLE 2-2. MEDICAL THERAPY FOR GASTROESOPHAGEAL REFLUX DISEASE

	Dosage	Side Effects
Topicals		
Antacids	1–2 tablets after meals and at bedtime, as needed	Diarrhea (magnesium-containing) and constipation (aluminum- and calcium-containing)
Sucralfate	1 g 4 times/day	Incomplete passage of pill, especially in patients with esophageal strictures; constipation; dysgeusia
H_2 Blockers		
Cimetidine	400–800 mg 2–4 times/day	Gynecomastia, impotence, psychosis, hepatitis, drug interactions with warfarin, theophylline
Ranitidine	150–300 mg 2–4 times/day	Same, less common
Famotidine	20–40 mg 1–2 times/day	Same, less common
PPIs		
Omeprazole	20–60 mg/day	Drug interaction due to cytochrome p-450 (warfarin, phenytoin, diazepam)
Lansoprazole	30 mg/day	CYP-1A2 inducer; decreases theophylline levels
Rabeprazole	20 mg/day	Probably none
Pantoprazole	40 mg/day	Probably none
Esomeprazole	20–40 mg/day	Probably none
Prokinetic Agents		
Bethanechol	10–25 mg 4 times/ day *or* at bedtime	Urinary retention in patients with detrusor-external sphincter dyssynergia or prostatic hypertrophy, worsening asthma
Metoclopramide	10 mg 3 times/ day *or* at bedtime	Extrapyramidal dysfunction, Parkinsonian-like reaction; cases of irreversible tardive dyskinesia have been reported
Cisapride	10–20 mg 3 times/day	FDA recall, because of potential fatal arrhythmia. Compassionate use available

TABLE 2-2.	MEDICAL THERAPY FOR GASTROESOPHAGEAL REFLUX DISEASE—CONT'D	
	Dosage	Side Effects
Tegaserod	2–6 mg b.i.d.	Clinical efficacy in GERD has not been proven and the drug is not FDA approved for this indication. Use should be confined to clinical research trials.

OPPIs = proton pump inhibitors; FDA = Food and Drug Administration.

5. What are some of the new endoscopic treatments for GERD?

- Endoluminal gastroplication (ELGP): Endocinch by CR Bard, Inc., or Endoscopic Suturing Device by Wilson Cook, Inc.
- Single full-thickness plication: NDO Endoplication System by NDO Surgical, Inc. (not FDA approved)
- Coagulation injury: Stretta by Curon Medical, Inc.
- Polymer injection: Enteryx by Boston Scientific Corp.

6. How should esophageal strictures be managed?

- Prevention of peptic stricture with early institution of effective medical or surgical therapy appears to be particularly important for patients with scleroderma.
- For patients suffering symptoms of dysphagia due to peptic stricture, esophageal dilation is effective. Dilation can be accomplished using mercury-filled, polyvinyl, Maloney bougies, wire-guided hollow Savary-Gilliard or American dilators, or through-the-scope (TTS) pneumatic balloons. Usually, the esophagus is dilated to a diameter of 14 mm or 44 Fr. After successful dilation of a peptic stricture, the patient should be placed on chronic PPI therapy to avoid recurrent stricture formation.
- Surgery is an effective method of managing esophageal strictures. Usually, preoperative and intraoperative dilation is combined with a definitive antireflux procedure.

KEY POINTS: GASTROESOPHAGEAL REFLUX

1. Gastroesophageal reflux is common, with 60 million American adults experiencing heartburn symptoms at least once per month and 15 million experiencing symptoms daily.

2. Endoscopic evidence of erosive esophagitis suggests likelihood of chronic GERD.

3. Patients with symptomatic peptic strictures should be treated with a proton pump inhibitor (PPI) indefinitely to prevent the need for repeated esophageal dilations.

4. Supra-esophageal manifestations of GERD include: asthma, cough, chest pain, hiccups, hoarseness, dental erosions (lingual surface), recurrent otitis in children, chronic throat clearing, and throat tightness.

27. **What is Barrett's esophagus? How is it managed?**
    Barrett's esophagus is a metaplastic degeneration of the normal esophageal lining, which is replaced with a premalignant, specialized columnar epithelium. It is seen in roughly 5–7% of patients with uncomplicated reflux but in up to 30–40% of patients with scleroderma or dysphagia.

    Currently, there is no proven method to eliminate Barrett's esophagus. Preliminary studies laser or bicap ablation of the metaplastic segment followed by alkalization of the gastroesophageal refluxate are encouraging. The need for cancer surveillance is discussed elsewhere this book.

28. **List some of the atypical symptoms and signs of GERD.**

Asthma	Lingual dental erosions
Chest pain	Recurrent otitis in children
Cough	Throat-clearing
Hiccups	Throat tightness
Hoarseness	

29. **Is there an association between obstructive sleep apnea (OSA) and GERD?**
    Yes. Nocturnal acid reflux is seen in 54–72% of persons with OSA. Administration of nighttim continuous positive airway pressure (CPAP) and/or proton pump inhibitor therapy have been shown to decrease apnea and acid reflux events.

30. **Does the presence of heartburn symptoms predict a GERD-related cough etiology?**
    No. There is poor correlation between symptoms of heartburn and cough. Between 43% and 75% of patients with GERD-related cough do not have heartburn symptoms. Both medical tre ment with PPIs and surgical antireflux procedures have been reported to be effective for GERL related cough. Caveats include:
    - 35% response rate to omeprazole 40 mg two times/day after 2 weeks
    - Results of surgical antireflux procedures are best when preoperative esophageal manometr is normal and response to PPI is positive.

31. **What is the best method to evaluate for possible GERD-related cough?**
    The first step is to exclude non–GERD-related etiologies: angiotensin-converting inhibitors, environmental irritants, smoking, parenchymal lung disease, allergic rhinitis and pneumonitis and asthma and sinusitis, which are often "silent." Symptom relief after a 2-week trial of Prilos (or equivalent), 40 mg two times/day, is a cost-effective approach. Patients who do not respon should be considered for further evaluation, including esophageal manometry/pH testing and EGD.

32. **What laryngeal conditions are associated with GERD?**
    The most common laryngeal manifestation of high reflux or esophagopharyngeal reflux (EPR) hoarseness. Other laryngeal conditions associated with EPR are listed below.

Arytenoid fixation	Laryngomalacia
Carcinoma of the larynx	Pachydermia laryngitis
Contact ulcers and granuloma	Paroxysmal laryngospasm
Globus pharyngeus	Recurrent leukoplakia
Hoarseness	Vocal cord nodules

33. **How often do people with EPR and hoarseness relate symptoms of heartburn?**
    The prevalence of GERD symptoms among patients with reflux laryngitis is low (6–43%).

. What is the most efficient, cost-effective method to evaluate hoarse patients for EPR?

The first step in the evaluation of hoarseness should be exclusion of structural ear, nose, and throat (ENT) disorders, including neoplasm. The next step is an empiric trial of double-dose PPI for 2–3 months. Most EPR-related hoarseness improves with acid suppression (60–96%). Patients responding to PPIs may stop the medication and be monitored for recurrence of symptoms. Hoarse patients with a negative ENT evaluation, who fail PPI therapy, should undergo formal esophageal pH analysis.

. Can gastroesophageal reflux worsen asthma?

Yes. Numerous studies have shown that reflux symptoms are common among asthmatics (65–72%) and that medical and surgical antireflux treatment may improve pulmonary function.

. How does gastroesophageal reflux worsen asthma?

Several mechanisms are theorized to explain GERD-induced bronchospasm:

- Asthmatics with GERD have been shown to have autonomic dysregulation with heightened vagal response, which is presumed to be responsible for the decrease in LES pressure and more frequent transient relaxations of the LES, which promote reflux.
- Esophageal reflux may incite a vagal-mediated esophagobronchial reflex of airway hyperreactivity.
- Microaspiration of gastric juice has been shown to activate a local axonal reflex involving release of substance P, which leads to airway edema. The finding of lipid-laden alveolar macrophages among asthmatics demonstrates aspiration of gastric material into the pulmonary tree.

. Which patients with GERD should be considered for a surgical antireflux procedure?

Any young, healthy patient with chronic GERD requiring lifelong PPI medical therapy may be considered for an antireflux procedure. Other indications include failed medical therapy, complicated GERD (e.g., bleeding, recurrent strictures), medical success at excessive cost in young, otherwise healthy patients, and problematic symptoms due to regurgitation (asthma, hoarseness, cough).

. Which patients are poor candidates for a surgical antireflux procedure?

- Elderly patients with substantial comorbid disease
- Patients with poor or absent esophageal peristalsis
- Patients with highly functional symptoms

Lack of available surgical expertise is also a contraindication for antireflux procedures.

. What is the best endoscopic or surgical antireflux procedure?

Rapid advances in endoscopic and laparoscopic surgery make this question unanswerable. Novel endoscopic suturing, burning, and injection techniques are exciting, but results are only preliminary. A comparative trial of endoscopic and surgical antireflux techniques is necessary.

. What cytochrome p-450 (CYP-450) systems are involved in the metabolism of PPIs?

All of the PPIs undergo some hepatic metabolism through the CYP-450 system. The CYP-2C19 and CYP-3A4 microsomal enzymes are responsible for the majority of PPI hepatic metabolism. Genetic polymorphism with CYP-2C19 is common; about 5% of Americans and 20% of Asians are deficient in this enzyme. Omeprazole decreases the metabolism of phenytoin and warfarin R-isomer (CYP-2C9), diazepam (CYP-2C19), and cyclosporine (CYP-3A4).

41. **How do esomeprazole (Nexium) and omeprazole (Prilosec) differ?**
Omeprazole is a racemic mixture of both the S- and R-isomers, whereas esomeprazole is a "pure" form of the S-isomer. Less esomeprazole (S-isomer) is metabolized by the CYP-2C19 pathway, leading to greater area under the curve and better intragastric acid suppression for 24 hours. Esomeprazole is the only PPI shown to be statistically superior to omeprazole in healing erosive esophagitis at 8 weeks (90–94% efficacy rate).

WEBSITES

1. http://www.vhjoe.com

2. http://www.reflux1.com

3. http://www.curonmedical.com/Physicians/stretta_gerd.html

4. http://www.ndosurgical.com/

5. http://www.endocinch.com/

BIBLIOGRAPHY

1. Bainbridge ET, Temple JG, Nicholas SP, et al: Symptomatic gastroesophageal reflux in pregnancy: A comparative study of white Europeans and Asians in Birmingham. Br J Clin Pract 37:53, 1983.

2. DeVault KR: Overview of therapy for the extraesophageal manifestations of gastroesophageal reflux disease. Am J Gastroenterol 95:S39–S44, 2000.

3. Gistout CJ. Endoscopic Antireflux. Visible Human Journal of Endoscopy (VHJOE). 2003;2:3:4. (http://www.vhjoe.com/Volume2Issue3/2-3-4.htm)

4. Green BT, Broughton WA, O'Connor JB: Marked improvement in nocturnal gastroesophageal reflux in a large cohort of patients with obstructive sleep apnea treated with continuous positive airway breathing. Arch Intern Med 163:41–45, 2003.

5. Harding SM, Sontag SJ: Asthma and gastroesophageal reflux. Am J Gastroenterol 95:S23–S32, 2000.

6. Irwin RS, Richter JE: Gastroesophageal reflux and chronic cough. Am J Gastroenterol 95:S9–S14, 2000.

7. Kellog TA, Oelschlanger BK, Pellegrini CA: Laparoscopic antireflux surgery. VHJOE 2:3, 2003. (http://www.vhjoe.com/Volume2Issue3/2-3-3.htm)

8. Lazarchick DA, Filler SJ: Dental erosion: Predominant oral lesion in gastroesophageal reflux disease. Am J Gastroenterol 95:S33–S38, 2000.

9. McNally PR: Eosinophilic esophagitis. VHJOE 3:1, 2004.

10. McNally PR, Maydonovitch CL, Prosek RA, et al: Evaluation of gastroesophageal reflux as a cause of idiopathic hoarseness. Dig Dis Sci 34:1900–1904, 1989.

11. Meier JH, McNally PR, Freeman SR, et al: Does omeprazole (Prilosec) improve asthma in patients with gastroesophageal reflux: A double blind crossover study. Dig Dis Sci 39:1900–1904, 1994.

12. Richter JE: Extraesophageal presentations of gastroesophageal reflux disease: An overview. Am J Gastroenterol 95:S1–S3, 2000.

13. Senior BA, Khan M, Schwimmer C, et al: Gastroesophageal reflux and obstructive sleep apnea. Laryngoscope 111:2144–2146, 2001.

14. Spencer CM, Faulds D: Esomeprazole. Drugs 60:321–327, 2000.

15. Tutuian R, Castell DO: Use of multichannel intraluminal impedance to document proximal esophageal and pharyngeal nonacidic reflux episodes. Am J Med 115(Suppl 3A):119S–123S, 2003.

16. Ward EM, Devault KR, Bouras EP, et al: Successful oesophageal pH monitoring with a catheter-free system. Aliment Pharmacol Ther 19:449–454, 2004.

17. Wong RKH, Hanson DG, Waring PJ, Shaw G: ENT manifestations of gastroesophageal reflux. Am J Gastroenterol 95:S15–S22, 2000.

CHAPTER 3

ESOPHAGEAL INFECTIONS

Dirk R. Davis, MD

Which organisms are most commonly identified in esophageal infections?
The most common etiologies are *Candida albicans*, herpes simplex virus (HSV), and cytomegalovirus (CMV). *C. albicans* and HSV can be seen in individuals with normal immunity, whereas CMV esophagitis is found in immunocompromised hosts.

What are the typical presenting symptoms in patients with infectious esophagitis?
Odynophagia and, to a lesser degree, dysphagia are the most common complaints. Heartburn, chest pain, nausea, dysgeusia, and bleeding can also be symptoms/signs.

What is the most common cause of infectious esophagitis in the general population?
Candida albicans. This yeast is virtually ubiquitous and is considered normal oral flora. Esophageal infection occurs by a two-step process. The first step is colonization, which involves adherence to the mucosal surface and proliferation. It is estimated that 20% of asymptomatic people have esophageal colonization with *Candida,* and this becomes more common with advanced age. The second step is often associated with impaired host defenses and is identified by mucosal invasion of budding yeast and the presence of mycelial forms on microscopic examination. Adherent creamy white plaques or exudates are the common appearance on endoscopic examination (Fig. 3-1).

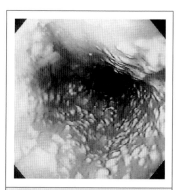

Figure 3-1. Endoscopic photograph showing creamy white exudates seen in candidal esophagitis *(Courtesy of Peter R. McNally, DO).*

List medical conditions known to predispose a person to candidal esophagitis.
Conditions compromising normal immune function, primarily HIV infection and hematologic malignancies, increase the incidence of fungal esophagitis. Nonhematologic malignancies, diabetes mellitus, adrenal dysfunction, alcoholism, and advanced age are risk factors as well. Radiation therapy for thoracic malignancies and immunosuppression required in organ transplant recipients are also associated with increased risk. Achalasia and scleroderma esophagus are associated with esophageal stasis and individuals with those conditions are prone to develop monilial esophagitis.

What commonly used drugs are associated with fungal esophagitis?
Antibiotics that affect normal oral flora change the competitive milieu, increasing colonization and the likelihood of fungal infection. Both systemic and inhaled topical corticosteroids increase risk of infection due to effects on mucosal immunity. Acid suppressive therapies, most significantly proton pump inhibitors but also H_2-receptor blockers, increase mucosal colonization with

C. albicans, probably as a result of the loss of the cleansing effect of spontaneous gastro-esophageal reflux events.

6. **How is Candida esophagitis treated?**
   The most commonly prescribed therapy for candidal esophagitis is fluconazole, 100–200 mg orally for 10–14 days. Other options for therapy include topical agents. Nystatin can be given as a liquid "swish-and-swallow" or as a dissolvable oral troche. Dosing of nystatin ranges from 200,000 to 500,000 units four or five times daily for 7–14 days. Clotrimazole nonabsorbable azole, can be given as a buccal troche, 10 mg five times daily for 1 week, or as a vaginal tablet, 100 mg dissolved in the mouth and swallowed five times daily. Oral suspensions of amphotericin B are also available but are usually reserved for azole-resistant infections. Topical agents have the advantage of being well tolerated, having no significant adverse effects or drug interactions. Topical therapy should be reserved for less severe infections in immunocompetent individuals. Other oral imidazole agents are itraconazole and voriconazole. Ketoconazole is no longer recommended for treatment of monilial esophagitis.

7. **How is candidal esophagitis treated in granulocytopenic patients?**
   Granulocytopenic patients should be treated with intravenous amphotericin B due to the high risk of fungal dissemination. Dose and duration of therapy are based on severity of infection; febrile patients with extensive esophagitis or evidence of systemic infection should receive 0.5 mg/kg/day, whereas milder cases may be treated with 0.3 mg/kg/day. Newer liposomal formulations of amphotericin B that are less nephrotoxic and have fewer systemic side effects are available and are dosed at 3–5 mg/kg/day.

8. **Should empiric therapy for candidal esophagitis be considered in an at-risk patient presenting with typical symptoms of esophageal infection?**
   Yes. A therapeutic trial of fluconazole for patients with presumed esophageal candidiasis is a cost-effective alternative to endoscopy. Patients not demonstrating symptomatic improvement within 3–5 days should undergo endoscopic evaluation.

9. **List the factors that predispose an individual to fluconazole-resistant candidiasis in the HIV-infected population, and discuss treatment options for azole-resistant candidal esophagitis.**
   The number of treated episodes and duration of therapy (azole-exposure) and lower CD_4 cell counts (more severe immunosuppression) make fluconazole-resistance a potential problem. One option for treatment in that situation is itraconazole solution 100–200 mg by mouth once twice daily, which has been shown to be effective in fluconazole-resistant candidal esophagitis. The solution has been shown to be superior to the tablet form likely due to an added topical effect. Another option is topical amphotericin B administered as a suspension or a lozenge. Intravenous amphotericin B is used in refractory disease; dosage is dictated by the severity of the infection. Cancidas (caspofungin) is reserved for imidazole and amphotericin-resistant fungal infections.

10. **What are recommendations for suppressive therapy to minimize recurrences of monilial esophagitis in HIV-infected patients?**
    Regimens of fluconazole, 100 mg by mouth once daily or 150 mg by mouth once weekly, have been shown to reduce reinfection rates.

11. **What other fungal organisms should be considered in esophageal infections?**
    Non-*albicans* species of *Candida* and other noncandidal fungi can be seen in severely immunocompromised patients. *Candida glabrata* and *Candida krusei* have been identified more frequently in recent years. Non-*albicans Candida* species are more resistant to imidazole

antifungals, requiring intravenous amphotericin B therapy. *Histoplasma, Cryptococcus, Blastomyces,* and *Aspergillus* species may also cause fungal esophagitis.

2. What is the most common viral pathogen-causing esophagitis?

CMV is the most common cause of viral esophagitis. This is because viral esophagitis occurs more frequently in immunocompromised patients, and CMV is identified as the pathogen in most cases. Other viral pathogens, including HSV, varicella-zoster virus (VZV), and Epstein-Barr virus (EBV), can also cause esophageal infections in patients with immune dysfunction.

3. What is the most common cause of viral esophagitis in patients with normal immunity?

HSV esophagitis, although rare, may cause viral esophagitis in an immunocompetent patient. The infection can be primary or due to reactivation of a latent infection. The finding of orolabial HSV may suggest the diagnosis in patients with acute esophageal symptoms but is present in only about 20% of cases. HSV esophagitis tends to be seen more commonly in males (male to female ratio >3:1).

4. How is viral esophagitis diagnosed?

In patients with esophageal ulcers presenting with symptoms of infectious esophagitis, multiple biopsies (10 biopsies are recommended to maximize diagnostic yield) of each ulcer should be obtained. Biopsies from the ulcer base and ulcer margins are evaluated for typical cytopathic changes microscopically. Tissue also needs to be sent in medium for viral cultures. Cultures are more sensitive than microscopic examination, and immunohistochemistry can increase the diagnostic sensitivity as well.

5. Differentiate herpes simplex virus (HSV) and cytomegalovirus (CMV) esophagitis endoscopically.

Early in HSV esophagitis, the typical small vesicles can be seen in the middle-distal esophagus. The vesicles may coalesce, forming well-circumscribed ulcers that have raised yellowish edges: the classic "volcano ulcers." HSV esophagitis can cause a diffusely ulcerated mucosa devoid of squamous epithelium in severe infections. CMV ulcers are more often linear, serpiginous lesions in the middle and/or distal esophagus. These ulcers may unite, forming giant ulcers, and may produce stricturing of the esophageal lumen. Concomitant infections with both organisms have been reported, and, in candidal esophagitis, a viral coinfection can be present in 20–50% of cases. Candidal plaques often obscure viral ulcers.

6. Differentiate HSV and CMV microscopically.

HSV infects squamous epithelium. Biopsies from the ulcer margins demonstrate multinucleated giant cells with ballooning degeneration of squamous cells, margination of chromatin, and characteristic ground-glass nuclei. Cowdry type A intranuclear inclusions are pathognomonic for HSV infections. The classic histologic features of CMV infection are large cells with both intracytoplasmic inclusions and amphophilic intranuclear inclusions. Biopsies should be placed in viral transport media; culture remains the standard for diagnosis.

7. How is HSV esophagitis treated?

HSV esophagitis is a self-limited infection in immunocompetent patients and may not require therapy. If the diagnosis is made early in the course of infection, initiating therapy may shorten duration of symptoms. In immunocompromised patients, infection is more serious, may disseminate, and requires treatment. Initial therapy is intravenous acyclovir, 250 mg/m^2 every 8 hours until the patient is able to swallow normally followed by valacyclovir, 100 mg three times daily for a total of 7–10 days. Acyclovir-resistant strains of HSV should be treated with foscarnet, 40 mg/kg three times daily for 2 weeks.

18. **Discuss the treatment of CMV esophagitis.**

    Both ganciclovir and foscarnet are effective drugs in treating CMV. Because of cost, ganciclovir is considered first-line therapy at a dose of 5 mg/kg intravenously for 2 weeks. Granulocytopenia is a potential side effect of ganciclovir. In patients who have failed ganciclovir, or when granulocytopenia is present, foscarnet, 90 mg/kg intravenously every 12 hours for 3–4 weeks, is recommended. The most significant adverse effect with foscarnet is renal toxicity. Recurrence of CMV is more common than not, and maintenance therapy at 90–120 mg/kg/day should be considered. Cidofovir is an alternative in ganciclovir/foscarnet-resistant strains. It is dosed at 5 mg/kg intravenously once weekly. Probenecid is given with cidofovir in an adequately hydrated patient to minimize renal toxicity.

19. **Does HIV cause esophageal ulceration?**

    Idiopathic esophageal ulcers (IEUs) have been reported in HIV-infected patients. HIV can be isolated from esophageal ulcers without evidence of other pathogens. It is thought that the mucosal injury is immunologically mediated and not a direct result of cytotoxic effects of HIV. IEUs do not respond to antiviral or antifungal treatment, but healing can be accomplished in approximately 90% of cases with corticosteroids or thalidomide. Because steroid use predisposes to candidiasis, prophylaxis with fluconazole is suggested. Recommended therapies include prednisone, 40 mg orally for 4 weeks, then tapering by 10 mg/week, or thalidomide, 200 mg/day for 4 weeks.

20. **Are immunocompromised patients at risk for bacterial esophagitis?**

    In HIV/AIDS patients, the risk of bacterial esophagitis is low due to preserved granulocyte function. Patients receiving chemotherapy for malignancy are at greatest risk. The use of acid suppressive medications is also considered a risk factor.

21. **How is the diagnosis of bacterial esophagitis established?**

    Gram stain of mucosal biopsies demonstrates invasion of the esophageal mucosa. Fungal/viral pathogens must be excluded to make a diagnosis of bacterial esophagitis. Cultures of biopsy material are not helpful because of the unavoidable contamination with oral flora. Infections are usually polymicrobial, typically with gram-positive organisms found in the normal oral flora, but gram-negative species may also be seen.

22. **Does it make sense to stain for acid-fast organisms in evaluating esophageal ulcers?**

    Yes. A shallow linear ulcer with smooth edges and a necrotic base, usually in the middle third of the esophagus, is suggestive of *Mycobacterium tuberculosis* (TB). TB is seldom a primary infection in the esophagus, but cases have been reported. It more often results from direct extension of adjacent mediastinal lymph nodes in patients with pulmonary tuberculosis. *Mycobacterium avium* complex is commonly reported in patients with AIDS and tends to be widely disseminated at the time of diagnosis. Esophageal involvement is rare but should be considered in the differential diagnosis; appropriate tissue stains and culture should be obtained. As is the case with TB, treatment is difficult, requiring multidrug regimens over months.

23. **Can the diagnosis of Chagas' disease be based on classic manometric findings and confirmed by histologic evaluation of deep mucosal biopsies from the distal esophagus?**

    Chagas disease is caused by infection with *Trypanosoma cruzi*, which is endemic in South America. The organism destroys ganglion cells, and multiple organs are involved. The esophageal abnormalities resemble achalasia, but the lower esophageal sphincter pressure is not elevated and, in fact, may be low. Symptoms occur typically years to decades after the acute infection. Diagnosis requires typical manometric findings, positive serologic tests for the parasite, and evidence of other organ involvement. Mucosal biopsies are of no value in the diagnosis

The esophagus in Chagas' disease is more responsive to nitrates and calcium channel antagonists, which improve esophageal emptying. Unlike primary achalasia, Chagas' disease is often associated with cardiac, renal, intestinal, and biliary abnormalities.

WEBSITES

1. http://www.gastroatlas.com/
2. http://www-medlib.med.utah.edu/WebPath/webpath.html

BLIOGRAPHY

Dietrich DT, Wilcox CM: Diagnosis and treatment of esophageal diseases associated with HIV infection. Am J Gastroenterol 91:2265, 1996.

Grim SA, Smith KM, Romanelli F, Ofotokun I: Treatment of azole-resistant candidiasis with topical amphotericin B. Ann Pharmacother 36:1383, 2002.

Kearney DJ, McDonald GB: Esophageal disorders caused by infection, systemic illness, medications, radiation and trauma. In Feldman M, Friedman LS, Sleisenger MH (eds): Gastrointestinal and Liver Disease, 7th ed. Philadelphia, W.B. Saunders, 2002, p 623.

Monkemuller KE, Wilcox CM: Diagnosis of esophageal ulcers in acquired immunodeficiency syndrome. Semin Gastrointest Dis 10:85, 1999.

Perez RA, Early DS: Endoscopy in patients receiving radiation therapy to the thorax. Dig Dis Sci 47:79, 2002.

Ramanathan J, Rammouni M, Baran J, Khatis R: Herpes simplex virus esophagitis in the immunocompetent host: An overview. Am J Gastroenterol 95:2171, 2000.

Rex JH, Walsh TJ, Sosel JD, et al: Practice guidelines for the treatment of candidiasis. Clin Infect Dis 30:662, 2000.

Vasquez JA: Options for the management of mucosal candidiasis in patients with AIDS and HIV infection. Pharmacotherapy 19:76, 1999.

CHAPTER 4

ESOPHAGEAL CAUSES OF CHEST PAIN

Brian T. Johnston, MD, and Donald O. Castell, MD

1. When should the clinician consider an esophageal cause of chest pain?

The concept of the esophagus as the origin of chest pain is not new. More than a century ago, Sir William Osler hypothesized that esophageal spasm represented one cause of chest pain in soldiers during wartime. A recent multicenter study reported that 55% of patients attending the emergency department for chest pain did not have cardiac pain. However, coronary artery disease (CAD) is the most serious and life-threatening cause of chest pain. It should therefore be excluded as a potential diagnosis prior to pursuing esophageal investigations.

2. Does history help to discriminate cardiac from esophageal chest pain?

Yes and no. A sharp pain localized by one finger at the fifth intercostal space in the midclavicular line with onset at rest in a 20-year-old woman is unlikely to be caused by coronary artery disease. Certain features in a patient's presenting history help clearly to differentiate between causes. However, many studies have shown sufficient overlap of all features to preclude certain diagnosis on the basis of symptoms alone. The description of pain by some patients with a known esophageal source and no cardiac disease mimics exactly the classic description of angina pectoris, including pain on exertion. One study from Belgium documented normal coronary angiograms in 25% of patients regarded by cardiologists as having myocardial ischemia on the basis of symptoms. In one half of these patients, a probable esophageal cause could be identified.

3. Does a normal coronary angiogram exclude all cardiac diagnoses?

No. Cardiac abnormalities other than CAD can be found in patients with chest pain, including mitral valve prolapse and microvascular angina. Exclusion of mitral valve prolapse requires echocardiography, whereas microvascular angina can be excluded only by the complicated procedure of measuring coronary artery resistance during stimulation with ergonovine and rapid atrial pacing.

However, studies suggesting that pain is no more common in patients with mitral valve prolapse or microvascular angina than in the general population question whether in fact these abnormalities produce pain. If they do, the mechanism is unclear. Furthermore, the prognosis is excellent, with the mortality rate being no different from that of the general population. Finally, positive association between these cardiac abnormalities and esophageal motility disorders suggests a common or associated cause—either a generalized smooth muscle defect or heightened visceral nociception. It is therefore appropriate to search for an esophageal cause, after excluding coronary artery disease.

4. What are the noncardiac causes of chest pain? How common are they?

Gastroesophageal reflux disease (GERD) is the most frequent esophageal cause of chest pain. most studies it accounts for up to 50% of all cases of unexplained chest pain (UCP). Esophageal dysmotility can be diagnosed in another 25–30% of cases. Of the remaining 20–30%, one third to one half can be explained by a musculoskeletal source, such as costochondritis (Tietze's syndrome) and chest-wall pain syndromes. Psychological disorders, acting either independently or as cofactors, are responsible for many of these pain syndromes. Panic disorder, in particular, must be considered.

Because gastroesophageal reflux disease is the most likely diagnosis, is a trial of acid suppression acceptable?

Yes. A therapeutic trial of acid suppression is relatively inexpensive, noninvasive, and easy to perform, and may avoid further investigation. However, adequate doses of appropriate medication must be used. Current studies suggest that a proton pump inhibitor (PPI; omeprazole, 20 mg; lansoprazole, 30 mg; rabeprazole, 20 mg; pantoprazole, 40 mg; or esomeprazole, 20 mg) be given twice daily before meals for a period of 4–8 weeks. This test produces both false-negative and false-positive results. In patients who do not have relief of symptoms, the tendency is to conclude that GERD is not the cause of the pain. This conclusion cannot be made with complete certainty without ambulatory monitoring of intragastric and intraesophageal pH, while the patient continues PPI therapy. False positives may occur because of a placebo response that can be particularly high in functional gastrointestinal disorders. One study of patients with presumed esophageal chest pain noted a placebo response of 36%.

What is the most useful esophageal investigation?

Because GERD is the most common cause of UCP, it should be the first diagnosis considered. Ambulatory pH monitoring of the esophagus is the gold standard for diagnosing GERD and is the test most likely to yield a positive result in patients with UCP. It remains the appropriate initial investigation, even when a trial of acid suppression has appeared ineffective.

If ambulatory pH monitoring is abnormal (see later text), esophagogastroduodenoscopy (EGD) may be indicated to exclude the more serious consequences of GERD, such as esophagitis and Barrett's esophagus. An EGD should be considered when the total esophageal acid exposure for a 24-hour period exceeds 10% or when supine acid exposure is above normal limits. However, diagnostic yield from EGD is low when the only symptom is chest pain. If ambulatory pH monitoring is negative, investigation for esophageal motility abnormalities is indicated.

Unexplained chest pain
↓
Exclude cardiac disease (of epicardial vessels)
↓
Trial of acid suppression
↓
Esophageal pH monitoring*
↓
Baseline manometry and provocation testing
(Bernstein, edrophonium, balloon distention)
↓
Consider other causes

*EGD is indicated for severe reflux on pH monitoring (see text).

Other more unusual causes of UCP, such as biliary tract disease and gastric or duodenal ulceration, have been reported. Therefore, further gastrointestinal investigation, including abdominal ultrasound, is occasionally warranted, especially if the history points to such diagnoses.

How is esophageal pH monitoring performed?

Esophageal pH monitoring is performed after an overnight fast. The level of acidity is measured by an intraesophageal electrode of either glass or antimony. The electrode is placed 5 cm above the upper border of the lower esophageal sphincter (LES), as previously determined by manometry.

An antimony electrode is thinner (2-mm diameter) but requires the use of a silver/silver chloride reference electrode either incorporated in the catheter or attached to the patient's chest. The electrode is passed transnasally, and pH is recorded for a minimum of 16 hours. Patients are encouraged to follow their usual routine. Data are recorded on a portable recording device with marker buttons that allow the patient to indicate timing of meals, bed rest, and symptoms A diary card is also completed to corroborate the timings. All information is transferred to a computer on completion of the study and analyzed both visually and by specialized software.

8. **What abnormalities may be found with pH monitoring?**
   Analysis of the tracing includes both duration of esophageal acid exposure (i.e., time when esophageal pH is < 4) and its association with symptoms. Objective GERD is diagnosed when th duration of acid exposure for the total time or for either the upright or recumbent periods excee the 95th percentile of normal values. In our laboratory, these limits are defined as exposures to a pH < 4 for 4.2% of the total time, 6.3% of the upright period, and 1.2% of the recumbent period.

   Although an abnormal degree of acid reflux suggests the cause of the patient's symptoms, the case is not proved. Thus, the occurrence of symptoms during the monitoring period is extremely valuable. If symptoms coincide frequently with episodes of acid reflux, the diagnosis can be made even when absolute levels of acid exposure do not exceed the 95th percentile of normal values. Similarly, failure of all symptoms to correlate with acid reflux is strong evidence against reflux-related chest pain.

   The situation is more difficult when some but not all symptoms are associated with episode of acid reflux. Various "symptom indices" have been introduced in an attempt to quantify the symptom-reflux association. The simplest index uses the total number of symptoms as its denominator and symptoms that coincide with acid reflux as its numerator:

   $$\text{Symptom index} = \frac{\text{No. of symptoms occurring during acid reflux}}{\text{Total no. of symptoms during pH monitoring}}$$

   A value of 50% or greater (e.g., two of four symptoms occurring during episodes of acid reflux is regarded as positive (Fig. 4-1). The approach to reflux-induced chest pain is no different fror the normal management of GERD (see Chapter 2, Gastroesophageal Reflux Disease).

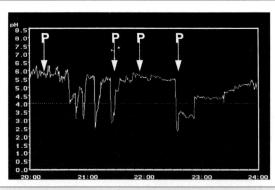

Figure 4-1. A 4-hour sample of esophageal pH monitoring. During this period, two of four symptoms (P) were associated with episodes of acid reflux, yielding a symptom index of 2/4 (50%).

9. **If reflux has been excluded, which esophageal motility abnormalities may be found in patients with chest pain?**
   Abnormal esophageal motility may be found in 25–30% of patients with UCP. The sooner this can be performed relative to an episode of chest pain, the higher its diagnostic yield. The relati frequency of different diagnoses in these patients with abnormal esophageal manometry is illu trated in Figure 4-2.

1. *Nutcracker esophagus* is the most common manometric abnormality. It has been so named because of the extremely high pressures generated during esophageal peristalsis. The diagnosis requires an average peristaltic amplitude >180 mmHg during 10 wet swallows over both distal channels (Fig. 4-3).
2. *Ineffective esophageal motility* is a diagnostic category that includes patients with weak or poorly conducted waves; it is the second most common manometric finding.
3. *Diffuse esophageal spasm* is diagnosed when at least 2 of 10 water swallows produce simultaneous contractions instead of normal peristalsis. It may also be associated with other abnormalities, such as multipeaked or prolonged duration contractions (Fig. 4-4).

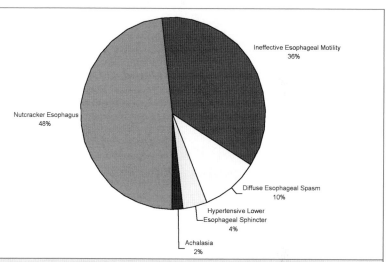

Figure 4-2. The relative frequencies of different diagnoses in patients with an esophageal dysmotility cause for chest pain.

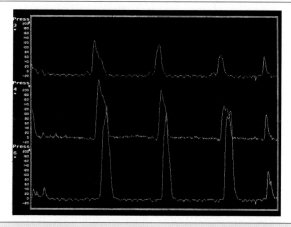

Figure 4-3. Nutcracker esophagus. The patient's average peristaltic amplitude was 250 mmHg. She experienced pain synchronous with most of her swallows.

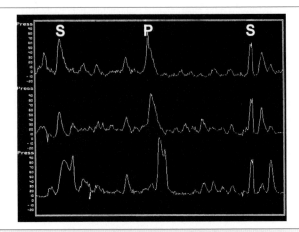

Figure 4-4. Diffuse esophageal spasm. Both simultaneous (S) and peristaltic (P) contractions occur in response to water swallows.

4. *An abnormally high basal LES pressure* is also associated, on occasion, with UCP— the "hypertensive LES."

5. *Achalasia* presents, occasionally, with chest pain and is further discussed in Chapter 5, Achalasi.

10. **How can esophageal motility abnormalities cause chest pain?**
    The mechanism or mechanisms by which motility abnormalities may cause chest pain are poorly understood. Specific mechanoreceptors have been identified in the esophageal mucosa and muscle layers. Abnormal contractions per se may be sufficient to stimulate these recep- tors and cause pain. Alternatively, the mechanoreceptors may be stimulated by esophageal distention, as a result of failed LES relaxation or retention of the bolus within the esophageal body. Yet another possibility is alteration of the threshold for esophageal sensation, which "tunes in" the patient to changes in esophageal pressure. A further theory is that high tension the esophageal wall inhibits esophageal blood flow, causing myoischemia. However, the esoph agus has an extensive blood supply, and contractions are unlikely to be sufficiently prolonged induce ischemia. It is also possible that dysmotility per se is not the cause of pain. Rather, it m represent an epiphenomenon that, like pain, is induced by another, unrecognized process. This emphasizes that simply diagnosing an esophageal motility disorder does not prove that it is th cause of the patient's pain. Occasionally, during routine manometry, a patient develops pain coincident with abnormal wave forms, demonstrating a closer link between the dysmotility an the pain. More typically, the patient remains asymptomatic.

11. **Can esophageal pain be provoked during testing?**
    Yes. In an attempt to provoke symptoms, additional measures analogous to the exercise stress test used by cardiologists may be used to stimulate the esophagus. Options include acid infusi pharmacologic stimulation, and intraesophageal balloon distention. For many years, it was believed that GERD caused chest pain by inducing dysmotility. Although this theory does not appear to be correct, acid perfusion (Bernstein test) is still used occasionally as a diagnostic tes in UCP. Typically, 60–80 mL of 0.1 N hydrochloric acid are infused into the esophagus at a rate 6–8 mL/min without the patient's knowledge, followed by a similar infusion of saline. The test is positive only if (1) it reproduces the patient's typical symptoms during acid infusion, and (2) the symptoms disappear or do not recur during saline infusion. Chemoreceptors are present in the esophageal mucosa. Patients with a positive Bernstein test demonstrate acid sensitivity and

should be treated for GERD-induced chest pain. Ambulatory pH monitoring with specific evaluation of symptom associations with pH decreases has largely made the Bernstein test obsolete.

Various pharmacologic agents have been used to stimulate the esophageal smooth muscle. The current choice is the cholinesterase inhibitor edrophonium (80 mg/kg intravenously). After injection, even in normal subjects, esophageal smooth muscle responds with increased peristaltic amplitude and duration during swallows. The test is regarded as positive only if it reproduces the patient's typical pain.

Intraesophageal balloon distention (IEBD) involves the graduated inflation of a latex balloon within the esophagus, until pain or a predetermined maximal volume is reached. This test has the advantage of being specific to the esophagus and may reproduce the pain by a mechanism not dissimilar to that of dysmotility. It is positive only if it induces a patient's typical pain at an inflation volume that does not induce pain in normal subjects. Balloon distention has been shown to be reproducible and has the highest yield of all available provocation tests. Of the three forms of provocation, acid and edrophonium typically induce symptoms in 20% of cases; balloon distention has double this yield (Fig. 4-5).

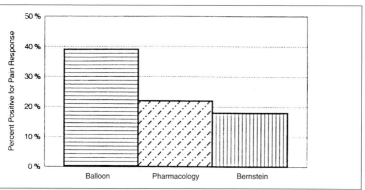

Figure 4-5. Mean values of seven reported studies of the percentage of positive pain response achieved by provocation with balloon distention, edrophonium, and acid in patients with unexplained chest pain.

2. **How does provocation testing compare with combined ambulatory monitoring of both motility and pH?**
All esophageal provocation tests have one major drawback—they are not physiologic. In an attempt to record the motility tracing during spontaneous chest pain, longer periods of manometry have been performed. However, this is little used outside research institutions.

3. **Are there any emerging technologies for investigation of unexplained chest pain?**
Yes. Multichannel intraluminal impedance (MII) is a new methodology that can detect intra-esophageal events, including the reflux or nonpassage of boluses of air or liquid. This has potential benefits for the diagnosis of both nonacid reflux and motility abnormalities.

Monitoring of brain activity in response to esophageal stimulation has advanced our understanding of the central processing of UCP. New technologies in this area include analysis of cerebral-evoked potentials, functional MRI, and PET scanning.

4. **What is visceral hypersensitivity? Define the "irritable esophagus."**
Many patients with UCP have lower thresholds to pain, in response to IEBD, than normal individuals. This finding is believed to be due to visceral hypersensitivity or altered nociception.

For some patients, the problem may not be due to abnormal contractions but rather to abnormal perception of normal events, including peristaltic muscle contractions, physiologic quantities of acid reflux, and luminal distention by air or food. Combined pH and manometric monitoring has identified patients who are sensitive to both acid and motility events. This condition is described as the *irritable esophagus*. Research analyzing cerebral-evoked potential responses to esophageal stimulation suggests that the abnormality is due to central interpretation rather than abnormal firing of the peripheral nociceptors.

15. Does unexplained chest pain have a psychological component?

Yes. All disease has a psychological element; illness is interpreted according to personality and previous experiences. This maxim appears to be particularly true for UCP. Psychological abnormalities have been documented in 34–59% of patients with UCP and are present in all of the causes described previously. Psychiatric diagnoses are probably most prevalent in patients with esophageal motility abnormalities (84% in one study). Psychological factors, therefore, must be considered in the management of patients with UCP, including the possibility of panic attacks. Patients with high psychological scores are particularly susceptible to an initial placebo response to medication, but, in the long-term, treatment is ineffective. If such patients are identified, specific therapies can address the problem. Patients with high psychological scores have a worse prognosis and experience increased disability attributed to the illness.

16. What are the treatment options for nonreflux esophageal chest pain?

Esophageal motility abnormalities. Calcium antagonists, nitrates, and anticholinergic agents are the primary treatments aimed at motility dysfunction, that is, the spastic component. If the pain is only occasional, short-acting nitrates or calcium antagonists may be taken sublingually as needed. More frequent episodes of chest pain are better managed by regular therapy with a long-acting preparation. Although such medications may have a dramatic effect on esophageal pressures, their symptomatic efficacy is often disappointing. Benzodiazepines both reduce skeletal muscular contractions and modify sensory pathways. They have had limited success in esophageal motility abnormalities. Management of achalasia is discussed separately in Chapter Achalasia.

Visceral hypersensitivity. Drugs used to modify sensory pathways include anxiolytics and antidepressants. The largest body of evidence is for imipramine and other tricyclic antidepressants. They have been shown to be effective in low doses, suggesting that the effect is not due primarily to antidepressant activity.

Psychological and behavioral therapies. Various psychological and behavioral therapies have been tried in small-scale studies. Relaxation therapy has met with some success and can be taught easily to patients who are willing to acknowledge the psychological element in their disease. Reassurance is an intervention that is available to all physicians. The ability to demonstrate a definite esophageal abnormality as an explanation for chest pain is of significant therapeutic benefit. The frequency of both pain and office visits for treatment of pain decreases after such reassurances.

Additional therapies. Both empiric dilatation with a bougie and more specific targeting of a hypertensive LES with pneumatic dilatation have had limited success in some patients. Surgical myotomy may be of benefit to some patients with diffuse esophageal spasm or nutcracker esophagus. However, such interventions have documented complications and should be reserved for the rare, severely disabled patient.

17. Are there any emerging treatment options?

Yes. Several studies have demonstrated good symptom response to botulinum toxin injection among patients with chest pain and hypermotility disorders. By contrast, chest pain patients with ineffective esophageal motility derived little benefit from the 5-HT1 agonist sumatriptan when it was used to improve muscle contractility. Theophylline significantly increased pain thresholds in patients with functional chest pain, possibly acting by altering adenosine-mediated nociception. Additional novel interventions can be anticipated with the increased understanding of how the brain processes visceral stimuli.

8. Can abnormal belching or aerophagia cause chest pain?
Esophageal distention, whether by reflux of gastric contents, impaction of a food bolus, or entrapment of air, can cause chest pain. In several well-documented cases, gaseous esophageal distention was secondary to an abnormal belch reflex. Normally, the upper esophageal sphincter relaxes in response to distention with air. When this response fails, pain may occur.

9. What is the prognosis for patients with unexplained chest pain?
Patients with UCP have a poor functional outcome. Their quality of life is poor compared with healthy controls. They continue to consult a physician or visit the emergency department an average of twice per year, with an average of one hospitalization per year. If the patient does not have coronary artery disease, making a positive esophageal diagnosis significantly reduces such behavior. Despite ongoing morbidity, the mortality rate of these patients (<1% per annum) is the same as for the general population.

BIBLIOGRAPHY

Bennett J: ABC of the upper gastrointestinal tract. Oesophagus: Atypical chest pain and motility disorders. Brit Med J 6(323):791–794, 2001.

Cannon RO, Cattau EL, Yakshe PN, et al: Coronary flow reserve, esophageal motility, and chest pain in patients with angiographically normal coronary arteries. Am J Med 88:217–222, 1990.

Cannon RO III, Quyyumi AA, Mincemoyer R, et al: Imipramine in patients with chest pain despite normal coronary angiograms. N Engl J Med 330:1411–1417, 1994.

Castell DO, Diederich LL, Castell JA (eds): Esophageal Motility and pH Testing, 3rd ed. Highlands Ranch, CO, Sandhill Scientific Inc., 2000.

Chambers J, Bass C: Chest pain and normal coronary anatomy: A review of natural history and possible etiologic factors. Progr Cardiovasc Dis 33:161–184, 1990.

Grossi L, Ciccaglione AF, Marzio L: Effect of the 5-HT1 agonist sumatriptan on oesophageal motor pattern in patients with ineffective oesophageal motility. Neurogastroenterol Motil 15(1):9–14, 2003.

Johnston BT, Castell DO: Intra-oesophageal balloon distension and oesophageal sensation in humans. Eur J Gastroenterol Hepatol 7(12):1221–1229, 1995.

Katz PO, Dalton CB, Richter JE, et al: Esophageal testing of patients with noncardiac chest pain or dysphagia: Results of three years' experience with 1161 patients. Ann Intern Med 106:593–597, 1987.

Kemp HG, Kronmal RA, Vlietstra RE, Frye RL: Seven year survival of patients with normal or near normal coronary arteriograms: A CASS registry study. J Am Coll Cardiol 7:479–483, 1986.

Lacima G, Grande L, Pera M, et al: Utility of ambulatory 24-hour esophageal pH and motility monitoring in noncardiac chest pain: Report of 90 patients and review of the literature. Dig Dis Sci 48(5):952–961, 2003.

Lantinga LJ, Sprafkin RP, McCroskery JH, et al: One-year psychosocial follow-up of patients with chest pain and angiographically normal coronary arteries. Am J Cardiol 62:209–213, 1985.

Miller LS, Pullela SV, Parkman HP, et al: Treatment of chest pain in patients with noncardiac, nonreflux, nonachalasia spastic esophageal motor disorders using botulinum toxin injection into the gastroesophageal junction. Am J Gastroenterol 97(7):1640–1646, 2002.

Prakash C, Clouse RE: Long-term outcome from tricyclic antidepressant treatment of functional chest pain. Dig Dis Sci 44:2372–2379, 1999.

Rao SS, Hayek B, Summers RW: Functional chest pain of esophageal origin: Hyperalgesia or motor dysfunction. Am J Gastroenterol 96:2584–2589, 2001.

Rao SS, Mudipalli RS, Mujica V, et al: An open-label trial of theophylline for functional chest pain. Dig Dis Sci 47:2763–2768, 2002.

Richter JE: Oesophageal motility disorders. Lancet 8(358):823–828, 2001.

Sarkar S, Aziz Q, Woolf CJ, et al: Contribution of central sensitisation to the development of non-cardiac chest pain. Lancet 30(356):1154–1159, 2000.

18. Shrestha S, Pasricha PJ: Update on noncardiac chest pain. Dig Dis 18(3):138–146, 2000.

19. Smout AJPM, DeVore MS, Dalton CB, Castell DO: Cerebral potentials evoked by oesophageal distension in patients with non-cardiac chest pain. Gut 33:298–302, 1992.

20. Tack J, Janssens J: The esophagus and noncardiac chest pain. In Castell DO, Richter JE (eds): The Esophagus Philadelphia, Lippincott Williams & Wilkins, 1999, pp 581–594.

21. Vantrappen G, Janssens J, Ghillebert G: The irritable oesophagus: A frequent cause of angina-like pain. Lancet I:1232–1234, 1987.

22. Ward BW, Wu WC, Richter JE, et al: Long-term follow-up of symptomatic status of patients with noncardiac chest pain: Is diagnosis of esophageal etiology helpful? Am J Gastroenterol 82:215–218, 1987.

CHAPTER 5

ACHALASIA

Xiaotuan Zhao, MD, PhD, and Pankaj Jay Pasricha, MD

1. Define *achalasia.*

The term *achalasia* (Greek = lack of relaxation) describes the pathophysiologic hallmark of the disease: failure of the lower esophageal sphincter (LES) to relax. This term has replaced the previous designation *cardiospasm*, which implies an exaggerated state of contraction. The second cardinal feature is aperistalsis of the body of the esophagus. However, LES dysfunction is more important because gravity appears to be able to compensate for the lack of pumping ability in the body of the esophagus, in most cases.

2. How common is achalasia?

Achalasia is a relatively uncommon disorder, with prevalence estimated at about 8 cases per 10,000 and an incidence rate approximately 0.5 new cases per year per 100,000. The incidence is increased with age, particularly after the seventh decade but equal between men and women.

3. Define *vigorous achalasia.*

The term *vigorous* is applied to cases of achalasia in which prominent contractions can be noticed in the body of the esophagus, either on radiography or by manometry. These contractions are simultaneous and therefore fulfill the manometric definition of aperistalsis required for the diagnosis of achalasia. They should be distinguished from isobaric waves, which can be seen in patients with achalasia and represent bolus-induced passive fluctuations in pressure within the common cavity of the dilated esophagus. Vigorous achalasia may represent an early stage of the disease.

4. What is the relationship between diffuse esophageal spasm (DES) and achalasia?

DES may be regarded as a "cousin" of achalasia. The primary manometric distinction between DES and vigorous achalasia is the presence of at least some normal peristalsis in the former. LES dysfunction is seen often in DES but to a lesser degree than in achalasia. Some evidence suggests that in a small subset (about 5% or less) of patients, DES may evolve into classic achalasia.

5. What is the major pathologic lesion in achalasia? How does it produce the disease?

Although other lesions have been described, including degeneration of the vagus nerve and changes in its dorsal motor nucleus, the myenteric plexus appears to be the major site of the disease. The characteristic finding is loss of ganglion cells, which appears to be selective for inhibitory neurons (those producing nitric oxide and/or vasoactive intestinal peptide [VIP]) with relative sparing of the cholinergic (stimulatory) nerves. Thus, the normal balance of excitatory and inhibitory neural input to smooth muscle is upset. The loss of inhibition, coupled with a relative preservation of the excitatory stimulus, may be responsible for the LES abnormalities. An inflammatory infiltrate, characteristically mononuclear, is also seen commonly in the myenteric plexus. It is speculated that unchecked inflammation at this site leads to neuronal destruction and, eventually, to the clinical manifestations of achalasia.

6. **What is the suspected cause of achalasia?**

   Earlier studies raised the possibility of a virus, particularly one belonging to the herpes family (because of the predilection of herpes viruses for squamous mucosa) and measles virus. A study with DNA hybridization techniques found evidence of the herpes virus in some myotomy specimens from achalasia patients. However, subsequent investigations, using the polymerase chain reaction to detect different markers, found no evidence for any known viral cause. More recently attention has focused on a possible autoimmune basis, with reports of circulating antineural antibodies. These suspicions are given further credence with the finding that achalasia may be particularly associated with certain class II human leukocyte antigens (HLAs), such as DQB1, DQA1, and DQw1. Neurodegeneration is also a possible cause. It has been speculated that the possible site primary involvement in achalasia is in the dorsal motor nucleus and the vagus nerve and that the myenteric abnormalities are secondary. Nevertheless, the cause of achalasia remains a mystery.

7. **Is achalasia an acquired or congenital disease?**

   Most cases of achalasia are acquired. Achalasia is uncommon before age 25, with a clear-cut age-related increase thereafter. Most commonly the disease occurs in middle adult life (ages 30–60) and affects both sexes and all races nearly equally. Rare cases of familial achalasia have been described. Occasionally, achalasia may be found as part of a congenital syndrome, such triple-A syndrome (achalasia, alacrima, and resistance to adrenocorticotropic hormone), also called *Allgrove's syndrome.* The gene mutated in triple A syndrome has now been identified an encodes a protein called ALADIN (also called Adracalin or AAAS). Although the function of this protein is not known, it localizes to nuclear pore complexes (NPCs), large multiprotein assemblies that are the sole sites of nucleocytoplasmic transport, and may play a role in the differentiation and maintenance of the involved issues.

8. **Describe the dysphagia associated with achalasia.**

   In general, the dysphagia due to motor disorder of the esophagus occurs with solids as well as liquids. However, many patients with achalasia complain predominately, if not exclusively, of solid food dysphagia. The converse, dysphagia for liquids only, is almost never seen. Patients often localize the dysphagia to the region of the LES. Regurgitation of food, either active or induced by the recumbent position or bending, should raise the suspicion of achalasia, particularly if it occurs early in the course of symptoms. Patients often complain of waking up in the mornings with remnants of the previous night's supper in their mouth.

9. **What other symptoms may be associated with achalasia?**

   Weight loss is common but not invariable. Pulmonary symptoms (e.g., pneumonia, lung abscesses from aspiration) are much less common than in the past because of earlier diagnosis and treatment. Two surprisingly common symptoms may lead to the wrong diagnosis: chest pain and heartburn (seen in up to 50% and 25% of patients, respectively). At least two different types of chest pain are experienced by patients with achalasia. The obstructive type is associated with swallowing a food bolus and resolves with passage of food into the stomach. The second type is unrelated to eating and is more often seen in patients with vigorous achalasia. However, it is not necessarily related to esophageal contractions and may reflect abnormalities in the sensory pathway, similar to those in patients with plastic motility disorders. Heartburn is indistinguishable from that in patients with gastroesophageal reflux disease (GERD), including response to antacids. In fact, some patients with achalasia have been mistakenly diagnosed with GERD for several years. Whether heartburn results from lactic acid production due to bacterial breakdown of retained food or true acid reflux is not clear.

10. **Does achalasia involve any other parts of the gastrointestinal tract?**

    Yes. The involvement of stomach and pyloric sphincter has been reported. Some studies also showed that a considerable number of patients with achalasia had dysfunction of the sphincter of Oddi.

. **What is the best way to diagnose achalasia?**

Achalasia should be considered in all patients with a history of dysphagia for both solids and liquids. A definitive diagnosis requires two steps: (1) confirmation of the underlying pathophysiology (best done by manometry) and (2) exclusion of cancer at the gastroesophageal (GE) junction, which can produce a similar picture (pseudo-achalasia); this requires endoscopy with particular emphasis on the retroflexed view.

. **What are the characteristic radiologic features of achalasia?**

An atonic and dilated body of the esophagus is often seen; however, occasional early cases present with a normal-sized esophagus and prominent (nonperistaltic) contractions. The "sigmoid esophagus" is an elongated, dilated organ seen in patients with long-standing disease. Epiphrenic diverticula may accompany this picture. In most cases of achalasia, the GE junction is narrowed smoothly, giving rise to the classic "bird's beak" and allowing only very small amounts of contrast to pass through to the stomach. Previous dilatation or surgery may alter this typical appearance. In early achalasia, these classic features may also be absent in about a third of patients.

. **What is required for the manometric diagnosis of achalasia?**

Two manometric features:

- Lack of peristalsis in the body (the smooth muscle portion) of the esophagus
- Abnormal or absent LES relaxation in response to swallowing (with normal relaxation being more than 90%)

. **What is the most important potential pitfall in the manometric diagnosis of achalasia?**

An occasional patient with otherwise typical features of achalasia may demonstrate complete or near-complete relaxation of the LES, but this appearance may be artifactual due to relative movement between the side-hole/point sensor in the manometry catheter and the LES. This problem can be avoided by the use of a Dent sleeve catheter, which incorporates a 6-cm long sensor device for measurement of LES pressures.

. **Describe the typical endoscopic features of achalasia.**

Endoscopy may be reported as normal in a surprising number of patients in whom achalasia is not suspected before the procedure. In more obvious cases, esophageal dilation, varying amounts of food material or secretions, and either a lack of contractions or multiple simultaneous contractions are seen. The esophageal mucosa may demonstrate various changes, from mild erythema to frank erosions or even ulceration. Candidiasis and retained medications may cause some of these lesions; in other cases, stasis of retained material may give rise to an edematous and nodular mucosa.

A tight but relatively elastic feel as the endoscope passes (or "pops") through the GE junction is characteristic of achalasia but may be easily overlooked if the diagnosis is not specifically entertained. The inability to pass the scope, despite moderate amounts of pressure, is highly suggestive of an inflammatory or neoplastic structure. Of interest, resistance may also be encountered at the pyloric outlet in patients with achalasia, giving rise to the "difficult pylorus" sign.

. **What is the difference between secondary achalasia and pseudo-achalasia?**

Although achalasia is most often idiopathic, it has been described in association with various diseases, such as cancer, Chagas' disease, amyloidosis and other infiltrative disorders, mixed connective tissue disorders, endocrine disorders, and intestinal pseudo-obstruction. Such cases are called *secondary achalasia*. Pseudo-achalasia refers to an achalasia-like syndrome that is produced by infiltrating cancer of the GE junction. Finally, in rare patients (typically those with small-cell lung cancer), a paraneoplastic noninfiltrative syndrome can cause the typical symptoms of achalasia.

17. **How can pseudo-achalasia be diagnosed?**

A high index of suspicion should be maintained in patients presenting with what looks like achalasia but with marked weight loss and short duration of symptoms. However, these and other features, such as the age of the patient, are not highly specific. Endoscopy remains the crucial diagnostic test because the clinical history, radiographic appearance of barium study, and even manometric analysis may not distinguish pseudo-achalasia from the idiopathic form. Failure to pass the endoscope into the stomach almost invariably rules out true achalasia. A careful examination of the GE region, including a retroflexed view from the stomach, is absolutely mandatory, and biopsies should be taken of any suspicious area or lesion. Even so, the sensitivity of this method in excluding underlying cancer is reported to be around 80% or less. Endoscopic ultrasound (EUS) may provide additional value, but this has yet to be convincingly demonstrated.

18. **Is achalasia a premalignant condition?**

Yes. Esophageal cancer may arise in achalasia, thought to result from long-standing stasis and secondary changes in the epithelium. When cancer develops, it is usually of the squamous variety and arises in the dilated middle part of the esophagus, rendering it relatively silent until a late stage. The overall prevalence of esophageal cancer in achalasia is about 3%, with an incidence of about 197 per 100,000 per year. This incidence significantly increases after 15 years of achalasia. A large population-based study demonstrated a 16-fold increase in cancer risk during years 2–24 after the diagnosis of achalasia. The risk of cancer in most patients with adequate treatment remains very small (see later text).

19. **Should patients with achalasia undergo periodic endoscopic surveillance?**

Yes and no. A surveillance strategy would require 406 endoscopies to detect one cancer in men and 2220 endoscopies to detect one cancer in women. The American Society of Gastrointestinal Endoscopy recommends the following guidelines for surveillance: (1) for the rare untreated patient, periodic endoscopic surveillance after 15 years is justified, (2) if effective dilation or myotomy was performed early in the course of the disease, there may be no need for endoscopic surveillance, and (3) patients who are treated later in the course of the disease may appear to be at increased risk for malignancy, and the role of endoscopic surveillance has not been determined.

20. **What treatment options are available for achalasia? Describe their rationale.**

All of the therapeutic options available for achalasia are palliative. Their goal is to decrease the resistance to bolus transit created by dysfunctional LES. Traditional pharmacologic therapy does so by inducing smooth muscle relaxation. Botulinum toxin injections block the excitatory neural inputs to the LES by inhibiting the release of acetylcholine from nerve endings. The theoretical rationale for balloon dilation is to achieve a partial tear of the LES muscle, but this option is somewhat speculative because the few animal studies that evaluate this method have shown no histologic evidence of damage, despite marked reductions in LES pressure. Surgical myotomy has the most straightforward rationale of all treatment options but comes at a price (see later text).

21. **Discuss the various pharmacologic options for palliation of achalasia.**

Nitrates are probably more effective than calcium channel blockers but have significant adverse side effects that lead to discontinuation of the drug in up to one third of patients. Isosorbide dinitrate (5–10 mg sublingually before meals) begins to act within 15 minutes, and its effect may persist for as long as 90 minutes. Symptoms are improved in 75–85% of patients. Nifedipine, which may be more effective than diltiazem or verapamil, lowers LES pressure by 30–40%. The effects peak within 30–45 minutes and last more than 1 hour. Contrary to popular belief, nifedipine is poorly absorbed sublingually. Oral doses of 10–20 mg have been reported to improve symptoms in 50–70% of patients. In most cases, however, the use of pharmacotherapy is at best temporizing. Most patients require additional forms of treatment after 6 months or so because of side effects, progression of disease, or development of tolerance.

What does Viagra have to do with achalasia?

Sildenafil (Viagra) blocks phosphodiesterase type 5 (the enzyme responsible for degradation of cyclic guanosine monophosphate [cGMP]), which results in increased cGMP levels within smooth muscle and consequent relaxation. It is effective in short-term reduction of LES pressures in patients with achalasia. A recent small number, randomized, double-blind clinical trial showed that sildenafil at 50 mg significantly decreased the LES pressure tone, residual pressure in patients with primary achalasia compared to placebo group. The effect lasted less than 60 minutes. However, sildenafil had no effect of improving propagation of pressure waves in esophageal body.

What is the single most permanent treatment of achalasia?

The answer is clearly surgery, with short-term (5 years or less) efficacy around 90%. Long-term results are less positive, with only about two thirds of patients reporting good-to-excellent outcomes. This is probably due, in large part, to the sequelae of the reflux disease that invariably accompanies successful myotomy (see later text).

What is the major problem with surgery?

In the past, surgery was associated with considerable morbidity, whether done via a thoracic or abdominal approach. Recent advances in laparoscopic techniques have enabled a minimally invasive approach to myotomy, with significant reductions in perioperative pain, morbidity, and length of hospitalization. However, the major problem remains unchanged: long-term GERD, which can be particularly damaging in an atonic esophagus. Although most surgeons using an abdominal approach incorporate a "loose" antireflux procedure along with the myotomy, its effectiveness in preventing GERD remains controversial. Two long-term studies using a thoracic approach, one with and one without an antireflux procedure, were comparable in that only two thirds of patients in either study were still doing well 10 years and beyond. Although the abdominal approach may be associated with less reflux, long-term results are not yet available after laparoscopic surgery, and patients and physicians should be on guard for this complication.

How can postoperative GERD be avoided?

The best advice to give patients after myotomy is that they need to be followed carefully for GERD. A very low threshold should be used for initiation of antireflux medications. Proton pump inhibitors are very effective in preventing postoperative GERD symptoms.

How is balloon dilation of the lower esophageal sphincter accomplished?

Using whalebone as a dilator, Sir Thomas Willis first described dilation of LES in a patient with achalasia. Forceful dilation of the LES is achieved by stretching it to at least 30 mm or more (for adults); this obviously requires more than a simple bougie and is best accomplished by using a specially designed balloon catheter. The most commonly available device (Rigiflex by Microvasive) is passed over a guidewire and requires fluoroscopic monitoring; a typical starting balloon size for most adults is 30 mm. A less common device is the Witzel dilator, which consists of a polyethylene balloon mounted on a forward viewing endoscope that is inflated under directed visualization (with the endoscope in the retroflexed position in the stomach). It has the advantage of not requiring fluoroscopy. Otherwise, there is little science to dilation. A good stretch requires obliteration of the balloon waist; however, consideration of durations, pressure, number of inflations, presence of blood on the dilator, or induction of chest pain, are of little, if any, importance in determining efficacy.

What can be done if symptoms do not respond to the first dilation?

A larger balloon (available in 5-mm increments from 25 mm up to 40 mm) may be used to attempt further stretching of the LES, the so-called progressive method. An alternative method, championed by van Trappen and colleagues but seldom practiced in the United States, is repeated dilation (regardless of the initial symptomatic response) until certain objective parameters of esophageal emptying (usually determined radiographically) are met. Regardless of the method used, if the patient fails three dilations, most authorities recommend surgery.

28. **What are the results of pneumatic dilation?**
The overall immediate response rate to pneumatic dilation is 75–80%; long-term results show that up to one half of patients require one or more dilations over a 5-year period. Beyond this time, about 50–70% of patients continue to do well; however, up to 20% or more may eventually need surgery.

29. **How does pneumatic dilation compare with surgery?**
A classic randomized, controlled trial of surgery and dilation clearly favored surgery in terms long-term results. However, it is not clear whether this is the most cost-effective approach, considering the long-term and cumulative costs of surgery (estimated at nearly 2.5 times more than the cost of pneumatic dilation), even in view of the perforation rate and need for retreatment associated with pneumatic dilation.

30. **What is the major disadvantage of forceful dilation? How can it be prevented?**
The major risk of dilation is perforation (estimated rate = 1–10% or even higher). Because of the empiric way in which dilation is performed, this risk appears to be inherent; there are few ways to prevent this complication. It is important to exclude stricture (malignant or benign), to ensure a near-empty esophagus, and to perform all manipulations of the balloon under fluoroscopic control. Relative contraindications cited in the literature include a tortuous sigmoid shape, previous myotomy, epiphrenic diverticula, and large hiatal hernias, but most experts do not view these as absolute. Larger balloons are expected to increase the risk for perforation. The overall perforation rate for Rigiflex dilation is about 3%, and for Witzel dilation the rate is about 6%. GERD is believed to be uncommon after forceful dilation, with an incidence of around 2%.

31. **How is perforation treated in patients with achalasia?**
Treatment is controversial. Perforations after achalasia dilation tend to be small and well contained. Thus, many authorities advocated conservative treatment (i.e., antibiotics and parenteral alimentation); good results are reported in the literature. However, it is difficult to predict the outcome with this form of treatment in individual cases. Surgery is definitely indicated in patients with large perforations and free flow of contrast into the mediastinum or with evidence of sepsis. When surgery is performed early, the clinical outcome and long-term course appear similar to elective myotomy.

32. **Which patients are particularly likely to respond to dilation?**
In general, older patients (over age 50) do significantly better after dilation than younger patients.

33. **What objective parameters should be followed after dilation?**
The most consistent and important parameter determining long-term response after pneumatic dilation is posttreatment LES pressure. The best results are obtained when LES pressure is < mmHg. It is theoretically possible that a treatment regimen based on "optimization" of esophageal emptying rather than symptomatic response alone may lead to better long-term results. A recent study showed that timed barium esophagram was an import tool to predict long-term results. In this study, about 30% of achalasia patients reported symptoms relieved after pneumatic dilatation had an abnormal timed barium esophagram study, while 90% of the patients failed within 1 year after treatment.

34. **How is botulinum toxin type A (Botox) injection administered?**
Botox is available through most hospital pharmacies in vials containing 100 units of the lyophilized powder. For use in achalasia, it can be diluted in 5 mL of normal saline to yield a

solution containing 20 U/mL. Flexible upper endoscopy is performed using routing sedation, and the toxin is injected via a 5-mm sclerotherapy needle into the LES region, piercing the mucosa about 1 cm above the Z-line and slanting the needle approximately 45 degrees. The injections are administered in four aliquots distributed circumferentially in four different quadrants. The original dose of 80 U/mL was chosen empirically; there is no good reason why the contents of an entire vial (100 U) cannot be administered. Precise location of the injection site may not be necessary because diffusion may take care of any minor variations. Others advocate the use of EUS to help guide injection; it is not clear whether EUS results in better outcomes than the traditional method.

. What are the results of Botox treatment?
Only about two third of patients sustained improvement (beyond the first month or so). Older patients do better, and patients with vigorous achalasia may have a more favorable response than those with the classic form. Patients who respond to an initial injection remain in remission for several months (range = 4 months to >1 year). When symptoms return, patients usually respond to repeat injections of botulinum toxin. Larger doses of Botox at the time of initial injection have not been proven to improve the response rate.

. Discuss the major drawbacks of botulinum toxin treatment?
Overall, Botox is a relatively safe and simple treatment with few, if any, major complications. The major drawback is cost, coupled with the need for multiple injections. Some surgical reports suggest that repeat injection of Botox is somewhat more difficult technically. However, outcomes after surgery appear not to be affected, whether or not Botox had been previously used.

. What is the overall best treatment for achalasia?
Because no treatment is curative, there is no real answer. It is best for the physician to become familiar with the advantages and disadvantages of each option and to present them to the patients. The final choice depends on several factors, including patient preference and risk tolerance as well as local availability of technical expertise. Regardless of the treatment, patients need to be followed carefully and therapeutic strategies revisited on a periodic basis.

WEBSITES

1. http://www.nlm.nih.gov/medlineplus/ency/article/000267.htm

2. http://www.clevelandclinicmeded.com/diseasemanagement

BLIOGRAPHY

Blam ME, Delfyett W, Levine MS, et al: Achalasia: A disease of varied and subtle symptoms that do not correlate with radiographic findings. Am J Gastroenterol 97:1916–1923, 2002.

Bortolotti M, Mari C, Lopilato C, et al: Effects of Sildenafil on esophageal motility of patients with idiopathic achalasia. Gastroenterology 118:253–257, 2000.

Brucher BL, Stein HJ, Bartels H, et al: Achalasia and esophageal cancer: Incidence, prevalence, and prognosis. World J Surg 25:745–749, 2001.

Cronshaw JM, Matunis MJ: The nuclear pore complex protein ALADIN is mislocalized in triple A syndrome. Proc Natl Acad Sci U S A 100:5823–5827, 2003.

Dunaway PM, Wong P: Risk and surveillance intervals for squamous cell carcinoma in achalasia. Gastrointest Endosc Clin N Am 11:425–434, 2001.

Goodgame RW, Graham DY: Manometry in classic and vigorous achalasia. Gastroenterology 103:1993, 1992.

7. Hoogerwerf WA, Pasricha PJ: Pharmacologic therapy in treating achalasia. Gastrointest Endosc Clin N Am 11:311–324, 2001.

8. Khelif K, De Laet MH, Chaouachi B, et al: Achalasia of the cardia in Allgrove's (triple A) syndrome: histopathologic study of 10 cases. Am J Surg Pathol 27:667–672, 2003.

9. Kobara H, Uchida N, Tsutsui K, et al: Abnormal bile flow in patients with achalasia. J Gastroenterol 38:327–331, 2003.

10. Mayberry JF: Epidemiology and demographics of achalasia. Gastrointest Endosc Clin N Am 11:235–248, 2001.

11. Parkman HP, Reynolds JC, Ouyang A, et al: Pneumatic dilatation or esophagomyotomy treatment for idiopathic achalasia: Clinical outcomes and cost analysis. Dig Dis Sci 38:75–85, 1993.

12. Pasricha PJ, Rai R, Ravich WJ, et al: Botulinum toxin for achalasia: Long-term outcome and predictors of response. Gastroenterology 110:1410–1415, 1996.

13. Pasricha PJ, Ravich WJ, Hendrix TR, et al: Intrasphincteric botulinum toxin for the treatment of achalasia. N Eng J Med 332:774–778, 1995.

14. Paterson WG: Etiology and pathogenesis of achalasia. Gastrointest Endosc Clin N Am 11:249–266, 2001.

15. Rajput S, Nandwani SK, Phadke AY, et al: Predictors of response to pneumatic dilatation in achalasia cardia. Indian J Gastroenterol 19:126–129, 2000.

16. Vaezi MF, Baker ME, Achkar E, Richter JE: Timed barium oesophagram: Better predictor of long term success after pneumatic dilation in achalasia than symptom assessment. Gut 50:765–770, 2002.

17. Zhao XT, Pasricha PJ: Botulinum toxin for spastic GI disorders: A systematic review. Gastrointest Endosc 57:219–235, 2003.

ESOPHAGEAL CANCER

CHAPTER 6

Nimish Vakil, MD

What is the incidence of esophageal cancer in the United States, and is it changing?

Esophageal cancer is relatively infrequent in the United States. The annual incidence is <10 of 100,000 population, whereas in some areas of China the annual incidence is >100 of 100,000. Over the past three decades, the incidence of distal esophageal adenocarcinoma has increased sharply in North America, whereas the incidence of squamous cell carcinoma of the esophagus has fallen. The rise in esophageal adenocarcinoma has been most marked in white men. Recent studies suggest that the incidence of esophageal adenocarcinoma is rising in African-American and Hispanic men. For unknown reasons, the disease remains rare in women. Although the absolute numbers of cases of esophageal cancer remain low, there has been a remarkable rise in the incidence of distal esophageal cancer over the past three decades in most developed countries, making it one of the most rapidly growing cancers in the United States. The decline in distal gastric cancers over the same period has been correlated with a decline in the prevalence of *Helicobacter pylori* infection in the United States.

What are the risk factors for the development of esophageal cancer?

Smoking and alcohol use have been associated with the development of squamous cell carcinoma of the esophagus, but they do not appear to be major risk factors for the development of esophageal adenocarcinoma. Squamous cell carcinoma is much more frequent in African Americans than in whites, whereas adenocarcinoma is much more frequent in whites. Frequent, long-standing heartburn is an important risk factor for the development of esophageal adenocarcinoma. In some studies, obesity has been shown to be an independent risk factor, and obese patients with reflux disease are at particularly high risk for the development of esophageal cancer. Recent studies have drawn an epidemiologic link between the widespread use of drugs that affect the lower esophageal sphincter and the increasing risk of esophageal cancer. A true cause-and-effect relationship has not been established. Diets low in fresh fruits and vegetables have also been associated with esophageal cancer.

What are the current recommendations for screening and surveillance of esophageal cancer in patients at risk?

Screening. Currently, there is no acceptable screening method for esophageal cancer in the United States. Some economic models have suggested that a one-time screening endoscopy to identify Barrett's esophagus may be cost-effective in patients with long-standing reflux esophagitis, but the assumptions for the risk of developing cancer in Barrett's esophagus in the model may be too high. The American College of Gastroenterology guidelines suggest that patients with chronic GERD are most likely to have Barrett's esophagus and should undergo endoscopy.

Surveillance. Surveillance is recommended in patients with Barrett's esophagus, and the grade of dysplasia determines the interval for surveillance. In patients with low-grade dysplasia as the highest grade after a 6-month follow-up endoscopy with concentrated biopsies in the area of dysplasia, annual endoscopy is recommended until there is no dysplasia. The finding of high-grade dysplasia requires a repeat endoscopy (after double-dose therapy with proton pump inhibitor). Special attention should be paid to any mucosal irregularity, and endoscopic mucosal resection should be considered. An intensive biopsy protocol should ideally be performed with a therapeutic endoscope and large-capacity biopsy forceps. An expert pathologist should confi[rm] the interpretation of high-grade dysplasia. Focal high-grade dysplasia (less than five crypts) ma[y] be followed with a 3-month surveillance. Intervention should be considered in a patient with co[n]firmed multifocal high-grade dysplasia. Surveillance endoscopy intervals are lengthening; whe[n] dysplasia is not found on two consecutive surveillance endoscopies, a 3-year interval for surve[il]lance is recommended by the American College of Gastroenterology guidelines.

4. **How is esophageal cancer diagnosed?**
    Endoscopy and biopsy are necessary for the diagnosis of esophageal cancer. Staging has become important in the management of patients with esophageal cancer. Staging helps dete[r]mine the choice of treatment and is an important determinant of prognosis. Computed tomog[ra]phy (CT) of the chest and abdomen is the recommended initial test for staging.

5. **Discuss the role of endoscopic ultrasound in the diagnosis and staging of esophageal cancer.**
    In patients who appear to have limited local disease on CT and no evidence of distant metastases, endoscopic ultrasound may be helpful in regional staging. Esophageal cance[r] is seen as a hypoechoic interruption of the layers of the esophagus. Endoscopic ultrasou[nd] is better than CT at staging the depth of insertion. This factor becomes important in deci[d]ing between different methods of curative therapy. For example, patients with cancer loc[al]ized to the mucosa can be considered for mucosal resection, but deeper levels of invasio[n] make this therapy inappropriate. Endoscopic ultrasound has better results in regional sta[g]ing than the newest spiral CT scanners. Magnetic resonance imaging (MRI) has not been particularly helpful in imaging the depth of local invasion. Endoscopic ultrasound may al[so] be helpful in the evaluation of mediastinal lymph nodes. Large nodes (>10 mm) that are [uni]formly hypoechoic are suspicious. Fine-needle aspiration under ultrasound guidance ma[y] help to establish lymph node involvement.

6. **How is esophageal cancer staged? Why is staging important?**
    Esophageal cancer staging is performed according to the tumor-node-metastasis (TNM) clas[si]fication (Table 6-1). Accurate staging is important to establish prognosis and treatment approach. Treatment, as in all malignant disorders, is based on the risk of the therapy balance[d] against the likelihood of a good outcome. Patient preference and local expertise may also dete[r]mine the choice of treatment. Rational choices can be based on the stage of esophageal canc[er] as discussed in later text.

7. **What curative therapies are available for esophageal cancer?**
    Treatment guidelines from the American College of Gastroenterology recommend stage-direc[ted] therapy. Treatment options are summarized by stage in the following text:
    Stages 0, I, IIA (early-stage disease). Patients with early-stage disease are generally treate[d] with curative surgery alone. Endoscopic mucosectomy, using a suction cap fitted with a snar[e] may be curative in stages 0 and I. Experience with this modality is increasing in the United States, but controlled data are lacking. Other ablative therapies have also been used, includin[g] electrocautery, argon plasma coagulation, and photodynamic therapy. Chemotherapy and rad[ia]tion are not used as adjuvants for early-stage disease. Surgical therapy consists of resection [of] the tumor with anastomosis of the stomach with the cervical esophagus (gastric pull-up) or interposition of the colon to reestablish gastrointestinal continuity. Results are better in hos[pi]tals that perform this surgery frequently and poorer in small hospitals that perform the sur[]gery infrequently. Photodynamic therapy (discussed later) is an alternative to surgery in patients with high-grade dysplasia or early cancer, particularly if the patient is unwilling or unfit for surgery. A recent study showed promising results in patients with high-grade dysp[la]sia and early cancer.

TABLE 6-1.   STAGING OF ESOPHAGEAL CANCER

Primary Tumor

T_x	Primary tumor cannot be assessed
T_0	No evidence of primary tumor
T_{is}	Carcinoma in situ
T_1	Tumor invades lamina propria or submucosa
T_2	Tumor invades muscularis propria
T_3	Tumor invades adventitia
T_4	Tumor invades adjacent structures

Regional Lymph Nodes

For the cervical esophagus, cervical and supraclavicular lymph nodes are considered regional; for the thoracic esophagus, mediastinal and perigastric lymph nodes (excluding celiac nodes) are considered regional.

N_x	Regional nodes cannot be assessed
N_0	No regional lymph node metastases
N_1	Regional lymph node metastases

Distant Metastases

M_x	Distant metastases cannot be assessed
M_0	No distant metastases
M_1	Distant metastases

Stages

Stage 0	T_{is}, N_0, M_0
Stage 1	T_1, N_0, M_0
Stage IIA	T_2, N_0, M_0; T_3, N_0, M_0
Stage IIB	T_1, N_1, M_0; T_2, N_1, M_0
Stage III	T_3, N_1, M_0; T_4, any N, M_0
Stage IV	Any T, any N, M_1

Stages IIB, III (regionally advanced disease). The results of single-modality (surgery, chemotherapy, or radiation) therapy are limited. Less than 10% of patients are cured by surgery alone. The results of radiation and chemotherapy alone are also limited. A recent meta-analysis has shown that a multimodality approach consisting of chemotherapy and radiation followed by surgery (triple therapy) offers the best likelihood of cure. Triple therapy is aggressive and expensive and has a high side-effect rate. Patients who are in poor general condition may elect to have palliative therapy after balancing the low probability of cure against the morbidity of treatment.

Stage IV (distant metastases). Distant metastases make esophageal cancer incurable; therapy is palliative. Radiation and chemotherapy are frequently used and may offer small increases in survival rates with the trade-off of systemic side effects. In patients with dysphagia, a number of palliative measures are possible but do not prolong survival.

8. **What are the endoscopic methods for the palliation of esophageal cancer?**

A number of endoscopic methods are available. Endoscopic dilation causes temporary relief of dysphagia and is not effective as long-term therapy. Expandable metal stents provide rapid palliation of dysphagia, but late complications can be a problem. Membrane-covered metal stents were developed to prevent the problems associated with tumor ingrowth and have been shown to be superior to uncovered stents. A number of tumor ablative therapies are also available. Injection of absolute alcohol into the tumor has been reported and is inexpensive. There is little control of the degree of necrosis, and tracking of the alcohol beyond the esophagus can cause perforation and chemical mediastinitis. Argon plasma therapy and Nd YAG laser can restore luminal patency by tumor ablation. Argon plasma coagulation is considerably less expensive than laser therapy and is equally effective. The principal disadvantage of these modalities is that they may require multiple treatments (and therefore multiple visits to the hospital), which is undesirable in patients who have a short time to live. Photodynamic therapy is a recent development in the treatment of esophageal cancer. A light-sensitive drug (Photofrin) is injected intravenously and selectively accumulates in the tumor tissue. Specially developed catheters are used to deliver light to the tumor and cause necrosis of the tumor. The procedure is relatively safe and generally well tolerated. Its principal disadvantages are cost, the development of cutaneous photosensitivity, and strictures in the esophagus. The procedure was recently approved by the Food and Drug Administration (FDA) and is an important alternative for patients who either do not wish to have surgery or are deemed poor risks for surgery.

9. **What does the future hold for patients at risk for development of esophageal cancer?**

The future of esophageal cancer lies in prevention. Symptoms develop late in the disease, and most patients are incurable at presentation. Because of the low absolute numbers of patients developing the disease, widespread screening programs in the general population are unlikely to be cost-effective. One-time endoscopic screening for Barrett's esophagus has been proposed in patients with chronic reflux disease as a method for identifying patients at risk, but timing, cost-effectiveness, and efficacy remain unproven. A systematic review of patients taking aspirin or nonsteroidal anti-inflammatory drugs (NSAIDs) suggested that these agents may be protective against adenocarcinoma and squamous cell carcinoma. Chemoprevention of esophageal cancer with aspirin or cyclooxygenase (COX-2) inhibitors is an exciting new dimension that is undergoing further study.

WEBSITES

1. http://www.cancer.gov/cancer_information/cancer_type/esophageal

2. http://www.nlm.nih.gov/medlineplus/ency/article/000283.htm

3. http://www.cancer.gov/cancertopics/pdq/treatment/esophageal

BIBLIOGRAPHY

1. Brown LM, Devesa SS: Epidemiologic trends in esophageal and gastric cancer in the United States. Surg Oncol Clin N Am 11(2):235–256, 2002.

2. Corley DA, Kerlikowske K, Verma R, Buffler P: Protective association of aspirin/NSAIDs and esophageal cancer: A systematic review and meta-analysis. Gastroenterology 124(1):47–569, 2003.

3. Ell C, May A, Gossner L, et al: Endoscopic mucosal resection of early cancer and high-grade dysplasia in Barrett's esophagus. Gastroenterology 118(4):670–677, 2000.

4. Inadomi JM, Sampliner R, Lagergren J, et al: Screening and surveillance for Barrett esophagus in high-risk groups: A cost-utility analysis. Ann Intern Med 138(3):176–186, 2003.

Lightdale C: Practice guidelines: Esophageal cancer. Am J Gastroenterol 94:20–29, 1999.

Overholt BF, Panjehpour M, Halberg DL: Photodynamic therapy for Barrett's esophagus with dysplasia and/or early stage carcinoma: Long-term results. Gastrointest Endosc 58(2):183–188, 2003.

Sampliner RE: Practice Parameters Committee of the American College of Gastroenterology. Updated guidelines for the diagnosis, surveillance, and therapy of Barrett's esophagus. Am J Gastroenterol 97(8):1888–1895, 2002.

Siersema PD, Marcon N, Vakil N: Metal stents for tumors of the distal esophagus and gastric cardia. Endoscopy 35(1):79–85, 2003.

Urschel JD, Vasan H: A meta-analysis of randomized controlled trials that compared neoadjuvant chemoradiation and surgery to surgery alone for resectable esophageal cancer. Am J Surg 185(6):538–543, 2003.

CHAPTER 7

PILL-INDUCED AND CORROSIVE INJUR OF THE ESOPHAGUS

Matthew Bachinski, MD

1. **Who is affected by pill-induced esophageal injury?**

   Anyone of any age who ingests caustic pills is susceptible to pill-induced injury. Reported cas range from ages 5–89. Women outnumber men by a ratio of 1.5:1. It is not uncommon for pi to stick in a normal esophagus during transit. One study showed that 36 of 49 normal subject who assumed a supine position after swallowing a round, nonsticky barium tablet with 15 mL water retained the tablet in the esophagus for 5–45 minutes. A more sticky gelatin tablet remained in the esophagus for more than 10 minutes in over one half of normal subjects who ingested the pill in a supine position. Esophageal dysmotility or structural abnormalities, such rings or strictures, are clearly not required for pill-induced injury.

2. **What factors contribute to esophageal retention of pills?**

   Esophageal clearance is determined by several factors, some of which can be modified to decrease the risk of pill-induced injury. Upright posture improves esophageal clearance of pill The volume of water ingested with pills also affects clearance, although no study has identifie the volume required to ensure passage through the esophagus. One study showed that 11 of patients retained a barium pill swallowed with 15 mL of water compared with 3 of 18 who swa lowed the pill with 120 mL of water. Other partially modifiable factors include structural abnor malities, such as rings or strictures, which can be dilated as needed. Abnormal esophageal motility is sometimes improved with pharmacologic agents, but motility is usually normal in patients with pill-induced injury. Taking the pill with inadequate fluid and lying down immediat afterward are often the only identifiable risk factors.

3. **What are the risk factors for pill-induced injury?**

   Anyone who takes a caustic pill is at risk, but some patients are at particular risk for severe pil induced esophageal injury, including those with structural abnormalities of the esophagus, bo pathologic (stricture, tumor, ring) and physiologic (hiatal hernia, narrowing of the esophagus secondary to compression from the left atrium, aortic arch, left mainstem bronchus). Cardiac disease is a risk factor because of esophageal compression by a dilated left atrium and freque use of inherently caustic medications (e.g., aspirin, potassium chloride, quinidine). Patients w have undergone thoracotomy are at increased risk because they are bedridden and may devel adhesions and fibrosis that trap the esophagus between the aorta and vertebral column, makir it more susceptible to compression by an enlarged left atrium and thus decreasing esophagea clearance. Supine positioning during pill ingestion impairs esophageal clearance and places patients at risk. The stickiness of the pill surface, the inherent caustic nature of certain drugs, and the volume of liquid consumed with pills affect risk. Elderly patients and patients with underlying gastroesophageal reflux disease (GERD) are at increased risk. GERD may cause a more acidic environment; because many drugs, including nonsteroidal anti-inflammatory dru (NSAIDs), are weak acids, their absorption into tissues is increased in an acidic environment.

4. **Describe the typical presentation of patients with pill-induced injury.**

   The typical patient has no prior history of esophageal disease and presents with the sudden onset of retrosternal pain, which may have awakened the patient from sleep (particularly if pill were ingested with little liquid just before or while lying down) and may be exacerbated by swallowing. The pain may be mild or so severe that swallowing is impossible. The pain increases typically over the first 3–4 days before gradually subsiding. Painless dysphagia is uncommon (20%) and may suggest an alternative diagnosis. Less common symptoms and signs include dehydration, weight loss, fever, and hematemesis. Patients with preexisting esophageal problems, such as GERD, frequently present with worsening symptoms of heartburn, regurgitation, and dysphagia.

How is the diagnosis of pill-induced esophageal injury made?
The diagnosis of pill-induced esophageal injury may be suspected on the basis of history alone when typical symptoms suddenly appear soon after the ingestion of a pill known to cause esophageal injury. In a typical and uncomplicated case, an invasive diagnostic test may not be required, and the diagnosis can be made on the basis of history and physical exam. A diagnostic study is indicated when symptoms are severe, persist longer than 3–4 days, have atypical features, or suggest a complication (stricture, hemorrhage), or when the history suggests an alternative diagnosis (e.g., foreign body obstruction, infectious esophagitis in an immunocompromised host). Upper endoscopy is the most sensitive test; results are abnormal in almost all cases of pill-induced esophageal injury. In addition, it allows the most accurate assessment of alternative diagnoses, such as severe GERD, infectious esophagitis, or malignancy.

What does the typical pill-induced lesion look like at time of endoscopy?
The typical lesion of pill-induced esophageal injury is one or more discrete ulcers with normal surrounding mucosa. Ulcers range in size from pinpoint to circumferential lesions that may be several centimeters long. Most ulcers involve the mucosa only, but deeper penetration can occur and localized perforations have been reported. Ulcers may have local surrounding inflammation. Pill fragments have been seen in ulcer craters.

What are the potential complications of pill-induced esophageal ulcers?
Typical ulcers involve the mucosa only, but deeper lesions may occur. Torrential hemorrhage has resulted from erosions into vascular structures, including the left atrium. Cases with penetration to the mediastinum have been reported. Deep circumferential ulceration may result in formation of a circumferential fibrotic stricture, but this occurs in less than 10% of reported cases. Probably the true incidence of stricture formation is much less, because severe or atypical cases are more likely to be reported.

What pills are frequently implicated or particularly injurious?
Antibiotic pills are frequent offenders, accounting for more than one half of all reported cases of pill-induced esophageal injury because of the large number of prescriptions written and the caustic nature of the pills themselves. Doxycycline and tetracycline accounted for 293 of 454 reported cases of pill-induced esophageal injury in one recent review. Although frequent offenders, antibiotics rarely cause complicated injury to the esophagus. Patients with antibiotic-associated injury almost always present with acute, severe pain and local, circumscribed tissue injury due to mucosal ulceration. The ulceration is believed to be secondary to a single trapped pill.

Cardiac and *vascular medications,* including antihypertensives and anti-arrhythmics, compose a large group of caustic drugs. Quinidine alone has been reported in 13 cases of pill-induced injury; 7 of the 13 patients later developed strictures, making quinidine a particularly injurious substance. An unusual feature of quinidine-induced injury is its tendency to form profuse, irregular exudate that is sufficiently thick and adherent, appearing as a filling defect suggestive of carcinoma on barium swallow. On endoscopy the exudate can be washed away and has not been shown to be predictive of late fibrotic stricture formation.

Anti-inflammatory medications are relatively uncommon agents in pill-induced esophageal injury. A recent review reported only 71 cases of injury attributable to this class of drugs. In part because they are so widely prescribed, 22 different anti-inflammatory agents have been reported to cause injury, but approximately 45% of these reports are secondary to aspirin, Doleron, and indomethacin, with aspirin the single most common anti-inflammatory medicine to cause pill esophagitis. No hallmark lesion is associated with NSAIDs.

9. **Do any new drugs on the market deserve special notice?**
   Alendronate sodium (Fosamax, Merck & Co., West Point, PA) is an oral aminobiphosphonate that inhibits osteoclast activity in the bones. It is used to treat and prevent osteoporosis in post-menopausal women. It can cause significant esophageal injury. The package insert for Fosamax advises how to administer the medication to maximize esophageal clearance. These factors include consuming 6–8 oz of water with the pill and staying upright for 30 minutes after taking the pill. In one study, a full 50% of patients who had complications with alendronate failed to follow these guidelines. The manufacturer advises that abnormalities of the esophagus that delay esophageal emptying and the inability to stand or sit upright for 30 minutes after ingestion are contraindications for prescription. Endoscopy reveals a classic esophageal lesion with Fosamax. Like quinidine it causes a circumscribed ulceration covered by a thick, white, loosely adherent exudate. Histology confirms a leukofibrinous exudate similar to pseudomembranous colitis. Current data suggest the actual incidence of severe or serious esophageal injury is actually well under 1% of patients using alendronate. A newer bisphosphonate, risedronate, is now available for the prevention and treatment of osteoporosis and appears to have minimal gastrointestinal toxicity.

10. **What other mechanisms have been proposed to explain pill-induced injury?**
    Animal studies have demonstrated that certain pills placed in direct contact with esophageal tissue can cause ulceration. This finding has been verified in humans by esophagogastroduo-denoscopy (EGD), which revealed an esophageal ulcer containing a retained pill and circum-scribed to the location of the pill. It is believed that pills must be inherently caustic to cause injury. Local acid burn is proposed for pills (e.g., doxycycline, tetracycline, ascorbic acid, ferrous sulfate) that produce an acidic solution with a pH < 3 when dissolved in 10 mL of water. Phenytoin dissolved in 10 mL of saliva raises the pH to 10.4, suggesting that it may cause an alkaline burn. Other proposed mechanisms of injury include induction of gastroesophageal reflux (theophylline and anticholinergics) and production of localized hyperosmolarity capable of tissue desiccation and vascular injury (potassium chloride). Finally, some medications appear to be absorbed locally into the esophageal mucosa, causing toxic intramucosal concentrations (doxycycline, NSAIDs, alprenolol).

11. **What are the postulated mechanisms of NSAID-induced injury?**
    Thirty million people use NSAIDs each day, and approximately 16% of patients report gastrointestinal side effects. Gastric injury is most common, although cases of esophageal injury are well documented. In one study, all patients with NSAID-induced esophageal injury, who were tested with 24-hour pH monitoring, had GERD. In the presence of GERD associated with a pH <4, NSAIDs may enter the mucosa and cause direct toxicity. NSAIDs may cause injury by inhibiting synthesis of mucosal prostaglandins. Prostaglandins are known to have a cytoprotective role in gastric mucosa, but it is unclear whether the same effect applies to esophageal mucosa. The role of the mucus and bicarbonate layer in protecting the esophagus is also unclear, but the deleterious effect of NSAIDs on the mucosal barrier of the stomach secondary to prostaglandin inhibition may also occur in the esophagus. Finally, NSAIDs may negatively affect lower esophageal sphincter pressure and function, thereby increasing GERD and potentiating their own absorption. Local acid injury may be caused by medications such as doxycycline, tetracycline, ascorbic acid, and ferrous sulfate. Each of these compounds has a pH of less than 3 when dissolved in distilled water or saliva.

12. **Where are the areas of physiologic narrowing of the esophagus?**
    The normal esophagus has areas, generally minor, of external compression and narrowing at the sphincters. Pills may be more likely to hang up and cause injury in these areas. Degenerative

arthritis of the cervical spine may cause external compression of the esophagus, which often worsens with age. The aortic arch and the left mainstem bronchus may cause compression of the esophagus. The left atrium varies in size, depending on underlying heart disease and may cause significant compression of the esophagus. Such compression is particularly troublesome because the medications often used to treat diseases associated with left atrial enlargement, such as potassium chloride in conjunction with diuretics and quinidine for atrial fibrillation, are particularly caustic agents.

3. Does alcohol consumption play a role in pill-induced esophageal injury?
Yes. Alcohol appears to act synergistically with caustic agents to induce esophageal injury. In one study, healthy volunteers took eight aspirin/day for 2 weeks. EGD showed no esophageal mucosal damage. After the same volunteers consumed a single dose of aspirin combined with alcohol, 33% had erythema and/or esophageal hemorrhage. Alcohol may affect the esophagus by interfering with esophageal clearance and thus prolonging aspirin contact with the mucosa. Alcohol is believed to decrease primary and secondary contractions of the esophagus.

4. What are the options for treating pill-induced esophageal injury?
Most cases of pill-induced injury heal without active intervention in 3 days to several weeks. Therapy starts with avoidance of the initial drug responsible for the injury and all other caustic drugs, when possible. When avoidance is not possible, every effort must be made to decrease the potential for reinjury by using elixir or other liquid preparations, administering medications in the upright position with at least 4 oz of liquid, and maintaining an upright posture for at least 10 minutes after ingestion.

Medications that buffer acid, decrease production of acid, or create a barrier coat for the esophagus are frequently prescribed (antacids, H_2-blockers, sucralfate) but are of questionable value unless GERD contributes to symptoms. The use of topical anesthetics in various combinations (Bemylid-Benadryl, Mylanta, and lidocaine in equal parts) may decrease symptoms, but their use is limited by potential systemic toxicity.

Patients with such severe symptoms that they cannot eat or drink require hydration. If symptoms persist, they may require parenteral nutrition and analgesia. Other supportive measures may also be required for treatment of complications (e.g., blood products for hemorrhage and antibiotics for bacterial superinfection).

Acute inflammatory stenosis may resolve spontaneously, but chronic stricture formation may require repeated esophageal dilation. Strictures that prove to be recalcitrant to repeated dilation may require surgical correction, but this complication is rare.

5. Discuss the epidemiology of caustic ingestion in the United States.
Chemical ingestion remains an important problem, despite improvements in packaging (e.g., child-proof containers), product labeling, and warnings. Approximately 26,000 caustic ingestions occur per year. Adolescents and adults who willfully ingest caustic agents as a suicidal gesture, in general, consume a larger volume and therefore have more serious injury than children, who ingest the agent accidentally and often expectorate most of it before swallowing. Children often have minimal esophageal damage, but their oral, pharyngeal, and laryngeal injury may be more severe. Approximately 80% of caustic ingestions occur accidentally in children younger than age 5, who most often consume household cleaners. Caustic ingestion is the leading cause of esophageal strictures in children.

6. What are the common caustic agents? Where are they found?
Caustic agents are present in many common household products (Table 7-1). The severity of the damage depends largely on the corrosive properties and concentration of the ingested agents. The caustic agents most often responsible for serious injury are strong alkaline cleaning products, such as drain cleaners and lye soaps. Severe alkaline burns also result from the ingestion of disk batteries that contain concentrated sodium or potassium hydroxide. Concentrated acid

compounds also cause severe injury but are not common household items; thus, they are encountered less often. The severity of esophageal and gastric injury secondary to caustic ingestion depends not only on the concentration and corrosive properties of the agent but also on the quantity consumed.

TABLE 7-1. CAUSTIC AGENTS FOUND IN COMMON HOUSEHOLD PRODUCTS		
Class	Caustic Agent	Product Containing Agent
Strong alkalis	Ammonia	Cleaning products
	Lye (sodium hydroxide,	Clinitest tablets
	potassium hydroxide)	Disk batteries
		Drain cleaners
		Nonphosphate detergents
		Paint removers
		Washing powders
Strong acids	Hydrochloric acid	Muriatic acid
		Soldering fluxes
		Swimming pool cleaners
		Toilet bowl cleaners
	Nitric acid	Gun barrel cleaners
	Oxalic acid	Antirust compounds
	Phosphoric acid	Toilet bowl cleaners
	Sulfuric acid	Battery acid
		Toilet bowl cleaners
Miscellaneous	Sodium hypochlorite	Liquid bleach

17. **Lye (sodium hydroxide) is a common caustic ingestion. How has its formulation changed over the past 30 years? How has this change affected the pattern of injury?**

Before the 1960s caustic ingestion frequently involved solid or crystalline lye products with concentrations >50%. Such products were extremely corrosive and caused extensive damage on contact with the mucosa, but the immediate burning pain on contact with the oral mucosa often caused the victim to spit out the solid material. Injury was limited usually to the mouth, pharynx and esophagus and rarely affected the stomach. Reports vary, but free esophageal perforation and mediastinitis were common complications. Such experiences led to the belief that lye injured the esophagus with relative sparing of the stomach compared with acids. This dictum did not hold true with concentrated liquid lye preparations, which can be swallowed more easily and quickly than solid lye. In the late 1960s such products were introduced as drain cleaners in concentrations of 25–36%. They caused devastating injury. Complications included respiratory compromise, esophageal and gastric perforations, septicemia, and death. Patients who survived often developed esophageal stricture as a later complication of ingestion. By the mid 1970s highly concentrated liquid products had been replaced in the United States by moderately concentrated (<10%) liquid drain cleaners. If ingested in sufficient quantity, such products are strong enough to cause severe esophageal and gastric injury, including visceral perforation. More often a smaller volume is ingested, and the patient recovers from the acute injury; later, however, strictures may develop. Caustic materials currently available for industrial usage are often much more concentrated than household products. Children occasionally encounter cleaning products containing highly concentrated lyes or acids, particularly around farms, construction sites, and swimming pools.

Describe the pathophysiology of acute alkali esophagitis.
When tissue is exposed to strong alkali, the immediate result is liquefactive necrosis, the complete destruction of entire cells and their membranes. Cell membranes are destroyed as their lipids are saponified and cellular proteins are denatured. Thrombosis of the local blood vessels also contributes to tissue damage. Tissue destruction and organ penetration progress rapidly until the alkali is diluted and neutralized by dilution with tissue fluids. Transmural necrosis of organs exposed to strong alkali occurs rapidly. Experimental exposure of cat esophagus to 5 mL of a 30.2% sodium hydroxide solution for only 3 seconds causes perforation and impending death.

The severity of caustic injury to the esophagus can be graded as first-, second-, or third-degree, using a system similar to that for classifying burns of the skin. Table 7-2 correlates the degree of burn with the endoscopic and pathologic findings. Endoscopy within the first 24 hours may underestimate the severity of esophageal injury.

TABLE 7-2.	DEGREE OF ESOPHAGEAL INJURY AND ASSOCIATED FINDINGS	
Degree	Endoscopic Findings	Pathology
First	Erythema and edema of mucosa only	Sloughing of superficial layers of mucosa
Second	Ulceration with membranous exudate	Ulcer extends through mucosa and submucosa to muscularis tissue
Third	Deep ulceration with penetration, black discoloration	Transmural injury, erosions into mediastinum or peritoneal structures

What are the three phases of injury and healing associated with lye?
Experimental lye injury may be divided into three phases: the acute or liquefaction phase (approximately days 1–4), the subacute or reparative phase (days 5–14), and the scar retraction or cicatrization phase. The acute phase is characterized by liquefactive necrosis, vascular thrombosis, and progressive inflammation. Mucosal erythema and edema are intense, but even severely injured tissue may not exhibit sloughing or ulceration during the first 24 hours. The hallmark of the subacute or reparative phase is sloughing of the necrotic areas with obvious ulceration and development of granulation tissue. Fibroblasts appear, and collagen deposition peaks during the second week but may continue for months. Mucosal re-epithelialization begins, and the wall of the esophagus is thinnest and most vulnerable during this period. The cicatrization phase, which begins about the end of the second week, is marked by continued proliferation of fibroblasts and further deposition of collagen. The recently formed collagen contracts both circumferentially and longitudinally, resulting in esophageal shortening and stricture formation. Re-epithelialization is generally complete by 1–3 months after lye ingestion. Table 7-3 summarizes the phases of lye injury. The evolution and outcome of a given lye ingestion involve a spectrum of events that may not follow the exact time course outlined earlier.

TABLE 7-3.   PHASES OF LYE INJURY

Phase	Pathology	Comments
Acute (days 1–4)	Liquefactive necrosis	Sloughing or ulcer not apparent <24
		Vascular thrombosis
		Increased inflammation
Subacute (days 5–14)	Sloughing of casts	Esophageal wall is thinnest
		Granulation tissue
		Fibroblast begun
		Collagen deposition
Cicatrization	Fibroblasts proliferate	Re-epithelialization in 1–3 months
(day 15–3 months)	Further collagen deposition	
	Stricture formation	

20. **Contrast the effects of acid ingestion with the effects of lye ingestion.**
    Concentrated acid solutions cause more severe pain on contact with the oropharyngeal mucosa than liquid alkalis, which are often swallowed before protective mechanisms can take effect. This property tends to limit the amount of acid that is ingested by accident. In past decades it was often noted that acid caused the greatest damage in the stomach, whereas alkali preferentially injured the esophagus. This observation was largely due to the fact that granular or solid lye was usually swallowed in small quantities and failed to reach the stomach in sufficient volume to cause serious gastric injury. The highly concentrated liquid alkalis introduced in the 1970s were likely to cause penetrating injury to both the esophagus and stomach. The moderately concentrated liquid acids and alkalis available today are less likely to cause acute perforation of either organ but often lead to late stricture formation.

    Histologic examination of tissue exposed to acid reveals coagulation necrosis with clumping and opacification of the cellular cytoplasm. The cell boundaries are usually recognizable in contrast to the complete cellular destruction of the liquefactive necrosis induced by strong alkali. The coagulum formed during coagulative necrosis consists, in part, of consolidated connective tissue, thrombosis of vessels, and clumping of blood proteins. This coagulum may limit the depth of penetration of the acid. However, esophageal perforations due to acid ingestion have been reported.

21. **Do acute signs and symptoms predict the severity and extent of caustic injury**
    Clinicians should be aware, when evaluating patients with caustic ingestion, that early signs and symptoms are not reliable indicators of the severity of caustic injury. Caustic agents (acids and crystalline lye) frequently cause immediate pain on contact with the mucosa of the oropharynx and may be expectorated before they are swallowed. Therefore, patients who ingest such agents may exhibit signs and symptoms of damage to the oropharynx with no injury to the esophagus. In contrast, lethal esophageal burns may occur with minimal evidence of oropharyngeal damage. Therefore, signs and symptoms of injury to the oropharynx do not reliably indicate the severity of damage to the esophagus or stomach. The distribution and severity of injury with acid or alkali depend as much on the physical characteristics of the product (solid versus liquid, volatility, titratable acid or base) as the volume ingested and the duration of exposure.

. Describe the presentation of a typical case of caustic ingestion.
The typical clinical course of uncomplicated caustic ingestion has three phases that closely parallel the phases of experimental caustic injury: acute, latent, and retractive. In the acute phase, immediate oral burning pain often limits the volume of ingestion. Caustic burns to the epiglottis and larynx may lead to immediate or delayed wheezing, cough, stridor, hoarseness, dyspnea, or aphonia. Dyspnea may also result from aspiration with damage to the bronchial tree and lung parenchyma. If a significant volume of the agent is swallowed, chest pain, dysphagia, or odynophagia may develop within minutes. Secretions may not be handled because of injury to and swelling of the posterior pharynx; drooling may occur. Retching and emesis may follow, and vomitus may contain blood or tissue. Pain and dysphagia in the uncomplicated course are due largely to dysmotility and edema and may subside over 3–4 days.

The patient with more complex injury may have additional symptoms and a worsening course. Persistent substernal pain or back pain may indicate a third-degree burn of the esophagus with mediastinitis. Perforation of the esophagus or stomach may cause peritonitis with abdominal rigidity and rebound tenderness. Perforation may evolve over the first few days and manifest as increasing pain, fever, and shock.

. Describe the common features of the patient's course after acute ingestion.
Initial pain and dysphagia may remit after a few days, ushering in the latent phase. Both physician and patient may be lulled into a false sense of security. The third phase, scar retraction, may begin as early as the end of the second week and last for several months. Clinically apparent esophageal strictures develop in 10–30% of patients with documented esophageal injury. Eighty percent of strictures become apparent during weeks 2–8, but, occasionally, patients may become symptomatic from stricture many months after the initial ingestion. Early strictures often progress rapidly, advancing from mild dysphagia to the inability to handle secretions in only a few days. The rapid progression of early strictures necessitates rapid evaluation and therapy to avoid the formation of dense, tight, constricting lesions. Therapy for such strictures is careful bougienage as needed to maintain esophageal patency.

. What is the mortality rate associated with caustic ingestion?
The mortality rate has decreased markedly over the past three decades from approximately 20% to 1–3%. The decreased mortality is due probably to improvements in supportive care (antibiotics and nutritional support), advances in surgery, anesthesia, and intensive care management as well as substitution of less concentrated alkali and acids for the highly concentrated products available in the 1950s and before.

. What is the cancer risk to a patient with stricture after lye ingestion?
The association between esophageal cancer and caustic ingestion is strong. The expected incidence of esophageal carcinoma is higher in patients with caustic ingestion than in the general population. Approximately 1–7% of patients with carcinoma of the esophagus have a history of caustic ingestion. The latent period is long and in one study was on average 41 years. Currently, no screening is recommended after lye ingestion.

. Describe the emergency department management of a patient with caustic ingestion.
The initial steps in the management of a suspected caustic injury are similar to those used on an emergency basis to manage any toxic ingestion. First, airway, breathing, and circulation (ABCs) must be controlled. Patients with caustic ingestion may present with respiratory compromise and require endotracheal intubation to protect the airway and to provide adequate oxygenation. Intubation should be performed only under direct visualization and should not be attempted in a blind manner. Next, hypotension must be addressed with adequate fluid support and resuscitation, as needed. If obvious signs of mediastinitis or peritonitis suggest perforation of a viscus, the patient should be prepared for surgery.

When respiratory and hemodynamic status have been addressed and the patient is stable, attempt should be made to determine the quantity and type of caustic agent and time of ingestion as well as any coingestions (more often with suicidal attempts than accidental ingestion). is helpful to obtain the container of the caustic agent, which lists all active substances as well concentrations of caustics. If the clinician is not familiar with management of poison ingestion or if the content of the caustic is in question, a poison control center should be contacted.

Emesis should not be induced because it will reexpose the esophagus, and perhaps larynx, to caustic materials. If a solid caustic has been ingested, a few sips of water may help to dislodge the solid particles from the esophageal mucosa and dissolve them in a larger volume of water the thicker-walled stomach. This, of course, should not be done in patients at risk of aspiration or with clinical evidence of perforation.

By the time victims of ingestion present to the physician, it is usually too late to intervene effectively to reduce internal burns. Because of the rapid action of alkali agents, efforts to neutralize caustic substances are not likely to be effective in limiting injury. In addition, an attempt neutralize the alkali agent may be dangerous. Neutralization may release significant amounts of heat and add thermal injury to chemical injury. Oral administration of any substance may also increase the risk of vomiting and aspiration. With acid injury, large volumes of water or milk within minutes of ingestion may dilute and neutralize the acid.

27. **Should gastric lavage be performed on patients with caustic ingestion?**
The answer is controversial. Patients most likely to benefit from gastric lavage present shortly after ingestion when a significant amount of caustic material may still be present in the stomach. In addition, patients with suspected coingestion of pills may benefit from lavage to decrease absorption. Such benefits must be weighed against the risks. Nasogastric intubation may induce retching and vomiting with recurrent exposure of the esophagus and oropharynx to caustics. Because the nasogastric tube may perforate the esophagus or stomach, strong consideration should be given to placement under fluoroscopic guidance. If the tube is placed, gastric contents should be aspirated before lavage. The stomach should be lavaged with cold water to dissipate any heat that is produced.

28. **What is the role of endoscopic evaluation in patients with caustic ingestion?**
Flexible upper endoscopy has a role in the early, emergent and later, subacute management of caustic ingestion. Patients in whom perforation (diagnosed either radiographically or clinically requires surgical exploration should undergo complete upper endoscopy to identify the extent disease. For example, in patients with a normal esophagus but injured stomach, surgery may limited to the abdomen. The risk of upper endoscopy is acceptable once the decision to operate has been made.

If surgery is not indicated, endoscopy should still be performed to identify uninjured patients who do not require prolonged hospital observation and to define the severity of burns in injured patients. Timing of endoscopy is based on clinical suspicion of severe injury. If significant esophageal injury is unlikely, EGD should be performed promptly to provide rapid reassurance and to avoid hospital observation. More than 50% of patients with a history of caustic injury are found on endoscopy to have no injury. If internal injury is likely but signs of perforation are absent, a delay of 48–72 hours permits development of the inflammatory reaction (little inflammation may be present in the first 24 hours) and easier assessment of the true extent of injury. Although endoscopic evaluation identifies the location of the mucosal injury, it may not accurately predict the depth of invasion.

29. **Can endoscopic findings help stratify the level of hospital care for patients suffering caustic injuries?**
Yes. Several endoscopic scoring systems have been shown to be helpful in predicting outcome and guiding management (Tables 7-4 and 7-5).

TABLE 7-4.	ENDOSCOPIC SCORING SYSTEM FOR SEVERITY OF DAMAGE	
Grade	Endoscopic Findings	Outcomes
Grade 0	Normal	Discharge
Grade 1	Mucosal edema and hyperemia	No risk of stricture
Grade 2A	Superficial ulcers, bleeding, exudates	Little risk of stricture
Grade 2B	Deep focal or circumferential ulcers	70–100% stricture
Grade 3A	Focal necrosis	70–100% stricture
Grade 3B	Extensive necrosis	65% early mortality, esophageal resection

TABLE 7-5.	CLASSIFICATION OF INJURY BY ENDOSCOPIC FINDINGS		
Endoscopic Findings	Hospital Stay	Risk of Stricture	Management
No injury	No observation in hospital	None	Discharge
Gastric only	Observe 24–48 h	None	
Linear esophageal injury, oriented longitudinally	Observe 24–48 h	Low	Liquid diet × 48 h
Circumferential esophageal injury	Observe at least 48 h	High	NPO, nasogastric tube

NPO = nothing orally.

. **What is the role of corticosteroids in the treatment of caustic ingestion?**
Patients in whom endoscopy demonstrates near-circumferential or circumferential esophageal burns are at risk for strictures. Since the 1950s, corticosteroids have been the mainstay of prophylaxis against stricture formation. The rationale for their use was based on animal studies showing that steroid therapy that begins within 24 hours after lye injury and continue for 6–8 weeks reduce the incidence of strictures by inhibiting formation of granulation tissue. This effect may be observed when corticosteroids are used as late as 4–7 days after caustic ingestion. Follow-up was short, however, and early death from septicemia was much more common in steroid-treated animals.

A prospective, randomized, controlled trial in children with caustic ingestion, performed by Anderson in 1990, showed that corticosteroids did not decrease stricture formation. The study, however, had a small number of patients and, although formation of esophageal stricture did not seem to be affected by corticosteroids, the need for total esophagectomy was decreased in the steroid-treated group (four vs. seven untreated patients).

Clearly there is no consensus. If steroids are to be used, they should be reserved for patients with circumferential esophageal burns, who are at greatest risk of stricture formation. The dosage and length of therapy for corticosteroids have not been defined. Prednisone, 1.5–2.0 mg/kg/day, with a tapering period of 2 months, has been recommended.

In patients with significant caustic ingestion and clinical evidence of impending airway compromise, corticosteroids may help to decrease inflammation of the bronchopulmonary tree. Dexamethasone (pediatric dosage = 0.5–1.0 mg/kg; adult dosage = 2.0–3.0 mg/kg) given intravenously to patients who have a high probability of impending airway compromise and may need intubation, cricothyrotomy, or tracheostomy for treatment of airway obstruction.

The negative aspects of corticosteroids, including increased risk of infection and systemic side effects, must also be considered.

31. **What is the role of antibiotics in the treatment of caustic ingestion?**

Empiric antibiotic therapy is even less established. It was originally advocated because antibiotics reduced the early mortality rate in animals treated with steroids for esophageal burns. addition, antibiotics were originally thought to decrease long-term stricture formation, but this effect has not been reproducible in animal or human studies. The patients most likely to benefit are those who are treated with corticosteroids and appear to be at increased risk of systemic infection. Gram-positive organisms are most commonly implicated, but broad-spectrum coverage is generally prescribed.

Empiric therapy has not been shown to be more efficacious than monitoring for clinical signs of infection and using broad-spectrum antibiotics at their first appearance. If empiric therapy chosen, antibiotics may be stopped after 5–7 days of infection-free observation.

32. **Discuss the prophylactic role of bougienage.**

Once the acute injury has resolved, the next complication is likely to be stricture of the esophagus in patients who had circumferential burns. If such patients are left untreated, a long narrow stricture may develop. Such strictures may not be amenable to dilation and may require surgery. To avoid stricture formation, patients may undergo prophylactic dilation with a Maloney dilator or esophageal stenting. Dilation should be avoided during the acute phase of injury because of the increased risk of perforation. Dilation should be initiated in patients with circumferential burns at about the third week, before the stricture becomes symptomatic. Dilation is accomplished with a single pass of a moderately large (42 Fr) dilator several times a week. If resistance is encountered, the dilator is not forced through. Instead, progressive dilations are initiated, starting with the largest dilator that passes without resistance. This method generally maintains patency of the esophageal lumen. Although some risk is associated with dilation, the procedure may prevent formation of the long, narrow stricture commonly associated with caustic ingestion. An alternative to prophylactic dilation is close personal observation and questioning so that therapeutic dilation can be instituted at the onset of symptomatic dysphagia. Unfortunately, many injured patients are too young or too unreliable to be managed with this wait-and-see approach.

33. **What is the role of computed tomography (CT) scanning?**

Available data support CT scan with contrast as a predictor of the number of sessions of dilation that will be required to maintain a patent esophagus. Maximal esophageal wall thickness (>9 mm) in the area of the stricture was shown on multivariate analysis to be independently associated with the number of sessions of dilation required by the patient.

34. **Discuss the role of esophageal stents.**

The use of prophylactic esophageal stents to maintain lumen patency during the healing process is controversial and should be limited to centers with experience in placing stents and ongoing research interests. Stents are placed endoscopically or surgically and left in place for approximately 3 weeks. The theory is that stenting allows esophageal healing without cicatrization and stenosis. After 3 weeks the stent is removed. The stents are uncomfortable, and appreciable risk is associated with placement and removal. No randomized data evaluate the efficacy of stents, but anecdotal data have shown that most patients require subsequent esophageal dilation.

5. **What factors contribute to the controversies associated with treatment of caustic ingestions?**

Currently, many sources promote different invasive and noninvasive therapies for caustic inges- tions. Fortunately, the number of severe caustic ingestions seems to be decreasing. Because of decreasing experience and ethical concerns about testing experimental therapies on humans, few well-controlled data are available to guide the clinician. Withholding therapy, however, is also an ethical concern.

6. **What are the advantages and disadvantages of nasogastric intubation?**

Advantages: Nasogastric tubes (NGTs) provide a mechanism to deliver adequate nutritional sup- port and needed medications. They also allow the esophagus to rest and prevent wound trauma that may be associated with bolus food ingestion. Finally, NGTs maintain a lumen that can be used to assist dilation.

Disadvantages: NGTs may cause continuous irritation and inflammation of the healing esoph- agus and lead to increased fibrosis and stricturing.

Overall recommendation: A fluoroscopically placed, flexible NGT seems to be beneficial for the first 2 weeks in patients who are seriously ill and unlikely to maintain adequate nutrition.

7. **What is the role of total parenteral nutrition (TPN)?**

TPN has been advocated to allow complete esophageal rest and maintain maximal nutrition for healing. No prospective data support TPN in all patients. Clear candidates are patients at high risk of aspiration and patients in whom passage of an NGT is contraindicated because of the severity of esophageal injuries.

8. **Why is prophylactic dilation controversial?**

The final area of controversy is the use and timing of prophylactic dilation. Most agree that oral esophageal dilation is the cornerstone of stricture prophylaxis. Others argue that repeated trauma to esophageal mucosa from dilation causes increased fibrosis and encourages stricture formation. Prophylactic dilation of all patients with caustic ingestion clearly subjects some patients to unneeded, potentially hazardous procedures. No data are available to resolve this issue. Because strictures rarely manifest before the second week after ingestion, it seems wise to wait 10–14 days before beginning bougienage.

BIBLIOGRAPHY

Anderson KD, Rouse TM, Randolph JG: A controlled trial of corticosteroids in children with corrosive injury of the esophagus. N Engl J Med 323:10, 1990.

Bozymski EM, London JF: Miscellaneous diseases of the esophagus. In Sleisinger MH, Fordtran JS (eds): Gastrointestinal Diseases, 5th ed. Philadelphia, W.B. Saunders, 1993.

Broor SL, Raju GS, Bore PP, et al: Long-term results of endoscopic dilation for treatment of corrosive esophageal strictures. Gut 34:1498–1501, 1993.

Browne JD, Thompson JN: Caustic injuries of the esophagus. In Castell DO (ed): The Esophagus. Boston, Little, Brown and Company, 1992.

Byrne WJ: Foreign bodies, bezoars, and caustic ingestions. Gastrointest Endosc Clin N Am 4:99–119, 1994.

Gumaste VV, Pradyuman BD: Ingestion of corrosive substances by adults. Am J Gastroenterol 87:1–5, 1991.

Kikendall JW: Caustic ingestion injuries. Gastroenterol Clin N Am 20:847–857, 1991.

Kikendall JW: Caustic injury of the esophagus and stomach. In Current Therapy in Gastroenterology and Liver Disease, 3rd ed. Philadelphia, B.C. Decker, 1990.

Kikendall JW, Johnson LF: Pill-induced esophageal injury. In Castell DO (ed): The Esophagus. Boston, Little, Brown and Company, 1995.

Kochhar R, Ray JD, Sriram PVJ, et al: Intralesional steroids augment the effect of endoscopic dilation in corro- sive esophageal strictures. Gastrointest Endosc 49:135–141, 1999.

11. Lahoti D, Broor SL, Basu PP, et al: Corrosive esophageal strictures: Predictors of response to endoscopic dilation. Gastrointest Endosc 141:86–91, 1995.

12. Lanza FL, Hunt RH, Thomson AB: Endoscopic comparison of esophageal and gastroduodenal effects of risedronate and alendronate in postmenopausal women. Gastroenterology 119:631–638, 2000.

13. Loeb PM, Eisenstein AM: Caustic injury to the upper gastrointestinal tract. In Scharschmidt BF (ed): Gastrointestinal Diseases, 5th ed. Philadelphia, W.B. Saunders, 1993, pp 293–301.

14. Minocha A, Greenbaum DS: Pill-esophagitis caused by nonsteroidal antiinflammatory drugs. Am J Gastroenterol 86:1086–1089, 1991.

15. Ribeiro A, DeVault KR, Wolfe J, Stark ME: Alendronate-associated esophagitis: Endoscopic and pathologic features. Gastrointest Endosc 47:216–221, 1998.

16. Semble EL, Wu WC, Castell DO: Nonsteroidal antiinflammatory drugs and esophageal injury. Semin Arthritis Rheum 19:99–109, 1989.

17. Spechler SJ: Caustic ingestions. In Taylor MB (ed): Gastrointestinal Emergencies. Baltimore, Williams & Wilk 1990, pp 13–21.

18. Taggart H, Bolognese MA, Lindsay R, et al: Upper gastrointestinal tract safety of risendronate: A pooled analy of 9 clinical trials. Mayo Clin Proc 77:262, 2002.

CHAPTER 8

BARRETT'S ESOPHAGUS

Richard E. Sampliner, MD

1. What is Barrett's esophagus?

Barrett's esophagus is a metaplastic change in the lining of the normally squamous-lined esophagus that is recognized at endoscopy. As a result of gastroesophageal reflux disease, the esophagus is lined with intestinal metaplasia, a premalignant epithelium.

2. How is Barrett's esophagus diagnosed?

The ultimate criterion for histologic diagnosis is the presence of goblet cells. Currently, two techniques are necessary: endoscopy to recognize abnormal-appearing esophageal epithelium and biopsy to detect intestinal metaplasia.

3. Why is Barrett's esophagus important?

It is a premalignant lesion for adenocarcinoma of the esophagus and presumably for a proportion of adenocarcinomas of the gastric cardia. The cancer continuing to have the most rapidly rising incidence in the United States and Western Europe over the past three decades has been adenocarcinoma of the esophagus in white men.

4. Does short-segment Barrett's esophagus need to be identified?

Yes. Barrett's esophagus ranges from short tongues of intestinal metaplasia in the distal esophagus to circumferential intestinal metaplasia of nearly the entire length of the esophagus. In the mid 1970s, before the recognition of the importance of intestinal metaplasia, Barrett's esophagus was defined as a "columnar-lined esophagus" of at least 3 cm in length. However, it is now recognized that short-segment Barrett's esophagus can develop dysplasia and adenocarcinoma and is more common than long-segment Barrett's.

5. What is the risk of cancer associated with Barrett's esophagus?

Recent prospective series have documented a lower risk for the development of cancer than former series. Rather than a 1–2% risk per year, the risk appears to be 0.4–0.5% per year. This difference may be due to the larger, prospective series with longer follow-up. This lower incidence has been documented in higher-risk patients—predominantly Caucasian men. However, the most important question for the individual patient is his or her specific risk. An evidence-based answer has not yet been developed.

6. Who should be screened for Barrett's esophagus?

People at highest risk for the development of adenocarcinoma should be screened. Clues are available from the epidemiology of adenocarcinoma: older white men, patients with long-standing reflux symptoms, smokers, and the obese. Specific criteria to select individual patients have not been defined by prospective studies. In clinical practice, however, the movement has been toward the concept of once-in-a-lifetime endoscopy for patients with chronic gastroesophageal reflux to detect Barrett's esophagus. Focusing on patients at highest risk of developing cancer would be more effective.

7. What is the therapy for Barrett's esophagus?

Standard clinical therapy is pharmacologic (proton pump inhibitor) and surgical (laparoscopic fundoplication). Both techniques are highly effective in controlling reflux symptoms and healing erosive esophagitis. For younger patients who are noncompliant or do not wish to take daily medication, surgery is an option. For patients with prominent regurgitation, inadequately controlled with proton pump inhibitors, surgery should be considered. A higher failure rate for laparoscopic fundoplication has been recognized in patients with Barrett's esophagus compared with non–Barrett's reflux.

Goals of therapy for Barrett's esophagus

- Control reflux symptoms.
- Heal erosive esophagitis.
- Prevent adenocarcinoma.

8. Does Barrett's esophagus reverse with medical therapy?

Rarely. In published series, which typically use high doses of proton pump inhibitors, Barrett's esophagus was eliminated in only 2% of 151 patients. Even if esophageal acid exposure is nearly eliminated, the estimated decrease in the area of Barrett's esophagus over an interval of 2 years is only 8%.

9. Does Barrett's esophagus reverse with surgical therapy?

Rarely. Barrett's esophagus has been eliminated in <4% of 449 patients having surgery in large series in the 1990s. If the elimination of all refluxate by successful fundoplication does not reverse Barrett's esophagus and eliminate the risk of cancer, it is unlikely that medical therapy other than chemoprevention will do so.

10. What is the appropriate surveillance of patients with Barrett's esophagus?

The database for developing guidelines for surveillance of this premalignant mucosa is limited but gastroenterologists must deal with this issue in everyday practice. Surveillance intervals are based on the detection of dysplasia with the goal of early intervention to improve the survival rates associated with adenocarcinoma. The surveillance intervals have been increasing and will probably continue to do so with improved understanding of the natural history of dysplasia. Currently, a patient with two endoscopies, with systematic biopsies showing no dysplasia, can be surveyed every 3 years. If low-grade dysplasia has no greater abnormality on follow-up endoscopy with biopsy, surveillance can be performed every year for 3 years, then every 2 years until no dysplasia is found.

11. Summarize the evolution of Barrett's esophagus to adenocarcinoma.

Intestinal metaplasia → low-grade dysplasia → high-grade dysplasia → adenocarcinoma.

12. Describe the management of high-grade dysplasia.

Management of high-grade dysplasia is one of the most controversial issues in the treatment of Barrett's esophagus. Current alternatives include more frequent surveillance (every 3 months) until cancer is detected, experimental endoscopic reversal therapy, and esophagectomy. The problems with conventional esophagectomy include operative mortality rate (especially in low-volume centers), the high frequency of morbidity, and the permanent impact on eating and nutrition. Many patients are elderly and are not good surgical candidates because of comorbidity. It is also not uncommon for patients to refuse surgery even after consulting with a surgeon.

13. Can the development of adenocarcinoma of the esophagus be prevented in patients with Barrett's esophagus?

Prevention is not clear. It is the major challenge to clinicians. Given the lack of reversal of Barrett's esophagus with standard medical and surgical therapy, it is not clear that we can prevent the development of adenocarcinoma. It has been argued that control of reflux into the esophagus will prevent the progression from metaplasia to dysplasia and subsequent adenocarcinoma. However, this argument is far from proven, and only retrospective data can be brought to bear upon the issue. There are exciting developments in experimental endoscopic therapy to eliminate the presence of intestinal metaplasia. Photodynamic endoscopic ablation therapy of patients with high-grade dysplasia can reduce the development of cancer over a minimum follow-up of 2 years. The overall reduction of the development of adenocarcinoma in patients with Barrett's esophagus remains a major challenge.

What advances can we anticipate in the management of Barrett's esophagus?
Progress in our understanding of the genetic changes involved in the progression of Barrett's esophagus to adenocarcinoma has been dramatic. The technical advances that continue to be made in endoscopy offer the opportunity for major advances in clinical management of Barrett's esophagus. We can look forward to unsedated endoscopy with smaller-caliber endoscopes or nonendoscopic techniques, for cheaper and easier detection of Barrett's esophagus. Optical methods for identifying dysplasia without biopsy add the possibility of real-time recognition. Newer endoscopic techniques to remove dysplastic and metaplastic epithelium will make our current attempts look primitive. Preventing adenocarcinoma may well require validation of biomarkers that define the subgroup of patients at highest risk for developing cancer. This approach will focus surveillance on patients at highest risk, leading to cost savings and greater clinical effectiveness. Chemoprevention may offer opportunities for cancer prevention that transcend the technical advances.

WEBSITES

1. http://www.cancer.gov/

2. http://www.cancer.gov/cancerinfo/wyntk/esophagus

BLIOGRAPHY

. Begg CB, Cramer LD, Hoskins WJ, Brennan MF: Impact of hospital volume on operative mortality for major cancer surgery. JAMA 280:1747–1751, 1998.

. Corley DA, Kerlikowske K, Verma R, Buffler PA: Protective association of aspirin/NSAIDs and esophageal cancer: A systematic review and meta-analysis. Gastroenterology 124:47–56, 2003.

. Devesa SS, Blot WJ, Fraumeni JF: Changing patterns in the incidence of esophageal and gastric carcinoma in the United States. Cancer 83:2049–2053, 1998.

. Drewitz DJ, Sampliner RE, Garewal HS: The incidence of adenocarcinoma in Barrett's esophagus: A prospective study of 170 patients followed 4.8 years. Am J Gastroenterol 92:212–215, 1997.

. Farrell TM, Smith CD, Metreveli RE, et al: Fundoplication provides effective and durable symptom relief in patients with Barrett's esophagus. Am J Surg 178:18–21, 1999.

. Fass R, Sampliner RE, Malagon IB, et al: Failure of oesophageal acid control in candidates for Barrett's oesophagus reversal on a very high dose of proton pump inhibitor. Aliment Pharmacol 14:597–602, 2000.

. Haag S, Nandurkar S, Talley NJ: Regression of Barrett's esophagus: The role of acid suppression, surgery, and ablative methods. Gastrointest Endosc 50:229–240, 1999.

. Hofstetter WL, Peters JH, DeMeester T, et al: Long-term outcome of antireflux surgery in patients with Barrett's esophagus. Ann Surg 234, 2001.

. O'Connor JB, Falk GW, Richter JE: The incidence of adenocarcinoma and dysplasia in Barrett's esophagus. Am J Gastroenterol 94:2037–2042, 1999.

. Ouatu-Lascar R, Triadafilopoloulos G: Complete elimination of reflux symptoms does not guarantee normalization of intraesophageal acid reflux in patients with Barrett's esophagus. Am J Gastroenterol 93:711–716, 1998.

11. Overholt B, Lightdale C, Wang K, et al: International, multicenter, partially blinded, randomised study of the eff cacy of photodynamic therapy (PDT) using porfimer sodium (POR) for the ablation of high-grade dysplasia (HGD) in Barrett's esophagus (BE): Results of 24-month follow-up. Gastroenterology 124:A20, 2003.

12. Peters FTM, Ganesh S, Kuipers EJ, et al: Endoscopic regression of Barrett's oesophagus during omeprazole treatment: A randomised double blind study. Gut 45:489–494, 1999.

13. Sampliner RE: Practice Parameters Committee ACG. Updated guidelines for the diagnosis, surveillance, and therapy of Barrett's esophagus. Am J Gastroenterol 97:1888–1895, 2002.

14. Sharma P, Morales TG, Bhattacharyya A, et al: Dysplasia in short segment Barrett's esophagus: A prospective 3 year follow-up. Am J Gastroenterol 92:2012–2016, 1997.

15. Sharma P, Morales TG, Sampliner RE: Short segment Barrett's esophagus: The need standardization of the def nition and of endoscopic criteria. Am J Gastroenterol 93:1033–1036, 1998.

16. Sharma P, Sampliner RE, Camargo E: Normalization of esophageal pH with high dose proton pump inhibitor therapy does not result in regression of Barrett's esophagus. Am J Gastroenterol 92:582–585, 1997.

CHAPTER 9

ESOPHAGEAL ANOMALIES

John H. Meier, MD

1. A patient with dysphagia is found to have a web by barium studies. What disorder must be considered?

Esophageal webs can be associated with iron deficiency anemia. This is called Plummer-Vinson syndrome. The Paterson-Brown-Kelly syndrome also consists of angular cheilitis and glossitis. Webs have also been associated with gastric inlet patches and graft-versus-host disease.

KEY POINTS: FOUR FEATURES OF PATERSON-BROWN-KELLY SYNDROME

1. Post-cricoid web

2. Iron deficiency

3. Glossitis

4. Angular cheilitis

2. What is the best therapy for dysphagia?

Esophageal bougienage is the preferred therapy, although many webs are probably ruptured unwittingly at endoscopy. Webs are thin, typically <2 mm in diameter.

3. What is the best way to confirm a suspected web?

Video fluoroscopy with lateral views. Standard barium swallow allows only brief visualization, and the lesion can be missed.

4. For which cancer are patients with esophageal webs reportedly at increased risk?

Esophageal webs are associated with squamous cell carcinoma of the hypopharynx and upper esophagus, although the degree of risk is not well defined.

5. When should one suspect an esophageal duplication cyst? How can it be diagnosed?

Esophageal duplication cysts are exceedingly rare but may present as a submucosal mass or extrinsic compression. Communication with the esophagus is unusual but can occur at either or both ends of the esophagus. Endoscopic ultrasound may be suggestive, but surgery is currently required to rule out cystic neoplasm.

6. Describe the three types of esophageal rings.

The three types of esophageal rings are cleverly named A, B, and C. The A ring occurs about 2 cm proximal to the gastroesophageal (GE) junction, is muscular in origin, and is usually asymptomatic. The B ring, also known as a Schatzki's ring, is mucosal and occurs at the squamocolumnar junction. The C ring is a nonpathologic radiographic anomaly caused by diaphragmatic indentation on the esophagus. C rings are never symptomatic.

7. **What causes esophageal A and B rings?**
   The precise cause of these is unknown. A rings may be associated with esophageal dysmotili
   B rings may be reflux-related, but the literature is contradictory. Recent radiology literature
   suggests that B rings may be more common in children than previously thought, which raise
   the possibility that they are congenital. Not many children are symptomatic, however, which
   remains unexplained.

8. **Are all Schatzki's rings symptomatic? What is the typical history of the symptomatic patient?**
   Schatzki's rings are usually symptomatic only when the luminal diameter is <13 mm.
   Symptomatic patients usually describe only intermittent solid-food dysphagia induced by hurr
   ing a meal or anxiety. Patients may present initially with foreign-body impaction.

9. **How are Schatzki's rings treated?**
   Usually with a large-diameter bougie. Repeat treatment may be needed over time.

10. **Describe the three types of esophageal diverticula.**
    1. Upper esophageal, also called *Zenker's diverticulum* (which is arguably a hypopharyngeal
       lesion; this could be a trick question).
    2. Mid-esophageal, also called *traction diverticulum.*
    3. Distal esophageal, also called *epiphrenic diverticulum.*

11. **What is the typical history of Zenker's diverticulum?**
    Patients may complain of regurgitation of undigested food, bad breath, a visible lump on the
    side of the neck, and dysphagia in the lower neck area.

12. **What causes Zenker's diverticulum?**
    This has been long debated, with initially contradictory studies. The lesion is more common in
    elderly patients. Impaired cricopharyngeal compliance, usually caused by fibrotic changes,
    causes increased intrabolus pressure with swallowing. Relaxation of the upper esophageal
    sphincter (UES) is usually normal. The result is increased hypopharyngeal pressure, with hernia
    tion at a weak point just above the cricopharyngeus.

13. **What is Killian's dehiscence?**
    The weak point just above the cricopharyngeus is called *Killian's dehiscence.* It is a triangu
    lar area where the oblique fibers of the inferior pharyngeal constrictors and the transverse
    fibers of the cricopharyngeus overlap.

14. **How is Zenker's diverticulum treated?**
    Symptomatic Zenker's diverticula require surgery. Most surgeons perform diverticulectomy
    because of the small risk of squamous cell carcinoma and persistent symptoms. Unilateral
    cricopharyngeal myotomy should also be done; otherwise, there is a significant recurrence rat
    (See the Key Points on p. 75.)

15. **Why are mid-esophageal diverticula called *traction diverticula?***
    It was previously thought that mid-esophageal diverticula were formed by adhesion of the
    esophagus to tuberculous mediastinal lymph nodes. Most are now thought to result from
    esophageal motility disorders or to represent a forme fruste of tracheoesophageal fistula. Few
    cause symptoms or need treatment.

16. **Should all epiphrenic diverticula be surgically treated?**
    No. Unusually large diverticula or those producing symptoms, such as regurgitation or aspira-
    tion, should be resected. Because of the high association with motility disorders, manometry
    should be performed. Results of manometry will often change the surgical approach to include

KEY POINTS: FOUR SYMPTOMS OF ZENKER'S DIVERTICULUM

1. Regurgitation of undigested food
2. Bad breath
3. Lump on side of neck
4. Dysphagia in lower neck

long myotomy or myotomy of the lower esophageal sphincter (LES). Recurrence is common with diverticulectomy alone.

Is surgery required for the cricopharyngeal "bar" or cricopharyngeal "achalasia" that radiologists sometimes describe?
No! This finding may or may not be the cause of symptoms. Because the bar can result from poor hypopharyngeal bolus propulsion, hypertrophy, or decreased opening capacity, caution must be exercised before recommending myotomy. Surgery occasionally causes severe reflux. Bougienage can be effective in relieving symptoms in some cases.

What is esophageal felinization? Does it cause symptoms?
This radiographic finding—with transient, delicate, transverse folds—is reminiscent of the cat esophagus. Although possibly related to reflux, it is usually asymptomatic. It may represent contractions of the muscularis mucosa.

Define dysphagia lusoria. What is the most common type?
Lusoria means "a trick of nature," and dysphagia lusoria refers to impingement of aberrant vasculature on the proximal esophagus. Most patients with aberrant vasculature are asymptomatic, but some have dysphagia. The most common type involves an aberrant right subclavian artery, which arises from the left side of the aortic arch and compresses the esophagus. Double aortic arch, right aortic arch, and several other anomalies are reported.

What sort of preoperative evaluation should be done in patients with dysphagia lusoria?
Magnetic resonance imaging (MRI) is believed to be the most accurate modality for defining the lesion. Patients should also undergo manometry and barium swallow with marshmallow or barium pill to be certain that the symptoms are caused by the vascular anomaly.

What causes esophageal atresia with tracheoesophageal fistula?
Atresia occurs when embryonic foregut fails to recanalize to form an esophagus. The tracheoesophageal (TE) fistula is due to lack of separation of lung bud from the foregut. The exact insult causing these anomalies is not known.

What is the most common type of esophageal atresia with tracheoesophageal fistula? Describe its presentation.
The most common type of TE fistula with atresia is the lower-pouch fistula. Because the esophagus has not fully formed (atresia), the upper and lower pouches are not in continuity. This anomaly may cause intrauterine polyhydramnios. After birth, regurgitation after feeding and weight loss are seen. The fistula between the distal part of the esophagus and the trachea can cause pneumonia due to reflux of stomach contents.

23. **What is the least common type of esophageal atresia with tracheoesophageal fistula? Describe its presentation.**

    The least common form is congenital esophageal stenosis, a forme fruste of atresia, which can present as late as adulthood. The differential diagnosis includes bullous skin disorders, radiation injury to the esophagus, caustic ingestion, and prolonged nasogastric suction. Congenital stenosis presents typically with lifelong dysphagia to solid foods and prolonged meals and low body weight. Barium radiographs may show a fixed segment of narrowing, usually mid-esophageal, whereas endoscopy may demonstrate multiple cartilaginous rings (Fig. 9-1). Recent studies suggest that the disorder may, in fact, be reflux-induced rather than congenital.

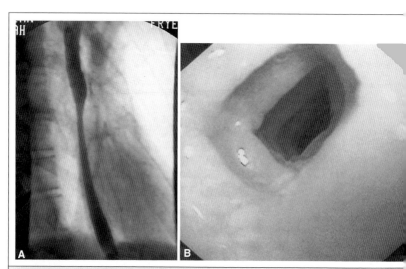

Figure 9-1. (A) Barium esophagram showing segmental narrowing consistent with congenital esophageal stenosis. (B) Endoscopic view of the same patient demonstrating cartilaginous rings at endoscopy.

24. **How is esophageal atresia with tracheoesophageal fistula treated?**

    For patients presenting in childhood, surgical repair is usually possible. With modern techniques, mortality is due to associated cardiac anomalies rather than to the surgery itself. Congenital esophageal stenosis is generally treatable with cautious bougienage.

25. **What is intramural pseudodiverticulosis?**

    Formed by dilation of submucosal esophageal glands, small pseudodiverticula are commonly associated with candidal esophagitis (50%). Many patients have esophageal motor disorders, and many have esophageal strictures. The inciting event is unknown, but the lesion has been seen after corrosive ingestion. Treatment with stricture dilation and medications can be effective. Some have identified an increased risk of esophageal cancer and recommend periodic surveillance, though the cost-effectiveness of this approach is not established.

WEBSITES

1. http://www.emedicine.com/ped/topic2934.htm

2. http://www.naspgn.org

BLIOGRAPHY

Achkar E: Esophageal diverticula. In Castell DO (ed): The Esophagus. Philadelphia, Lippincott, Williams & Wilkins, 1999, pp 301–314.

Beekman RP, Hazekamp MG: A new diagnostic approach to vascular rings and pulmonary slings: The role of MRI. Magn Reson Imaging 16:137–145, 1998.

Boyce GA, Boyce HW: Esophagus: Anatomy and structural anomalies. In Yamada T (ed): Textbook of Gastroenterology, 3rd ed. Philadelphia, J.B. Lippincott, 1999, pp 1180–1195.

Buckley K, Buonomo C, Husain K, Nurko S: Schatzki ring in children and young adults: Clinical and radiologic findings. Pediatr Radiol 28(11):884–886, 1998.

Harford W: Diverticula of the hypopharynx and esophagus, the stomach, and the small bowel. In Feldman M, Scharschmidt B, Sleisenger M (eds): Sleisenger and Fordtran's Gastrointestinal and Liver Disease, 6th ed. Philadelphia, W.B. Saunders, 1998, pp 309–316.

Long J, Orlando R: Anatomy and developmental and acquired anomalies of the esophagus. In Feldman M, Scharschmidt B, Sleisenger M (eds): Sleisenger and Fordtran's Gastrointestinal and Liver Disease, 6th ed. Philadelphia, W.B. Saunders, 1998, pp 457–466.

McNally PR, Lemon JC, Goff JS, Freeman SR: Congenital esophageal stenosis presenting as noncardiac, esophageal chest pain. Dig Dis Sci 38(2):369–373, 1993.

McNally PR, Rak KM: Dysphagia lusoria caused by persistent right aortic arch with aberrant left subclavian artery and diverticulum of Kommerell. Dig Dis Sci 37(1):144–149, 1992.

Pokieser P, Schima W, Schober E, Levine M: Congenital esophageal stenosis in a 21-year-old man: Clinical and radiographic findings. AJR 170:147–148, 1998.

Shand A, Papachrysostomou M, Ghosh S: Dysphagia in oesophageal intramural pseudo-diverticulosis: Fibrosis, dysmotility, or web? Eur J Gastroenterol Hepatol 11(11):1331–1333, 1999.

Tobin R: Esophageal rings and webs. In Castell DO (ed): The Esophagus, 3rd ed. Philadelphia, Lippincott Williams & Wilkins, 1999, pp 295–300.

Tobin R: Esophageal rings, webs, and diverticula. J Clin Gastroenterol 27(4):285–295, 1998.

Tsai JY, Berkery L, Wesson DE, et al: Esophageal atresia and tracheoesophageal fistula: Surgical experience over two decades. Ann Thorac Surg 64(3):778–783, 1997.

Uygur-Bayramicli O, Tuncer K, Dolapcioglu C: Plummer-Vinson syndrome presenting with an esophageal stricture. J Clin Gastroenterol 29(3):291–292, 1999.

Waring JP, Wo JM: Cervical esophageal web caused by an inlet patch of gastric mucosa. South Med J 90(5):554–555, 1997.

Wilkinson JM, Euinton HA, Smith LF, et al: Diagnostic dilemmas in dysphagia aortica. Eur J Cardiothorac Surg 11(2):222–227, 1997.

GASTRITIS

Frank L. Lanza, MD

CHAPTER 10

1. What is gastritis?

Gastritis is best defined, in most cases, as inflammation of the gastric mucosa.

2. What are the symptoms of gastritis?

The symptoms of gastritis are also the symptoms of many other upper gastrointestinal (GI) problems. Patients may complain of epigastric burning, nausea, postprandial fullness, or "bloating," as well as other nonspecific upper GI-type complaints. Unfortunately, these are also the symptoms of other upper GI disorders (e.g., gallbladder disease, gastric neoplasm, gastroesophageal reflux disease [GERD], gastroparesis). These diagnoses need to be excluded in patients with these symptoms before a diagnosis of symptomatic gastritis can be considered.

3. How is gastritis diagnosed?

Gastritis is usually diagnosed endoscopically, both visually and microscopically. However, some types of gastritis require endoscopic ultrasound (Ménétrièr's disease) or serologic studies (chronic autoimmune gastritis) to confirm the diagnosis.

4. How is gastritis classified?

Gastritis may be acute or chronic. Table 10-1 lists the most common causes of both types.

5. Describe the endoscopic and histologic appearance of acute and chronic gastritis.

The endoscopic changes seen with acute gastritis due to toxic agents are quite characteristic. Round or flame-shaped intramucosal hemorrhages are seen throughout the stomach, and erosions are commonly found in the antrum. The erosions appear typically as white-based flat

TABLE 10-1. CLASSIFICATION OF GASTRITIS	
Acute Gastritis	**Chronic Gastritis**
Toxic agents	*Helicobacter pylori*
NSAIDs, including COX-2	Autoimmune
inhibitors and aspirin	Nonspecific
Bisphosphonates	Lymphocytic
Potassium	Bile reflux
Macrolides	Ménétrier's disease
Alcohol	Eosinophilic
Stress	Granulomatous
Viruses	
Bacteria	

lesions surrounded by a margin of intense erythema. The intervening mucosa is usually norm
or simply erythematous. Continued use of the offending substance leads to an increase in the
number of erosive lesions, and hemorrhages disappear gradually. The mucosa can then beco
more erythematous, friable, and granular in appearance, and may visually resemble chronic g
tritis. Microscopically, there is a diminished number of inflammatory cells associated with fov
olar hyperplasia and increased numbers of smooth muscle fibers in the lamina propria. The
endoscopic appearance of chronic gastritis is that of an atrophic mucosa with a clearly visible
vascular pattern, primarily in the fundus, where the usual rugal folds have often completely di
appeared. In chronic superficial gastritis the mucosa can typically exhibit a patchy erythema,
scattered areas of submucosal hemorrhage, and/or superficial erosion with adherent exudate.
This is the usual appearance in the antrum. Less often, raised areas of discrete erythema with
central erosion are present, and these lesions can appear polypoid in nature.

6. **What is the treatment of acute gastritis secondary to toxic agents, and how ca
it be prevented?**

The most common cause of acute gastritis is nonsteroidal, anti-inflammatory drug (NSAID)
therapy. In most cases, cessation of the offending agent leads to rapid normalization of the ga
tric mucosa. However, in many patients, especially in certain high-risk individuals (Table 10-2),
NSAID gastritis can progress to gastric ulcer and its complications (perforation and hemorrhage
If NSAID therapy must be continued in these patients, concomitant treatment with misoprost
or high doses of proton pump inhibitors should be instituted. This applies to the selective
cyclooxygenase-2 (COX-2) inhibitors as well as the older, nonselective NSAIDs. Recent evider
shows that low-dose aspirin, when taken concurrently with a COX-2 inhibitor, increases the le
of gastric toxicity seen with these agents to that of the older drugs. This is important because
large number of patients who take low-dose aspirin also use NSAIDs, especially the newer CO
2 inhibitors. The acute gastritis seen with bisphosphonates, potassium, and macrolides is usu
ally mild and limited to the duration of the use of these agents and rarely leads to complication
Acute alcoholic gastritis can be accompanied by upper GI hemorrhage, but this is more likely
be related to the portal gastropathy often seen in these patients.

TABLE 10-2.   RISK FACTORS FOR COMPLICATIONS OF ACUTE NSAID GASTRITIS

1. Prior history of ulcer or upper GI bleeding
2. Age >65 years
3. High-dose NSAID therapy, especially in low-body-weight patients
4. Concurrent use of other gastrotoxic agents, including a second NSAID or low-dose
   aspirin
5. Anticoagulants
6. Corticosteroids
7. *Helicobacter pylori*
8. Debilitation

GI = gastrointestinal, NSAID = nonsteroidal anti-inflammatory drug.

---

7. **What are the characteristics of stress gastritis, and how should it be treated?**

Stress gastritis usually occurs in an ICU setting in patients with central nervous system injury
severe burns, sepsis, or extensive surgery, especially those requiring mechanical ventilation.
Gastric ulceration can occur, especially in burn patients, which often leads to severe GI hemor

rhage or perforation. The best treatment is prophylaxis in high-risk patients. The recent availability of intravenous proton pump inhibitors has made it possible to raise gastric luminal pH to more than 4 on a 24-hour basis. This degree of acid inhibition inactivates the proteolytic enzyme pepsin and effectively prevents mucosal injury.

What is the most common etiology of chronic gastritis?

By far, the most common cause of chronic gastritis is *Helicobacter pylori* infection. This organism is acquired usually in infancy or early childhood and is more common in people from underdeveloped countries. In Western nations, the percentage of infected individuals is much higher in the older population, reflecting sanitary conditions existent during their youth. Symptoms rarely occur until later in life.

How is chronic gastritis secondary to *Helicobacter pylori* infection diagnosed?

The diagnosis of *H. pylori* gastritis can be made histologically, biochemically, or serologically. Patients chronically infected with *H. pylori* usually have circulating IgG antibodies to that organism. IgA antibodies are found in some patients who are IgG-negative, and IgM antibodies are seen in early cases. Many clinicians feel that a positive serology in a symptomatic patient with no history of treatment for *H. pylori* infection is presumptive evidence of active infection and warrants therapy. Endoscopic biopsy with special staining (Giemsa or Warthin-Starry) for *H. pylori* organisms is the gold standard for diagnosis. Culture is unnecessary except in cases where resistant organisms are suspected. Because *H. pylori* produces large amounts of urease, which converts urea to ammonia, a small biopsy specimen placed in a gel containing phenol red will cause an increase in the pH of the gel, yielding a red color and indicating the presence of the organism (CLO-test). This is also the basis for a breath test utilizing radiolabeled urea to detect the organisms. Both of these tests have a high degree of specificity and sensitivity. Unfortunately, all of these tests, except the serology, require that the patient refrain from the use of antibiotics and acid-suppressing drugs for 7–14 days.

How is chronic gastritis secondary to *Helicobacter pylori* infection treated?

H. pylori infection is treated with antibiotics combined with acid suppression. Quadruple therapy with bismuth, tetracycline, metronidazole, and b.i.d. proton pump inhibitor therapy for 14 days is 90% effective in eradicating *H. pylori* infection. Triple therapy with amoxicillin, clarithromycin, and b.i.d. proton pump inhibitors for 14 days is also 80–90% effective. Numerous other antibiotic regimens with acid suppression have been reported with varying degrees of effectiveness and are useful in patients demonstrating antibiotic resistance to metronidazole or amoxicillin.

What are the long-term implications of *Helicobacter pylori* infection?

Patients chronically infected with *H. pylori* frequently develop gastric and duodenal ulcer disease, especially the latter. Although less common, B-cell lymphoma and adenocarcinoma of the stomach are also associated with chronic gastritis due to *H. pylori*. Antral-predominant corpus sparing chronic gastritis due to *H. pylori* is more often associated with duodenal ulcer. Gastritis involving the entire stomach with intestinal metaplasia and achlorhydria is associated with gastric ulcer and cancer. B-cell lymphoma is often seen in conjunction with *H. pylori* infection and very often resolves with eradication of the bacteria.

What are the other types of chronic gastritis?

The other types of chronic gastritis are listed in Table 10-1. Autoimmune gastritis, lymphocytic gastritis, and nonspecific gastritis are similar in their endoscopic appearance to the chronic gastritis seen with *H. pylori*. These entities, along with the others listed in Table 10-1, are diagnosed by histology and/or other special studies.

13. **What is autoimmune gastritis?**

Autoimmune gastritis (AIG) is a relatively rare type of chronic gastritis that is diagnosed usually during the evaluation of patients with the megaloblastic anemia of pernicious anemia (PA). Although the presence of parietal cell and intrinsic factor antibodies strongly suggests this diagnosis, the combination of high serum gastrin levels and low pepsinogen I is a specific characteristic and is more sensitive than the parietal cell antibody study. AIG per se is asymptomatic. The endoscopic appearance of AIG with or without PA is that of severe gastric atrophy with marked rugal flattening and clearly visible submucosal vasculature. The most typical histologic changes are found in the fundus, where there is marked gastric atrophy with loss of almost all specialized glands of the upper stomach. Intestinal metaplasia is often present in the late stages of the disease. In the early cases there is chronic inflammation, again primarily in the corpus of the stomach. However, later in the course of the disease the degree of inflammation is minimal. Asymptomatic AIG not associated with PA does not require therapy. Patients with gastric atrophy and parietal cell or intrinsic factor antibodies should be followed carefully for the development of PA and also by endoscopy for gastric polyps and/or carcinoma. Endoscopy should be performed at 3–5 year intervals.

KEY POINTS: GASTRITIS

1. NSAIDs are the most common cause of acute gastritis and its complications.

2. COX-2 inhibitors, when given in association with low-dose aspirin, are not safe, especially in high-risk patients.

3. The most common cause of chronic gastritis is *Helicobacter pylori* infection.

4. Chronic untreated *H. pylori* infection is associated with peptic ulcer disease and can lead to B-cell lymphoma or gastric carcinoma.

5. Autoimmune gastritis is associated with autoantibodies and pernicious anemia.

14. **Describe lymphocytic gastritis.**

Lymphocytic gastritis (LG) is a special form of gastritis, which is characterized by the accumulation of intraepithelial lymphocytes (IELs) containing cytotoxic granules in the surface and foveolar epithelium. The number of IELs in normal gastric mucosa is between 3 and 8 per 100 epithelial cells; a minimal number of 30 IELs per 100 epithelial cells is usually accepted for the diagnosis of LG. LG is usually asymptomatic. Patients occasionally present with epigastric pain or anorexia. It often occurs in association with *H. pylori* infection and celiac disease. However, only 2–4% of patients with *H. pylori* infection will develop LG. There is no specific therapy for LG. However, patients who are serologically positive for *H. pylori,* but negative by all other diagnostic techniques, may still respond to antimicrobial therapy for that organism.

15. **What is chronic nonspecific gastritis?**

Despite the discovery of *H. pylori* and advances in other forms of chronic gastritis, there remains a small group of undiagnosed patients with the endoscopic and histologic features of chronic gastritis. These are usually elderly patients with atrophic gastritis in which autoantibodies or *H. pylori* cannot be found. These patients may represent late-stage *H. pylori* infection-associated gastritis, but no proof of this has been forthcoming.

16. **What is Ménétrier's disease, and how does it differ from the other special forms of chronic gastritis?**

Ménétrier's disease differs from the other forms of chronic gastritis in that it is not associated with any significant degree of mucosal inflammation. The disease is seen usually in middle-age adults. They often present with weight loss, diarrhea, and hypoproteinemic edema. Low acid secretion, loss of parietal cell mass, and protein-losing gastropathy are typical of this disease. The degree of symptomatology varies greatly between patients. Its most severe manifestation is severe wasting secondary to GI protein loss. The endoscopic appearance is that of large folds in the upper stomach, and maximal inflation does not bring about the disappearance of these thick fundal rugae. Diagnosis is by endoscopic biopsy. Loop biopsy from the top of a large fold is usually necessary to obtain adequate tissue for diagnosis. Full-thickness mucosal biopsies show the characteristic massive foveolar hyperplasia seen with this disease. Regular or jumbo forceps biopsies are not adequate for the diagnosis. Endoscopic ultrasound has greatly enhanced the ability of the clinician to differentiate between the various pathologic entities presenting with large or giant gastric folds. This technique defines five distinct layers of the gastric wall. Ménétrier's disease typically produces thickening in the **second layer only,** corresponding to the mucosa, whereas carcinoma and lymphoma will also usually involve the third and fourth layers (i.e., the submucosa and muscularis propria). Lymphoma and simple rugal hyperplasia typically involve the second and third layers and can thus be differentiated from Ménétrier's disease. The treatment of Ménétrier's disease with H_2-blockers, prostaglandins, and proton pump inhibitors has generally been unsatisfactory. High doses of anticholinergics have reduced albumin loss. Subtotal or total gastrectomies have been performed in patients with severe and intractable symptomatology.

Describe bile reflux gastritis.

Bile reflux gastritis is most commonly seen after gastrectomy, pyloroplasty, or cholecystectomy. Endoscopically, the gastric mucosa is granular and intensely erythematous with a brick red color or greenish-yellow discoloration. Large amounts of bile are often found in the stomach. Histologic examination of the gastric mucosa reveals elongation and serration of the foveolae, which, in some ways, resemble the histologic picture seen with patients chronically on NSAIDs or using alcohol. Diversionary surgery is probably the best treatment of patients with this condition who fail to respond to symptomatic therapy.

In what circumstances do granulomatous and eosinophilic gastritis occur?

Granulomatous and eosinophilic gastritis probably do not exist as diseases isolated to the stomach. They are more often associated with other systemic diseases. Granulomatous gastritis, when it involves the stomach, is usually part of the spectrum of Crohn's disease. Because the antrum is the portion of the stomach most often involved with this disease, the most common clinical presentation is gastric outlet obstruction. Endoscopically, the entire antrum feels firm, and the pylorus is small and rigid. Aphthous ulcers are often seen in the antrum, but the deep crevice-like ulcers seen elsewhere in the gastrointestinal tract are not normally noted in the stomach. Histologic confirmation is difficult to obtain; however, biopsies taken with jumbo forceps are sometimes diagnostic. Other diseases that can produce this picture are sarcoidosis, Wegener's granulomatosis, and systemic granulomatosis. Eosinophilic gastritis is part of the overall syndrome of eosinophilic gastroenteritis. The most common areas of involvement, however, are the stomach and small bowel. The most common clinical presentation of this entity is antral ulceration, and the patient often presents with the typical symptoms of ulcer disease. Biopsies are diagnostic. No definite therapy is recommended, except treatment for the ulcers; however, there are empiric reports of success with corticosteroid therapy.

BIBLIOGRAPHY

1. Cello JP: Eosinophilic gastroenteritis: A complex entity. Am J Med 67:1097–1104, 1979.

2. Cook D, Heyland D, Griffith L, et al: Risk factors for clinically important upper gastrointestinal bleeding in patients requiring mechanical ventilation. Crit Care Med 27:2812–2817, 1999.

3. Dixon MF, O'Connor HJ, Axon AT: Reflux gastritis: Distinct histopathological entity? J Clin Pathol 39(5):524–530, 1986.

4. Dubois RW, Melmed GY, Henning JM, Laine L: Guidelines for the appropriate use of nonsteroidal anti-inflammatory drugs, cyclo-oxygenase-2-specific inhibitors and proton pump inhibitors in patients requiring chronic anti-inflammatory therapy. Aliment Pharmacol Ther 19:197–208, 2004.

5. Graham DY: H. pylori infection in the pathogenesis of duodenal ulcer and gastric cancer: A model. Gastroenterology 113:1983–1991, 1997.

6. Hansson LE, Nyren O, Hsing AW, et al: The risk of stomach cancer in patients with gastric or duodenal ulcer disease. N Engl J Med 335(4):242–249, 1996.

7. Hayat M, Arora DS, Dixon MF: Effects of *Helicobacter pylori* eradication on the natural history of lymphocytic gastritis. Gut 45(4):495–498, 1999.

8. Hsing AW, Hansson LE, McLaughlin JK, et al: Pernicious anemia and subsequent cancer: A population-based cohort study. Cancer 71:745–750, 1993.

9. Lanza FL, Aspinall RL, Swabb EA, et al: Double-blind, placebo-controlled endoscopic comparison of the mucosal protective effects of misoprostol versus cimetidine on tolmetin-induced mucosal injury to the stomach and duodenum. Gastroenterology 95(2):289–294, 1988.

10. Lanza F, Schwartz H, Sahba B: An endoscopic comparison of the effects of alendronate and risedronate on upper gastrointestinal mucosae. Am J Gastroenterol 95(11):3112–3117, 2000.

11. Larkai EN, Smith JL, Lidsky MD, Graham DY: Gastroduodenal mucosa and dyspeptic symptoms in arthritic patients during chronic nonsteroidal anti-inflammatory drug use. Am J Gastroenterol 82(11):1153–1158, 1987.

12. Loffeld BC, van Spreeuwel JP: The gastrointestinal tract in pernicious anemia. Dig Dis 9(2):70–77, 1991.

13. Madura JA: Primary bile gastritis: Which treatment is better, Roux-en-Y or biliary diversion? Am Surg 179:618–627, 1974.

14. Meuwissen SG, Ridwan BU, Hasper HJ, Innemee G: Hypertrophic protein-losing gastropathy: A retrospective analysis of 40 cases in the Netherlands. The Dutch Menetrier Study Group. Scand J Gastroenterol Suppl 194:1–7, 1992.

15. Oberhuber G, Bodingbauer M, Mosberger I: High proportion of granzyme B-positive (activated) intraepithelial and lamina propria lymphocytes in lymphocytic gastritis. Am J Surg Pathol 22(4):450–458, 1998.

16. Parsonnet J, Issacson PG: Bacterial infection and MALT lymphoma. N Engl J Med 350:213–215, 2004.

17. Scolapio JS, DeVault K, Wolfe JT: Eosinophilic gastroenteritis presenting as a giant gastric ulcer. Am J Gastroenterol 91(4):804–805, 1996.

18. Shapiro JL, Goldblum JR, Petras RE: A clinicopathologic study of 42 patients with granulomatous gastritis. Is there really an "idiopathic" granulomatous gastritis? Am J Surg Pathol 20(4):462–470, 1996.

19. Stemmermann GN, Hayashi T: Intestinal metaplasia of the gastric mucosa: A gross and microscopic study of distribution in various disease states. J Natl Cancer Inst 41(3):627–634, 1968.

20. Terdiman JP, Ostroff JW: Gastrointestinal bleeding in the hospitalized patient: A case-controlled study to assess risk factors and outcomes. Am J Med 104:349–354, 1998.

21. Wolfsen HC, Carpenter HA, Talley NJ: Ménétrièr's disease: A form of hypertrophic gastropathy or gastritis? Gastroenterology 104:1310–1319, 1993.

CHAPTER 11

GASTRIC CANCER

John C. Deutsch, MD

What are the histologic types of gastric cancer?
Over 80% of gastric cancers are adenocarcinomas. Less common are gastric lymphomas, gastric stromal tumors, leiomyosarcomas, carcinoid tumors, and metastatic tumors (e.g., melanoma, breast cancer).

What is the ethnic and geographic distribution of distal gastric adenocarcinoma?
Distal gastric adenocarcinoma is one of the most common malignancies worldwide. Approximately 600,000 deaths per year are due to gastric cancer worldwide. There is a high incidence in Asia and South America. Scandinavian countries have a higher incidence than the United States.

What is the role of diet in the development of gastric cancer?
Dietary factors appear to be important in the development of gastric cancer. In general, the incidence of gastric cancer is higher when a higher proportion of the diet is obtained from salted or smoked meats or fish. Fruits and vegetables appear to be protective. Tobacco smoking appears to increase the risk of gastric cancer. Dietary factors are thought to explain a large part of the variation in incidence of gastric cancers from country to country. Immigration from high-incidence countries to lower-incidence countries decreases the risk of gastric cancer risk.

What is the role of *Helicobacter pylori* in gastric adenocarcinoma?
The medical literature generally supports the notion that *H. pylori* infection appears to increase the lifetime risk of gastric cancer. Infected persons have about a twofold increase in the risk of acquiring gastric adenocarcinoma. However, the chance of an *H. pylori*-infected person contracting cancer is very low.

What mechanism is proposed for *Helicobacter pylori* causing an increased risk of gastric cancer?
H. pylori infection results in a rather marked inflammatory state in the stomach, which can eventually lead to atrophic gastritis and achlorhydria. Some reports suggest that host factors, including a "proinflammatory host genotype," favor achlorhydria and gastric cancer development.

What is the role of achlorhydria in gastric cancer?
Achlorhydria is generally caused by immune destruction of the parietal cells. Antiparietal cell antibodies and elevated gastrin levels can be found in the serum, and patients have associated B_{12} deficiency. Other causes include destruction after long bouts of infection with *H. pylori*. People with achlorhydria have a fourfold to sixfold increase in the incidence of gastric cancers, possibly related to the associated elevation in gastrin levels as well as the inflammation that leads to the parietal cell destruction.

Should *Helicobacter pylori* infection be eradicated to prevent gastric cancer from occurring?
Despite the epidemiologic link between *H. pylori* infection and gastric cancer, the data do not appear to support *H. pylori* eradication as a cancer preventive strategy at this point in time.

The reasons for this include the relatively low incidence of cancer development in *H. pylori* infected individuals and the variety of other factors related to cancer development, including host's genetic propensity and the genetic makeup of different *H. pylori* strains. Furthermore, there seem to be important environmental factors, such as tobacco use and diet, that modulate the potential carcinogenic effects of *H. pylori*.

8. **Who should be screened for gastric cancer?**
Screening is performed in Japan in middle-aged people and is recommended on an annual basis for those over age 50. There are no screening recommendations for distal gastric adenocarcinoma in the United States, and no recommendations are widely accepted for the screening of immigrants from high-risk areas. Screening for proximal gastric cancer is probably warranted people with a long-standing history of reflux symptoms.

9. **What is gastric stump cancer?**
After partial gastric resection, the incidence of gastric cancers at the sight of the intestinal-gastric anastomosis appears to be increased by about twofold. However, this increase is not apparent until at least 15 years after surgery. In the initial 5 years after partial gastrectomy, there may be an actual decrease in cancer risk. These data suggest a certain background rate of gastric cancer formation. If part of the stomach is removed, less mucosa is at risk for malignant transformation. However, the surgery then imparts a procancer effect, and over time more and more cancers start to form in the remaining mucosa.

10. **How is the incidence of gastric adenocarcinoma changing?**
Gastric adenocarcinoma has two major sights of presentation—either proximally in the stomach near the esophagogastric junction or distally in the stomach in the antrum. Worldwide, adenocarcinoma of the distal stomach is one of the most common malignancies; in the United States however, this presentation has markedly decreased over the past several decades. Conversely proximal gastric adenocarcinoma has been increasing rapidly in the United States, probably in relation to reflux of gastric contents.

11. **What is the staging scheme for gastric adenocarcinoma?**
Tumor-node-metastasis (TNM) staging is generally used. T-stage is determined primarily by the relation of the tumor to the muscularis propria (above, into, or through). N-stage is determined by the number and location of affected nodes (local versus distant). M-stage is determined by whether distant metastases are present.

12. **How does staging help in treating gastric cancer?**
Survival after gastrectomy for gastric cancer is directly correlated with stage. For instance, stage-stratified 5-year and 10-year relative survival rates in a study of over 50,000 cases of gastric cancer in the United States were as follows: stage IA, 78%/65%; stage IB, 58%/42%; stage II, 34%/26%; stage IIIA, 20%/14%; stage IIIB, 8%/3%; and stage IV, 7%/5%. Therapy, prognosis, and follow-up can be tailored based on the initial staging.

13. **What is the role of endoscopic ultrasonography in staging gastric cancer?**
Endoscopic ultrasonography (EUS) is a technique in which an ultrasound probe is attached to endoscope. As a rule, it is the most accurate method of T- and N-staging gastrointestinal tumors and has the advantage of biopsy capability. EUS can detect small amounts of ascites in staging gastric cancer, which suggests unresectability.
   However, the accuracy of EUS in staging gastric cancer is still relatively low for certain tumor stages, including T_2 lesions, which tend to be overstaged. Lymph node staging is about 80% accurate in most studies and may be lower with the general application of EUS in the medical community. EUS imaging can provide a road map, but, in general, biopsy proof or surgical staging should be performed.

What is the role of surgery in treating localized gastric adenocarcinoma?
Surgery is a potential curative therapy for localized gastric adenocarcinoma. The prognosis is based on TNM staging. The extent of resection is somewhat controversial. Japanese literature suggests that an extended lymphadenectomy plus omentectomy (D_2 operation) is superior to a limited lymphadenectomy with omentectomy (D_1 procedure) or limited lymphadenectomy (D_0 procedure). In a randomized European study, patients undergoing D_2 resection had twice the operative mortality as those undergoing D_1 resection. There was no survival benefit.

What is the role of neoadjuvant therapy in gastric adenocarcinoma?
Neoadjuvant therapy is treatment given prior to an attempt at curative surgical resection to make the primary tumor smaller and to possibly treat small foci of disease outside the operative field. Although the concept is attractive, definitive studies demonstrating the utility of neoadjuvant therapy for gastric cancer have not been performed.

What is the role of adjuvant therapy in gastric adenocarcinoma?
Adjuvant therapy is additional treatment given to patients after attempted curative surgery. Adjuvant treatment is given if there is no evidence of remaining disease. A recent report has shown the effectiveness of neoadjuvant therapy in treating gastric cancer in American patients. In this large randomized study, fluorouracil, leucovorin, and radiation therapy provided a significant survival advantage over observation following surgery. There was a 33% increase in median survival.

What is the usual therapy for metastatic gastric adenocarcinoma?
Chemotherapy can be used with modest benefits. Several regimens have activity in gastric adenocarcinoma, using drugs such as 5-fluorouracil, etoposide, platinum-containing drugs, and taxanes.

What is a MALT lymphoma?
Mucosal-**a**ssociated **l**ymphoid **t**umor. It can occur in any mucosal location, both within and outside the gastrointestinal tract. MALT lymphomas are often low-grade B-cell lymphomas but may also be high-grade aggressive tumors.

What is special about gastric MALT lymphomas?
Gastric MALT lymphomas, unlike MALT lymphomas in other locations, are often associated with infection by *Helicobacter pylori*. Lymphoid tissue is not a normal part of gastric epithelium, and infection with *H. pylori* seems to drive lymphoid proliferation and tumor development.

What is the role of antibiotic therapy in gastric MALT lymphomas?
Treatment of *H. pylori* infection leads usually to regression of low-grade B-cell gastric MALT lymphomas. It is believed that the low-grade tumors retain responsiveness to *H. pylori* antigen stimulation. Complete responses can take up to 18 months after antibiotic therapy. In general, high-grade gastric MALT lymphomas and those with more acquired chromosomal abnormalities do not respond well to antibacterial therapy.

Describe the staging scheme for gastric lymphoma.
Several staging systems are used for gastric lymphoma, including TNM staging (as for gastric adenocarcinoma). A clinical staging system used for non-Hodgkin's lymphoma (the Ann Arbor Classification) is also available. The Ann Arbor system identifies the primary site of lymphoma as nodal or extra nodal and assesses extent of disease based on number of sites involved, relation of the tumor to the diaphragm, and whether the disease has metastasized to nonlymphoid organs. In the Ann Arbor system, a lymphoma involving both the stomach and a lymph node may be stage IIE (two sites with extra nodal primary) or stage IV (nodal primary with metastasis to the stomach). A new staging system that combines TNM staging with Ann Arbor criteria has recently been recommended for gastrointestinal lymphomas.

22. **What is the best therapy for aggressive (non-MALT) gastric lymphoma?**

    Therapy is determined somewhat by stage. For most cases of Ann Arbor stages I and II, surg
    can be curative. However, recent data suggest that chemotherapy, with or without radiation t
    apy, can be equally effective. T-stage is also important because of the possibility of perforatio
    when chemotherapy is used for T_3 or T_4 tumors. The trend is away from surgery for all stage

23. **What are gastric carcinoid tumors?**

    Gastric carcinoid tumors are growths of neuroendocrine cells that may be benign or maligna
    They stain for chromogranin. As a rule, even the malignant tumors are slow growing.
    Tumors >1 cm in diameter are generally more aggressive, whereas smaller tumors are not
    and may represent endochromagraffin cell hyperplasia. Tumors >2 cm often have metastasiz
    Management depends on whether an elevated gastrin level is present and the size of the
    primary tumor. High gastrin levels confer a more benign prognosis than tumors in patients
    with low gastrin levels. As a rule, large tumors often require gastrectomy, whereas smaller
    tumors can be managed endoscopically.

24. **What causes gastric carcinoid tumors?**

    Two processes appear to lead to gastric carcinoid: de novo malignant transformation and los
    normal growth regulation in response to chronic elevation of serum gastrin levels. Tumors a
    ing from de novo malignant transformation are usually single, larger, and more aggressive,
    whereas those arising from elevated gastrin levels are often multiple and smaller. It is import
    to distinguish between the two types.

25. **What are gastric GISTs?**

    GISTs, or **g**astro**i**ntestinal **s**tromal **t**umors, are tumors that develop in the gastric wall from th
    interstitial cells of Cajal. They can be benign or malignant. Generally, malignancy correlates w
    size and histologic features, such as the number of mitoses per 10 high power fields. These
    tumors resemble leiomyomas, and the distinction between gastric leiomyomas and GISTs ca
    be difficult. GISTs mark with an antibody against surface KIT, which is a tyrosine kinase. KIT
    otherwise known as CD117. It has recently been shown that a GIST responds to a specific ty
    sine kinase inhibitor, imatinib mesylate, or STI571.

WEBSITES

1. http://www.vhjoe.com

2. http://www.nlm.nih.gov/medlineplus/stomachcancer.html

3. http://www.carcinoid.org/

4. http://www.stomachcancer.org/

5. http://www.cancer.gov/cancerinfo/types/stomach/

BIBLIOGRAPHY

1. American Joint Committee on Cancer: Handbook for staging of cancer. In Greene FL, Page DL, Fleming ID (e
   The Manual for Staging of Cancer, 6th ed. New York, Springer Publishers, 2002, pp 111–116.

2. Bretagne JF: Could Helicobacter pylori treatment reduce stomach cancer risk? Gastroenterol Clin Biol 27(3 F
   2):440–452, 2003.

3. Chen CH, Yang CC, Yeh YH: Preoperative staging of gastric cancer by endoscopic ultrasound: The prognostic
   usefulness of ascites detected by endoscopic ultrasound. J Clin Gastroenterol 35(4):321–327, 2002.

Crump M, Gospodarowicz M, Shepherd FA: Lymphoma of the gastrointestinal tract. Semin Oncol 26:324–337, 1999.

Cuschieri A, Fayers P, Fielding J, et al: Postoperative morbidity and mortality after D1 and D2 resections for gastric cancer: Preliminary results of the MRC randomised controlled surgical trial. The Surgical Cooperative Group [see comments]. Lancet 347:995–999, 1996.

De Silva CM, Reid R: Gastrointestinal stromal tumors (GIST): C-kit mutations, CD117 expression, differential diagnosis and targeted cancer therapy with imatinib. Pathol Oncol Res 9(1):13–19, 2003.

Devesa SS, Blot WJ, Fraumeni JF Jr: Changing patterns in the incidence of esophageal and gastric carcinoma in the United States. Cancer 83:2049–2053, 1998.

El-Omar EM, Rabkin CS, Gammon MD, et al: Increased risk of noncardia gastric cancer associated with proinflammatory cytokine gene polymorphisms. Gastroenterology 1193–1201, 2003.

El-Serag HB, Sonnenberg A: Ethnic variations in the occurrence of gastroesophageal cancers [see comments]. J Clin Gastroenterol 28:135–139, 1999.

Eslick GD, Lim LL, Byles JE, et al: Association of *Helicobacter pylori* infection with gastric carcinoma: A meta-analysis. Am J Gastroenterol 94:2373–2379, 1999.

Granberg D, Wilander E, Stridsberg M, et al: Clinical symptoms, hormone profiles, treatment, and prognosis in patients with gastric carcinoids. Gut 43:223–228, 1998.

Hundahl SA, Phillips JL, Menck HR: The National Cancer Data Base Report on poor survival of U.S. gastric carcinoma patients treated with gastrectomy: Fifth Edition American Joint Committee on cancer staging, proximal disease, and the "different disease" hypothesis. Cancer 921–932, 2000.

Isaacson PG: Gastric MALT lymphoma: From concept to cure. Ann Oncol 10:637–645, 1999.

Kulke MH, Mayer RJ: Carcinoid tumors [see comments]. N Engl J Med 340:858–868, 1999.

Lauffer JM, Zhang T, Modlin IM: Review article: Current status of gastrointestinal carcinoids. Aliment Pharmacol Ther 13:271–287, 1999.

Moradi T, Delfino RJ, Bergstrom SR, et al: Cancer risk among Scandinavian immigrants in the US and Scandinavian residents compared with US whites, 1973–89. Eur J Cancer Prev 7:117–125, 1998.

Pisani P, Parkin DM, Bray F, Ferlay J: Estimates of the worldwide mortality from 25 cancers in 1990. Int J Cancer 83:18–29, 1999.

Reed PI: Diet and gastric cancer. Adv Exp Med Biol 348:123–132, 1993.

Safatle-Ribeiro AV, Ribeiro U Jr, Reynolds JC: Gastric stump cancer: What is the risk? Dig Dis 16:159–168, 1998.

Svendsen JH, Dahl C, Svendsen LB, Christiansen PM: Gastric cancer risk in achlorhydric patients: A long-term follow-up study. Scand J Gastroenterol 21:16–20, 1986.

Vanagunas A: Eradication of *Helicobacter pylori* and regression of B-cell lymphoma. Biomed Pharmacother 51:156–160, 1997.

Vaquerano J, Esemuede N, Odocha O, Leffall LD: Gastric carcinoma in African Americans: A 10-year single center analysis. In Vivo 10:233–235, 1996.

Zinzani PL, Magagnoli M, Galieni P, et al: Nongastrointestinal low-grade mucosa-associated lymphoid tissue lymphoma: Analysis of 75 patients. J Clin Oncol 17:1254–1260, 1999.

CHAPTER 12

PEPTIC ULCER DISEASE AND HELICOBACTER PYLORI

Khalouck M. Abdrabbo, MD, and David A. Peura, MD

1. **Why is *Helicobacter pylori* a unique bacterium?**

   H. pylori is a spiral-shaped, gram-negative bacterium, 0.5 microns in width and 2–6.5 microns in length. It is distinguished by its multiple sheathed, unipolar flagella and potent urease activity urease accounts for more than 1% of the organism's protein weight. Its shape and flagella allow penetration of and movement through the gastric mucus layer while its urease activity appears essential for colonization and survival. *H. pylori* is unique in its ability to survive within the hostile acid environment of the stomach. Although gastric bacteria were described as early as the turn of the 20th century, their importance in peptic ulcer disease and chronic gastritis was not appreciated until the 1980s. *H. pylori* was first successfully cultured in 1982 by Marshall and Warren.

2. **Do any other *Helicobacter*-like organisms cause disease?**

   Several other *Helicobacter* species have been implicated in human disease. *H. pullorum* and *H. winghamensis* have been isolated from adults and children with symptoms of gastroenteritis fever, stomach pain, and diarrhea. A *Helicobacter* species has been isolated from gallbladder mucosa of patients with chronic cholecystitis, and *H. heilmannii* has been shown to cause gastritis, gastric ulcers, and, rarely, mucosa-associated lymphoid tissue (MALT) lymphoma. Finally *H. hepaticus* and *H. bilis* have been associated with hepatic and biliary tract malignancies and primary biliary cirrhosis. Substantiation of these observations is an area of ongoing research and clinical interest.

3. **What is the prevalence of *Helicobacter pylori*?**

   H. pylori is estimated to infect 60% of the world's adult population, possibly making it the most common chronic human bacterial infection. Its geographic distribution correlates closely with socioeconomic development (Fig. 12-1). In developing countries, the prevalence of infection may reach levels of 80–90% by age 20, and this prevalence remains constant for the rest of adult life. In contrast, in developed countries the prevalence of *H. pylori* infection is less than 20% in people below age 25 and increases about 1% per year to about 50–60% by age 70. Incidence data from developing countries appear to be subject to generational bias; primary infection is acquired during childhood, but each successive birth cohort is less likely to develop infection. Within a given geographic area, incidence appears to be affected by racial, ethnic, and economic factors. For example, in the United States, African Americans and Hispanics acquire infection earlier in life and more frequently than Caucasians, and living in poverty increases the likelihood of infection.

4. **Are children infected by *Helicobacter pylori*?**

   Yes. Most infection is acquired during childhood, usually by age 5 years in both developing and developed countries. Anti-*Helicobacter* antibodies have been demonstrated in neonates, but they probably represent placental transfer of maternal antibodies rather than primary infection. Familial clustering of *H. pylori* infection is common, and siblings and parents of infected children are more likely to be infected. Members of the same family have been demonstrated to be infected with the same strain of *H. pylori*.

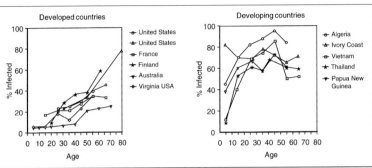

Figure 12-1. Seroprevalence of *Helicobacter pylori* infection in developed and developing countries. (From Marshall BJ, McCallum RW, Guerrant RL: *H. pylori* in Peptic Ulceration and Gastritis. Boston, Blackwell, 1991, pp 46–58. Reprinted with permission of the American Digestive Health Foundation.)

5. What are the risk factors for *Helicobacter pylori* infection?

Lower socioeconomic status, crowded living conditions, and exposure to suboptimal sanitation appear to be major risk factors. Gastroenterologists have a higher than expected prevalence of infection, possibly from occupational contact with infected gastric secretions and endoscopic equipment. Such transmission is less likely now that most physicians adhere to universal pre-cautions during endoscopic procedures, and instruments are adequately decontaminated. Dental plaque has been implicated as a possible reservoir for infection and source of transmis-sion, yet dentists are not at higher infection risk. No evidence links *H. pylori* infection to gender, smoking, alcohol, or particular diet. Studies in monozygotic and dizygotic twins raised in the same and different environments have supported genetic susceptibility to infection.

6. How is infection transmitted?

The exact method of transmission is not known, but most data support fecal-oral or oral-oral routes and best explain the high rate of infection in young children. The bacterium has been cul-tured from the stool of individuals with acute diarrheal disease. The higher than anticipated prevalence in institutionalized individuals, familial clustering of infection, association with crowded living conditions, and documented transmission from contaminated devices, such as endoscopes, also support person-to-person spread. Humans appear to be the major reservoir of *H. pylori*, although the organism has been isolated from domestic cats and primates. The organism remains viable in water for several days and thus municipal water supplies may serve as a source of infection. Although *H.* pylori can be isolated from houseflies, insect transmission remains unproven and unlikely. There is also no evidence to support sexual transmission of infection.

7. Where in the gastrointestinal (GI) tract does *Helicobacter pylori* live?

The organism lives within or beneath the gastric mucous layer, somewhat protected from stom-ach acid. *H. pylori* has potent urease activity, which hydrolyzes urea to ammonia and bicarbon-ate and increases its resistance to the stomach's low pH environment. *H. pylori* recognizes and binds to specific receptors expressed by gastric epithelial cells and, therefore, is able to adhere tightly to the epithelial cell surface. This attachment process may morphologically or function-ally alter the epithelial cell. The organism has been found adherent to ectopic gastric epithelium throughout the GI tract, that is, esophagus (Barrett's), duodenum (gastric metaplasia), small intestine (Meckel's diverticulum), and rectum (ectopic patches of gastric mucosa).

8. How does *Helicobacter pylori* produce mucosal damage?

The organism generally does not directly invade the epithelial cells but indirectly makes the gas-tric mucosa more vulnerable to acid peptic damage by disrupting the mucous layer, liberating a variety of enzymes and toxins, and adhering to and altering the gastric epithelium. In addition, the host immune response to *H. pylori* incites an inflammatory reaction that further perpetuate tissue injury. This chronic inflammation upsets gastric acid secretory physiology to varying degrees and leads to chronic gastritis, which, in most individuals, is asymptomatic but, in som will lead to ulcers and even gastric cancer.

9. **What endoscopy-based (invasive) tests can be used to diagnose *Helicobacter pylori* infection?**

Histopathologic examination is widely available, and specimens are easy to store. Organisms can be detected with standard hematoxylin and eosin stains or special stains, such as Giemsa Warthin-Starry, which make the organisms easier to identify. The sensitivity and specificity of histopathology for *H. pylori* are greater than 95% but may be influenced by sampling error, nu ber of organisms present, use of proton pump inhibitors, and experience of the pathologist.

Rapid urease testing relies on the potent urease activity of *H. pylori,* when a gastric biopsy specimen is placed in medium containing urea and a colored pH indicator. If the organism is present in the specimen, its urease hydrolyzes urea to bicarbonate and ammonia, increasing th pH and changing the color of the pH indicator. The number of organisms present, use of certai medications, and sampling error may influence urease testing. The sensitivity of the rapid ure-ase test is approximately 90%; its specificity is 100%.

10. **Is there a role for culture of *Helicobacter pylori*?**

Culture of gastric biopsy specimens for *H. pylori* is performed occasionally but is difficult, requiring incubation for 3–5 days in special medium in a controlled microaerophilic environ-ment. With easier diagnostic methods available, culture is not clinically useful for diagnosis ar is reserved for determining antibiotic sensitivities in treatment resistant infections.

11. **How is *Helicobacter pylori* diagnosed noninvasively?**

Serology—IgG or IgA antibodies directed at various bacterial antigens can be detected by enzyme-linked immunosorbent assay (ELISA) in serum of infected individuals. In addition, sev eral office-based serologic methods are commercially available. Serologic methods detect evi-dence of primary *H. pylori* infection in untreated people with sensitivity and specificity >90%. Although antibody levels may fall after successful bacterial eradication, they remain elevated fo up to 3 years. This "serologic scar" limits the usefulness of serology in assessing treatment an determining reinfection as well as reduces the positive predictive value of the test, especially ir areas of the world (such as the United States) where prevalence of infection is low. For this rea son a positive serology result should be confirmed with a test of active infection, such as a sto or urea breath test before treatment is initiated.

Urea breath or *blood tests* are ideally suited to make a primary diagnosis of infection, to mo itor treatment response, and to assess reinfection, because they are positive only in a setting c active infection. The patient ingests a small amount of carbon-labeled (13C or 14C) urea. The urease of *H. pylori* hydrolyzes the urea and liberates labeled carbon dioxide, which is absorbed and exhaled in the breath. Labeled carbon dioxide can be collected and quantified in breath or blood samples. Sensitivity and specificity of urea breath or blood testing are >95%. Certain medications can influence test results.

Stool antigen testing is becoming increasingly popular. It is accurate (sensitivity and speci-ficity = 90% and 98%, respectively) and inexpensive. The test is based on polymerase chain reaction amplification of specific *H. pylori* antigens in stool samples. Stool antigen testing is useful in primary diagnosis and confirmation of eradication of the organism after antibiotic tre ment. Certain medications can influence test results (see Table 12-1).

12. **Do any medications affect diagnostic *Helicobacter pylori* testing?**

Yes. Use of antibiotics, bismuth-containing compounds, or proton pump inhibitors (PPIs) can suppress *H. pylori*, leading to false-negative results with rapid urease testing, histopathology,

TABLE 12-1.   DIAGNOSTIC TESTS FOR HELICOBACTER PYLORI

Test	Sensitivity (%)	Specificity (%)	Relative Cost
Noninvasive (nonendoscopic)			
Serology	88–99	86–95	$
Urea breath test	90–97	90–100	$$
Stool antigen test	90	98	$
Invasive (endoscopic)			
Rapid urease assay	89–98	93–98	$$$$*
Histology	93–99	95–99	$$$$$*
Culture	77–92	100	$$$$$*

*Includes cost of endoscopy.
Data from the Foundation for Digestive Health and Nutrition.

urea breath or blood testing, and stool antigen testing. Ideally, diagnostic testing should be performed at least 4 weeks after the discontinuance of any antibiotics and 2 weeks after the discontinuation of PPIs. Multiple biopsies from two or more regions of the stomach can improve the sensitivity of histologic examination or rapid urease testing when patients are taking any of these agents at the time of testing.

What is the association of *Helicobacter pylori* with histologic gastritis?
Infection with *H. pylori* produces an active chronic gastritis with intraepithelial and interstitial neutrophils, in addition to lymphocytes and plasma cells. In most people, gastritis remains confined to the antrum. In others, however, it may progress to involve the entire stomach. Patients with antral gastritis alone are more likely to produce more acid and develop subsequent duodenal ulcers, whereas patients with pangastritis, especially in association with atrophy and intestinal metaplasia, produce less acid and are at risk for gastric ulcers and adenocarcinoma. Genetic differences in the host's inflammatory cytokine profile appear to determine which pattern of gastritis and which potential clinical outcome results from infection.

Does *Helicobacter pylori* play a role in gastric ulcers?
Yes. Many gastric ulcers (>60%) occur in the setting of *H. pylori* gastritis. *H. pylori* makes the gastric mucosal layer more susceptible to acid injury through various mechanisms. Direct adherence of the organism to epithelial cells, ammonia produced by the urease enzyme, and bacterial cytotoxins may damage epithelial cell membranes. Other bacterial enzymes disrupt the protective mucous barrier, rendering the underlying mucosal surface more susceptible to acid injury. Further damage may result from the local and systemic inflammatory response to infection.

What is the association of *Helicobacter pylori* with duodenal ulcer disease?
The association is quite strong. Infection increases serum gastrin levels, which results in increased gastric acid production by parietal cells. Excessive acid production leads to damage of duodenal mucosa over time with subsequent development of duodenal gastric metaplasia. *H. pylori* may infect these duodenal "patches" of gastric mucosa, leading to duodenitis and

eventual duodenal ulceration. Elimination of either gastric acid or infection can prevent duode
ulcers due to *H. pylori*.

16. **Does *Helicobacter pylori* play a role in gastric cancer?**
    Yes. Gastric cancer is the second most common cancer in the world. Unfortunately, it still car
    ries a poor prognosis, and treatment options are limited. Patients with *H. pylori* infection have
    been repeatedly reported to have a threefold to sixfold higher incidence of gastric cancer. The
    World Health Organization (WHO) has classified *H. pylori* as a group I carcinogen. The chroni
    gastritis produced by *H. pylori* results in increased DNA turnover and free radical generation.
    Infection with *H. pylori* also results in decreased secretion of vitamin C, a known antioxidant,
    gastric juice. Over time these factors can lead to mutation of gastric epithelial cells and develc
    ment of adenocarcinoma. Recent studies suggest that eliminating *H. pylori* in high-risk peopl
    can obviate development of subsequent gastric cancer.

17. **Describe the association of *Helicobacter pylori* with mucosa-associated
    lymphoid tissue (MALT) lymphoma.**
    The association is strong. It is believed that the chronic inflammation produced by the organi
    (T-cell response to bacterial antigens) can lead to a monoclonal (B-cell) neoplasm of inflamm
    tory cells. Eradication of *H. pylori* infection results in regression of or cure of this type of tum
    in 90% of patients, when it is superficial and of low histologic grade.

18. **What may cause ulcers besides *Helicobacter pylori*?**
    Most *H. pylori*-negative gastric ulcers are associated with nonsteroidal anti-inflammatory dru
    (NSAIDs). However, both adenocarcinoma and lymphoma can cause gastric ulceration and
    should be excluded. As the prevalence of *H. pylori* decreases, *H. pylori*–negative duodenal ulc
    are more commonly encountered and now account for 40–60% of duodenal ulcers in the Uni
    States. They are often caused by NSAIDs, hypersecretory conditions, such as Zollinger-Ellisc
    syndrome, or unusual manifestations of conditions, such as Crohn's disease. True idiopathic
    duodenal ulcers may be genetically determined and are characterized by hypersecretion of ac
    rapid gastric emptying, poor response to traditional treatment, frequent recurrence, and clini
    complications.

19. **Can infected people develop symptoms, even without a detectable ulcer?**
    Functional (or nonulcer) dyspepsia is a poorly defined clinical entity, probably with multiple
    causes. Evidence that *H. pylori* gastritis causes dyspepsia in the absence of an ulcer has beer
    difficult to obtain, because no specific symptoms separate *H. pylori*–related dyspepsia from
    other forms of functional dyspepsia. In addition, the effect of treatment for *H. pylori* infection
    dyspeptic symptoms has been inconsistent. Nevertheless, a subset of patients with functiona
    dyspepsia has symptoms certainly related to infection and responds to treatment. Unfortuna
    at present, we cannot reliably identify such patients.

20. **Why do only a few infected people develop clinical disease?**
    All infected people develop histologic evidence of active chronic gastritis. However, only a
    minority develop clinically obvious symptoms. At present, it is unknown whether host factors
    such as immune response or genetic susceptibility or infection with more virulent bacterial
    strains, are the major determinants of clinical illness. Recent data suggest that specific
    pleomorphisms of inflammatory cytokines, such as IL1-B, can confer a genetic risk for those
    infected with *H. pylori*, resulting in low acid output and subsequent development of gastric
    cancer.

21. **In what situation is it appropriate to eradicate *Helicobacter pylori* infection?**
    Anyone with active or past ulcer disease should be tested for *H. pylori* and treated, if positive.
    Those who experience any ulcer-related complication should also be tested and treated, if posit

Patients with low-grade MALT lymphoma should be tested and treated because eradication of *H. pylori* may result in a cure of the lymphoma. More controversial yet reasonable treatment situations include young patients with dyspepsia prior to proceeding with invasive diagnostic studies, patients at increased risk of gastric cancer (i.e., positive family history or gastric metaplasia on prior biopsies), or older patients beginning NSAID therapy. Treatment decisions in these situations should be made on a case-by-case basis. Current data are insufficient to recommend screening and treating asymptomatic people to prevent subsequent ulcer disease or gastric neoplasia.

What role does treatment of *Helicobacter pylori* infection play in complicated ulcer disease?

Complications, such as bleeding from peptic ulcers, are associated with significant morbidity and mortality. Data suggest that once complicated ulcers have healed, maintenance antisecretory therapy reduces the likelihood of recurrent complication; eradicating *H. pylori* may also be effective in preventing ulcer complications. However, many complicated ulcers are due to NSAIDs and not *H. pylori* alone; therefore, patients who require chronic NSAID therapy may be at risk for recurrent complications, despite the eradication of *H. pylori*. Such patients may be best treated with *H. pylori* eradication and chronic antisecretory therapy or with the new Cox-2 inhibitors.

What treatment regimens have been used to eradicate *Helicobacter pylori*?

The preferred initial treatment for *H. pylori* infection is a 10- to 14-day course of PPI triple therapy (PPI, amoxicillin 1000 mg, and clarithromycin 500 mg, all given twice daily), and this can successfully cure infection in >80% of individuals. Metronidazole 500 mg can be substituted for amoxicillin, but this should be done only in penicillin-sensitive individuals because of the high rate of metronidazole resistance (Table 12-2). Those in whom this treatment fails (positive stool, breath, or endoscopic test after treatment) should not be retreated with clarithromycin because of presumed acquired macrolide resistance. An appropriate second treatment regimen is a 2-week course of quadruple therapy (PPI b.i.d. plus bismuth subsalicylate [PeptoBismol] two tabs, tetracycline 500 mg, and metronidazole 500 mg four times daily). Although third and even fourth courses of this quadruple therapy are sometimes successful in curing persistent infection, rifabutin, quinolone, or furazolidone-based therapies may be more suitable for particularly refractory cases.

TABLE 12-2.   THERAPY FOR HELICOBACTER PYLORI INFECTION

First-line triple therapy (10–14 days)

Drug 1 (PPI)	Drug 2	Drug 3
Omeprazole 20 mg b.i.d.	Clarithromycin 500 mg bid	Amoxicillin 1000 mg b.i.d.
or lansoprazole 30 mg b.i.d.		(can be replaced by
or pantoprazole 40 mg b.i.d.		metronidazole 500 mg
or rabeprazole 20 mg b.i.d.		b.i.d. in patient sensitive
or esomeprazole 40 mg b.i.d.		to penicillin)

Quadruple therapy (14 days)

Drug 1	Drug 2	Drug 3	Drug 4
PPI	Tetracycline	Metronidazole	Bismuth subsalicylate
(b.i.d.)	500 mg q.i.d.	500 mg q.i.d.	2 tablets q.i.d.

24. **How should eradication of *Helicobacter pylori* be confirmed?**

    Once therapy for *H. pylori* eradication is complete, cure of the infection should be confirmed noninvasively, unless confirmation of ulcer healing is clinically necessary as well. Urea blood breath testing and stool antigen testing are appropriate for this purpose.

25. **What happens to peptic ulcer disease when *Helicobacter pylori* infection is eradicated?**

    The annual recurrence rate of healed gastric ulcers in *H. pylori*–infected patients is approximately 60%. The rate of recurrence of duodenal ulcers after healing is approximately 70%. These can be reduced to <25% with chronic acid suppression therapy. But, when *H. pylori* is eradicated, recurrence of gastric and duodenal ulcers has been reported to be approximately per year. However, data from United States trials suggest that the true recurrence rate after cu of infection may be closer to 20%, at least for duodenal ulcer.

26. **Is reinfection a common problem?**

    Rates of reinfection after eradication vary geographically, but even in developing countries the annual recurrence rate is typically <5%. In developed countries, such as the United States, on infection has been eliminated, the annual rate of reinfection is very low (<1%).

27. **What is the role of vaccination in the prevention of *Helicobacter pylori*?**

    Vaccines against *H. pylori* have proved effective in preventing infection in animals, but no safe vaccine is available for large-scale human use. Development of a preventive or therapeutic va cine remains an important area of research.

28. **What role does *Helicobacter pylori* play in gastroesophageal reflux disease (GERD)?**

    There is no evidence that *H. pylori* causes GERD; in fact, it may be protective or reduce its severity. The bacteria also appear to augment the effect of antisecretory drugs, H_2 blockers ar PPIs used to treat reflux. Some patients who have no reflux symptoms and peptic ulcer disea may actually develop GERD once treated with an eradication regimen for *H. pylori*.

29. **Is *Helicobacter pylori* associated with any diseases outside the gastrointestin tract in humans?**

    Yes. Many studies report an association between *H. pylori* and ischemic heart disease. Althou the studies vary in methods and results, there appears to be a small but consistent excessive risk of ischemic heart disease in patients infected with *H. pylori*. It is theorized that higher ser cytokine levels induced by *H. pylori* infection lead to increased systemic inflammatory responses and atherosclerosis. Idiopathic chronic urticaria, as well as acne rosacea and alope areata, have been linked to *H. pylori* infection. In some patients, urticaria has improved with th eradication of *H. pylori*, but the results with alopecia and rosacea are less striking. Raynaud's phenomenon and migraine headaches have been observed to improve with treatment of *H. pylori,* although no controlled studies have been performed in these or any other extraintestinal conditions.

WEBSITES

1. http://www.consensus.nih.gov

2. http://www.consensus.nih.gov/cons/094/094_intro.htm

BLIOGRAPHY

1. Blecker U, Lanciers S, Mahta D, et al: Familial clusters of *Helicobacter pylori* infections. Clin Pediatr 33:307–308, 1994.

2. Chang MC, Wu MS, Wang Hp, Lin JT: *Helicobacter pylori* stool antigen (HpSA) test: A simple, accurate, and non-invasive test for detection of *Helicobacter pylori* infection. Hepatogastroenterology 46:299–302, 1999.

3. Ciocola AA, McSorley DJ, Turner K, et al: *Helicobacter pylori* infection rates in duodenal ulcer patients in the U.S. may be lower than previously estimated. Am J Gastroenterol 94:1834–1840, 1999.

4. Cremonini F, Di Caro S, Delagado-Aros S, et al: Meta-analysis: The relationship between *Helicobacter pylori* infection and oesophageal reflux disease. Aliment Pharmacol Ther 18:279–289, 2003.

5. El-Omar EM, Carrington M, Chow WH, et al: Interleukin-1 polymorphisms associated with increased risk of gastric cancer. Nature 404:398–402, 2000.

6. Fallone CA, Barkun AN, Friedman G, et al: Is *Helicobacter pylori* eradication associated with gastroesophageal reflux disease? Am J Gastroenterol 95:914–920, 2000.

7. Gasbarrini A, Franceschi F, Armuzzi A, et al: Extra digestive manifestations of *Helicobacter pylori* gastric infection. Gut 45(Suppl 1):I9–I12, 1999.

8. Go MF: Review article: Natural history and epidemiology of *Helicobacter pylori* infection. Aliment Pharmacol Ther 16(Suppl 1):3–15, 2002.

9. Huang JQ, Sridhar S, Hunt RH: Role of *Helicobacter pylori* infection and non-steroidal anti-inflammatory drugs in peptic-ulcer disease: A meta-analysis. Lancet 359:14–22, 2002.

10. Laine L, Estrada R, Trujillo M, et al: Effect of proton-pump inhibitor therapy on diagnostic testing for *Helicobacter pylori*. Ann Intern Med 129:547–550, 1998.

11. Marshall BJ, Warren JR: Unidentified curved bacilli in the stomach of patients with gastritis and peptic ulceration. Lancet 1:1311–1315, 1984.

12. McColl L, El-Omar E, Gillen D: *Helicobacter pylori* gastritis and gastric physiology. Gastroenterol Clin North Am 29:687–703, 2000.

13. McMahon BJ, Hennessy TW, Bensler JM, et al: The relationship among previous antimicrobial use, antimicrobial resistance, and treatment outcomes for *Helicobacter pylori* infections. Ann Intern Med 139:463–469, 2003.

14. Moayyedi P, Soo S, Deeks J, et al: Systematic review and economic evaluation of *Helicobacter pylori* eradication treatment for non-ulcer dyspepsia. Brit Med J 321:659–664, 2000.

15. Sanders MA, Peura DA: *Helicobacter pylori*-associated diseases. Curr Gastroenterol Rep 4:448-454, 2002.

16. Spiegel B, Vakil N, Ofman J: Dyspepsia management strategies in primary care: A decision analysis of competing strategies. Gastroenterology 122:1270–1285, 2002.

17. Sutton P, Lee A: Review article: *Helicobacter pylori* vaccines—the current status. Aliment Pharmacol Ther 14:1107–1118, 2000.

18. Uemora N, Okamoto S, Yamamoto S, et al: *Helicobacter pylori* infection and the development of gastric cancer. N Engl J Med 345:784–789, 2001.

19. Vaira D, Gatta L, Ricci C, Miglioli M: Review article: Diagnosis of *Helicobacter pylori* infection. Aliment Pharmacol Ther 16(Suppl 1):16–23, 2002.

20. Van Leerdam ME, Tytgat GN: Review article: *Helicobacter pylori* infection in peptic ulcer haemorrhage. Aliment Pharmacol Ther 16(Suppl 1):66–78, 2002.

CHAPTER 13

GASTRIC POLYPS AND THICKENED GASTRIC FOLDS

Gregory G. Ginsberg, MD

1. **What are gastric polyps?**

   Gastric polyps are any abnormal growth of epithelial tissue arising from the otherwise smooth surface of the stomach. Gastric polyps may be sessile or pedunculated. *Fundic gland* polyps (Fig. 13-1) are now the most commonly observed gastric polyp in Western populations, superceding *hyperplastic* gastric polyps in prevalence (Fig. 13-2). Together they account for >90% of gastric polyps. *Adenomatous* and *hamartomatous* polyps make up the remainder. Early *gastric cancers* may present as polypoid lesions. Gastric polyps may be singular or multiple. Although endoscopic features may predict histology, accurate discrimination of polyp type can be achieved with tissue sampling only and, in some cases, only after complete resection of the polyp.

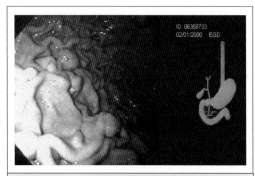

Figure 13-1. Two fundic gland polyps are seen among normal-appearing gastric rugae in the fundus.

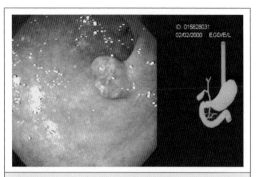

Figure 13-2. Sessile hyperplastic polyp with superficial inflammatory changes is seen in the antrum.

2. Describe the endoscopic features typical of each type of gastric polyp.

Fundic gland polyps are typically numerous (greater than five, often too numerous to count), small (3–5 mm), and hemispherical arising in the gastric fundus. Larger fundic gland polys may develop a pedicle. *Hyperplastic* polyps are typically pedunculated, vary more in number (one to many) and size (5–20 mm), and may occur anywhere throughout the stomach. *Adenomatous* gastric polyps are more apt to be singular and 5–20 mm in size. They may be sessile or pedunculated. Endoscopic appearance-wise, *hamartomatous* polyps are indistinguishable from hyperplastic and adenomatous polyps.

3. Describe the histologic features of each type of gastric polyp.

Fundic gland polyps are composed of hypertrophied fundic gland mucosa. *Hyperplastic* polyps consist of hyperplastic, elongated gastric glands with abundant edematous stroma. There is often cystic dilation of glandular portions but no alteration of the original cellular configuration. *Adenomatous* polyps are true neoplastic growths composed of dysplastic epithelium not normally present in the stomach. They are composed of cells with hyperchromatic, elongated nuclei arranged in picket-fence patterns with increased mitotic figures. *Hamartomatous* polyps have branching bands of smooth muscle surrounded by glandular epithelium; the lamina propria is normal.

KEY POINTS: GASTRIC EPITHELIAL POLYPS

1. Fundic gland

2. Hyperplastic

3. Adenomatous

4. Hamartomatous

4. What is the risk of malignancy associated with gastric polyps?

Adenomas are true neoplasms. The risk of malignant transformation is as high as 75% and size-dependent; size >2.0 cm is critically significant, although carcinoma arising in adenomatous polyps <2.0 cm is well reported. The risk of malignant transformation in *hyperplastic* polyps is low (0.6–4.5%). Because hyperplastic and adenomatous gastric polyps occur against a background of chronic gastritis, the risk of cancer in the gastric mucosa apart from the polyp is increased. Therefore, in addition to removing all polyps, a careful exam should be performed to evaluate the remaining mucosa for early gastric cancer. *Fundic gland* polyps and gastric *hamartomas* are thought to have no malignant potential.

5. How should gastric polyps be managed?

Because polyp histology cannot be reliably distinguished by endoscopic appearance, gastric epithelial polyps should be excised endoscopically when feasible. Forceps biopsy alone may result in a sampling error. Small gastric epithelial polyps (diameter 3–5 mm) may be removed entirely by forceps biopsy resection. Sessile and pedunculated polyps >5.0 mm in diameter should be excised by *snare resection* and tissue retrieved for histologic inspection. Large polyps that cannot be safely removed endoscopically should undergo surgical excision. When gastric polyps are too numerous to count, resection or biopsy should be performed on the largest lesions and a sufficient number sampled to confirm benignity and uniformity of histology.

6. Is surveillance indicated for patients with gastric polyps?

Although data are insufficient to demonstrate a long-term benefit from endoscopic surveillance, in selected patients it is appropriate. The detection of intestinal metaplasia in the surrounding gastric mucosa—and even more so atypia or dysplasia—should be taken into consideration. Endoscopic surveillance, if undertaken, should be considered at *2-3–year intervals* in the absence of dysplasia.

7. **Describe the relationships between gastric polyps and other conditions.**
Fundic gland polyps are promoted by the long-term use of proton pump inhibitors; however, th causal mechanism is unclear. Gastric adenomas and hyperplastic polyps appear commonly against a background of chronic gastritis and are late manifestations of *Helicobacter pylori* infection or type A chronic gastritis (pernicious anemia). Mucosal biopsies should be obtained to determine the presence and severity of underlying gastritis and the presence and type of intestinal metaplasia. *H. pylori* eradication should be undertaken for patients with *H. pylori* gas tritis and gastric polyps. *H. pylori* eradication may reduce polyp recurrence. Gastric hyperplast adenomatous, and fundic gland polyps have an increased prevalence in patients with familial adenomatous polyposis (FAP) and attenuated FAP syndromes.

8. **What is meant by thickened gastric folds?**
Thickened gastric folds appear larger than normal and do not flatten with insufflation of air at endoscopy. Radiographically, large gastric folds are >10 mm in width after distention of the stomach with contrast material during upper gastrointestinal (GI) series.

9. **List the differential diagnosis for intrinsic causes of thickened gastric folds.**
See Table 13-1.

TABLE 13-1. INTRINSIC CAUSES OF THICKENED GASTRIC FOLDS	
Lymphoma	Lymphocytic gastritis
Mucosa-associated lymphoid tissue (MALT)	Eosinophilic gastritis
Linitis plastica	Granulomatous gastritis
Gastric adenocarcinoma	Gastritis cystica profunda
Ménétrier's disease	Gastric anisakiasis
Gastric antral vascular ectasia (GAVE) syndrome	Kaposi's sarcoma
Helicobacter pylori gastritis (acute)	Gastric varices
Zollinger-Ellison syndrome	Sentinel fold

10. **What systemic diseases may be associated with thickened gastric folds or granulomatous gastritis?**
Gastric Crohn's disease and sarcoidosis are the most commonly encountered granulomatous gastropathies. Other potential causes of granulomatous gastritis include histoplasmosis, cand dal infection, actinomycosis, and blastomycosis. Secondary syphilis may present with *Treponema pallidum* infiltration, producing a perivascular plasmacytic response in the gastric mucosa. Disseminated mycobacteria in tuberculosis may result in gastric infiltration. Systemic mastocytosis, in addition to facial flushing, may be associated with hyperemic, thickened gastric folds. Rarely, amyloidosis may cause gastric wall infiltration with thickened gastric folds. (See Key Points on p. 101.)

11. **Endoscopic ultrasound (EUS) displays the gastric wall in five alternating hyperechoic and hypoechoic bands. Histologically, to which wall layers do the correlate?**
See Table 13-2.

TABLE 13-2.   CORRELATION OF ENDOSCOPY ULTRASOUND (EUS) BANDS AND WALL LAYERS

Wall Layer	EUS Bands	Histologic Correlation
1st	Hyperechoic	Superficial mucosa
2nd	Hypoechoic	Deep mucosa, including the muscularis mucosa
3rd	Hyperechoic	Submucosa
4th	Hypoechoic	Muscularis propria
5th	Hyperechoic	Serosa

KEY POINTS: DIFFERENTIAL DIAGNOSIS FOR THICKENED GASTRIC FOLDS

1. Inflammation

2. Neoplasia

3. Infiltration

4. Infection

5. Congestion

6. Variceal

7. Hyperplasia

2. Describe the role of endoscopic ultrasound in the evaluation of thickened gastric folds.
EUS is the most accurate diagnostic imaging study for the evaluation of thickened gastric folds. EUS allows selection of patients in whom further investigation is warranted with large-particle endoscopic biopsy, snare biopsy, EUS-guided fine-needle aspiration, or full-thickness biopsy at laparotomy. Gastric varices are readily recognized. When EUS demonstrates thickening limited to the superficial layers, multiple large-capacity forceps biopsies are apt to provide a histologic diagnosis. Conversely, when EUS documents thickening and wall-layer disruption of the deeper layers (i.e., the submucosa or muscularis propria), endoscopic biopsies are not apt to be diagnostic. This appearance on EUS is highly suggestive for malignancy, and full-thickness biopsy is recommended when endoscopic tissue sampling is negative (Fig. 13-3).

3. What are the clinical features of high-grade non-Hodgkin's gastric lymphoma?
High-grade non-Hodgkin's gastric lymphomas account for 3% of all gastric malignancies but make up the largest group second to adenocarcinoma. The stomach is the most common site of extra nodal lymphoma, accounting for 10%. B-cell lymphomas make up the largest pathologic group of gastric lymphomas, followed by T-cell phenotype and other varieties. Endoscopically, they may present as a discrete polypoid lesion, an ulcerated mass, or a diffuse submucosal infiltration with enlarged rugal folds. The most common presenting symptoms are abdominal pain, weight loss, nausea, anorexia, and bleeding. When gastric lymphoma is suspected, large-particle

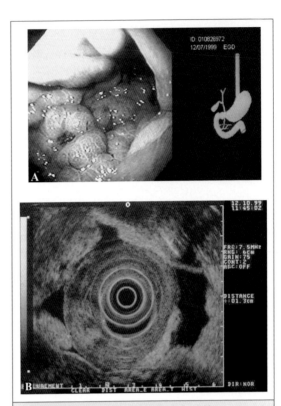

Figure 13-3. Thickened gastric folds in a patient with linitis plastica. (A) The gastric lumen fails to distend on insufflation, and the folds do not flatten out. (B) EUS may show wall-thickening (13 mm), elimination of the normal wall-layer pattern, and ascites, as seen here.

biopsies should be attempted. EUS is useful in identifying abnormalities of the submucosal wall layers and in establishing nodal involvement. When endoscopic biopsy techniques are unrevealing, full-thickness biopsy should be obtained (Fig. 13-4).

14. **Define MALToma.**
Low-grade gastric mucosa-associated lymphoid tissue (MALT) lymphoma is classified as an extra nodal marginal zone lymphoma. MALT is characterized histologically by numerous enlarged lymphoid follicles, a dense B-cell lymphocytic infiltrate, infiltrates of plasma cells, and the presence of lymphoepithelial lesions. Gastric MALTomas may present with bleeding due to ulceration or simply as thickened folds seen on endoscopy or computed tomography (CT) scan. Mucosal biopsies, preferably from large-particle forceps, are usually satisfactory for diagnosis. The majority (>80%) of gastric MALT lymphomas are associated with *H. pylori* infection. The median age of detection is in the fifth decade, but it can occur at any age. The majority of MALTomas are low-grade and run an indolent course; however, they may bleed and/or progress to invasive lymphoma (Fig. 13-5).

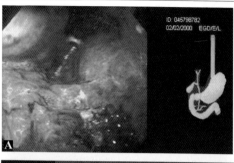

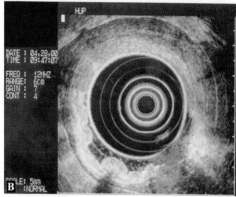

Figure 13-4. (A) In a patient with gastric lymphoma, endoscopy demonstrates expansive focal thickening of folds, erosions, and hyperemia. (B) EUS demonstrates focal mural thickening (12 mm) and disruption of the normal wall-layer pattern superiorly. The normal wall-layer pattern and thickness (5.4 mm) are preserved inferiorly.

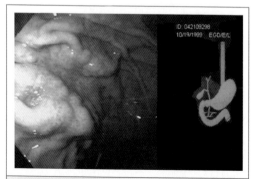

Figure 13-5. MALToma detected on endoscopy in a patient with dyspeptic symptoms. There is focal thickening of the folds in contrast to normal surrounding gastric mucosa.

15. **How are MALTomas managed?**
Gastric mapping should be done to assess for *H. pylori* and distribution of the MALT. EUS shou be performed to assess the depth of wall-layer involvement and presence of wall-layer disrup- tion. Low-grade MALTomas demonstrate only focal thickening of the mucosal and submucosa layers without wall-layer disruption or surrounding adenopathy. Transmural thickening and wa layer disruption indicate high-grade MALToma. Treatment options include surgery, radiation, chemotherapy, and *H. pylori* eradication. Numerous studies indicate that if *H. pylori* infection is eradicated in low-grade disease limited to the submucosa, regression of tumor occurs in 60–75% of patients. EUS is useful to measure regression of disease objectively.

16. **Define Ménétrier's disease.**
Ménétrier's disease is a rare condition characterized by giant gastric rugal folds that often spar the antrum. The histologic features are marked foveolar hyperplasia with cystic dilations that may penetrate into the submucosa. Symptoms include abdominal pain, weight loss, gastroin- testinal blood loss, and hypoalbuminemia. The cause is unclear. The diagnosis can be confirme by EUS findings of thickening of the deep mucosal layer and large-particle biopsy specimens demonstrating the characteristic histology. Treatment with H_2 receptor antagonists benefits some patients (Fig. 13-6).

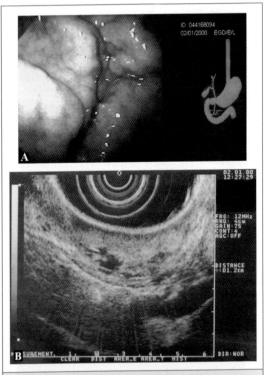

Figure 13-6. In Ménétrier's disease, giant gastric folds are com- monly seen. (A) They are soft and pliable on palpation with a probe. (B) EUS demonstrates marked thickening of the submucosa (12 mm) with cystic dilations.

17. **How is Ménétrièr's disease different in children and adults?**

Unlike Ménétrièr's disease in adults, which is characterized by chronicity of symptoms, Ménétrièr's disease in children is generally self-limited. Recurrence and sequelae are rare. Clinically, pediatric patients present with abrupt onset of vomiting associated with abdominal pain, anorexia, and hypoproteinemia. Gradual onset of edema and ascites results from this protein-losing enteropathy. Hypoalbuminemia, peripheral eosinophilia, and mild normochromic, normocytic anemia are often seen. Radiographic findings include thickened gastric folds in the fundus and body of the stomach, often with antral sparing. Such findings are confirmed by an upper GI barium meal, ultrasonography, and endoscopy. Histologically, the gastric mucosa is hypertrophic with elongation of gastric pits and glandular atrophy. In children, however, intranuclear inclusion bodies consistent with cytomegalovirus (CMV) infection are common; culture of gastric tissue is often positive for CMV. Pediatric patients respond generally to supportive, symptomatic treatment with complete resolution.

18. **What is the differential diagnosis for a subepithelial mass seen on endoscopy?**

Extrinsic compression by normal or abnormal liver, spleen, gallbladder, lymph nodes, or surrounding vasculature occurs in 30% of cases (Table 13-3).

TABLE 13-3. DIFFERENTIAL DIAGNOSIS FOR A SUBEPITHELIAL MASS SEEN ON ENDOSCOPY

Common	Less Common	Rare
Gastrointestinal stromal tumor (GIST)	Leiomyoma	Leiomyoblastoma
Lipoma	Granular cell tumor	Liposarcoma
Pancreatic rest	Leiomyosarcoma	Schwannoma
Carcinoid	Duplication cyst	Fibroma
Submucosal cyst	Neurofibroma	Glomus tumor

19. **What role does endoscopy ultrasound play in evaluating submucosal lesions?**

EUS is accurate in differentiating intramural lesions from extraluminal compression. Although EUS does not provide a histopathologic diagnosis, it can suggest the nature of certain submucosal lesions based on their wall layer location and echotexture (Fig. 13-7). Cysts and varices are anechoic, fatty tumors are hyperechoic, and stromal tumors are hypoechoic. Gastrointestinal stromal tumors (GISTs) are seen as hypoechoic structures arising, most commonly, from the fourth (hypoechoic) sonographic layer, which corresponds to the muscularis propria. Although no unique sonographic differences in size, shape, or appearance distinguish benign from malignant GISTs, the risk of malignancy is considered low if the lesion is <3 cm in diameter. Gastric lipomas appear as hyperechoic lesions within the submucosal layer. Gastric wall cysts are seen as echo-free structures within the submucosa. Varices are serpiginous. Less common submucosal lesions, such as pancreatic rests, carcinoids, fibromas, and granular cell tumors, can also be recognized.

20. **What is a gastrointestinal stromal tumor (GIST)?**

GISTs are the most commonly identified intramural subepithelial mass in the upper GI tract, and the stomach is the most common location. GISTs were once thought to smooth muscle tumors (leiomyoma and leiomyosarcoma); however, they are now believed to arise from the interstitial cells of Cajal and express C-kit protein (CD117) on immunohistochemical staining. GISTs arise most commonly in the muscularis propria layer and are usually asymptomatic. All GISTs have malignant potential. Large (>3 cm) and symptomatic lesions should be resected, as should

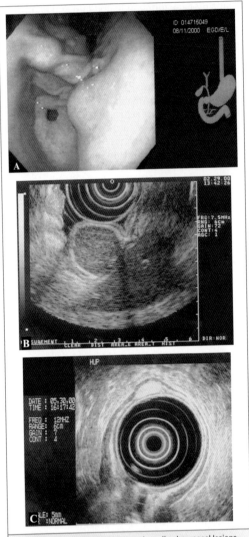

Figure 13-7. (A) Multiple large and small submucosal lesions are seen on endoscopy. EUS demonstrates typical characteristics of (B) leiomyoma and (C) lipoma.

lesions that increase in size or invade surrounding tissue. When the lesion is well circumscribed, small (<3 cm), and without evidence of surrounding tissue invasion or adenopathy, it may be followed for interval stability.

21. **A 65-year-old woman presents with self-limited, coffee-ground emesis. Endoscopy reveals a single, pedunculated, 1-cm polyp in the gastric body. What is the best option for management?**
Although most gastric epithelial polyps are asymptomatic, gastric polyps may cause abdominal pain or bleeding. Complete removal of the lesion by snare polypectomy for histologic evaluation

is both diagnostic and curative. Snare polypectomy is generally safe and well tolerated, though bleeding occurs more commonly than with colonoscopic polypectomy. Glucagon may be used to inhibit peristalsis, aiding in specimen retrieval. An overtube or Roth net (US Endoscopy, Mentor, OH) should be used to avoid accidental dislodgement of the polyp into the airway during retrieval. A 6- to 8-week course of a proton pump inhibitor is generally recommended to promote healing.

KEY POINTS: MOST COMMON SUBEPITHELIAL GASTRIC LESIONS

1. Gastrointestinal stromal tumor (GIST)

2. Extrinsic compression

3. Lipoma

4. Carcinoid

5. Pancreatic rest

2. **A patient with FAP has multiple gastric polyps on surveillance endoscopy. What is the most likely histology of such polyps? What is their malignant potential? What other significant upper gastrointestinal lesions may be detected at the time of upper endoscopy?**
Nearly all patients with FAP have polyps in the upper GI tract. Most polyps are found in the proximal stomach or fundus; they are small, multiple, and hyperplastic. Although they carry no risk for carcinomatous conversion, they may cause bleeding. Forty to 90% of patients, however, have adenomatous polyps in the distal stomach, antrum, or duodenum, particularly in the periampullary region. Risk of adenocarcinoma of the gastric antrum is not increased in U.S. families with adenomatous polyposis but appears to be increased in Japanese families. The relative risk of duodenal, particularly periampullary, cancer is markedly increased in patients with FAP and duodenal or ampullary adenomas.

3. **Describe the manifestations of gastric polyps in the other hereditary gastrointestinal polyposis syndromes.**
Patients with Gardner's syndrome have a preponderance of hyperplastic polyps in the proximal stomach. Patients with Peutz-Jeghers syndrome and juvenile polyposis syndromes may have hamartomatous polyps in the stomach. Although hamartomas may cause bleeding, an increased cancer risk is not apparent.

. **A 40-year-old man has a history of chronic pancreatitis complicated by pseudocysts requiring drainage. He presents with a self-limited upper gastrointestinal bleed. Endoscopy demonstrates a normal esophagus and duodenum. What is the most likely diagnosis? What therapeutic options should be considered?**
The patient has isolated gastric varices secondary to splenic vein thrombosis. Splenic vein thrombosis is a potential complication of acute and chronic pancreatitis, pancreatic carcinoma, lymphoma, trauma, and hypercoagulable states. The left gastric veins empty via the splenic vein. Esophageal venous flow is unaffected. Gastric varices are submucosal or deep to the submucosa, whereas the esophageal varices lie superficial in the lamina propria. Gastric variceal bleeding accounts for 10–20% of acute variceal hemorrhage. The incidence of gastric variceal bleeding is 10–20% among patients with bleeding from esophagogastric

varices. Acute bleeding may be treated endoscopically. However, rebleeding is the rule, and the mortality rate is as high as 55%. When endoscopic therapy is not effective, splenectomy is required.

25. **A 65-year-old woman is referred for evaluation of chronic iron deficiency anemia and Hemoccult-positive stool. Colonoscopy and upper gastrointestinal series are negative. Findings of an upper endoscopy are noted in Figure 13-8. Identify the immediately apparent diagnosis and appropriate treatment.**

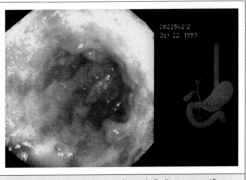

Figure 13-8. What do these endoscopic findings suggest?

The raised red folds that radiate spoke-like from a pylorus displaying friable vascular malforma-tions is characteristic of gastric antral vascular ectasia (GAVE), also known as "watermelon stomach." GAVE is a source of chronic occult GI bleeding. It occurs more frequently in women and is often associated with autoimmune or connective tissue disorders. Underlying atrophic gastritis with hypergastrinemia and pernicious anemia may be present. The pathogenesis is unclear. Histologic features include dilated mucosal capillaries with focal thrombosis; dilated, tortuous submucosal venous channels; and fibrous fibromuscular hyperplasia. Chronic GI blood loss responds to endoscopic contact or noncontact coagulation therapy. Lesions may recur but respond usually to repeat endoscopic therapy.

WEBSITE

http://www.vhjoe.com

BIBLIOGRAPHY

1. Amer MH, el-Akkad S: Gastrointestinal lymphoma in adults: Clinical features and management of three hundr cases. Gastroenterology 106:846, 1994.
2. Caletti GC, Brocchie E, Baraldini M, et al: Assessment of portal hypertension by endosonography. Gastrointes Endosc 34:154–155, 1988.
3. Choudhry U, Boyce HW Jr, Coppola D: Proton pump inhibitor-induced gastric polyps: A retrospective analysis their frequency, and endoscopic, histologic, and ultrastructural characteristics. Am J Clin Pathol 110:615–62 1998.
4. Cristallini E, Ascani S, Bolis G: Association between histologic type of polyp and carcinoma of the stomach. Gastrointest Endosc 38:481–484, 1992.

D'Amore F, Brincker H, Gronback K: Non-Hodgkin's lymphoma of the gastrointestinal tract: A population-based analysis of incidence, geographic distribution, clinical pathologic presentation features, and prognosis. J Clin Oncol 12:1673, 1994.

Deppish LM, Rona VT: Gastric epithelial polyps: A ten year study. J Clin Gastroenterol 11:110–115, 1989.

el-Zimaity HM, Jackson FW, Grahm DY: Fundic gland polyps developing during omeprazole therapy. Am J Gastroenterol 92:1858–1860, 1997.

Friedman SL, Wright TL, Altman DF: Gastrointestinal Kaposi's sarcoma in patients with AIDS: Endoscopic and autopsy findings. Gastroenterology 89:102, 1985.

Frucht H, Howard JM, Slaff JL, et al: Secretin and calcium provocative tests in Zollinger-Ellison syndrome. Ann Intern Med 111:697–699, 1989.

Gilliam JH, Geisinger KR, Wu WC, et al: Endoscopic biopsies diagnostic of gastric antral vascular ectasia: The watermelon stomach. Dig Dis Sci 34:885–888, 1989.

Ginsberg GG, Al-Kawas FH, Fleischer DE, et al: Gastric polyps: Relationship of size and histology to cancer risk. Am J Gastroenterol 91(4):714–717, 1996.

Gostout CJ, Ahlquist DA, Radford CM, et al: Endoscopy laser therapy for watermelon stomach. Gastroenterology 96:1462–1465, 1989.

Hughes R: Diagnosis and treatment of gastric polyps. Gastrointest Endosc Clin North Am 2:457–467, 1993.

Hwang JH, Kimmey MB: The incidental upper gastrointestinal subepithelial mass. Gastroenterology 126:301–307, 2004.

Kimmey ND, Martin RW, Haggit RC, et al: Histologic correlates of gastrointestinal ultrasound imaging. Gastroenterology 94:433, 1989.

Mendis RE, Gerdes H, Lightdale CJ, Botete JF: Large gastric folds: A diagnostic approach using endoscopic ultrasonography. Gastrointest Endosc 40:437–441, 1994.

Nobre-Leitao C, Lage P, Cravo S, et al: Treatment of gastric MALT lymphoma by *Helicobacter pylori* eradication: A study controlled by endoscopic ultrasonography. Am J Gastroenterol 93:732–736, 1998.

Ohkusa T, Takashimizu I, Fujiki K, et al: Disappearance of hyperplastic polyps in the stomach after eradication of *Helicobacter pylori*. A randomized clinical trial. Ann Intern Med 129:712–715, 1998.

Okada M, Lizuka Y, Oh K, et al: Gastritis cystica profunda presenting as giant gastric mucosal folds: The role of endoscopic ultrasonography and mucosectomy in the diagnostic work-up. Gastrointest Endosc 40:640–644, 1994.

Rustgi AK: Hereditary gastrointestinal polyposis in non-polyposis syndromes. N Engl J Med 331:1694–1702, 1994.

Scharschmidt B: The natural history of hypertrophic gastropathy (Ménétrier's disease). Am J Med 63:644–652, 1997.

Steinbach G, Ford R, Glober G, et al: Antibiotic treatment of gastric lymphoma-associated lymphoid tissue: An uncontrolled trial. Ann Intern Med 131:88–95, 1999.

Tio TL, Tytgat GN, der Hartog Jager FC: Endoscopic ultrasonography for the evaluation of smooth muscle tumors in the upper gastrointestinal tract: An experience with 42 cases. Gastrointest Endosc 36:343–350, 1990.

CHAPTER 14

GASTROPARESIS

Erik G. Kerekes, MD, and Michael H. Walter, MD

1. **Define *gastroparesis.***
   Literally, *gastroparesis* means incomplete or partial paralysis of the stomach. It is a disorder delayed gastric emptying in the absence of mechanical obstruction. Symptoms result from faure of the stomach to properly empty its contents into the duodenum.

2. **What are the factors that determine gastric motility and emptying?**
   There is an interplay of multiple factors, such as meal composition, neuroregulators, and hormonal regulators that determine gastric motility and emptying. Once in the stomach, liqui tend to empty without a lag phase. On the other hand, prior to emptying through the pylorus, solids must undergo trituration (grinding) until approximately 1 mm in size.

Slow emptying:	Fatty meals and certain proteins
	Secretin and cholecystokinin
Accelerated emptying:	Motilin and neurotensin

3. **Describe the electric pacesetter in the stomach.**
   The rate of contraction of the stomach is controlled by an area called the pacesetter, which is located in the proximal corpus along the greater curvature of the stomach. Throughout the entire gastrointestinal (GI) tract, a repetitive, highly regular electrical pattern, known as *slow waves,* occurs at different frequencies. In the stomach, these slow waves are generated from pacesetter at three cycles per minute. Gastric contractions can occur only at the peak of one c these slow waves.

4. **What is the migrating motor complex?**
   In the fasting state, the stomach and small bowel in humans undergo cyclical contractions wi cycle lengths of 90–120 minutes. There is little activity in the quiescent phase (phase I). Durir the dominant phase II, irregular muscle contractions begin to appear and crescendo to a poir maximal contractility (phase III), which lasts about 5 minutes. Phase III is a forceful burst of uninterrupted phasic contractions that sweep the antrum and continue along the entire GI tra to the ileocecal valve. Each repetition of phases I, II, and III is known as the *migrating motor complex* (MMC). The key function of the MMC is to eliminate the small intestine of food, bact ria, and debris between meals.

5. **Describe gastric motility and emptying.**
   Gastric emptying is controlled by activities in the proximal and distal halves of the stomach as well as in the pyloric outlet, all of which act in sequence. The stomach serves as a food reserv that allows controlled emptying into the duodenum. In the fundus and the upper body of the stomach, receptive relaxation occurs with distention of the esophagus and/or stomach to accommodate food. In the distal two thirds of the stomach, forceful contractions by circumfe ential bands of muscles culminate in terminal antral contractions that grind food into 1-mm pieces (trituration). Liquid emptying is volume-dependent and follows first-order kinetics, whereas solid emptying is volume-independent. Once solids are reduced in size, a prolonged ear phase of emptying occurs.

6. **What are the causes of gastroparesis?**
    - Peptic ulcer disease
    - Endocrine disorders (thyroid, diabetes, parathyroid)
    - Collagen vascular disease
    - Psychogenic cause

    Greater than 70% of cases are secondary to diabetes mellitus (DM), postsurgical, and idiopathic gastroparesis.

7. **What is idiopathic gastroparesis?**

    These patients may present with sudden or insidious onset of postprandial pain, nausea, vomiting, and bloating. Despite normal endoscopic exams and no history of previous surgeries or any identifiable primary cause, these patients have delayed gastric emptying. Women younger than age 50 comprise 80–90% of these patients. Nausea, fever, myalgia, and diarrhea may be present prior to onset in some cases, suggesting a viral etiology.

8. **Describe the natural history of idiopathic gastroparesis.**

    Although some patients with idiopathic gastroparesis exhibit persistent symptoms, a subset of them improves spontaneously to a point in which medical therapy is no longer required. A viral etiology is believed to play a role in these patients. On the other hand, those without a viral prodrome experience a more progressive course with worsening pain, early satiety, anorexia, and overall lower quality of life.

9. **What is diabetic gastroparesis?**

    The most common cause of delayed gastric emptying is diabetic gastroparesis with a prevalence of 27–58% in long-standing DM type 1. Although advanced DM may affect small intestinal motility, impaired gastric motor function is more common. Previously, it was thought that diabetic gastroparesis was a complication seen more often after 10 years of DM type 1 and in those with concomitant autonomic neuropathy. However, it is also seen commonly in the first 10 years of DM type 2, and, although neuropathy is not always present, this complication of DM significantly increases the risk of gastroparesis.

10. **What is the pathogenesis of diabetic gastroparesis?**

    Under normal circumstances, intramural nerves under the influence of the vagus predominantly control gastric motility. A diseased vagus nerve is thought to be the cause of impaired gastric motility in diabetics. For example, diabetics produce only one third of the normal gastric acid output in response to sham feeding, a vagally mediated reflex. However, periods of hyperglycemia in the absence of neuropathy have been correlated with delays in emptying, suggesting that the motor defect is not fixed. A strong correlation exists with delayed gastric emptying of liquids and when the blood glucose exceeds 270 mg/dL. Likewise, delays in solid emptying are observed during periods of hyperglycemia in type I diabetics, which improve during euglycemia.

11. **Which surgical procedures are associated with postoperative gastroparesis?**

    Gastroparesis can be seen after the following surgical procedures:
    - *Gastric atony after vagotomy:* Approximately 5% of patients who undergo vagotomy and drainage for peptic ulcer disease or malignancy experience nausea, vomiting, and early satiety caused by postoperative gastric stasis in the absence of an anatomic obstruction. Even some patients who undergo highly selective vagotomy develop gastroparesis.
    - *Roux stasis syndrome:* Some patients may experience intractable nausea, vomiting, and abdominal pain after construction of a Roux-en-Y gastrojejunostomy. Symptoms of retention may result from either gastric, spastic, or retroperistaltic Roux limb motor abnormalities.
    - *Delayed gastric emptying in association with fundoplication:* Nausea and bloating may develop after laparoscopic or open antireflux surgery.

- *Gastric stasis after gastric bypass surgery:* Gastroplasty and gastric bypass are performed in some morbidly obese patients who fail lifestyle and dietary methods of weight control. Gastroplasty creates a 50-mL fundic pouch that is continuous with the distal stomach through a 10-mm stoma. Gastric bypass divides the stomach in two with the proximal compartment draining through a 12-mm gastroenterostomy. Both procedures produce delayed gastric emptying of solids and fundic distention, which leads to early satiety, loss of appetite, and weight reduction.

- *Gastroparesis after other surgeries:* Esophagectomy with gastric pull-through into the thoracic cavity may be curative for esophageal malignancy, but with colonic interposition, delays in gastric emptying are reported. Pylorus-preserving Whipple procedures, performed for pancreatic cancer and chronic pancreatitis, are complicated by delayed gastric emptying in up to 50% of cases. Gastroparesis is a common sequela of lung and heart-lung transplantation and may predispose to microaspiration into the transplanted lung.

12. **Which conditions cause selective gastric motor dysfunction leading to gastroparesis?**
    - *Gastroparesis in association with gastroesophageal reflux disease:* Delays in solid or liquid phase gastric emptying can be seen in some patients with gastroesophageal reflux. This often correlates poorly with symptoms, lower esophageal sphincter pressure, and 24-hour pH monitoring results.
    - *Radiation-induced gastric stasis:* Severe nausea, vomiting, and intolerance of both liquid and solid meals are common after abdominal irradiation.
    - *Delayed gastric emptying with atrophic gastritis:* Delayed gastric emptying of solids, but not liquid meals, may be seen in patients with atrophic gastritis, with or without pernicious anemia. This may be caused, in part, by poor intragastric processing of food due to decreased secretion of digestive enzymes, which, in turn, prolongs the time needed to fragment solid foods.

13. **Which disorders with diffuse abnormalities of gastrointestinal motor activity cause gastroparesis?**
    - *Rheumatologic disorders:* Gastrointestinal symptoms, such as dysphagia, heartburn, nausea and vomiting, are common in patients with scleroderma and result from motility abnormalities of the upper gut. Characteristic manometric findings are observed in both the stomach and small intestine. Either delayed gastric emptying or gastric atony is seen in other rheumatologic diseases, such as polymyositis, dermatomyositis, and systemic lupus erythematosus.
    - *Chronic intestinal pseudo-obstruction:* Chronic idiopathic intestinal pseudo-obstruction presents with nausea, vomiting, bloating, and early satiety from gastric and small intestinal motor impairment. Idiopathic chronic pseudo-obstruction is familial in many cases, resulting from an inherited visceral myopathy or neuropathy. The diagnosis is suggested by delayed transit and luminal dilation on barium radiography as well as characteristic neuropathic or myopathic patterns on manometry. A full-thickness biopsy of the small intestinal wall is needed to make a definitive diagnosis.
    - *Infectious disorders:* Gastrointestinal motor activity is disrupted in Chagas' disease, because the myenteric plexus is damaged by *Trypanosoma cruzi* infection. Gastroparesis, megaduodenum, and chronic intestinal pseudo-obstruction may be seen in Chagas' disease. Other infections that disrupt gut motor activity include the following: Varicella zoster, Epstein-Barr virus, and *Clostridium botulinum.* Gastric emptying is often markedly delayed in patients with human immunodeficiency virus who have pathogenic gastrointestinal infections.
    - *Miscellaneous conditions with diffuse motor abnormalities:* Delayed gastric emptying is seen also in smooth muscle disorders, such as myotonic dystrophy and progressive muscular dystrophy. Primary or secondary amyloidosis can cause neuropathic or myopathic intestinal pseudo-obstruction. Solid phase gastric emptying may be delayed in patients with idiopathic slow transit constipation, idiopathic megarectum, and achalasia. Furthermore, voluntary suppression of defecation can delay gastric emptying in healthy volunteers.

Which drugs affect gastric emptying?

Numerous prescription and over-the-counter medications can modify gastric emptying rates (Table 14-1).

TABLE 14-1. EFFECTS OF MEDICATIONS ON GASTRIC EMPTYING		
Accelerate Gastric Emptying		
Beta blockers	Diazepam	Metoclopramide
Bulk laxatives	Domperidone	Tegaserod
Cisapride	Erythromycin	
Delay Gastric Emptying		
Alcohol	Dopamine	Phenothiazine
Aluminum hydroxyl antacids	Glucagon	Potassium
Anticholinergics	L-dopa	Progesterone
Beta agonist	Lithium	Sucralfate
Calcitonin	Omeprazole	Theophylline
Calcium channel blockers	Ondansetron	Tobacco
Diphenhydramine	Opiates	Tricyclic antidepressants

List the conditions that have an established association with delayed gastric emptying.

- *Diabetes mellitus*
- *Anorexia nervosa:* Delayed gastric emptying is common in anorexia nervosa. Nausea, vomiting, gastric dilation, and even perforation on feeding have been reported.
- *Gastric surgery:* Gastric atony may occur after gastric surgery. This uncommon complication affects from 1.25% of patients who undergo vagotomy and pyloroplasty to 9% of patients who undergo vagotomy and subtotal gastrectomy. Surgery should not be done acutely on a dilated, obstructed stomach because atony is more likely to occur.

What associations are likely to be important in gastroparesis?

- *Gastric dysrhythmias:* Usually of an idiopathic nature, these may delay gastric emptying. Various dysrhythmias have been described and may be measured with electrogastrography (Fig. 14-1).
- *Tachygastria* is associated with delayed gastric emptying. During periods of tachygastria, contractions do not occur. Secondary gastric dysrhythmias are associated with anorexia nervosa and motion sickness. They have also been reported in gastric ulcers and gastric cancers.
- *Obesity:* This seems to slow gastric emptying. An inverse relationship between body size and gastric emptying has been observed.
- *Various kinds of stress:* Through the central nervous system (CNS), these can modulate gastric emptying, including stress from pain or anxiety.
- *Neurologic disorders,* including strokes, brain tumors, headaches, and high intracranial pressures, can alter gastric emptying.
- *Diseases involving the gastric wall:* Scleroderma, amyloidosis, systemic lupus erythematosus, and dermatomyositis may slow gastric emptying.
- *Abdominal cancers:* Direct involvement of the stomach wall or invasion of surrounding nerves may delay gastric emptying. Gastroparesis may also be a paraneoplastic effect.

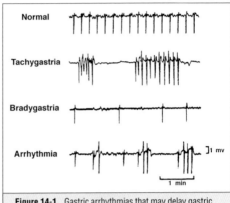

Figure 14-1. Gastric arrhythmias that may delay gastric emptying are measured with electrogastrography.

17. **What is the differential diagnosis of chronic nausea and vomiting?**

New onset of nausea and vomiting is generally associated with new medications (i.e., antibiotics, narcotics), acute infections, pregnancy, pain from myocardial ischemia (MI) and acute brain injury, pain from inflammation (i.e., pancreatitis, cholecystitis), or pain from trauma, especially to the head. Chronic nausea and vomiting should make one consider motility disorders (i.e., gastroparesis, scleroderma) or mechanical obstruction (i.e., peptic ulcer disease, malignancy, previous surgery). Furthermore, endocrinopathies (i.e., hyperthyroidism, hypothyroidism, adrenal insufficiency) or psychogenic disorders (i.e., bulimia) need to be considered

18. **What are the symptoms of gastroparesis?**
    - Early satiety
    - Nausea, especially postprandial
    - Postprandial bloating
    - Postprandial emesis or delayed emesis
    - Abdominal pain

19. **Which part of the history and physical exam is important in establishing a diagnosis of gastroparesis?**

The nonspecific symptoms listed in question 18 suggest gastroparesis. Nausea may be insidious, and vomiting may not even be present. When present, the timing of vomiting is important because patients with gastroparesis tend to vomit undigested food several hours after eating. Associated symptoms, such as pain, fever, and diarrhea, may be indicative of other causes. Review of the surgical history is crucial. Medication lists need to be reviewed because many slow gastric emptying. Furthermore, taking a psychological history is also helpful in identifying patients with bulimia and anorexia nervosa. Ruling out gastric outlet obstruction and its cause is necessary before making a diagnosis of gastroparesis.

20. **What modalities are available for diagnosing gastroparesis?**

The mainstay of diagnosing delayed gastric emptying is gastric scintigraphy. The patient ingests a radiolabeled low-fat egg meal, after which its retention or elimination from the stomach is observed over time with serial images. Because gastric emptying of solids is a better indicator disease, a solid-meal study is the method of choice. A convenient measure is the time it takes half of the test meal to leave the stomach. A 2-hour test is sometimes used, but a recent study showed that a 4-hour test significantly increases sensitivity. Electrogastrography (EGG) is becoming more readily available and measures the pacesetter potential in the stomach.

KEY POINTS: GASTROPARESIS

. Symptoms include nausea, vomiting, bloating, early satiety, and pain.

. Diabetes is the most common cause, followed by idiopathic gastroparesis.

. Nuclear scintigraphy correlates poorly with symptoms of gastroparesis.

. Management includes lifestyle modification as well as medical and surgical therapies.

. **Outline an approach to the diagnosis of gastroparesis.**
A pregnancy test, along with tests to rule out Addison's disease and thyroid disease, should be done. An upper endoscopy is necessary to exclude gastric outlet obstruction. Work-up for partial small-bowel obstruction should also be performed, if clinically indicated. Next, a quantitative gastric emptying study should be done. Although there are several options, gamma scintigraphy is the procedure of choice because of its precision, simplicity, and reproducibility.

. **Once gastroparesis is diagnosed, how should it be treated?**
It is necessary to correct any reversible causes of gastroparesis. Electrolyte abnormalities should be corrected, and drugs that potentially slow gastric emptying should be stopped. With diabetics, good glycemic control is imperative and needs to be emphasized. A diet consisting of small, frequent, low-fat meals should be started. Several prokinetic drugs that facilitate gastric motility are also available.

- *Bethanechol:* A cholinergic drug that stimulates muscarinic receptors. There is a slight increase in amplitude but a slight decrease in frequency of antral contractions (Gut 1999 Sept; 45[3]: 346). Its usefulness in gastroparesis is limited.
- *Metoclopramide:* A dopamine antagonist with potent cholinergic effects. It acts mainly on the proximal GI tract. In the stomach, it increases antral contractions and relaxes the pylorus. The usual dosage is 10 mg four times a day, and it may be given orally or intravenously. Dose adjustments must be made for those with renal impairment. Side effects, such as drowsiness, dystonic reactions, and nervousness, are common and can limit its use.
- *Cisapride:* A benzamide derivative that facilitates acetylcholine release at the myenteric plexus. It affects the entire GI tract and does not have the CNS side effects of metoclopramide. Cisapride was taken off the market due to life-threatening arrhythmias in some patients but may be obtained directly from Janssen Pharmaceutical, if certain criteria are met.
- *Domperidone:* A benzimidazole derivative with clinical effects similar to metoclopramide. It acts primarily on the proximal GI tract and has been shown to be more efficacious and has fewer side effects than metoclopramide. It is not available in the United States.
- *Erythromycin:* A motilin receptor agonist, given in doses of 50 mg IV, induces phase III contractions in the antrum and upper small bowel. Tachyphylaxis occurs within 4 weeks.
- *Tegaserod:* A serotonin (5-HT$_4$) receptor partial agonist was found to improve gastric emptying compared to placebo in healthy men. It also improved gastric emptying in patients with gastroparesis complaining of dyspeptic symptoms.

. **What are the prokinetic medication options for medically refractory gastroparesis?**
A few patients may be unresponsive to, or may not tolerate, oral prokinetic pills. Because liquid emptying may be near normal in gastroparesis, a liquid form of a prokinetic agent can be prescribed. Metoclopramide can also be efficacious in gastroparesis when given subcutaneously, but injections are painful.

24. **What are the complications of gastroparesis?**

Gastroparesis can have a significant impact on a patient's quality of life. Severe nausea and vomiting may lead to significant weight loss, malnutrition, gastrointestinal hemorrhage from Mallory-Weiss tears, and aspiration pneumonia. A common complication is the development of phytobezoar in the stomach, which can lead to ulcerations, small intestinal obstruction, and gastric perforation.

25. **What is the surgical management for medically refractory gastroparesis?**

Surgery is reserved as the last resort in patients with gastroparesis. Surgical jejunostomy with enteric feeding can improve overall health, gastrointestinal symptoms, nutritional status, and reduce hospitalizations. Adding a gastrostomy tube can also help drain gastric secretions during severe symptom flares. Diabetic patients with gastroparesis and renal failure have shown greater improvement in gastric function after combined pancreas-kidney transplantation than after kidney transplantation alone, thus supporting the argument that the enhancement of glycemic control provided by the pancreatic graft provides significant beneficial effects. Surgical placement of electrical leads on the gastric wall for electrical stimulation has been performed for the treatment of gastroparesis. Studies show that gastric electrical stimulation reduces the frequency of nausea and vomiting, accelerates liquid emptying, improves nutritional parameters, and has variable effects on gastric emptying of solids.

WEBSITES

1. http://www.medscape.com/viewarticle/460632

2. http://www.medtronic.com/neuro/gastro/enterra/enterra.html

BIBLIOGRAPHY

1. Abell T, Lou J, Batista O, et al: Gastric electrical stimulation for gastroparesis improves nutritional parameters a short, intermediate and long-term follow-up. J Parenter Enteral Nutr 27:277, 2003.

2. Abell T, McCallum R, Hocking M, et al: Gastric electrical stimulation for medically refractory gastroparesis. Gastroenterology 125:421, 2003.

3. Bardhan PK, Salam MA, Molla AM: Gastric emptying of liquid in children suffering from acute rotaviral gastroenteritis. Gut 33:26, 1992.

4. Bitytskiy LP, Soykan I, McCallum RW: Viral gastroparesis: A subgroup of idiopathic gastroparesis clinical characteristics and long-term outcomes. Am J Gastroenterol 92:1501, 1997.

5. Cucchiara S, Salvia G, Borrelli O, et al: Gastric electrical dysrhythmias and delayed gastric emptying in gastroesophageal reflux disease. Am J Gastroenterol 92:1103, 1997.

6. Degen L, Matzinger D, Merz M, et al: Tegaserod, a 5-HT$_4$ receptor partial agonist, accelerates gastric emptying and gastrointestinal transit in healthy male subjects. Aliment Pharmacol Ther 15:1745, 2001.

7. Foltynova V, Brousil J, Velatova A, et al: Swallowing function and gastric emptying in patients undergoing replacement of the esophagus. Hepatogastroenterol 40:48, 1993.

8. Fujiwara Y, Nakagawa K, Tanaka T, Utsunomiya J: Relationship between gastroesophageal reflux and gastric emptying after distal gastrectomy. Am J Gastroenterol 91:75, 1996.

9. Guo JP, Maurer AH, Fisher RS, et al: Extending gastric emptying scintigraphy from two to four hours detects more patients with gastroparesis. Dig Dis Sci 46:24, 2001.

10. Hathaway DE, Abell T, Cardoso S, et al: Improvement in autonomic and gastric function following pancreas-kidney versus kidney-alone transplantation and the correlation with quality of life. Transplantation 57:816, 199

11. Hunter RJ, Metz DC, Morris JB, Rothstein RD: Gastroparesis: A potential pitfall of laparoscopic Nissen fundoplication. Am J Gastroenterol 91:2617, 1996.

12. Jones MP, Maganti K: A systematic review of surgical therapy for gastroparesis. Am J Gastroenterol 98:2122, 2003.

Konturek JW, Fischer H, van der Voort IR, Domschke W: Disturbed gastric motor activity in patients with human immunodeficiency virus infection. Scand J Gastroenterol 32:221, 1997.

Lyrenas EB, Olsson EH, Arvidsson UC, et al: Prevalence and determinants of solid and liquid gastric emptying in unstable type I diabetes. Relationship to postprandial blood glucose concentrations. Diabetes Care 20:413, 1997.

McCallum RW, Champion MC: Gastrointestinal motility disorders: Diagnosis and treatment. Baltimore, Williams & Wilkins, 1990.

McCallum RW, Chen JD, Lin Z, et al: Gastric pacing improves emptying and symptoms in patients with gastroparesis. Gastroenterology 114:456, 1998.

Parkman HP, Fisher RS: Disorders of gastric emptying. In Yamada T, Alpers DH, Laine L, et al (eds): Textbook of Gastroenterology, 4th ed. Philadelphia, Lippincott Williams & Wilkins, 2003.

Patterson D, Abell T, Rothstein R, et al: A double-blind multicenter comparison of domperidone and metoclopramide in the treatment of diabetic patients with symptoms of gastroparesis. Am J Gastroenterol 94:1230, 1999.

Quigley EM: Gastric motor and sensory function, and motor disorders of the stomach. In Feldman M, Friedman LS, Sleisenger MH (eds): Sleisenger & Fortran's Gastrointestinal and Liver Disease: Pathophysiology, Diagnosis, Management, 7th ed. Philadelphia, W.B. Saunders, 2002, pp 691–713.

Tobi M, Holtz T, Carethers J, Owyang C: Delayed gastric emptying after laparoscopic anterior highly selective and posterior truncal vagotomy. Am J Gastroenterol 90:810, 1995.

EVALUATION OF ABNORMAL LIVER TESTS

Kenneth E. Sherman, MD, PhD

CHAPTER 15

What are liver tests?

Usually, the term refers to the routine chemistry panel that includes alanine aminotransferase (ALT), aspartate aminotransferase (AST), gamma glutamyl transpeptidase (GGT), alkaline phosphatase (AP), bilirubin, albumin, and protein. Other terms for the same tests are liver function tests (LFTs) and liver-associated enzymes (LAEs), but neither is totally accurate. Only the first four are properly called enzymes, and only the last two provide a measure of liver function. These tests help to characterize injury patterns and provide a crude measure of the synthetic function of the liver. Various combinations can be helpful in diagnosing specific disease processes, but, generally, these tests are not diagnostic. Other LFTs are described later. Finally, certain tests help to define specific causes of liver disease. They may be serologic (e.g., hepatitis C antibody) or biochemical (e.g., alpha-1 antitrypsin level) but, generally, are not used as screening assays or as part of general health profiles.

What are the true liver function tests?

True LFTs evaluate the liver's synthetic capacity or measure the ability of the liver, either to uptake and clear substances from the circulation or to metabolize and alter test reagents. *Albumin* is the most commonly used indicator of synthetic function, although it is not highly sensitive and may be affected by poor nutrition, renal disease, and other factors. In general, low albumin levels indicate poor synthetic function. The *prothrombin time* (PT) is another simple measure of the liver's capacity to synthesize clotting factors. The PT may be related to decreased synthetic ability or vitamin K deficiency. A high PT that does not correct with oral administration of vitamin K (5–10 mg for 3 days) may indicate liver disease, unless ductal obstruction or intrahepatic cholestasis prevents bile excretion into the duodenum and thus limit absorption of vitamin K. Administration of a subcutaneous or intravenous injection of vitamin K (10 mg) may correct the defect and suggests that vitamin K absorption rather than synthetic dysfunction is responsible for the PT abnormality.

Various uptake and excretion tests profess to define liver function, including bromosulfophthalein (BSP), indocyanine green, aminopyrine, caffeine, and monoethylglycinexylidide (MEGX). Research laboratories frequently use such tests to determine severity of liver disease and to predict survival outcomes, but, currently, they are not part of routine clinical practice.

What is the difference between cholestatic and hepatocellular injury?

The two main mechanisms of liver injury are damage, or destruction, of liver cells, which is classified as *hepatocellular*, and impaired transport of bile, which is classified as *cholestatic*. Hepatocellular injury is most often due to viral hepatitis, autoimmune hepatitis, and various toxins and drugs. Transport of bile may be impaired by extrahepatic duct obstruction (e.g., gallstone, post-surgical stricture), intrahepatic duct narrowing (e.g., primary sclerosing cholangitis), bile duct damage (e.g., primary biliary cirrhosis), or failed transport at the canalicular level (e.g., chlorpromazine effect). In some cases, elements of both types of damage are involved; this scenario is often called a "mixed injury" pattern.

4. **What is the most specific test for hepatocellular damage?**
The most specific test for hepatocellular damage is the ALT level. The AST level may also be e[levated] but is not as specific.

5. **How is cholestatic injury best diagnosed?**
Cholestatic injury is best diagnosed by an elevated AP level. Bile acids stimulate AP productio[n] but duct obstruction or damage prevents bile acid excretion into the duodenum. Therefore, th[e] AP level in serum rises dramatically. Serum AP levels may be slightly increased in early hepat[o]cellular disease, but this increase is due to the release of cellular enzyme without excessive st[im]ulation of a new enzyme. Because AP can be derived from other body tissue (e.g., bone, intestine), a concurrent elevation of GGT or 5′-nucleotidase helps to support a cholestatic me[ch]anism.

6. **What are serum transaminases?**
The two serum transaminases commonly assayed in clinical practice are ALT and AST. Many laboratories still use older terminology that refers to ALT as serum glutamic pyruvate transam[i]nase (SGPT) and to AST as serum glutamic oxaloacetic transaminase (SGOT). The newer ter[ms] reflect more accurately their enzymatic action, which involves the transfer of amino groups fr[om] one structure to another. As noted earlier, elevation of ALT and/or AST reflects the presence o[f] hepatocellular injury. It is important to understand how the assays are performed and what c[on]founding factors may alter interpretation of test results.

7. **How is alanine aminotransferase assessed?**
The most commonly used test reaction for ALT is as follows:

$$\text{Alanine} + \text{alpha-ketoglutarate} \rightarrow \text{pyruvate} + \text{L-glutamate}$$

This reaction requires ALT and pyridoxal phosphate (vitamin B_6). A crucial point is that enzyme assays do not measure how much enzyme is present; instead, they indirectly measur[e] the catalytic activity of the enzyme in performing a particular function. Therefore, the assay d[oes] not indicate how much ALT is present but how quickly it causes the previously mentioned rea[c]tion to take place. The assumption is that the faster the reaction, the greater the amount of AL[T.] To complicate matters further, the assay does not measure the amount of reaction product th[at] is created. Instead, a linked enzyme reaction is used:

$$\text{Pyruvate} \rightarrow \text{lactic acid}$$

This reaction occurs in the presence of another enzyme, lactate dehydrogenase. The reacti[on] requires the oxidation of reduced nicotinamide adenine dinucleotide (NADH) and creates the unreduced form (NAD^+) as an additional reaction product. NAD^+ absorbs light at a 340-nm wavelength. This absorption, as measured by a spectrophotometer, is used to determine ALT activity. Therefore, the endpoint measurement is several steps removed from the quantitative measurement of interest. The speed of a reaction, however, may be affected by several compo[o]nents of the process, including temperature, substrate concentration, amount of enzymes or cofactors, interfering substances in the reaction mix, and sensitivity of the spectrophotomete[r.] For example, if a patient is deficient in pyridoxal phosphate, and this cofactor is not added in excess of the amount needed for the test reaction, the reaction rate is slowed, and the final res[ult] is a falsely low ALT activity. This confounding effect is common in malnourished alcoholics an[d] other patients with end-stage liver disease, in whom deficiency of vitamin B_6 rather than ALT level is the limiting step in the reaction.

8. **How are normal and abnormal levels of alanine aminotransferase determined[?]**
This determination is made generally by the local laboratory in an arbitrary manner. A small se[t] of so-called healthy patients is selected, often from a blood bank. The ALT is determined in all members, and a mean and standard deviation are calculated. Arbitrary cutoffs are assigned,

usually at values representing the top and bottom 2.5% of the sample population. This technique is unfortunate, because many demographic factors play a role in ALT level. Men have higher ALT levels than women, obese women have higher ALT levels than people close to their ideal body weight, and certain racial groups have higher ALT activity. In addition, patients who donate blood may not, in fact, be free of liver disease. In clinical practice, failure to use gender-specific cutoff values for ALT has led to decreased diagnosis of hepatitis C and other liver diseases in women. This problem applies to all of the enzyme tests described in this chapter. Therefore, the further a test result is from normal, the more likely that disease, in fact, exists. Conversely, patients with significant silent liver disease may have normal ALT levels.

The ALT level, therefore, is an imperfect marker of the liver process. In diseases that involve massive liver damage, such as acute viral hepatitis, acetaminophen or solvent toxicity, or amanita mushroom poisoning, ALT may be increased to very high levels. For example, an ALT $\geq$2000 IU/L (50 times the upper limit of normal) is seen frequently in significant acetaminophen overdoses. This value reflects significant leakage of ALT from damaged hepatocytes. In patients with chronic viral hepatitis, levels tend to be lower and are frequently 2–10 times normal.

9. **What makes the alkaline phosphatase level rise?**
AP is a group of enzymes that catalyzes the transfer of phosphate groups. Different isoenzymes can be identified from multiple sites in the body, including liver, bone, and intestine. Most hospital labs do not have the facilities to identify the source. This inability may pose a problem for clinicians. In one large study of hospitalized patients, only about 65% of elevated AP was from the liver. When the source is the liver, the mechanism appears to be related to stimulation of enzyme synthesis associated with local increases in bile acids. This finding results from drug-associated cholestasis and intrahepatic and extrahepatic obstruction. The problems associated with determining enzyme activity and establishing a normal range are analogous to those described for serum transaminases. The association of elevated AP with either GGT or 5'-nucleotidase helps to establish a liver source and suggests the presence of a cholestatic process.

10. **What does an elevated bilirubin mean?**
Bilirubin, a breakdown product of red blood cells, exists in two forms: conjugated and unconjugated. Unconjugated bilirubin appears in the serum when blood is broken down at a rate that overwhelms the processing ability of the liver. This finding is most common in patients with hemolysis. Several genetically acquired enzyme deficiencies result in improper or incomplete bilirubin conjugation in the liver. The most common is Gilbert's syndrome, which is characterized by a relative deficiency of glucuronosyltransferase. Recently, the specific gene defect that accounts for a significant proportion of the observed phenotypic abnormality has been described and the heterozygotic carrier state may be present in 30–40% of the U.S. population. Patients often have high-normal to borderline-elevated bilirubin levels. When they fast or decrease caloric intake (e.g., patients with viral gastroenteritis), the bilirubin rises, primarily because of increases in the unconjugated form. If a bilirubin fractionation is not done, a patient with abdominal pain, nausea and vomiting, and an elevated bilirubin may be misdiagnosed as having cholecystitis. The resulting cholecystectomy could have been easily avoided by obtaining the fractionation.

11. **How is the bilirubin level determined?**
The most common test for bilirubin involves a biochemical reaction over time. Most labs report only total bilirubin. By stopping the reaction at a particular time and subtracting the result from the total bilirubin, the lab arrives at the indirect bilirubin, which is an approximation of unconjugated bilirubin. Exact measurement requires the use of chromatography, which is not routinely performed in clinical labs. Conjugated bilirubin is elevated in many diseases, including viral,

chemical, and drug- and alcohol-induced hepatitis; cirrhosis; metabolic disorders; and intrahepatic and extrahepatic biliary obstruction.

12. **What tests are used to evaluate hemochromatosis?**
Hemochromatosis is a disease of iron overload in the liver and other organs. The defect is in a regulatory mechanism for iron absorption in the small intestine. Over many years, patients build up stored iron in the liver, heart, pancreas, and other organs. The most common screening test for hemochromatosis is *serum ferritin;* an elevated level suggests the possibility of iron overload. Unfortunately, ferritin is also an acute-phase reactant and may be falsely elevated in various inflammatory processes. If ferritin is elevated (usually >400 mg/L), serum iron and total iron-binding capacity (TIBC) should be assessed. If the serum iron divided by TIBC is >50–55%, hemochromatosis should be strongly suspected instead of secondary iron overload (hemosiderosis).

Until recently, the definitive test was a quantitative assessment of iron. A *liver biopsy* specimen is used to determine the amount of iron in liver tissue. From a calculation based on the patient's age and iron content in liver, an index, called the *iron-age index*, was used to determine the presence or absence of hemochromatosis. This test may not be as reliable as previously thought, based on the recent availability of genetic testing. Three major *gene defects* have been described. They involve single amino acid mutations, which result in altered iron absorption. The most important gene is designated C282Y; H63D may also have a role in some populations. These genes are bi-allelic; that is, each parent contributes one half of the patient's complement. Therefore, patients may be homozygote wildtype, heterozygote, or homozygote with mutation. Only patients with both mutated alleles are thought to have genetic hemochromatosis.

Studies suggest that *magnetic resonance imaging (MRI)* of the liver may also be helpful in evaluating hepatic iron content and, in the future, may reduce the need for liver biopsy. However most radiologists are not trained to interpret the results.

13. **Describe the role of alpha-1 antitrypsin.**
Alpha-1 antitrypsin is an enzyme, made by the liver, that helps to break down trypsin and other tissue proteases. Multiple variants are described in the literature. The variant is expressed as an allele from both parents. Therefore, a person may have one or two forms of alpha-1 antitrypsin in the blood. One particular variant, called Z, because of its unique electrophoretic mobility on gel, is the product of a single amino acid gene mutation from the wild-type protein (M). The Z protein is difficult to excrete from the liver cell and causes local damage that may result in hepatitis and cirrhosis.

14. **What three tests are used to diagnose alpha-1 antitrypsin deficiency?**
   1. Serum protein electrophoresis (SPEP). When blood proteins are separated on the basis on electrical migration in gel, several bands are formed. One of these, the alpha-1 band, consis of mostly alpha-1 antitrypsin. Therefore, an alpha-1 antitrypsin deficiency results in a flatten ing of the alpha-1 band on SPEP.
   2. Direct assay that uses a monoclonal antibody against alpha-1 antitrypsin. The degree of bin ing can be measured in a spectrophotometer by rate nephelometry.
   3. Alpha-1 antitrypsin phenotype. Only a few labs in the United States run this test, which des nates the allelic protein types in the serum (e.g., MM, ZZ, MZ, FZ). Patients with protein of t ZZ type are said to be homozygotic for Z-type alpha-1 antitrypsin deficiency. This is the forr most frequently associated with significant liver disease. If Z protein is trapped in hepatocytes, it can be seen in liver tissue as small globules that stain with the periodic acid-Schiff (PAS) reaction and resist subsequent digestion with an enzyme called *diastase.* An immuno stain is also available in some institutions and may be more sensitive than the PAS-diastase staining technique.

15. **What is Wilson's disease?**

Wilson's disease, a disorder of copper storage, is associated with deficiency of an enzyme derived from liver cells. Like iron, copper may accumulate in many tissues in the body. Its storage sites are somewhat different, however. Deposition may be seen in the eye (Kayser-Fleischer rings) and parts of the brain. Many cholestatic diseases of the liver (e.g., primary biliary cirrhosis) also result in aberrant copper storage but not to the degree seen in true Wilson's disease.

16. **How is Wilson's disease diagnosed?**

The main screening test is the serum ceruloplasmin level, which is low in over 95% of patients with Wilson's disease. Ceruloplasmin is also an acute-phase reactant and may be falsely elevated into a low-normal range in patients with an inflammatory process. Follow-up tests include assessments of urine and serum copper levels. A quantitative assessment of copper in liver tissue from liver biopsy provides definitive diagnosis. Copper is stained in the tissue with special stain processes (e.g., rhodanine stain).

17. **Summarize the tests for common metabolic disorders of the liver.**

There are numerous other hereditary diseases of the liver, including Gaucher's disease, Niemann-Pick disease, and hereditary tyrosinemia. These rare diseases are usually diagnosed in children. Specific tests are beyond the scope of this chapter (Table 15-1).

TABLE 15-1.   TESTS FOR COMMON METABOLIC DISORDERS OF THE LIVER

Disease	Primary Test	Supportive Test	Definitive Test
Hemochromatosis	Serum ferritin >400 mg/L	Iron saturation >55% Iron age index >2	C282Y, H63D homozygosity
Alpha-1 antitrypsin deficiency	SPEP or A1-AT level	Phenotype (Pi type)	Liver biopsy with PAS-positive diastase-resistant granules
Wilson's disease	Ceruloplasmin <10 mg/dL	Urine/serum copper >80 mg/24 h	Liver biopsy with quantitative copper >250 µg/g dry weight

SPEP = serum protein electrophoresis; PAS = periodic acid-Schiff test.

8. **What are autoimmune markers?**

Autoimmune markers are tests used to determine the presence of antibodies to specific cellular components that have been epidemiologically associated with the development of specific liver diseases. Autoimmune markers include antinuclear antibody (ANA), antismooth muscle antibody (ASMA; also called anti-actin antibody), liver-kidney microsomal antibody type 1 (LKM-1), anti-mitochondrial antibody (AMA), soluble liver antigen (SLA), and antiasialoglycoprotein receptor antibody. ANA, ASMA, and AMA are the most readily available tests and help define the probability of the more common classes of autoimmune liver disease. Currently, SLA is not easily obtained in the United States.

19. How are the common antibody tests performed and interpreted?

The common antibody tests are performed by exposure of the patient's serum to cultured cell and labeling with a fluorescein-tagged antibody against human antibodies. The cells are examined by fluorescent microscopy and graded according to intensity of the signal and which part the cell binds the antibody. Therefore, reading of antibody levels and determination of positive negative results are highly subjective, and most hepatologists require positive results in dilution titers >1:80 or 1:160 before considering the tests as part of a diagnostic algorithm. ANA and ASMA are particularly common in older people, women, and patients with a wide spectrum of liver diseases. Therefore, the diagnosis of autoimmune liver disease depends on a broad clinical picture that takes into account age, sex, presence of other autoimmune processes, gamma globulin levels, and liver biopsy findings. In addition, the overlap in antibodies in different autoimmune liver diseases is considerable. Table 15-2 provides a crude representation of one classification scheme. A newer scoring system that tries to take into account the variables not earlier has also been proposed.

TABLE 15-2. CLASSIFICATION OF AUTOIMMUNE LIVER DISEASE	
Disease	**Antibody**
Type I classic lupoid hepatitis	Antinuclear antibody and/or antismooth muscle antibody (anti-actin antibody)
Type II autoimmune hepatitis	Liver-kidney microsomal antibody type I
Type III autoimmune hepatitis	Soluble liver antigen
Primary biliary cirrhosis	Anti-mitochondrial antibody

20. When should screening or diagnostic tests be ordered for patients with suspected liver disease?

The transaminases, bilirubin, and alkaline phosphatase serve as screening tests when liver disease is suspected. The history, physical exam, and estimation of risk factors help to determine which specific diagnostic tests should be ordered. Some patients have occult liver disease with normal or near-normal enzymes, and, occasionally, patients with isolated enzyme elevations have no identifiable disease. In general, patients should have at least two sets of liver enzyme tests to eliminate lab error before a full work-up for liver disease is begun. Many diseases (e.g., hepatitis B) generally require proof of chronicity (abnormality >6 months) before therapy is initiated or confirmatory and staging liver biopsies are obtained. The severity of enzyme abnormality and the likelihood of finding a treatable process may modify the typical waiting period. For example, a female patient with transaminase levels 10 times the normal, a history of autoimmune thyroid disease, and an elevated globulin fraction probably has a flare of previously unrecognized chronic autoimmune hepatitis. An autoimmune profile and early liver biopsy may help to support this hypothesis and lead to prompt treatment with steroids and other immunosuppressants.

WEBSITES

1. http://www.aasld.org/

2. http://www.liverfoundation.org

3. http://www.eurowilson.org/

BLIOGRAPHY

Bacon BR, Olynyk JK, Brunt EM, et al: HFE genotype in patients with hemochromatosis and other liver disease. Ann Intern Med 130:953–962, 1999.

Bassett ML, Halliday JW, Powell LW: Value of hepatic iron measurements in early hemochromatosis and determination of the critical iron level associated with fibrosis. Hepatology 6:24–29, 1986.

Brensilver HL, Kaplan MM: Significance of elevated liver alkaline phosphatase in serum. Gastroenterology 68:1556–1562, 1975.

Buffone GS, Beck JR: Cost-effectiveness analysis for evaluation of screening programs: Hereditary hemochromatosis. Clin Chem 40:1631–1636, 1994.

Eriksson S, Carlson J, Velez R: Risk of cirrhosis and primary liver cancer in alpha-1 antitrypsin deficiency. N Engl J Med 314:736–739, 1983.

Kaplan MM: Laboratory Tests in Diseases of the Liver, 6th ed. Philadelphia, J.B. Lippincott, 1987, pp 219–260.

Scharschmidt BF, Goldberg HI, Schmid R: Approach to the patient with cholestatic jaundice. N Engl J Med 308:1515–1519, 1983.

Sherman KE: Alanine aminotransferase in clinical practice: A review. Arch Intern Med 151:260–265, 1991.

Wroblewski F: The clinical significance of transaminase activities of serum. Am J Med 27:911–923, 1959.

CHAPTER 16

VIRAL HEPATITIS

Kenneth E. Sherman, MD, PhD

1. **What are the types of hepatitis viruses?**
   There are currently five identifiable forms of viral hepatitis: A, B, C, D, and E (Table 16-1). All o
   these viruses are hepatotrophic; that is, the liver is the primary site of infection. Other viruses
   also infect the liver, but it is not their primary site of replication and cellular damage. Example
   include cytomegalovirus (CMV), herpes simplex virus (HSV), Epstein-Barr virus (EBV), and
   many of the arthropod-borne flaviviruses (e.g., dengue virus, yellow fever virus). Other viruse
   may be hepatotrophic, but their pathogenic potential is unclear. Examples include the TT virus
   and GB virus C. The latter agent has been associated with improved survival in patients with
   human immunodeficiency virus (HIV) infection.

TABLE 16-1.	KEY CHARACTERISTICS OF THE HEPATITIS VIRUSES			
Type	Nucleic Acid	Gene Shape	Envelope	Size (nm)
A	RNA	Linear	No	28
B	DNA	Circular	Yes	42
C	RNA	Linear	Yes	(?) 40–50
D	RNA	Circular	Yes	43
E	RNA	Linear	No	32

2. **What is the difference between acute and chronic hepatitis?**
   All hepatitis viruses can cause acute infection, which is defined as the presence of clinical,
   biochemical, and serologic abnormalities for up to 6 months. Hepatitis A and E are cleared fro
   the body within 6 months and do not cause persistent infection for a longer period. In contras
   hepatitis B, C, and D can lead to chronic infection, which is more likely to be associated with
   development of cirrhosis. An increased risk of primary hepatocellular carcinoma occurs in
   patients who are chronically infected with hepatitis B, C, and D.

3. **How common is chronicity in hepatitis B?**
   The risk of chronicity for hepatitis B is highly dependent on the person's age at infection and
   immunologic status. Neonates infected with hepatitis B have a chronicity rate approaching
   100%. The rate decreases to about 70% for young children. Healthy young adults probably ha
   chronicity rates less than 1%, but patients who take steroids or experience chronic illness
   (e.g., renal disease) are less likely to clear the viral infection.

4. **When does chronic hepatitis D develop?**
   Hepatitis D chronicity occurs only in the presence of simultaneous hepatitis B infection. In
   patients with chronic hepatitis B who become superinfected with hepatitis D, the risk of
   chronicity approaches 100%.

How common is chronic hepatitis C?

Hepatitis C chronicity may occur in up to 85% of patients. It is frequently associated with the development of histologically identifiable hepatitis. A small number of patients may have a chronic, nonfibrotic carrier state. A liver biopsy is essential to determine whether fibrogenic potential is present.

How are hepatitis viruses transmitted?

Hepatitis A and E are transmitted via a fecal-oral route. Both agents are prevalent in areas where sanitation standards are low. Large epidemics of both diseases occur frequently after floods and other natural disasters that disrupt already marginal sanitation systems. Hepatitis A is endemic in the United States and in much of the world, whereas hepatitis E is not endemic in the United States. Large outbreaks of hepatitis E have been seen in Central and South Americas, Bangladesh, and India. The fecal-oral transmission route includes not only direct contamination of drinking water and food, but also viral concentration and enteric acquisition by eating raw shellfish from sewage-contaminated waters.

The hepatitis B, C, and D viruses are transmitted by percutaneous contact with infected blood or body fluids. Risk factors include unprotected sexual activity, IV drug use, accidental needle stick, blood transfusion, hemodialysis, and mother-to-infant transmission through childbirth.

Describe the symptoms of hepatitis.

The classic symptoms of acute hepatitis include anorexia, nausea, vomiting, severe fatigue, abdominal pain, mild fever, jaundice, dark urine, and light stools. Some patients may have a serum sickness–like presentation that includes arthralgia, arthritis, and skin lesions; this presentation is more common in *hepatitis B* than in other forms of acute viral hepatitis and may be seen in up to 20% of infected patients. It is associated with the formation of immune complexes between antigen and antibody. Many patients with acute viral hepatitis do not have disease-specific symptoms. All forms of viral hepatitis may present as a mild-to-moderate flu-like illness. In a recent national survey of the U.S. population, approximately 30% of participants had serologic evidence of past *hepatitis A* infection, but few were diagnosed with hepatitis A or reported an illness with classic hepatitis features.

Patients with chronic *hepatitis B* or *C* report fatigue as the leading symptom. Other common manifestations include arthralgia, anorexia, and vague, persistent right upper quadrant pain. Jaundice, easy bruisability, or prolonged bleeding after shaving or other small skin breaks usually mark the development of end-stage liver disease and often signify the presence of scarring and irreversible liver dysfunction.

What biochemical abnormalities are associated with viral hepatitis?

Elevation of serum transaminases (alanine aminotransferase [ALT], aspartate aminotransferase [AST]) is the hallmark of acute liver damage and identifies the presence of various processes caused by viral hepatitis. ALT is more specific than AST because AST may be elevated in association with muscle injury. In patients with acute hepatitis A, B, D, or E, elevations of transaminases to ≥1000–2000 IU/L are not uncommon; they are usually accompanied by more modest increases in alkaline phosphatase and gamma-glutamyl-transferase (GGT). As the disease progresses, the transaminases decrease. As the levels decrease slowly over a period of weeks, bilirubin often rises and may peak weeks after the transaminases peak. Bilirubin levels usually subside by 6 months after infection. Hepatitis C is not associated as frequently with a notable acute hepatitis, and transaminases rarely exceed 1000 IU/L. An important subset of hepatitis C virus (HCV) patients have persistently normal serum ALT levels. This is more common among women than men. Many of these patients have active liver disease on liver biopsy.

9. **What biochemical findings indicate chronic infection?**
   Abnormalities that persist for longer than 6 months define the process as chronic. In this stage of disease, transaminases range from mildly elevated to 10–15 times the upper limit of normal. Bilirubin is often normal or mildly elevated, as are alkaline phosphatase and GGT. Sudden elevations of transaminases in the chronic period often signify a viral flare rather than development of a new process superimposed on the preexisting chronic viral state. However, superinfection with hepatitis D in a patient with chronic hepatitis B is frequently observed.

10. **How is hepatitis A diagnosed?**
    The diagnosis of hepatitis A depends on identifying a specific immunoglobulin M (IgM) antibody directed against the viral capsid protein. This is often identified as a hepatitis A viral antibody-IgM (HAVAB-M) class test on lab order sheets. The IgM antibody appears early in infection and persists for 3–6 months. The other available lab test detects the immunoglobulin (IgG) form of the antibody, which provides diagnosis of past infection and does not have a role in routine clinical practice. Some laboratories offer a combined (total) IgM + IgG, which complicates interpretation of positive results.

KEY POINTS: HEPATITIS A VIRUS

1. Fecal-oral transmission
2. Common in both United States and developing countries
3. Diagnosed with IgM antibody
4. Supportive treatment
5. Self-limited infection

11. **How is hepatitis B diagnosed?**
    The incorrect interpretation of hepatitis B serologic markers is common and leads to many inappropriate laboratory tests and specialty consultations. It is important to understand the sequence of marker appearance and disappearance and the information that each marker provides. Tests of hepatitis B include both serologic and molecular markers: hepatitis B surface antigen (HBsAg) and hepatitis B surface antibody (HBsAb), hepatitis B anticore antibody (HBcAb), hepatitis B e antigen (HBeAg) and hepatitis B e antibody (HBeAb), DNA polymerase assay, hybridization assays, bDNA assays, and polymerase chain reaction (PCR).

12. **Describe the hepatitis B surface antigen (HBsAg) and hepatitis B surface antibody (HBsAb) tests.**
    HBsAg, a protein that forms the outer coat of the hepatitis B virus, is produced in great excess during viral replication and aggregates to form noninfectious spherical and filamentous particles in the serum. It is detected by a radioimmunoassay (RIA) or enzyme-linked immunosorbent assay (ELISA) and indicates the presence of either acute or chronic infection. Its disappearance from the serum indicates viral clearance.
    The *HBsAb* test detects an antibody directed against the surface antigen. This neutralizing antibody binds with and helps to clear the virus from the circulation. Its presence, therefore, indicates past infection with hepatitis B, which has been cleared successfully. The surface antibody may also appear in patients who are vaccinated successfully with the currently

available recombinant hepatitis B vaccines. Its presence at a titer >10 mIU/mL of serum confers protection against active infection.

13. **How is the hepatitis B anticore antibody (HBcAb) test interpreted?**
This test detects antibody formation against the core protein of the hepatitis B virus. The core protein surrounds the viral DNA and is surrounded by HBsAg in the complete virion, which is called the *Dane particle*. No commercial assay for HB core antigen is available. An ELISA assay is used to detect the antibody (HBcAb). The specific test comes in three forms, which must be differentiated to understand the meaning of the results: an IgG form, an IgM form, and a total form that measures both IgG and IgM. Most laboratories include the total test in hepatitis screening profiles, but it is important to find out which test is run routinely. A positive total HBcAb indicates either current or past hepatitis B infection. A positive HB anti-HBc IgM usually indicates an acute hepatitis B infection, although it also may indicate viral reactivation associated with immunosuppression or chronic illness. In contrast, a positive HB anticore IgG is consistent with either resolved past infection or, if present in conjunction with HBsAg, a chronic carrier state. Rarely, the presence of anti-HBc, without anti HBs, suggests an occult infectious process. This finding requires futher evaluation with an HBV DNA assay.

14. **What do the hepatitis B e antigen (HBeAg) and hepatitis B e antibody (HBeAb) tests indicate?**
The e antigen is a soluble protein encoded by a portion of the core coding domain. Its presence suggests active replication. Therefore, HBeAg is seen in both acute infection and actively replicating chronic hepatitis B. In patients with acute infection, ordering of this test is not necessary. In patients with chronic infection, a positive result indicates a replicative form of the disease. Only when HBsAg is present and chronic liver disease is suspected does this test help in decision-making related to treatment and treatment outcomes. In a patient with resolved acute infection or relatively inactive (nonreplicative) chronic hepatitis B infection, HBeAg disappears and anti-HBe appears. Some patients, with a point mutation in the precore coding region of the hepatitis B genome, cannot make HBe and therefore do not develop an antibody response after resolution. The clinical significance of this mutation remains unclear, but it is quite prevalent in certain parts of the world.

15. **Describe the DNA polymerase assay.**
The polymerase assay was one of the earliest molecular assays used to detect hepatitis B DNA in serum. It was based on the finding that the hepatitis B virus carries its own DNA polymerase enzyme within the core. The assay measures the enzyme activity as it directs the incorporation of radioactive-tagged nucleotides into new viral DNA. The test is not highly sensitive and is not in routine clinical use. However, it is referenced frequently in research about hepatitis B from the 1970s and 1980s as a marker of viral activity.

KEY POINTS: HEPATITIS B VIRUS

1. Sexual and percutaneous transmission

2. Chronicity uncommon, except in infants and children

3. Treatment with interferon or nucleoside analogs

4. Screening for hepatocellular carcinoma needed in chronic disease

16. **What are hybridization assays?**

Hybridization assays include various specific techniques that use a probe complementary to specific portions of the hepatitis B DNA genome. The actual hybridization may be performed on a filter paper matrix (dot blot) or in a column filled with beads that are impregnated with the probe material. The assay detects a marker substance on the probe that sticks to the viral DNA. The marker is often a radioactive tracer (e.g., radioactive phosphorus [^{32}P]) but may also be a chemical reactant (e.g., horseradish peroxidase). The sensitivity of these assays is not as great as amplification techniques, but most detect HBV DNA in a range of 1.5–20 pg/mL of serum. This range seems to provide a good marker for distinguishing replicative from nonreplicative disease.

17. **Describe the bDNA assay.**

In this hybridization assay the viral nucleic acid hybridizes with complementary bDNA (branched-chain DNA) attached to a microtiter well. The hybridized viral DNA is then further hybridized to specific complementary DNAs in a reaction mixture, which are arrayed in a manner analogous to a multibranched tree. On the tree are pods of a marker molecule that emit light in a chemiluminescent reaction that can be detected by a luminometer. Because the light emission is proportionate to the amount of bound DNA, the test provides a highly reliable quantitative assay that is more sensitive than standard hybridization assays.

18. **What are PCR assays?**

Whereas the bDNA assay amplifies the signal generated by hybridization, PCR amplifies a portion of the DNA itself and makes it more detectable. PCR is the most sensitive technique available for detection of hepatitis DNA; the commercial version of this assay is a highly sensitive quantitative marker of infection. Although all HB chronic carriers are positive by this assay, the titer for those with nonreplicative disease is low. Current assay sensitivity is approximately 200 copies/mL. New generations of real-time PCR with a large dynamic range and high sensitivity are under clinical evaluation.

19. **How is hepatitis C diagnosed?**

The screening assay for hepatitis C is an ELISA (also called EIA) assay that detects the presence of antibody to two regions of the hepatitis C genome. The currently available assay is in its third generation, and future modifications are likely. The test is highly sensitive but not specific; therefore, it gives many false-positive reactions. In populations with a low pretest probability of carrying hepatitis C, more than 40% of repeatedly reactive specimens are false positives. The antibody that is detected is nonneutralizing; that is, its presence does not confer immunity. If antibody is detected and the reaction is not a false positive, the patient almost always has active viral infection. Clearly, it is important to separate false positives from true positives. The cause of most false-positive reactions is binding of nonspecific immunoglobulin on the ELISA well surface. To avoid the use of serum, which requires obtaining drawn blood, oral fluid collection has been demonstrated to be an alternative screening modality to screen populations for HCV.

20. **How is a positive result on the ELISA confirmed?**

To support a true-positive reaction, the most commonly used test is a recombinant immunoblot assay (RIBA), which involves exposing the patient's serum to a nitrocellulose strip impregnated with bands of antigen. The currently available version (HCV RIBA 3.0, Chiron Corp, Emeryville CA) has multiple antigens on the test strip as well as controls for nonspecific immunoglobulin binding and superoxide dismutase antibodies, which may confound the test results. The RIBA not as sensitive as the ELISA, however, and therefore should not be used as a screening test for hepatitis C infection.

KEY POINTS: HEPATITIS C VIRUS

1. Percutaneous exposure or blood transfusion risk should lead to HCV antibody screening

2. High risk of chronicity

3. Treatment with pegylated interferon plus ribavirin leads to greater than 50% sustained viral response

4. Screening for hepatocellular carcinoma in patients with cirrhosis

21. What nucleic acid assays are available for hepatitis C?

Other assays in specialized laboratories include a bDNA quantitative assay for hepatitis C RNA and a PCR assay (see hepatitis B tests). The PCR is more sensitive but less amenable to clinical laboratory testing. In the past, both bDNA assays and PCR-based assays were reported in terms of copies of HCV RNA/mL. Now, a World Health Organization (WHO) standard defined as an international unit (IU) is used for reporting purposes. The presence of hepatitis C RNA in serum or liver tissue is the gold standard for diagnosis of hepatitis C infection. Quantitative evaluation of hepatitis C RNA levels in serum has prognostic value in determining who is likely to respond to therapeutic intervention and in following the course of a treatment cycle. The most sensitive nucleic acid assay is performed by a method called *transcription mediated amplification* (TMA). This technique is sensitive to approximately 5 IU/mL. Development of real-time PCR should approach this sensitivity and permit a broad quantitative dynamic range.

22. How is hepatitis D diagnosed?

Hepatitis D is diagnosed by an ELISA assay that detects the presence of antibody to hepatitis D in serum or plasma. The presence of the antibody in serum correlates with ongoing hepatitis D replication in the liver. Detection of hepatitis D antigen in liver tissue generally adds little to the diagnostic process. Early in the course of infection, acute hepatitis D may be detectable only by performing a test for the IgM form of the antibody. A PCR-based assay may also be performed to detect the presence of RNA from hepatitis D in serum or tissue. This assay is not commercially available, and its use seems to add little to the antibody testing. Because hepatitis D occurs only with concurrent acute hepatitis B infection or as a superinfection of chronic hepatitis B, there is little use in testing for its presence at the initial work-up for viral causes of liver enzyme abnormalities.

23. How is hepatitis E diagnosed?

The original assays relied on a technique called *antibody-blocking assay,* in which freshly infected primate tissue was exposed first to serum from the patient and then to serum from a known positive patient. If antibody is present in the unknown serum, it binds to the tissue and blocks the attachment of the second-known antibody. This technique was difficult and was supplanted by a commercial ELISA. Hepatitis E does not seem to occur naturally in the United States. However, there should be a high index of suspicion in patients who have an acute hepatitis A–like illness, test negative for hepatitis A antibody IgM, and have traveled to an endemic area.

24. Are there other hepatitis viruses not yet discovered?

Probably. Several lines of evidence suggest that there are more hepatotrophic viruses than are currently recognized. Epidemiologic studies suggest that a small percentage of posttransfusion cases and a higher percentage of community-acquired cases of hepatitis have no identifiable viral infection, even when molecular detection techniques are used. Forms of liver disease (e.g., giant cell hepatitis) have been associated with paramyxovirus infection, although its role remains speculative at best. The cause of fulminant hepatic failure, hepatitis-associated aplastic anemia, and cryptogenic cirrhosis cannot be defined in a significant proportion of cases. Such findings point to the presence of one or more as yet unidentified agents. In recent years, three new agents have been extensively studied: the TT virus, GB-C virus, and SEN-V. All may be associated with serum transaminase abnormalities in certain circumstances, but their exact role in acute and chronic diseases has not been delineated.

25. **What is the treatment of acute viral hepatitis?**
The primary treatment of acute hepatitis of any type is mainly supportive. In general, patients do not require hospitalization unless the disease is complicated by significant hepatic failure, as evidenced by encephalopathy, coagulopathy with bleeding, renal failure, or inability to maintain adequate nutrition and fluid intake. Efforts must be made to identify the form of hepatitis and, if necessary, to ensure that the patient is removed from situations in which he or she is a high risk to others. For example, a food handler should be removed from the workplace when hepatitis A is diagnosed, and health authorities must be notified.

26. **Are specific antiviral agents available?**
Yes. Specific antiviral treatment has been attempted in acute hepatitis cases. In well-documented acute HCV infection, early intervention (3–6 months post-exposure) with interferon plus ribavirin seems to be associated with a decreased carrier rate. Alpha interferon has also been studied in patients with acute hepatitis D infection and fulminant hepatitis caused by either coinfection or superinfection with hepatitis B. It appears to have little value in this setting.

27. **Is chronic viral hepatitis treatable?**
Yes. The chronic forms of hepatitis B, C, and D have been studied with regard to a number of treatment modalities. Alpha interferon has been tested in multiple randomized, controlled trials and has been found to be effective for all three agents. Interferon plus ribavirin is the most effective approved therapy for chronic hepatitis C. Lamivudine (3TC) and adefovir are nucleotide analogs that are highly effective in suppression of hepatitis B and are also FDA approved. Tenofovir is also highly active against HBV but is not FDA approved for this indication. Other nucleoside/nucleotide analogs are under evaluation.

28. **Which patients with chronic hepatitis B are candidates for therapy?**
Patients with chronic hepatitis B, well-compensated liver disease, and evidence of viral replication (HBV DNA or HBeAg) are candidates for therapy. The goal of therapy is to reduce the level of replication and to change the infection to a relatively inactive disease. The clearance of HBsAg is not the immediate goal of therapy, although some evidence suggests that this may occur more frequently in successfully treated patients than in those who do not respond over subsequent years. Patients with decompensated liver disease caused by hepatitis B may also benefit for nucleoside analog treatment, but this should be provided under the direction of an experienced hepatologist in a transplant center setting.

29. **Describe the standard treatment and its side effects.**
The standard treatment may be interferon or nucleoside analog based. Alpha interferon 2b at a dose of 30–35 MU/week for 16 weeks is approved by the FDA. Longer treatment regimens are under evaluation. Patients seem to tolerate a dosing of 5 MU 6 days/week better than other dosing schemes. Side effects include a flu-like syndrome, which is, occasionally, quite severe. Often platelet count and absolute neutrophil count decrease significantly; thus, the patient must be monitored closely and dose adjustments made. Alternatively, 1 year of treatment with lamivudine 100 mg orally once a day or adefovir 10 mg orally once a day may be used. Side effects of this treatment are minimal.

What is the response rate to treatment of chronic hepatitis B?
Response rates range up to 60%, although in some groups it may be as low as 5%. Poor response is seen in patients with chronic, long-standing infection since childhood and in patients with HIV infection or other immunosuppression. The ideal patients, in terms of response outcomes, are women with recent chronic infection, ALT >200 IU/L, and viral load <100 pg/mL. Treatment with lamivudine at a dose of 100 mg/day results in complete viral suppression in nearly 100% of treated patients within a few months. Unfortunately, mutant virus emerges at a rate of 10–20% per year. Adefovir appears to be associated with a much lower (<2% per year) mutational breakthrough rate. Multidrug regimens are under evaluation. Adefovir and tenofovir appear to be effective for treatment of lamivudine-resistant mutants.

Describe the treatment of chronic hepatitis C. How effective is it?
Treatment of chronic hepatitis C is also interferon-based. Current treatment standards include use of pegylated interferon alpha 2a or 2b weekly plus ribavirin 1000–1200 mg daily for 24 to 48 weeks, depending upon the HCV viral genotype. Treatment response rates in large multicenter trials range from 54–63% sustained viral response (SVR). The SVR is determined by absence of HCV RNA by a sensitive (PCR or TMA) assay at end of treatment and 6 months following treatment. It is now believed that most patients who achieve SVR are cured of HCV infection. If one stratifies response by HCV genotype, patients with genotype 2 or 3 have SVR rates in excess of 70%. Lower rates (approximately 40%) are seen in those with genotype 1.

Describe the side effects of ribavirin.
Certain patients may be at risk of complications with ribavirin use. Ribavirin causes a dose-dependent hemolysis in approximately 80% of treated patients. This anemia may be ameliorated with use of epopoietin or other growth factors. Patients with underlying cardiac disease, who cannot tolerate anemia, may not be suitable candidates. Furthermore, ribavirin is teratogenic. Adequate birth control should be used during, and for 6 months after, treatment.

What is polyethylene glycol (PEG) interferon?
Addition of a PEG moiety to interferon results in a PEG-interferon product that has a prolonged half-life with higher potency against the hepatitis C virus.

What alternative therapies for hepatitis C are under investigation?
Newer-generation therapies are under development, including protease/helicase inhibitors; RNA-dependent, RNA-polymerase inhibitors; ribozymes; and antisense therapy. Immune modulation therapy, with agents including thymosin alpha-1, and study of antifibrotic therapy (gamma IFN) are under active evaluation.

How is hepatitis D treated?
Hepatitis D may also be treated with interferon. Doses of 9 MU three times per week for 48 weeks were associated with a 50% response rate in one randomized, controlled trial. Relapse at the end of therapy was common, however.

How can hepatitis A be prevented?
Hepatitis A infection can be prevented by the use of pooled gamma globulin after acute exposure or a vaccine for long-term protection. A vaccine previously used in Europe, Canada, and elsewhere became available in the United States in 1995. The vaccine is prepared from an attenuated strain of the virus grown on tissue culture cells. It is chemically inactivated and seems to confer immunity in 80–90% of treated subjects. The vaccine has not been tested in young (<age 2) children but is recommended for people who travel to hyperendemic areas with poor sanitation, child-care workers, deployable military personnel, and other high-risk individuals. Universal vaccination has not been studied adequately to determine its cost-benefit ratio. For individuals exposed in local outbreaks (shellfish, food handler), gamma globulin

should be adequate for short-term protection. It is also recommended that all patients with chronic liver disease or HIV be screened for hepatitis A antibody and vaccinated, if absent.

37. **Describe the vaccine for hepatitis B.**
A vaccine for hepatitis B has been available since the early 1980s. It was originally prepared by isolation of the surface antigen protein. The current forms most widely used in the United States are surface antigen proteins made by recombinant techniques. The vaccine is more than 90% effective in providing long-term immunity after three doses. In 20–30% of vaccinated people, antibody titers drop to <10 mIU/mL within 5 years. This titer is believed to be the critical protective level. Current Public Health Service recommendations do not mandate either follow-testing or boosters, except in dialysis patients. These recommendations may change as future data become available. Acute hepatitis B exposure in nonvaccinated individuals requires treatment with hepatitis B immunoglobulin (HBIG). This hyperimmune gamma globulin has high titer antibodies against hepatitis B surface antigen. It may be administered simultaneously with the first dose of vaccine; this regimen is often followed in infants of HBsAg-positive mothers.

38. **Can hepatitis C be prevented?**
No vaccine is available for hepatitis C. Because of rapid mutation in the envelope region of the genome, a multivalent vaccine will probably be required and may take several years to develop and test before it is available for routine use. There is some interest in development of virus-free pooled globulin products, which may mediate the infectious process, particularly in patients infected with hepatitis C virus after liver transplant.

CONTROVERSY

39. **Should all patients with hepatitis C undergo liver biopsy?**
For: Liver biopsy is the gold standard for evaluation of inflammatory activity and fibrosis in the liver. Surrogate markers, including imaging with liver-spleen scan, single photon emission-computed tomography (SPECT), computed tomography (CT), magnetic resonance (MR), and ultrasound as well as lab tests for procollagen, have not been reliable markers. Standard liver tests are also frequently not helpful. A liver biopsy helps (1) determine whether treatment should be started, (2) decide aggressiveness of therapy, and (3) provide factual evidence of an otherwise often asymptomatic condition, which encourages patients to continue treatment. The risk of biopsy in experienced hands is low, and until treatments are highly effective in all treated patients, it should be a mandatory part of the work-up.
Against: Almost all patients with HCV infection deserve at least one course of therapy, regardless of the level of activity or fibrosis. Biopsies are a barrier to treatment, relegating patient care to a limited pool of practitioners who perform liver biopsies. Therefore, liver biopsy is not indicated in routine management.

WEBSITES

1. http://www.aasld.org/
2. http://www.aasld.org/eweb/docs/hepatic.pdf
3. http://www.aasld.org/eweb/docs/hepatitisc.pdf
4. http://www.aasld.org/eweb/docs/chronichep_B.pdf
5. http://www.aasld.org/eweb/docs/update_chronichep_B.pdf

BIBLIOGRAPHY

Alter MJ, Margolis HS, Krawczynski K, et al: The natural history of community-acquired hepatitis C in the United States. N Engl J Med 327:1899–1905, 1992.

Centers for Disease Control: Hepatitis B virus: A comprehensive strategy for eliminating transmission in the United States through universal childhood vaccination: Recommendations of the Immunization Practices Advisory Committee (ACIP). MMWR 40(no. RR-13), 1991.

Choo QL, Richman KH, Han JH, et al: Genetic organization and diversity of the hepatitis C virus. Proc Natl Acad Sci U S A, 88:2451–2455, 1991.

Davis GL, Balart LA, Schiff E, et al: Treatment of chronic hepatitis C with recombinant interferon alpha. N Engl J Med 321:1501–1506, 1989.

Dawson GJ, Chau KH, Cabal CM, et al: Solid phase enzyme linked immunosorbent assay for hepatitis E virus IgG and IgM antibodies utilizing recombinant antigens and synthetic peptides. J Virol Methods 38:175–186, 1992.

Di Bisceglie AM, Martin P, Kassianides C, et al: Recombinant interferon alpha therapy for chronic hepatitis C: A randomized, double-blind, placebo-controlled trial. N Engl J Med 321:1506–1510, 1989.

Di Bisceglie AM, Shindo M, Fong T-L, et al: A study of ribavirin therapy for chronic hepatitis C. Hepatology 16:649–654, 1992.

Dienstag JL, Schiff ER, Wright TL, et al: Lamivudine as initial treatment for chronic hepatitis B in the United States. N Engl J Med 341:1256–1263, 1999.

Farci P, Mandas A, Coina A, et al: Treatment of chronic hepatitis D with interferon alpha-2a. N Engl J Med 330:88–94, 1994.

Fried MW, Shiffman ML, Reddy KR, et al: Peginterferon alpha-2a plus ribavirin for chronic hepatitis C virus infection. N Engl J Med 347(13):975–982, 2002.

Houghton M, Weiner A, Han J, et al: Molecular biology of the hepatitis C viruses: Implications for diagnosis, development and control of viral disease. Hepatology 14:381–388, 1991.

Jaeckel E, Cornberg M, Wedemeyer H, et al: Treatment of acute hepatitis C with interferon alpha-2b. N Engl J Med 345(20):1452–1457, 2001.

Kaneko S, Miller RH, Di Bisceglie AM, et al: Detection of hepatitis B virus DNA in serum by polymerase chain reaction: Application for clinical diagnosis. Gastroenterology 99:799–804, 1990.

Koretz RL, Abbey H, Coleman E, Gitnick G: Non-A, non-B post-transfusion hepatitis: Looking back in the second decade. Ann Intern Med 119:110–115, 1993.

Krawczynski K, Bradley DW: Enterically transmitted non-A, non-B hepatitis. Identification of virus-associated antigen in experimentally infected cynomolgus macaques. J Infect Dis 159:1042–1049, 1989.

Laras A, Koskinas J, Avigidis K, Hadziyannis SJ: Incidence and clinical significance of hepatitis B precore gene translation initiation mutants in e antigen-negative patients. J Viral Hepat 5:241–248, 1988.

Manns M, McHutchison JG, Gordon SC, et al: Peginterferon alpha-2b plus ribavirin compared with interferon alpha-2b plus ribavirin for initial treatment of chronic hepatitis C: A randomised trial. Lancet 358(9286): 958–965, 2001.

Perrillo RP, Regenstein FG, Peters MG, et al: Prednisone withdrawal followed by recombinant alpha interferon in the treatment of chronic type B hepatitis: A randomized, controlled trial. Ann Intern Med 109:95–100, 1988.

Seeff LB, Ruskell-Bales Z, Wright EC, et al: Long-term mortality after transfusion-associated non-A, non-B hepatitis. N Engl J Med 327:1906–1911, 1992.

Sherman KE, Creager RL, O'Brien J, et al: The use of oral fluid for hepatitis C antibody screening. Am J Gastroenterol 89:2025–2027, 1994.

Zaaijer HL, ter Borg F, Cuypers HT, et al: Comparison of methods for detection of hepatitis B virus DNA. J Clin Microbiol 32:2088–2091, 1994.

CHAPTER 17

ANTIVIRAL THERAPY FOR HEPATITIS C INFECTION

Jorge L. Herrera, MD

1. **What are the indications for antiviral therapy in patients with chronic hepatitis C?**

   Hepatitis C progresses in all chronically infected patients but at different rates. The average time for development of cirrhosis is 30 years, but there is a wide range of variability. Only about 20% of patients progress to cirrhosis. Because it is difficult to predict who will progress, everyone who is chronically infected should be evaluated for possible treatment. Many factors can speed progression of fibrosis, including alcohol consumption, coinfection with hepatitis B or human immunodeficiency virus (HIV), iron overload, and concomitant liver disease, such as alpha$_1$ antitrypsin deficiency, Wilson's disease, or autoimmune hepatitis.

   Patients with extrahepatic manifestations of hepatitis C infection should be considered for antiviral treatment. Mixed cryoglobulinemia, leading to leukocytoclastic vasculitis, may be a systemic manifestation of hepatitis C infection and may respond to antiviral therapy. Renal disease, joint inflammation, or central nervous system complications may result from microvascular injury.

2. **What is the recommended evaluation of patients with chronic hepatitis C before therapy is begun?**

   The initial history and physical should include identification of possible risk factors in an effort to assess the duration of infection. Laboratory evaluation is geared toward confirming the infection, excluding other possible causes of liver disease, and detecting coinfection. Recommended laboratory tests are listed in Table 17-1.

TABLE 17-1.   RECOMMENDED PRETREATMENT EVALUATION OF PATIENTS WITH CHRONIC HEPATITIS C INFECTION

Test	Purpose
HCV-RNA by PCR	Confirm viremia
Serum albumin, bilirubin, PT	Assess liver function
Iron, transferrin, ferritin	Assess for iron overload
Antinuclear antibody	Detect autoimmune hepatitis
Alpha$_1$ antitrypsin phenotype	Detect alpha$_1$ antitrypsin deficiency
Ceruloplasmin (age <45 years)	Detect Wilson's disease
HBsAg, HIV antibody test	Detect viral coinfection
Hepatitis C genotype	Assess likelihood of response to therapy
Liver biopsy	Determine severity of disease and urgency for therapy

HCV = hepatitis C virus; PCR = polymerase chain reaction; PT = prothrombin time; HBsAg = hepatitis B surface antigen; HIV = human immunodeficiency virus.

Some experts recommend testing for immunity against hepatitis B (hepatitis B surface antibody [HBsAb]) and hepatitis A (anti-HAV); in patients who are not immune, vaccination to prevent hepatitis A and B should be considered. In the absence of obvious advanced disease, a liver biopsy is advised to assess severity of disease, estimate prognosis, and determine urgency of antiviral therapy.

3. **Should hepatitis C genotype testing be performed before initiation of therapy?**
Yes. Based on genomic sequencing of the hepatitis C virus, several genotypes (or strains) have been identified. They are classified as genotypes 1 through 6, with several subtypes denoted as 1a, 1b, 2a, and so forth. The various genotypes exhibit geographic variability. In the United States, genotype 1 accounts for approximately 70% of infections. Genotypes 2 and 3 account for the remaining 30%. In Europe, the proportion of genotype 2 and 3 infections is greater than in the United States. In the Middle East, genotype 4 predominates, and genotype 6 is seen most commonly in Asia.

Determining the genotype before therapy is important because it helps to predict the likelihood of response and length of antiviral therapy. For example, patients infected with genotypes 2 or 3, without cirrhosis, have a greater than 80% chance of achieving a sustained response and need to be treated for 6 months only. In contrast, the probability of response to therapy is less likely in genotype 1 infections, which require treatment for 1 year to maximize the chance of sustained remission. The genotype, however, has no value in predicting severity of disease or likelihood of progression to cirrhosis.

4. **Is a liver biopsy mandatory before initiation of antiviral therapy?**
A liver biopsy is not required to diagnose chronic hepatitis C but evaluates the level of hepatic inflammation and fibrosis. No other test makes this determination accurately. Liver function tests, such as prothrombin time and albumin or bilirubin level, become abnormal only when extensive damage has occurred. Likewise, liver enzymes, viral load, and genotype do not correlate with severity of liver disease. An adequate biopsy sample is the best way to assess the severity of liver disease and helps the patient and clinician in deciding whether or not to proceed with therapy. In patients with genotype 2 or 3 infection, the likelihood of sustained response with short-term therapy is relatively high and a liver biopsy may not be necessary in many patients.

5. **What are the treatment options for hepatitis C infection?**
The immune modulator interferon (IFN) was the first medication approved by the Food and Drug Administration (FDA) for treatment of hepatitis C. Three different types—IFN α-2a, IFN α-2b, consensus IFN—differing in amino acid configuration are available. They require subcutaneous administration three or more times per week, and the antiviral efficacy is lower than newer forms of interferon therapy.

To increase the half-life of the interferon molecule, increase its antiviral efficacy, and reduce the number of injections per month, a polyethylene glycol (PEG) molecule was covalently attached to interferon. The size and shape of the PEG molecule affects the biologic properties of the interferon. Currently, two types of pegylated interferon are approved by the FDA for the treatment of chronic hepatitis C infection. Pegylated interferon α-2b is attached covalently to a linear 12 kDa PEG molecule. Pegylated interferon α-2a is attached to a larger, branched 40 kDa PEG molecule. Both of these compounds are self-administered by patients as a once-a-week subcutaneous injection.

Ribavirin, an oral nucleoside analog, is approved for the treatment of hepatitis C. Used alone, it is not effective as an antiviral agent against hepatitis C; however, in combination with IFN alpha, the antiviral activity of interferon is greatly enhanced.

At present, combination therapy with PEG-interferon and ribavirin is the treatment of choice for patients who have not been treated previously. Selected patients who failed to respond to interferon monotherapy or to combination interferon-ribavirin therapy may also benefit from a trial of PEG-interferon-ribavirin combination therapy.

6. **How are the antiviral agents dosed?**
    Pegylated interferon α-2b is dosed by weight and administered as a single subcutaneous injection once a week. Pegylated interferon α-2a is administered as 180 µg subcutaneously once a week regardless of the patient's weight. Ribavirin should also be dosed by weight. Patients who weigh <75 kg should receive 1000 mg/day of ribavirin, and those who weigh ≥75 kg should receive 1200 mg/day. Currently, the FDA has approved only a fixed dose of 800 mg daily of ribavirin with PEG-interferon α-2b; however, extensive research indicates that a higher, weight-based dose increases efficacy. PEG-interferon α-2a is FDA approved for use with the weight-based ribavirin dose. The duration of therapy is determined by the patient's genotype and early virologic response.

7. **How is response to antiviral therapy assessed?**
    A decrease or normalization of liver enzymes usually indicates a positive response and is classified as a biochemical response to treatment. Such changes correlate with decreased hepatic inflammation, as assessed by repeat liver biopsy. A biochemical response to treatment is not always associated with a virologic response. Liver enzymes should be monitored monthly, and viral load should be assessed at 3 and 6 months of treatment. Early virologic response is measured at 12 weeks of therapy and is defined as a loss of detectable virus or a decrease in viral load of ≥2 logs from baseline. At 6 months, a favorable response to therapy is defined as no detectable virus in blood using a qualitative or highly sensitive, quantitative HCV-RNA assay. Patients who do not achieve these milestones have a <2% chance of achieving a sustained response to antiviral therapy, and discontinuation of therapy should be considered. In contrast, those who achieve the expected response have a >65% chance of sustained viral response. Patients who have no detectable virus at the end of treatment are considered virologic responders. If detectable virus appears after treatment is stopped, the patient is considered a relapser. In contrast, if virus remains undetectable 6 months after discontinuation of therapy, the patient is considered a sustained responder and has a very high likelihood of remaining virus-free for the foreseeable future.

8. **How often should viral load be measured during treatment?**
    Baseline quantitation of HCV-RNA should be performed before initiation of therapy. Because of marked variability among laboratories measuring viral load, it is recommended that the same laboratory and assay be used to monitor response to therapy over time. At 12 weeks of therapy, repeat quantitative HCV-RNA assay should be obtained to assess for early viral response. If the expected response is achieved, antiviral therapy should be continued. At 24 weeks of therapy, a qualitative HCV-RNA PCR assay, or a highly sensitive quantitative HCV-RNA assay, should be obtained. If no detectable virus is found, a repeat assay should be obtained at the end of therapy document a positive end of treatment response. Six months after discontinuation of therapy, a repeat, highly sensitive HCV-RNA assay should be obtained to determine whether a sustained virologic response was achieved.

9. **What pretreatment characteristics predict a favorable response to antiviral therapy?**
    1. Infection with genotype 2 or 3
    2. Low viral load
    3. Liver biopsy with little or no fibrosis
    4. Age <40 years at time of treatment
    5. Low body weight
    6. Caucasian ethnicity

    Genotype is the most important predictive factor of response to therapy. Patients infected with genotype 2 or 3 without fibrosis on liver biopsy need to receive combination therapy for 6 months only.

10. **What is the efficacy of PEG-interferon monotherapy for chronic hepatitis C?**

Considering all patients treated for hepatitis C, approximately 25–36% achieve sustained response after 12 months of PEG-interferon monotherapy. The response rate is lower in patients infected with genotype 1 or in patients with substantial fibrosis on liver biopsy. For this reason, PEG-interferon monotherapy should only be used in those patients who have a contraindication to ribavirin therapy.

11. **What is the efficacy of combination PEG-interferon and ribavirin?**

Combining ribavirin with PEG-interferon markedly increases the rate of virologic sustained response; 47–56% of treated patients achieve this response. Among genotype 1 patients, 45–55% can achieve a sustained response when treated for 48 weeks. Non-genotype 1 patients achieve a sustained response in about 80–85% of cases, and in most, 24 weeks of therapy is sufficient to achieve this response. Patients infected with genotype 3, however, are more likely to relapse after completion of therapy, compared with genotype 2 infection.

12. **How can response to antiviral therapy be maximized?**

To maximize sustained response rates, the ribavirin should be dosed by weight, and adherence to medications should be promoted. Patients who are unable to take 80% of their medications for 80% of the time are much less likely to achieve a sustained response. To minimize dose reduction and dose interruptions, it is crucial that side effects be monitored and treated aggressively. Whenever possible, dose reduction should be avoided.

13. **What are the side effects of interferon therapy? How should the patient be monitored?**

Interferon suppresses the bone marrow, potentially resulting in leukopenia or thrombocytopenia. Complete blood counts are monitored periodically, and the dose is adjusted as needed. To avoid dose reductions, use of growth factors, such as filgrastim for neutropenia, is strongly recommended. Other side effects that can diminish quality of life include flu-like symptoms, headaches, fever, depression, anxiety, sexual dysfunction, hair loss, insomnia, and fatigue. Evening administration and preinjection acetaminophen or ibuprofen can reduce the flu-like symptoms.

Depression requires close monitoring. Patients with a history of severe depression or suicidal ideation or attempts should not be treated with interferon. Patients who have required pharmacologic therapy for mild depression in the past may benefit from initiation of antidepressants before treatment with interferon. Selective serotonin reuptake inhibitors are usually successful in reversing interferon-associated depression. Close monitoring for suicidal ideation is mandatory.

Hypothyroidism is an irreversible side effect of interferon. Levels of thyroid-stimulating hormone (TSH) should be determined before initiation of therapy and at regular intervals during treatment.

14. **What are the side effects of ribavirin therapy? How should the patient be monitored?**

Ribavirin can cause hemolysis and may lead rapidly to symptomatic anemia. A reduction in hemoglobin of >4 gm/dL from baseline or to 10 gm/dL or less should trigger a decrease in the daily dose. Aggressive use of epoetin alfa for anemia is preferred to ribavirin dose reduction to maximize treatment efficacy. If the hemoglobin decreases to 8.5 gm/dL or less, discontinuation of therapy is advised. For patients with known ischemic cardiac disease, closer monitoring is recommended, with reduction or discontinuation of therapy, if the hemoglobin decreases by more than 2 gm/dL compared with baseline.

Other side effects from ribavirin include rash, shortness of breath, nausea, sore throat, and glossitis. The rash may be severe and require discontinuation of the medication. The other side effects are generally not life threatening and can be treated symptomatically.

Because ribavirin is teratogenic, male and female patients should be advised to **practice effective contraception during therapy and for 6 months after completion.**

15. **What are the contraindications to interferon therapy?**
    1. Interferon should not be used in patients who already have leukopenia or thrombocytopen[ia] because of the potential for bone marrow suppression. It is not recommended for patients with decompensated cirrhosis because it is rarely effective and may cause further decompensation of liver disease.
    2. Patients with severe depression, history of suicide attempt or ideation, psychosis, or personality disorders should not be treated or should receive treatment only under the clo[se] monitoring of a psychiatrist. Patients with manic depression do poorly with interferon therapy and should not be treated unless they are under the care of a psychiatrist and the psychiatric disease has remained stable for the last 12–24 months.
    3. Patients who continue to drink alcohol on a daily basis respond less to antiviral therapy. Complete abstinence from alcohol during therapy is recommended. For patients who drin[k] excessive amounts of alcohol, abstinence for a minimum of 6 months before initiation of therapy is required to maximize benefits of therapy.
    4. Autoimmune diseases, such as rheumatoid arthritis and systemic lupus erythematosus (S[LE]) pose a relative contraindication to therapy. Psoriasis can worsen during therapy.
    5. Interferon therapy should not be administered during pregnancy. If hepatitis C infection is diagnosed during pregnancy, treatment should be initiated after delivery and breastfeedin[g] has been completed.
    6. Patients with advanced comorbid conditions should not be offered antiviral therapy for hepatitis C. Hepatitis C infection progresses slowly over time. If the patient has a serious comorbidity that is likely to be fatal within 5–10 years, treating the hepatitis C infection is [un]likely to be of benefit.

16. **What are the contraindications to ribavirin therapy?**
    Because ribavirin must be used with interferon, all contraindications to interferon apply to treatment with ribavirin. In addition, there are specific contraindications to ribavirin:
    1. Pregnancy is an absolute contraindication because of the teratogenic potential.
    2. Anemia and hemoglobinopathies should be considered relative contraindications. Extrem[e] care should be exercised in treating such patients. As a rule, women with a hemoglobin <12 gm/dL, or men with <13 gm/dL before therapy, are at high risk of developing severe anemia during therapy.
    3. Patients with known ischemic heart disease should be treated with caution and monitored closely.
    4. Patients with renal insufficiency should not be treated with ribavirin because the development of severe, long-lasting, and life-threatening hemolysis is common.

17. **Should patients with cirrhosis resulting from hepatitis C infection be treated with antiviral therapy?**
    Yes. Patients with compensated cirrhosis (normal albumin and bilirubin levels; normal prothrombin time; and no ascites, encephalopathy, or history of variceal bleeding) are excelle[nt] candidates for antiviral therapy. They are most likely to benefit from viral eradication. Once li[ver] insufficiency develops or complications of portal hypertension become clinically evident, antiviral therapy is relatively contraindicated. Evaluation for liver transplantation is a better option for such patients.

    For patients with compensated disease, the main concern about antiviral therapy is worsening of preexisting thrombocytopenia or leukopenia caused by hypersplenism. Althoug[h] sustained viral response in patients with cirrhosis is less common than in noncirrhotic patien[ts] normalization of liver enzymes and reduction in viral load during treatment may result in overall improvement of liver disease and possibly a delayed need for liver transplantation or development of hepatocellular carcinoma. Long-term treatment with interferon to minimize inflammation and improve fibrosis is being explored in this group of patients.

Should patients with hepatitis C and normal liver enzyme levels be treated with antiviral therapy?

As a group, patients who test positive for HCV-RNA in blood and have persistently normal levels of alanine aminotransferase over time tend to have mild disease on liver biopsy. Such is not the case in all patients, however, and up to 20% may have evidence of significant necroinflammatory disease on biopsy or even fibrosis. For this reason, the approach should be individualized. In general, the natural history of the disease should be discussed with the patient. A liver biopsy should be offered to stage severity of disease. If the liver biopsy shows mild or minimal disease, continued observation without therapy is a reasonable option. For patients with more advanced disease on liver biopsy, or for those who choose to be treated regardless of findings on liver biopsy, antiviral therapy has been shown to be as effective as in patients with elevated liver enzymes.

Should patients with HCV/HIV coinfection receive antiviral therapy for hepatitis C infection?

Yes. Coinfection with HIV and HCV results in marked acceleration of progression of liver disease. With the advent of newer, more effective antiretroviral agents, patients infected with HIV are living longer, and more are developing end-stage liver disease from HCV infection. For this reason, patients coinfected with HIV and HCV should be considered candidates for antiviral therapy against HCV.

Anti-HCV therapy is most likely to be effective if the patient is first placed on antiretroviral therapy, the HIV viral load is controlled, and the CD4 count is reconstituted. In general, patients with a CD4 count <250/mm and high HIV viral load are less likely to respond to antiviral therapy for HCV.

Anti-HCV therapy in patients receiving anti-HIV medications is complicated by the additive bone marrow suppression as well as other gastrointestinal side effects. Interactions between ribavirin and several anti-retroviral agents may increase the risk of lactic acidosis. Close monitoring of blood counts and chemistries is needed. Monitoring of HIV blood levels is also recommended because of concern about a possible negative interaction between ribavirin and some antiretroviral medications.

How should patients with HCV/HBV coinfection be treated?

Because most patients with HCV/HBV coinfection have quiescent hepatitis B infection, the antiviral therapy needs to be directed at the hepatitis C virus only. If active hepatitis B and C infection is present, as evidenced by a positive HCV-RNA and high-level viremia by HBV-DNA PCR assay, the patient should be treated with the recommended dose of interferon for hepatitis B in conjunction with ribavirin for hepatitis C. A flare of hepatitis is not unusual when treating patients with hepatitis B infection. Alternatively, treatment with pegylated interferon, ribavirin, and lamivudine or adefovir could be considered.

What are the options for patients who do not respond to combination therapy with interferon and ribavirin?

Currently, PEG-interferon and ribavirin therapy is not FDA approved for prior nonresponders. Research has shown that patients who responded to interferon and ribavirin therapy and then relapsed have a 45–55% chance of a sustained response, if retreated with PEG-interferon and ribavirin therapy for 48 weeks; these patients should be offered retreatment. In contrast, those patients who did not achieve a virologic response with interferon and ribavirin have only a 10–15% chance of sustained response after retreatment with PEG-interferon and ribavirin. Decision to retreat prior nonresponders should be individualized, taking into consideration the histologic severity of disease, the side effects experienced by the patient during the initial therapy, and the patient's enthusiasm for retreatment. Antiviral products aimed directly at the hepatitis C virus genome, such as proteases, helicases, and ribozymes, are currently under development and may increase the percentage of patients who achieve a sustained response to therapy.

22. **What is the role of antiviral therapy in acute hepatitis C?**

The role for antiviral therapy in acute hepatitis C is unclear. Acute infections are usually asymptomatic and found incidentally, such as needlestick injuries in health care workers. It is not clear what percentage of these cases become chronic. Some studies have shown that early treatment with IFN or combination therapy decreases the chronicity rate in patients with acute hepatitis C. More recent data suggest that as many as 50% of acute hepatitis C cases acquired via a needlestick injury may clear virus within 6 months. Although the current antiviral regimens for hepatitis C are not FDA approved for the treatment of acute hepatitis C, strong consideration should be given to early initiation of antiviral therapy when acute hepatitis C is diagnosed, particularly if the virus has not cleared within 6 months.

WEBSITES

1. http://www.aasld.org
2. http://www.aasld.org/eweb/docs/hepatitisc.pdf
3. http://www.cheo-foundation.on.ca/americanliverfoundation
4. http://www.cdc.gov/ncidod/diseases/hepatitis

BIBLIOGRAPHY

1. Dieterich DT, Purow JM, Rajapaksa R: Activity of combination therapy with interferon alpha-2b plus ribavirin chronic hepatitis C patients co-infected with HIV. Semin Liver Dis 19:(Suppl 1):87–94, 1999.
2. Fried MW, Shiffmann ML, Reddy R, et al: Peg-interferon alpha-2a plus ribavirin for chronic hepatitis C virus infection. N Engl J Med 347:975–982, 2002.
3. Gish RG: Standards of treatment in chronic hepatitis C. Semin Liver Dis 19(Suppl 1):35–47, 1999.
4. Herrine SK: Approach to the patient with chronic hepatitis C virus infection. Ann Intern Med 136:747–757, 2002.
5. Lindsay KL, Trepo C, Heintges T, et al: A randomized, double-blind trial comparing pegylated interferon alpha to interferon alpha-2b as initial treatment for chronic hepatitis C. Hepatology 34:395–403, 2001.
6. Maddrey WC: Safety of combination interferon alpha-2b/ribavirin therapy in chronic hepatitis C-relapsed and treatment-naïve patients. Semin Liver Dis 19(Suppl 1):67–75, 1999.
7. Manns MP, McHutchison JG, Gordon SC, et al: Peg-interferon alpha-2b plus ribavirin compared with interferon alpha-2b plus ribavirin for initial treatment of chronic hepatitis C: A randomised trial. Lancet 358:958–965, 2001.
8. McHutchison JG, Manns MP, Patel K, et al: Adherence to combination therapy enhances sustained response genotype 1 infected patients with chronic hepatitis C. Gastroenterology 123:1061–1069, 2002.
9. Morishima C, Gretch DR: Clinical use of hepatitis C virus tests for diagnosis and monitoring during therapy. Clin Liver Dis 3:717–740, 1999.
10. Reddy KR, Wright TL, Pockros PJ, et al: Efficacy and safety of pegylated (40-kd) interferon alpha-2a compared with interferon alpha-2a in noncirrhotic patients with chronic hepatitis C. Hepatology 33:433–438, 2001.
11. Rossine A, Ravaggi A, Biasi L, et al: Virological response to interferon treatment in hepatitis C virus carriers with normal aminotransferase levels and chronic hepatitis. Hepatology 26:1012–1017, 1997.
12. Vogel W: Treatment of acute hepatitis C virus infection. J Hepatol 31(Suppl 1):189–192, 1993.
13. Zarski JP, Bohn B, Bastie A: Characteristics of patients with dual infection by hepatitis B and C viruses. J Hepatol 28:27–33, 1998.
14. Zeuzem S, Feinman V, Rasenack J, et al: Peg-interferon alpha-2a in patients with chronic hepatitis C. N Engl J Med 343:1666–1672, 2000.

CHAPTER 18

ANTIVIRAL THERAPY FOR HEPATITIS B

Jorge L. Herrera, MD

Is antiviral therapy recommended for acute hepatitis B?

No. Acute hepatitis B, defined as a positive test for hepatitis B surface antigen (HBsAg) and the presence of hepatitis B core antibody-immunoglobulin M (HBcAb-IgM), is a self-limited disease in 90–95% of adults and resolves without specific antiviral therapy within 3–6 months after the onset of clinical symptoms. For this reason, only supportive care is offered to patients with acute hepatitis B infection. Antiviral therapy is considered only for patients with chronic hepatitis B (positive HBsAg test for more than 6 months).

Do all patients with chronic hepatitis B benefit from therapy?

No. Only patients with high viral load (>10^5 copies/mL) and evidence of ongoing hepatic necrosis, such as elevated liver enzyme levels or liver biopsy demonstrating active inflammation, should be considered for therapy. Typical candidates for antiviral therapy test positive for hepatitis B e antigen (HBeAg) and negative for HBe antibodies (HBeAb); they also have high levels of hepatitis B virus DNA by polymerase chain reaction (HBV-DNA PCR) assays. In contrast, chronic hepatitis B carriers (HBsAg-positive)—who are characterized by normal levels of liver enzymes, negative HBeAg, positive HBeAb, and nondetectable or low levels of HBV-DNA by PCR—do not require antiviral therapy. Table 18-1 summarizes the approach to antiviral therapy.

How should the HBV-DNA PCR assay results be interpreted?

In contrast to other chronic viral illnesses, total eradication of the virus to achieve a nondetectable level of HBV-DNA by PCR is desirable but not required for successful therapy. Low levels of HBV-DNA are not associated with progressive liver disease and do not require therapy. The upper limit of HBV-DNA levels that are consistently associated with inactive disease has not been clearly established. The National Institutes of Health (NIH) workshop on management of hepatitis B recommended that antiviral treatment be considered in patients with HBeAg-positive or HBeAg-negative chronic hepatitis B and HBV-DNA PCR levels >10^5 copies/mL. This threshold was arbitrarily chosen based on prior data obtained using nonamplified assays. Recent work suggests that patients with HBeAg-negative infection may have active disease at lower HBV-DNA levels, and that viral levels of 10,000 to 100,000 copies/mL may require therapy if associated with elevated liver enzymes and/or histologic evidence of active liver disease, regardless of the hepatitis B e antigen status.

Should patients with chronic hepatitis B who test negative for HBeAg be treated with antiviral therapy?

Yes. Traditionally, a positive HBeAg has been used as the hallmark of high viral load and an indication for antiviral therapy; thus, the absence of HBeAg implies a low viral load and no need for therapy. To complicate matters, an increasing number of patients who are HBeAg-negative and HBeAb-positive is found to have high levels of viremia due to mutation of the virus. The mutant strains are incapable of producing the e-antigen. The only way to identify patients infected with e-mutant strains of the hepatitis B virus is to find elevated levels of HBV-DNA by PCR in association with elevated alanine aminotransferase (ALT) levels and/or histologic evidence of active disease. Patients infected with the HBeAg mutants should be treated, but they

TABLE 18–1.   ANTIVIRAL THERAPY FOR PATIENTS WITH HEPATITIS B INFECTION

Serologic Pattern	Interpretation	Course of Action
HBsAg-positive, HBcAb-IgM-positive	Acute hepatitis B	Observe; resolution likely in 90–95% of adults
HBsAg-positive >6 mo, HBeAg-positive, HBeAb-negative, HBV-DNA–positive, elevated ALT level	Chronic infection with high-grade viremia	Initiate antiviral therapy
HBsAg-positive >6 mo, HBeAg-negative, HBeAb-positive, ALT normal HBV-DNA–negative, or low-level viremia (<100,000 copies/mL)	Chronic carrier	Observe
HBsAg-positive >6 mo, HBeAg-negative, HBeAb-positive, HBV-DNA–positive, elevated ALT level	Chronic infection with HBeAg mutant	Initiate antiviral therapy

HBsAg = hepatitis B surface antigen; HBcAb-IgM = hepatitis B core antibody-immunoglobulin M; HBeAg = hepatitis B e antigen; HBeAb = hepatitis e antibody; HBV-DNA = hepatitis B virus DNA by PCR; ALT = alanine aminotransferase; mo = month(s).

are more resistant to therapy. Long-term remission is less common compared with patients infected with the HBeAg-producing or "wild" strain, and many require lifelong therapy. In contrast, patients who test negative for HBeAg, positive for HBeAb, and test either negative for HBV-DNA by PCR or have low levels of virus (<10^5 copies/mL) may not require therapy.

5. **Is liver biopsy required before therapy is started?**
   No. A liver biopsy is not needed to establish the diagnosis of hepatitis B infection; however, it is the only tool available to determine severity of disease. Because the treatment of hepatitis B with interferon can exacerbate hepatic inflammation, it is important to know the severity of liver disease before initiating therapy. Patients who already have extensive fibrosis or cirrhosis on biopsy are less likely to tolerate a flare of hepatitis during treatment than patients with milder histologic disease. In addition, the detection of cirrhosis on liver biopsy selects a group of patients who require closer observation as well as screening for hepatocellular carcinoma and esophageal varices.

6. **What are the options for treating chronic hepatitis B infection?**
   Currently, three medications have been approved for the treatment of chronic hepatitis B infection: interferon alpha-2b, lamivudine, and adefovir dipivoxil (Table 18-2). Interferon alpha-2b is an injectable immunomodulatory medication that enhances clearance of the hepatitis B

virus by improving the immune response. Interferon is dosed at either 10 million units subcutaneously three times/week or 5 million units subcutaneously daily for 16 weeks. The new form of pegylated interferons are not yet FDA approved for the treatment of hepatitis B. Recent clinical research suggests that treatment of chronic HBV with PEG-interferon for 48 weeks achieves a higher percent of virologic response compared with oral nucleosides. Side effects, however, are more common with interferon than with nucleoside therapy. Lamivudine is an oral nucleoside analog that directly inhibits viral replication without stimulating an immune response. Lamivudine inhibits the reverse transcriptase activity of HBV-DNA polymerase and halts viral replication. Lamivudine is given as one 100-mg tablet by mouth once a day for 1–2 years. Adefovir dipivoxil is an oral nucleotide analog of adenosine monophosphate. It inhibits both the reverse transcriptase and DNA polymerase activity and is incorporated into viral DNA, causing chain termination. Adefovir is given as a single 10-mg daily dose.

A fourth medication, tenofovir, has been FDA approved for the treatment of HIV infection but not hepatitis B infection. Studies in HIV subjects coinfected with hepatitis B suggest that this agent is quite active against the HBV virus. Because tenofovir is not FDA approved for the treatment of hepatitis B infection, it will not be discussed further in this chapter.

TABLE 18–2. COMPARISON OF APPROVED ANTIVIRAL TREATMENTS FOR CHRONIC HEPATITIS B

	INF-α	Lamivudine	Adefovir Dipivoxil
Indications			
HBeAg-positive normal ALT	Treatment is *not* indicated	Treatment is usually *not* indicated	Treatment is usually *not* indicated
HBeAg-positive chronic hepatitis	Treatment *is* indicated	Treatment *is* indicated	Treatment *is* indicated
HBeAg-negative chronic hepatitis	Treatment *is* indicated	Treatment *is* indicated	Treatment *is* indicated
Duration of Treatment			
HBeAg-positive chronic hepatitis	16–48 weeks	$\geq$1 yr	$\geq$1 yr
HBeAg-negative chronic hepatitis	1 yr	>1 yr	>1 yr
Route	Subcutaneous	Oral	Oral
Dose	Variable depending on product used	100 mg daily*	10 mg daily
Side Effects	Numerous and expected	Uncommon, well tolerated	Nephrotoxicity
Drug Resistance	—	approx. 20% yr 1; approx. 70% yr 5	Approx. 3% at year 2 of therapy

*For persons coinfected with HIV 150 mg twice daily along with other antiretroviral medications.
INF = interferon; ALT = alanine aminotransferase; mo = month(s); yr = year(s); MU = million units.

7. **What are the endpoints of antiviral therapy?**

The goals of antiviral therapy are to eradicate or drastically reduce viremia, and to induce e-antigen seroconversion (defined as achieving HBeAg-negative, HBeAb-positive status). On e-antigen seroconversion is achieved and maintained for 3–6 months, antiviral therapy may discontinued. Remission is usually long-lasting, but as long as the patient continues to test positive for HBsAg, he or she is at risk of reactivation and should be monitored closely.

HBsAg rarely, if ever, clears during antiviral therapy. With continued follow-up after successful antiviral therapy, however, a percentage of patients lose HBsAg and develop HBsA HBsAg clearance occurs in 10–15% of patients within the first year after treatment. After 4 ye of observation, as many as 65% lose HBsAg and acquire HBsAb. Once HBsAg is cleared and surface antibody appears, long-lasting remission and immunity to hepatitis B are likely. HBsA clearance appears to be more common after successful therapy with interferon compared wit oral nucleoside or nucleotide therapy.

8. **What is the expected response to interferon therapy?**

Because interferon stimulates the immune response, increased clearance of the hepatitis B virus is expected during therapy. Clearance of the virus is achieved by necrosis of infected hepatocytes. Thus, a flare of hepatitis is common during treatment with interferon. Usually occurs soon after initiation of interferon therapy and is manifested by elevated levels of ALT and aspartate aminotransferase (AST). The flare may be accompanied by jaundice and sign and symptoms typical of acute viral hepatitis but is usually associated with reduction or disappearance of HBV-DNA in blood. As the liver enzyme levels return to normal, the HBeA assay becomes negative, followed by seroconversion to positive HBeAb. Once seroconvers is achieved, therapy can be discontinued. The virologic response is usually long-lasting. If e-antigen seroconversion has not been achieved after 16 weeks of interferon therapy, response to further interferon therapy is unlikely and it should be discontinued. Positive predictors of response to interferon therapy include HBeAg-positive patients, low viral leve elevated ALT levels (over 150 IU), and absence of cirrhosis. Seroconversion to HBeAg negative and HBeAb positive occurs in 25–40% of patients treated with interferon; the majority of responders have a durable response. Recent research using PEG interferon for treatment of hepatitis B infection indicates that the ideal length of therapy is 48 weeks inste of 16 weeks.

9. **What is the expected response to lamivudine or adefovir therapy?**

In contrast to interferon, lamivudine and adefovir inhibit viral replication but do not stimulate immune clearance of the virus. For this reason, immune-mediated hepatocyte necrosis is unusual, and biochemical flare of hepatitis is rarely seen with lamivudine or adefovir therapy. most patients, the HBV-DNA serum levels decrease dramatically or become undetectable soo after initiating therapy. This decrease is associated with normalization of liver enzyme levels. Seroconversion from HBeAg-positive to HBeAg-negative and from HBeAb-negative to HBeAb positive is less common and often requires prolonged therapy for 1–3 years. During lamivudi therapy, HBeAg becomes negative in 32% of patients treated for 1 year and induces a positive HBeAb in about 17% after 1 year. With adefovir therapy, approximately 12% of patients achie e-antigen seroconversion after the first year of therapy.

Prolonged therapy with lamivudine has been associated with the emergence of escape mutants, also known as YMDD or M552 mutants. The incidence of lamivudine escape muta increases with duration of therapy and is estimated to occur in 16–32% of patients during first year, 38–50% after 2 years of therapy, and 49% or higher after the third year. The emergence of these mutants is usually signified by a resurgence of detectable HBV-DNA lev as measured by hybridization detection of HBV-DNA; this event is often associated with ALT elevation, which is usually asymptomatic. Patients who develop lamivudine-resistant muta should be changed to an alternative therapy. Adefovir is active against lamivudine-resistant strains and currently is the medication of choice for lamivudine-resistant strains.

Adefovir resistance is less common, but occurs at a rate of 1–2% per year. Fortunately, adefovir-resistant mutants are sensitive to lamivudine. Patients who develop adefovir-resistant mutants should have lamivudine added to their therapy, and treatment with adefovir should be continued to minimize the risk of lamivudine-resistant mutants.

10. **What are the advantages of interferon therapy for chronic hepatitis B infection?**

Successful response is durable and relapses are rare, once interferon is discontinued. Once the HBV infects the liver cell, the HBV genome localizes to the nucleus of the hepatocyte and is converted to covalently closed circular DNA (cccDNA). Clearance of this HBV-DNA is needed to achieve HBsAg seroconversion and can be achieved only by immune-mediated lysis of infected hepatocytes. Cases of HBsAg seroconversion (HBsAg becomes negative and HBsAb becomes positive) have been documented years after inducing e-antigen seroconversion by interferon. Finally, "interferon escape mutants" have not been described.

11. **What are the disadvantages of interferon therapy?**

Interferon therapy is associated with significant side effects, including flu-like syndrome, fever, depression, insomnia, irritability, and bone marrow suppression (see Chapter 17, Antiviral Therapy for Hepatitis C Infection). The interferon-induced flare of hepatitis may be severe and is particularly dangerous in patients with advanced liver disease and cirrhosis, who may not be able to tolerate a flare of hepatitis. For this reason, interferon therapy is relatively contraindicated in patients with cirrhosis caused by chronic hepatitis B infection. Another disadvantage is that patients with persistently normal liver enzyme levels, and those who acquired the disease at birth, are unlikely to respond to interferon therapy.

12. **Which parameters predict a good response to interferon therapy?**

Patients likely to respond to interferon therapy are characterized by elevated liver enzymes (ALT >150 U/dL), low viral load (HBV-DNA <200 pg/mL), female sex, and acquisition of infection during adulthood. Such patients have a 30–40% chance of achieving e-antigen seroconversion after a 16-week course of interferon. In contrast, patients with normal or minimal elevations of liver enzymes have a <5% chance of achieving sustained remission.

13. **What is the role of "prednisone priming" before initiation of interferon therapy?**

To enhance response to interferon among patients with normal ALT levels, prior treatment with prednisone has been proposed. The rationale for this approach is based on the observation that withdrawal of corticosteroid therapy frequently results in an acute hepatitis-like elevation of serum aminotransferases that is thought to represent an immunologic rebound against the virus. This flare is associated with a transient decrease in HBV-DNA and elevations of ALT, two features that predict a good response to interferon therapy. Increased likelihood of response to interferon has been noted among patients with normal ALT levels who receive corticosteroids before receiving interferon therapy. With the advent of nucleoside and nucleotide therapy, prednisone priming is rarely used.

14. **What are the advantages of lamivudine therapy?**

Lamivudine is taken orally once daily and is associated with minimal to no side effects. Lamivudine therapy rarely induces a flare of hepatitis and can be used in patients with cirrhosis. Lamivudine is particularly attractive for patients with advanced disease and complications from cirrhosis. In some, a response to lamivudine may produce dramatic improvement in liver function with resolution of some of the complications of cirrhosis. In most patients, it significantly reduces HBV-DNA levels and normalizes liver enzymes. Patients with normal ALT levels appear to respond to lamivudine therapy as well as those with elevated ALT. Patients infected with HBeAg mutants also appear to respond well to lamivudine.

15. **What are the disadvantages of lamivudine therapy?**

    The treatment course is long, lasting 1–3 years. To approach the efficacy rates of interferon in inducing e-antigen seroconversion, treatment for longer than 1 year is needed. The durability of the response is not as good as with interferon. The development of resistant lamivudine escape mutants increases with longer duration of therapy, and patients infected with lamivudine-resistant strains will have progressive disease even if lamivudine therapy is continued. Finally, because lamivudine acts at the reverse transcriptase level in the cytoplasm and does not affect the cccDNA in the nucleus, HBsAg seroconversion is less likely.

16. **What are the advantages of adefovir therapy?**

    Adefovir, like lamivudine, is an oral agent associated with minimal side effects. The main advantage of adefovir is the relatively low-resistance rate of 1–2% per year, making it an ideal agent for long-term therapy. Adefovir is also effective in suppressing lamivudine-resistant strains of HBV, making this the drug of choice for treating lamivudine-resistant hepatitis B infection. After 1 year of adefovir therapy, e-antigen seroconversion was achieved in 12% of patients. Significant histologic improvement was noted in 53% of patients. Adefovir is also active in treating e-antigen mutant strains of the hepatitis B virus.

17. **What are the disadvantages of adefovir therapy?**

    The major concern with adefovir is nephrotoxicity, which is frequent when doses of 30 mg or higher are used. With the approved dose of 10 mg daily, nephrotoxicity is extremely rare, but it is recommended that blood urea nitrogen (BUN) and creatinine levels be monitored during therapy. Cost is another concern; adefovir is significantly more expensive than lamivudine. Although resistant mutations are rare, they do occur and patients must be monitored with periodic HBV-DNA assays to detect emergence of resistance.

18. **Should patients with advanced, decompensated cirrhosis resulting from hepatitis B receive antiviral therapy or be referred for liver transplantation without a trial of therapy?**

    Yes. Although patients with decompensated disease cannot be treated with interferon, treatment with lamivudine is beneficial and often life-saving. In many such patients, evidence of severe decompensation reverses, and patients no longer need to be listed for liver transplantation after response to lamivudine therapy. In addition, lamivudine therapy, when continued after transplantation, is associated with a decreased chance of recurrence of infection in the graft. In general, patients with severe liver disease resulting from hepatitis B infection, even if listed for transplantation, should be considered potential candidates for treatment with lamivudine. Once a response is achieved, lifelong therapy is recommended because flares induced by discontinuation of antiviral therapy could be fatal in these patients. It is likely that adefovir will also be safe for use in these patients; however, current data have not established the safety of adefovir in patients with decompensated cirrhosis, and there is concern about possible nephrotoxicity in this group of patients.

19. **How are lamivudine escape mutants detected? What should be the course of action if they develop?**

    Mutations that cause HBV resistance to lamivudine develop frequently and usually begin to appear after 8–9 months of treatment, with a progressive increase in rate of detection over time. Mutations develop in approximately 16–50% of patients treated for 1–3 years. The development of the mutant strain can be detected clinically by the reappearance of HBV-DNA in serum in a patient who had become HBV-DNA-negative upon initiation of lamivudine therapy. Occasionally, mild elevation of ALT is noted with the emergence of the mutant strain. Although the mutant strain replicates less efficiently and is less virulent than the "wild" strain, progressive disease will occur if the infection is not controlled. New antiviral agents, including adefovir dipivoxil, are effective in controlling lamivudine-resistant mutants, and patients with lamivudine-resistant mutant infection should receive adefovir therapy.

What is the role of famciclovir in the treatment of hepatitis B?
Famciclovir is effective in reducing HBV-DNA levels; however, less than 10% of patients achieve e-antigen seroconversion after 1 year of therapy with famciclovir. Fortunately, famciclovir-resistant strains appear to be sensitive to lamivudine, but famciclovir is not effective against lamivudine-resistant strains. Famciclovir is likely to be more effective, if used as part of a multidrug cocktail to treat HBV infection. The combination of famciclovir and lamivudine appears to be additive in its ability to suppress viral load, but preliminary studies have not shown an increased e-antigen seroconversion rate.

What is the role of antiviral therapy after liver transplantation?
Oral nucleoside or nucleotide therapy are the agents of choice for the treatment of hepatitis B after transplant. Interferon is not effective in this setting, because the immune suppression needed to prevent rejection makes interferon ineffective in clearing the virus. In contrast, lamivudine induces a sustained inhibition of viral replication and normalizes serum transaminases in the majority (>70%) of post-transplant patients with hepatitis B. Loss of HBsAg can be achieved in a substantial number of patients treated soon after transplantation. Most of these patients also require long-term therapy with hepatitis B immune globulin (HBIG) (see Table 18-2).

WEBSITES

. http://www.aasld.org/

. http://www.aasld.org/eweb/docs/chronichep_B.pdf

. http://www.aasld.org/eweb/docs/update_chronichep_B.pdf

. http://www.hbvadvocate.org

BLIOGRAPHY

Chu CH, Hussain M, Lock ASF: Quantitative serum HBV DNA levels during different stages of chronic hepatitis B infection. Hepatology 36:1408–1415, 2002.

Conjeevaram HS, Lok AS: Management of chronic hepatitis B. J Hepatol 38:S90–S103, 2003.

Cooksley WG: Treatment with interferons (including pegylated interferons) in patients with hepatitis B. Sem Liv Dis 24(Suppl1):45–53, 2004.

Dienstag JL, Schiff ER, Mitchell M, et al: Extended lamivudine retreatment for chronic hepatitis B: Maintenance of viral suppression after discontinuation of therapy. Hepatology 30:1082–1087, 1999.

Hussain M, Lok AS: Mutations in the hepatitis B virus polymerase gene associated with antiviral treatment for hepatitis B. J Viral Hepat 6:183–194, 1999.

Kapoor D, Guptan RC, Wakil SM, et al: Beneficial effects of lamivudine in hepatitis B virus related decompensated cirrhosis. J Hepatol 33:308–312, 2000.

Lai CL, Chien RN, Leung NW, et al: A one-year trial of lamivudine for chronic hepatitis B. N Engl J Med 339:61–68, 1998.

Locarnini S, Birch C: Antiviral chemotherapy for chronic hepatitis B infection: Lessons learned from treating HIV-infected patients. J Hepatol 30:536–550, 1999.

Marcellin P, Lau GK, Ferruccio B: Peg interferon alfa-2a alone, lamivudine alone, and the two in combination in patients with HBeAg-negative chronic hepatitis B. N Engl J Med 351:1206–1217, 2004.

Pawlotsky JM: Molecular diagnosis of viral hepatitis. Gastroenterology 122:1554–1568, 2002.

Perillo R, Rakela J, Dienstag J, et al: Multicenter study of lamivudine therapy for hepatitis B after liver transplantation. Hepatology 29:1581–1586, 1999.

12. Perillo R, Schiff E, Yoshida E, et al: Adefovir dipivoxil for the treatment of lamivudine-resistant hepatitis B mutants. Hepatology 32:129–134, 2000.

13. Perillo R, Schiff ER, Davis GL, et al: A randomized, controlled trial of interferon alpha-2b alone and after prednisone withdrawal in the treatment of chronic hepatitis B. N Engl J Med 232:295–301, 1990.

14. Perillo RB, Mason AL: Therapy for hepatitis B virus infection. Gastroenterol Clin North Am 23:581–601, 199

15. Perillo RP, Regenstein FG, Peters M, et al: Prednisone withdrawal followed by recombinant alpha interferon the treatment of chronic type B hepatitis. A randomized, controlled trial. Ann Intern Med 109:98–100, 1988.

16. Tassopoulos NC, Volpes R, Patore Giuseppe, et al: Efficacy of lamivudine in patients with hepatitis B e-antigen negative/hepatitis B virus DNA-positive (precore mutant) chronic hepatitis B. Hepatology 29:889–896, 1999

17. Villeneuve JP, Condreay LD, Willems B, et al: Lamivudine treatment for decompensated cirrhosis resulting fr chronic hepatitis B. Hepatology 31:207–210, 2000.

18. Wong DK, Cheung AM, O'Rourke K, et al: Effect of alpha-interferon treatment in patients with hepatitis B e antigen-positive chronic hepatitis B: A meta-analysis. Ann Intern Med 119:312–323, 1993.

19. Xion X, Flores C, Ynag H, et al: Mutations in hepatitis B DNA polymerase associated with resistance to lamivudine do not confer resistance to adefovir in vitro. Hepatology 28:1669–1673, 1998.

20. Yang H, Westland CE, Delaney WE, et al: Resistance surveillance in chronic hepatitis B patients treated with a fovir dipivoxil for up to 60 weeks. Hepatology 36:464–473, 2002.

CHAPTER 19

AUTOIMMUNE HEPATITIS: DIAGNOSIS

Albert J. Czaja, MD

1. **What is autoimmune hepatitis?**

   Autoimmune hepatitis is an unresolving inflammation of the liver of unknown cause that is characterized by interface hepatitis on histologic examination, autoantibodies, and hypergammaglobulinemia. Cirrhosis, portal hypertension, liver failure, and death are possible consequences. Diagnosis requires the exclusion of chronic viral hepatitis, Wilson disease, alpha$_1$ antitrypsin deficiency, genetic hemochromatosis, drug-induced hepatitis, alcoholic and nonalcoholic fatty liver disease, and other immune-mediated liver diseases, such as autoimmune cholangitis, primary biliary cirrhosis, and primary sclerosing cholangitis. A careful clinical history, selected laboratory tests, and expert histologic examination establish the diagnosis in most instances (Table 19-1).

2. **What are its predominant features?**

   Autoimmune hepatitis affects mainly women (71%). It may occur at any age (9 months to 77 years), but, typically, it is diagnosed before the fourth decade. An acute, even fulminant, presentation is possible, and the disease may be mistaken for acute viral or toxic hepatitis. Concurrent immunologic diseases are present in 38% of cases (Table 19-2). Cirrhosis is present in 25% of patients at presentation, and the disease can have an indolent, subclinical stage. Smooth muscle antibodies (SMA) and antinuclear antibodies (ANA) are the most common serologic markers. In 64% of patients, SMA and ANA are present together. Autoantibody titers fluctuate and may disappear. Patterns of seropositivity also change during the disease, and one autoantibody may disappear as another appears. There is no minimum titer of significance, but autoantibody titers in adults should be >1:40. Serum titers >1:80 increase diagnostic confidence.

   Hypergammaglobulinemia, especially elevation of the serum immunoglobulin G level, is a hallmark of the disease, and the diagnosis is suspect without it. Marked cholestatic features are incompatible with the diagnosis, and a predominant serum alkaline phosphatase abnormality, pruritus, hyperpigmentation, and/or bile duct lesions on histologic examination suggest other diseases, such as primary biliary cirrhosis, primary sclerosing cholangitis, or autoimmune cholangitis. Similarly, serologic evidence of active infection with hepatitis A, B, or C viruses, Epstein-Barr virus, or cytomegalovirus argues against the diagnosis.

3. **What are the characteristic histologic findings in autoimmune hepatitis?**

   Interface hepatitis ("piecemeal necrosis" or periportal hepatitis) implies disruption of the limiting plate of the portal tract by inflammatory infiltrate, and it is a requisite finding (Fig. 19-1). Interface hepatitis, however, is not pathognomonic, and this same pattern may be seen in acute and chronic hepatitis associated with viruses, drugs, alcohol, and toxins. Acinar ("lobular") hepatitis, which is characterized by prominent cellular infiltrates that line sinusoidal spaces in association with degenerative or regenerative changes, is another common but nondiagnostic histologic manifestation (Fig. 19-2). Marked plasma cell infiltration of the portal tracts is also a histologic change that characterizes the disease (Fig. 19-3). In contrast, prominent portal lymphoid aggregates and steatosis suggest the diagnosis of chronic hepatitis C (Fig. 19-4); ground-glass hepatocytes are characteristic of chronic hepatitis B; and marked bile duct damage or loss connotes a cholangiopathy. Unusual histologic features associated with autoimmune hepatitis include centrilobular or "perivenular" (Rappaport zone 3) necrosis and hepatocytic giant cells.

TABLE 19-1.   DIFFERENTIAL DIAGNOSIS AND DISCRIMINATIVE TESTS

Possible Diagnoses	Diagnostic Tests	Diagnostic Findings
Wilson disease	Copper studies	Low ceruloplasmin
		Low serum copper level
		High urinary copper
		Increased hepatic copper
	Slit-lamp eye exam	Kayser-Fleischer rings
Primary sclerosing cholangitis	Cholangiography	Focal biliary strictures
	Liver biopsy	Fibrous obliterative cholangitis
Primary biliary cirrhosis	Antimitochondrial antibodies	AMA ≥1:40
		Antipyruvate dehydrogenase-E2
	Liver biopsy	Florid duct lesion
		Increased hepatic copper
Autoimmune cholangitis	Liver biopsy	Cholangitis
		Ductopenia
Chronic hepatitis C	Viral markers	Anti-HCV positive
		HCV RNA present
	Liver biopsy	Portal lymphoid aggregates
		Steatosis
Drug-induced hepatitis	Clinical history	Exposure to minocycline, isoniazid, nitrofurantoin, propylthiouracil, α-methyldopa
Hemochromatosis	Genetic testing	C282Y, H63D mutations
	Transferrin saturation	Increased
	Liver biopsy	Iron overload
		Hepatic iron index >1.9
Alpha$_1$ antitrypsin deficiency	Phenotype	ZZ or MZ
	Liver biopsy	Hepatic inclusions
Nonalcoholic steatohepatitis	Clinical findings	Obesity, diabetes, drugs, hyperlipidemia
	Ultrasonography	Hepatic hyperechogenicity
	Liver biopsy	Macrosteatosis

AMA = antimitochondrial antibodies; HCV = hepatitis C virus; RNA = ribonucleic acid; C282Y = substitution of tyrosine for cysteine at amino acid position 282 in alpha$_3$ loop; H63D = substitution of histidine for aspartate at amino acid position 63 in alpha$_1$ loop; ZZ or MZ = major protease inhibitor (P$_L$) deficiency phenotypes.

4. **What are the different types of autoimmune hepatitis?**
    The two major types of autoimmune hepatitis are based on distinctive serologic markers (Table 19-3). These classifications do not clinically define valid subgroups of different etiology or prognosis. The designations have entered the clinical jargon as descriptive terms, but they do not identify independent pathologic entities, and they should not be used as formal diagnoses.

TABLE 19-2.	IMMUNOLOGIC DISEASES ASSOCIATED WITH AUTOIMMUNE HEPATITIS
Autoimmune thyroiditis*	Lichen planus
Celiac disease	Myasthenia gravis
Coombs' positive hemolytic anemia	Neutropenia
Cryoglobulinemia	Pericarditis
Dermatitis herpetiformis	Peripheral neuropathy
Erythema nodosum	Pernicious anemia
Fibrosing alveolitis	Pleuritis
Focal myositis	Pyoderma gangrenosum
Gingivitis	Rheumatoid arthritis*
Glomerulonephritis	Sjögren's syndrome
Graves' disease*	Synovitis*
Idiopathic thrombocytopenic purpura	Systemic lupus erythematosus
Insulin-dependent diabetes	Ulcerative colitis*
Intestinal villous atrophy	Urticaria
Iritis	Vitiligo

*Most common association.

Type 1 autoimmune hepatitis is characterized by SMA and/or ANA, and it is the most common form in the United States and Western Europe. Antibodies to actin (antiactin), a subgroup of SMA, may also be present and support the diagnosis.

Type 2 autoimmune hepatitis is characterized by antibodies to liver/kidney microsome type 1 (anti-LKM1). These antibodies rarely coexist with SMA or ANA. Patients with type 2 autoimmune hepatitis are typically young (ages 2–14 years). They frequently have concurrent immunologic diseases, such as autoimmune thyroiditis, vitiligo, insulin-dependent diabetes, and ulcerative colitis, and they commonly express organ-specific antibodies, such as antibodies to thyroid, islets of Langerhans, and parietal cells.

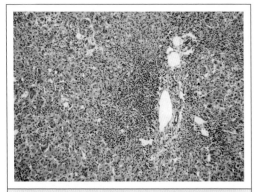

Figure 19-1. *Interface hepatitis.* The limiting plate of the portal tract is disrupted by inflammatory infiltrate (H & E; original magnification × 100).

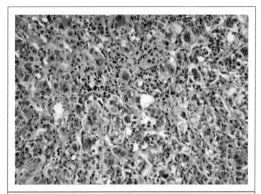

Figure 19-2. *Acinar hepatitis.* Inflammatory cells line the sinusoidal spaces in association with liver cell regenerative or degenerative changes (H & E; original magnification × 200).

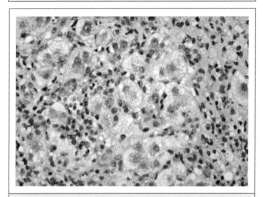

Figure 19-3. *Plasma cell infiltration.* Plasma cells infiltrate the periportal region (H & E; original magnification × 400).

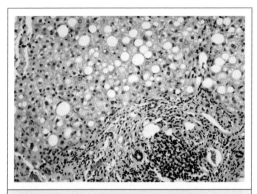

Figure 19-4. *Chronic hepatitis C.* Small lymphocytes aggregate in the portal tract and vacuoles of lipid are present within the cytoplasm of hepatocytes (H & E; original magnification × 200).

Type 3 autoimmune hepatitis is the least established form. It is characterized by the presence of antibodies to soluble liver antigen/liver pancreas (anti-SLA/LP). Eleven percent of patients with type 1 autoimmune hepatitis have anti-SLA/LP, and they cannot be distinguished from seronegative counterparts by age, gender, frequency, and nature of concurrent autoantibodies and immune diseases, laboratory findings, and treatment response. Type 3 autoimmune hepatitis, as defined by anti-SLA/LP, may be a variant of type 1 autoimmune hepatitis rather than a separate entity.

TABLE 19-3.	TYPES OF AUTOIMMUNE HEPATITIS	
Features	Type 1	Type 2
Autoantibodies	Smooth muscle	Liver/kidney microsome 1
	Nucleus	Liver cytosol type 1
	Actin	Recombinant P450 IID6
	Asialoglycoprotein receptor	254-271 core motif
	Perinuclear antineutrophil cytoplasm	Asialoglycoprotein receptor
Organ-specific antibodies	Possible (especially antibodies to thyroid)	Common (antibodies to thyroid, parietal cells, islets of Langerhans)
Autoantigen	Unknown	CYP2D6 (P450 IID6)
HLA phenotype	B8, DR3, DR4	DR7, B14, DR3, *C4A-Q0*
Susceptibility alleles	*DRB1*0301, DRB1*0401* (North American and Northern Europe) *DRB1*04* alleles (Japan, Mexico) *DRB1*1301* (South America)	*DRB1*0701*
Predominant age	Adult	Child
Fulminant onset	Possible	Possible
Concurrent immune disease	38%	34%
Low IgA level	No	Possible
Progression to cirrhosis	36%	82%
Corticosteroid responsive	Yes	Yes

HLA = human leukocyte antigen; IgA = immunoglobulin A.

. **What are the diagnostic criteria?**
The diagnostic criteria for autoimmune hepatitis have been codified by an international panel. The *definite diagnosis* requires histologic evidence of interface hepatitis with or without acinar (lobular) hepatitis or bridging necrosis and absence of biliary lesions, granulomas, copper deposits, or other changes suggestive of a different etiology. The serum aminotransferase level must be abnormally increased, and it must dominate the biochemical profile. Total serum globulin, gamma globulin, or immunoglobulin G levels must be greater than 1.5-fold the upper limit of normal, and

serum titers of SMA, ANA, or anti-LKM1 must be greater than 1:80. There must be no history of parenteral exposure to blood or blood products, recent use of hepatotoxic drugs, or excessive alcohol consumption (<35 gm/day in men and <25 gm/day in women). Active viral infection must be excluded, and serum levels of alpha$_1$ antitrypsin and ceruloplasmin must be normal. The *probable diagnosis* is made when there are similar findings that are less pronounced. A cholestatic form of autoimmune hepatitis is not recognized. A scoring system has been developed and recently revised by the International Autoimmune Hepatitis Group (Table 19-4).

TABLE 19-4. SCORING SYSTEM FOR THE DIAGNOSIS OF AUTOIMMUNE HEPATITIS[*]			
Clinical Features	**Score**	**Clinical Features**	**Score**
Female	+2	Average alcohol intake	
		<25 g/day	+2
Alkaline phosphatase:		>60 g/day	−2
Aspartate		Histologic findings	
Aminotransferase ratio		Interface hepatitis	+3
<1.5	+2	Lymphoplasmacytic infiltrate	+1
1.5–3.0	0	Rosette formation	+1
>3.0	−2	None of above	−5
Serum γ-globulin or		Biliary changes	−3
immunoglobulin G		Other changes	−3
level above normal limit		Concurrent immune disease	+2
>2.0	+3	Novel autoantibodies	+2
1.5–2.0	+2	HLA DR3 or DR4	+1
1.0–1.5	+1		
<1.0	0	Response to corticosteroids	
ANA, SMA or anti-LKM1		Complete	+2
>1:80	+3	Relapse after drug withdrawal	+3
1:80	+2		
1:40	+1	**Aggregate score pre-treatment**	
<1:40	0	Definite autoimmune hepatitis	>15
		Probable autoimmune hepatitis	10–15
AMA positive	−4		
		Aggregate score post-treatment	
Hepatitis markers		Definite autoimmune hepatitis	>17
Positive	−3	Probable autoimmune hepatitis	12–17
Negative	+3		
Drug history			
Positive	−4		
Negative	+1		

[*]Revised proposal of the International Autoimmune Hepatitis Group, J Hepatol 31:929–938, 1999.
ANA = antinuclear antibodies; SMA = smooth muscle antibodies; LKM1 = liver kidney/microsome type 1; AMA = human leukocyte antigen; AMA = antimitochondrial antibodies.

What is the standard serologic battery used for diagnosis?

Antinuclear antibodies, smooth muscle antibodies, and antibodies to liver/kidney microsome type 1 are the standard serologic markers of autoimmune hepatitis, but they do not have pathogenic properties (Table 19-5). They are useful in diagnosis, but they do not have diagnostic specificity. Autoantibody behavior does not correlate with disease activity or treatment response, and determinations of ANA, SMA, and anti-LKM1 should be used for diagnostic purposes only.

What other autoantibodies may have diagnostic and prognostic importance?

Multiple autoantibodies have been described in autoimmune hepatitis, but none has been shown to be pathogenic or clinically versatile. Their characterization may help identify the autoantigens responsible for the disease, and some may prove to be valuable diagnostic and prognostic instruments. Commercial assays are available for anti-SLA/LP, antichromatin, antiactin, and perinuclear antineutrophil cytoplasmic antibodies (pANCA).

- *Antibodies to soluble liver antigen/liver pancreas* are directed against a 50 kDa cytosolic protein that has been identified as a transfer ribonucleoprotein complex (tRNP$^{ser(sec)}$) involved in selenocysteine metabolism. Anti-SLA/LP have high specificity (99%) for autoimmune hepatitis, but they occur in only 16% of individuals with the disease.
- *Antibodies to chromatin (antichromatin)* are found in 39% of patients with autoimmune hepatitis, and they occur more commonly in men than women (33% vs.15%, respectively; p = .0008). They commonly disappear during corticosteroid therapy, and they are more frequent during active than inactive disease (32% vs. 19%, respectively; p = .01).
- *Antibodies to liver cytosol type 1* (anti-LC1) have specificity for autoimmune hepatitis, and they were used initially to differentiate anti-LKM1-positive patients with and without HCV infection. They occur mainly in young patients, typically less than age 20, and their presence has been associated with more severe disease.
- *Antibodies to asialoglycoprotein receptor* (anti-ASGPR) are specific for autoimmune hepatitis. They are present in all types of autoimmune hepatitis, including 82% of patients with SMA and/or ANA, 67% of patients with anti-LKM1, and 67% of patients with anti-SLA/LP. The autoantibodies are directed against a transmembrane hepatocytic glycoprotein that can capture, display, and internalize potential antigens, induce T-cell proliferation, and activate cytotoxic T-cells.
- *pANCA* are commonly present (50–93%) in patients with type 1 autoimmune hepatitis. Preliminary studies have suggested that the pANCA of autoimmune hepatitis differ from those of primary sclerosing cholangitis by being higher in titer and of the IgG1 isotype. A variety of antigens—including actin, cathepsin G, catalase, elastase, bacterial permeability increasing protein, lactoferrin, and enolase—have been implicated as the targets of pANCA, but none has been established.

What investigational antibodies have promise as clinical tools?

Investigational efforts continue to characterize novel immune reactions in autoimmune hepatitis in the hope of discovering pertinent target antigens, improving diagnostic algorithms, and providing accurate prognostic indices. Key immune reactions are primarily reflective of the underlying pathogenic mechanisms. Other immune reactions may reflect "cryptic" antigens that can extend and/or perpetuate the disease after being uncovered by the inflammatory process. Last, the autoantibodies may be nonspecific collateral responses to the nonselective release of liver cell constituents, and they may have no clinical value. Autoantibodies in the early phases of characterization are investigational, and they may never be incorporated into conventional diagnostic strategies. Antibodies to lactoferrin and *Saccharomyces cerevisiae* are of this genre.

Antibodies to lactoferrin are directed against an iron-binding protein with putative anti-inflammatory and immunomodulatory actions that is expressed at mucosal surfaces and cleared by the liver. Antibodies to lactoferrin occur in ulcerative colitis, primary sclerosing cholangitis, rheumatoid arthritis, primary biliary cirrhosis, autoimmune hepatitis, and autoimmune cholangitis. Lactoferrin is present in the granules of granulocytes, and it prevents complement

TABLE 19-5. AUTOANTIBODIES ASSOCIATED WITH AUTOIMMUNE HEPATITIS

Autoantibody Species	Implication(s)
Nuclear	Type 1 autoimmune hepatitis
	Not disease specific
	Reactive to multiple nuclear antigens
Smooth muscle	Type 1 autoimmune hepatitis
	Reactive to actin and nonactin components
	Frequently concurrent with antinuclear antibodies
Actin	Type 1 autoimmune hepatitis
	Diagnostic specificity
	Commonly young patients
	Possibly more aggressive disease
	Unsettled assay
Liver/kidney microsome 1	Type 2 autoimmune hepatitis
	Inhibits P450 IID6 *in vitro*
	May occur in chronic hepatitis C
Asialoglycoprotein receptor	Generic marker of autoimmune hepatitis
	Correlates with inflammatory activity
	Possible barometer of treatment response
	Persistence identifies propensity to relapse
	Possible marker of important autoantigen
Liver cytosol type 1	Type 2 autoimmune hepatitis
	Young patients
	Possibly worse prognosis
	Commonly discounts hepatitis C virus infection
	Directed against formiminotransferase cyclodeaminase
Soluble liver antigen/ liver pancreas	Type 3 autoimmune hepatitis
	Antigenic target is tRNP$^{ser(sec)}$
	Useful in evaluating seronegative autoimmune hepatitis
	Associated with *DRB1*0301* and relapse after treatment
	High specificity but low sensitivity
Chromatin	Prognostic index in ANA-positive patients
	Reactivity against macromolecular octameric immunogen
	Associated with relapse after treatment
Perinuclear antineutrophil cytoplasm	Common in type 1 autoimmune hepatitis
	Absent in type 2 autoimmune hepatitis
	Mainly IgG1 isotope
	Useful in evaluating seronegative autoimmune hepatitis
	Unknown antigenic target

ANA = antinuclear antibodies; IgG = immunoglobulin G.

activation by inhibiting the C3 pathway. It may also be a target of pANCA. The role of antilactoferrin in the pathogenesis, diagnosis, and management of autoimmune hepatitis remains uncertain.

Antibodies to S. cerevisiae *(ASCA)* are directed against a species of baker's or brewer's yeast, and they occur mainly in Crohn disease (35–80%), ulcerative colitis (2–24%), and celiac disease (43%). Patients with primary sclerosing colitis (20%), primary biliary cirrhosis (19%), and autoimmune hepatitis (22–28%) also express these antibodies, and they may reflect disruption of the gastrointestinal mucosal barrier and sensitization against an environmental agent. Recent studies in autoimmune hepatitis have not demonstrated their value in detecting concurrent inflammatory bowel disease or celiac disease, but they have been associated with higher serum IgA levels than seronegative patients with autoimmune hepatitis. This laboratory distinction may reflect heightened mucosal immunity within the gastrointestinal tract, and ASCA may yet be shown to contribute to the diagnosis of concurrent mucosal diseases in autoimmune hepatitis.

9. **What is the significance of antimitochondrial antibodies in autoimmune hepatitis?**

Antimitochondrial antibodies (AMA) can be demonstrated by indirect immunofluorescence in 20% of patients with autoimmune hepatitis, but serum titers are typically low (<1:160 in 88% of instances). The histologic findings in such patients are indistinguishable from those of patients without AMA, and tissue copper stains by rhodanine are negative or only mildly positive. Responsiveness to corticosteroids can also be anticipated.

Patients with high titer AMA may have primary biliary cirrhosis, an overlap syndrome between autoimmune hepatitis and primary biliary cirrhosis, or anti-LKM1 that has been mistaken for AMA. Recognition of AMA by indirect immunofluorescence requires reactivity to the distal tubules of the murine kidney and parietal cells of the murine stomach. Recognition of anti-LKM1 requires reactivity to the proximal tubules of the murine kidney and murine hepatocytes. An exuberant reaction against the renal tubule may obscure these distinctions, and anti-LKM1 reactivity may be reported as AMA positivity. Enzyme-linked immunosorbent assays (ELISAs) based on recombinant mitochondrial and LKM1 antigens have reduced the interpretative errors associated with assays dependent on indirect immunofluorescence.

The antibodies that are specific against the mitochondrial autoantigens of primary biliary cirrhosis are the E2 subunits of pyruvate dehydrogenase and/or branched-chain ketoacid dehydrogenase. These occur in only 8% of patients with autoimmune hepatitis, and they may indicate an incorrect original diagnosis, a disorder with mixed features (overlap syndrome), or a rare instance of false seropositivity.

0. **Can autoimmune hepatitis exist in the absence of conventional autoantibodies?**

Yes. Thirteen percent of patients with severe chronic hepatitis lack a confident etiologic diagnosis. These patients are classified as cryptogenic chronic hepatitis, but they may have an autoimmune hepatitis that has escaped diagnosis by conventional serologic testing. Patients with cryptogenic chronic hepatitis are frequently similar by age, gender, human leukocyte antigen (HLA) phenotype, laboratory findings, and histologic features to patients with autoimmune hepatitis. They also respond well to corticosteroid therapy, entering remission as commonly (83% vs. 78%) and failing treatment as rarely (9% vs. 11%) as patients with conventional markers. These individuals may have "autoantibody-negative autoimmune hepatitis." Some patients may express SMA and/or ANA later in their course or have less conventional autoantibodies, such as anti-SLA/LP, anti-LC1, or pANCA. The scoring system is the best method of securing the diagnosis, and they should be treated, if indicated, with corticosteroids. Celiac disease may be associated with chronic hepatitis, and IgA antibodies to endomysium (EMA) and/or tissue transglutaminase (anti-tTG) should be performed in all patients with cryptogenic chronic hepatitis to exclude this diagnosis.

11. **What antibodies should be tested in patients who are seronegative at presentation?**

Twenty-five percent of seronegative patients will later express ANA and/or SMA and satisfy criteria for autoimmune hepatitis. pANCA may identify another 25% with autoimmune hepatitis and a similar number may be classifiable after testing for anti-SLA/LP. Immunoglobulin A EMA have a sensitivity of 94% and specificity of 99% for celiac disease, and IgA EMA should be sought in all patients with cryptogenic chronic hepatitis to exclude a gluten-responsive form liver disease. Tissue transglutaminase is a calcium-dependent enzyme that cross-links fibronectin and other collagens, and IgA anti-tTG can be nonspecifically increased in inflammatory conditions associated with fibrogenesis. Accordingly, testing for IgA EMA rather than IgA anti-tTG is the preferred method of excluding celiac disease as a cause of the liver dysfunction. The appropriate second battery of serologic tests in patients with seronegative cryptogenic chronic hepatitis at presentation includes ANA, SMA, and anti-LKM1 (repeat studies); pANCA; anti-SLA/LP; and IgA EMA. Celiac disease can be asymptomatic except for the liver disease. Furthermore, true seronegativity for IgA EMA requires exclusion of IgA deficiency.

12. **What are the pathogenic mechanisms?**

The pathogenic mechanisms of autoimmune hepatitis are unknown, but two theories prevail (Fig. 19-5). One theory proposes an *antibody-dependent cell-mediated form of cytotoxicity.* A defect is postulated in the modulation of B-cell production of immunoglobulin G. The

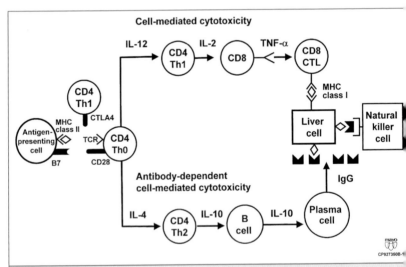

Figure 19-5. *Putative pathogenic mechanisms.* Activation of CD4 T-helper cells requires ligation of its T-cell antigen receptor (TCR) with the antigenic peptide displayed by the class II molecule of the major histocompatibility complex (MHC) (first signal) and coupling of B7 and CD28 (second signal). The activated CD4 T-helper cell (Th0) then differentiates in accordance with the predominant cytokine milieu. Cell-mediated cytotoxicity is favored by a type 1 (Th1) cytokine response mediated by interleukin (IL)-12, IL-2, and tumor necrosis factor-α (TNF-α). Cytotoxic T-lymphocytes (CD8 CTL) undergo activation by interaction with processed antigenic peptides presented by class I MHC molecules. Sensitized cytotoxic T-lymphocytes accomplish liver cell injury by the release of lymphokines. Antibody-dependent cell-mediated cytotoxicity is favored by a type 2 (Th2) cytokine response mediated by IL-4 and IL-10. Plasma cells are activated to produce immunoglobulin G (IgG), which forms complexes with normal membrane constituents of the hepatocyte. The Fc receptors of natural killer cells bind to the antigen-antibody complexes and cause cytolysis.

immunoglobulin adheres to normal hepatocytic membrane proteins and creates an antigen-antibody complex on the hepatocyte surface. This complex is then targeted by natural killer cells that have Fc receptors for the immunoglobulin. The natural killer cells do not require previous exposure to the target antigen for activation, and they accomplish liver cell injury by cytolysis.

The other theory proposes a *cellular form of cytotoxicity.* A disease-specific autoantigen is displayed on the surface of antigen-presenting cells in association with HLA class II antigens. Immunocytes that are HLA restricted are sensitized to the self-antigen, and clonal expansion of the antigen-primed lymphocytes follows. Activated cytotoxic T-lymphocytes infiltrate the liver tissue and destroy the hepatocytes displaying the target autoantigen. Lymphokines facilitate cell-to-cell communication, promote neo-expression of HLA class II antigens, enhance autoantigen presentation, activate the immunocytes, and intensify tissue damage by direct action.

Common to both theories are (1) a host predisposition for heightened immunoreactivity that is genetically determined and (2) uncertainty about the nature or need of a triggering agent. Viral infections, drug exposures, and environmental factors have been evoked as triggering mechanisms that can activate a final common pathway of pathogenesis. Molecular mimicry between foreign and self antigens is the most popular hypothesis for loss of self-tolerance, and antibodies that cross react against foreign and host antigens have been demonstrated. Molecular mimicry, however, has not been established as a cause of human autoimmune disease, and the humoral cross-reactivities found in autoimmune hepatitis have not been pathogenic. Liver-infiltrating immunocytes that are cross-reactive to foreign and self-antigens have not been found.

3. What are the autoantigens?

Cytochrome mono-oxygenase, CYP2D6 (P450 IID6), is the target autoantigen of type 2 autoimmune hepatitis. The target autoantigen of type 1 autoimmune hepatitis is unknown, but asialoglycoprotein receptor is an excellent candidate. Each antigen is expressed on the hepatocyte surface, and each is associated with tissue-infiltrating, antigen-sensitized lymphocytes. CD4 T-helper cells predominate in the portal tracts and scar tissue, antigen-sensitized suppressor/cytotoxic lymphocytes congregate near areas of interface hepatitis, and B-cells and natural killer cells are scant in all regions. These findings suggest that a cell-mediated form of cytotoxicity is the most important mechanism of liver cell injury in autoimmune hepatitis, and they implicate CD8 cytotoxic T-lymphocytes as the most likely effectors.

CYP2D6 (P450 IID6) is a 50-kDa microsomal enzyme that metabolizes at least 25 different drugs, including antihypertensive agents, beta blockers, antiarrhythmic drugs, and antidepressants. Asialoglycoprotein receptor is a transmembrane hepatocytic glycoprotein that can process and display multiple intrinsic and extrinsic antigens. Each is capable of transforming a variety of peptides into immunoreactive molecules. Other candidate autoantigens may exist, and they should be sought in the periportal regions of the liver tissue, where the inflammatory infiltrate predominates.

4. Do viruses cause autoimmune hepatitis?

Yes. Multiple viruses can trigger autoimmune hepatitis, including hepatitis A virus, hepatitis B virus, and hepatitis C virus. The lack of a confident animal model for the disease, the long lag time between exposure and clinical manifestation, and the likely persistence of autoimmune hepatitis after disappearance of its trigger have hampered efforts to fully define etiologic factors. Currently, the definite diagnosis of autoimmune hepatitis requires the exclusion of viral infection, and patients with true viral infection and low-titer autoantibodies are considered to have viral disease with nonspecific features of autoimmunity. The multiplicity of viruses that have been implicated as triggers suggests that there is a final common pathway of pathogenesis that can be initiated by a variety of agents. The triggering epitope must be small and commonly shared.

15. **Do drugs cause autoimmune hepatitis?**
Yes. Drugs can produce the clinical syndrome of autoimmune hepatitis, and they must be excluded at the time of presentation. An important drug that has recently been implicated as a cause for the disease is minocycline. Other medications that can mimic the syndrome are nitrofurantoin, isoniazid, propylthiouracil, and L-methyldopa. Identification of a drug-induced syndrome is important because discontinuation of the medication ameliorates the disease.

16. **Why does autoimmune hepatitis affect mainly women?**
The basis for the female propensity for autoimmune hepatitis is unknown. The predisposition women for autoimmune disease, in general, may reflect synergisms between the sex hormone immunoregulatory cytokine profiles, and HLA DR4 alleles.

17. **Are there genetic predispositions for autoimmune hepatitis?**
Yes. Susceptibility in caucasoid Northern Europeans and North Americans relates to HLA DR3 and DR4. HLA DR3 is the principal risk factor, and HLA DR4 is a secondary but independent risk factor. Eighty-five percent of North American patients with type 1 autoimmune hepatitis are positive for HLA DR3, HLA DR4, or both. HLA DR7 characterizes patients with type 2 autoimmune hepatitis (Table 19-6). The HLA phenotype identifies patients with a predisposition for

TABLE 19-6. EFFECTS OF CLASS II MHC ALLELES ON DISEASE EXPRESSION AND BEHAVIOR		
	Associated Class II MHC Alleles	
Disease Expression and Behavior	*DRB1*0301*	*DRB1*0401*
Earlier age onset	+	−
More frequent confluent necrosis and/or cirrhosis	+	−
Lower frequency of remission during therapy	+	−
Higher frequency of treatment failure	+	−
Higher frequency of relapse after drug withdrawal	+	−
More frequent liver transplantation	+	−
Associated with tumor necrosis factor-α polymorphism (TFNA*2)	+	−
Associated with cytotoxic T lymphocyte antigen-4 polymorphism involving guanine for alanine substitution	+	−
Older age onset	−	+
More commonly women	−	+
More commonly associated with concurrent immune disorders	−	+
Higher frequency of remission during therapy	−	+
Higher serum levels of γ-globulin and immunoglobulin G	−	+
More frequently associated with smooth muscle antibodies	−	+
More frequently associated with high titer antinuclear antibodies	−	+

MHC = major histocompatibility complex.

autoimmune hepatitis, but it does not predict emergence of the disease. Autoimmune hepatitis does not have a strong penetrance in families, and familial occurrence is rare.

Fifteen percent of patients with autoimmune polyendocrinopathy-candidiasis-ectodermal dystrophy (APECED) have autoimmune hepatitis, and the gene responsible for this syndrome is located on chromosome 21q22.3. The gene encodes an autoimmune regulator that modulates the negative selection of autoreactive T-cells by the thymus. Deficiencies in this regulator can result in the escape of autoreactive T-cells that can cause the syndrome by targeting CYP1A2 and CYP2A6. Autoimmune hepatitis can be a consequence of this autosomal recessive disease. APECED is most common among individuals of Finnish and Sardinian ancestry.

18. Is there a single susceptibility gene?

No. A single susceptibility gene has not been described for nonsyndromic disease, and autoimmune hepatitis is probably a polygenic disorder. The principal susceptibility alleles reside on the *DRB1* gene. High-resolution DNA-based techniques have indicated that the class II allele, *DRB1*0301*, of the major histocompatibility complex (MHC) is the principal risk factor, and the allele *DRB1*0401* is the secondary risk factor in caucasoid Northern Europeans and North Americans. In contrast, *DRB1*1501* protects against the disease in this population. Susceptibility alleles for type 1 autoimmune hepatitis in various ethnic groups are different, and they include *DRB1*0405* in Japanese patients and Argentine adults, *DRB1*1301* in Argentine children and Brazilian patients, and *DRB1*0404* in Mestizo Mexicans.

19. How do different susceptibility alleles produce the same disease?

Each susceptibility allele for autoimmune hepatitis encodes an amino acid sequence in the antigen-binding groove of the HLA DR molecule, and this sequence influences recognition of the autoantigen by the T-cell antigen receptor (TCR) of CD4 T-helper cells. The sequence is six amino acids long and in a critical position on the lip of the antigen-binding groove. The sequence encoded by *DRB1*0301* and *DRB1*0401* in caucasoid Northern Europeans and North Americans is denoted as LLEQKR at positions 67-72 of the DRβ polypeptide chain. Lysine (K) at position DRβ71 is the critical residue. Different susceptibility alleles that encode the same or similar short amino acid sequence in this critical location carry the same risk for autoimmune hepatitis ("shared motif hypothesis").

*DRB1*0404* in the Mestizo Mexicans and *DRB1*0405* in the Japanese encode an arginine for a lysine at position DRβ71. Arginine is positively charged like lysine, and its substitution would have little effect on the presentation of antigenic peptide. Both alleles, therefore, would be predicted to confer similar susceptibilities to autoimmune hepatitis. In contrast, *DRB1*1501* encodes an alanine for a lysine at DRβ71, and the substitution of this neutral nonpolar amino acid for either lysine or arginine at DRβ71 would have a major effect on antigen binding and TCR recognition. As a result, *DRB1*1501* is protective against autoimmune hepatitis.

The "shared motif hypothesis" does not account for all ethnic differences in susceptibility, and the association between *DRB1*1301* and type 1 autoimmune hepatitis in South America is unexplained by this theory. *DRB1*1301* encodes a negatively charged glutamic acid (E) for the positively charged lysine (K) at DRβ71.

20. How do regional factors affect susceptibility?

The association between *DRB1*1301* and autoimmune hepatitis in South American patients suggests that certain geographic and ethnic factors may affect susceptibility to autoimmune hepatitis. Certain regions may have indigenous agents that can trigger the disease, and individuals within that environment may have certain genetic predispositions that favor an immune response to that agent. *DRB1*1301* has been associated with protracted hepatitis A virus infection, and the hepatitis A virus has been implicated as a cause of autoimmune hepatitis. Hepatitis A virus infection is endemic in South America, and the high association between autoimmune hepatitis and children with *DRB1*1301* in this region may reflect the protracted exposure of these patients to viral and hepatic antigens. Other geographic regions may have other indigenous etiologic agents that select patients with different genetic phenotypes. In thi fashion, autoimmune hepatitis may be associated with multiple susceptibility genes that are region- and/or ethnic-dependent, and the genetic phenotype associated with autoimmune hepatitis in any one region may be a clue to the etiologic agent indigenous to that region ("molecular footprint hypothesis").

21. **What other factors promote autoimmune hepatitis?**
Multiple autoimmune promoters contribute to disease expression and severity. These may be genetically acquired and not disease specific. A polymorphism of the gene governing product of TNF-α, *TNFA***2*, has been described in type 1 autoimmune hepatitis. This polymorphism m result in high inducible and constitutive levels of TNF-α and thereby favor a type 1 cytokine response and expansion of cytotoxic T-cells.

Similarly, a polymorphism involving substitution of a guanine for an alanine at position 49 the gene encoding cytotoxic T-lymphocyte antigen-4 (CTLA-4) has been described in type 1 autoimmune hepatitis. This polymorphism may impair down-regulation of the immunocyte response and foster cellular hyperreactivity. Other autoimmune promoters, including those governing cytokine levels, autoantibody production, adhesion molecule display, and Fas-Fas ligand interactions are unstudied.

22. **Do the HLA phenotypes influence disease expression and outcome?**
Yes. In Caucasoid patients with type 1 autoimmune hepatitis, both HLA DR3 and HLA DR4 ha been associated with different clinical manifestations and outcomes. Patients with HLA DR3 a younger, and they have more active disease, as assessed by serum aminotransferase levels. They also have histologic findings of confluent necrosis and cirrhosis more often than other patients. Similarly, they relapse more frequently after drug withdrawal, enter remission less commonly, deteriorate more often, and require liver transplantation more frequently than patients with other phenotypes. In contrast, patients with HLA DR4 are older and more commonly women than patients with HLA DR3. They have higher serum levels of gamma globulin, a greater frequency of concurrent immunologic diseases, and a greater likelihood o entering remission during therapy. The expression of SMA and high-titer ANA may also be associated with HLA DR4, whereas the production of anti-SLA/LP is associated with HLA DR High-resolution DNA-based techniques have indicated that the same alleles, *DRB1***0301* and *DRB1***0401*, that affect susceptibility also affect outcome.

23. **What are the determinants of prognosis?**
The severity of inflammatory activity. Sustained serum aspartate aminotransferase (AST) activity of at least 10-fold normal or more than 5-fold normal in conjunction with a hypergammaglobulinemia of at least twice normal is associated with a 3-year survival of 50% and 10-year survival of 10%. Lesser degrees of biochemical activity are associated with bette prognoses. In such patients, the 15-year survival exceeds 80%, and the probability of progression to cirrhosis is less than 50%.

Histologic findings at presentation. Extension of the inflammatory process between portal tracts or between portal tracts and central veins (bridging necrosis) is associated with a 5-ye mortality of 45% and an 82% frequency of cirrhosis. Similar consequences occur in patients who have destruction of entire lobules of liver tissue at presentation (multilobular necrosis). 5-year mortality of cirrhosis is 58%, and 20% die of variceal hemorrhage within 2 years.

In contrast, patients with interface hepatitis ("piecemeal necrosis" or periportal hepatiti on histologic examination have a normal 5-year life expectancy and a low frequency of cirrhosis (17%). Spontaneous resolution of inflammatory activity may occur unpredictably 13–20% of patients, regardless of disease activity at accession, and no findings at presentation, including hepatic encephalopathy and ascites, preclude a satisfactory respon to corticosteroid therapy.

WEBSITES

. http://www.aasld.org/

. http://www.aasld.org/eweb/docs/autoimmune_hepatitis.pdf

BLIOGRAPHY

Czaja AJ: Autoimmune hepatitis after liver transplantation and other lessons of self-intolerance. Liver Transpl 8:505–513, 2000.

Czaja AJ: Frequency and nature of the variant syndromes of autoimmune liver disease. Hepatology 28:360–365, 1998.

Czaja AJ: Treatment of autoimmune hepatitis. Semin Liver Dis 22:365–377, 2002.

Czaja AJ: Treatment strategies in autoimmune hepatitis. Clin Liver Dis 6:799–824, 2002.

Czaja AJ, Carpenter HA: Histological features associated with relapse after corticosteroid withdrawal in type 1 autoimmune hepatitis. Liver Int 23:116–123, 2003.

Czaja AJ, Cookson S, Constantini PK, et al: Cytokine polymorphisms associated with clinical features and treatment outcome in type 1 autoimmune hepatitis. Gastroenterology 117:645–652, 1999.

Czaja AJ, Doherty DG, Donaldson PT: Genetic bases of autoimmune hepatitis. Dig Dis Sci 47:2139–2150, 2002.

Czaja AJ, Freese DK: Diagnosis and treatment of autoimmune hepatitis. Hepatology 36:479–497, 2002.

Czaja AJ, Menon KVN, Carpenter HA: Sustained remission after corticosteroid therapy for type 1 autoimmune hepatitis: A retrospective analysis. Hepatology 35:890–897, 2002.

Czaja AJ, Norman GL: Antibodies in the diagnosis and management of liver disease. J Clin Gastroenterol 37:315–329, 2003.

CHAPTER 20

AUTOIMMUNE HEPATITIS: TREATMENT

Albert J. Czaja, MD

1. **What therapies are effective?**

   Prednisone in combination with azathioprine and a higher dose of prednisone alone are the established therapies (Tables 20-1 and 20-2). Both regimens are equally effective in inducing clinical, biochemical, and histologic remission and prolonging immediate life expectancy. The combination regimen is associated with a lower frequency of drug-related side effects than the regimen using higher doses of prednisone alone (10% vs. 44%), and it is preferred.

   Postmenopausal women and patients with labile hypertension, brittle diabetes, emotional instability, exogenous obesity, acne, or osteoporosis are ideal candidates for the combination regimen. Women who are pregnant or contemplating pregnancy, and patients with active neoplasia or severe cytopenia, are candidates for the single-drug regimen. The single-drug regimen may also be used in patients in whom a short treatment trial (6 months or less) is anticipated.

   The treatment schedules have been established only in patients with type 1 autoimmune hepatitis, but the same regimens are applied to all types.

2. **What are the indications for treatment?**

   The benefits of corticosteroid therapy have been demonstrated only in patients with severe inflammatory activity. Therapy in patients with less active disease has an uncertain benefit-risk ratio. The absolute indications for treatment are incapacitating symptoms, bridging necrosis or multilobular necrosis on histologic examination, and/or sustained severe biochemical abnormalities. Other findings do not compel therapy, and in patients with mild-moderate disease, the treatment decision must be individualized. Treatment is not indicated in patients with inactive or minimally active cirrhosis, patients with decompensated liver disease and mild or no inflammatory activity, and patients who are asymptomatic with histologic features of mild interface hepatitis.

3. **Are there any predictors of response to treatment?**

   No findings at presentation predict response to treatment, and no patient with absolute indications for therapy should be denied treatment, even in the presence of cirrhosis, ascites,

TABLE 20-1. RECOMMENDED TREATMENT REGIMENS

Interval Adjustments	Prednisone (mg daily)	Combination	
		Prednisone (mg daily)	Azathioprine (mg daily)
Week 1	60	30	50
Week 2	40	20	50
Week 3	30	15	50
Week 4	30	15	50
Daily maintenance until endpoint	20	10	50

TABLE 20–2.   INDICATIONS FOR CORTICOSTEROID THERAPY AND CRITERIA FOR TREATMENT SELECTION

Indications for Treatment	Criteria for Treatment Selection
Absolute	**Prednisone Regimen**
AST ≥10-fold normal	Severe cytopenia
AST ≥5-fold normal and γ-globulin ≥2-fold normal	Thiopurine methyltransferase deficiency
	Pregnancy or contemplation of pregnancy
Histologic findings of bridging necrosis or confluent necrosis	Active neoplasia
Incapacitating symptoms	Short-term (≤6 months) trial
Relative	**Combination Regimen**
Persistent symptoms	Preferred therapy
Disease progression	Postmenopausal women
Mild-moderate laboratory changes	Obesity
	Osteopenia
	Brittle diabetes
None	Labile hypertension
Interface hepatitis and no symptoms	Acne
AST <5-fold normal	Long-term (>6 months) treatment
Inactive or minimally active cirrhosis	
Liver failure with minimal inflammatory activity	

AST = aspartate aminotransferase.

hepatic encephalopathy. The principal indices of response are the serum levels of aspartate aminotransferase (AST), bilirubin, and gamma globulin. At least 90% of patients demonstrate improvement in at least one parameter within 2 weeks of therapy, and this improvement predicts immediate survival with 98% accuracy. Failure to improve a pretreatment hyperbilirubinemia within 2 weeks of therapy in a patient with multilobular necrosis invariably predicts death within 6 months. These patients should be assessed for liver transplantation. Patients who fail to enter remission within 2 years of treatment have a 43% frequency of subsequent hepatic decompensation, and the frequency of decompensation increases to 69% after 4 years of continuous therapy without remission. Typically, the first feature of decompensation is the formation of ascites, and this finding compels evaluation for liver transplantation. Long-term prognosis relates to the ability to induce remission and prevent features of liver failure.

What are the results of corticosteroid therapy?
Sixty-five percent of patients achieve clinical, biochemical, and histologic remission within 3 years of treatment (Fig. 20-1). The average duration of therapy until remission is 22 months. The probability of entering remission increases at a constant annual rate during the first 3 years of therapy, and the majority of individuals who enter remission (87%) do so within this period. Patients with and without histologic cirrhosis at presentation have 10-year life expectancies that exceed 90%. Their survival is similar to that of age- and sex-matched normal individuals from the same geographic region.

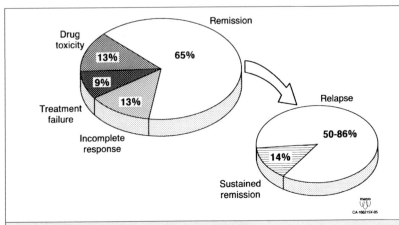

Figure 20-1. Responses to initial course of corticosteroid therapy.

Thirteen percent of patients develop drug-related side effects that prematurely limit treatment (drug toxicity). The most common serious complication is intolerable obesity or cosmetic change (47%). Osteoporosis with vertebral compression (27%), brittle diabetes (20%), and peptic ulceration (6%) restrict therapy less frequently. Patients with cirrhosis develop serious side effects more commonly than others, possibly because they have higher serum levels of unbound prednisolone as a consequence of prolonged hyperbilirubinemia and/or hypoalbuminemia. No findings at presentation predict a serious side effect, and all previously untreated patients with absolute indications for therapy, including postmenopausal women, should be managed aggressively. Serum thiopurine methyltransferase levels may be valuable assessing candidates for azathioprine therapy, especially those who have preexistent or evolving cytopenia.

Deterioration, despite compliance with therapy (treatment failure), develops in 9% of patients, and an incomplete response occurs in 13% (Fig. 20-2). Cirrhosis develops in 36% of patients within 6 years. Relapse after drug withdrawal occurs in as many as 86% of individuals who enter remission, and only 14% of patients have sustained inactivity after cessation of therapy. The risk of extrahepatic malignancy in patients receiving long-term immunosuppress therapy is 1.4-fold greater than that in an age- and sex-matched normal population (95% confidence limits, 0.6- to 2.9-fold normal). This realization underscores the importance of adhering to rigid criteria for treatment.

5. **What are the endpoints of conventional treatment?**
All therapies in treatment-naive patients should have a predefined endpoint. Therapy should n be instituted with the intention of never stopping. Conventional treatment should be continued until remission, drug toxicity, clinical deterioration (treatment failure), or confirmation of an incomplete response. Remission connotes absence of symptoms, resolution of laboratory indices of active inflammation, and histologic improvement to normal, inactive cirrhosis, or portal hepatitis. Improvement of the serum AST level to twice normal or less is compatible with remission, if the other criteria are met. Liver biopsy assessment before drug withdrawal is essential to establish remission because histologic activity may be present in 55% of patients who satisfy other requirements. Typically, histologic improvement lags behind clinical and biochemical resolution by 3–8 months, and treatment should be extended for at least this period.

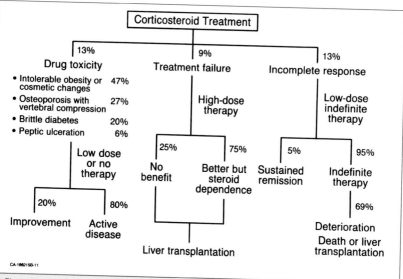

Figure 20-2. Frequency and consequences of suboptimal responses to corticosteroid therapy.

Treatment failure connotes progressive worsening of laboratory tests, persistent or recurrent symptoms, ascites formation, or features of hepatic encephalopathy, despite compliance with therapy. These changes justify an alternative treatment strategy.

The emergence of serious drug-related side effects and failure to induce remission after protracted treatment also compel modifications in therapy. The risk of serious drug toxicity exceeds the likelihood of inducing remission after 3 years of continuous administration. In these patients, an incomplete response is established, and a decreasing benefit-risk ratio justifies termination of conventional treatment.

6. When should liver biopsy be performed?

Liver biopsy should be performed at presentation to establish the diagnosis and stage of the disease. Liver biopsy is also indicated after clinical and biochemical resolution has been achieved during therapy. It is typically done 3–8 months after disappearance of the clinical and laboratory features and prior to drug withdrawal. The presence of interface hepatitis justifies continuation of treatment for another 6 months. Reversion of liver architecture to normal is the ideal treatment endpoint, and it is associated with the lowest frequency of relapse after drug withdrawal (20%). The presence of portal plasma cells in the remission biopsy specimen augurs relapse after drug withdrawal. Similarly, progression to cirrhosis during therapy identifies patients who commonly relapse after the termination of treatment. A long-term maintenance strategy with low-dose prednisone or azathioprine should be considered in these high-risk patients. Liver biopsy is justified at any time that there is worsening, despite compliance with treatment. The tissue examination may disclose a superimposed insult or the emergence of a variant syndrome.

. Does corticosteroid treatment prevent or reverse cirrhosis?

Maybe. Cirrhosis develops in 36% of patients within 6 years, despite corticosteroid treatment. Typically, it eventuates during the early, most active stages of disease, and it is less likely after induction of remission. The mean annual incidence of cirrhosis is 11% during the first 3 years of illness and 1% thereafter, despite relapse and retreatment. The presence of histologic cirrhosis during or after treatment does not diminish survival or increase morbidity. The 10-year life expectancy of such patients is 93%, the probability of esophageal varices is 13%, and the likelihood of upper gastrointestinal bleeding is 6%. Progression to cirrhosis undoubtedly reflects the difficulty in obtaining complete, rapid, and sustained suppression of inflammatory activity.

Corticosteroids have been reported to reverse cirrhosis in autoimmune hepatitis, and the medication does have antifibrogenic effects. By suppressing inflammatory activity, corticosteroids eliminate metalloproteinase inhibitors, stimulate degradation of the fibrotic liver matrix, and enhance apoptosis of hepatic stellate cells. Treatment can decrease fibrosis scores in the liver tissue, and it may decrease fibrosis in cirrhosis. Cirrhosis, however, is a complex anatomic transformation, and its disappearance during corticosteroid therapy remains controversial.

8. **Does hepatocellular carcinoma occur?**
Yes. Hepatocellular cancer may develop in patients with autoimmune hepatitis who have cirrhosis, but its occurrence is rare. Only 1 of 212 patients who have been adequately screened for viral infection (0.5%) has developed hepatocellular cancer during 1732 patient years of follow-up. Among patients with cirrhosis at presentation or subsequently, the incidence of hepatocellular cancer has been only 1 per 1002 patient years of observation, and among patients with histologic cirrhosis for at least 5 years, the incidence of primary hepatic malignancy has been only 1 per 965 patient years. The efficacy of a surveillance program in detecting early treatable tumors is uncertain, and implementation of such a program is empiric. Serum alpha-fetoprotein levels are abnormally increased in 35% of patients with severe autoimmune hepatitis, but these abnormalities are typically mild (range = 19.6–262 ng/mL). Furthermore, the abnormalities commonly resolve during corticosteroid therapy. High elevation of the serum alpha-fetoprotein level suggests neoplasm, whereas normal level never exclude the diagnosis.

9. **What is the most common treatment problem?**
Relapse after drug withdrawal is the most common management problem. Fifty percent of patients who enter remission relapse within 6 months after termination of treatment, and 70% relapse within 3 years. The frequency of relapse can be as high as 86%, and it increases after each subsequent retreatment and drug withdrawal. The risk of relapse diminishes with duration of sustained remission, but it never disappears. A sustained remission of at least 6 months is associated with only an 8% frequency of relapse.

The principal cause of relapse is premature withdrawal of medication resulting from anxiety about drug-related side effects or reliance on clinical and laboratory indices to define the endpoin of treatment. Patients who have interface hepatitis at termination of therapy, and patients who hav developed cirrhosis during treatment, invariably relapse after drug withdrawal. Relapse occurs in 50% of patients with portal hepatitis at remission and 20% of patients with normal liver tissue.

The inability to prevent relapse probably reflects failure of corticosteroid therapy to eliminat the pathogenic mechanisms. Patients with the human leukocyte antigen (HLA) A1-B8-DR3 phenotype, and those with persistence of antibodies to asialoglycoprotein receptor, antichromatin, or anti-SLA/LP may relapse more commonly than counterparts without these findings.

10. **How should relapse be managed?**
The major consequence of relapse and retreatment is the development of drug-related sid effects. The frequency of complications after the first relapse and retreatment is similar to that after the original treatment (33% vs. 29%). This frequency increases to 70% after a second relapse and retreatment. Two regimens have been used successfully in the management of multiple relapse. The objective of *indefinite low-dose prednisone therapy*

to control symptoms and maintain serum AST levels below fivefold normal on the lowest dose of medication possible. The daily dose of prednisone is reduced by 2.5 mg each month until these goals are achieved. Eighty-seven percent of patients can be managed on 10 mg of prednisone daily or less (median dose = 7.5 mg daily). Side effects that occurred during conventional therapy improve in 85%; new side effects do not develop; and mortality is similar to that of patients treated with full-dose conventional regimens (9% vs. 10%).

The objective of *indefinite azathioprine therapy* is to sustain the remission achieved during conventional corticosteroid treatment by using nonsteroidal medication. Azathioprine (2 mg/kg/day) is sufficient to control clinical and biochemical manifestations of the disease as prednisone is withdrawn. Cytopenia compels dose reduction in only 9% of patients; corticosteroid-induced side effects improve; and arthralgia associated with steroid withdrawal eventually resolves (but may be protracted). Malignancy develops in 7%, and the risk of tetragenicity is probably low. Both regimens have not been compared head-to-head, and there is no objective basis for preference. The nonsteroidal nature of azathioprine contributes to its greater popularity.

11. Do patients who have relapsed ever get off treatment?

Yes, sometimes. Previous relapse and retreatment does not preclude a sustained remission without drug. Twenty-eight percent of patients who are retreated after relapse can achieve a sustained remission. There are no predictors of sustained remission after relapse, and this outcome can only be assessed by periodic treatment withdrawal. Fifty-nine percent of patients retreated with conventional drug regimens, and 12% of patients retreated with low-dose prednisone or azathioprine maintenance regimens achieve this endpoint. The probability of entering a sustained remission after initial treatment or after relapse and retreatment is 47% after 10 years. Because the consequences of relapse in a closely monitored patient is well tolerated and effectively treated, drug withdrawal should be attempted in all patients with inactive disease. Withdrawal attempts can be repeated each year of treatment, if necessary.

2. How should treatment failure be managed?

High-dose prednisone (60 mg/day) or prednisone (30 mg/day) in conjunction with azathioprine (150 mg/day) induces clinical and biochemical remission in 75% of patients within 2 years. The doses of medication are reduced each month of clinical and biochemical improvement until conventional maintenance doses are achieved. Histologic remission occurs in less than 20% of patients, and the majority who fail treatment become corticosteroid-dependent and at risk for disease progression and drug-related complications. Limited studies have suggested the advantage of 6-mercaptopurine (6-MP) over azathioprine in treatment failure. The drug may have different absorption characteristics or metabolic pathways that favor its use. The initial dose of 12.5–25 mg/day can be increased as tolerated to 1.5 mg/kg/day. Pharmacokinetic studies in patients with cirrhosis have not demonstrated a sufficient disturbance in the conversion of prednisone to prednisolone to justify use of the latter drug. Decompensations unresponsive to high-dose corticosteroid therapy justify liver transplantation evaluation.

3. How effective is liver transplantation?

Liver transplantation is an excellent treatment for patients with decompensated disease. The 5-year life expectancy of the patient and graft after transplantation ranges from 83–92%, and the actuarial 10-year survival after transplantation is 75%. The autoantibodies and hypergammaglobulinemia disappear within 2 years. Disease recurs in at least 17% of patients, usually as a result of inadequate immunosuppression, and it is controlled by adjustments in this regimen. Progression to cirrhosis and graft failure have been reported, and patients with autoimmune hepatitis may be at increased risk of developing acute rejection, steroid-resistant rejection, and chronic rejection. Corticosteroid withdrawal may be difficult in patients transplanted for autoimmune hepatitis, and one strategy has been to continue corticosteroids for at least 1 year after surgery.

14. **When should autoimmune hepatitis be considered after transplantation?**
Autoimmune hepatitis should be considered in all patients with graft dysfunction after liver transplantation. Recurrent autoimmune hepatitis is possible within 1–8 years after transplantation, and de novo autoimmune hepatitis occurs in 3–5% of patients transplanted for nonautoimmune liver diseases. De novo autoimmune hepatitis develops typically in children, especially in those receiving cyclosporine, but adults can also be afflicted. Recurrent and de novo disease respond to corticosteroid therapy. The prognosis of de novo autoimmune hepatitis is poor, if untreated.

15. **What strategy is best for patients with drug toxicity or incomplete response?**
There are no confident treatment guidelines for patients with drug toxicity or incomplete response. Management is empirical, and outcomes must be monitored closely. In the former instance, the dose of the offending medication is reduced to the lowest possible level or withdrawn fully. Disease activity is controlled by the alternative, presumably tolerated, medication (prednisone or azathioprine), and its dose is adjusted in accordance with the response. In the latter instance, the medication is reduced to the lowest level possible to prevent symptoms and maintain serum AST levels below fivefold normal. Patients may eventually decompensate and require liver transplantation. Novel therapies for steroid intolerance, such as cyclosporine (5–6 mg/kg/day) and mycophenolate mofetil (2 gm/day), have been used empirically, and preliminary results have been encouraging. Empirical treatments with such drugs lack predefined endpoints, and they have an uncertain risk for serious long-term complications.

16. **What are the variant syndromes?**
Codification of the diagnostic criteria for autoimmune hepatitis has highlighted the presence of many conditions with autoimmune features that lack classical findings or that have mixed manifestations. Disorders with features of two different diseases are designated "overlap syndromes," and they include patients with autoimmune hepatitis and primary biliary cirrhosis and patients with autoimmune hepatitis and primary sclerosing cholangitis. Disorders with features that are inconsistent with the diagnosis of autoimmune hepatitis or insufficient for classification in another diagnostic category are "outlier syndromes," and they include patients with autoimmune cholangitis and cryptogenic chronic hepatitis ("autoantibody-negative autoimmune hepatitis"). The variant syndromes are detectable in 18% of patients with autoimmune liver disease, and they should be sought in all individuals with autoimmune features who respond poorly to corticosteroid therapy.

The principal manifestation of a variant syndrome is cholestasis in conjunction with hepatitis. Antimitochondrial antibodies, inflammatory bowel disease, pruritus, disproportionate elevation of the serum alkaline phosphatase level, hyperlipidemia, and/or histologic changes that suggest bile duct destruction and/or loss are clues to its presence. The cholestatic findings justify cholangiography and a management strategy suited for the predominant manifestations. Marked hepatocellular disease should be treated with corticosteroids; prominent cholestatic features should be treated with ursodeoxycholic acid (13–15 mg/kg/day); and comparably mixed hepatocellular and cholestatic findings warrant combination therapy with corticosteroids and ursodeoxycholic acid. Treatments are empirical and continued as a 3- to 6-month trial. None has been shown effective, especially in reversing the histologic findings, and serum alkaline phosphatase levels greater than twofold normal identify individuals who are unlikely to benefit from corticosteroids.

17. **What about patients with mixed autoimmune and viral features?**

Most patients with mixed autoimmune and viral features have true viral infection and low-titer autoantibodies that have no diagnostic, clinical, or therapeutic relevance. These patients have chronic viral hepatitis with autoimmune features, and antiviral therapy should be instituted as indicated (Fig. 20-3). Rarely, patients with autoimmune hepatitis have either false positive markers for viral infection or true coincidental viral infection. Patients with false-positive viral markers respond well to corticosteroids, and the false-positive virologic reactions usually disappear. Patients with true viral infection and high titers of smooth muscle antibodies (SMA) and/or antinuclear antibodies (ANA) (titers ≥1:320) and histologic changes of moderate-to-severe interface hepatitis with portal lymphoplasmacytic infiltration have autoimmune hepatitis with coincidental viral infection. Treatment must be directed against the predominant disorder, and corticosteroids are justified, if the diagnosis is autoimmune hepatitis. Antiviral therapy may be instituted later, if viral-predominant manifestations emerge and corticosteroids are withdrawn.

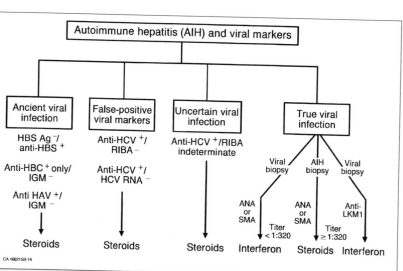

Figure 20-3. Treatment strategies for patients with autoimmune hepatitis (AIH) and viral markers. Patients with true viral infection require liver biopsy assessment to establish the presence of histologic patterns consistent with viral infection (viral biopsy) or AIH. Clinical, laboratory, and histologic changes of AIH, including high-titer autoantibodies, suggest AIH with coincidental viral infection. Empirical treatment of the predominant syndrome with corticosteroids can be instituted and monitored closely.

8. **What new immunosuppressant therapies are promising?**

Drugs have evolved from the transplantation arena, which provide better blanket immunosuppression than prednisone and azathioprine (Table 20-3).

9. **What new site-specific treatment interventions are promising?**

Greater knowledge about the pathogenesis of autoimmune hepatitis has suggested certain site-specific interventions that require further testing (Table 20-4).

TABLE 20–3. PROMISING NEW THERAPIES OFFERING BLANKET IMMUNOSUPPRESSION

Agent	Putative Actions	Experience
Cyclosporine	Inhibits lymphokine release Prevents cytotoxic T-cell expansion	Anecdotal in steroid-intoleran or recalcitrant disease
Tacrolimus	Prevents effector cell expansion Inhibits IL-2 receptor Impairs antibody production	Limited open trial beneficial Never used to remission Stimulates experimental fibrogenesis
Ursodeoxycholic acid	Suppresses class I HLA display Impairs cytokine production Inhibits apoptosis	Anecdotal benefit in treatment-naïve mild diseas No advantage in problematic patients
Budesonide	2nd generation steroid High hepatic 1st pass clearance Metabolites devoid of steroid activity	Anecdotal benefit in treatment-naïve mild diseas No advantage in problematic patients Steroid side effects
Deflazacort	Prednisolone derivative Less diabetogenic	Efficacy comparable to prednisone in open-label trial Uncertain side-effect profile
Mycophenolate mofetil	"Prodrug" metabolized to mycophenolic acid Prevents purine synthesis during lymphocyte activation Lymphocyte-specific actions	Anecdotal success in steroid recalcitrance
Rapamycin	Similar to tacrolimus Blocks IL-2, IL-4, and IL-6 signals Prevents effector cell expansion	Theoretical value Untested
6-mercaptopurine	Metabolite of azathioprine Possibly better absorption Different metabolic pathways	Anecdotal success in treatmen failure and steroid intolerance

HLA = human leukocyte antigen, IL = interleukin.

TABLE 20–4.   PROMISING NEW THERAPIES BASED ON SITE–SPECIFIC INTERVENTIONS

Agent	Putative Actions	Experience
Blocking peptides	Displaces autoantigenic peptide from antigen-binding groove of class II HLA DR molecule	Theoretical Untested
Soluble CTLA-4	Blocks ligation of B7 to CD28 and prevents CD4 T-helper cell activation	Successful in preventing rejection after mismatched bone marrow transplantation
T-cell vaccination	Eliminates cytotoxic T-cell clones	Effective in prevention and treatment of experimental hepatitis
Oral tolerance	Induces nonresponsiveness to fed antigen Causes suppression or clonal anergy, depending on antigen dose	Limited success in experimental and human autoimmune encephalitis, diabetes, rheumatoid arthritis
Recombinant interleukin-10	Bolsters type 2 cytokine response May down-regulate cytotoxic type 1 cytokine response	Theoretical Untested
Antibodies to TNF-alpha	Suppresses pro-inflammatory cytokine May impair cytotoxic type 1 cytokine response	Theoretical Untested
Gene therapy	Replaces or counteracts critical susceptibility gene, autoimmune promoter gene, or immunocyte activator gene Delivers genes to promote regeneration and resistance to fibrosis	Theoretical value Untested

TNF = tumor necrosis factor, HLA = human leukocyte antigen, CTLA = cytotoxic T lymphocyte antigen.

WEBSITES

1. http://www.aasld.org/

2. http://www.aasld.org/eweb/docs/autoimmune_hepatitis.pdf

BIBLIOGRAPHY

1. Czaja AJ: Autoimmune hepatitis after liver transplantation and other lessons of self-intolerance. Liver Transp 8:505–513, 2002.

2. Czaja AJ: Frequency and nature of the variant syndromes of autoimmune liver disease. Hepatology 28:360– 1998.

3. Czaja AJ: Treatment of autoimmune hepatitis. Semin Liver Dis 22:365–377, 2002.

4. Czaja AJ: Treatment strategies in autoimmune hepatitis. Clin Liver Dis 6:799–824, 2002.

5. Czaja AJ, Carpenter HA: Histological features associated with relapse after corticosteroid withdrawal in type autoimmune hepatitis. Liver Int 23:116–123, 2003.

6. Czaja AJ, Cookson S, Constantini PK, et al: Cytokine polymorphisms associated with clinical features and tre ment outcome in type 1 autoimmune hepatitis. Gastroenterology 117:645–652, 1999.

7. Czaja AJ, Doherty DG, Donaldson PT: Genetic bases of autoimmune hepatitis. Dig Dis Sci 47:2139–2150, 20

8. Czaja AJ, Freese DK: Diagnosis and treatment of autoimmune hepatitis. Hepatology 36:479–497, 2002.

9. Czaja AJ, Menon KVN, Carpenter HA: Sustained remission after corticosteroid therapy for type 1 autoimmur hepatitis: A retrospective analysis. Hepatology 35:890–897, 2002.

10. Czaja AJ, Norman GL: Antibodies in the diagnosis and management of liver disease. J Clin Gastroenterol 37:315–329, 2003.

CHAPTER 21

PRIMARY BILIARY CIRRHOSIS AND PRIMARY SCLEROSING CHOLANGITIS

Jayant A. Talwalkar, MD, MPH, and Nicholas F. LaRusso, MD

1. **Define *primary biliary cirrhosis* and *primary sclerosing cholangitis*.**

   Primary biliary cirrhosis (PBC) and primary sclerosing cholangitis (PSC) are chronic cholestatic liver diseases of unknown etiology in adults. PBC affects mainly women in the sixth decade of life and is characterized by destruction of interlobular and septal bile ducts. PSC affects mainly men in the fifth decade of life and is characterized by diffuse inflammation and fibrosis of the intrahepatic and extrahepatic bile ducts. Both PBC and PSC may progress eventually to end-stage liver disease requiring consideration for liver transplantation.

2. **Is primary biliary cirrhosis an autoimmune disorder?**

   Yes. The underlying cause of PBC is unknown. Evidence for an autoimmune etiology includes the following:

   - Frequent association with other autoimmune diseases, such as Sjögren's syndrome, rheumatoid arthritis, scleroderma/CREST (the syndrome consisting of *c*alcinosis, *R*aynaud's phenomenon, *e*sophageal disease, *s*clerodactyly, and *t*elangiectasia), thyroiditis, lichen planus, discoid lupus, and pemphigoid
   - Presence of circulating serum autoantibodies, such as antimitochondrial antibody (AMA), antinuclear antibody (ANA), antismooth muscle antibody (ASMA), extractable nuclear antigen (ENA), rheumatoid factor, thyroid-specific antibodies, and elevated serum immunoglobulin M (IgM) levels
   - Histologic features, including lymphoplasmacytic cholangitis with portal tract expansion indicative of immunologic bile duct destruction
   - Familial clustering among patients with PBC
   - Increased prevalence of circulating serum autoantibodies in relatives of patients with PBC
   - Increased frequency of class II major histocompatibility complex (MHC) antigens in PBC.

3. **Is primary sclerosing cholangitis an autoimmune disorder?**

   Yes. The evidence supporting an immunogenic origin for PSC includes the following:

   - 70–80% prevalence of inflammatory bowel disease among patients with PSC in Europe and North America
   - Increased incidence of PSC and chronic ulcerative colitis in families of patients with PSC
   - Evidence for immune system dysregulation, including increased serum levels of IgM, serum autoantibodies such as ANA, ASMA, and peripheral antineutrophil cytoplasmic antigen (pANCA), circulating immune complexes, and abnormalities in peripheral blood lymphocyte subsets
   - Increased frequency of human leukocyte antigens (HLAs) B8, DR3a, and DR4
   - Aberrant expression of HLA class II antigen on bile duct epithelial cells.

4. **Do viral infections have a role in the development of primary sclerosing cholangitis?**

   Yes. Viral agents such as respiratory enteric orphan (REO) virus type III and cytomegalovirus, which are capable of infecting the biliary tree, have been implicated in the development of PSC. Therefore, a hypothesis of viral-mediated immune system activation with subsequent immunologically mediated bile duct destruction has been proposed. However, no direct evidence has linked these or other viruses to the development of PSC.

5. **What are the clinical features of primary biliary cirrhosis and primary sclerosing cholangitis?**

The clinical presentations of both PBC and PSC may be similar, although some demographic clinical characteristics differ. Between 85% and 90% of patients with PBC are women present in the fourth to sixth decades of life, whereas 70% of patients with PSC are men with an approximate age of 40 years at diagnosis. Despite an increasing frequency of asymptomatic subclinical disease, affected patients with either condition present generally with the gradual onset of fatigue and pruritus. Right upper quadrant pain and anorexia may also be observed diagnosis. Although uncommon, steatorrhea in PBC and PSC is due usually to bile salt malabsorption, pancreatic exocrine insufficiency, or coexisting celiac disease. Jaundice as a primary manifestation of PBC is uncommon but strongly associated with the presence of advanced histologic disease. In PSC, the development of bacterial cholangitis characterized b recurrent fever, right upper quadrant pain, and jaundice may occur. A history of previous reconstructive biliary surgery, the presence of dominant extrahepatic biliary strictures, or the development of a superimposed cholangiocarcinoma may be responsible. The symptoms of end-stage liver disease, such as gastrointestinal bleeding, ascites, and encephalopathy, occur late in the course of both diseases.

6. **What are the common findings on physical examination?**

Physical examination may reveal jaundice and excoriations from pruritus in both disorders. Xanthelasmas (raised lesions over the eyelids from cholesterol deposition) and xanthomas (lesions over the extensor surfaces) are occasionally seen in the late stages of both diseases, particularly PBC. Hyperpigmentation (especially in sun-exposed areas) and vitiligo may be present. The liver is usually enlarged and firm to palpation. The spleen may also be palpable, portal hypertension from advanced disease has developed. Characteristics of end-stage liver disease, including muscle wasting and spider angiomata, appear in the advanced stages of bc diseases.

7. **What diseases are associated with primary biliary cirrhosis?**

Up to 80% of patients with PBC also have coexistent extrahepatic autoimmune diseases. The most common extrahepatic autoimmune disease is sicca (Sjögren's) syndrome. Other conditions described in association with PBC include autoimmune thyroiditis, scleroderma/CREST, rheumatoid arthritis, dermatomyositis, mixed connective tissue disease, systemic lupus erythematosus, renal tubular acidosis, and idiopathic pulmonary fibrosis.

8. **What diseases are associated with primary sclerosing cholangitis?**

Chronic ulcerative colitis (CUC) and, less frequently, Crohn's colitis are present in at least 70–80% of patients with PSC. The disease activity of CUC in PSC is usually quiescent; in 80% patients, CUC is either asymptomatic or mildly symptomatic when PSC is diagnosed. CUC ma also be diagnosed after the recognition of PSC. Although reports of CUC have been described association with PBC, this is still considered quite uncommon.

9. **What important biochemical abnormalities are associated with primary biliary cirrhosis and primary sclerosing cholangitis?**

In both disorders, serum alkaline phosphatase is elevated at least three to four times the uppe limit of normal with mild-to-moderate elevations in alanine aminotransferase (ALT) and aspartate aminotransferase (AST). In PBC, total serum bilirubin values are usually within norn limits at diagnosis. In PSC, serum bilirubin values are modestly increased in up to 50% of patients at the time of diagnosis. Tests reflective of synthetic liver function, including serum albumin and prothrombin time, remain normal unless advanced liver disease is present. Serum immunoglobulin M (IgM) levels are elevated in 90% of patients with PBC. Tests related to copper metabolism are virtually always abnormal in both diseases, reflecting the influence of chronic cholestasis. Based on the widespread use of automated blood chemistries, an increasing number of asymptomatic patients with PBC and PSC are being diagnosed.

10. **What is the lipid profile in patients with primary biliary cirrhosis? Are they at increased risk for developing coronary artery disease?**
Serum cholesterol levels are usually elevated in PBC. In the early stages of disease, increases in high-density lipoprotein (HDL) cholesterol exceed those of low-density lipoprotein (LDL) and very-low-density lipoprotein (VLDL). With liver disease progression, the concentration of HDL decreases while LDL concentrations become markedly elevated. An increased risk for atherosclerotic disease has not been demonstrated among patients with persistent hyperlipidemia in association with PBC.

11. **What serum autoantibodies are associated with primary biliary cirrhosis?**
Serum AMA is found in up to 95% of patients with PBC. Although considered nonorgan-specific as well as nonspecies-specific, serum AMA is usually detected by an enzyme-linked immunosorbent assay (ELISA). However, antibodies directed against a specific group of antigens on the inner mitochondrial membrane (M2 antigens) are present in 98% of patients with PBC. This subtyping of serum AMA increases the sensitivity and specificity for disease detection.

Other AMA subtypes related to PBC react with antigens on the outer mitochondrial membrane. Anti-M4 occurs in association with anti-M2 in patients with overlap syndromes of autoimmune hepatitis and PBC. Anti-M8, when present with anti-M2, may be associated with a more rapid course of disease progression in selected patients. Anti-M9 has been observed with and without anti-M2 and may be helpful in the diagnosis of early-stage PBC.

12. **What serum autoantibodies are associated with primary sclerosing cholangitis?**
In PSC, serum AMA is rare and, if present, is usually seen in very low titers. However, detectable titers of serum ANA, ASMA, and antithyroperoxidase antibodies have been found in up to 70% of patients with PSC.
Periantineutrophil cytoplasmic antibody (pANCA) has been observed in up to 65% of patients with PSC. However, the finding of pANCA among patients with ulcerative colitis and no evidence of PSC limits its diagnostic utility. Anticardiolipin antibodies are also increased in patients with PSC.

13. **What are the cholangiographic features of the biliary tree in primary sclerosing cholangitis?**
Evaluation of the biliary tree in PSC by endoscopic or percutaneous transhepatic cholangiography may reveal diffuse stricturing of both intrahepatic and extrahepatic ducts with saccular dilatation of intervening areas. These abnormalities result in the characteristic "beads-on-a-string" appearance seen with PSC (Fig. 21-1). Exclusive intrahepatic and hilar involvement occurs in only 20% of patients. Hepaticolithiasis is observed in 10–20% of cases.

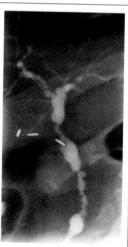

Figure 21-1. Retrograde cholangiogram exhibiting classic features of PSC, including diffuse stricturing and beading of intrahepatic and extrahepatic bile ducts. (From LaRusso NF, Wiesner RH, Ludwig J, et al: Current concepts. Primary sclerosing cholangitis. N Engl J Med 310:899–903, 1984, with permission.)

The presence of a dominant stricture should raise the question of cholangiocarcinoma as a complication of PSC. Increasing experience with magnetic resonance cholangiography (MRC) suggests that this noninvasive diagnostic approach is accurate in over 90% of cases diagnosed as PSC compared to invasive cholangiography.

14. **Is it important to evaluate the biliary tree in primary biliary cirrhosis?**
Sometimes. In PBC, an ultrasound examination of the biliary tree is usually adequate to exclude the presence of extrahepatic biliary obstruction. However, in patients with atypical features, such as male sex, AMA seronegativity, or associated inflammatory bowel disease, a cholangiogram should be considered to distinguish PBC from PSC and other disorders causing biliary obstruction.

15. **What are the hepatic histologic features of primary biliary cirrhosis and primary sclerosing cholangitis?**

Histologic abnormalities on liver biopsy are highly characteristic of both PBC and PSC in the early stages of disease. In PBC, the diagnostic finding is described as a "florid duct lesion," which reveals bile duct destruction and granuloma formation (Fig. 21-2). A severe lymphoplasmacytic inflammatory cell infiltrate in the portal tracts is accompanied by the segmental degeneration of interlobular bile ducts (also termed *chronic nonsuppurative destructive cholangitis*).

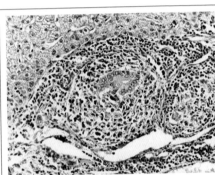

Figure 21-2. Florid duct lesion (granulomatous bile duct destruction) in PBC. A poorly formed granuloma surrounds and destroys the bile duct in an eccentric fashion.

Early histologic changes in PSC include enlargement of portal tracts by edema, increased portal and periportal fibrosis, and proliferation of interlobular bile ducts (Fig. 21-3). The diagnostic morphologic abnormality in PSC is termed *fibrous obliterative cholangitis*, which leads to the complete loss of interlobular and adjacent septal bile ducts from fibrous chord and connective tissue deposition. This histologic feature, however, occurs in only 10% of known cases. The histologic findings of end-stage liver disease for PBC and PSC are characterized by a paucity of bile ducts and biliary cirrhosis.

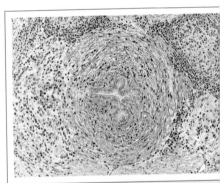

Figure 21-3. Fibrous obliterative cholangitis in PSC. The interlobular bile duct shows a typical fibrous collar, and epithelium seems undamaged.

16. **Do asymptomatic patients with primary biliary cirrhosis have a normal life expectancy?**
No. Most patients with PBC experience a progressive clinical course resulting in eventual cirrhosis. Asymptomatic patients have a longer median survival than symptomatic patients. However, a reduced median survival in asymptomatic PBC patients compared to age- and se

matched healthy populations is observed. Estimates of overall median survival without liver transplantation range between 10 and 12 years from the time of diagnosis; advanced histologic disease imparts a median survival approaching 8 years. Elevations of total bilirubin above 8–10 mg/dL have been associated with a median life expectancy of 2 years without liver transplantation.

17. **Do asymptomatic patients with primary sclerosing cholangitis have a normal life expectancy?**

No. Although some patients with PSC show no evidence for disease progression for many years, most published investigations support the contention that PSC is a progressive disease that ultimately can lead to liver failure and death without liver transplantation. A median survival of 9–12 years from the time of diagnosis in all patients with PSC appears to be independent of geographic and environmental influences.

18. **What is the role of mathematical models in estimating survival for primary biliary cirrhosis and primary sclerosing cirrhosis?**

The development of mathematical models for both PBC and PSC has improved the ability to predict rates of disease progression and survival without liver transplantation. They are useful for stratifying patients by survival risk, developing endpoints of treatment failure, and designing therapeutic trials. The use of these models in defining the optimal selection of patients and timing for liver transplantation has been the subject of several investigations.

A prognostic model for PBC developed at the Mayo Clinic relies on clinical and biochemical parameters, including total serum bilirubin, albumin, prothrombin time, presence or absence of peripheral edema, and the patient's age. In PSC, the important variables that predict survival include the patient's age, total serum bilirubin, presence of splenomegaly, and histologic stage by liver biopsy. A revision of the Mayo Clinic PSC model (substituting a history of variceal bleeding for histologic stage) continues to provide similar prognostic information without the need for invasive procedures, such as a liver biopsy.

19. **What vitamin deficiencies are associated with primary biliary cirrhosis and primary sclerosing cholangitis?**

Patients with PBC and PSC are susceptible to fat-soluble vitamin deficiencies, especially in advanced stages of disease. The occurrence of diminished visual acuity at night can be attributed to vitamin A deficiency. Vitamin D deficiency occurs commonly in association with marked steatorrhea, which is related to a decrease in duodenal bile acid concentration. The development of metabolic bone disease in PBC and PSC is associated, in part, with vitamin D deficiency. Prolongation of serum prothrombin time is associated with vitamin K deficiency. Finally, vitamin E deficiency occurs uncommonly but, when severe, may result in neurologic abnormalities affecting the posterior spinal columns, leading to areflexia, loss of proprioception, and ataxia.

20. **What bone disease is associated with primary biliary cirrhosis and primary sclerosing cholangitis?**

Metabolic bone disease (i.e., hepatic osteodystrophy) is a serious complication of both PBC and PSC. Clinical manifestations include osteopenia, osteoporosis, and fracture. Both vitamin D deficiency and smoking have been implicated as risk factors for metabolic bone disease. Risk factors for osteoporosis include advancing age, low body mass index, previous history of fractures, and advanced histologic disease. Severe bone pain in an acute or chronic setting related to avascular necrosis (AVN) may also occur in PBC and PSC.

. **What liver-related complications are specific to primary sclerosing cholangitis?**

Complications specific to PSC include recurrent bacterial cholangitis, dominant stricturing of the extrahepatic bile ducts, and cholangiocarcinoma. Bacterial cholangitis is frequent in patients with a history of previous biliary surgery or dominant stricture formation. Dominant strictures

occur in approximately 15–20% of patients with PSC during the natural course of disease. Th
often involve the hilum but can equally affect the common bile duct. Dominant strictures are
frequently associated with asymptomatic elevations in serum liver biochemistries or the acut
onset of symptoms, including jaundice, pruritus, and bacterial cholangitis.

Between 10% and 15% of patients with PSC will develop cholangiocarcinoma during the
course of disease. The annual risk for cholangiocarcinoma is estimated between 1% and 1.
per year. Between 30% and 50% of patients are diagnosed with cholangiocarcinoma within
2 years of identifying PSC. Early detection of cholangiocarcinoma remains difficult, based
the insensitivity of mucosal biopsy and brush cytology. The detection of elevated serum
CA19-9 levels >100 U/L may herald the existence of clinically detectable cholangiocarcinom
in patients with PSC.

22. **What is the differential diagnosis of primary biliary cirrhosis and primary
sclerosing cholangitis?**
The differential diagnosis of PBC and PSC includes other causes of chronic cholestasis,
including extrahepatic biliary obstruction due to choledocholithiasis, iatrogenic strictures, ar
tumors. Although ultrasound or computed tomography may suggest the presence of biliary
dilation, the performance of cholangiography is required to render a definitive diagnosis of P
Drug-induced cholestasis secondary to phenothiazines, estrogens, azoles, and a number of
other drugs should also be considered as alternative diagnoses.

23. **Define *autoimmune cholangitis*. How is it related to primary biliary cirrhosis**
Recent observations have documented a group of patients with PBC and no detectable serur
AMA. The presence of significant titers (>1:40) of serum ANA and/or ASMA is observed in th
setting as well. The terms *autoimmune cholangitis* and *AMA-negative PBC* have been applie
such patients. The clinical course and response to therapy with ursodeoxycholic acid (UDCA
however, are the same as in patients with AMA-positive PBC.

24. **What is meant by an *overlap syndrome* in primary biliary cirrhosis and prima
sclerosing cholangitis?**
The presence of features consistent with both autoimmune hepatitis (AIH) and PBC is define
an overlap syndrome. Both serum ANA and AMA are present with increased titers by serolog
testing. Lymphocytic piecemeal necrosis and plasma cell infiltration with bile duct destructi
are commonly seen. This group appears to benefit from immunosuppressive treatment. Usi
strict criteria, less than 20% of patients with PBC actually have objective evidence for an ove
syndrome with AIH.

Similar overlap occurs in PSC in both adult and pediatric populations. The multifocal bilia
stricturing and dilation typical of PSC is often accompanied by histologic lesions seen in AIF
patients with features of AIH and inflammatory bowel disease, cholangiography is recommen
to exclude PSC, especially in the presence of abnormal serum liver biochemistries reflective
cholestasis. Patients with AIH-PSC overlap syndrome may benefit from immunosuppressive
therapy. Using strict criteria, less than 5% of patients with PSC will have objective evidence f
overlap syndrome with AIH.

25. **What is meant by *small duct* primary sclerosing cholangitis?**
Small duct PSC is defined by the presence of chronic cholestatic liver test abnormalities, liv
histology compatible with PSC, and a normal biliary tree by cholangiography. Most patients
have a concurrent diagnosis of inflammatory bowel disease, but this may not be absolutely
required in some cases. Approximately 10–40% of patients will progress to typical PSC ove
time. Histologic disease progression may occur without biliary tract involvement and can le
hepatic failure necessitating liver transplantation. The median survival of patients with sma
duct PSC is favorable compared to individuals with typical PSC but reduced compared to th
general population.

Describe the treatment of pruritus in patients with primary biliary cirrhosis and primary sclerosing cholangitis.

Pruritus is a frequent complication of both diseases and creates difficult management options for patients with moderate to severe involvement. Cholestyramine relieves the itching associated with PBC and PSC in patients with cholestasis. In addition, it increases the intestinal excretion of bile acids by preventing their absorption. It is administered in 4-gm doses (mixed with liquids) with meals or after breakfast for a total daily dose of 12–16 gm. Cholestyramine should be given 1.5 hours before or after other medications to avoid nonspecific binding and diminished intestinal absorption. Once the itching remits, the dosage should be reduced to the minimal amount that maintains relief.

Rifampin at a dose of 300–600 mg/day also has been effective in relieving pruritus due to either p450 enzyme induction or inhibition of bile acid uptake. Novel approaches for the treatment of severe or refractory pruritus include phototherapy and charcoal hemoperfusion for the removal of bile acids. Intractable pruritus resolves following liver transplantation.

How is osteopenia treated in patients with primary biliary cirrhosis and primary sclerosing cholangitis?

There is no identified effective therapy for metabolic bone disease associated with PBC and PSC. As mentioned earlier, this is due most often to osteoporosis and, infrequently, to osteomalacia. However, low serum vitamin D levels can be corrected by administering 50,000 U up to three times/week with calcium 1000–1200 mg/day.

Estrogen replacement therapy (ERT), especially when instituted soon after menopause, has been associated with the slowing of bone loss in women. In cholestatic patients, ERT was thought previously to be contraindicated because of the risk for drug-induced cholestasis. However, this problem does not appear to be associated with standard ERT, which was shown to improve osteoporosis in a recent retrospective study. It is prudent, however, to institute clinical and biochemical monitoring of treated patients within 2–3 months after starting estrogen therapy. Recent concerns about the safety of ERT, however, have resulted in diminished enthusiasm for its use. A number of studies have described improvements or stability in bone mineral density with the use of bisphosphonate therapy. However, none of these studies has used fracture rate as a primary endpoint.

Describe the treatment of fat-soluble vitamin deficiency in primary biliary cirrhosis and primary sclerosing cholangitis.

Problems with night vision due to vitamin A deficiency may be alleviated by oral replacement therapy. Decreased serum levels can be corrected with the oral administration of vitamin A (25,000–50,000 U) two or three times/week. Because excessive vitamin A intake has been associated with hepatotoxicity, serum levels should be monitored frequently. In patients with low vitamin E levels, oral replacement therapy with 400 U/day can be instituted. If prothrombin time (PT) levels improve after a trial of water-soluble vitamin K (5–10 mg/day for 1 week), patients should be maintained on this regimen indefinitely. Prolongation of PT may be associated with hepatic failure in treatment unresponsive cases.

Do lipid-lowering agents have a role in treatment of primary biliary cirrhosis and primary sclerosing cholangitis?

No. Because patients with PBC and PSC do not appear to have an increased risk of atherosclerotic disease, despite high serum cholesterol levels, lipid-lowering agents are not usually recommended. In some patients with xanthelasma, cholestyramine may stabilize or even decrease the size of subcutaneous lipid deposits.

Describe the treatment of bacterial cholangitis in primary sclerosing cholangitis.

Bacterial cholangitis in PSC should be treated with broad-spectrum parenteral antibiotics. This results in high biliary concentrations and has broad gram-negative and gram-positive coverage.

Prophylactic therapy with oral fluoroquinolone, such as ciprofloxacin may reduce the freque
recurrent cholangitis, although no controlled trial has been performed to support this conclu

31. **What are the therapeutic options for biliary strictures in primary sclerosing cholangitis?**

Balloon dilation of dominant strictures by either transhepatic or endoscopic approaches
relieve biliary obstruction in PSC. Balloon dilation is most effective in patients with acu
elevations of total serum bilirubin level or recent onset of bacterial cholangitis. It appe
less effective in patients with long-standing jaundice or a history of recurrent bacterial
cholangitis. The role for long-term endoscopic stent placement and exchange for recur
PSC-related strictures, however, has not been assessed in a prospective controlled tria
setting. Concerns regarding an increased rate of stent-related infection suggest their
cautious use at this time.

32. **Describe the role of transjugular intrahepatic portosystemic shunt (TIPS) i
primary biliary cirrhosis and primary sclerosing cholangitis.**

TIPS rapidly decompresses the portal system with subsequent reduction in local venous
pressure within both esophageal and gastric varices. TIPS placement is indicated for refra
variceal bleeding or recalcitrant ascites from end-stage liver disease. In patients with PSC
have undergone proctocolectomy because of CUC, the development of peristomal varices
subsequent transfusion-dependent bleeding has been shown to resolve after TIPS placem
Serial Doppler ultrasound examinations every 3–6 months are required to exclude the pos
of TIPS shunt stenosis or occlusion.

33. **What medical agents have been tried for the treatment of primary biliary cirrhosis?**

A number of potential treatments for PBC have been evaluated to date with the primary goa
stabilizing or halting disease progression. Pharmacologic agents (such as colchicine,
corticosteroids, cyclosporine, azathioprine, and methotrexate) have demonstrated margin
clinical benefit and significant adverse effects. Currently, UDCA (13–15 mg/kg/day) is the
FDA-approved medical therapy for PBC. The efficacy of UDCA as medical therapy for PBC
recently been questioned in a meta-analysis of randomized, controlled trials. However, in f
the largest randomized, placebo-controlled clinical trials, UDCA in doses of 13–15 mg/kg/
associated with an estimated 30% risk reduction in the time to treatment failure or liver
transplantation compared to placebo or inactive therapy. However, an estimated 30–40% c
patients do not achieve a complete biochemical response after 6 months of UDCA, which p
them at increased risk for histologic disease progression.

34. **What medical agents have been tried for the treatment of primary sclerosing cholangitis?**

Because of the variable nature of disease progression in PSC, the development of randomi
clinical trials for the assessment of medical therapies in PSC has been difficult. As a
consequence, no identified effective treatment is available. As with PBC, the use of
pharmacologic agents (such as D-penicillamine, colchicine, corticosteroids) have not confe
significant clinical benefit. UDCA in standard doses (13–15 mg/kg/day) appears to improve
biochemical parameters, but no significant effect on histology or survival has been observe
Higher doses of UDCA (20–30 mg/kg/day) were observed to improve biochemical,
cholangiographic, and Mayo risk scores in two pilot investigations. Subsequent randomize
controlled trials of high-dose UDCA are currently underway.

35. **Describe the mechanism of action for ursodeoxycholic acid in primary bilia cirrhosis.**

UDCA is a hydrophilic, nonhepatotoxic compound that acts by attenuating the effect of
endogenous hydrophobic bile acids, some of which are believed to be hepatotoxic. Alteratio

the bile acid pool may occur by competition for ileal uptake sites or by direct action at the hepatocyte level. In addition, UDCA may reduce class I and class II HLA expression on hepatocytes and biliary epithelial cells.

What is the role of reconstructive biliary tract surgery in primary sclerosing cholangitis?
Choledochoduodenostomy and choledochojejunostomy are palliative measures to alleviate symptoms related to biliary obstruction. Reconstructive surgery does not have a beneficial effect on the natural history of PSC, particularly in patients with advanced liver disease. The development of postoperative bacterial cholangitis occurs in greater than 60% of patients. In addition, an increased risk for technical difficulty, increased blood product use, and mortality during liver transplantation have been associated with previous biliary reconstructive surgery. At most centers, however, reconstructive biliary tract surgery is rarely performed for PSC because of improvements in endoscopic approaches to therapy.

Does proctocolectomy in patients with primary sclerosing cholangitis and chronic ulcerative colitis favorably affect hepatobiliary disease?
No. Proctocolectomy has not been shown to have a beneficial effect on clinical outcome or survival in PSC. Currently, there is no indication to remove the colon in a patient with PSC in anticipation of a beneficial effect on liver disease. If carcinoma or precancerous lesions in the colon develop, a proctocolectomy is indicated. The development of peristomal varices after ileostomy creation is associated with considerable morbidity after proctocolectomy. Creation of an ileal pouch-anal anastomosis is recommended to avoid this significant complication.

Do patients with primary biliary cirrhosis and primary sclerosing cholangitis have an increased risk for hepatocellular carcinoma?
Yes. Recent information suggests a higher-than-expected rate of hepatocellular carcinoma (HCC) in male patients with end-stage liver disease from PBC. Screening and surveillance procedures, including abdominal ultrasound with serum alpha-fetoprotein (AFP) levels every 6 months, may be useful for the early detection of HCC. An increased risk for HCC in patients with PSC also occurs in the setting of end-stage liver disease.

What is the role of liver transplantation in primary biliary cirrhosis and primary sclerosing cholangitis?
The treatment of choice for patients with end-stage PBC and PSC is liver transplantation. Five- and 10-year survival rates of 85% and 70%, respectively, are among the highest for all individuals after liver transplantation. Factors that influence the consideration for liver transplantation are deteriorating hepatic synthetic function (defined as a Child-Turcotte-Pugh score ≥7), intractable symptoms, and diminished quality of life. Refractory ascites, progressive hepatic encephalopathy, uncontrolled or recurrent variceal bleeding, spontaneous bacterial peritonitis, and hepatorenal syndrome are also indications for consideration of liver transplantation. Patients with PSC may also be considered for liver transplantation, based on the development of recurrent bacterial cholangitis, despite maximum medical therapy. In addition to increased survival, a number of published reports have documented improvements in health-related quality of life after liver transplantation for patients with PBC and PSC.

Do primary biliary cirrhosis and primary sclerosing cholangitis recur after liver transplantation?
Sometimes. The cumulative incidence of recurrent PBC is between 15% and 30% over 10 years, based on strict clinical and histologic criteria. No significant impact on survival, however, has been associated with recurrent histologic disease. The role of UDCA in preventing disease progression among liver transplant recipients with early-stage, recurrent PBC remains unknown.

Recurrent allograft disease with PSC has been reported, yet its true prevalence depends establishing well-defined diagnostic criteria and the rigor of excluding patients with chroni ischemic biliary tract strictures from other causes. These include the presence of chronic ductopenic rejection, ABO incompatibility, prolonged cold ischemia time, cytomegalovirus infection, and hepatic artery thrombosis. Nevertheless, recent data suggest that approxima 20% of patients transplanted for PSC will develop recurrent disease with some individuals requiring consideration for hepatic retransplantation.

41. **What are the complications in primary sclerosing cholangitis patients after transplantation?**
    Patients with PSC appear to have an increased incidence of chronic ductopenic rejection ar ischemic biliary duct stricturing. Individuals with concurrent inflammatory bowel disease a higher risk for increased colonic disease activity, colonic dysplasia, and carcinoma.

WEBSITES

1. http://www.aasld.org/

2. http://www.guideline.gov

BIBLIOGRAPHY

1. Angulo P, Maor-Kendler Y, Lindor KD: Small-duct primary sclerosing cholangitis: A long-term follow-up st Hepatology 35:1494–1500, 2002.

2. Batts KP, Ludwig J: Histopathology of autoimmune chronic active hepatitis, primary biliary cirrhosis, and p mary sclerosing cholangitis. In Krawitt EL, Wiesner RH (eds): Autoimmune Liver Diseases. New York, Rav Press, 1991, pp 75–92.

3. Boberg KM, Bergquist A, Mitchell S, et al: Cholangiocarcinoma in primary sclerosing cholangitis: Risk fact and clinical presentation. Scand J Gastroenterol 37:1205–1211, 2002.

4. Cangemi JR, Wiesner RH, Beaver SJ, et al: Effect of proctocolectomy for chronic ulcerative colitis on the n history of primary sclerosing cholangitis. Gastroenterology 96:790–794, 1989.

5. Crippin JS, Lindor KD, Jorgensen R, et al: Hypercholesterolemia and atherosclerosis in primary biliary cirr What is the risk? Hepatology 15:858–862, 1992.

6. Dickson ER, Grambsch PM, Fleming TR, et al: Prognosis in primary biliary cirrhosis: Model for decision m Hepatology 10:1–7, 1989.

7. Fulcher AS, Turner MA, Franklin KJ, et al: Primary sclerosing cholangitis: Evaluation with MR cholangiogra A case-control study. Radiology 215:71–80, 2000.

8. Graziadei IW, Wiesner RH, Batts KP, et al: Recurrence of primary sclerosing cholangitis following liver tran tation. Hepatology 29:1050–1056, 1999.

9. Graziadei IW, Wiesner RH, Marotta PJ, et al: Long-term results of patients undergoing liver transplantation primary sclerosing cholangitis. Hepatology 30:1121–1127, 1999.

10. Hay JE, Lindor KD, Wiesner RH, et al: The metabolic bone disease of primary sclerosing cholangitis. Hepat 14:257–261, 1991.

11. Harnois DM, Angulo P, Jorgensen RA, et al: High-dose ursodeoxycholic acid as a therapy for patients with mary sclerosing cholangitis. Am J Gastroenterol 96:1558–1562, 2001.

12. Kim WR, Therneau TM, Wiesner RH, et al: A revised natural history model for primary sclerosing cholangit Mayo Clin Proc 75:688–694, 2000.

13. LaRusso NF, Wiesner RH, Ludwig J, MacCarty RL: Primary sclerosing cholangitis. N Engl J Med 310:899–903, 1

14. Liermann Garcia RF, Evangelista Garcia C, McMaster P, et al: Transplantation for primary biliary cirrhosis: Retrospective analysis of 400 patients in a single center. Hepatology 33:22–27, 2001.

15. Lindor KD: Ursodiol for primary sclerosing cholangitis. Mayo Primary Sclerosing Cholangitis-Ursodeoxycholic Acid Study Group. N Engl J Med 336:691–695, 1997.

16. Lindor KD, Dickson ER, Baldus WP, et al: Ursodeoxycholic acid in the treatment of primary biliary cirrhosis. Gastroenterology 106:1284–1290, 1994.

17. Menon KV, Angulo P, Weston S, et al: Bone disease in primary biliary cirrhosis: Independent indicators and rate of progression. J Hepatol 35:316–323, 2000.

18. Mitchell SA, Bansi DS, Hunt N, et al: A preliminary trial of high-dose ursodeoxycholic acid in primary sclerosing cholangitis. Gastroenterology 121:900–907, 2001.

19. Nichols JC, Gores GJ, LaRusso NF, et al: Diagnostic role of CA 19-9 for cholangiocarcinoma in patients with primary sclerosing cholangitis. Mayo Clin Proc 68:874–879, 1993.

20. Talwalkar JA, Keach JC, Angulo P, et al: Overlap of autoimmune hepatitis and primary biliary cirrhosis: An evaluation of a modified scoring system. Am J Gastroenterol 97:1191–1197, 2002.

21. Talwalkar JA, Lindor KD: Primary biliary cirrhosis. Lancet 362:53–61, 2003.

22. Wiesner RH: Liver transplantation for primary biliary cirrhosis and primary sclerosing cholangitis: Predicting outcomes with natural history models. Mayo Clin Proc 73:575–588, 1998.

CHAPTER 22

HEPATITIS VACCINES AND IMMUNOPROPHYLAXIS

Col. Maria H. Sjögren, MD, and Marcos Amorim, MD

1. **Discuss the concept of immunization (vaccination).**

   During the past century major progress in the control of infectious diseases has become possible because of the remarkable developments in microbiology. The success of immunization in humans rests on one major concept—humans have specific immunologic mechanisms that can be programmed to provide a defense against infectious agents. The body's immune mechanism is stimulated by direct introduction of infectious agents or smaller components in the form of vaccines.

2. **Outline briefly the history of vaccination.**

   In 1798 Edward Jenner described his work with cowpox vaccination. He demonstrated that a person inoculated and infected with cowpox was protected against smallpox. The procedure, which he termed "vaccination," represented the first use of a vaccine for prevention of disease. The word *vaccine* is derived from the Latin word for *cow;* cows were host to the first true vaccine virus, cowpox. The evolution into the golden era of vaccine development began in 1949 with the discovery of virus propagation in cell culture. The first product developed by using the new cell culture technique was the Salk trivalent formalin-inactivated polio vaccine. After its success, vaccines to prevent human hepatitis A and B were developed rapidly, considering that the viral agents were discovered in 1973 and 1965, respectively.

3. **Distinguish between active and passive immunizations.**

   Active immunization involves the introduction of a specific antigen to provoke an antibody response that will prevent disease. *Passive immunization* or *immunoprophylaxis* is the introduction of antibodies produced by immunization or prior natural infection (of a suitable animal or human host) to prevent or modify the natural infection in a susceptible person.

4. **What are the major categories of vaccines?**

   Two categories of vaccines are widely available: (1) *inactivated* or *killed vaccines,* in which the infectious agent is incapable of multiplying in the host but retains antigenic properties and evokes an antibody response, and (2) *live, attenuated vaccines,* which are prepared with live, viable agents. Because of attenuation, however, the agents are incapable of inducing clinical disease. The end result is development of antibody and prevention of infection. The live vaccines generally contain relatively low concentrations of the infectious agent. Ideally, only one administration is required with live vaccines, and the immunity is long-lasting. With killed vaccines, the immunologic response correlates with the concentration of the antigenic component. Inactivated vaccines commonly require a series of doses to stimulate a long-lasting immunologic response.

5. **Describe the basic characteristics of immunoprophylaxis.**

   Immunoprophylaxis affords a relatively brief period of protection (weeks to a few months). Before the development of hepatitis A and B vaccines, immunoprophylaxis was the mainstay of preventing infection. Passive immunization occurs naturally in humans when maternal antibodies of the immunoglobulin G (IgG) class are passed to neonates. Such antibodies provide protection against many communicable bacterial and viral diseases for a period of months, during the time when the immune system has not yet fully developed. They disappear within the first year of life.

At the beginning of passive immunization therapy, the antibody-containing serum (e.g., horse serum) was administered directly. Currently, the antibody of interest is isolated and concentrated by means of fractionation of serum.

6. **Which immunoglobulins are available for human use?**
   See Table 22-1.

TABLE 22–1. IMMUNOGLOBULINS FOR HEPATITIS PROPHYLAXIS		
Product	Source	Use
Immune serum globulin	Pooled human plasma	Prevents measles
		Prevents hepatitis A virus
Measles immunoglobulin	Pooled human plasma	Prevents measles
Hepatitis B immunoglobulin	Pooled plasma donors with high antibody titer	Used in accidental needlestick or sexual exposure
Rabies immunoglobulin	Pooled plasma from hyper-immunized donors	Immunotherapy for rabies
Botulism	Specific equine antibody	Treatment and prophylaxis for botulinum toxin

7. **Which viral agents are responsible mainly for acute and chronic viral hepatitis?**
   See Table 22-2.

TABLE 22–2. VIRAL AGENTS RESPONSIBLE FOR ACUTE AND CHRONIC HEPATITIS			
Acute Hepatitis	Chronic Hepatitis	Main Route of Transmission	Vaccine Status
Hepatitis A virus	No	Fecal-oral	Commercially available
Hepatitis B virus	Yes	Bloodborne	Commercially available
Hepatitis C virus	Yes	Bloodborne	Not available
Hepatitis D virus	Yes	Bloodborne	Not available
Hepatitis E virus	No	Fecal-oral	IND status

IND = investigational new drug.

- **What kind of immunoprophylaxis is available for hepatitis A?**
  Although hepatitis A vaccine is the first line of preventive therapy, administration of serum IgG is still of value to prevent hepatitis A infection in certain circumstances. Immunoglobulin may be used to provide short-term protection in persons who require immediate immunity and in children who are too young to receive the vaccine. The recommended dose of IgG for adults is 0.02 mL/kg for preexposure when the period of exposure will not exceed 3 months.

If the period of exposure is prolonged, 0.06 mL/kg every 5 months is recommended. IgG affords excellent prophylaxis but is impractical because protection lasts only a few months. Although considered safe, it may cause fever, myalgia, and considerable pain at injection sites

9. **What vaccines are available for hepatitis A?**
Two vaccines are commercially available in the United States: VAQTA (Merck, Sharp, and Dohme West Point, PA) and HAVRIX (Glaxo SmithKline, Rixensart, Belgium). A single dose of VAQTA ha 100% protective efficacy. The initial trial included 1037 children aged 2–16 years and took place an upstate New York community with a 3% annual incidence of acute hepatitis A. Children were randomized to receive one intramuscular injection of a highly purified, formalin-inactivated HAV vaccine or placebo. From day 50 until day 103 after injection, 25 cases of clinically apparent hep tis developed in the placebo group and 0 in the vaccine group ($p<.001$). The vaccine gave a calc lated 100% efficacy rate. HAVRIX, when tested against placebo in more than 40,000 Thai childre gave a calculated 97% rate of protective efficacy after three doses. Two doses of either vaccine provide long-term immunity. Both are approved in the United States for subjects older than age

10. **Compare the major characteristics of VAQTA and HAVRIX.**
See Table 22-3.

TABLE 22-3.   COMPARISON OF VAQTA AND HAVRIX VACCINES

	VAQTA	HAVRIX
Type	Inactivated Vaccine	Inactivated Vaccine
HAV strain	Attenuated CR326F	Attenuated HM175
Cell culture	Cultured in MRC-5 cells	Cultured in MRC-5 cells
Adjuvant	Aluminum hydroxide	Aluminum hydroxide
Standards met	FDA, WHO	FDA, WHO
Immunity	Promotes anti-HAV in serum	Promotes anti-HAV in serum
Route of administration	Intramuscular	Intramuscular
Adult doses	1 mL (50 U) at 0 and 6 mo	1 mL (1440 U) at 0 and 6–12 m
Pediatric doses (2–17 yr)	0.5 mL (25 U) at 0 and 6–18 mo	0.5 mL (720 U) at 0 and 6–12 mo

HAV = hepatitis A virus, FDA = Food and Drug Administration, WHO = World Health Organization.

11. **Who should be immunized against hepatitis A?**
   - Travelers to countries with high endemicity for hepatitis A virus (HAV) infection
   - Military personnel
   - Persons with chronic liver diseases of any etiology
   - Homosexually active men
   - Users of illicit drugs
   - Residents of communities experiencing a hepatitis A outbreak
   - Persons with clotting factor disorders
   - Certain institutional workers
   - Employees of child day-care centers
   - Laboratory workers who handle live HAV

- Handlers of primates that may harbor HAV
- Children and adolescents living in states with historically elevated rates of hepatitis A: Alaska (cyclical epidemics), Arizona, California, Idaho, Nevada, New Mexico, Oklahoma, Oregon, South Dakota, Utah, and Washington; routine vaccination should be considered in Arkansas, Colorado, Missouri, Montana, Texas, and Wyoming.

What side effects have been observed with the hepatitis A vaccine?

- *1–10%:* local reactions at injection site, such as induration, redness, and swelling; systemic reactions, such as fatigue, fever, or malaise; anorexia; nausea.
- *<1%:* hematoma at injection site, pruritus, skin rash, pharyngitis, upper respiratory tract infections, abdominal pain, diarrhea, vomiting, arthralgia, myalgia, lymphadenopathy, insomnia, photophobia, vertigo.
- Hepatitis A vaccine should not be administered to persons with a history of hypersensitivity reactions to alum or, for HAVRIX, to the preservative 2-phenoxyethanol. The safety of hepatitis A vaccination during pregnancy has not been determined.

Do nonresponders to hepatitis A vaccine exist?

Yes. HAV vaccines are highly immunogenic in most healthy people. Some nonhealthy populations have shown a lower anti-HAV titer after immunization, such as HIV-infected people and people with chronic liver disease.

What is the lowest protective anti-hepatitis A virus serum level after immunization?

The lowest anti-HAV protective titer has not been established, but the Advisory Committee on Immune Practices defines the minimum as 20 mIU/mL.

Does the concurrent administration of hepatitis A vaccine influence the immune response to other traveler's vaccines?

No. Recent studies of 396 travelers who received vaccines against hepatitis A, poliomyelitis, hepatitis B, diphtheria, tetanus, yellow fever, Japanese encephalitis, typhoid fever, or rabies (according to individual needs) showed that concurrent administration of hepatitis A vaccine did not compromise the immune response to the hepatitis A or other vaccines.

What kind of immunoprophylaxis is available for hepatitis B virus?

1. *Active immunization:* hepatitis B vaccine, first licensed in the United States in 1981, is recommended for both preexposure and postexposure prophylaxis.
2. *Passive immunization:* hyperimmune globulin (HBIG) provides temporary passive protection and is indicated in certain postexposure situations.

What is the recommended dose of hyperimmune globulin for adults and children?

HBIG contains high concentrations of anti-HBs, whereas regular immunoglobulin is prepared from plasma with varying concentrations of anti-HBs. In the United States, HBIG has an anti-HBs titer >1:100,000 by radioimmunoassay (*see* Table 22-4).

How many hepatitis B vaccines are available in the United States? Are they comparable?

Three vaccines have been licensed in the United States. For practical purposes, they are comparable in immunogenicity and efficacy rates, although the preparations are different:
1. *Heptavax-B* (Merck, Sharp & Dohme; West Point, PA) became available in 1986 and is no longer manufactured in the United States. It consists of hepatitis B surface antigen (HBsAg) purified from the plasma of chronically infected humans and evokes antibodies to the group a determinant of HBsAg, effectively neutralizing the various subtypes of hepatitis B virus

TABLE 22-4. RECOMMENDED TREATMENT AFTER EXPOSURE TO HEPATITIS B VIRUS

	HBIG		Vaccine	
Exposure	Dose	Timing	Dose	Timing
Perinatal	0.5 mL IM	Within 12 hr of birth	0.5 mL at birth	Within 12 hr of birth; repeat at 1 and 6 mo
Sexual	0.6 mL/kg IM	Single dose within 14 days of sexual contact	Same time as HBIG	Start immunization at once

IM = intramuscularly, HBIG = hyperimmune globulin.

(HBV). Abundant evidence supports its efficacy, but it is expensive to prepare, and a number of physical and chemical inactivation steps are needed for purification and safety. Because of these problems, alternative approaches based on recombinant DNA technology were developed. Each milliliter of plasma-derived vaccine has 20 mg of HBsAg.

2. *Recombivax-HB,* also manufactured by Merck, Sharp & Dohme, became available in 1989. It is a noninfectious, nonglycosylated HBsAg vaccine, subtype adw, made by recombinant DNA technology. Yeast cells (*Saccharomyces cerevisiae*) expressing the HBsAg gene are cultured collected by centrifugation, and broken by homogenization with glass beads. HBsAg particle are purified and absorbed in aluminum hydroxide. Each milliliter has 10 mg of HBsAg.

3. *Engerix-B,* manufactured by SmithKline Biologicals (Rixensart, Belgium), is a noninfectious recombinant DNA vaccine. It contains purified HBsAg obtained by culturing genetically engineered *S. cerevisiae* cells, which carry the surface antigen gene of HBV. This surface antigen is purified from the cells and adsorbed on aluminum hydroxide. Each milliliter has 20 mg of HBsAg.

19. **What is the immunization schedule for hepatitis B virus vaccine in adults and children?**
See Table 22-5.

TABLE 22-5. IMMUNIZATION SCHEDULE FOR HEPATITIS B VIRUS VACCINE IN ADULTS AND CHILDREN

Recombivax-HB Vaccine				
Group	Formulation	Initial	1 month	6 month
Birth to 10 yr	Pediatric dose: 0.5 mL	0.5 mL	0.5 mL	0.5 mL
Adults and older children	Adult dose: 10 mg/1.0 mL	1.0 mL	1.0 mL	1.0 mL
Dialysis patients	Special dose: 40 mg/1.0 mL	1.0 mL	1.0 mL	1.0 mL
Engerix-B Vaccine				
Group	Formulation	Initial	1 month	6 month
Birth to 10 yr	Pediatric dose: 10 mg/0.5 mL	0.5 mL	0.5 mL	0.5 mL
Adults and older children	Adult dose: 20 mg/1.0 mL	1.0 mL	1.0 mL	1.0 mL
After needlestick injury	20 mg/1.0 mL	1.0 mL at 0, 1, and 2 mo		
Hemodialysis patients	40 mg/2.0 mL	2.0 mL at 0, 1, 2, and 6 mo		

What is the recommended regimen for infants born to hepatitis B surface antigen-positive mothers?

Infants born to HBsAg-positive mothers should receive HBIG (0.5 mL) and the first dose of hepatitis B vaccine ≤12 hours of birth. Women admitted for delivery without HBsAg test results should have blood drawn for testing. While test results are pending, the infant should receive hepatitis B vaccine without HBIG within 12 hours of birth (standard practice) (*see* Table 22-6).

TABLE 22-6.	RECOMMENDED REGIMEN FOR INFANTS BORN TO HEPATITIS B SURFACE ANTIGEN–POSITIVE MOTHERS			
Treatment	Birth	Within 7 days	1 month	6 months
Recombivax-HB (pediatric dose)	0.5 mL	0.5 mL	0.5 mL	0.5 mL
Hyperimmune globulin	0.5 mL	None	None	None

Is a booster needed after immunization? If so, how often?

No. Booster shots are not recommended for healthy adults or children. For immunocompromised patients (e.g., hemodialysis patients), a booster dose should be administered when anti-HBs levels drop to 10 mIU/mL or less.

Summarize the evidence for long-term immunization after vaccination.

The persistence of antibody correlates directly with the peak level achieved after the third dose. Follow-up of adults who were immunized with plasma-derived hepatitis B vaccine demonstrated that the antibody levels had fallen to undetectable or very low levels in 30–50% of recipients. Long-term studies of adults and children indicate that protection lasts at least 9 years, despite loss of anti-HBs in serum. After 9 years of follow-up, anti-HBs loss ranged from 13–60% in a group of homosexual men and Alaskan Eskimos, two groups at high risk of infection. However, vaccine recipients were virtually 100% protected from clinical illness, despite the absence of booster immunization. Among people without detectable anti-HBs, breakthrough infections have been noted in later years, based on the detection of hepatitis B core antibody. However, clinical illness did not occur, and HBsAg was not detected. The infection is assumed to be without consequence and to confer permanent immunity.

Is it possible that the vaccine will not protect against hepatitis B virus infection?

Hepatitis B vaccines effectively evoke neutralizing antibodies to the group a determinant of HBsAg, which is believed to be formed by the highly conformational structure between amino acids 124 and 127. Some diversity has been demonstrated but probably does not affect neutralization of HBsAg. Hepatitis B mutants have been reported. They probably arose randomly and were not corrected because of an intrinsic failure of the polymerase enzyme. Significant variants have been described in HBV vaccines, initially in Italy but also in Japan and Gambia. Italian investigators reported that 40 of 1600 immunized children showed evidence of HBV infection, despite adequate antibody response to the HBV vaccine. The mutant virus had substitutions in amino acids 145 (Italy), 126 (Japan), and 141 (Gambia). Whether HBV mutants have substantial clinical significance is not known. Large-scale epidemiologic studies of the incidence, prevalence, and clinical correlation have not been performed.

Is it harmful to give hepatitis B vaccine to known hepatitis B carriers?

No deleterious effects were observed in 16 chronic carriers of HBsAg who received at least six monthly injections of hepatitis B vaccine. The vaccine was administered in an attempt to eliminate the chronic carrier status. However, no such result was observed. None of the volunteers lost HBsAg or developed anti-HBs. This finding simplified the design of hepatitis B vaccination programs.

25. Is it appropriate to use the therapeutic vaccines to hepatitis B virus?

No. A recent study with inactive HBsAg carriers (patients had never received prior antiviral therapies) showed that the recombinant HBV vaccine had no great effect in enhancing the rate of HBsAg seroconversion in inactive HBsAg carriers.

26. Is it possible to immunize people simultaneously against hepatitis A and B viruses?

Yes. To date, over 1000 subjects have received a combined product of both vaccines. Twinrix (SmithKline Biologicals), which is commercially available in the United States and Europe, elicits antibodies to HAV and HBV in more than 80% of recipients by month 2. Limited long-term follow-up reports a 100% anti-HAV and a 95% anti-HBV response by 2 years after immunization. The combined vaccine appears to be safe, well tolerated, and highly immunogenic. The side-effect profile is reportedly similar to that of the individual vaccines.

27. Is immunoprophylaxis advisable for hepatitis C virus?

No firm recommendation can be made for postexposure prophylaxis for hepatitis C virus (HCV). Study results are equivocal. Some experts recommend administration of immunoglobulin (0.6 mg/kg) after a bona fide percutaneous exposure. The immunoglobulin should be administered as soon as possible. However, work in chimpanzees has shown a lack of protectiveness when animals that received prophylaxis with immunoglobulin were challenged with HCV. Moreover, recent data show that in humans the neutralizing antibody evoked after infection with HCV is short-lived and does not protect against reinfection. Immunoprophylaxis for hepatitis C seems to be quite difficult. To date, there is no effective vaccine against HCV infection. Efforts to develop an HCV vaccine are complicated by the extensive genetic and possible antigenic diversity among HCV strains, the absence of a robust immunity after natural infection, and the lack of tissue culture systems and small animal models.

28. Is a vaccine available for hepatitis E virus?

No. At present, no commercially available vaccines exist for the prevention of hepatitis E virus (HEV). However, several studies for the development of an effective vaccine against HEV are in progress:

Recombinant vaccines: A 56 Kda recombinant HEV-derived ORF2 protein has been used to vaccinate rhesus monkeys against different strains of HEV. Recent studies demonstrated that recombinant hepatitis E vaccine suitable for clinical evaluation was highly immunogenic and efficacious in preventing HEV and even infection in rhesus monkeys following intravenous challenge with three different genotypes of HEV. Two doses of vaccine were essential for optimal protection. The titers of anti-HEV that were protective in this study were quantified against a World Health Organization (WHO) standard. The results of this preclinical trial of a candidate hepatitis E vaccine strongly suggest that it will be highly efficacious for preventing HEV in the field trial of this vaccine that is currently in progress in Nepal (an endemic setting).

29. Should patients with chronic liver disease be immunized against hepatitis A and hepatitis B viruses?

Yes. Acute HAV has resulted in higher morbidity and mortality rates in healthy people over age 40 and in people with chronic HCV. HAV vaccine is safe and effective in people with chronic liver disease and may prevent additional injury to an already compromised liver. Acute HBV has not been shown to induce high mortality rates in people with chronic liver disease; however, preventing further hepatic injury seems logical and wise. A recent review showed that the cost-effective analyses have yielded encouraging results regarding the immunization to prevent HAV infection in all patients with chronic liver disease.

WEBSITES

- http://www.cdc.gov/ncidod/diseases/hepatitis/b/
- http://www.cdc.gov/ncidod/diseases/hepatitis/a/index.htm

BIBLIOGRAPHY

Bock HL, Kruppenbacher JP, Bienzle U, et al: Does the concurrent administration of an inactivated hepatitis A vaccine influence the immune response to other travelers' vaccines? J Travel Med 7:74–78, 2000.

Carman WF, Zanetti AR, Karayaiannis P, et al: Vaccine-induced escape mutants of hepatitis B virus. Lancet 336:325–329, 1990.

Centers for Disease Control and Prevention: Hepatitis B virus: A comprehensive strategy for eliminating transmission in the United States through universal childhood vaccination. MMWR 40/RR-13:10, 1991.

Centers for Disease Control and Prevention: Prevention of hepatitis A through active or passive immunization. MMWR 48/RR-12, 1999.

Centers for Disease Control and Prevention: Update: Recommendations to prevent hepatitis B virus transmission—United States. MMWR 48:33–34, 1999.

Chen HL, Chang MH, Ni YH, et al: Seroepidemiology of hepatitis B virus infection in children: Ten years of mass vaccination in Taiwan. JAMA 276:906–908, 1996.

Fan PC, Chang MH, Lee PI, et al: Follow-up immunogenicity of an inactivated hepatitis A vaccine in healthy children: Results after 5 years. Vaccine 16:232–235, 1998.

Hadler SC, Francis DP, Maynard J, et al: Long-term immunogenicity and efficacy of hepatitis B vaccine in homosexual men. N Engl J Med 315:209–214, 1986.

Keefe EB, Iwarson S, McMahon BJ, et al: Safety and immunogenicity of hepatitis A vaccine in patients with chronic liver disease. Hepatology 27:881–886, 1998.

Lee PI, Chang LY, Lee CY, et al: Detection of hepatitis B surface gene mutation in carrier children with or without immunoprophylaxis at birth. J Infect Dis 176:427–430, 1997.

Parkman PD, Hopps HE, Meyer HM: Immunoprevention of infectious diseases. In Nohmias AJ, O'Reilly RJ (eds): Immunology. New York, Plenum, 1982, pp 561–583.

Plotkin S, Plotkin S: A short history of vaccine. In Plotkin S, Mortimer E (eds): Vaccines, 2nd ed. Philadelphia, W.B. Saunders, 1988, pp 1–7.

Prevention and control of infections with hepatitis viruses in correctional settings. MMWR 52/RR-18, 34, 2003.

Purcell RH, Nguyen H, Shapiro M, et al: Pre-clinical immunogenicity and efficacy trial of a recombinant hepatitis E vaccine. Vaccine 21(19-20):2607–2615, 2003.

Qiao M, Murata K, Davis AR, et al: Hepatitis C virus-like particles combined with novel adjuvant systems enhance virus-specific immune responses. Hepatology 37:52, 2003.

Ryan ET, Kain K: Health advice and immunization for travelers. N Engl J Med 342:1716–1725, 2000.

Sjögren M: Immunization and the decline of viral hepatitis as a cause of acute liver failure. Hepatology 38:554–556, 2003.

Taliani G, Gaeta GB: Hepatitis A: Post-exposure prophylaxis. Vaccine 21(19-21): 2234–2237, 2003.

Thoelen S, Van Damme P, Leentvaar-Kuypers A, et al: The first combined vaccine against hepatitis A and B: An overview. Vaccine 17:1657–1662, 1999.

Wainwright RB, McMahon B, Bulkow L, et al: Duration of immunogenicity and efficacy of hepatitis B vaccine in a Yupik Eskimo population. JAMA 261:2362–2366, 1989.

Whittle HC, Inskip H, Hall AJ, et al: Vaccination against hepatitis B and protection against viral carriage in Gambia. Lancet 337:747–750, 1991.

Yalcin K, Acar M, Degertekin H: Specific hepatitis B vaccine therapy in inactive HBsAg carriers: A randomized controlled trial. Infection 31(4):221–225, 2003.

CHAPTER 23

LIVER PROBLEMS IN PREGNANCY

Anca I. Pop, MD, and Caroline A. Riely, MD

1. **What are the structural and functional hepatic adaptations during pregnancy**
   Liver size and histology do not change. Maternal blood volume and cardiac output increase si
   nificantly, without a corresponding increase in hepatic blood flow, but with a net decrease in
   fractional blood flow to the liver. An enlarging uterus makes venous return via the inferior ven
   cava progressively more difficult toward term. Blood is shunted via the azygous system with
   possible development of esophageal varices.

2. **Does liver function change during pregnancy?**
   No. Hepatic function remains normal during pregnancy, but the normal range of laboratory va
   ues changes because of hormonal changes and an increase in blood volume with subsequent
   hemodilution. Aspartate aminotransferase (AST), alanine aminotransferase (ALT), gamma-gl
   tamyl transpeptidase (GGTP), bilirubin, and prothrombin remain within normal limits. Total al
   line phosphatase (AP) is elevated. The placenta is the major source of AP; levels return to
   normal within 20 days after delivery. Increased fibrinogen synthesis leads to a significant rise
   serum levels, which is attributed to the action of estrogens, along with increases in other coa
   lation proteins (factors VII, VIII, IX, and X), a gradual increase in ceruloplasmin levels, and
   increased serum-binding proteins for thyroxine, vitamin D, folate, corticosteroids, and testos
   terone. Also attributed to estrogen effects are the significant increases in serum concentratio
   major lipid classes (triglycerides, low-density and very-low-density lipoproteins, and cholesterol), which may be twice the normal limit for nonpregnant women of the same age. Serum
   albumin decreases slightly, contributing to the approximate 20% decline in total serum prote
   concentration.

3. **Is the serum ceruloplasmin level a good diagnostic marker in pregnant wome**
   at term, who are suspected of having Wilson's disease?
   No. Ceruloplasmin levels increase gradually during pregnancy, reaching the maximum at tern
   The patient's usual low level may be misleadingly normal (>20 mg/dL during pregnancy).

4. **Can we assume the presence of chronic liver disease in a pregnant patient wi**
   angiomas and palmar erythema on physical examination and small esophage
   varices detected endoscopically?
   No. Spider angiomas and palmar erythema are common and appear in about two thirds of pre
   nant women without liver disease. Small esophageal varices are present in approximately 50%
   of healthy pregnant women without liver disease because of the increased flow in the azygou
   system.

5. **What is the most common liver disorder unique to pregnancy?**
   Intrahepatic cholestasis of pregnancy.

6. **What is the most common cause of jaundice in pregnancy?**
   Viral hepatitis.

7. **What is the expected clinical and biochemical course after delivery for patients with intrahepatic cholestasis of pregnancy?**
Pruritus should improve promptly after delivery (within 24 hours). Jaundice is rare and, if present, may persist for days. Biochemical abnormalities may persist for months.

8. **What biochemical changes are noted in cholestasis of pregnancy?**
Serum bile acids, often measured as cholylglycine, increase by 10- to 100-fold. Serum levels of AP rise by 7- to 10-fold, along with a modest rise in serum levels of 5′-nucleotidase (confirming the hepatic source of AP). AST, ALT, and direct bilirubin also rise. No evidence of hemolysis is found. GGTP is usually normal, as is prothrombin time (PT), unless cholestyramine treatment leads to malabsorption.

9. **What is the major clinical manifestation of intrahepatic cholestasis of pregnancy?**
Severe pruritus with onset in the second or, more commonly, third trimester (>70% of cases).

10. **What is a possible cause for abnormal bleeding in a postpartum woman previously diagnosed with intrahepatic cholestasis of pregnancy? What is the treatment?**
Malabsorption of liposoluble vitamins, including vitamin K, especially in patients treated with cholestyramine for pruritus. The international normalized ratio (INR) corrects with parenteral administration of vitamin K.

11. **What is the effect of intrahepatic cholestasis of pregnancy on the fetus?**
Fetal distress requiring caesarean section develops in about 30–60% of cases. Prematurity occurs in about 50% of cases and fetal death in up to 9% of affected pregnancies. All of these effects are more likely if the disorder begins early in pregnancy.

12. **What is the therapy for intrahepatic cholestasis of pregnancy?**
Alleviating pruritus is the main goal. Therapeutic agents include:
- Ursodeoxycholic acid, approximately 15 mg/kg/day; up to 24 mg/kg/day studied with good results
- Cholestyramine, 4 gm four or five times/day (bile acid-binding resin)
- Hydroxyzine hydrochloride (Atarax) or pamoate (Vistaril) (antihistamines)
- Phenobarbital, 100 mg/day (choleretic and centrally acting sedative)
- Phototherapy with ultraviolet B light

Vitamin K before delivery is highly recommended to minimize the risk of postpartum hemorrhage. Mother and fetus should be observed closely. Elective induction is recommended at 36 weeks (severe cases) or 38 weeks (average cases), if the fetal lungs have matured.

13. **Can intrahepatic cholestasis of pregnancy recur?**
Yes. About 40–70% of subsequent pregnancies show evidence of mild intrahepatic cholestasis. The same pattern can be seen with use of estrogen-containing contraceptives.

14. **What atypical signs and symptoms make the diagnosis of intrahepatic cholestasis of pregnancy doubtful?**
Fever, hepatosplenomegaly, pain, jaundice preceding or without pruritus, and pruritus after delivery or before 21 weeks of pregnancy (especially with a singleton pregnancy) should prompt the search for an alternate diagnosis.

15. **What biochemical changes suggest an alternate diagnosis?**
- Normal AST and ALT levels
- Elevated AP and GGTP
- Predominantly unconjugated hyperbilirubinemia

16. **What are the clinical and laboratory features of acute fatty liver of pregnancy?**
    Acute fatty liver of pregnancy (AFLP) is a rare disorder with an incidence of 1:13,000–1:16,000 pregnancies. Onset occurs in the second half of pregnancy, usually during the third trimester, although, occasionally, postpartum onset is reported. Clinical manifestations include nausea and vomiting, jaundice, malaise, thirst, and altered mental status. Severe cases progress rapidly to hypoglycemia, disseminated intravascular coagulation (DIC), renal insufficiency, coma, and death. Signs of coexistent preeclampsia may be present, such as moderately increased arterial blood pressure, proteinuria, and hyperuricemia. Laboratory abnormalities consist of moderate AST/ALT elevations (usually <1000), conjugated hyperbilirubinemia, elevated PT, fibrin split products, and D-dimers, along with low platelet count, elevated levels of ammonia and serum uric acid, and leukocytosis. Hypoglycemia is a sign of extreme severity; blood glucose levels must be monitored closely.

17. **Is biopsy pathognomonic for acute fatty liver of pregnancy?**
    No. Biopsy is confirmatory but not pathognomonic or indispensable in making the diagnosis. Histology is characterized by microvesicular fatty infiltration, mostly in centrilobular zones. In general, lobular and trabecular architecture is preserved, and inflammatory infiltrates and cell necrosis are mild, if present at all. AFLP is a systemic disorder. Similar fatty changes have been noted in pancreatic acinar cells and tubular epithelial cells of the kidneys. The same prominent microvesicular steatosis is seen in other conditions, such as Reye's syndrome, sodium valproate toxicity, Jamaican vomiting sickness, and congenital defects of urea cycle enzymes or betaoxidation of fatty acids.

18. **How do we diagnose and treat acute fatty liver of pregnancy?**
    High clinical suspicion is crucial for early recognition and appropriate management. AFLP is suggested by hepatic failure at or near term or shortly after delivery in the absence of risk factors or serology, suggesting viral hepatitis. Thirst, a symptom of underlying vasopressin-resistant diabetes insipidus, is characteristic to AFLP or hemolysis, elevated liver enzymes, low platelets (HELLP) syndrome. Biopsy, if feasible, is diagnostic in the appropriate clinical context. Treatment consists of admission to hospital, close monitoring by a multidisciplinary team (hepatologist, maternal-fetal medicine specialist, intensive care specialist) and immediate delivery. Recovery is usually complete, although it may be delayed in patients with significant clinical complications before delivery (e.g., DIC, renal failure, infections).

19. **Describe the pathogenesis of acute fatty liver of pregnancy.**
    Pathogenesis remains somewhat unclear. AFLP seems to be a fetal–maternal interaction. In some cases the fetus has an isolated deficiency of long chain 3-hydroxyacyl-CoA dehydrogenase (LCHAD), which leads to a disorder of mitochondrial fatty-acid oxidation. The inheritance pattern is recessive and involves a mutation from glutamic acid to glutamine at amino-acid residue 474 (Glu474Gln) on at least one allele. It is hypothesized that in the presence of this mutation in homozygous or compound heterozygote fetuses, long-chain fatty acid metabolites produced by the fetus or placenta accumulate in the mother and are highly toxic to the maternal liver. The mother is phenotypically normal; her genotype does not correlate with development of AFLP.

20. **Does acute fatty liver of pregnancy recur in subsequent pregnancies?**
    Yes. In the cases associated with LCHAD defects, the disorder is recessive, affecting 1:4 fetuses. The rate of recurrence of maternal liver disease is 15–25%.

21. **What is the outcome of a child whose mother has acute fatty liver of pregnancy?**
    Previously reported fetal mortality rates of 75–90% have been significantly reduced by better awareness, earlier diagnosis, availability of neonatal intensive care units, and institution of c

monitoring and dietary treatment through childhood. In pregnancies associated with LCHAD defects, children present at a mean age of 7.6 months (range = 0–60 months) with acute hepatic dysfunction (incidence of 79%). They may experience hypoketotic hypoglycemia, hypotonia, hepatomegaly, hepatic encephalopathy, high transaminases, and fatty liver. The condition may progress rapidly to coma and death. Frequent feedings of a low-fat diet in which the fats are medium-chain triglycerides prevent hypoketotic hypoglycemic liver dysfunction. According to recent studies, 67% of children treated with dietary modification are alive, and most attend school.

2. Is genetic testing indicated in women diagnosed with acute fatty liver of pregnancy?

Yes. All women with AFLP, as well as their partners and children, should be advised to undergo molecular diagnostic testing. Testing for Glu474Gln in the mother only is not sufficient to rule out LCHAD deficiency in the fetus or other family members.

3. Is prospective screening necessary in pregnancies complicated by liver disease?

Yes. Fifteen percent to 20% of pregnancies complicated by AFLP and less than 2% of pregnancies complicated by HELLP syndrome are associated with fetal LCHAD deficiency. Newborns should be screened prospectively at birth in all pregnancies complicated by AFLP. Homozygosity and heterozygosity for Glu474Gln would indicate the need for avoidance of prolonged fasting and replacement of dietary long-chain fatty acids with medium-chain fatty acids. Parents and physicians should be educated in the risk of metabolic crises and sudden death and instructed in the need for early intervention with intravenous glucose during episodes of vomiting, lethargy, and even minor illnesses.

Recent results do not justify routinely screening newborns in pregnancies complicated by HELLP syndrome. Molecular diagnostic testing should, however, be considered in women with recurrent HELLP syndrome in multiple pregnancies.

4. What is the spectrum of liver involvement in preeclampsia?

Liver involvement in preeclampsia ranges from subclinical, with biopsy evidence of fibrinogen deposition along hepatic sinusoids, to several possibly severe disorders. In patients with HELLP syndrome, the chief complaint is abdominal pain, which presents usually in the second half of gestation but may occur up to 7 days after delivery (almost 30% of affected women). Hepatic infarction is another rare manifestation of liver involvement in preeclampsia. Patients present in the third trimester or early after delivery with unexplained fever, leukocytosis, abdominal or chest pain, and extremely elevated aminotransferases (>3000). The diagnosis depends on visualization of hepatic infarcts on computed tomographic (CT) contrast images or magnetic resonance imaging (MRI). Subcapsular hematomas and hepatic rupture are life-threatening complications with high morbidity and mortality rates. A high index of suspicion and early CT imaging allow diagnosis and prompt intervention.

5. How common is hemolysis, elevated liver enzymes, low platelets syndrome?

The incidence of HELLP syndrome is 0.2–0.6% in all pregnancies and 4–12% in preeclamptic patients. The incidence is higher in multiparous, white, and older women, but the mean age of occurrence is around age 25.

6. Describe the incidence and prognosis of spontaneous intrahepatic hemorrhage.

Spontaneous intrahepatic and subcapsular hemorrhage occurs in about 1–2% of patients with preeclampsia, with an estimated incidence of 1 in 45,000 live births. Prognosis improves with awareness, early diagnosis by imaging studies, and aggressive surgical management. Recent reported maternal mortality rates range from 33–49%. Fetal mortality remains high (approximately 60%).

27. **What findings lead typically to the diagnosis of hemolysis, elevated liver enzymes, low platelets syndrome?**
    Diagnosis relies on typical laboratory evidence of liver involvement with associated thrombocytopenia. Not all patients have clinical hypertension or proteinuria at presentation. Liver test abnormalities are hepatocellular. Liver function is normal. Thrombocytopenia is present, usually <100,000/mm^3. Hemolysis is mild, with microangiopathic findings on peripheral smear. Biopsy is characteristic but may be extremely risky and is not needed for diagnosis. It shows periportal hemorrhage, fibrin deposition, and necrosis, possibly with steatosis and/or deposition of fibrinogen along sinusoids with focal parenchymal necrosis. A normal biopsy does not exclude the diagnosis because involvement may be patchy.

28. **What is the treatment for severe preeclamptic liver disease?**
    The initial priority is to stabilize the mother by administering intravenous fluids, correcting any concurrent coagulopathy, administering magnesium for seizure prophylaxis, and treating severe hypertension. Early hepatic imaging is indicated to rule out infarcts or hematomas. Fetal functional status should be determined. Fetal outcome is related mostly to gestational age. Beyond 34 weeks of gestation with evidence of fetal lung maturity, delivery is the recommended therapy. If fetal lungs are immature, the fetus can be delivered 48 hours after administration of two doses of steroids. Termination of pregnancy should be attempted immediately with evidence of fetal or maternal distress. In cases of ruptured subcapsular hematoma, massive transfusions and immediate surgical intervention are required.

29. **Does hemolysis, elevated liver enzymes, low platelets syndrome recur in subsequent pregnancies?**
    Possibly. Studies report recurrence risks as low as 3.4% and as high as 25%.

30. **What information helps to differentiate acute fatty liver of pregnancy from hemolysis, elevated liver enzymes, low platelets syndrome?**
    At presentation, AFLP and HELLP may be difficult to differentiate. Hypertension is usually, but not invariably, associated with HELLP syndrome. Patients with HELLP have mild, predominantly unconjugated hyperbilirubinemia due to hemolysis, along with severe thrombocytopenia, but the laboratory values are suggestive of hepatic failure. Laboratory abnormalities are significantly more severe in AFLP; evidence of hepatic synthetic failure manifests as prolonged PT and significant hypoglycemia in advanced stages. Fibrinogen is low, and ammonia is elevated. Biopsy shows microvesicular steatosis, predominantly in the central zone, in patients with AFLP, whereas patients with HELLP show predominantly periportal fibrin deposition, necrosis, and hemorrhage.

31. **Can gestational age differentiate between different liver diseases in pregnancy?**
    Most definitely. Hyperemesis gravidarum presents in the first trimester of pregnancy. Patients have severe nausea and vomiting, and about one half have associated elevations of bilirubin, AST, or ALT. Cholestasis of pregnancy, viral hepatitis, and abnormal liver chemistries due to cholelithiasis may present at any point in gestation, from the first to the third trimesters. Acute fatty liver of pregnancy and preeclamptic liver disease (HELLP, hepatic infarct, and hepatic rupture) are specifically encountered in the third trimester of pregnancy. Herpes simplex virus or hepatitis E virus is exacerbated in pregnancy and presents usually with or without hepatic failure in the third trimester, close to term. Budd-Chiari syndrome presents from the second half of pregnancy to 3 months after delivery.

32. **What signs and symptoms suggest the diagnosis of Budd-Chiari syndrome?**
    The clinical triad of sudden onset of abdominal pain, hepatomegaly, and ascites, near term or shortly after delivery. Ascitic fluid shows a high protein content in about one half of cases.

Biopsy shows typically centrilobular hemorrhage and necrosis, along with sinusoidal dilation and erythrocyte extravasation into the space of Disse. Hepatic scintigraphy and CT show typically compensatory hypertrophy of the caudate lobe due to its separate drainage into the inferior vena cava. Doppler analysis of portal and hepatic vessels and MRI establish hepatic vein occlusion.

How severe is the course of viral hepatitis acquired during pregnancy?
Hepatitis A, B, and C viruses run a similar course in pregnant and nonpregnant patients. On the other hand, hepatitis E virus runs a different course in pregnancy. It is fulminant in up to 20% of patients, compared with less than 1% of nonpregnant women. The fatality rate is 1.5% during the first trimester, 8.5% during the second trimester, and up to 21% during the third trimester, compared with 0.5–4% in nonpregnant women. Fetal complications and neonatal deaths are increased if infection is acquired in the third trimester of pregnancy. Herpes simplex hepatitis can also be fulminant in pregnancy and associated with high mortality rates. Patients in the third trimester present with fever, systemic symptoms, and possibly vesicular cutaneous rash. Associated pneumonitis or encephalitis may be present. Liver biopsy is characteristic, showing necrosis and inclusion bodies in viable hepatocytes, along with few or no inflammatory infiltrates. Response to acyclovir therapy is prompt; there is no need for immediate delivery of the baby.

Can a woman with Wilson's disease be maintained on therapy during pregnancy?
Absolutely. Therapy must continue during pregnancy; otherwise, the mother is at risk for hemolytic episodes associated with fulminant hepatic failure. Agents approved by the Food and Drug Administration are D-penicillamine, trientine, and zinc. Evidence indicates that penicillamine and trientine (tissue copper-chelating agents) are teratogenic in animal studies, and there are reports of penicillamine effects in humans, including cutis laxis syndrome or micrognathia, low-set ears, and other abnormalities. According to the current consensus, penicillamine and trientine are safe in doses of 0.75–1 gm/day during the first two trimesters; the dose should be reduced to 0.5 gm/day during the last trimester and in nursing mothers. Zinc therapy is an attractive alternative with a different mechanism of action; it induces synthesis of metallothionein, which sequesters copper in enterocytes, blocking its absorption. No teratogenic effects have been reported in animals or humans. The recommended doses are 50 mg three times/day for patients with 24-hour urinary copper values over 0.1 mg and 25 mg three times/day for patients with lower urinary copper values. Close monitoring of urinary copper and zinc levels is suggested; the zinc dose should be adjusted accordingly.

What methods of contraception are available for patients with liver disease?
Patients with advanced or untreated liver disease commonly experience amenorrhea and infertility. If clinical improvement leads to restoration of fertility, multiple methods of contraception are available, including barrier methods and intrauterine devices. Tubal ligation may be used in women who have completed their families. Estrogen-based contraceptive agents are generally contraindicated, especially for patients with acute liver disease, but progestin contraceptives are safe alternatives. Combination contraceptives are absolutely contraindicated in patients with cholestatic jaundice of pregnancy or jaundice with prior use, and the World Health Organization is listing them as category 4 type of drugs for patients with decompensated cirrhosis of any etiology. Numerous formulations and delivery systems are available.

How should patients with preexistent liver disease be managed if pregnancy occurs?
Patients are best managed by a multidisciplinary team that includes a maternal-fetal medicine specialist, perinatologist, and hepatologist. Patients have an increased risk for maternal complications along with a higher incidence of fetal wastage and prematurity. In general, patients should be maintained on the previous therapy that was successful in controlling liver disease and restoring fertility. Women with autoimmune hepatitis should be continued on corticosteroids alone or in combination with azathioprine, which is not teratogenic at the usual dose.

Patients with Wilson's disease should be continued on the anticopper agent. Patients with portal hypertension should have a baseline endoscopy. If they have never bled and medium or large varices are present, they are at increased risk for variceal hemorrhage during pregnancy. Primary prophylaxis with a nonselective beta blocker or isosorbide mononitrate should be instituted. The fetus should be monitored for bradycardia or growth retardation the mother is maintained on beta blockers. Variceal bleeding is safely managed with varice band ligation or sclerotherapy. Octreotide in customary doses is safe in pregnancy. Performing surgical portacaval shunts for patients with well-preserved liver function is po sible. Placement of a transjugular intrahepatic portosystemic shunt and splenectomy (in patients with massive splenomegaly, varices, and thrombocytopenia) have also been reported.

37. **What are the effects of pregnancy on the mother with portal hypertension?**
The morbidity rate is 30–50% because of possible onset of hepatic encephalopathy, spontaneous bacterial peritonitis, and progressive liver failure. The incidence of variceal hemorrhage 19–45%, especially in the second trimester and during labor. Postpartum hemorrhage is seen 7–10% of women, most frequently in those with cirrhotic portal hypertension; thrombocytope nia plays a major role. The mortality rate of the previously mentioned complications is 4–7% noncirrhotic and 10–18% in cirrhotic patients with portal hypertension. Data regarding this to originate mostly from case series, and prospectively acquired data are few.

38. **What is the effect of the maternal portal hypertension on pregnancy?**
Spontaneous abortion rates for patients with cirrhosis range from 15–20%. Most cases occu the first trimester. Of interest, patients with extrahepatic portal hypertension and patients with well-compensated cirrhosis, who underwent surgical shunting before conception, have abort rates similar to the general population. The incidence of premature termination of pregnancy the second and third trimesters is similar in all of the previously mentioned groups. Fetal mor ity rates are around 50% if the mother requires emergent surgical intervention for variceal he orrhage. Perinatal mortality rates in cirrhotic mothers are as high as 11–18% because of premature delivery, stillbirth, and neonatal death, but they are similar to those for the general population in noncirrhotic patients with portal hypertension and in patients who underwent p vious portal surgical decompressive procedures.

39. **When can a liver transplant recipient actively seek conception?**
A waiting period of at least 1 year is advisable. Case reports suggest that conception close to transplant date may result in increased maternal and fetal morbidity and mortality. Contraception should be instituted before resuming sexual relations, preferably with barrier methods.

40. **Is pregnancy possible after liver transplantation?**
Yes. Pregnancy will become possible once normal menstrual cycles resume. In women with chronic liver disease, most pretransplant amenorrhea resolves in approximately 3 to 10 mont following liver transplantation.

41. **What are the possible complications of pregnancies occurring after liver transplantation?**
Hypertensive complications, preterm delivery, infection, and fetal growth restriction. Immunosuppressive agents used, such as cyclosporine and FK506, cause hypertension and renal insufficiency, as well as impairment of placental amino acid transport systems, leading fetal growth restriction. Cytomegalovirus (CMV) infection can cause congenital anomalies and liver disease, if the mother was infected early in the pregnancy. Risk for CMV infection is greate immediately after transplant or in cases of increased immunosuppression caused by rejection episodes.

Rejection is a very rare complication; only about 10% of reported pregnancies have been complicated by biopsy proven rejection.

What is recommended in the management of a pregnancy occurring post liver transplantation?

Management of high risk pregnancy by a specialist in maternal-fetal medicine is preferred. Immunosuppression should be continued with close monitoring of blood levels. Abnormal liver function tests should be evaluated aggressively. Percutaneous liver biopsy is not contraindicated but should be performed under ultrasound guidance. Monitoring for maternal and fetal CMV infection is indicated. Quantitative CMV immunoglobulins or detection of CMV viremia and viuria in the mother are adequate tests, and even amniotic fluid analysis could be used if there is suspicion of fetal infection. Deliveries should be by caesarean section if there are active herpes simplex lesions present. Prophylactic antibiotics should be used for deliveries, in general.

What is pregnancy safety data regarding maintenance immunosuppressive agents used in orthotopic liver transplantation?

- *Category B* (no evidence of risk in humans): prednisone
- *Category C* (risks cannot be ruled out): cyclosporine, tacrolimus (FK506), mycophenolate mofetil (CellCept), rapamycin (Sirolimus), OKT3, antithymocyte globulin, antilymphocyte globulin
- *Category D* (evidence of risk): azathioprine

Is breastfeeding permitted after delivery in a liver transplant recipient?

At this time, it is believed that breastfeeding should be discouraged. A woman with administered immunosuppressive drugs should not breastfeed. Calcineurin inhibitors could cause immuno-suppression and nephrotoxicity, and no recommendation can be made, at this time, regarding azathioprine-based regimens because there is extremely limited experience. Manufacturer recommends against breastfeeding in mothers with administered interferon therapy, ribavirin, ganciclovir, lamivudine. No specific recommendation can be made regarding foscarnet. No data are available regarding ursodeoxycholic acid excretion in breast milk.

Are immunosuppressive agents safe during pregnancy?

No. Corticosteroids, azathioprine, cyclosporine, tacrolimus, and OKT3 have no apparent teratogenic potential. All may contribute to low birth weights and fetal prematurity. Tacrolimus crosses the placenta and may contribute to transient perinatal hyperkalemia and mild, reversible renal impairment. There are no reports of allograft loss as a result of pregnancy in the tacrolimus-treated group of 35 patients at the University of Pittsburgh. The Philadelphia-based cyclosporine registry reports an allograft rejection rate of 17% and a graft loss rate of 5.7% in 35 patients taking cyclosporine.

How may vertical transmission of viral hepatitis A be prevented?

Maternal infection with the hepatitis A virus (HAV) is not associated with fetal wastage or teratogenic effects. Vertical transmission of HAV is rare. There are no restrictions concerning breastfeeding. Passive immunization with immunoglobulin for urgent postexposure prophylaxis and HAV vaccine is safe and recommended in pregnant women at risk for acquiring the disease, such as women traveling to endemic areas.

How may vertical transmission of viral hepatitis B be prevented?

The hepatitis B virus (HBV) may be transmitted vertically. If the mother acquires HBV in the first trimester of pregnancy, there is a 10% risk that the infant will test positive for hepatitis B surface antigen (HBsAg) at birth. The percentage increases dramatically to 80–90% if the acute maternal infection develops during the third trimester. In mothers who have chronic HBV and test positive for the hepatitis Be antigen (HBeAg), 90% of neonates develop chronic HBV without prophylaxis. If the mother has HBeAg- and HBeAb-negative chronic HBV, 40% of neonates develop chronic HBV infection without prophylaxis. The rate decreases to <5% if th mother is HBeAg-negative and HBeAb-positive. Antepartum serum HBsAg testing is manda Neonates of HBsAg-positive mothers or HBsAg-unknown mothers are treated with HBV hum hyperimmune globulin (HBIG), 0.5 mL intramuscularly, at delivery. At the same time, they ar given the first dose of HBV vaccine. The second dose is administered at age 1 month and the third dose at age 6 months. If the mother is HBsAg-negative, the child should be vaccinated the three-dose regimen only, with the first inoculation at birth. The regimen is about 85% eff tive in preventing chronic HBV in neonates and is ineffective in cases of hematogenous trans cental transmission, which are seen in about 15% of pregnancies as a result of small placen tears. Active and passive immunization at birth also reduces possibility of viral transmission breastfeeding. Hepatitis B vaccination is safe in pregnant women. Lamivudine administered the last month of pregnancy was recently shown to be safe and efficacious in decreasing risk vertical transmission.

48. **What about vertical transmission of viral hepatitis C?**
The risk of perinatal transmission is approximately 2% for infants of anti-hepatitis C vir (HCV) seropositive women. When a pregnant woman is HCV RNA positive at delivery, th risk increases to 4–7%. Higher HCV RNA levels appear to be associated with a greater r Levels of RNA ≥1,000,000 copies/mL are reportedly associated with vertical transmissi rates as high as 50%. HCV transmission increases up to 20% in women coinfected with HCV and HIV. There are currently no data to determine whether antiviral therapy reduces perinatal transmission. Immunoglobulin therapy is ineffective. Rate of infection is simila among first- and second-born children.

49. **Is it possible to prevent vertical transmission of viral hepatitis D and G?**
Perinatal transmission of the hepatitis D virus (HDV) is rare. There are no documented cases vertical transmission of HDV in the United States. No clinical data about hepatitis G virus infe tion during pregnancy are available, and no studies of vertical transmission have been done. Because of lack of data on HDV, recommendations regarding breastfeeding are unknown.

50. **Are hepatitis C virus-infected women allowed to breastfeed?**
Yes. HCV-infected women should be told that hepatitis C transmission via breastfeeding has been documented. Current available studies show that the average rate of infection is 4%, si larly for breastfed and bottlefed infants. According to the Centers for Disease Control and Prevention (CDC) and to a 1997 consensus statement from the National Institutes of Health (NIH), "Breastfeeding is not contraindicated for HCV-positive mothers," and "the maternal to baby transmission of HCV infection through breast milk has not been documented." Risk of transmission by breastfeeding was not found to be significant, unless coinfection with HIV v present.

51. **Does the mode of delivery influence hepatitis C virus transmission?**
No. Current data are limited but indicate that infection rates are similar in infants delivered va nally and caesarean-delivered infants. There are no prospective studies evaluating the use of elective caesarean section for the prevention of mother-to-infant transmission of HCV. Howe avoiding fetal scalp monitoring and prolonged labor after rupture of membranes may reduce risk of transmission to the infant.

52. **How can perinatal hepatitis C virus infection be diagnosed?**
Infants passively acquire maternal antibodies that can persist for months. Anti-HCV antibodi after age 15 months or positive HCV-RNA, which can be detected as early as 1 or 2 months, diagnostic of perinatal transmission of HCV. Recent NIH consensus conference recommends that infants born to HCV-positive mothers should be tested for HCV infection by HCV RNA te

on two occasions between ages 2 and 6 months and/or have tests for anti-HCV after age 15 months. Positive anti-HCV in infants prior to age 15 months may be due to transplacental transfer of maternal anti-HCV antibody.

WEBSITES

1. http://www.aasld.org
2. http://www.liverfoundation.org

BIBLIOGRAPHY

Armenti VT, Herrine SK, Radomski JS, Moritz MJ: Pregnancy after liver transplantation. Liver Transpl 6(6):671–685, 2000.

Barton JR, Sibai BM: HELLP and the liver diseases of preeclampsia. Clin Liver Dis 3:31–49, 1999.

Barton JR, Sibai BM: Care of the pregnancy complicated by HELLP syndrome. Gastroenterol Clin North Am 21:937–950, 1992.

Borgelt-Hansen L: Oral contraceptives: An update on health benefits and risks. J Am Pharm Assoc 41(6):875–886, 2001.

Brewer GJ, Johnson VD, Dick RD, et al: Treatment of Wilson's disease with zinc. XVII: Treatment during pregnancy. Hepatology 31:364–370, 2000.

Carr DB, Larson AM, Schmucker BC, et al: Maternal hemodynamics and pregnancy outcome in women with prior orthotopic liver transplantation. Liver Transpl 6(2):213–221, 2000.

Centers for Disease Control and Prevention: Recommendations for prevention and control of hepatitis C virus (HCV) infection and HCV-related chronic disease. MMWR 47(RR-19), 1998.

Connoly TJ, Zuckerman AL: Contraception in the patient with liver disease. Semin Perinatol 22:178–182, 1998.

European Pediatric Hepatitis C Virus Network: Effects of mode of delivery and infant feeding on the risk of mother-to-child transmission of hepatitis C virus. Br J Obstet Gynaecol 108:371–377, 2001.

Everson GT: Liver problems in pregnancy: Distinguishing normal from abnormal hepatic changes. Medscape Women's Health 3(2):3, 1998.

Ibdah JA, Bennett MJ, Rinaldo P, et al: A fetal fatty-acid oxidation disorder as a cause of liver disease in pregnant women. N Engl J Med 340:1723–1731, 1999.

Ibdah JA, Yang Z, Bennett MJ: Liver disease in pregnancy and fetal fatty acid oxidation defects. Mol Genet Metab 71(1-2):182–189, 2000.

Jain A, Venkataramanan R, Fung JJ, et al: Pregnancy after liver transplantation under tacrolimus. Transplantation 64:559–565, 1997.

Knox TA: Evaluation of abnormal liver function in pregnancy. Semin Perinatol 22:98–103, 1998.

Kochrar R, Kumar S, Goel R, et al: Pregnancy and its outcome in patients with noncirrhotic portal hypertension. Digest Dis Sci 44:1356–1361, 1999.

Misra S, Sanyal AJ: Pregnancy in a patient with portal hypertension. Clin Liver Dis 3:147–163, 1999.

Molmenti EP, Jain AB, Marino N, et al: Liver transplantation and pregnancy. Clin Liver Dis 3:163–173, 1999.

National Institutes of Health Consensus Development Conference Statement: Management of hepatitis C, June 10–12, 2002.

Parolin MB, Coelho JC, Balbi E, et al: Normalization of menstrual cycles and successful pregnancy after orthotopic liver transplantation. Arq Gastroenterol 37(1):3–6, 2000.

Polywka S, Schroter M, Feucht HH, et al: Low risk of vertical transmission of hepatitis C virus by breast milk. Clin Infect Dis 29:1327–1329, 1999.

Radomski JS, Ahlswede BA, Jarrell BE, et al: Outcomes of 500 pregnancies in 335 female kidney, liver and heart transplant recipients. Transplant Proc 27:1089, 1995.

Radomski JS, Moritz MJ, Munoz SJ, et al: National Transplantation Pregnancy Registry: Analysis of pregnancy outcomes in female liver transplant recipients. Liver Transplant Surg 1:281, 1995.

23. Reinus JF, Leikin EL: Viral hepatitis in pregnancy. Clin Liver Dis 3:115–131, 1999.

24. Riely CA: Contraception and pregnancy after liver transplantation. Liver Transpl 7(11Suppl 1):S74–S76, 200

25. Riely CA, Fallon HJ: Liver diseases. In Burrow GN, Duffy TP (eds): Medical Complications During Pregnancy, ed. Philadelphia, W.B.Saunders, 1999, pp 269–294.

26. Riely CA: Liver diseases in pregnancy. In Reece EA, Hobbins JC (eds): Medicine of the Fetus and Mother, 2nd Philadelphia, Lippincott-Raven, 1999, pp 1153–1163.

27. Rinaldo P, Raymond K, Al-Odaib A, Bennett MJ: Clinical and biochemical features of fatty acid oxidation diso ders. Curr Opin Pediatr 10:615–621, 1998.

28. Rosa FW: Teratogen update: Penicillamine. Teratology 33:127–131, 1986.

29. Sandhu BS, Sanyal AJ: Pregnancy and liver disease. Gastroenterol Clin North Am 32(1):407–436, 2003.

30. Sheikh RA, Yasmeen S, Pauly MP, Riegler JL: Spontaneous intrahepatic hemorrhage and hepatic rupture in t HELLP syndrome. J Clin Gastroenterol 28:323–328, 1999.

31. Solomon L, Abrams G, Dinner M, Berman L: Neonatal abnormalities associated with D-penicillamine treatme during pregnancy. N Engl J Med 296:54–55, 1977.

32. Sternlieb I: Wilson's disease and pregnancy [Editorial]. Hepatology 31:531–532, 2000.

33. van Nunen AB, De Man RA, Heijtink RA, et al: Lamivudine in the last 4 weeks of pregnancy to prevent perinat transmission in highly viremic chronic hepatitis B patients. J Hepatol 32:1040–1041, 2000.

34. World Health Organization: Hepatitis B and breastfeeding. J Int Assoc Physicians AIDS Care 4:20–21, 1998.

35. Yang Z, Yamada J, Zhao Y, et al: Prospective sceening for pediatric mitochondrial trifunctional protein defect pregnancies complicated by liver disease. JAMA 288:2163–2166, 2002.

36. Zanetti AR, Ferroni P, Magliano EM, et al: Perinatal transmission of the hepatitis B virus and of the HBV-assoc ated delta agent from mothers to offspring in Northern Italy. J Med Virol 9:139–148, 1982.

CHAPTER 24

RHEUMATOLOGIC MANIFESTATIONS OF HEPATOBILIARY DISEASES

Sterling G. West, MD

VIRAL HEPATITIS

How often is viral hepatitis associated with rheumatic manifestations?
Approximately 25% of patients with hepatitis B antigenemia develop a rheumatic syndrome. Up to 50% of patients with hepatitis C virus (HCV) develop an autoimmune syndrome. Transient arthralgia can occur in 10% of patients during acute hepatitis A viral infection.

What are the most common extrahepatic rheumatologic manifestations of hepatitis B virus infection?
- Acute polyarthritis–dermatitis syndrome
- Polyarteritis nodosa
- Membranous glomerulonephritis
- Cryoglobulinemia—usually associated with hepatitis C. Only 5% of all essential mixed cryoglobulinemia is due to hepatitis B alone.

Describe the clinical characteristics of the polyarthritis–dermatitis syndrome associated with hepatitis B virus infection.
In the preicteric prodromal period of acute hepatitis B virus infection, 25% of patients develop a polyarthritis that is acute, severe, and symmetric, involving both small (fingers) and large (knees, ankles) joints. A classically urticarial rash frequently (40%) accompanies the arthritis. Both the arthritis and rash precede the onset of jaundice and/or elevated liver-associated enzymes by several days. The arthritis improves with nonsteroidal anti-inflammatory drugs (NSAIDs) and subsides usually soon after the onset of jaundice. Patients who develop chronic hepatitis B viremia may subsequently have recurrent arthralgia/arthritis. The etiology of this syndrome is due to deposition of circulating hepatitis B surface antigen–hepatitis B surface antibody (HBsAg–HBsAb) immune complexes in the joints and skin.

What is the typical presentation of hepatitis B–associated polyarteritis nodosa (PAN)?
Up to 25% of all patients with PAN have positive hepatitis B serologies and evidence of viral replication. They may present with a combination of fever, arthritis, mononeuritis multiplex, abdominal pain, renal disease, and/or cardiac disease. Although liver-associated enzymes may be abnormal, symptomatic hepatitis is not a prominent feature.

How is polyarteritis nodosa, associated with hepatitis B antigenemia, diagnosed?
The diagnosis is made on the basis of a consistent clinical presentation coupled with an abdominal or renal angiogram showing vascular aneurysms and corkscrewing of blood vessels (Fig. 24-1). The gold standard is a tissue biopsy showing medium-vessel vasculitis.

What is the treatment of hepatitis B-associated polyarteritis nodosa?
Patients are typically very ill and will die without aggressive therapy. Antiviral agents and plasmapheresis are used early to control the acute symptoms and antigenemia. Corticosteroids are also

used early to control inflammation acutely. Once the acute process is controlled, corticosteroids are tapered because they alone, or in combination with cytotoxic drugs, can enhance viral replication. Patients over age 50 and those with renal insufficiency, cardiac, gastrointestinal, or central nervous system involvement have the worst prognosis. Overall, 5-year survival rate is 50–70%.

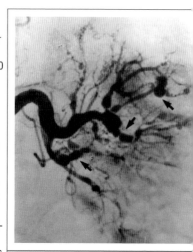

Figure 24-1. Renal angiogram showing vascular aneurysms in a patient with hepatitis B-associated polyarteritis nodosa (*arrows*).

7. **What are the most common hepatitis C virus related autoimmune disorders?**
   - Mixed cryoglobulinemia (60–90% of HCV patients have cryoglobulins, but only 15% get vasculitis)
   - Systemic polyarteritis-nodosa-like vasculitis (1% of HCV patients)
   - Membranoproliferative glomerulonephritis
   - Nonerosive polyarthritis (5–10%): typically intermittent, monoarthritis or oligoarthritis affecting large and medium-sized joints. However, rarely, patients with acute HCV infection can have an acute polyarthritis resembling rheumatoid arthritis with involvement of hands, wrists, shoulders, knees, and hips symmetric
   - Autoantibody production: rheumatoid factor, antinuclear antibodies, anticardiolipin antibodies, antismooth muscle, anti-LKM-1, and antithyroid antibodies
   - Porphyria cutanea tarda: metabolic disorder due to reduced hepatic activity of uroporphyrinogen decarboxylase
   - Sjögren's-like syndrome with dry eyes and dry mouth (5–19% of HCV patients)

8. **What is the relationship between viral hepatitis and cryoglobulinemia?**
   Approximately 80–90% of patients with essential mixed cryoglobulinemia (type II and type III) are positive for HCV. HCV is concentrated up to 1000-fold in the cryoprecipitate. HCV-infected patients are prone to develop autoimmune and lymphoproliferative diseases due to HCV predilection to infect B cells resulting in proto-oncogene, bcl-2, recombination that inhibits apoptosis leading to extended lymphocyte survival. This results in increased autoantibody formation, cryoglobulinemia, and/or neoplastic transformation (non-Hodgkin's B-cell lymphoma).

KEY POINTS: VIRAL HEPATITIS AND RHEUMATIC MANIFESTATIONS

1. Essential mixed cryoglobulinemia is due to chronic hepatitis C infection in over 90% of patients.

2. All patients with a systemic medium and/or small vessel vasculitis should be evaluated for chronic hepatitis B and C infections.

3. The treatment of vasculitis due to hepatitis B or C infection must include antiviral therapy to eliminate the antigenemia.

4. All patients with an inflammatory small joint arthritis, positive rheumatoid factor, and elevated liver-associated transaminase levels should have chronic hepatitis C infection ruled out before receiving the diagnosis of rheumatoid arthritis.

Describe the typical clinical features of cryoglobulinemia associated with hepatitis C infection.

Cryoglobulins are one or more immunoglobulins that precipitate at temperatures below 37°C and redissolve with rewarming. They precipitate in blood vessels in patients causing a variety of symptoms. Patients present with a combination of fever, arthritis (that can be confused with rheumatoid arthritis), renal disease, paresthesia from peripheral neuropathy, and a predominantly lower extremity petechial rash, positive rheumatoid factor, and low complement levels (especially C4). Hepatitis is not a prominent feature. Patients have been successfully treated with combined corticosteroids, interferon α/ribavirin combination, and plasmapheresis. Recently, rituximab (anti-CD20) has been used successfully to deplete the B-cell population making the cryoglobulins.

AUTOIMMUNE AND OTHER LIVER DISEASES

What is lupoid hepatitis?

Lupoid hepatitis is now called *type I autoimmune hepatitis* (AIH). Patients are middle-aged, predominantly female (70%), and have clinical (arthralgia [50%]) and laboratory manifestations that resemble systemic lupus erythematosus (SLE). Patients commonly have positive antinuclear antibodies (ANA), antibodies against smooth muscle antigen (80%) frequently with specificity against F1 actin, and, occasionally, lupus erythematosus (LE) cells. They do not have antibodies against double-stranded (ds) DNA.

To what degree is type I autoimmune hepatitis similar to systemic lupus erythematosus?

See Table 24-1.

TABLE 24-1.	COMPARISON OF TYPE I AUTOIMMUNE HEPATITIS (AIH) AND SYSTEMIC LUPUS ERYTHEMATOSUS (SLE)	
	SLE	Type I AIH
Young women	+	+
Polyarthritis	+	+
Fever	+	+
Rash	+	+
Nephritis	+	−
Central nervous system disease	+	−
Photosensitivity	+	−
Oral ulcers	+	−
ANA	99%	70–90%
LE cells	70%	40–50%
Polyclonal gammopathy	+	+
Anti-Smith antibodies	25%	0
+ anti-ds DNA	70%	Rare
+ anti-F1 actin	Rare	60–95%

ANA = antinuclear antibody, LE = lupus erythematosus.

12. **What is the difference between anti-Sm antibody and anti-SM antibodies?**
Anti-Sm antibodies are antibodies against the Smith antigen, which is an epitope on small nuclear ribonuclear proteins. It is highly diagnostic of SLE. Anti-SM antibody is an antibody against the smooth muscle antigen (which is frequently F1 actin). It is highly diagnostic of type autoimmune hepatitis (Table 24-2).

TABLE 24-2. ANTI-SM VERSUS ANTI-SM ANTIBODIES		
	SLE	Type I AIH
Anti-Smith (Sm) antibodies	Yes	No
Antismooth muscle (SM) antibodies	No	Yes

13. **List the common autoimmune diseases associated with primary biliary cirrhosis (PBC).**
Up to 80% of patients with PBC have one or more of the following disorders:
- Keratoconjunctivitis sicca (Sjögren's syndrome)   66%
- Autoimmune thyroiditis (Hashimoto's disease)   20%
- Scleroderma/Raynaud's disease*   20%
- Rheumatoid arthritis   10%

*Limited scleroderma (calcinosis, Raynaud's phenomenon, esophageal disease, sclerodactyly, and telangiectasia [CREST]) occurs in 4% of PBC patients and antedates PBC by 14 years.

14. **Compare and contrast the arthritis that may occur with primary biliary cirrhosis and rheumatoid arthritis.**
See Table 24-3.

TABLE 24-3. PRIMARY BILIARY CIRRHOSIS ARTHRITIS VERSUS RHEUMATOID ARTHRITIS		
	PBC Arthritis	Rheumatoid Arthritis
Frequency in patients	10% get RA	10% get PBC
Number of joints*	Polyarticular	Polyarticular
Symmetry	Symmetric	Symmetric
Inflammatory	Yes	Yes
Rheumatoid factor	Sometimes	Yes (85%)
Erosions on radiograph	Rare	Common

*PBC can involve distal interphalangeal joints of fingers, whereas rheumatoid arthritis does not involve these joints.
RA = rheumatoid arthritis, PBC = primary biliary cirrhosis.

15. **What other musculoskeletal manifestations may occur in patients with primary biliary cirrhosis?**
- Osteomalacia due to fat-soluble vitamin D malabsorption (low 25-OH vitamin D level)
- Osteoporosis due to renal tubular acidosis
- Hypertrophic osteoarthropathy

What autoantibodies occur commonly in patients with primary biliary cirrhosis?

- Antimitochondrial antibodies   80%
- Anticentromere antibodies   20%*

   *Most patients also have manifestations of the CREST variant of scleroderma.

How commonly does arthritis occur in patients with hemochromatosis?
Approximately 40–75% of patients have a noninflammatory degenerative arthritis, most commonly involving the second and third metacarpophalangeal joints (MCPs), proximal interphalangeal joints (PIPs), wrists, hips, knees, and ankles. Of importance, this arthropathy may be the presenting complaint (30–50%) of patients with hemochromatosis and is misdiagnosed frequently in young men as seronegative rheumatoid arthritis.

Describe the radiographic features suggestive of hemochromatotic arthropathy.
Suggestive radiographic features include subchondral sclerosis, cyst formation, irregular joint space narrowing, and osteophyte formation consistent with degenerative arthritis of involved joints. The key is finding degenerative changes in the MCP joints (typically 2nd and 3rd) with hook-like osteophytes (Fig. 24-2). This finding is important, because the MCPs and wrists rarely develop degenerative joint disease without an underlying cause, such as hemochromatosis.

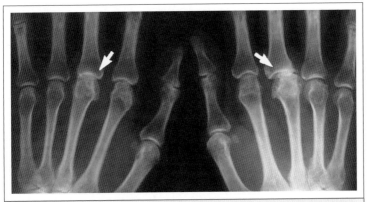

Figure 24-2. Radiograph of hands showing degenerative arthritis with hook-like osteophytes of the second and third metacarpophalangeal joints in a patient with hemochromatosis (*arrows*).

What is the relationship between calcium pyrophosphate disease and hemochromatosis?
Chondrocalcinosis of the triangular fibrocartilage at the ulnar side of the wrist and the hyaline cartilage of the knees is seen in 20–50% of patients with hemochromatosis. Crystals of calcium pyrophosphate may shed into the joints, causing superimposed flares of inflammatory arthritis (i.e., pseudogout).

Discuss the genetics of hemochromatosis.
Hemochromatosis is among the most common genetic disorders in Caucasians of Northern European descent. Nearly 90% of patients with hereditary hemochromatosis are homozygous for the same mutation (C 282Y) in the hemochromatosis (HFE) gene. The homozygote frequency in this Caucasian population is 0.3–0.5% and carrier frequency is 7–10% (i.e., heterozygotes). The HFE gene is located on chromosome 6 near the major histocompatibility complex

(MHC) locus. It encodes for an MHC class-I like protein that complexes with beta$_2$-microglob and the transferrin receptor. This protein complex on the surface of duodenal crypt cells can bind to transferrin-bound iron in the circulation, enabling these cells to sense body iron store The mutation of HFE gene results in a protein that does not bind well to the transferrin recepto resulting in a protein complex that does not bind well to transferrin. Consequently, the duode crypt cells sense that the body is low in iron and, in turn, upregulate their divalent transporter protein that facilitates iron absorption from the intestinal lumen.

KEY POINTS: AUTOIMMUNE HEPATITIS, HEMOCHROMATOSIS, AND RHEUMATIC MANIFESTATIONS

1. All patients with symptoms compatible with systemic lupus erythematosus, who have elevated liver-associated transaminase levels, should be evaluated for type I autoimmune hepatitis with antismooth muscle antibody testing.

2. Primary biliary cirrhosis, Sjögren's syndrome, and limited scleroderma (CREST) can occur together or separately.

3. The majority of patients with hemochromatosis present with musculoskeletal complaints (arthritis, osteoporosis due to hypogonadism) before other manifestations of the disease.

4. All Caucasian male patients less than age 50, with degenerative arthritis involving their metacarpophalangeal joints, should be evaluated for hemochromatosis.

5. All patients with chronic liver diseases should be screened for osteoporosis and be evaluated for vitamin D deficiency causing osteomalacia.

21. **Compare and contrast the features of hemochromatotic arthropathy (HA) and rheumatoid arthritis (RA).**
See Table 24-4.

TABLE 24-4. COMPARISON OF HEMOCHROMATOTIC ARTHROPATHY AND RHEUMATOID ARTHRITIS

	HA	RA
Sex	M>F (10:1)	F>M (3:1)
Age of onset	>35 yr	All ages
Joints	Polyarticular	Polyarticular
Symmetry	Symmetric	Symmetric
Inflammatory signs/symptoms	Only if pseudogout attack	Yes
Rheumatoid factor	Negative	Positive (85%)
Gene	HFE (90%)	HLA DR4 (70%)
Synovial fluid	Noninflammatory	Inflammatory
Radiographs	Degenerative changes	Inflammatory, erosive disease

HA = hemochromatotic arthropathy, RA = rheumatoid arthritis, M = male, F = female, yr = year(s), HLA = human leukocyte antigen.

How effective is phlebotomy in halting the progression of hemochromatotic arthropathy?
Phlebotomy does not halt the progression of the arthropathy.

What is the correlation between the severity of arthropathy and severity of liver disease in hemochromatosis?
There is no correlation.

Why does hemochromatosis cause a degenerative arthritis?
The arthropathy is characterized by hemosiderin deposition in synovium and chondrocytes. The presence of iron in these cells may lead to increased production of destructive enzymes (e.g., collagenase) that cause cartilage damage. Other mechanisms may also be possible; the precise pathway by which chronic iron overload leads to tissue injury has not been fully established.

What other musculoskeletal problems may occur in patients with hemochromatosis?

- Osteoporosis due to gonadal dysfunction from pituitary insufficiency caused by the iron over-load state (low follicle-stimulating hormone [FSH], leutinizing hormone [LH], and testos-terone).
- Osteomalacia due to vitamin D deficiency due to liver disease (low 25-OH vitamin D level).
- Hypertrophic osteoarthropathy: cirrhosis of any cause, including hemochromatosis, can be associated with periosteal reaction involving shafts of long bones.

BLIOGRAPHY

Bothwell TH, MacPhail AP: Hereditary hemochromatosis: Etiologic, pathologic, and clinical aspects. Semin Hematol 35:55–71, 1998.

Cacoub P, Poynard T, Ghillani P, et al: Extrahepatic manifestations of chronic hepatitis C. Arthritis Rheum 42:2204–2212, 1999.

Culp KS, Fleming CR, Duffy J, et al: Autoimmune associations and primary biliary cirrhosis. Mayo Clin Proc 57:365–370, 1982.

Duffy J: Arthritis and liver disease. In Koopman W (ed): Arthritis and Allied Conditions, 14th ed. Philadelphia, Lea & Febiger, 2001, pp 1383–1399.

Fleming RE, Sly WS: Mechanisms of iron accumulation in hereditary hemochromatosis. Annu Rev Physiol 64:663–680, 2002.

Gayroud M, Guillevin L, le Toumelin P, et al: Long-term follow-up of polyarteritis nodosa, microscopic polyangi-itis, and Churg-Strauss syndrome: Analysis of four prospective trials including 278 patients. Arthritis Rheum 44:666–675, 2001.

Hall S, Czaja AJ, Kaufman DK, et al: How lupoid is lupoid hepatitis? J Rheumatol 13:95–98, 1986.

Inman RD: Rheumatoid manifestations of hepatitis B infections. Semin Arthritis Rheum 11:406–420, 1982.

Lamprecht P, Gause A, Gross WL: Cryoglobulinemic vasculitis. Arthritis Rheum 42:2507–2516, 1999.

Lunel F, Cacoub P: Treatment of autoimmune and extrahepatic manifestations of hepatitis C virus. J Hepatol 31:210–216, 1999.

Marx WJ, O'Connell DJ: Arthritis of primary biliary cirrhosis. Arch Intern Med 139:213–216, 1979.

Olsson KS: Hemochromatosis. In Hochberg MC (ed): Rheumatology, 3rd ed. London, Mosby, 2003, pp 2005–2010.

Rivera J, Garcia-Monforte A, Pineda A, Millan Nunez-Cortes J: Arthritis in patients with chronic hepatitis C virus infection. J Rheumatol 26:420–424, 1999.

Trepo C, Guillevin L: Polyarteritis nodosa and extrahepatic manifestations for HBV infection. J Autoimmun 16:269–274, 2001.

Vassilopoulos D, Calabrese LH: Hepatitis C virus infection and vasculitis: Implications of antiviral and immuno-suppression therapies. Arthritis Rheum 46:585–597, 2002.

CHAPTER 25

EVALUATION OF FOCAL LIVER MASSES

Steven P. Lawrence, MD

1. **Describe the initial work-up for a patient with a liver mass.**
   The first step is an accurate history and physical examination. Age, sex, and birthplace are important clues to etiology. Risk factors for viral hepatitis or a history of cirrhosis increases t possibility of a primary malignant process. A previously diagnosed neoplasm heightens suspicion for metastatic disease. Use of oral contraceptives or anabolic steroids, alcohol inta and potential occupational exposure to carcinogens should be noted. Hepatomegaly and/or splenomegaly, abdominal pain, or stigmata of chronic liver disease (such as palmar erythema spider angiomata, or gynecomastia) may be present.

   Liver-associated enzymes, with the exception of gamma-glutamyl transpeptidase (GGT), a usually normal with benign liver tumors. Serum alkaline phosphatase levels are often elevate with hepatic metastases, but not in all cases. An increase in serum transaminases may signif chronic hepatitis or cirrhosis. Positive hepatitis B or C serologies or iron studies may identify underlying cause of liver dysfunction or cirrhosis (Table 25-1).

TABLE 25-1. DIFFERENTIAL DIAGNOSIS OF FOCAL LIVER MASSES IN ADULTS	
Benign	**Malignant**
Epithelial tumors	
Hepatic adenoma	Hepatocellular carcinoma
Bile duct adenoma	Cholangiocarcinoma
Biliary cystadenoma	Biliary cystadenocarcinoma
Mesenchymal tumors	
Cavernous hemangioma	Angiosarcoma
	Primary hepatic lymphoma
Other lesions	
Focal nodular hyperplasia	Metastatic tumors
Liver abscess	
Macroregenerative nodules in cirrhosis	
Focal fatty infiltration	
Simple hepatic cyst	

Modified from Kew MC: Tumors of the liver. In Zakim D, Boyer TD (eds): Hepatology: A Textbook of Liver Disease, 2nd ed. Philadelphia, W.B. Saunders, 1990, pp 1206–1239.

2. **What tumor markers are useful in the evaluation of focal liver lesions?**

Serum α-fetoprotein (AFP) and tumor-associated antigen CA19-9 are markers of primary hepatic malignancy and are used when radiographic studies indicate a focal neoplasm originating in the liver.

AFP is the best diagnostic marker for hepatocellular carcinoma (HCC) and also plays a role in screening programs of at-risk populations. AFP levels above 200 ng/mL are highly suggestive of HCC, whereas lesser elevations may be due to benign chronic hepatitis. A universally accepted cutoff value for AFP in the diagnosis of HCC has not been established, and some authorities use a level >500 ng/mL. Not all hepatomas secrete AFP, and approximately one third of patients have a normal AFP value, especially when the tumor is smaller than 2 cm. AFP levels should decrease or normalize with successful treatment.

CA19-9 is used in the diagnosis of cholangiocarcinoma, a malignancy originating in the bile ducts. CA19-9 levels >100 U/mL are found in over 50% of patients and values >1000 U/mL suggest unresectability. This marker is more sensitive in patients with primary sclerosing cholangitis, a risk factor for cholangiocarcinoma. Significant false-positive elevations in CA19-9 can occur with bacterial cholangitis. CA19-9 also serves as a tumor marker for pancreatic carcinoma.

3. **What imaging modalities are used in the detection and characterization of focal liver masses?**

Recent advances in computed tomography (CT) and magnetic resonance imaging (MRI) allow detailed assessment of focal liver lesions. These imaging studies have largely supplanted previously used nuclear medicine-based protocols for the characterization of liver masses.

Triphasic CT, which is now widely available, offers substantial improvement in hepatic imaging because of its rapid scan time within a single breath-hold. This feature eliminates respiratory motion and allows contrast injection to be viewed in unenhanced, arterial (early), and portal venous phases of perfusion. Lesions that derive their vascular supply from the hepatic artery, such as HCC and hypervascular metastases, are prominent during the arterial phase. The venous or portal phase of helical CT provides maximal enhancement of normal liver parenchyma and optimizes detection of hypovascular lesions, such as colon, gastric, and pancreatic metastases.

MRI scanning has undergone similar refinements, with breath-hold T1-weighted images and fast (turbo) spin-echo T2-weighted sequences that eliminate motion artifacts and make use of contrast agents in a manner analogous to triphasic CT. Gadolinium-enhanced MRI should be considered in patients with contraindications to iodine-based CT, such as contrast allergies or renal insufficiency.

Many focal liver masses are found, incidentally, on *ultrasound* examination of the abdomen. Although liver ultrasound often cannot fully characterize the lesion, it has a role in verifying simple hepatic cysts, which may have nonspecific radiographic patterns on CT or MRI. Intraoperative ultrasound remains the best modality for defining hepatic metastases.

4. **What is the most common benign cause of a focal liver lesion?**

Cavernous hemangiomas are the most common benign hepatic tumor, occurring in up to 20% of the population. They occur in all age groups, more commonly in women, as solitary (60%) or multiple asymptomatic masses. Most are <3 cm and occur usually in the posterior segment of the right hepatic lobe. The term *giant hemangioma* is sometimes used when the size exceeds 5 cm. Microscopically, hemangiomas consist of blood-filled vascular sinusoids separated by connective-tissue septae. Occasionally, hemangiomas are large enough to cause abdominal pain, but the risk of tumor growth or bleeding is minimal and does not justify surgical removal unless the patient is significantly symptomatic.

. **Why is oral contraceptive use important in the differential diagnosis of focal liver masses?**

Most cases of hepatic adenomas relate directly to the use of oral contraceptive pills (OCPs). This benign tumor was seen rarely before oral contraceptive agents came into common usage in the

1960s. Risk correlates with duration of use and age >30 years. Hepatic adenomas occur most commonly in young and middle-aged women, with an incidence of 3–4 per 100,000. Men infrequently develop adenomas, although cases have been reported with anabolic steroid use.

Hepatic adenomas are well-demarcated, fleshy tumors with prominent surface vasculature. Microscopically, they consist of monotonous sheets of normal or small hepatocytes with no bile ducts, portal tracts, or central veins.

6. **Why is surgical resection of hepatic adenomas recommended?**
Spontaneous rupture and intra-abdominal hemorrhage can occur in up to 30% of patients with hepatic adenoma, especially during menstruation or pregnancy. HCC can also develop within adenomas. Approximately 50% of patients with these tumors have abdominal pain, sometimes as a result of bleeding within the adenoma. Adenomas have been known to regress with discontinuation of birth control pills, which should be recommended, but surgical resection remains the management of choice.

7. **What is focal nodular hyperplasia?**
Focal nodular hyperplasia (FNH) is a round, nonencapsulated mass, usually exhibiting a vascular central scar. Fibrous septae radiate from the scar in a spoke-like fashion. Hepatocytes are arranged in nodules or cords between the septae, and the mass includes bile ductules, Kupffer cells, and chronic inflammatory cells. FNH is theorized to result from a hyperplastic tissue response to a congenital arterial malformation.

FNH is the second most common benign liver tumor. Over 90% occur in women and are usually diagnosed between ages 20 and 60. Oral contraceptives are not considered a causative agent of FNH but, occasionally, may enhance their growth; therefore, some authorities recommend discontinuing OCPs in women if FNH is diagnosed.

8. **List the differences between hepatic adenomas and focal nodular hyperplasia.**
See Table 25-2.

TABLE 25-2. HEPATIC ADENOMAS VERSUS FOCAL NODULAR HYPERPLASIA

	Hepatic Adenoma	Focal Nodular Hyperplasia
Size (mean)	10 cm	<5 cm
Kupffer cells	No	Yes
Central scar	Rare	Common
Symptoms	Common	Rare (only with large lesions)
Complications	Bleeding, malignancy	Rare lesions may grow in size
Treatment	Surgical resection	Resection not necessary
Sulfur-colloid liver scan	Cold defect	Positive uptake in 60–70%

9. **What is the most frequent malignancy in the liver?**
Metastatic disease to the liver is much more common than primary hepatic tumors in the United States and Europe. Cancers arising in the colon, stomach, pancreas, breast, and lung are the most likely to metastasize to the liver. Esophageal, renal, and genitourinary neoplasms should also be considered when searching for the primary site. Multiple defects in the liver suggest a metastatic process: only 2% present as solitary lesions. Involvement of both lobes is most common; 20% are confined to the right lobe alone and 3% to the left lobe.

10. **What is the most common primary liver cancer?**
Hepatocellular carcinoma is, by far, the most common malignancy originating in the liver, accounting for approximately 80% of primary liver cancers. The incidence in the United States

ranges from 2–3 cases per 100,000. The recent increase in HCC in the United States over the past decade is directly attributable to the rising incidence of hepatitis C. Geographic location influences both the age of peak occurrence (> age 55 in the United States) and male-to-female incidence ratios. High-incidence areas in Asia and Africa, related to hepatitis B, have a much younger average age of onset and a higher male predominance. Worldwide, men are more likely than women to develop HCC by a factor of 4:1. HCC occurs usually within a cirrhotic liver; approximately 80% of patients diagnosed with HCC have cirrhosis.

KEY POINTS: ITEMS TO SEARCH FOR AT THE INITIAL EVALUATION OF A FOCAL LIVER LESION

1. A history of liver disease, hepatitis, or cirrhosis

2. A history of cancer

3. Past use of oral contraceptives

4. Risk factors for viral hepatitis

5. Right upper or epigastric pain

1. **Describe the various presenting forms of hepatocellular carcinoma.**
   Nodular: most common; multiple nodules of varying size scattered throughout the liver.
   Solitary (or massive): occurs in younger patients; large, solitary mass, often in the right lobe.
   Diffuse: rare; difficult to detect on imaging; widespread infiltration of minute tumor foci.

2. **What types of cirrhosis are most commonly associated with hepatocellular carcinoma?**
   Autopsy studies indicate that 20–40% of patients dying with cirrhosis harbor HCC. The etiologies of cirrhosis related most commonly to HCC, in order of decreasing risk, are as follows:
   1. Chronic hepatitis C (over 5 years, 7% of patients with HCV cirrhosis develop HCC)
   2. Chronic hepatitis B
   3. Hemochromatosis
   4. Alpha$_1$-antitrypsin deficiency
   5. Alcoholic cirrhosis (alcohol potentiates the carcinogenic risk in viral cirrhosis)

3. **What clinical and laboratory findings should raise suspicion for hepatocellular carcinoma?**
   1. New abdominal pain or weight loss
   2. Hepatomegaly
   3. Hepatic bruit
   4. Acute hemoperitoneum
   5. Blood-tinged ascitic fluid
   6. Persistent fever
   7. Sudden increase in serum alkaline phosphatase
   8. Increasing ratio of aspartate aminotransferase to alanine aminotransferase
   9. Polycythemia or persistent leukocytosis
   10. Hypoglycemia
   11. Hypercalcemia
   12. Hypercholesterolemia
   Findings 9–12 are paraneoplastic syndromes associated with HCC.

14. **What primary liver tumor occurs in young adults without underlying cirrhosis?**

The fibrolamellar variant of HCC is a distinctive, slow-growing subtype of hepatic neoplasm, occurring at a mean age of 26 years. Patients seldom have a history of prior liver disease. Unlike typical HCC, men and women are equally affected. Fibrolamellar tumors present usually with abdominal pain due to a large, solitary mass, most often in the left lobe (75%). The AFP level is normal.

The term *fibrolamellar* characterizes the microscopic appearance of this lesion; thin layers of fibrosis separate the neoplastic hepatocytes. A *fibrous central scar* may be seen on imaging studies. Recognition of this variant is important because nearly one half are resectable at the time of diagnosis.

15. **What factors predispose to the development of cholangiocarcinoma?**

Cholangiocarcinomas, which account for about 10% of primary liver cancers, arise as adenocarcinomas from bile duct epithelium. Jaundice is the most frequent clinical presentation of this tumor. Risk factors for cholangiocarcinoma include:

- Primary sclerosing cholangitis
- Liver fluke infestation
- Chronic ulcerative colitis
- Congenital cystic liver diseases
- Choledochal cysts

16. **What is a Klatskin's tumor?**

Cholangiocarcinomas at the hilar bifurcation of the hepatic ducts are referred to as Klatskin's tumors. Peripheral (or intrahepatic) and extrahepatic bile duct cholangiocarcinomas are other subtypes. The characteristic desmoplastic reaction accompanying these tumors often makes them poorly visible on imaging studies and difficult to diagnose on biopsy. Delayed tumor enhancement on CT after IV contrast is noted in approximately 75% of intrahepatic cholangiocarcinomas. Only about 25% of cholangiocarcinomas occur in the setting of cirrhosis. Most are unresectable when diagnosed and thus require palliative drainage of obstructive jaundice by endoscopic, percutaneous, or surgical methods.

17. **When should liver transplantation be considered in patients with hepatocellular carcinoma?**

Solitary lesion <5 cm or <3 nodules, each <3 cm; no metastatic or regional lymph node involvement; and no major vascular invasion.

18. **When should resection be considered in patients with hepatocellular carcinoma?**

HCC is resectable in only approximately 10% of patients in the United States. Five-year survival rates with surgical treatment range between 17% and 40%. Most patients succumb to intrahepatic recurrence of tumor. The multifocal nature of HCC carcinogenesis explains this poor prognosis. Selection criteria for resectability of HCC include:

- Child-Pugh class A cirrhosis
- Solitary lesion <5 cm
- Hepatic wedge pressure gradient <10 mmHg
- Lack of vascular invasion or extrahepatic spread

19. **What palliative therapies are available for the management of hepatocellular carcinoma?**

Radiofrequency ablation is a direct application of thermal energy by percutaneous or surgical means, which destroys unresectable areas of HCC. Radiofrequency ablation appears to offer some benefit over percutaneous ethanol injection by decreasing local recurrence rates and enhancing directed tissue necrosis, although both modalities are now commonly used.

Transarterial chemoembolization involves the selective administration of chemotherapy, followed by embolization, into the hepatic artery branch feeding the tumor. Recent reports suggest that this technique may improve survival as well as local tumor control. It is used frequently to delay tumor progression in patients awaiting liver transplantation.

20. **Who should be screened for hepatocellular carcinoma? Describe a typical screening strategy.**
Patients with cirrhosis, especially those at high risk of HCC, should be screened. Screening is done routinely in people with viral-induced cirrhosis (hepatitis B and C) and cirrhosis-related to metabolic liver disease.

Serial AFP measurements and hepatic ultrasound studies are the most commonly used screening tools. Optimal screening intervals are not established, but AFP levels and ultrasound every 6 months are common practice. Although surveillance may not have a definite impact on mortality rate, it allows more tumors to be amenable to curative resection.

21. **What benign tissue abnormality may simulate a focal liver mass?**
Focal fatty infiltration may appear similar to the focal hepatic lesions described previously. Focal fatty liver is often seen in alcoholism, obesity, diabetes mellitus, malnutrition, corticosteroid excess or therapy, and AIDS. MRI may be necessary to fully characterize this entity. An interesting aspect of focal fat is its rapid disappearance, once the inciting disease process is corrected.

22. **What new imaging techniques are under development to evaluate focal liver masses?**
MRI angiography, which permits the rapid acquisition of arterial and venous sequences, has shown promise in the detection of small HCCs missed by triphasic CT scanning.

Positron emission tomography (PET scan) is currently being studied to improve the difficult detection of cholangiocarcinoma. PET scans are also playing an increasing role in the detection of hepatic metastases from colorectal cancer, when liver resection is contemplated.

Endoscopic ultrasound with fine needle aspiration has also been reported to aid in the diagnosis of suspected cholangiocarcinoma, when other tissue sampling methods, such as intraductal cytology, have failed to provide a diagnosis.

23. **Why is fine-needle biopsy of hepatic masses controversial?**
Establishing a diagnosis for a focal liver mass by fine-needle aspiration (FNA) cytology is more problematic than one would think, owing to subtle histopathologic differences between normal hepatocytes and benign lesions or even well-differentiated hepatomas. The literature reveals a wide range of sensitivity for FNA-based diagnosis of primary hepatic lesions. The most optimistic studies report sensitivities and specificities >90%. Hemangiomas, FNH, and HCC appear to be more difficult to diagnose accurately by FNA; sensitivity ranges between 60% and 70% in many series. Rigorous protocols, making use of two or more imaging studies to characterize a benign lesion, can have an accuracy and sensitivity as high as 80–90%. When HCC is suspected, the use of MRI, CT, and angiography (in selected cases) can confirm the diagnosis in >95% of patients, without the use of FNA.

Another controversy about the use of FNA in HCC is the risk of needle-tract seeding and tumor spread into the circulation, a risk that may be as high as 5%. With the increasing use of liver transplantation in the treatment of HCC, this complication can have grave consequences.

FNA plays a dominant role in the setting of suspected metastatic disease to the liver and inoperable primary cancers. When surgical resection of a lesion, based on clinical and imaging findings, is deemed necessary, preoperative biopsy is generally not advocated.

24. **What should be done when small incidental liver lesions are found?**
Lesions <1 cm are common incidental findings on liver imaging. In the vast majority of cases, they represent benign entities, such as small cysts or hemangiomas. Their small size makes

further characterization by other radiographic studies or percutaneous biopsy problematic and, usually, impossible.

Simple, thin-walled hepatic cysts, regardless of size, need no further follow-up when definitively documented by ultrasound. Otherwise, clinical follow-up by repeating the imaging study in 6 months is recommended. This provides verification that the lesion has not grown in size. Interval growth of such lesions should prompt further work-up.

25. **Outline a logical approach to the evaluation of a focal hepatic mass.**
The work-up of a focal liver mass must occur in the context of a carefully considered differential diagnosis. Associated symptoms, presence of underlying liver disease or extrahepatic malignancy, drug and occupational exposures, and laboratory abnormalities must be assessed before proceeding with further radiographic studies. Symptomatic lesions and lesions noted incidentally are likely to have different etiologies. The patient's age and sex are important clues. Cirrhosis requires a modified approach because of the increased likelihood of HCC.
Incidental lesions
    Small lesions <1 cm → repeat study in 6 months
    Simple cysts → verify with ultrasound
    Hemangiomas → triphasic CT with contrast → 99Tc-labeled red blood cell scan (for lesions >2 cm) or gadolinium-enhanced MRI
    FNH → triphasic CT with contrast → gadolinium-enhanced MRI → ? biopsy
    Hepatic adenoma → history of OCPs → rule out hemangioma and FNH → resection (outlined previously)
Symptomatic lesions
    Hepatic adenoma → history of OCPs → rule out hemangioma/FNH → resection
    Liver abscess → sepsis → ultrasound → triphasic CT (rim enhancement)
Cirrhosis or risk factors for cholangiocarcinoma
    HCC → AFP → triphasic CT → MRI with contrast or MRI angiography
    Cholangiocarcinoma → CA19-9 → triphasic with delayed-phase CT → ? MRCP or PET scan
History of malignancy
    Metastases → triphasic CT with contrast → if resection is considered → PET scan (to rule out multiple metastasis)

BIBLIOGRAPHY

1. Bennett WF, Bova JG: Review of hepatic imaging and a problem-oriented approach to liver masses. Hepatology 12:761–775, 1990.
2. Chopra S: Focal nodular hyperplasia. In Rose BD (ed): Up To Date. Wellesley, MA, 2004.
3. Craig JR, Peters RL, Edmondson HA, Omata M: Fibrolamellar carcinoma of the liver: A tumor of adolescents and young adults with distinctive clinico-pathologic features. Cancer 46:372–379, 1980.
4. Curley SA, Stuart KE, Schwartz JM, Carithers RL Jr: Nonsurgical therapies for localized hepatocellular carcinoma. In Rose BD (ed): Up To Date. Wellesley, MA, 2004.
5. de Groen PC, Gores GJ, LaRusso NF, et al: Biliary tract cancers. N Engl J Med 341:1368–1378, 1999.
6. Fernandez MP, Redvanly RD: Primary hepatic malignant neoplasms. Radiol Clin North Am 36:333–348, 1998.
7. Kerlin P, Davis GL, McGill DB, et al: Hepatic adenoma and focal nodular hyperplasia: Clinical, pathologic, and radiologic features. Gastroenterology 84:994–1002, 1983.
8. Kew MC: Tumors of the liver. In Zakim D, Boyer TD (eds): Hepatology: A Textbook of Liver Disease, 2nd ed. Philadelphia, W.B. Saunders, 1990, pp 1206–1239.
9. Mergo PJ, Ros PR: Benign lesions of the liver. Radiol Clin North Am 36:319–331, 1998.
10. Mor E, Kaspa RT, Sheiner P, Schwartz M: Treatment of hepatocellular carcinoma associated with cirrhosis in the era of liver transplantation. Ann Intern Med 129:643–653, 1998.
11. Patel AH, Harnois DM, Klee GG, et al: The utility of CA 19-9 in the diagnosis of cholangiocarcinoma in patients without primary sclerosing cholangitis. Am J Gastroenterol 95:204–207, 2000.

Peng YC, Chan CS, Chen GH: The effectiveness of serum α-fetoprotein level in anti-HCV positive patients for screening hepatocellular carcinoma. Hepatogastroenterology 46:3208–3211, 1999.

Reddy KR, Schiff ER: Approach to a liver mass. Semin Liver Dis 13:423–435, 1993.

Ros PR, Davis GL: The incidental focal liver lesion: Photon, proton, or needle? Hepatology 27:1183–1190, 1998.

Schwartz JM, Outwater EK: Approach to the patient with a focal liver lesion. In Rose BD (ed): Up To Date. Wellesley, MA, 2004.

Schwartz LH, Gandras EJ, Colangelo SM, et al: Prevalence and importance of small hepatic lesions found at CT in patients with cancer. Radiology 210:71–74, 1999.

Souto E, Gores GJ: When should a liver mass suspected of being a hepatocellular carcinoma be biopsied? Liver Transpl 6:73–75, 2000.

Takamori R, Wong LL, Dang C, Wong L: Needle-tract implantation from hepatocellular cancer: Is needle biopsy of the liver always necessary? Liver Transpl 6:67–72, 2000.

Torzilli G, Minagawa M, Takayama T, et al: Accurate preoperative evaluation of liver mass lesions without fine-needle biopsy. Hepatology 30:889–893, 1999.

Weimann A, Ringe B, Klempnauer J, et al: Benign liver tumors: Differential diagnosis and indications for surgery. World J Surg 21:983–991, 1997.

CHAPTER 26

DRUG-INDUCED LIVER DISEASE

Peter R. McNally, DO

1. **How common is drug-induced liver disease?**

   More than 600 medicines have been reported to cause liver injury. Drug-induced hepatic injur
   is the most frequent reason cited for the withdrawal from the market of an approved drug, and
   also accounts for 2–5% of hospital admissions for jaundice and more than 50% of the cases
   acute liver failure in the United States today.

2. **How are the three patterns of drug-induced liver injury distinguished?**

   Hepatocellular, cholestatic, and mixed injury patterns are typically distinguished by alanine
   aminotransferase (ALT) and alkaline phosphatase (AP) values and ratios (Table 26-1).

   TABLE 26-1. PATTERNS OF DRUG-INDUCED LIVER DISEASE

	ALT	ALK PHOS	ALT: ALK PHOS RATIC
Hepatocellular injury	≥ Twofold increase	Normal	High (≥5)
Cholestatic injury	Normal	≥ Twofold increase	Low (≤2)
Mixed injury	≥ Twofold increase	≥ Twofold increase	2–5

   ALT = alanine aminotransferase, ALK PHOS = alkaline phosphatase.

3. **Describe the typical chronologic association between drug exposure and ons
   of hepatitis or cholestasis.**

   Cholestatic or hepatocellular liver injury occurs typically 5–90 days after initial exposure. On
   withdrawal of the drug, biochemical improvement in hepatocellular injury is seen usually with
   2 weeks, whereas cholestatic or mixed injury may not improve for 4 weeks. Persistence of
   abnormal liver biochemistries beyond these intervals suggests a coexistent or independent
   cause of liver disease (e.g., viral or autoimmune liver disease, primary biliary cirrhosis, prima
   sclerosing cholangitis).

4. **What is the differential diagnosis of drug-induced liver disease?**

   Diagnosis of a drug-induced cause of liver injury requires exclusion of viral, toxic,
   cardiovascular, inheritable, and malignant causes. Careful history, review of past laboratory
   testing, and physical examination are often helpful. When drug-induced liver injury is suspecte
   withdrawal of the offending agent and close observation often provide adequate circumstantia
   evidence for the diagnosis. Liver biopsy should be reserved for situations in which
   discontinuation of the medication is not followed by prompt improvement, the cause of liver
   disease remains in question, or the severity necessitates intervention (e.g., organ
   transplantation, corticosteroids).

5. **Explain the two most common mechanisms of drug-induced liver injury.**
   1. *Intrinsic* (hepatotoxin with direct or indirect toxicity to hepatocytes). Examples include phosphorus, carbon tetrachloride, acetaminophen, and chloroform. Intrinsic hepatotoxins cause direct damage to the liver by covalently binding to cellular macromolecules, such as hydrogen peroxide, hydroxyl radicals, or lipid peroxides. These, in turn, interrupt cell membranes or inactivate critical cellular enzyme systems.
   2. *Idiosyncratic* hyperimmune reaction. Examples include phenytoin, isoniazid, ticrynafen, halothane, and valproic acid. Idiosyncratic hepatotoxins are dose-independent, and hepatic injury cannot be reproduced in animal models. Clinical features of hypersensitivity (i.e., rash, fever, and eosinophilia) are common.

6. **What variables appear to influence susceptibility to drug-induced hepatic injury?**
   Age. Young people are more susceptible to aspirin and valproic acid. Old people are more susceptible to isoniazid, halothane, and acetaminophen.
   Sex. Women are more susceptible to all drug-induced liver disease, probably because of lower body mass and susceptibility to autoimmune hepatitis (e.g., alcohol, methyldopa, nitrofurantoin).
   Inducers of hepatic enzymes. Phenobarbitol, phenytoin, ethanol, cigarette smoke, and grapefruit juice have all been shown to induce the hepatic cytochrome P-450 system, causing either rapid or competitive metabolism of drugs.
   Route of administration. Tetracycline toxicity occurs primarily with the parenteral route.
   Drug–drug interactions. Valproic acid increases chlorpromazine-induced cholestasis. Rifampin potentiates isoniazid hepatotoxicity. Chronic alcohol ingestion potentiates acetaminophen and isoniazid hepatotoxicity.
   Malnutrition. Low glutathione level potentiates acetaminophen hepatotoxicity.

7. **Name the two most common causes of drug-induced liver disease.**
   Alcohol and acetaminophen.

8. **How is acetaminophen toxic to the liver?**
   Acetaminophen is toxic to the liver in excessive doses only or when the protective-detoxifying pathway (cytochrome P-450 2E1) in the liver is overwhelmed. Accumulation of the toxic metabolite, N-acetyl-p-benzoquinone-imine (NAPQI), is responsible for the death of hepatocytes. Acetaminophen is the second most common cause of death from poisoning in the United States.

9. **At what dose is acetaminophen toxic?**
   Acetaminophen is hepatotoxic in nonalcoholic patients at doses >7.5 gm. A potentially lethal effect is seen with ingestion of >140 mg/kg (10 gm in a 70-kg man). Chronic alcoholics are at greater risk of acetaminophen injury because of alcohol induction of the cytochrome P-450 2E1 system and attendant malnutrition with low levels of glutathione, an intracellular protectant found naturally in hepatocytes.

10. **How is acetaminophen toxicity treated?**
    The Rumack-Matthew nomogram helps to predict the likelihood of liver injury from acetaminophen and to direct therapy. The antidote for acetaminophen overdose is *N*-acetylcysteine (NAC). The oral dose of NAC is 140 mg/kg, followed by 17 maintenance doses of 70 mg/kg every 4 hours. NAC can be administered intravenously for 48 hours with equal or better efficacy than the oral route. Ipecac is given if the time of ingestion can be verified to be <4 hours. Use of activated charcoal is controversial, because it can interfere with the adsorption of oral NAC.

11. **Describe the clinical features of allergic hepatitis.**
    Phenytoin causes allergic hepatitis, cholestasis, granulomatous liver disease, and even frank fulminant hepatic failure. Symptoms of hepatotoxicity occur usually within the first 8 weeks of

administration. The incriminated metabolite is arene oxide. Systemic symptoms include pharyngitis, lymphadenopathy, and atypical lymphocytosis (so-called pseudolymphoma syndrome). There are some favorable reports of treating acute phenytoin hepatitis with corticosteroids.

12. **What drugs have been reported to cause chronic hepatitis and cirrhosis?**
Isoniazid, methotrexate, methyldopa, nitrofurantoin, oxyphenisatin, perhexiline maleate, and trazodone.

13. **Name the two types of cholestatic drug-induced hepatic injury.**
Inflammatory and bland cholestasis.

14. **List the common causes of drug-induced cholestasis.**

Inflammatory cholestasis	*Bland cholestasis*
Allopurinol	Anabolic steroids
Amitriptyline	Androgens
Azathioprine	Estrogens
Captopril	Oral contraceptives
Carbamazepine	Phenytoin

15. **List the drugs associated with mixed cholestatic-hepatitis type of liver injury.**

Amitriptyline	Flutamide	Ranitidine
Amoxicillin	Ibuprofen	Sulfonamides
Ampicillin	Imipramine	Sulindac
Captopril	Nitrofurantoin	Toxic oil syndrome
Carbamazepine	Phenylbutazone	Trimethoprim-sulfamethoxazole
Cimetidine	Quinidine	Naproxen

16. **Which drugs cause the three types of drug-induced steatosis ("fatty liver")?**
See Table 26-2.

TABLE 26-2. THREE TYPES OF DRUG-INDUCED STEATOSIS		
Microvesicular Steatosis	**Macrovesicular Steatosis**	**Phospholipidosis**
Aspirin (Reye's syndrome)	Acetaminophen	4,4'-Diethylamino ethyl hexestrol
Ketoprofen	Cisplatin	Perhexiline maleate
Tetracycline	Corticosteroids	Amiodarone
Valproic acid	Methotrexate	Trimethoprim-sulfamethoxazole
Zidovudine (AZT)	Tamoxifen	Parenteral nutrition

17. **Which three vascular injuries to the liver can be caused by drugs?**

Hepatic VOD	Pyrrolizidine alkaloids, antineoplastic drugs
Peliosis hepatis	Anabolic steroids, oral contraceptives
Hepatic vein thrombosis	Oral contraceptives

18. **What are the three most common drug-induced hepatic neoplasms?**
- *Hepatocellular carcinoma:* anabolic steroids, oral contraceptives, thorium oxide (Thorotrast vinyl chloride

- *Angiosarcoma:* thorium oxide (Thorotrast), vinyl chloride, arsenic, anabolic steroids
- *Hepatic adenoma:* oral contraceptives, anabolic steroids

Before the availability of oral contraceptives, hepatic adenomas were rare. After 5 years of oral contraceptive use, the relative risk of developing a hepatic adenoma has been estimated to increase 116-fold. Hepatic adenomas often regress when exogenous estrogen is removed and can recur during pregnancy. Anabolic steroids have also been reported to cause hepatic adenomas. Hepatic adenomas are usually asymptomatic but can be associated with abdominal fullness, pain, hepatomegaly, and hemorrhage.

19. **Over 50 drugs have been cited as causing hepatic granulomas. List the most common.**

Allopurinol	Phenylbutazone	Isoniazid	Chlorpromazine
Quinidine	Nitrofurantoin	Diazepam	Sulfonamides
Penicillin	Gold	Aspirin	Phenytoin
Mineral oil	Oral contraceptives	Quinine	Oxicillin
Diltiazem	Tolbutamide		

20. **What antiarthritic drugs have been reported to cause liver injury?**

Aspirin. Dose-dependent hepatocellular injury. Risk factors include high salicylate levels, female, youth, underlying rheumatoid arthritis, systemic lupus erythematosus (SLE), and, possibly, coexistent liver disease.

Sulindac (Clinoril). Over 400 cases of sulindac-induced hepatitis have been reported. A cholestatic hepatitis is seen in most patients. Common clinical manifestations include fever, rash, and Stevens-Johnson syndrome. A "trapped" common bile duct causing cholestasis has been reported after sulindac-induced pancreatitis.

Bromfenac (Duract). Acute hepatitis and liver failure. More common in women, age > 50; treatment longer than 90 days. Food and Drug Administration (FDA) removal from U.S. market in June 1998.

Diclofenac (Voltaren). The pattern of injury, uniquely more common in women than men, is primarily hepatitis. Fulminant hepatitis and death have been reported. Steroids may be helpful in severe cases.

Phenylbutazone (Butazolidin). An immunologic type of injury is usually seen with fever, rash, and eosinophilia. Illness starts usually within 6 weeks of initiating the drug. The hepatic injury seen is variable; acute hepatitis, cholestasis, and granulomatous hepatitis have been reported.

Ibuprofen (Motrin, Advil). Hepatic injury caused by ibuprofen is relatively uncommon. Over-the-counter doses of ibuprofen have not been reported to cause clinically apparent liver injury.

Piroxicam (Feldene). Lethal hepatitis and cholestasis have been reported, but overall liver injury appears to be uncommon.

Celecoxib (Celebrex). Acute pancreatitis and hepatitis have been reported. Women are more susceptible, and an increased risk for those with preexisting sulfa allergy is controversial.

1. **How should patients receiving chronic methotrexate (MTX) be monitored for chronic hepatitis and cirrhosis?**

MTX has been used in patients with refractory psoriasis and rheumatoid arthritis. In patients with psoriasis, many advocate an index liver biopsy after 2–4 months of MTX therapy, followed by serial repeat biopsies after every 1.0–1.5 gm of cumulative dose. In patients with rheumatoid arthritis, MTX appears to be somewhat less hepatotoxic. The American College of Rheumatology does not recommend a pretreatment liver biopsy in the absence of preexisting liver disease, but liver-associated enzymes should be monitored. Reevaluation of MTX safety is advised when aspartate aminotransferase (AST) or ALT levels exceed three times the baseline values. Liver biopsies are advised every 2 or 3 years (or every 1.5 gm of cumulative dose).

22. **What are the histologic grades of methotrexate liver injury?**
   See Table 26-3.

Grade	Fibrosis	Fatty Infiltration	Nuclear Variability	Portal Inflammation
		TABLE 26-3. HISTOLOGIC GRADES OF METHOTREXATE LIVER INJURY		
I	None	Mild	Mild	Mild
II	None	Moderate to severe	Moderate to severe	Portal expansion, lobular necrosis
IIIA	Mild (septa extending into lobules)	Moderate to severe	Moderate to severe	Portal expansion, lobular necrosis
IIIB	Moderate to severe	Moderate to severe	Moderate to severe	Portal expansion, lobular necrosis
IV	Cirrhosis			

23. **Outline the recommendations for change in methotrexate therapy, based on liver biopsy findings.**

   I   Continue therapy; repeat biopsy after 1–1.5 gm of cumulative dose.
   II   Continue therapy; repeat biopsy after 1–1.5 gm of cumulative dose.
   IIIA   Continue therapy, but repeat biopsy in 6 months.
   IIIB   No further MTX; exceptional cases need close histologic follow-up.
   IV   No further MTX; exceptional cases need close histologic follow-up.

24. **What are the clinical findings of chlorzoxazone hepatotoxicity?**
   Chlorzoxazone (Parafon Forte) is a centrally acting muscle relaxant. Hepatotoxic effects are ra[re]
   but severe hepatitis, including fulminant hepatic failure, has been reported. Onset of injury ma[y]
   occur within 1 week of initiation or up to several years later. The transaminase elevation may
   exceed 1000 IU/L. Most patients also exhibit hyperbilirubinemia. Discontinuation of the
   medication is usually the only intervention necessary.

25. **Which drugs commonly used to treat endocrine disease have been reported t[o] cause liver injury?**
   Thiazolidinediones (TZDs) are a class of compounds specifically designed to reduce insulin
   resistance by increasing peripheral glucose disposal and decreasing glucose production. The
   TZDs include troglitazone, rosiglitazone, and proglitazone. Ninety-four cases of acute liver
   failure were reported to be caused by troglitazone, causing the drug to be removed from the U[S]
   market in March 2000. Case reports of hepatotoxicity caused by rosiglitazone and pioglitazone
   have been published, but the rate of hepatotoxicity is far less common than with troglitazone.
   FDA recommendations for baseline and then monthly monitoring of liver tests during the first
   year of treatment with glitazone agents is of unproven value and infrequently performed by
   health care providers.
   Sulfonylureas include chlorpropamide, glipizide, tolazamide, tolbutamide, acetohexamide,
   and glyburide. The pattern of injury is cholestatic for chlorpropamide, glipizide, tolazamide, an[d]
   tolbutamide and hepatocellular or mixed with the remainder. A hypersensitivity reaction is
   thought to be responsible. Hypersensitivity to chlorpropamide does not predict the same
   response to tolbutamide.

Thiourea derivatives (propylthiouracil, methimazole) may cause hepatocellular or cholestatic injury.

Steroid derivatives (anabolic steroids, oral contraceptives, tamoxifen, danazol, glucocorticoids) are reported to cause cholestasis or canalicular type of liver injury.

Lipid-lowering agents include niacin and HMG-CoA reductase inhibitors. Niacin (nicotinic acid) may cause mixed cholestatic-hepatic injury. Injury is more common with the sustained-release form or at doses >3 gm/day for the regular-release form. Serial monitoring of liver enzymes is recommended, and the drug should be discontinued if elevations are detected. Lovastatin is the most commonly prescribed of the HMG-CoA reductase inhibitors used to treat hypercholesterolemia. Mild elevations in aminotransferases are common, but levels usually return to normal on drug withdrawal.

KEY POINTS: DRUG-INDUCED LIVER DISEASE

1. Drug-induced hepatic injury is the most frequent reason cited for the withdrawal from the market of an approved drug. Serious drug-induced hepatotoxicity is responsible for 4.7% of hospital admissions, 2.1% of hospitalized patients suffer an adverse drug reaction (ADR), and 0.32% of hospitalized patients die of an ADR.

2. Idiosyncratic drug-induced liver disease is characterized by a latency period ranging from 5–90 days from the initial ingestion of the drug, and is frequently fatal if the causative drug is continued once the reaction has begun.

3. For unclear reasons, the majority of drug-induced liver injury occur in women—73% of all reported cases.

4. Substances such as phenobarbitol, phenytoin, ethanol, cigarette smoke, and grapefruit juice can induce hepatic enzymes and potentiate drug-induced hepatotoxicity.

5. Complementary and alternative medicines (CAMs) are used by 3% of the adult U.S. population. Many have been shown to cause potent drug interactions or hepatotoxicity. Careful inquiry of the use of over-the-counter CAMs should be initiated in all patients with unexplained elevations in liver enzyme tests.

6. **What commonly used cardiovascular drugs have been reported to cause liver injury?**

Quinidine. Liver injury has been reported after a single dose. The predominant injury is hepatocellular with focal necrosis, but diffuse granulomas have also been seen.

Procainamide. Injury to the liver is rare, but hepatocellular, cholestatic, and granulomatous injuries have been reported.

Verapamil and *nifedipine*. Hepatitis has been reported to develop within 2–3 weeks of drug administration. Cholestatic, hepatocellular, and mixed injuries have been reported. A pseudoalcohol pattern of steatosis and Mallory's hyaline has been reported with use of nifedipine.

Hydralazine. Hepatocellular and granulomatous injury have been reported.

Captopril. Hypersensitivity symptoms usually herald jaundice. Cholestasis usually ameliorates rapidly after drug removal.

Enalapril. Scattered cases of hepatitis and cholestasis have been reported.

Ticrynafen. This uricosuric diuretic was removed from the U.S. market shortly after its introduction because of the significant incidence of liver injury. The hepatitis can be fatal.

Amiodarone. This iodine-containing benzofuran, used as an antianginal and antiarrhythmic agent, accumulates within the hepatic lysosome, where it complexes with phospholipids and inhibits lysosomal phospholipases.

27. **What are the clinical features of methyldopa (Aldomet) hepatocellular injury?**
Liver injury occurs usually within 6–12 weeks of initiation of methyldopa therapy. Aminotransferase values should be obtained periodically during the first 4 months of drug administration. Women appear to be more susceptible to methyldopa hepatotoxicity, and the clinical presentation may mimic autoimmune "lupoid" hepatitis.

28. **What commonly used antimicrobial agents have been shown to cause liver injury?**
Tetracycline. Liver injury is seen almost exclusively with parenteral administration and is more common in women, especially during pregnancy. Microvesicular steatosis is the characteristic histologic finding.
Erythromycin estolate. Initially, liver injury was thought to occur only with the estolate form but the ethylsuccinate form has recently been implicated as a cause of cholestatic hepatitis. A hypersensitivity picture is usually seen within days to 2 weeks after exposure.
Chloramphenicol. Rare cases of cholestasis and jaundice have been reported.
Penicillin. Both cholestatic and hepatitis-like patterns have been reported. Hypersensitivity the mechanism of injury.
Amoxicillin, clavulanic acid. Cholestatic hepatitis has been seen during or within weeks of administration.
Sulfonamides cause mixed hepatocellular injury that is usually heralded by rash, fever, and eosinophilia.
Pyrimethamine-sulfadoxine. Hepatocellular injury is most common, but fulminant hepatitis and death have been reported.
Sulfasalazine, which is used to treat inflammatory bowel disease, may cause the same injury as sulfonamides.
Nitrofurantoin. Hallmarks of hypersensitivity are common, with both cholestatic and hepatocellular injury reported. Chronic active hepatitis has been reported, usually in women older than age 40 with HLA-B8 histocompatibility.
Rifampin potentiates the hepatotoxity of isoniazid, presumably by induction of cytochrome P450. Women older than 50 years are especially susceptible.
Griseofulvin. Hepatitis is rare, but the drug can precipitate attacks of acute intermittent porphyria.
Ketoconazole. Toxic hepatitis is more common in women older than age 40. Fulminant hepatitis has been reported. Periodic monitoring of liver enzymes is recommended to detect early injury.
Flucytosine. Transaminase elevations are common; significant hepatitis is rare.

29. **Who is at risk for liver toxicity from isoniazid (INH) therapy?**
INH hepatitis may present insidiously from 4–6 months after initiation of therapy. Some patients experience influenza-like symptoms. Abnormal AST and ALT elevations develop in up to 20% patients taking INH, but aminotransferase activity usually subsides to normal spontaneously. The risk for frank hepatitis is 0.3% at ages 20–34 years, 1.2% at ages 35–49, and 2.3% at ages >50. Coadministration of rifampin increases the likelihood of INH toxicity. Acetaminophen toxicity is increased by INH because it induces the cytochrome P450 enzyme system.

30. **How is INH toxicity prevented?**
Current recommendations include screening patients for ethanol abuse and preexisting liver or renal disease. The presence of chronic liver disease is not an absolute contraindication to the use of INH, but the indications should be scrutinized and therapy monitored more closely. The American Thoracic Society recommends dispensing only one month's supply of INH to ensure close monitoring. Patients should be advised to report prodromal symptoms immediately. All patients older than 35 years should have serial monitoring of ALT, and the use of INH should be reconsidered when ALT elevations persist or remain >100 IU/L.

31. **What commonly used recreational drugs are associated with hepatotoxicity?**

Cocaine. An estimated 30 million Americans have experimented with cocaine, and 5 million Americans abuse it habitually. Patients with cocaine hepatotoxicity may present with jaundice or fatigue and generalized malaise. The aminotransferase elevations can be in the 5000-IU/L range. Cocaine toxicity may also cause coagulopathy, rhabdomyolysis, and disseminated intravascular coagulation (DIC). The mechanism of hepatotoxicity is unknown. Liver biopsy typically shows zone III injury, suggesting related ischemia. In this setting, liver injury may be multifactorial and include coexistent viral liver disease (hepatitis B, C, and D) and acetaminophen or alcohol use.

Ecstasy. This synthetic amphetamine (3,4-methylene dioxymethamphetamine) is commonly used as a "weekend" drug. It makes users euphoric and more sociable and eliminates fatigue. Initially thought to have little toxicity, Ecstasy has been reported to cause various systemic effects, including cardiac arrhythmias, DIC, acute renal failure, hyperthermia, and fulminant hepatitis. Physicians should suspect Ecstasy use in a young adult with acute hepatitis but no identifiable cause.

32. **What anesthetic agents are associated with hepatocellular injury?**

Halothane, enflurane, methoxyflurane, and isoflurane. Whenever hepatitis occurs postoperatively, nonanesthetic causes must be considered (e.g., viral hepatitis, drug-induced hepatitis, bile duct injury, cholestasis of total parenteral nutrition or sepsis, transfusion hepatitis, ischemic hepatopathy).

The risk for halothane hepatitis is 1/10,000 patients but increases to 7/10,000 after two or more exposures. Over 75% of patients with halothane liver injury present within 2 weeks of exposure with fever, nausea, rash, arthralgia, and diffuse abdominal discomfort. Laboratory abnormalities include eosinophilia, AST and ALT elevations in the range of 500–1000-IU/L, and AP elevation (usually <2 times normal). The mechanism appears to be related to development of sensitization to both the oxidative metabolite of halothane, trifluoroacetyl halide, and autoantigens (including CYP2D6). Prognostic factors for poor outcome include short latent period from exposure to jaundice, obesity, age >40 years, hepatic encephalopathy, and prolongation of the prothrombin time. Corticosteroids and exchange transfusions are not helpful, and the mortality rate of fulminant halothane hepatitis is nearly 80% without liver transplantation.

33. **Can herbal therapies injure the liver?**

Yes and no. Because the composition of herbal remedies is variable and unregulated, persons with preexisting liver disease should be cautious and consult their doctor and repudabile Websites, such as http://www.nccam.nih.gov.

"Safe herbs": milk thistle (*Silybum marianum*) is a safe substance that has been used for centuries to remedy liver disease. Many patients with liver disease self-medicate with milk thistle. Although aminotransferase levels commonly improve, no good evidence suggests that it improves the liver disorder. Silymarin plus thioctic acid and penicillin has been successfully used in the treatment of *Amanita* mushroom poisoning.

Potentially hepatotoxic herbs: Autoimmune hepatitis: syo-saiko-to, ma-huang, germander; cirrhosis: syo-saiko-to, chaparral, greater celandine, jin bu huan; cholestasis hepatitis: *Cascara sagrada*, chaparral, greater celandine, kava, syo-saiko-to; fulminant hepatic failure: *Atractylis gummifera*, chaparral, cocaine, germander, kava; and veno-occlusive disease: pyrollizidine alkaloids (teas), skullcap.

WEBSITES

1. http://www.livertransplant.org

2. http://www.fda.gov/cder/livertox/

BIBLIOGRAPHY

1. Blumberg HM, Hopewell PC, O'Brien RJ: Treatment of tuberculosis: Recommendations and reports. MMWR 52(RR-11):1–77, 2003.
2. Bromer MQ, Black M: Acetaminophen hepatotoxicity. Clin Liver Dis 7:351–367, 2003.
3. Burgquest SR, Felson DT, Prashker MJ, Freedberg KA: The cost of liver biopsy in rheumatoid arthritis patients treated with methotrexate. Arthritis Rheum 38:326–333, 1995.
4. Cunha BA: Antibiotic therapy: Antibiotic side effects. Med Clin North Am 85:149–185, 2001.
5. Kremer JM, Alaarcon GS, Lightfoot RW, et al: Methotrexate for rheumatoid arthritis: Suggested guidelines for monitoring liver toxicity. Arthritis Rheum 37:316–328, 1994.
6. Lee WM: Drug-induced hepatotoxicity. N Engl J Med 349:474–485, 2003.
7. Liu ZX, Kaplowitz N: Immune-mediated drug-induced liver disease. Clin Liver Dis 6:467–486, 2002.
8. Nolan CM, Goldberg SV, Buskin SE: Hepatotoxicity associated with isoniazid preventive therapy: A 7-year survey from a public health tuberculosis clinic. JAMA 281:1014–1018, 1999.
9. Para JL, Reddy KR: Hepatotoxicity of hypolipemic drugs. Clin Liver Dis 7:415–433, 2003.
10. Schiano TD: Hepatotoxicity and complementary and alternative medicines. Clin Liver Dis 7:453–473, 2003.
11. Teoh NC, Farrell GC: Hepatotoxicity associated with non-steroidal anti-inflammatory drugs. Clin Liver Dis 7:401–413, 2003.
12. Tolman KG, Chandramouli J: Hepatotoxicity of the thiazolidinediones. Clin Liver Dis 7:369–379, 2003.
13. West SG: Methotrexate hepatotoxicity. Rheum Dis Clin North Am 23:883–915, 1997.
14. Zimmerman HJ, Maddrey WC: Toxic and drug-induced hepatitis. In Schiff L, Schiff ER (eds): Diseases of the Liver, 7th ed. Philadelphia, J.B. Lippincott, 1993, pp 707–783.

CHAPTER 27

ALCOHOLIC LIVER DISEASE

Thomas E. Trouillot, MD

1. **How does one identify a patient with a pathologic pattern of alcohol consumption?**

   Alcohol is ubiquitous in Western society. Over 95% of people have tried an alcoholic beverage in their lifetime. The overall prevalence of alcohol abuse in the general population is 9.4%. The clinician is challenged with identifying the pathologic patterns of alcohol consumption in his or her patients before long-term consequences develop. Ultimately, the total amount of alcohol consumed per weight determines who is at risk for alcohol-related disease. Identifying patients who have developed tolerance to alcohol is often facilitated by the *CAGE* question mnemonic. A positive answer to any of the four questions helps identify a patient who is at risk for alcohol abuse and may require further counseling or intervention:

   C   Have you ever felt you should **c**ut down on your drinking?
   A   Did you ever get **a**ngry when someone asked you about your alcohol consumption?
   G   Did you ever feel **g**uilty about your drinking habits?
   E   Did you ever have an **e**ye-opener in the morning to steady your nerves or get rid of a hangover?

2. **Describe the pathologic patterns of alcohol consumption.**

   The pathologic patterns of alcohol consumption include episodic or binge drinking associated with periods of inebriation followed by extended periods of sobriety. Daily consumption of alcohol amounting to >45 gm/day is associated with progressive liver injury. It is postulated that women require less daily alcohol to develop liver injury due, in part, to a lower body mass compared with men.

3. **What terms for alcohol-related disease are included in the *Diagnostic and Statistical Manual of Mental Disorders,* Fourth Edition, Text Revision, of the American Psychiatric Association (DSM-IV-TR)?**

   Alcohol dependency is a maladaptive pattern of substance abuse leading to clinically significant impairment or distress, as manifested by three or more of the following within the same 12-month period: (1) tolerance; (2) withdrawal; (3) alcohol taken in larger amounts or for longer periods than intended; (4) persistent desire to cut down use; (5) great deal of time spent in activities surrounding alcohol; (6) giving up important social, occupational, or recreational activities; and (7) continued use, despite knowledge of adverse physical or psychological problems related to alcohol.

   Alcohol abuse is a maladaptive pattern of substance abuse leading to clinically significant impairment or distress, as manifested by one or more of the following within the same 12-month period: (1) recurrent use resulting in a failure to fulfill major role obligations at work, school, or home, (2) recurrent use in situations in which alcohol is physically hazardous, (3) recurrent substance-related legal problems, and (4) continued use, despite having persistent or recurrent social or interpersonal problems caused or exacerbated by the effects of alcohol.

4. **How does the body metabolize alcohol?**

   Alcohol is metabolized primarily through the liver. Once alcohol is ingested, it is metabolized by both gastric and hepatic alcohol dehydrogenase to acetaldehyde. This, in turn, is oxidized by the

liver, using aldehyde dehydrogenase and the microsomal ethanol-oxidizing system, cytochrom
P450 2E1 (CYP2E1).

5. **What liver enzyme is a potential target for drug intervention to discourage alcohol consumption?**

Aldehyde dehydrogenase (ALDH) is the enzyme responsible for variable rates of alcohol cleara
based on the genetic inheritance of an aberrant allele. It enables oxidation of acetaldehyde to
acetate. Certain Asian populations carry an aberrant allele that results in impaired enzyme activi
accumulations of acetaldehyde, and secondary symptoms of flushing, tachycardia, and severe
nausea and vomiting. To take advantage of this reaction, disulfiram (Antabuse), a competitive
inhibitor of ALDH, is used as a deterrent to consume alcohol. Accumulation of acetaldehyde
results in the typical reaction of skin flushing, anxiety, nausea, and vomiting.

6. **What is considered heavy alcohol consumption?**

Beer (12 oz), wine (5 oz), and hard liquor (1.5 oz of 80-proof) contain approximately 8–12 gm
ethanol. Moderate alcohol consumption is considered <20 gm/day in women and <40 gm/day
men. Heavy alcohol consumption is considered >20 gm/day in women and >80 gm/day in men
The incidence of cirrhosis is significantly increased in men who consume >40–60 gm/day.
Approximately 20% of men drinking >12 beers/day develop cirrhosis in 10 years.

7. **How does acute alcohol toxicity manifest?**

Large quantities of alcohol consumed over a short period can result in acute liver toxicity as w
as a more general syndrome called *acute alcohol poisoning*. Patients usually have evidence of
recent alcohol ingestion with clinically relevant behavioral and psychological changes. The
average alcoholic beverage raises blood alcohol concentration by 15–20 mg/dL, the amount
metabolized by the liver in 1 hour (*see* Table 27-1).

TABLE 27-1. EXPECTED EFFECTS OF BLOOD ALCOHOL LEVELS	
Blood Alcohol Level (mg/dL)	**Expected Effect**
20–99	Impaired coordination, euphoria
100–199	Ataxia, decreased mentation, poor judgment, labile mood
200–299	Marked ataxia and slurred speech, poor judgment, labile mood, nausea and vomiting
300–399	Stage I anesthesia, memory lapse, labile mood
>400	Respiratory failure, coma, death

8. **Describe the most common form of alcoholic liver disease and its clinical manifestations.**

Fatty liver or hepatic steatosis is the most common form of alcoholic liver disease and is
reversible with abstinence from alcohol intake. Its first clinical manifestation is typically
asymptomatic hepatomegaly. As a consequence of preferential alcohol oxidation, the liver
develops fatty deposition. In turn, there is a slight-to-moderate elevation in liver transaminase
with a typical ratio of aspartate aminotransferase to alanine aminotransferase (AST:ALT) of 2:1
This transaminitis usually resolves after several days of abstinence.

9. **Describe the features of alcoholic hepatitis.**

The clinical manifestations of alcoholic hepatitis range from anicteric hepatomegaly to fulminar
liver failure. Alcoholic hepatitis is usually associated with heavy alcohol consumption for more

than 10 years. The clinical features include jaundice, fever, elevated white blood cell count, hepatomegaly, frequent infection, and moderate elevation of AST to two to five times the upper limits of normal. The pathophysiology of alcoholic hepatitis is related to the toxic effects of acetaldehyde production from the hepatic metabolism of alcohol. Liver histology is characterized by hepatocellular disarray; polymorphonuclear cell infiltration in the parenchyma; Mallory's hyaline bodies (approximately 30% of cases), which are clumps of intermediary cytokeratin filaments due to tubulin-acetaldehyde adducts; and some degree of steatosis cholestasis, fibrosis, and necrosis. Approximately 25% of patients with alcoholic hepatitis present with infection and manifestations of portal hypertension (ascites or varices) without cirrhosis. In addition, an estimated 30% of patients with alcoholic hepatitis are infected with hepatitis C virus.

When is it appropriate to use corticosteroids for alcoholic hepatitis?
The use of corticosteroids to treat patients with acute alcoholic hepatitis has been studied in a number of clinical trials. Although the pathophysiology to explain their efficacy is not well understood, their use may attenuate immune processes that activate or perpetuate alcohol hepatitis, possibly by decreasing cytokine production. Most studies support the use of corticosteroids when a patient develops severe alcoholic hepatitis characterized by hepatic encephalopathy and/or a high discriminant function (DF) value.

KEY POINTS: FEATURES OF ALCOHOL HEPATITIS

1. Jaundice

2. Hepatomegaly

3. Moderate elevations of AST and ALT

4. Hepatic steatosis, neutrophilic inflammation and Mallory's bodies

How is discriminant function value calculated?
  [4.6 × (prothrombin time seconds – control time)] + serum bilirubin mg/dL
   or
  [4.6 × (prothrombin time seconds – control time)] + serum bilirubin mmol/L/17.

A DF value >32 is associated with severe alcoholic hepatitis and a high short-term mortality rate (within approximately 1 month). The usual treatment is prednisolone or prednisone, 40 mg once daily for 30 days. Patients with mild alcoholic hepatitis or more severe clinical manifestations complicated by significant gastrointestinal (GI) bleeding or sepsis are **not** likely to benefit from corticosteroids. An early change in the serum bilirubin within the first week of corticosteroid therapy may also identify a group of patients who will most likely benefit from the therapy.

What other treatments may be used for alcoholic hepatitis?
Pentoxifylline, a nonselective phosphodiesterase inhibitor of tumor necrosis factor production, was recently shown in a randomized, placebo-controlled trial to decrease mortality by 40% in patients with severe alcoholic hepatitis (DF >32), particularly by decreasing the incidence of hepatorenal syndrome. Other inhibitors of tumor necrosis factor, such as infliximab, are currently under study.

 Other medications, such as polyenylphosphatidylcholine, colchicine, and propylthiouracil, may decrease the inflammatory response to alcoholic liver injury and inhibit or reverse hepatic fibrosis. Antioxidants, such as S-adenosylmethionine, may also be of benefit.

 Nutritional support is important because many alcoholic patients are malnourished with depleted vitamin stores and low hepatic glutathione levels (an important liver compound used to metabolize drugs and toxins).

Note: All treatment for alcoholic hepatitis is predicated on complete abstinence from alcoh●
No therapy shows any benefit in patients who continue to drink heavily.

13. **Why can moderate doses of acetaminophen be toxic to patients with alcoholi●
liver disease?**
Because alcohol induces the cytochrome P-450 system, hepatic metabolism of acetaminophe●
can result in the development of toxic intermediates. Normally, these toxic intermediates are
conjugated with glutathione, which protects against oxidative injury. Typically, alcoholics hav●
poor nutrition and depleted glutathione stores. Alcohol-induced cytochrome P-450 and deple●
glutathione stores probably explain why alcoholics are more susceptible to acetaminophen
hepatotoxicity.

14. **What is the most advanced form of chronic alcoholic liver disease?**
Cirrhosis, which accounts for approximately 75% of deaths due to alcoholism. It is characteriz●
by the formation of severe hepatic fibrosis (scarring), typically in a micronodular pattern. This,
turn, leads to (1) loss of liver cell mass, which impairs liver synthetic function (development of
hepatic encephalopathy, hypoalbuminemia, and coagulopathy), and (2) development of portal
hypertension and its clinical complications (esophageal and gastric varices, ascites, and
spontaneous bacterial peritonitis). Patients who develop these clinical complications are
considered to have decompensated liver function. The 5-year survival rate is upward of 90% in●
patients with alcoholic liver disease and cirrhosis when they have compensated liver disease a●
maintain abstinence. When patients develop hepatic decompensation and continue to drink
heavily, the 5-year survival rate drops to approximately 30%. Life-threatening complications of
cirrhosis include infection, variceal bleeding, and hepatorenal syndrome.

15. **List the important extrahepatic manifestations of alcoholic liver disease.**

Ascites	Spider angiomata	Dupuytren's contractures	Peripheral neuropathy
Splenomegaly	Asterixis	Korsakoff's syndrome	Hypogonadism
Caput medusae	Palmar erythema	Wernicke's encephalopathy	Gynecomastia

16. **When is a patient with advanced alcoholic liver disease a suitable candidate f●
liver transplantation?**
When a patient with alcoholic liver disease and cirrhosis develops hepatic decompensation, li●
transplantation should be considered. Manifestations of chronic liver failure that are consider●
indications for liver transplant evaluation include hepatic encephalopathy, ascites, spontaneo●
bacterial peritonitis, bleeding esophageal or gastric varices, and/or liver biochemical
deterioration with a prolonged protime or international normalized ratio, elevated total bilirub●
or low serum albumin. Patients with alcoholic liver disease who actively consume alcohol are
not immediate liver transplant candidates. However, a somewhat arbitrary rule of 6-month
sobriety has been used as a guideline by most liver transplant centers. Definitive data are lack●
to determine the ideal candidates, intervention, and period of abstinence to ensure sobriety a●
liver transplantation.

WEBSITES

1. http://www.liverfoundation.org/cgi-bin/dbs/articles.cgi?db=articles&uid=default

2. http://www.niaaa.nih.gov/publications/harm-al.htm

BIBLIOGRAPHY

1. Abittan CS, Lieber CS: Alcoholic liver disease. In Clinical Perspectives in Gastroenterology. 1999, pp 257–263.

2. Akriviadis E, Botla R, Briggs W, et al: Pentoxifylline improves short-term survival in severe acute alcoholic hepatitis: A double-blind, placebo-controlled trial. Gastroenterology 199:1637–1648, 2000.

3. Gish RG, Olden K: Alcohol and liver disease: Should liver transplantation be offered? Pract Gastroenterol 9–23, 1997.

4. Imperiale TF, McCullough AJ: Do corticosteroids reduce mortality from alcoholic hepatitis? A meta-analysis of the randomized trials. Ann Intern Med 113:299–307, 1990.

5. Keeffe EB: Assessment of the alcoholic patient for liver transplantation: Comorbidity, outcome, and recidivism. Liver Transpl Surg 2:12–20, 1996.

6. Maher JJ: Treatment of alcohol hepatitis. J Gastroenterol Hepatol 17:448–455, 2002.

7. Matfield D, McLeod G, Hall P: The CAGE questionnaire: Validation of a new alcoholism screening instrument. Am J Psychiatry 131:1121–1123, 1974.

8. Mathurin P, Abdelnour M, Ramond MJ: Early change in bilirubin levels is an important prognostic factor in severe alcoholic hepatitis treated with prednisolone. Hepatology 38:1363–1369, 2003.

9. Mathurin P, Duchatelle V, Ramond MJ, et al: Survival and prognostic factors in patients with severe alcoholic hepatitis treated with prednisolone. Gastroenterology 110:1847–1853, 1996.

10. Raymond MJ, Poynard T, Reuff B, et al: A randomized trial of prednisolone in patients with severe alcoholic hepatitis. N Engl J Med 326:507–512, 1992.

11. Schuckit MA: Drug and Alcohol Abuse. A Clinical Guide to Diagnosis and Treatment, 4th ed. New York, Plenum, 1995.

12. Weinrieb RM, Van Horn DH, McLellan AT, Lucey MR: Interpreting the significance of drinking by alcohol-dependent liver transplant patients: Fostering candor is the key to recovery. Liver Transpl 6:769–776, 2000.

CHAPTER 28

VASCULAR LIVER DISEASE

Augustin R. Attwell, MD, and Marcelo Kugelmas, MD

1. **Describe the principal vascular anatomy of the liver.**

   The liver constitutes 5% of body weight in adults and receives 20% of cardiac output via the hepatic artery and portal vein. The *hepatic artery* is a branch of the celiac artery via the hepaticoduodenal artery. It delivers approximately 30% of the hepatic afferent flow but more than 50% of the necessary oxygen in the resting state. Oxygen delivery to the biliary tree deri[ves] almost exclusively from the hepatic artery.

   Conversely, the *portal vein* carries nearly 70% of total liver blood flow and delivers less tha[n] 50% of the needed oxygen. The portal vein derives its name from being one of two portal systems in the human body, the other located in the pituitary gland. Its first set of venules dra[ins] blood from intestinal and splenic capillaries, forming the superior and inferior mesenteric vei[ns] and the splenic vein. These veins join to form the portal vein that, in turn, divides into tributar[ies] and a net of fenestrated capillaries (sinusoids) in the liver. Despite its low oxygen content, portal venous blood delivers intestinal nutrients, drugs, and inflammatory mediators directly to the liver.

   At the end of the sinusoid, blood enters the central venules, which drain directly into the ri[ght], middle, and left *hepatic veins*. The right hepatic vein drains directly into the inferior vena cava (IVC), whereas the left and middle hepatic veins usually merge before draining into the IVC vi[a a] common trunk. Vascular anatomy divides the liver into eight segments, each with its own afferent and efferent blood flow (Fig. 28-1). This anatomy is particularly important in the surg[ical] resection of liver masses. The caudate lobe drains directly into the vena cava through dorsal hepatic veins, which explains its compensatory hypertrophy in hepatic outflow obstructive states, such as Budd-Chiari syndrome.

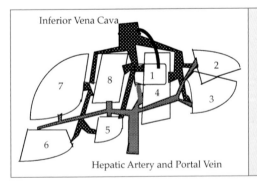

Figure 28-1. Vascular and surgical anatomy of the liver. According to Couinaud, there are eight functional segments in the liver that receive blood supply via the portal vein and hepatic artery. Efferent drainage is through the right, middle, and left hepatic veins. The caudate lobe (segment 1) has a separate and direct outflow into the vena cava via the dorsal hepatic veins.

2. **Describe the microcirculation of the liver.**

   The basic element in the liver architecture is the cell plate, which consists of 15–20 hepatocyt[es] between the portal area and central (hepatic) vein lined up between sinusoids (Fig. 28-2). Blo[od] flows unidirectionally from the portal venule and hepatic arteriole through the sinusoid and bathes hepatocytes before emptying into the central venule.

Rappaport's concept of the liver lobule divides it into three zones (Fig. 28-3). Zone I refers to hepatocytes surrounding the portal triad, zone III refers to perivenular hepatocytes, and zone II refers to the intermediate hepatocytes between the periportal and perivenular areas. There are no absolute boundaries between these zones; however, the metabolic function and susceptibility to injury significantly varies according to the zone. For example, in congestive diseases such as right-sided heart failure or Budd-Chiari syndrome, the outflow is impeded and zone III hepatocytes are the first to be damaged, as a result of their relative hypoxia.

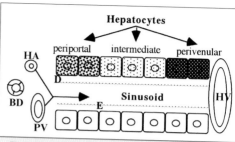

Figure 28-2. Hepatic microarchitecture. Blood *(BD)* from the portal vein *(PV)* and hepatic artery *(HA)* traverses the sinusoids, eventually leaving the liver from the hepatic veins *(HV)*. The low-pressure circulation in the sinusoids allows plasma to pass through the fenestrated epithelium *(E)* and reach the space of Disse *(D)*, where exchange of nutrients and metabolites occurs. The hepatocytes near the portal triad are called *periportal* and those near the hepatic vein are called *perivenular* or *pericentral*.

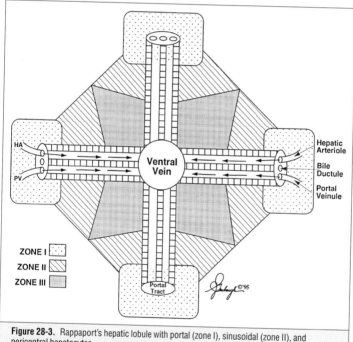

Figure 28-3. Rappaport's hepatic lobule with portal (zone I), sinusoidal (zone II), and pericentral hepatocytes.

What makes the liver resistant to ischemic and vascular disease?

The liver benefits from an extremely rich blood supply of fully oxygenated blood from the hepatic artery and partially oxygenated blood from the portal vein. Between these sources the liver receives over 20% of the cardiac output, one third of which comes from the hepatic artery.

The liver can autoregulate its blood flow in the setting of portal venous or hepatic artery insufficiency via vasoconstriction of the affected vessel, closure of intrasinusoidal sphincters and vasodilation of the other vessel. Oxygen extraction is also enhanced and autoregulated in the liver, probably because of short diffusion distances and properties of the hepatocyte itself. Finally, the regenerative capacity of hepatocytes allows liver function to continue and recover rapidly after severe ischemia.

4. **What is Budd-Chiari syndrome (BCS)?**
BCS results from obstruction of the hepatic venous outflow tract from any etiology, including thrombosis, tumor, abscess, or vascular anomaly. Obstruction of at least two of three hepatic veins is generally required to cause clinical symptoms. (Hepatic veno-occlusive disease and congestive heart failure are not included in this category.) IVC webs are the leading causes in developing countries, whereas thrombosis is the predominant cause in Europe and the United States. The majority of thrombotic cases are associated with an underlying coagulation disorder such as polycythemia rubra vera, factor V Leiden deficiency, or paroxysmal nocturnal hemoglobinuria. Less common inheritable disorders include protein C/S deficiencies, antithrombin III deficiency, and the antiphospholipid antibody syndrome. Additional risk factors include oral contraceptives, cancer, and trauma.

5. **How is Budd-Chiari syndrome diagnosed?**
The onset of ascites, abdominal pain, hepatosplenomegaly, or unexplained liver failure in a patient should raise the suspicion of BCS, particularly if there are risk factors for thrombosis. Doppler ultrasonography usually shows hepatomegaly and decreased or absent flow in the hepatic veins. Contrast-enhanced computed tomography (CT) or magnetic resonance imaging (MRI) may additionally show nonvisualization of the main hepatic veins or a mosaic perfusion pattern of the liver parenchyma. Another key imaging finding is caudate lobe hypertrophy (Fig. 28-4).

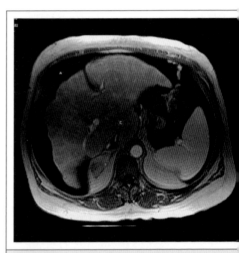

Figure 28-4. MRI showing features of BCS, including hepatomegaly with caudate lobe hypertrophy, ascites, splenomegaly. A = ascites, C = caudate lobe.

Transjugular hepatic venography confirms the site and extent of thrombosis, may demonstrate collateral formation in a "spider web" distribution, allows for biopsy, and may direct intravascular therapy. Typically, pressure readings reveal increased wedged hepatic venous pressure, portal pressure, and gradient.

6. **Why do some patients with Budd-Chiari syndrome have an enlarged caudate lobe?**
Approximately one half of patients with BCS develop hypertrophy in the caudate lobe of the liver (see Fig. 28-4). This finding occurs because dorsal hepatic veins drain the caudate lobe and empty directly into the IVC. Usually, the obstruction does not affect these veins, and the caudate lobe hypertrophies in a compensatory fashion. The hypertrophy may be marked, cause a characteristic indentation in the inferior venogram, or result in significant IVC stenosis.

Describe the histopathologic findings in Budd-Chiari syndrome.

A nearly universal finding on liver biopsy is centrilobular congestion with dilation of the perivenular sinusoids. In severe and chronic forms, hepatocyte necrosis may occur, most prominently in zone III. Ongoing hepatic venous outflow obstruction may lead to centrilobular fibrosis after 4–6 weeks, with fibrosis and/or cirrhosis developing later. As fibrosis becomes more extensive, it may contribute to occlusion of the outflow tract and liver failure. Examination of the hepatic veins and IVC may reveal concentric thickening in the vessel wall, but intravascular thrombosis is uncommon.

What is the treatment for Budd-Chiari syndrome?

Except for occasional reports of cases improving with medical therapy alone, BCS is generally progressive without definitive therapy. Diuretics may control ascites, and anticoagulants are useful to limit clot burden. The underlying hematologic disorder should be treated accordingly. Ultimately, most patients require decompression of the hepatic veins to preserve liver function. In the acute setting, percutaneous transluminal angioplasty, stenting, and thrombolytic therapy have been used successfully, although the evidence is limited to case reports and uncontrolled series.

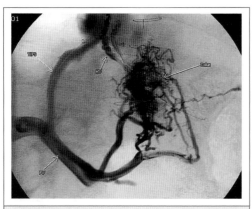

Figure 28-5. Hepatic venography with TIPS insertion. HV = hepatic vein; PV = portal vein; Collat = venous collateral formation within liver; TIPS = transjugular intrahepatic portosystemic shunt.

Portosystemic shunt surgery (portocaval, mesocaval, or mesoatrial) is effective in improving symptoms, parameters of liver function, and liver histology. However, there is significant surgical morbidity, and shunts may become thrombosed in the long-term. Patients with cirrhosis or liver failure may have limited benefit.

Transjugular intrahepatic portosystemic shunting (TIPS) (Fig. 28-5) has been used to stabilize liver function and bridge patients to transplantation. Occasionally, patients have long-term, symptomatic benefit with compensated liver function, but they often need periodic shunt revisions and/or replacements to maintain patency.

KEY POINTS: CLINICAL FEATURES OF BUDD-CHIARI SYNDROME

1. Classic triad of abdominal pain, hepatomegaly, and ascites (>60%).

2. Mild elevations of liver enzymes and bilirubin are common.

3. Acute (<2 weeks) or subacute (<6 months) onset of symptoms is typical.

4. Minority present with chronic liver disease or cirrhosis.

5. Fulminant liver failure is rare (5%).

9. **Which patients with Budd-Chiari syndrome should be considered for liver transplantation?**

Patients with BCS and signs of liver failure should be evaluated for liver transplantation. Fulminant liver failure is an indication for urgent transplantation, and patients with this presentation may benefit from TIPS, thrombolytics, or angioplasty until an allograft is available. Patients with persistent symptoms or liver dysfunction, despite shunting or intravascular therapy, should also be considered for liver transplantation. Patients with a known clotting factor deficiency may be cured by liver transplantation. The presence of cirrhosis on biopsy generally warrants a transplant evaluation; however, patients with cirrhosis may have long-term benefit from other therapies. Often the choice between surgical shunt, TIPS, or transplantation remains challenging.

10. **What is the pathogenesis of hepatic veno-occlusive disease (VOD)?**

A better term for VOD may be *sinusoidal obstruction syndrome* because the initial injury involves the perivenular endothelium and hepatocytes. Although no specific mechanism has been identified, risk factors include chemotherapy (particularly cyclophosphamide and busulfan-containing regimens), stem cell transplantation, hepatic irradiation, and ingestion of pyrrolizidine alkaloids. Initially, the sinusoidal endothelium becomes leaky with extravasation of red blood cells into the space of Disse and edema in zone III hepatocytes. Perivenular necrosis, fibrosis, and fibrin deposition usually follow, causing outflow obstruction and congestion. The central vein may not be involved. Histologically, sinusoidal dilation and pericentral necrosis are typical, which can mimic BCS or congestive hepatopathy.

11. **What are the clinical features of veno-occlusive disease?**

The typical presentation of right upper quadrant pain and weight gain 1–5 weeks after chemotherapy or bone marrow transplantation may be subtle. Alternatively, patients can develop rapidly progressive jaundice. Physical exam may reveal jaundice, tender hepatomegaly, and/or ascites. The most common lab abnormality is a conjugated hyperbilirubinemia, although thrombocytopenia and elevated prothrombin time may also occur from spleen and liver congestion. Mild-moderate elevations in aspartate aminotransferase (AST) and alanine aminotransferase (ALT) suggest hepatocyte necrosis. A serum AST greater than 750 or rapidly rising bilirubin portends a poor prognosis. Elevated creatinine occurs in less than 50% of patients.

12. **How is veno-occlusive disease diagnosed?**

Any patient with risk factors and unexplained weight gain, abdominal pain, hepatomegaly, or jaundice should raise the suspicion for VOD. Ultrasonography may show ascites, hepatomegaly, or venous dilation, although it is most helpful for excluding other diseases, such as BCS or gallstones. MRI and CT add little information if the sonogram is adequate. Liver biopsy remains the gold standard for diagnosis of VOD and should complement the clinical picture. It is usually done by the transjugular route to minimize bleeding risk and to allow measurement of hepatic venous pressures. Histologic findings typically include edema and/or necrosis of zone III hepatocytes and sinusoidal congestion. Centrilobular fibrosis is uncommon.

13. **Describe the clinical features of ischemic hepatitis.**

Also known as shock liver, ischemic hepatitis is clinically diagnosed by a sudden, profound elevation in liver enzymes shortly after a drop in cardiac output and/or blood pressure. It mostly affects elderly patients with underlying cardiac disease, often in the setting of surgery, trauma, or sepsis. Tender hepatomegaly and anorexia are common exam findings. The elevation in serum transaminases may be abrupt and marked (>1000), reflecting hepatocyte necrosis. Serum bilirubin and prothrombin time are modestly elevated, and many patients have elevated creatinine, usually from acute tubular necrosis (ATN). The liver function tests and coagulopathy improve over the ensuing days as the patient's hemodynamic status is restored.

14. **What is the pathogenesis of ischemic hepatitis?**
A drop in cardiac output may result from various etiologies, including sepsis, hypovolemia, cardiac tamponade, pulmonary embolism, and left or right ventricular failure. Hypoperfusion mostly affects the perivenular hepatocytes because they receive oxygen-poor blood. Histologically, the typical finding of centrilobular necrosis reflects mechanism. Because many patients have chronic underlying heart disease, hepatic congestion or fibrosis may be present.

15. **What are the clinical manifestations of congestive hepatopathy?**
The underlying cardiac disease dominates the presentation with dyspnea, fatigue, edema, and weight gain. Many patients will report right upper quadrant pain and/or fullness, which is thought to result from distension of Glisson's capsule. Jaundice is less common, and encephalopathy and variceal bleeding are rare. Physical exam may reveal ascites, hepatosplenomegaly, or hepatojugular reflux.

16. **What liver chemistry abnormalities are found in congestive hepatopathy?**
Elevated prothrombin time is the most common lab abnormality. Chronic passive congestion alone rarely causes significant elevations of ALT or AST. Markedly increased transaminases in the setting of heart disease suggest acute ischemia caused by low cardiac output rather than congestion. Unconjugated hyperbilirubinemia and mildly elevated alkaline phosphatase occur in less than half of patients. The biochemical abnormalities tend to improve with treatment of the underlying cardiac disease.

17. **Describe the pathologic changes associated with congestive hepatopathy.**
Grossly, the liver is enlarged and darkened. The classic cross-sectional appearance, termed "nutmeg liver," represents lighter, less affected periportal areas surrounding the darkened, congested areas around central venules. Microscopically, there is centrilobular and sinusoidal dilation. Adjacent hepatocytes usually appear atrophic, compressed, or necrotic. Fibrosis occurs in the majority of patients with chronic disease, but cardiac cirrhosis is uncommon.

KEY POINTS: PATHOLOGIC FEATURES OF CONGESTIVE HEPATOPATHY

1. "Nutmeg" appearance on cross section owing to darkened perivenular areas surrounded by less affected portal areas.

2. Centrilobular and sinusoidal dilation.

3. Centrilobular hepatocyte atrophy and/or necrosis.

4. Pericentral fibrosis occurs in most patients.

5. (Cardiac) cirrhosis is rare but may occur in chronic disease.

18. **What is the most frequent vascular complication following liver transplantation?**

Hepatic artery thrombosis occurs with an incidence of 2–10% following orthotopic liver transplantation and carries over 50% mortality. Roughly half of cases present early (<1 week), although some may present after months to years. Risk factors include old donor age, prolonged cold ischemia time, and the use of an aortic conduit. Although a minority of patients are asymptomatic with abnormal liver tests or imaging, most develop cholestasis and cholangitis secondary to ischemic bile duct injury. Imaging by Doppler ultrasound may suggest the diagnosis, although confirmatory angiography is usually necessary. Surgical thrombectomy and revascularization may salvage selected grafts but they do not always reverse the underlying cholangiopathy. Otherwise, retransplantation remains the treatment of choice.

19. **What are the risk factors for portal vein thrombosis (PVT)?**

Cirrhosis with or without hepatocellular carcinoma is the most common risk factor for portal vein thrombosis today, presumably by causing sluggish portal blood flow and/or decreased synthesis of clotting inhibitors. Inherited or acquired prothrombotic disorders, such as protein C/S deficiencies, the antiphospholipid syndrome, polycythemia vera, and estrogen use or pregnancy, are independent risk factors. Cancer, particularly pancreatic and hepatocellular carcinomas, predisposes the portal vein to thrombosis through extrinsic compression, direct invasion, or an underlying thrombophilia. Surgery or trauma involving the portal or splenic veins similarly increases the risk.

20. **What treatment options are available for portal vein thrombosis?**

In the acute setting, thrombolytics, angioplasty, or surgical thrombectomy may restore portal flow, although controlled studies demonstrating their safety and long-term efficacy are lacking. Otherwise, heparinization and long-term warfarin therapy usually allow repermeation in acute PVT. The first-line treatment of chronic PVT involves endoscopic and medical obliteration of esophageal varices. Shunt surgery and splenectomy carry surgical risk but may be helpful in patients with preserved liver function and refractory complications of portal hypertension. Long-term anticoagulation may benefit noncirrhotic patients with underlying thrombophilia, although the benefit needs to be weighed carefully against the risk of bleeding.

21. **What is the most common vascular tumor of the liver?**

Cavernous hemangioma is the most common benign liver tumor with autopsy series indicating a prevalence of 2–20%. It is typically small (<5 cm), asymptomatic, and found incidentally in adults during hepatic imaging. However, larger lesions are not uncommon and may cause significant abdominal pain. Hemangiomas larger than 10 cm are at risk for rupture, internal bleeding, or causing disseminated intravascular coagulation (Kasabach-Merritt syndrome). Tumors tend to be more common and larger in females, so estrogen sensitivity may play a role. Ultrasound, CT scan, or red blood cell scans may suggest the diagnosis, but MRI has evolved into the most specific and sensitive test. Fine-needle biopsy may confirm the diagnosis but carries a significant risk of bleeding. Treatment options, including surgical enucleation, resection, or liver transplantation, are reserved for large, painful tumors or complications (Fig. 28-6).

22. **What is hepatic hemangioendothelioma?**

It is a rare vascular neoplasm with variable malignant potential that may occasionally involve the liver. It grows more commonly in soft tissue or bone. Histologic examination with endothelium-specific (FVIII-rAg) staining is diagnostic. It is nearly always multifocal and slow growing; however, it is resistant to chemotherapy and may recur following liver transplantation. The overall prognosis is poor.

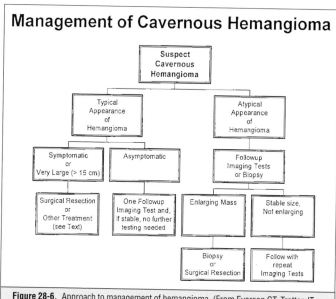

Figure 28-6. Approach to management of hemangioma. (From Everson GT, Trotter JT: Benign focal lesions of the liver. Clin Liver Dis 5:17–42, 2001. Reprinted with permission.)

BIBLIOGRAPHY

1. Bacon BR, Joshi SN, Granger DN: Ischemia, congestive failure, Budd-Chiari syndrome, and veno-occlusive disease. In Kaplowitz N: Liver and Biliary Diseases, 2nd ed. Baltimore, Williams & Wilkins, 1992, pp 469–481.

2. Bynum TE, Biotnott JK, Maddrey WC: Ischemic hepatitis. Dig Dis Sci 24:129–135, 1979.

3. Chalasani N, Cummings OW: The liver in systemic illness. In Boyer TD, Zakim D (eds): Hepatology: A Textbook of Liver Disease, 4th ed. Philadelphia, W.B. Saunders, 2003, pp 1561–1565.

4. DeLeve LD, Shulman HM, McDonald GB: Toxic injury to hepatic sinusoids: Sinusoidal obstruction syndrome. Semin Liver Dis 22:27–41, 2002.

5. Eid A, Lyass S, Venturero M, et al: Vascular complications post orthotopic liver transplantation. Transplant Proc 31:1903–1904, 1999.

6. Fuchs S, Bogomolski-Yahalom V, Paltiel, et al: Ischemic hepatitis: Clinical and laboratory observations in 34 patients. J Clin Gastroenterol 26:183–186, 1998.

7. Kugelmas M: Budd-Chiari syndrome. Treatment options and the value of liver transplantation. Hepatogastroenterology 45:1381–1386, 1998.

8. Kumar S, DeLeve LD, Kalamath PS, et al: Hepatic veno-occlusive disease after hematopoietic stem cell transplantation. Mayo Clin Proc 78:589–598, 2003.

9. Mahmoud AE, Mendoza A, Meshikhes AN, et al: Clinical spectrum, investigations, and treatment of Budd-Chiari syndrome. Q J Med 89:37–43, 1996.

10. MuCuskey RS, Reilly FD: Hepatic microvasculature: Dynamic structure and its regulation. Semin Liver Dis 13:1–12, 1993.

11. Myers RP, Cerini R, Sayegh R, et al: Cardiac hepatopathy: Clinical, hemodynamic, and histologic characteristics and correlations. Hepatology 37:393–400, 2003.

12. Orloff MJ, Daily PO, Orloff SL, et al: A 27-year experience with surgical treatment of Budd-Chiari syndrome. Ann Surg 3:340–352, 2000.

13. Ross RM: Hepatic dysfunction secondary to heart failure. Am J Gastroenterol 7:511–517, 1981.

14. Sanyal AJ: Budd-Chiari syndrome: Is TIPS tops? Am J Gastroenterol 94:559–561, 1999.

15. Sarin SK, Agarwal SR: Extrahepatic portal vein obstruction. Semin Liver Dis 22:43–55, 2003.

16. Seeto RK, Fenn B, Rockey DC: Ischemic hepatitis: Clinical presentation and pathogenesis. Am J Med 109:109–113, 2000.

17. Sobhonslidsuk A, Reddy KR: Portal vein thrombosis: A concise review. Am J Gastroenterol 97:535–541, 200C

18. Tesser TS, Sze DY, Jeffrey RB: Imaging and intervention in the hepatic veins. Am J Radiol 180:1583–1591, 2003.

19. Tilanus HW: Budd-Chiari syndrome. Br J Surg 82:1023–1030, 1995.

20. Torras J, Lladó L, Figueras J, et al: Diagnostic and therapeutic management of hepatic artery thrombosis after liver transplantation. Transplant Proc 31:2405, 1999.

21. Trotter JF, Everson GT: Benign focal lesions of the liver. Clin Liver Dis 5:17–42, 2001.

22. Uchimara K, Nakamuta M, Osoegawa M, et al: Hepatic epithelioid hemangioendothelioma. J Clin Gastroenter 32:431–434, 2001.

23. Valla DC: Hepatic vein thrombosis. Semin Liver Dis 22:5–14, 2002.

24. Valla DC, Condat B: Portal vein thrombosis in adults: Pathophysiology, pathogenesis, and management. J Hepatol 32:865–871, 2000.

CHAPTER 29

NONALCOHOLIC FATTY LIVER DISEASE

Steven Zacks, MD, MPH, and Roshan Shrestha, MD

. **Define *nonalcoholic fatty liver disease* (NAFLD).**

NAFLD is fat accumulation in the liver exceeding 5–10% by weight, but it is practically estimated as the percentage of fat-laden hepatocytes observed by light microscopy. Whether a minimum amount of hepatic fat is truly a disease (hence the "D" in its acronym) or simply a benign condition is debated. A subset of NAFLD, nonalcoholic steatohepatitis (NASH), has macrovesicular fatty changes (steatosis) and lobular inflammation in the absence of alcoholism. NAFLD is a spectrum ranging from steatosis (fatty infiltration without inflammation) to steatosis with inflammation (NASH) to NASH with fibrosis and cirrhosis. Primary NAFLD is idiopathic. Secondary NAFLD is due to a number of causes (see later).

How is nonalcoholic fatty liver disease diagnosed?

The diagnosis of primary NAFLD depends on convincing evidence of negligible (<20 gm/day) alcohol consumption and must include a negative evaluation for chronic hepatitis C virus infection (antibody to hepatitis C virus) and hepatitis B virus infection (hepatitis B surface antigen). Ceruloplasmin and alpha$_1$-antitrypsin levels are usually normal. Idiopathic genetic hemochromatosis must be excluded because, in one series, elevated levels of serum ferritin and transferrin saturation were found in up to 58% of patients with NAFLD. Autoimmune serology (antimitochondrial antibody, antinuclear antibody, antismooth muscle antibody, and antiliver/kidney microsomal antibody) should remain negative, although some patients may have low titers of antinuclear antibodies (ranging from 1:40 to 1:320). A substantial portion of cases of cryptogenic cirrhosis may be "burnt-out" NAFLD, because high proportions are associated with obesity, type 2 diabetes, and/or hyperlipidemia.

. **Discuss the prevalence of nonalcoholic fatty liver disease.**

There are few data on the prevalence of NAFLD in the United States. In the recent National Health and Nutrition Examination Survey (NHANES-3), 2.6% of the U.S. population had raised values of serum alanine aminotransferase (ALT) for which no cause of chronic liver disease could be found, suggesting a diagnosis of NAFLD. Raised ALT concentration was significantly associated with increased waist-to-hip ratio and indices of insulin resistance.

Using the presence of a hyperechoic liver on ultrasound as a diagnostic criterion, 14% of 2574 randomly selected Japanese subjects had fatty liver. Because ultrasound can detect fat only, not all of these patients had the inflammation necessary for a diagnosis of NAFLD. Autopsy studies demonstrate NAFLD in 18.5% of obese subjects and 2.7% of normal-weight people. In the United States, 20% of apparently normal people evaluated as donors for living-related liver transplant had fatty liver and 7.5% had NASH. In Japan, fatty liver was detected in 9.2% subjects assessed for living donation.

NAFLD is possibly the most prevalent liver disorder. Steatosis was seen in 70% of obese and 35% of lean patients and NASH in 18.5% of obese and 2.7% of lean patients in a consecutive autopsy study. Among obese patients, the prevalence of type 1 NAFLD (simple steatosis) is about 60%. True NASH is found in 20–25%, and 2–3% have cirrhosis. Among those with type 2 diabetes, as many as 75% have some form of NAFLD.

4. **Are there any gender, ethnic, or genetic predispositions to nonalcoholic f** **liver disease?**

   Yes. There may be an equal distribution of NAFLD among men and women, although the be gender variation among the specific histologic classes (see later). Published reports o patients with more advanced disease have generally had more women, suggesting wome a more aggressive course. There may be a lower prevalence of NAFLD among African Am compared with European and Hispanics. These variations may represent selection bias in referral patterns or genetic differences in body fat distribution or metabolism. Description families with NAFLD suggest that genetic factors predispose to the development of NAFL

5. **What causes nonalcoholic fatty liver disease?**

   Patients with NAFLD may have insulin resistance as the predisposing metabolic abnorma The fraction of NAFLD patients with insulin resistance has yet to be established. Other abnormalities (e.g., defects in apolipoprotein B or microsomal triglyceride transfer protei alone or with insulin resistance, may also contribute to hepatic fat accumulation. Excess fat predisposes some individuals to hepatocellular injury. The injury may be caused by th cellular toxicity of excess free fatty acids, oxidant stress and lipid peroxidation, or other mechanisms. Hepatocellular injury may cause an inflammatory response with progressiv fibrosis in a subset of patients. The extent of this adverse outcome most likely depends o variety of environmental and genetic influences (Fig. 29-1). Portions of this model of NAF have been referred to as the "two-hit hypothesis." The accumulation of fat is the first hit a hepatocellular injury in the fatty liver is the second hit.

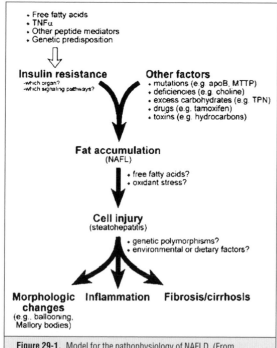

Figure 29-1. Model for the pathophysiology of NAFLD. (From Neuschwander-Tetri BA, Caldwell SH: Nonalcoholic steatohepatitis: Summary of an AASLD single topic conference. Hepatology 37:1202–1219, 2003, with permission.)

How can one distinguish between nonalcoholic fatty liver disease and alcoholic steatohepatitis?

An alcohol history is the key to distinguishing the two entities. Because patients may not be honest about alcohol consumption, a number of tests have been devised to detect excessive alcohol consumption. Among several indicators of excessive alcohol consumption, the ratio of desialyted transferrin to total transferrin is the best single marker.

Describe the natural history of nonalcoholic fatty liver disease.

In the past, NAFLD was thought to have a benign course, with few patients progressing to decompensated cirrhosis. Recent studies suggest that up to 40% of patients with fibrosis may develop cirrhosis. Prognosis correlates with the amount of inflammatory change seen on biopsy. Patients with significant inflammatory activity on biopsy are more likely to progress to cirrhosis. In patients who developed cirrhosis and/or had a liver-related death, 90% had ballooning degeneration or ballooning degeneration with polymorphonuclear cell infiltration, Mallory's hyaline, or fibrosis.

NAFLD may be less serious than alcoholic hepatitis. During a follow-up period of 1–7 years, the progression to cirrhosis occurred in approximately 8–17% of patients with NAFLD compared with 38–50% of patients with alcoholic hepatitis.

Among these, age greater than 40–50 years and the severity of obesity, diabetes, or hyperlipidemia (especially hypertriglyceridemia) are some of the most reliable predictors of advanced histology. The role of female gender is less clear. The apparently increased prevalence of women among patients with more advanced disease supports female gender as a risk for progression. Other reported predictors of advanced disease include elevation of aspartate aminotransferase (AST) and alanine aminotransferase (ALT) and an AST:ALT ratio greater than 1. However, it is well known that significant liver disease may exist with liver enzymes in the normal range among NAFLD patients.

The 5- and 10-year survivals in NASH have been estimated at 67% and 59%, respectively. Death is often from comorbid conditions. Longitudinal studies of NASH are few in number. Compiling 32 patients from several reports, the risk of developing increased fibrosis in histologic classes 3 and 4 NAFLD over approximately 5 years is 25% and for developing cirrhosis is 15%. Although even simple steatosis may progress to cirrhosis, preliminary studies suggest a more benign course for histologic class 2 NAFLD. Obese, diabetic patients who develop cirrhosis are at increased risk for complications of portal hypertension and hepatocellular carcinoma.

What factors predict the presence of steatosis and fibrosis in nonalcoholic fatty liver disease?

In one retrospective study of 144 patients with NAFLD, older age, obesity, presence of diabetes mellitus, and an aspartate aminotransferase (AST)/ALT ratio >1 were significant predictors of severe liver fibrosis (bridging fibrosis or cirrhosis). Body mass index was the only independent predictor of the degree of fat infiltration. Increased transferrin iron saturation correlated positively with the severity of fibrosis in univariate analysis. Female patients tended to have more advanced fibrosis. Neither iron transferrin saturation nor gender was significant after controlling for age, obesity, diabetes, and AST/ALT ratio in the multivariate analysis.

What conditions are associated with nonalcoholic fatty liver disease?

Morbid obesity is the most common. Non–insulin-dependent diabetes mellitus occurs in 20–75% of patients with NAFLD. Hyperlipidemia is seen in 20–80% of patients. An increasing number of patients have been described with normal body mass index, although these individuals may have central obesity and insulin resistance. Other features of metabolic syndrome can be seen in association with NAFLD (e.g., hypertension, hyperuricemia, and polycystic ovarian syndrome [hirsutism, oligomenorrhea, or amenorrhea]).

Less commonly, short bowel syndrome and long-term use of total parenteral nutrition are associated with NAFLD. Jejunoileal and gastric bypass for obesity are also associated with NAFLD. Jejunal diverticulosis with bacterial overgrowth can cause NAFLD. In children, galactosemia, abetalipoproteinemia, Weber-Christian disease, fructose intolerance, and cholesterol ester storage disease are associated with fatty infiltration.

10. **Describe the clinical features of nonalcoholic fatty liver disease.**
Most patients with primary NAFLD are women (65–83%), and most are obese (69–100%). The majority of patients are 10–40% heavier than ideal body weight. Non–insulin-dependent diabetes mellitus is present in 25–75% of patients. The mean age at diagnosis is 50 years, but ages range from 16–80 years. A high proportion of patients (48–100%) have no symptoms of liver disease. A small proportion may have right upper quadrant discomfort. Many patients come to light when liver tests are done as part of the management of other conditions associated with NAFLD (e.g., dyslipidemia). Although patients may not have any signs of liver disease, some may have hepatomegaly. A few patients may present with signs and symptoms of decompensated cirrhosis.

KEY POINTS: NONALCOHOLIC FATTY LIVER DISEASE

1. NAFLD is probably the most prevalent liver disorder in the United States.

2. Steatosis of the liver is seen in 70% of obese and 35% of lean patients; NAFLD is seen in 18.5% of obese and 2.7% of lean patients.

11. **What is the most common laboratory abnormality in patients with nonalcoholic fatty liver disease?**
A twofold to threefold elevation of serum levels of ALT and AST. The AST/ALT ratio appears to be a useful index for distinguishing nonalcoholic steatohepatitis from alcoholic liver disease. Although values <1 suggest NAFLD, a ratio of ≥2 is strongly suggestive of alcoholic liver disease.

12. **What other laboratory abnormalities may be found?**
Bilirubin levels are usually normal. In 12–17% of patients, the bilirubin barely exceeds 1.5–2. mg/dL. Alkaline phosphatase levels are modestly elevated in 39–59% of patients. Hypoalbuminemia and hypoprothrombinemia are less common. Hemosiderosis with elevated iron saturations may be seen.

Immunoserologic findings compatible with autoimmune hepatitis are commonly present in primary NAFLD. Hypergammaglobulinemia is present in 13–30% of patients with primary NAFLD. Although smooth muscle antibodies are absent, antinuclear antibodies, ranging in titer from 1:40 to 1:320, are observed in 40% of patients.

Hyperlipidemia (hypertriglyceridemia and hypercholesterolemia) is found in about 20% of patients. In a group of overweight patients (150–300% of ideal weight for height), lipoprotein abnormalities, particularly type IV hyperlipidemia, are common (54%). The lipoprotein abnormalities are found mostly in patients with less fibrotic NAFLD. Abnormal results of iron tests (elevated levels for serum ferritin and transferrin saturation) were seen in 58% of a series of patients. Elevations in serum ferritin levels as great as fivefold have been reported in the absence of histologic evidence for idiopathic genetic hemochromatosis.

The lack of specificity of standard liver tests limits their usefulness in diagnosing NAFLD and differentiating it from fatty liver without inflammation. If all of the serologic tests for other causes of liver diseases are negative and the patient has a risk factor for NAFLD (e.g., obesity, diabetes mellitus) a diagnosis of fatty liver or NAFLD as a cause of the elevated liver tests can usually be made with some degree of certainty.

13. **List the four types of biopsy findings in patients with fatty liver disease, and give the prevalence of each.**
Type 1: fatty liver alone (37%)
Type 2: fat accumulation and lobular inflammation (7.5%)
Type 3: fat accumulation and ballooning degeneration (14%)
Type 4: fat accumulation, ballooning degeneration, and either Mallory's hyaline or fibrosis (41%: highest proportion of cirrhosis and liver-related death)

14. **What medications are associated with nonalcoholic fatty liver disease?**
Chloroquine, diltiazem, nifedipine, amiodarone, glucocorticoids, tamoxifen, and estrogens.

15. **Summarize the classification of nonalcoholic fatty liver disease.**
Primary NAFLD
    Obesity
    Diabetes
    Hyperlipidemia
Secondary NAFLD
    Drug treatments
        Amiodarone
        Glucocorticoids
    Synthetic estrogens
        Tamoxifen
    Surgical procedures
        Jejunal bypass
        Gastroplasty for morbid obesity
        Biliopancreatic diversion
        Extensive small bowel resection
Other metabolic factors
    Total parenteral nutrition
    Acute starvation
    Rapid weight loss
Miscellaneous
    Bacterial overgrowth (jejunal diverticulosis)
    Limb lipodystrophy
    Abetalipoproteinemia
    Weber-Christian disease

16. **Describe the typical radiologic features of nonalcoholic fatty liver disease.**
The most specific tests for the diagnosis of fatty liver, and therefore NAFLD, appear to be imaging techniques. Ultrasound is a relatively specific method for the identification of fat in the liver (a hyperechoic or bright liver). The sensitivity of ultrasound in diagnosing small amounts of fat is unclear. On a computed tomography (CT) scan, the liver appears less dense than the spleen with a ratio of densities <0.9. On magnetic resonance imaging (MRI), the changes of NAFLD are most pronounced on T1-weighted images. The liver appears very hypointense (dark). Neither MR nor CT imaging is more sensitive than ultrasound in the diagnosis of fatty liver, and neither helps in distinguishing fatty liver from NAFLD. Tumors of the liver can have the appearance of focal fat, especially on ultrasound. Additional imaging by either CT or MRI may be necessary in this group of patients to be certain that the findings represent focal fat and not a malignancy.

17. **Is liver biopsy necessary to establish the diagnosis?**

Yes. The definitive diagnosis of steatohepatitis can be made by liver biopsy only. Sonography may suggest the presence of a fatty liver, but it cannot detect hepatitis. The histologic stage (prefibrotic versus fibrotic versus cirrhotic) can also be definitively identified by liver biopsy only. Staging is useful in assessing prognosis and potential therapeutic interventions.

However, firm recommendations of whether to perform a liver biopsy in the routine clinical setting have not yet been developed. The decision to biopsy requires assessment of the risks and benefits to each patient. A pragmatic approach in younger patients without clinical evidence of more advanced disease is a trial period of increased exercise and improved dietary habits before performing a liver biopsy.

18. **Can nonalcoholic fatty liver disease patients receive "statins"?**

Yes. The lipid lowering HMG CoA reductase inhibitors, or "statins," are associated with liver test abnormalities. On the other hand, one of the driving factors behind NAFLD may be dyslipidemia. Many patients with NAFLD will have dyslipidemia that physicians will want to treat. The question of whether it is safe to use the "statins" is not completely resolved. The role of baseline or serial biopsy in patients with liver abnormalities while using "statins" has yet to be established. However, hepatologists generally recommend using "statins" while monitoring of liver tests, provided the transaminases are less than two times the upper limit of normal.

19. **What histologic changes are associated with nonalcoholic fatty liver disease?**

Histologic changes of NAFLD may mirror those of alcoholic steatohepatitis. The main findings are macrovesicular and microvesicular fatty changes within the centrilobular hepatocytes (zone 3). Polymorphonuclear and mononuclear leukocyte and lymphocyte infiltration of portal tracts and parenchyma are also present. Although the changes are most often seen in zone 3, fatty changes within the hepatocytes and inflammatory changes may occur in all zones of the hepatic lobule. Histologic exam may show focal necrosis of centrilobular hepatocytes and hyaline (Mallory's bodies) within these hepatocytes. The hyaline bodies are usually sparse, small, and centrilobular. The ultrastructure of Mallory's bodies in patients with NAFLD is similar to those in patients with alcoholic hepatitis (Fig. 29-2).

One of the key histopathologic features of NAFLD in adults is the presence of perisinusoidal fibrosis, whereas in children portal fibrosis may be more characteristic. In adults the fibrosis begins typically in the centrilobular region. The wide spectrum of fibrosis ranges from mild to cirrhotic. The prevalence of mild-to-moderate fibrosis is 76–100%; of severe fibrosis, 15–50%. Cirrhosis is described less frequently in adults (7–16%) and is absent in children. Approximatel 10–20% of patients may have cirrhosis. Iron may be found within hepatocytes and Kupffer cells but the hepatic iron index is <1.9.

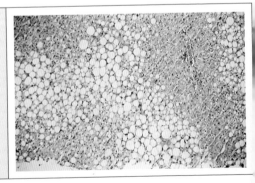

Figure 29-2. Nonalcoholic steatohepatitis with inflammatory cells, fat cells, and necrosis (hematoxylin-eosin stain).

20. What grading and staging system is used to describe the histologic features of nonalcoholic fatty liver disease?

The following system was proposed by Brunt, Janney, and Bisceglie:

Necroinflammatory activity

- Grade 1: Steatosis (predominantly macrovesicular) involving up to 66% of biopsy; occasional ballooned zone 3 hepatocytes; scattered amount of intra-acinar polymorphonuclear neutrophils (PMNs), with or without intra-acinar lymphocytes; no or mild portal chronic inflammation.
- Grade 2: Steatosis of any degree; obvious ballooning of hepatocytes (predominantly zone 3); intra-acinar PMNs; may be associated with zone 3 pericellular fibrosis; portal and intra-acinar chronic inflammation (mild to moderate).
- Grade 3: Panacinar steatosis; obvious ballooning and disarray, predominantly in zone 3; intra-acinar inflammation noted as scattered PMNs; PMNs associated with ballooned hepatocytes, with or without mild chronic inflammation; portal chronic inflammation mild or moderate, not marked.

Fibrosis

- Stage 1: Zone 3 perisinusoidal/pericellular fibrosis; focally or extensively present.
- Stage 2: Zone 3 perisinusoidal/pericellular fibrosis with focal or extensive periportal fibrosis.
- Stage 3: Zone 3 perisinusoidal/pericellular fibrosis and portal fibrosis with focal or extensive bridging fibrosis.
- Stage 4: Cirrhosis

21. How is nonalcoholic fatty liver disease treated?

Although there are no established treatments for NAFLD, empiric treatment strategies have been proposed. Gradual weight reduction can improve laboratory abnormalities, histologic changes, and hepatomegaly. However, improvements can be achieved, even if the patient remains obese. On the other hand, striking weight loss has been associated with progression of NAFLD. The long-term benefit of weight loss is difficult to evaluate because patients with NAFLD would have to maintain sustained reductions in weight. Obese patients with NAFLD rarely achieve or maintain sustained reductions in weight. Moreover, the effect of weight loss on liver disease is not consistent. The effects of many popular diets on the fatty liver are not known. For patients with significant obesity (75% overweight) who are not successful at dieting, gastric bypass or gastroplasty may significantly reduce steatosis. Several studies have reported beneficial effects of bariatric surgery, although precipitous weight loss can exacerbate NAFLD.

Despite its lipid-lowering properties, clofibrate therapy for 1 year in patients with NAFLD and hypertriglyceridemia was not found to be beneficial. A small trial suggests that gemfibrozil improves transaminases and serum lipids after 1 month's treatment, possibly by inhibiting free fatty acid mobilization from adipose tissue. The "statins" have not shown promise to date. Betaine has shown encouraging results in adults. Vitamin E showed promise for NAFLD in a pediatric population. Vitamin E may reduce the efficacy of the "statins." Small, short-duration studies suggest that alpha-tocopherol and combinations of lecithin, vitamin C, low-dose vitamin E, beta-carotene, selenium, and vitamin B complex can produce some improvements in liver tests. Some of these studies failed to show an improvement in histology.

The thiazolidinediones have shown promise. These agents activate the PPARγ (peroxisome proliferator-activated receptor-gamma) nuclear transcription factor, altering skeletal muscle glucose uptake, decreasing central adiposity, promoting adipocyte differentiation, altering mitochondrial mass, and altering thermogenesis. Metformin has also attracted the interest of NAFLD researchers.

Patients with decompensated cirrhosis from NAFLD can undergo successful liver transplantation, but it is possible for NAFLD to recur in the graft after transplantation. The weight gain and dyslipidemia seen after successful liver transplantation may contribute to the recurrence of NAFLD.

22. **What proportion of patients with nonalcoholic fatty liver disease undergo liver transplantation?**

Although the vast majority of patients with NAFLD exhibit a benign course, progressive disease has been reported in 15–20% of patients. However, few patients with NAFLD develop cirrhosis and liver failure and require transplantation.

Follow-up of patients transplanted for NAFLD has been limited, but recurrence has been noted as early as 6–10 weeks after transplantation. Rapid weight gain and the presence of a functioning jejunoileal bypass seem to be the most reliable predictors of recurrent NAFLD. No therapy has been reported to be of value in treating recurrent NAFLD after transplantation, with the exception of reversing a jejunoileal bypass. Weight loss in obese patients transplanted for primary NAFLD has been proposed as important in preventing recurrent disease.

23. **Are there any other liver diseases, besides alcoholic liver disease, in which fat is seen on biopsy?**

Yes. Fatty changes can be seen in hepatitis C, Wilson's disease, Weber-Christian disease, Mauriac's syndrome, Madelung's lipomatosis, celiac disease, chemical solvent exposure, medications (amiodarone, tamoxifen, nucleoside analogs, and methotrexate), and abetalipoproteinemia. Many of these disorders have either abnormal lipid metabolism and/or mitochondrial injury or dysfunction.

WEBSITES

1. http://www.liverfoundation.org

2. http://www.aasld.org/

3. http://www.liverfoundation.org/images/articles/1027/NAFLD.pdf

BIBLIOGRAPHY

I. Angulo P, Keach JC, Batts KP, Lindor KD: Independent predictors of liver fibrosis in patients with nonalcoholic steatohepatitis. Hepatology 30:1356–1362, 1999.

2. Bacon BR, Farahvash MJ, Janney CG, et al: Nonalcoholic steatohepatitis: An expanded clinical entity. Gastroenterology 107:1103–1109, 1994.

3. Brunt EM, Janney CG, Di Bisceglie AM, et al: Nonalcoholic steatohepatitis: A proposal for grading and staging the histological lesions. Am J Gastroenterol 94:2467–2474, 1999.

4. Caldwell SH, Oelsner DH, Iezzoni JC, et al: Cryptogenic cirrhosis: Clinical characterization and risk factors for underlying disease. Hepatology 29:664–669, 1999.

5. Diehl AM: Nonalcoholic steatohepatitis. Semin Liver Dis 10:221–229, 1999.

6. Kim WR, Poterucha JJ, Porayko MK, et al: Recurrence of nonalcoholic steatohepatitis following liver transplantation. Transplantation 62:1802–1805, 1996.

7. Matteoni CA, Younossi ZM, Gramlich T, et al: Nonalcoholic fatty liver disease: A spectrum of clinical and pathological severity. Gastroenterology 116:1413–1419, 1999.

8. Neuschwander-Tetri BA, Caldwell SH: Nonalcoholic steatohepatitis: Summary of an AASLD single topic conference. Hepatology 37:1202–1219, 2003.

Powell EE, Cooksley WG, Hanson R, et al: The natural history of nonalcoholic steatohepatitis: A follow-up study of forty-two patients for up to 21 years. Hepatology 11:74–80, 1990.

Sheth SG, Gordon FD, Chopra S: Nonalcoholic steatohepatitis. Ann Intern Med 126:137–145, 1997.

Sorbi D, Boynton J, Lindor KD: The ratio of aspartate aminotransferase to alanine aminotransferase: Potential value in differentiating nonalcoholic steatohepatitis from alcoholic liver disease. Am J Gastroenterol 94:1018–1022, 1999.

Teli MR, James OF, Burt AD, et al: The natural history of nonalcoholic fatty liver: A follow-up study. Hepatology 22:1714–1719, 1995.

Tilg H, Diehl AM: Cytokines in alcoholic and nonalcoholic steatohepatitis. N Engl J Med 343:1467–1476, 2000.

Wanless IR, Lentz JS: Fatty liver hepatitis (steatohepatitis) and obesity: An autopsy study with analysis of risk factors. Hepatology 12:1106–1110, 1990.

CHAPTER 30

LIVER TRANSPLANTATION

Kevin S. Sieja, MD, and James F. Trotter, MD

PATIENT REFERRAL AND SELECTION

1. **What is the current basis for prioritizing patients for cadaveric transplantation?**
    Priority for liver transplantation is currently determined by the MELD (Model for Endstage Liver Disease) score, which incorporates laboratory values for serum creatinine, bilirubin, and Internationalized Normalized Ratio (INR) in a mathematical equation to derive a probability of 90-day survival.

    $$\text{MELD score: R} = (0.957 \times \text{Log}_e[\text{creatinine mg/dL}] + 0.378 \times \text{Log}_e[\text{total bilirubin mg/dL}] + 1.120 \times \text{Log}_e[\text{INR}] + 0.643) \times 10$$

    The MELD equation excludes subjective assessments of the degree of ascites and encephalopathy that were components of the previous allocation system. In addition, time on the waiting list plays a minor role in the MELD system, serving only to break ties between patients with the same score. A high MELD score correlates with higher 90-day mortality and higher priority for transplantation. Patients with a MELD score <9 experienced a 1.9% mortality 90-day mortality rate, whereas patients with a MELD score ≥40 had a mortality rate of 71.3% 90 days.

2. **Why was the MELD score developed?**
    Under the previous allocation system, the Child-Turcotte-Pugh (CTP) score as well as waiting time were used to prioritize patients for transplantation. CTP score had several weaknesses, including subjective clinical measures and lack of validation as a measure of disease severity as an estimate of mortality risk in patients awaiting transplantation. Waiting time was also found to be a poor predictor of need for transplantation. As a result, the MELD score was developed allow the sickest patients to receive the highest priority for transplantation and to deemphasize waiting time as a determinant in prioritizing patients. Finally, only objective variables are used prioritize patients, which prevents the use of subjective criteria to increase transplantation priority.

3. **For patients with chronic liver disease, when is the appropriate time to refer for liver transplantation?**
    The decision to list a patient for transplantation rests, ultimately, with the transplant center. In general, patients should be considered for listing for transplantation if they have a MELD score ≥14 or life-threatening complications of end-stage liver disease, including ascites, encephalopathy, portal hypertensive bleeding, jaundice, or significant weight loss. Coexistent medical disorders such as coronary artery disease or chronic obstructive lung disease may jeopardize successful liver transplantation, especially in the elderly. Consequently, many transplant centers will not list elderly patients (>age 65), especially if significant comorbidities exist. There is no advantage gained by early listing of patients for liver transplantation, because waiting time no longer determines priority for transplantation.

Which patients with hepatocellular carcinoma (HCC) are considered for transplantation?

Overall survival for carefully selected patients with HCC is similar to that for patients undergoing transplantation for nonmalignant causes. The most consistent variable associated with prognosis appears to be tumor size and absence of metastasis. Patients with large HCC (>5 cm) or carcinoma outside the liver have prohibitively high recurrence rates to warrant transplantation. Acceptable candidates are patients with limited tumor size (one tumor ≤5 cm or three or fewer tumors where each tumor is <3 cm); no macrovascular involvement; and no identifiable extrahepatic spread to lymph nodes, lungs, abdominal organs, or bone. Under these criteria, 3- to 4-year actuarial survival is 75–85%, and recurrence-free survival is estimated at 83–92%.

How is HCC handled in the MELD system?

HCC is given special consideration in the MELD system. Patients with stage T2 (solitary tumor ≤5 cm or three or fewer tumors where each tumor is <3 cm) are awarded 24 points. For each month the patient remains listed without evidence of metastasis, he or she is awarded an additional 10 points. A biopsy is not mandatory to document HCC. However, in the absence of a biopsy, the diagnosis of HCC is established by specific imaging criteria. Patients must have a chest CT and bone scan to rule out metastatic lesions and at least one of the following: a tumor >1 cm in size with a blush corresponding to the area of suspicion seen on abdominal CT or MRI; an alpha-fetoprotein level of >200; an arteriogram confirming a tumor; a biopsy confirming HCC; chemo-embolization of the lesion; or radiofrequency, cryoablation, or chemical ablation of the lesion.

What can be done to improve the availability of donor organs?

A recent report estimated that only 15–20% of potential donors in the United States ultimately donated their organs. The most important impediment to donation is the inability to gain consent for donation from the donor family. Although logistic issues undoubtedly contribute to this low rate, many families refuse consent for donation. Several strategies have been used to improve the donor consent rate, including: public awareness campaigns, driver license registry for donation, payment of donor families to offset funeral costs, and mandatory reporting of brain death to organ procurement agencies. Reports have found that rates of consent for donation are significantly lower among minority groups. A Howard University survey of the African-American community found five principal reasons for refusal of donation:

- Lack of awareness of the status of organ transplantation
- Religious beliefs and misconceptions regarding transplantation
- Distrust of the medical establishment
- Fear of premature death among potential organ donors
- Desire for recipients to be African American

Public education programs conducted by African-American organ procurement coordinators have decreased apprehension about organ donation and increased minority participation.

Given the high waiting list mortality, is living donor liver transplantation (LDLT) an option?

Yes. Approximately 10% of patients listed for liver transplantation in the United States die each year awaiting a suitable donor organ. To help reduce this high mortality rate, many transplantation centers now offer LDLT for selected patients. Most adult-to-adult LDLTs in the United States use the right hepatic lobe from the donor. A recent series found the procedure effective and safe for both the donor and the recipient when performed at an experienced transplant center.

What are the advantages and disadvantages of LDLT?

The most important advantage of LDLT is a reduction in waiting time for the recipient. Once the recipient and the donor have been approved, surgery can occur within days. An expedited transplantation may allow the surgery to occur prior to clinical decompensation, which could jeopardize the success of the transplantation. Other advantages include: the ability to optimize recipient's condition given that the transplant is scheduled; a reduction in cold ischemia time (time between removal of the donor liver and its implantation in the recipient); and obtaining a graft from a healthy person who has undergone extensive testing. Disadvantages of LDLT include risk to the donor and lack of long-term outcome data for the LDLT recipient. Initial results suggest that recipients of LDLT may have more biliary complications than recipients of cadaveric organs.

9. **What potential recipients and donors are candidates for LDLT?**
The selection of appropriate recipients is an evolving process. The most appropriate recipients are patients in urgent need of transplantation, mainly those at substantial risk of dying prior to anticipated cadaveric transplantation. The most appropriate candidates for LDLT are patients with decompensated liver disease and/or hepatoma. There is controversy about whether patients with stable chronic liver disease should be evaluated for LDLT, but many centers consider that the risks to the donor outweigh the benefits to the recipient in these patients. Patients with multiple coexisting conditions, previous major abdominal surgery, or extensive mesenteric-vein thrombosis have increased risk for postoperative complications and may not be candidates for LDLT.

Donor selection requires a thorough medical and psychological evaluation to ensure that the patient can tolerate the procedure and understands the risks. Donors should be similar in size to the recipient, between 18 and 55 years of age, have a long-term significant relationship with the recipient, and have an identical or compatible blood type. The discovery of significant medical problems in the donor may preclude organ donation. A recent study showed that donors could be excluded on the basis of body-mass index (BMI) because 76% of potential donors with BMI >28 had substantial hepatic steatosis.

10. **List the diseases for which liver transplantation is performed.**
Acute liver failure (8%)
Cryptogenic
Viral hepatitis (A, B, other)
Drug-induced (acetaminophen, isoniazid, disulfiram, halothane, other)
Metabolic liver disease (Wilson's disease, Reye's syndrome)
Vascular (ischemic liver failure)
Toxin (Amanita mushroom)

Chronic liver disease (82%)
Chronic viral hepatitis (hepatitis C, hepatitis B)
Cryptogenic cirrhosis
Autoimmune hepatitis
Primary biliary cirrhosis
Primary sclerosing cholangitis
Nonalcoholic steatohepatitis
Budd-Chiari syndrome
Drug-induced cirrhosis (methotrexate, amiodarone)
Sarcoidosis
Alcoholic liver disease
Polycystic liver disease

Congenital/metabolic liver disease (8%)
Hemochromatosis
Wilson's disease
Alpha$_1$-antitrypsin deficiency
Cystic fibrosis

Amyloidosis

Other (2%)
Hepatic adenoma
Carcinoid tumor

11. **A 21-year-old woman is admitted following an overdose of acetaminophen. How does one determine whether she should be referred for liver transplantation?**

Acetaminophen is the most common cause of drug-induced liver failure. Acute ingestion of ≥12 gm of acetaminophen is predictive of hepatic injury, usually severe. The toxic metabolite of acetaminophen, N-acetyl-p-benzoquinoneimine is the result of metabolism by the cytochrome P450 system.

Chronic alcohol ingestion and the use of many medications (phenytoin, carbamazepine, isoniazid, and rifampin) may induce the cytochrome P450 system, which will reduce the amount of acetaminophen required to induce hepatotoxicity. The acetaminophen level is highly predictive of hepatotoxicity. Without treatment, an acetaminophen level above 300 mcg/mL at 4 hours or above 45 mcg/mL at 15 hours is associated with a 90% risk of hepatotoxicity. All patients with elevated liver enzymes and a history consistent with acetaminophen overdose should be considered for treatment. In patients who present within 4 hours of ingestion, activated charcoal can reduce acetaminophen absorption. N-acetylcysteine (Mucomyst), a glutathione precursor, remains the treatment of choice for acetaminophen-induced hepatotoxicity. The loading dose is 150 mg/kg and then 70 mg/kg every 4 hours for 17 doses. Although more effective when given within 10 hours of ingestion, benefits may occur with administration up to 24 hours.

Over the last 15 years, a number of criteria have been developed to identify those patients with fulminant hepatic failure caused by acetaminophen poisoning who are most likely to benefit from a liver transplant. The most widely used criteria are the King's College Criteria, which are an arterial blood pH <7.30 or a combination of prothrombin time (PT) >100 seconds, serum creatinine >3.3 mg/dL, and grade III or IV encephalopathy. These two cohorts of patients had 90% and 81% mortality rates, respectively, without liver transplantation.

12. **A 33-year-old man was diagnosed with acute hepatitis A 3 weeks ago. His jaundice has progressively worsened. Today, his wife found him to be mildly confused, and she brought him to the emergency room. What is the definition of *fulminant hepatic failure?***

Fulminant hepatic failure is defined as acute hepatitis with the onset of encephalopathy within 8 weeks of the development of symptoms in a patient with no preexisting liver disease. Patients will typically present with a history of progressive lethargy and jaundice over the course of several days. Common causes include viral hepatitis, drugs or toxins, Wilson's disease, Budd-Chiari syndrome, and hepatic ischemia. The largest series of fulminant hepatitis patients (n = 308) reported in the United States identified the following etiologies:

- Acetaminophen (39%)
- Indeterminate (17%)
- Drug reactions (13%)
- Hepatitis B (7%)
- Hepatitis A (4%)
- Other (20%)

Patients with fulminant hepatic failure require prompt referral to a liver transplant center. Patients may progress from stage II encephalopathy to full coma within a matter of hours. The King's College Criteria also address fulminant hepatic failure from causes other than acetaminophen. Patients fulfilling these criteria had greater than 90% risk of mortality and would benefit from liver transplantation:

- PT >100 seconds

Or any three of the following:

- Age <10 years or >40 years
- Etiology: non-A, non-B hepatitis; halothane; drug reaction
- Duration of jaundice before onset of encephalopathy >7 days
- PT >50 seconds
- Serum bilirubin >18 mg/dL

13. **What other options are available to support a patient with fulminant hepatic failure?**

Artificial and bioartificial support systems have been used to "bridge" patients with liver failure to transplantation or recovery. Liver support must include removal of toxins, synthesis of products, and treatment of inflammation. The first artificial support systems removed toxins through hemodialysis, hemofiltration, or hemoperfusion. Newer systems combine hemodialysis with adsorption to charcoal or albumin, whereas others use living hepatocytes that add synthetic functions to detoxification (bioartificial support systems). Several versions of bioartificial liver are currently in clinical trials to examine their ability to support patients with fulminant hepatic failure until a donor liver is available or regeneration occurs. The artificial livers use either porcine- or hepatoblastoma-derived hepatocytes as a Biofilter over which either plasma or whole blood is perfused.

A recent systematic review of 12 randomized trials of artificial and bioartificial support systems in acute liver failure found no significant mortality reduction when compared with standard medical therapy. The review did suggest that artificial support systems reduce mortality in acute-on-chronic liver failure compared with standard medical therapy. The evidence regarding bioartificial systems in acute liver failure was less conclusive. There was, however, significant heterogeneity between the studies included and the studies were limited size, so randomized trials on artificial and bioartificial support systems are still justified.

14. **Is human immunodeficiency virus (HIV) infection a contraindication to liver transplantation?**

Yes. In general terms, HIV infection is a contraindication for transplantation. However, select centers have transplanted small series of HIV-infected patients with outcomes similar to non–HIV-infected patients. Transplantation can be considered for HIV-infected patients because of the efficacy of HAART therapy. In a recently published series of 19 patients, 1-year patient survival was 79% compared with 87.9% in non-HIV patients undergoing liver transplantation.

KEY POINTS: PRETRANSPLANTATION

1. Approximately 5000 liver transplants are performed each year. One year survival is ~ 88%.

2. Orthotopic liver transplantation is limited by organ shortage. Ten percent of patients die each year on the waiting list.

3. Hepatitis C infection is the most common indication for liver transplantation.

4. Priority for transplantation is currently determined by the MELD score.

15. **What are contraindications to liver transplantation?**

The decision to perform a liver transplant in a given patient is made by the individual transplant center based on its judgment and experience. In general, the contraindications for transplantation are as follows:

Absolute contraindications
- Extrahepatic malignancy (excluding squamous cell carcinoma of the skin)
- Uncontrolled sepsis/infection
- Active alcohol or drug use
- Inadequate social support
- Hepatocellular carcinoma (stage T3 or higher)
- Advanced cardiopulmonary disease (including coronary artery disease, congestive heart failure, and severe chronic obstructive pulmonary disease)

Relative contraindications
- Portal vein and/or mesenteric vein thrombosis
- Cholangiocarcinoma
- Advanced age (≥65)
- Pulmonary hypertension (uncontrolled)
- HIV infection

6. **A 45-year-old man with end-stage liver disease is evaluated for liver transplantation. What features of the patient's psychosocial profile connote a good prognosis for continued abstinence from alcohol?**

For patients with a history of alcohol abuse, most centers require a period of abstinence (usually 6–12 months) and evaluation by a substance abuse professional prior to transplantation. Recognition of the alcoholism by the patient and family members is especially important, and the patients demonstrate this through adherence to an alcohol rehabilitation program. Other features associated with a low rate of recidivism include lack of comorbid substance abuse, social function, and lack of family history. The long-term post-transplant survival of appropriately selected alcoholics is typically higher than comparable nonalcoholic patients.

7. **Which factors measured prior to transplant correlate with reduced patient survival after liver transplantation?**

Previous reports have suggested that clinical factors, including Child-Pugh class, are not good predictors of survival after transplantation. However, poor renal function prior to transplant does predict poorer survival. Advanced age, re-transplantation, and extensive stage HCC are also associated with worse outcome. A recent study found that HCV infection significantly impairs long-term patient and allograft survival because of recurrent HCV in the transplanted liver.

EARLY POST-TRANSPLANT PERIOD (1–4 WEEKS)

8. **Which immunosuppressants are used in liver transplantation? What are their mechanisms of actions and side effects?**

See Table 30-1.

9. **What is the typical immunosuppressive regimen?**

The specific immunosuppressive regimen varies from center to center. Current immunosuppressive therapy usually involves multiple agents. These agents operate through different mechanisms to increase the immunosuppressive effect while minimizing the side effect from any one agent. The two most common regimens use either cyclosporine or tacrolimus. Cyclosporine and tacrolimus prevent T-cell activation through inhibition of calcineurin, a calcium-dependent phosphatase involved in intracellular signal transduction. Additional agents used with tacrolimus include prednisone and/or mycophenolate, and additional agents used with cyclosporine include prednisone, azathioprine, and mycophenolate.

TABLE 30-1. MECHANISM OF ACTION AND SIDE EFFECTS OF IMMUNOSUPPRESSANTS

	Mechanism of Action	Toxicities
Tacrolimus	Calcineurin inhibitor: suppresses IL-2–dependent T-cell proliferation	Renal, neurologic, diabetes mellitus
Cyclosporine	Same as tacrolimus	Renal, neurologic, hyperlipidemia, hypertension, hirsutism
Azathioprine	Inhibits T- and B-cell proliferation by interfering with purine synthesis	Bone marrow depression, hepatotoxicity
Mycophenolate mofetil	Selective inhibition of T- and B-cell proliferation by interfering with purine synthesis	Bone marrow depression, diarrhea
Prednisone	Cytokine inhibitor (IL-1, IL-2, IL-6, TNF, and IFN gamma)	Diabetes mellitus, obesity, hypertension, osteoporosis, infection
Sirolimus	Inhibits signal transduction from IL-2 receptors, decreasing T- and B-cell proliferation	Neutropenia, thrombo-cytopenia, hyperlipidemia, hepatic artery thrombosis in acute rejection
OKT3	Blocks T-cell CD3 receptor, preventing stimulation by antigen	Cytokine release syndrome, pulmonary edema, increased risk of infections/lymphoproliferative disorders
Daclizumab/ Basiliximab	Monoclonal antibody that blocks IL-2 receptor, inhibiting T-cell activation	Hypersensitivity reactions with basiliximab

There is increasing evidence that long-term maintenance corticosteroids may not be necessary to prevent rejection. Therefore, most transplant centers perform transplantation without corticosteroids or wean corticosteroids completely by 6 months. Direct comparisons of tacrolimus and cyclosporine suggest that both are effective in a strategy of early steroid withdrawal.

20. **A liver transplant patient has just sustained a grand mal seizure 36 hours pos' transplant. The cyclosporine level is within acceptable limits. The patient is in postictal state but has no obvious focal neurologic deficits. Which factors contribute to an increased risk of seizures post-transplant?**
Both cyclosporine and tacrolimus (FK506) have been associated with neurotoxicity, including seizures, paresthesia, ataxia, and delirium. Tremor is common with both medications and may improve with time. In general, these side effects were more common with intravenous tacrolimus. In addition, they are usually reversible with a reduction in dosage or discontinuation.

A patient who is 3 weeks post-transplant receives erythromycin for atypical pneumonia. Does this drug affect immunosuppressive therapy?

Cyclosporine and tacrolimus are metabolized by the cytochrome $P450_{3A4}$ system. Medications that inhibit $P450_{3A4}$ will raise cyclosporine and tacrolimus levels and place the patient at risk for toxicity or over-immunosuppression. Medications that induce $P450_{3A4}$ will lower levels and increase the risk of rejection or require higher doses (with increased costs) of the immunosuppressant. If these medications are necessary, dose adjustment and monitoring of cyclosporine and tacrolimus may be necessary. Medications that commonly interact with cyclosporine and tacrolimus include:

Increase cyclosporine/tacrolimus levels	Reduce cyclosporine/tacrolimus levels
Erythromycin	Phenytoin
Clarithromycin	Carbamazepine
Ketoconazole	Phenobarbital
Fluconazole	Rifampin
Itraconazole	
Verapamil	
Diltiazem	
Amiodarone	

A patient who had an uncomplicated transplant is noted to have rising liver enzymes on day 10 after transplantation. What is the differential diagnosis, and which tests should be obtained?

Elevated liver enzymes within the first 7–14 days after transplantation may be the first indication of a significant problem with the hepatic allograft. One of the most common causes of elevated liver enzymes is acute allograft rejection. Approximately 20–50% of all liver transplant recipients experience acute cellular rejection within the first 3 months after transplant. Early diagnosis is critical to ensure prompt initiation of immunosuppressive therapy (corticosteroid pulse or OKT3) to prevent graft loss. Liver biopsy remains the gold standard for the diagnosis of cellular rejection. The differential should include thrombus of the hepatic artery or portal vein, biliary leak, cholangitis, drug toxicity, recurrent viral hepatitis, and opportunistic infection. In general, opportunistic infections and recurrent viral hepatitis appear later than day 10. Appropriate tests may include cyclosporine or tacrolimus level, Doppler ultrasound, cholangiogram, and liver biopsy. If these are unrevealing, infectious etiologies should be considered.

KEY POINTS: POSTTRANSPLANTATION

. The two most common immunosuppressive regimens use either cyclosporine or tacrolimus.

. Cytomegalovirus (CMV) infection is the most common infection after transplantation.

. Differentiation between recurrent hepatitis C and acute cellular rejection is one of the most problematic areas in clinical transplantation.

. Recurrence of hepatitis C occurs almost universally and hepatitis C infection is associated with higher allograft failure and mortality rates.

A patient with cirrhosis from chronic hepatitis C undergoes liver trans-plantation. Ten days later his liver enzymes increase. What are the histologic findings of acute rejection versus post-transplant hepatitis C on liver biopsy?

The differentiation between recurrent hepatitis C and acute cellular rejection is one of the most problematic areas in clinical transplantation. In many cases, the histologic findings on the liver biopsy are inconclusive in differentiating these two clinical disorders. The histologic features of acute cellular rejection include (1) mixed cellular infiltrate (including eosinophils) in the portal tri (2) inflammation of the bile ducts presenting as either apoptosis or intraepithelial lymphocytes; and (3) endothelialitis of the central or portal veins. Recurrent hepatitis C can be difficult to distinguish from rejection. The histology may demonstrate a predominantly lymphocytic infiltra in the portal areas rather than the mixed cellular infiltrate of rejection. Other histologic findings include spotty parenchymal inflammation and vacuolization of the biliary epithelium.

24. **Describe the other post-transplant complications manifested by elevated live enzymes.**

Hepatic artery thrombosis remains a serious complication following transplant. The clinical presentation may be variable but is usually associated with elevated transaminases. Other sig include decreased bile output, persistent elevation of the PT or bilirubin, and/or bacteremia. Cessation of hepatic artery blood flow preferentially causes ischemic damage to the biliary tre resulting in breakdown of the biliary tree and development of biloma, bile leaks, and, eventuall strictures. Early hepatic artery thrombosis may be amenable to interventional radiologic intervention but usually warrants reoperation. In hepatic artery thrombosis, retransplantation usually required for successful long-term outcome.

In the early post-transplant period, portal vein thrombosis may present with signs of graft dysfunction and require immediate revascularization or retransplantation. Late thrombosis ma be well tolerated or may lead to graft dysfunction and/or portal hypertension. Balloon angioplas stent placement, and thrombolytic infusion have been used to reestablish the portal circulation

Biliary leaks or strictures may be asymptomatic but can also lead to jaundice, bacteremia, sepsis. Biliary leaks can occur at the biliary anastomosis and within the liver as a result of bile duct destruction. Ischemic damage from hepatic artery thrombosis may be a contributing fact

Medications may also lead to elevated liver enzymes. A cholestatic pattern may occur with cyclosporine, tacrolimus, azathioprine, sulfa drugs, and various antibiotics. A hepatocellular pattern may occur with azathioprine, nonsteroidal anti-inflammatory drugs, and some antibioti

The most common opportunistic infection of the hepatic allograft is cytomegalovirus (CMV infection, and the infection may present as elevated liver enzymes. However, CMV infection is uncommon in the first month after transplant (Fig. 30-1).

Recurrent hepatic disease may also first present with abnormal liver enzymes. Almost all patients with hepatitis C will have recurrence of hepatitis C infection. Most patients will have

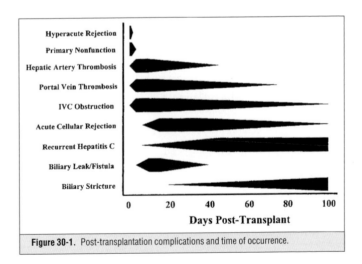

Figure 30-1. Post-transplantation complications and time of occurrence.

mild to moderate transaminase elevations and mild to moderate inflammation on biopsy. In a minority of patients, both hepatitis B and C infections may lead to fibrosing cholestatic hepatitis, which can lead to cirrhosis and graft loss during the first year. Recurrent disease may also occur with autoimmune hepatitis, primary biliary cirrhosis, and sclerosing cholangitis.

LONG-TERM TRANSPLANT PERIOD (>4 WEEKS)

A patient having early allograft rejection is treated with a 7-day course of OKT3 and returns 1 week later with headache, mild fatigue, low-grade fever, and increased liver enzymes. Is this OKT3 toxicity?
This is unlikely to be OKT3 toxicity. Most reactions occur during the initial few days of OKT3 therapy and include rigors, flash pulmonary edema, bronchospasm, arthralgia, nausea, vomiting, and diarrhea. One concern would be aseptic meningitis, which can present during or after OKT3 toxicity and can present with headache, fever, fatigue, and meningismus.

If it isn't OKT3 toxicity, what is the most likely diagnosis?
The differential would include CMV infection, incomplete treatment of rejection, postsurgical complications (hepatic artery thrombosis, hepatic abscess, biliary leak), cyclosporine or tacrolimus toxicity, and other opportunistic infections, including Epstein-Barr virus and fungal infections.

CMV is the most likely diagnosis in the patient described in question 25. In fact, CMV is the most common infection following liver transplantation. Most CMV infections occur within 1 to 4 months after liver transplantation. Patients who are initially seronegative for CMV and received a graft from a seropositive donor are at greatest risk. Other risk factors include the use of anti-lymphocyte antibodies and the occurrence of acute cellular rejection. Patients at high risk for CMV infection should receive prophylaxis with ganciclovir for 4–12 weeks after surgery. Patients at lower risk for CMV infection, including those who are seropositive for CMV prior to transplant, may receive ganciclovir or acyclovir for prophylaxis. Signs of CMV infection include fever, malaise, leukopenia, thrombocytopenia, and organ involvement (hepatitis, gastroenteritis, pancreatitis, pneumonia, and retinitis). The CMV DNA assay correlates well with viremia and has gained wide acceptance as a diagnostic tool. In addition, the liver biopsy is diagnostic, if the viral inclusions are present in the hepatic parenchyma or if the immunohistochemical stains are positive. Treatment requires a 2- to 4-week course of intravenous ganciclovir.

What are the clinical, biochemical, and histologic features of chronic rejection?
Chronic allograft rejection is generally characterized by an insidious, but progressive, rise in alkaline phosphatase and bilirubin. Patients are usually asymptomatic, and synthetic function remains intact until the late stages. The pathogenesis of this syndrome remains unclear, but the evidence favors an impressive loss of bile ducts and the development of obliterative arteriopathy in the small hepatic arteries. Histologic findings include a normal-appearing parenchyma with few mononuclear infiltrates in the portal areas but absence of bile ducts in almost all of the portal triads. Later in the course, patients develop strictures and dilations in the larger bile ducts, resembling primary sclerosing cholangitis. In these cases, the clinical course may be complicated by recurrent attacks of biliary sepsis. The differential diagnosis at this stage includes hepatic artery thrombosis, CMV cholangitis, anastomotic strictures of the biliary tree, and recurrent primary sclerosing cholangitis.

How is chronic rejection treated?
The process frequently progresses to graft failure, but recent reports indicate that 20–30% of patients may respond to additional immunosuppressive therapy. Patients with chronic rejection may also need evaluation for retransplantation.

29. **How often is it necessary to perform a second liver transplant, and for what reasons are retransplants performed?**

Approximately 10% of the liver transplants performed in the United States are retransplants. Early retransplants are performed usually for primary nonfunction and hepatic artery thrombosis. Improved immunosuppression and improved surgical techniques have reduced the early retransplant rate. Late retransplants may occur for recurrence of the original disease or chronic rejection. Recurrent disease may occur with viral hepatitis, autoimmune hepatitis, primary biliary cirrhosis, and primary sclerosing cholangitis.

30. **Describe the long-term metabolic complications that occur in the liver transplant recipient.**

Although patients experience a dramatic improvement in their quality of life following liver transplant, they are at risk for complications associated with the use of immunosuppressive regimens. The most common metabolic complications following liver transplantation include weight gain, diabetes, hypertension, and renal insufficiency. Most patients gain weight following transplant because of corticosteroids as well as their liberation from the pretransplant diet. Weight gain is more frequent in patients receiving cyclosporine than tacrolimus. Diabetes may occur following transplant because of the corticosteroids and in patients receiving calcineurin inhibitors. Hypertension is common with cyclosporine and tacrolimus, and the associated renal insufficiency may exacerbate this problem. Hyperlipidemia also occurs following transplant because of corticosteroids and cyclosporine. Although improvement may occur as immunosuppression is lowered, persistent hyperlipidemia needs aggressive treatment. All of these factors may place patients at greater risk for cardiovascular or cerebrovascular disease, and patients should receive counseling regarding appropriate diet, exercise, and smoking cessation. The incidence of post-transplant diabetes, hypertension, and hypercholesterolemia are significantly reduced by rapid corticosteroid weaning immediately after transplantation. Renal insufficiency occurs frequently after liver transplantation and is more frequent in patients receiving cyclosporine than tacrolimus. Up to 24% of patients develop end-stage renal disease. Other risk factors for developing ESRD include advanced age, hypertension, diabetes, hepatitis C, renal disease prior to liver transplantation, and postoperative acute renal failure.

Patients may be at risk for osteoporosis associated with corticosteroid use, particularly if they received significant steroids prior to transplant. A low threshold for measurement of bone density prior to transplantation may be appropriate in high-risk populations, such as patients with cholestatic liver disease. Patients at risk should receive calcium and vitamin D supplementation.

31. **Are liver transplant recipients at increased risk to develop cancer?**

Immunosuppression significantly increases the risk of malignancy and complicates approximately 2% of liver transplants. The most common malignancy following liver transplantation is squamous cell carcinoma of the skin. Therefore, patients should avoid exposure to ultraviolet light and wear protective clothing and sunscreen, if they participate in activities leading to sun exposure.

Post-transplant lymphoproliferative disorder (PTLD) is also a common malignancy after liver transplantation. Most are B-cell type, and the pathogenesis is related to Epstein-Barr virus (EBV) infection. The two most important risk factors for PTLD are the degree of immunosuppression (including OKT3 use) and EBV donor mismatch (negative recipient and positive donor). The clinical presentation includes fever, lymphadenopathy, and symptoms related to the organ involved. Extra nodal masses are common, and organs involved typically include the gastrointestinal tract, liver, lung, skin, and central nervous system. Treatment is a marked reduction in immunosuppression, which may result in complete resolution of disease. Referral for oncology consultation is also necessary for consideration of chemotherapy or radiation, which is required in many patients.

A liver transplant patient comes to the emergency room complaining of cough and shortness of breath. How does one suspect, diagnose, and treat *Pneumocystis carinii* infection?

Pneumocystis carinii pneumonia (PCP) is an opportunistic infection. The clinical presentation can be variable, but typical symptoms include fever, shortness of breath, and nonproductive cough. If left untreated, PCP may have a rapid course to respiratory failure. As a result, patients typically receive prophylaxis with trimethoprim/sulfamethoxazole. In the event of noncompliance, a high index of suspicion remains appropriate. Definitive diagnosis often requires bronchoscopy or bronchoalveolar lavage and should not delay treatment in the appropriate setting. Fortunately, PCP is a relative rare complication after liver transplantation. This is likely due to prophylaxis with trimethoprim/sulfamethoxazole and the reduction of immunosuppression compared to 10 years ago. Most transplant centers recommend at least 1 year of prophylactic trimethoprim/sulfamethoxazole for PCP. With institution of PCP prophylaxis and more conservative immunosuppressive regimens, the incidence of PCP at most transplant centers is less than 1%.

What factors contribute to metabolic bone disease after transplantation?

Chronic liver diseases, particularly cholestatic liver diseases, are associated with osteopenia. The pathogenesis was originally thought to be related to decreased bile salt flow and vitamin D malabsorption, but plasma vitamin D levels are normal. Instead, these patients appear to have inhibition of bone formation and low or normal bone resorption. Prior to transplant, therefore, these patients may already have significant bone loss. Following transplant, glucocorticoids worsen the condition and place the patients at risk for fractures. One study measured the bone density of 20 women with primary biliary cirrhosis. At 3 months after transplant, their bone density fell at a mean rate of 18.1% per year. The nadir in bone density appeared to occur within the first 6 months. As glucocorticoid use decreased, bone density improved and, ultimately, surpassed the pre-transplant density at 2 years.

A patient who underwent liver transplantation for cirrhosis resulting from hepatitis C returns with persistently elevated liver enzymes. Liver biopsy reveals chronic active hepatitis but no cirrhosis. Should he be treated with interferon-alpha and/or ribavirin?

Virtually all patients who receive a liver transplant for hepatitis C will have recurrent disease. Diagnosis of recurrence requires presence of HCV RNA and biopsy findings consistent with hepatitis C. A small minority develop fibrosing cholestatic hepatitis that may have an aggressive course and lead to graft loss within a year. Most patients will have mild to moderate elevations in transaminases and mild to moderate fibrosis on biopsy, and the optimal management of these patients is less clear. A recent study found that HCV infection in liver transplant recipients was associated with a 23% increased mortality rate and a 30% increased allograft failure rate.

Treatment of recurrent hepatitis C is pegylated-interferon-alpha and ribavirin. Experience in the post-transplant setting is limited, and trials are ongoing. Most transplant centers avoid treatment within the first 6 months because of concern that interferon-alpha may promote rejection. Current experience suggests that viral eradication may be difficult after transplantation, but treatment may decrease inflammation and improve histology. Consequently, patients with biochemical and histologic evidence of aggressive hepatitis C are considered for treatment at most transplant centers 6 months after transplantation. Side effects of therapy are more common and more severe in patients on immunosuppressive therapy. Therefore, patients on therapy must be monitored carefully and frequently require reductions in ribavirin and interferon. Long-term sustained viral response rates are, at best, about one half compared with non-transplant patients.

At this time, no prophylactic treatment is available for recurrent hepatitis C. Studies are in progress to examine the role of interferon-alpha and ribavirin in preventing recurrent disease. Aggressive early treatment may have a role in preventing or blunting the infection. However, the

concern remains of increasing the risk of rejection, and the ongoing trials should provide mor
assistance in this area.

35. **Is retransplantation for recurrent hepatitis C recommended?**
Yes, however, not without controversy. The prevalence of HCV infection in patients undergoin
retransplantation has significantly increased since 1990. Approximately one half of all liver
transplant recipients in the United States are infected with HCV. Because recurrent hepatitis C
causes graft failure in an increasing number of patients, retransplantation is considered in mo
and more patients. However, retransplantation for patients with graft failure caused by recurre
hepatitis C is quite controversial for two reasons: (1) long-term survival rates for
retransplantation recipients with graft failure caused by HCV are only 50%, and (2) the critica
shortage of deceased-donor livers forces clinicians to select patients with the best chance of
survival after transplantation. As a result, many transplantation centers do not offer
retransplantation to patients with graft loss caused by recurrent hepatitis C. However, outcom
may be improved if retransplantation can occur prior to the onset of hyperbilirubinemia and
renal failure.

BIBLIOGRAPHY

1. Beresford TP, Turcotte JG, Merion R, et al: A rational approach to liver transplantation for the alcoholic. Psychosomatics 31:241–254, 1990.
2. Bray GP, Harrison PM, O'Grady JG, et al: Long-term anticonvulsant therapy worsens paracetamol-induced ful nant hepatic failure. Hum Exp Toxicol 11:265–270, 1992.
3. Curley S, Carlton B, Abdalla E: Liver transplantation for hepatocellular carcinoma. UpToDate 11.1, 2003.
4. Deschenes M, Villeneuve JP, Dagenais M, et al: Lack of relationship between the severity of cirrhosis and sho term survival after transplantation. Liver Transpl Surg 3:532–537, 1997.
5. Eastell R, Dickson ER, Hodgson SF, et al: Rates of vertebral bone loss before and after liver transplantation in women with primary biliary cirrhosis. Hepatology 14:819–827, 1996.
6. Eckhoff DE, Pirsch JD, D'Alessandro AM, et al: Pretransplant status and patient survival following liver transplantation. Transplantation 60:920–925, 1995.
7. Figueras J, Jaurrieta E, Valls C, et al: Survival after liver transplantation in cirrhotic patients with and without hepatocellular carcinoma: A comparative study. Hepatology 25:1485, 1997.
8. Forman LM, Lewis JD, Berlin JA, et al: The association between hepatitis C infection and survival after orthotc liver transplantation. Gastroenterology 122:889–896, 2002.
9. Foster PF, Fabrega F, Karademir S, et al: Prediction of abstinence from ethanol in alcoholic recipients following liver transplantation. Hepatology 25:1469–1477, 1997.
10. Freeman R, Wiesner R: The new liver allocation system: Moving toward evidence-based transplantation polic Liver Transplantation 8:851–858, 2002.
11. Golling M, Safer A, Kriesche B, et al: Transplant survival following liver transplant: A multivariate analysis. Transplant Proc 30:3239–3240, 1998.
12. Gonzalez E, Rimola A, Navasa M, et al: Liver transplantation in patients with non-biliary cirrhosis: prognostic value of preoperative factors. J Hep 28:320–328, 1998.
13. Gralnek IM, Liu H, Shapiro MF, Martin P: The United States liver donor population in the 1990s: A descriptive, population-based comparative study. Transplantation 67:1019–1023, 1999.
14. Greig P, Lilly L, Scudamore C, et al: Early steroid withdrawal after liver transplantation: the Canadian tacrolimu versus microemulsion cyclosporine A trial: 1-year follow-up. Liver Transpl 9:587–595, 2003.
15. Kjaergard LL, Liu J, Als-Nielsen B, Gluud C: Artificial and bioartificial support systems for acute and acute-on-chronic liver failure. JAMA 289:217–222, 2003.
16. Makin AJ, Wendon J, Williams R: A 7-year experience of severe acetaminophen-induced hepatotoxicity (1987-1993). Gastroenterology 109:1907–1916, 1995.
17. Marcos A, Fisher RA, Ham JM, et al: Right lobe living donor liver transplantation. Transplantation 68:798–903 1999.

Nolan CM, Sandblom RE, Thummel KE, et al: Hepatotoxicity associated with acetaminophen usage in patients receiving multiple drug therapy for tuberculosis. Chest 105:408–411, 1994.

O'Grady JG, Alexander GJM, Hayllar KM, Williams R: Early indicators of prognosis in fulminant hepatic failure. Gastroenterology 97:439–445, 1989.

Ojo A, Held P, Port F, et al: Chronic renal failure after transplantation of a nonrenal organ. N Engl J Med 349:931–940, 2003.

Ostapowicz G, Fontana R, Schiodt F, et al: Results of a prospective study of acute liver failure at 17 tertiary care centers in the United States. Ann Int Med 137:947–954, 2002.

Prescott LF: Paracetamol overdosage: Pharmacological consideration and clinical management. Drugs 25:290–314, 1983.

Prottas JM, Batten HL: The willingness to give: The public and the supply of transplantable organs. J Health Polit Policy Law 16:121–124, 1991.

Rinella ME, Alonso E, Rao S, et al. Body mass index as a predictor of hepatic steatosis in living liver donors. Liver Transpl 7:409–414, 2001.

Roland ME, Stock PG: Review of solid-organ transplantation in HIV-infected patients. Transplantation 75:425–429, 2003.

Rosen HR, Martin P: Hepatitis C infection in patients undergoing liver retransplantation. Transplantation 66:1612–1616, 1998.

Shafer T, Wood RP, Van Buren CT, et al: A success story in minority donation: The LifeGift/Ben Taub General Hospital In-House Coordinator Program. Transpl Proc 29:3753–3755, 1997.

Sheil AGR, Disney APS, Mathew TH, et al: Lymphoma incidence, cyclosporine, and the evolution and major impact of malignancy following organ transplantation. Transpl Proc 29:825–827, 1997.

Trotter JF, Wachs M, Everson GT, Kam I: Adult to adult transplantation of the right hepatic lobe from a living donor. N Engl J Med 346:1074–1082, 2002.

Vale JA, Proudfoot AT: Paracetamol (acetaminophen) poisoning. Lancet 346:547–552, 1995.

Wiesner R, Edwards E: Model for end-stage liver disease (MELD) and allocation of donor livers. Gastroenterology 124:91–96, 2003.

Wiesner RH, Batts KP, Krom RA: Evolving concepts in the diagnosis, pathogenesis, and treatment of chronic hepatic allograft rejection. Liver Transpl Surg 5:388–400, 1999.

Wong T, Devlin J, Rolando N, et al: Clinical characteristics affecting the outcome of liver retransplantation. Transplantation 64:878–882, 1997.

CHAPTER 31

ASCITES

Carlos Guarner, MD, and Bruce A. Runyon, MD

1. What are the most common causes of ascites?

Ascites is the accumulation of fluid within the peritoneal cavity. More than 80% of patients with ascites have decompensated chronic liver disease. However, it is important to know the other possible causes of ascites, because treatment and prognosis may be quite different. Peritoneal carcinomatosis is the second most common cause of ascites, followed by acute alcoholic hepatitis, heart failure, fulminant or subacute hepatic failure, pancreatic disease, dialysis ascites, nephrotic syndrome, hepatic vein obstruction, chylous ascites, bile ascites, and miscellaneous disorders of the peritoneum.

2. Should a diagnostic tap be performed routinely on all patients with ascites at the time of admission to the hospital?

Yes. Ascites is readily diagnosed when large amounts of fluid are present in the peritoneal cavity. If clinical examination is not definitive in detecting or excluding ascites, ultrasonography may be helpful. In addition, ultrasonography may provide information about the cause of ascites, for instance, by documenting parenchymal liver disease, splenomegaly, and an enlarged portal vein. Abdominal tap may be performed easily and safely, and analysis of ascitic fluid provides useful data for differentiating causes of ascites. Prior to the era of prevention of infection by selective intestinal decontamination, up to 30% of patients with cirrhosis and ascites had ascitic fluid infection at the time of admission to the hospital or developed it during hospitalization. This infection is less common now but still remains a preventable cause of death in these patients. As a rule, therefore, diagnostic abdominal tap should be performed routinely (1) in all patients with new-onset ascites and (2) at the time of admission in patients with ascites. In addition, it should be repeated in patients whose clinical condition deteriorates during hospitalization, especially when they develop signs or symptoms of bacterial infection, hepatic encephalopathy, gastrointestinal hemorrhage, or deterioration of renal function. Patients with refractory ascites are currently submitted to repeated large-volume paracentesis in the outpatient clinic. Recent studies have demonstrated that the incidence of ascitic fluid infection or bacterascites is very low in these patients. Therefore, it seems reasonable to obtain a cell count and differential on samples of ascitic fluid in the paracentesis clinic setting and to culture only samples of ascitic fluid of symptomatic outpatients.

3. How should a diagnostic paracentesis be performed?

Although paracentesis is a simple and safe procedure, precautions should be taken to avoid complications. Paracentesis should be performed under sterile conditions. The abdomen should be cleaned and disinfected with an iodine solution, and the physician should wear sterile gloves during the entire procedure. The needle should be inserted in an area that is dull to percussion. The midline between the umbilicus and symphysis pubis was the preferable site of needle insertion in the past. However, three factors have changed this philosophy: (1) the frequency of therapeutic paracentesis, (2) the thickness of the panniculus in the midline in the obese patient, and (3) the frequency of obesity in patients with cirrhosis. Now the left lower quadrant appears to be the best site for needle insertion. Because the panniculus is less thick in this area, the needle traverses less tissue. Occasionally, even a 3.5-inch needle will not reach ascitic fluid in the midline in obese patients. Therapeutic taps in the lower quadrants drain more fluid than midline taps. Patients on lactulose tend to have a distended cecum. Therefore, the left lower quadrant is chosen over the right lower quadrant. A site is chosen in the left lower quadrant two fingerbreadths cephalad from the anterior superior iliac spine and two fingerbreadths medial to this landmark.

Scars should be avoided, because they are often sites of collateral vessels and adherent bowel. Between 30 and 50 mL of ascitic fluid should be withdrawn for analysis. After paracentesis, patients should recline for 30 minutes on the opposite side of the paracentesis to avoid leakage of ascitic fluid.

4. **What tests should be ordered routinely on ascitic fluid?**
Analysis of ascitic fluid is useful for the differential diagnosis of ascites. However, it is not necessary to order all tests on every specimen. The most important tests are cell count, bacterial culture, albumin, and total protein.

The *white blood cell count* is probably the single most important test performed on ascitic fluid, because it provides immediate information about possible bacterial infection. An absolute neutrophil count ≥250 cells/mm^3 provides presumptive evidence of bacterial infection of ascitic fluid and warrants initiation of empiric antibiotics. An elevated white blood cell count with a predominance of lymphocytes strongly suggests peritoneal carcinomatosis or tuberculous peritonitis.

Albumin concentration of ascitic fluid allows calculation of the serum-ascites albumin gradient to classify specimens into high- or low-gradient categories (see question 6).

Ascitic fluid should be cultured by inoculating *blood culture* bottles at the bedside. The sensitivity of this method is higher than that of the conventional technique in detecting bacterial growth. Automated systems for bacterial growth culture, such as BacT/ALERT, provide an earlier microbiologic diagnosis of ascitic fluid infection (usually <12 hours). Specific culture for tuberculosis should be ordered when tuberculous peritonitis is suspected on clinical grounds, and the ascitic fluid white blood cell count is elevated with a predominance of lymphocytic cells.

Total protein concentration of ascitic fluid has been used to classify ascitic fluid into transudates and exudates. Presently, this classification is not particularly helpful, because >30% of cirrhotic ascites samples are exudates. Nevertheless, total protein concentration of ascitic fluid should be ordered routinely, because it is useful for determining which patients are at high risk of developing spontaneous bacterial peritonitis (SBP) (total protein <1.0 gm/dL) and for differentiating spontaneous from secondary bacterial peritonitis. Measurement of glucose and lactate dehydrogenase (LDH) in ascitic fluid has also been found to be helpful in making this distinction (see question 11).

Amylase activity of ascitic fluid is markedly elevated in pancreatic ascites and gut perforation into ascites.

Gram stain of ascitic fluid is usually negative in cirrhotic patients with early SBP, but it may be helpful in identifying patients with gut perforation, in whom multiple types of bacteria are seen.

Cytology of ascitic fluid is useful in detecting malignant ascites when the peritoneum is involved with the malignant process. Unfortunately, ascitic fluid cytology is not useful in detecting hepatocellular carcinoma, which seldom metastasizes to the peritoneum.

Other tests proposed as helpful in detecting malignant ascites, such as fibronectin, cholesterol, ferritin, transferrin, lactate, ceruloplasmin, alpha$_2$ microglobulin, alpha$_1$ antitrypsin, interleukin-8, and carcinoembryonic antigen, have limited, if any, value in ascitic fluid analysis.

5. **Should a diagnostic thoracocentesis be performed in cirrhotic patients with pleural hydrothorax?**
Hepatic hydrothorax is defined as the accumulation of ascitic fluid in the pleural space in a patient with cirrhosis, in whom a cardiac, pulmonary, or pleural cause has been excluded. Between 5% and 10% of cirrhotic patients with ascites develop hepatic hydrothorax, mainly in the right side (almost 70% of the cases), but it can also be in the left side and bilateral. In a

recent study, almost 10% of cirrhotic patients admitted to the hospital with hepatic hydrothorax had a spontaneous bacterial empyema, and 40% of these episodes were not associated to spontaneous bacterial peritonitis. In consequence, a diagnostic thoracocentesis in cirrhotic patients with ascites could be useful to evaluate other causes of pleural effusion in selected patients and to diagnose spontaneous bacterial empyema in cirrhotic patients with a suspected bacterial infection and negative studies of urine, ascitic fluid, and blood specimens.

6. **Why is it useful to measure serum-ascites albumin gradient?**
Serum-ascites albumin gradient (SAAG) is more useful than the total protein concentration of ascitic fluid in the classification of ascites. This gradient is physiologically based on oncotic-hydrostatic balance and is related directly to portal pressure. The serum-ascites albumin gradient is calculated by subtracting the albumin concentration of ascitic fluid from the albumin concentration of serum obtained on the same day:

$$SAAG = albumin_{serum} - albumin_{ascites}$$

Patients with gradients ≥1.1 gm/dL have portal hypertension, whereas patients with gradients <1.1 gm/dL do not:

≥1.1 gm/dL	<1.1 gm/dL
↓	↓
Portal hypertension	Normal portal pressure

7. **What are the causes of high (≥1.1 gm/dL) serum-ascites albumin gradients?**
The most common cause of a high serum-ascites albumin gradient is cirrhosis, but any cause of portal hypertension (e.g., alcoholic hepatitis, cardiac ascites, massive liver metastases, fulminant hepatic failure, Budd-Chiari syndrome, portal vein thrombosis, veno-occlusive disease, myxedema, fatty liver of pregnancy, "mixed" ascites) leads to a high gradient. Mixed ascites are due to two different causes, including one that causes portal hypertension (e.g., cirrhosis and tuberculous peritonitis).

8. **What are the causes of low (that is, <1.1 gm/dL) serum-ascites albumin gradients?**
Low-gradient ascites are found in the absense of portal hypertension and are usually due to peritoneal disease. The most common cause is peritoneal carcinomatosis. Other causes are tuberculous peritonitis, pancreatic disease, biliary ascites, nephrotic syndrome, serositis, and bowel obstruction or infarction.

9. **What are the variants of ascitic fluid infection?**
Ascitic fluid infection can be spontaneous or secondary to an intra-abdominal, surgically treatable source of infection. More than 90% of ascitic fluid infections in cirrhotic patients are spontaneous. According to the characteristics of ascitic fluid culture and polymorphonuclear (PMN) cell count, four different variants of ascitic fluid infection have been described in cirrhotic patients. *SBP* is defined as an ascitic fluid infection with PMN count ≥250 cells/mm^3 and positive culture (usually for a single organism). *Culture-negative neutrocytic ascites* (CNNA) defined as an ascitic fluid PMN count ≥250 cells/mm^3 with a negative culture. *Bacterascites* is defined as an ascitic fluid PMN count <250 cells/mm^3 with a positive culture for a single organism. *Polymicrobial bacterascites* is defined as an ascitic fluid with PMN count <250 cells/mm^3 with a positive culture for more than one organism. This condition is usually caused by gut puncture by the needle during attempted paracentesis.

10. **What are the diagnostic criteria of spontaneous bacterial empyema?**
Current diagnostic criteria of spontaneous bacterial empyema is a positive pleural fluid with a pleural fluid polymorphonuclear leukocyte count ≥250 cells/μL and the exclusion of

parapneumonic infections. Culture-negative spontaneous bacterial empyema is defined when the patient has a negative pleural fluid culture and a polymorphonuclear leukocyte ≥500 cells/μL, without a parapneumonic infection.

11. **How does one differentiate spontaneous from secondary peritonitis?**
It is important to differentiate spontaneous from secondary peritonitis in cirrhotic patients, because treatment for SBP is medical, whereas treatment for secondary peritonitis is usually surgical. Although secondary peritonitis represents <10% of ascitic fluid infections, it should be considered in any patient with neutrocytic ascites. Analysis of ascitic fluid is helpful in differentiating the two entities. Secondary bacterial peritonitis should be suspected when ascitic fluid analysis shows two or three of the following criteria (Runyon's criteria): total protein >1 gm/dL, glucose <50 mg/dL, and LDH >225 mU>/mL (or higher than the upper limit of normal for serum). Most of the ascitic fluid cultures in such patients are polymicrobial, whereas in patients with SBP the infection is usually monomicrobial. Patients with suspected secondary peritonitis must be evaluated by emergency radiologic techniques to confirm and localize the possible visceral perforation. In patients with nonperforation secondary peritonitis, these criteria are not as useful; however, PMN cell count after 48 hours of treatment increases beyond the pretreatment value, and ascitic fluid culture remains positive. Conversely, ascitic fluid PMN cell count decreases rapidly in appropriately treated patients with SBP, and ascitic fluid culture becomes negative. Determination of ascitic fluid carcinoembryonic antigen and alkaline phosphatase levels (>5 ng/mL and/or >240 U/L, respectively) may be helpful to diagnose secondary bacterial peritonitis due to occult intestinal perforation (higher specificity than Runyon's criteria).

12. **Who is at high risk of developing SBP?**
- Cirrhotic patients with gastrointestinal hemorrhage
- Cirrhotic patients with ascitic fluid total protein <1 gm/dL, especially those with high bilirubin (>3.2 mg/dL) or low platelet count (<98,000 cells/mm^3)
- Cirrhotic patients who have survived an episode of SBP
- Patients with fulminant hepatic failure

13. **What is the pathogenesis of SBP?**
Gram-negative bacteria are the most common causative agents isolated in bacterial infections in cirrhotic patients. Therefore, it has been suggested that the gut may be the source of the bacteria. Direct passage of intestinal bacteria to portal blood or ascitic fluid has not been documented in cirrhotic patients, if the gut mucosa has not lost its integrity. Bacterial translocation, defined as the passage of viable bacteria from gastrointestinal tract to mesenteric lymph nodes, has been demonstrated in an experimental model of cirrhotic rats with ascites and in cirrhotic patients submitted to a laparotomy. In fact, genetic identity has been observed between bacteria isolated in the gut, mesenteric lymph nodes, and ascitic fluid in cirrhotic rats. Intestinal bacterial overgrowth seems to be the main mechanism of bacterial translocation in cirrhotic rats. Reducing the quantity of intestinal flora has been shown to decrease the incidence of bacterial translocation and SBP. A recent experimental study has observed that cirrhotic rats, with severe intestinal oxidative damage in ileum and cecum, have a higher incidence of bacterial translocation, suggesting a possible role of functional mucosal alterations in the pathogenesis of SBP. Several immune deficiencies, especially decreased activity of the reticuloendothelial system and low serum complement levels, lead to frequent and prolonged bacteremia in cirrhotic patients and to colonization of body fluids, such as ascitic fluid. The development of a bacterial infection depends on the capacity of ascitic fluid to kill the bacteria. In vitro, the capacity of ascitic fluid to kill bacteria (i.e., opsonic activity) is related directly to total protein and C3 concentration of ascitic fluid. Cirrhotic patients with low ascitic fluid opsonic activity have low C3, low total protein, and thus a higher incidence of SBP. In contrast, patients with high ascitic fluid opsonic activity have high C3 and high total protein; thus, bacterial colonization may resolve spontaneously.

14. **What single test provides early information about possible ascitic fluid infection?**

The decision to start empiric antibiotic treatment must be made as soon as possible, because the survival rate depends, in part, on early diagnosis and treatment. Gram stain is positive in only 5–10% of patients, and bacterial culture of ascitic fluid takes at least 12 hours to demonstrate growth. The ascitic fluid neutrophil count is highly sensitive in detecting bacterial infection of peritoneal fluid, and the result should be available in a matter of minutes. An absolute neutrophil count ≥250 cells/mm^3 warrants empiric antibiotic treatment. Ascitic fluid cell count should be immediately injected into a tube containing an anticoagulant (i.e., "purple top" tube) to avoid clotting of the specimen. The laboratory should perform the cell count in less than 60 minutes, but this is unusual. Recent data have demonstrated that the use of urine "dipsticks" to detect neutrophils in ascitic fluid has a high sensitivity, specificity, and negative predictive value and reduces the time from paracentesis to a presumptive diagnosis of SBP from a few hours to as little as 90 seconds. A standard cell count and differential should be performed by the laboratory to confirm the results, but empiric antibiotics can be started immediately in patients with a positive urine "dipstick."

Other tests, such as ascitic fluid pH or lactate or arterial-ascitic fluid gradient of pH or lactate, are significantly less sensitive than ascitic fluid neutrophil count and are currently not used in clinical practice.

15. **What is the treatment of choice for suspected spontaneous bacterial peritonitis?**

A relatively broad-spectrum antibiotic combination, such as an aminoglycoside plus ampicillin, was used routinely in the past for treatment of suspected SBP. However, most cirrhotic patients treated with an aminoglycoside developed nephrotoxicity, even when serum levels were controlled. Third-generation cephalosporins cover most of the flora responsible for SBP; they are more effective than the combination of ampicillin and aminoglycoside and lack nephrotoxicity. Cefotaxime or a similar cephalosporin should be started when SBP is suspected. A recent demonstration showed that 2.0 gm of cefotaxime, given intravenously every 8–12 hours, is as effective as dosing every 6 hours. A short course of therapy (5 days) has been shown to be as effective as a long course (10 days). Amoxicillin-clavulanic acid, initially intravenously (0.2–1.0 gm/8 h) and then orally (125–500 mg/8 h), has been shown to be as effective as cefotaxime but less expensive. Unfortunately, intravenous amoxicillin-clavulanic acid is not available in the United States. A short course of intravenous ciprofloxacin (200 mg/12 h for 2 days followed by oral ciprofloxacin (500 mg/12 h for 5 days) is also an effective treatment of SBP. Patients with uncomplicated SBP (i.e., those without shock, ileus, gastrointestinal hemorrhage, or hepatic encephalopathy) can be treated safely with oral ofloxacin (400 mg/12 h). However, oral or intravenous quinolones should not be used as empiric treatment of patients on quinolone prophylaxis with suspected bacterial infection. These patients develop infections caused by gram-negative cocci or quinolone-resistant gram-negative bacilli. Empiric cefotaxime or amoxicillin-clavulanic acid is also effective in such patients. One recent study has shown that intravenous albumin administration, at a dose of 1.5 gm/kg at the time of diagnosis of SBP and 1 gm/kg on day 3 of treatment, reduces the incidence of renal impairment and death. Albumin should be considered, especially in patients with SBP and blood urea nitrogen (BUN) >30 mg/dL and/or serum bilirubin >4 mg/dL (Fig. 31-1).

16. **When should antibiotic treatment be started in a patient with cirrhosis and suspected ascitic fluid infection?**

Empiric antibiotic treatment must be started as soon as possible to improve survival rates. Therefore, it is important to perform routine bacterial cultures of ascitic fluid, blood, urine, and sputum as well as an ascitic fluid cell count and differential when a hospitalized patient with ascites develops clinical signs of possible infection (e.g., fever, abdominal pain, encephalopathy) or shows deterioration in clinical or laboratory parameters. In addition, ascitic fluid and urine

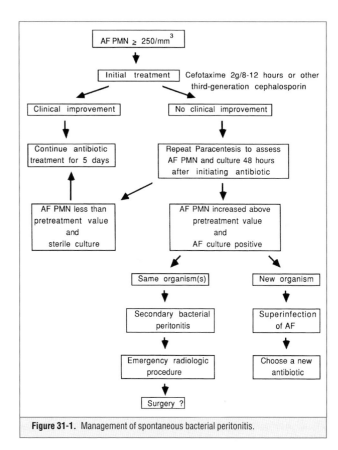

Figure 31-1. Management of spontaneous bacterial peritonitis.

should be analyzed when cirrhotic patients with ascites are admitted to the hospital; about 20% are infected at this time. A high level of suspicion for bacterial infection is appropriate, because it is a reversible cause of deterioration and a frequent cause of death in patients with cirrhosis. Empiric antibiotics should be started immediately after performing cultures and ascitic fluid analysis whenever (1) bacterial infection is suspected based on abdominal pain or fever or (2) ascitic fluid neutrophils are ≥250 cells/mm^3 (*see* Fig. 31-1).

Should the PMN cell count in ascitic fluid be monitored during treatment of SBP?
Ascitic fluid culture becomes negative after a single 2-gm dose of cefotaxime in 86% of patients with SBP. The neutrophil count also decreases rapidly to normal values during therapy in 90%. Superinfection or early recurrence after treatment with third-generation cephalosporins is uncommon. Repeat paracentesis is not necessary if the setting (advanced cirrhosis) is typical, one organism is cultured, and the patient has the usual dramatic response to treatment. However, 2 or 3 days after starting antibiotic treatment, repeat paracentesis can be considered to confirm the decrease in PMNs in the fluid and sterility of the fluid.

Does bacterascites represent a real peritoneal infection? Should it be treated?
Recent studies have documented the short-term natural history of monomicrobial nonneutrocytic bacterascites. A repeat paracentesis of patients with bacterascites before starting antibiotic

therapy showed that, in 62–86% of them, the episode of bacterascites resolved spontaneously. interest, all patients who progressed to SBP had symptoms of bacterial infection at the time of first tap. Such data demonstrate that bacterascites is a dynamic process; its evolution may depend on several factors, including systemic and ascitic fluid defenses as well as organism virulence. According to these studies, symptomatic patients with bacterascites should be treat with antibiotics. Asymptomatic patients need not receive antibiotic treatment but should be reevaluated with a second tap. If the PMN count is $\geq 250/mm^3$, antibiotics should be started.

19. **Which subgroups of patients with liver disease should receive treatment to prevent bacterial infection?**

Because enteric aerobic gram-negative bacteria are the most frequent causative agents isolat in bacterial infections in cirrhosis, and because bacterial translocation seems to be an import. step in pathogenesis, inhibition of intestinal gram-negative bacteria should be an effective method of preventing bacterial infections. Patients with liver disease who are at high risk of developing bacterial infection and/or SBP should be considered for selective intestinal decontamination (SID). SID consists of the inhibition of the gram-negative flora of the gut wit preservation of gram-positive cocci and anaerobic bacteria. Preservation of the anaerobes is important in preventing intestinal colonization, overgrowth, and subsequent translocation of pathogenic bacteria.

Several trials have shown that SID with oral norfloxacin is highly effective in preventing bacterial infections and/or SBP in cirrhotic inpatients with (1) gastrointestinal hemorrhage (4 mg twice daily) or (2) low ascitic fluid protein (400 mg/day) and (3) in patients with fulminant hepatic failure (400 mg/day). Long-term antibiotic therapy has been used in preventing the fi episode of SBP as well as recurrences. Long-term prophylactic treatment decreases the incidence of SBP in both conditions but increases the appearance of quinolone-resistant bacteria and infections. Secondary prophylaxis is generally well accepted, especially in patien awaiting liver transplantation. Long-term primary prophylaxis is currently being evaluated in more restrictive groups of patients, such as those with low ascitic fluid total protein and high serum bilirubin (>3.2 mg/dL) or low platelet count (<98,000 cells/mm³).

20. **Do we have alternative prophylactic treatments to quinolones for preventing bacterial infections in cirrhosis?**

Prophylaxis with oral quinolones or trimethoprim/sulfamethoxazole promotes infections caus by quinolone-resistant gram-negative bacilli; this reduces the efficacy of the preventive treatment, especially in patients submitted to long-term prophylaxis. Therefore, it is very important to evaluate nonantibiotic drugs for preventing bacterial infections in cirrhosis. Seve experimental studies in cirrhotic rats have demonstrated the efficacy of short-term prevention bacterial translocation and SBP with different drugs, such as beta blockers, probiotics, antioxidants, and bile salts. Unfortunately, no clinical trials have been published demonstratin any effect of these drugs in cirrhotic patients.

21. **What is the treatment of spontaneous bacterial empyema?**

Microbiologic studies of pleural fluid have shown that gram-negative bacteria are present in almost 50% of patients with spontaneous bacterial empyema—the others being culture-negative. Therefore, patients with spontaneous bacterial empyema should be treated with brc spectrum antibiotics, as in patients with SBP. A chest tube is not necessary and should be avoided. Patients surviving a spontaneous bacterial empyema should be evaluated for liver transplantation.

22. **Why is it important to know the sodium balance in patients with cirrhosis and ascites?**

Ascites formation in cirrhosis is due to renal retention of sodium and water. The aim of medic treatment of ascites in patients with cirrhosis is to mobilize the ascitic fluid by creating a net negative balance of sodium. This goal is accomplished by reducing sodium intake in the diet and increasing urinary sodium excretion. Therefore, knowledge of urinary excretion of sodium allows the clinician to plan initial treatment. In addition, urinary sodium excretion is an easily determined prognostic indicator. Patients with cirrhosis and a urinary sodium excretion <10 mEq/day have a 2-year survival rate of 20%, whereas those with sodium excretion >10 mEq/day have a 2-year survival rate of 60%.

Describe the initial treatment of patients with cirrhosis and ascites.
Cirrhotic patients with ascites should be treated initially by dietary sodium restriction (50–88 mEq/day) and diuretics. A more severe restriction of sodium intake may worsen anorexia and malnutrition. Water restriction is usually not necessary if serum sodium concentration is above 120 mEq/L. In 15–20% of patients, a negative sodium balance may be obtained with dietary sodium restriction in the absence of diuretics. However, because 80–85% of patients need diuretics, it is reasonable to start diuretics in all patients. The initial dose of diuretics should be 100 mg of spironolactone and 40 mg of furosemide; both drugs are given orally in a single morning dose. If the body weight does not decrease, or the urinary sodium excretion does not increase after 2–3 days of treatment, the dose of both diuretics should be progressively increased, usually in simultaneous increments of 100 mg/day and 40 mg/day, respectively. Serial monitoring of urinary sodium excretion and daily weight is the best way to determine the optimal dose of diuretics. Doses should be increased until a negative sodium balance is obtained (i.e., urinary excretion is greater than dietary intake) with corresponding weight loss. The ceiling doses of spironolactone and furosemide are 400 mg/day and 160 mg/day, respectively. Once ascites has been mobilized, diuretic dosage should be adjusted individually to keep the patient free of ascites. Patients with tense ascites should be treated initially with a therapeutic paracentesis of 4 or more liters (Fig. 31-2).

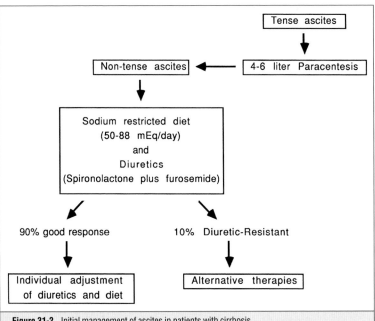

Figure 31-2. Initial management of ascites in patients with cirrhosis.

24. **What is refractory ascites?**

Refractory ascites is an inadequate response to sodium-restricted diet (<90 nmoles/day) high-dose diuretic treatment (400 mg/day of spironolactone and 160 mg/day furosemide inadequate response is manifested by the absence of weight loss (<0.8 kg over 4 days) or development of complications of diuretics, such as hepatic encephalopathy, renal impairr hyponatremia, or hypokalemia or hyperkalemia. Excessive sodium intake, bacterial infecti occult gastrointestinal hemorrhage, and intake of prostaglandin inhibitors (e.g., aspirin or nonsteroidal anti-inflammatory drugs) should be excluded before labeling patients as refr Early ascites recurrence (within 4 weeks after initial mobilization) is also considered refra ascites. Less than 10% of cirrhotic patients are refractory to standard medical therapy. Th small group should be evaluated for other therapeutic options, such as liver transplantati chronic outpatient paracentesis (usually every 2 weeks), peritoneovenous shunt, or trans intrahepatic portosystemic stent-shunt (TIPS).

25. **Which patients should be treated with large-volume paracentesis?**

Large-volume paracentesis is an old but safe and effective procedure to mobilize ascitic flui in cirrhotic patients. Interest in this procedure has been renewed in the past decade. Recentl therapeutic paracentesis has shown to be not only safe but also may have additional benefic effects on the hemodynamic status of patients with tense ascites. However, repeated large-volume paracentesis causes depletion of proteins and, theoretically, may predispose to SBP. Therefore, therapeutic paracentesis should not be used as a routine treatment of all cirrhotic patients with ascites and should be reserved for treating patients with tense and/or refractor ascites.

26. **Should volume expanders be infused after large-volume paracentesis?**

Plasma volume expansion after large-volume paracentesis is controversial. Volume expanc were introduced to avoid theoretic hemodynamic disturbances that may develop in cirrhoti patients after therapeutic paracentesis of 5 or more liters of ascitic fluid. One study reporte that patients receiving albumin infusion after large-volume paracentesis had less hyponatre and azotemia than patients who did not receive albumin. However, albumin infusion did no decrease symptomatic complications or hospital readmissions or increase survival rates. Because albumin infusion is expensive, less costly volume expanders have been tried. Paracentesis-induced circulatory dysfunction, defined as an increase in plasma renin activi more than 50% of the preparacentesis value to a level of more than 4 ng/mL/h, is observed with a higher incidence in cirrhotic patients not submitted to volume expansion or treated v nonalbumin expanders after a large-volume paracentesis. A study has observed that patien developing paracentesis-induced circulatory dysfunction have a worse long-term prognosi A recent study has demonstrated that the incidence of paracentesis-induced circulatory dysfunction is similar in patients treated with albumin or saline (170 mL of 3.5% saline solu per liter of ascites removed at 999 mL/h) after total paracentesis, when less than 6 L of asci fluid was evacuated. The cost of saline infusion was 100-fold cheaper than albumin infusio These data suggest that repeated paracentesis of less than 6 L does not require albumin inf and can be safely substituted with saline infusion. However, infusion of saline may lead to t recurrent, rapid need for another large-volume paracentesis. At this time, albumin should b viewed in patients submitted to a large-volume paracentesis of 6 L or more as optional unti demonstrated that volume expansion after therapeutic paracentesis has a beneficial effect c morbidity or survival. More recent data have observed that an early decrease in systemic vascular resistances after total paracentesis is due to an increase in arterial vasodilation th may be related to an abrupt decrease in intra-abdominal pressure after fast paracentesis. T data suggest that hemodynamic disturbances after total paracentesis could be prevented l reducing the flow rate of ascites extraction, making volume expansion unnecessary. More are required.

Is there currently any indication for peritoneovenous shunt?

Peritoneovenous shunt was introduced for the treatment of cirrhotic patients with refractory ascites in 1974 by LeVeen and associates. After initial enthusiasm, many complications were reported, and the enthusiasm decreased progressively. The number of complications is especially high in patients with severe hepatocellular insufficiency. Obstruction of the shunt, especially at the venous end, despite the collocation of a titanium tip, is the main complication and requires the implantment of a new stent. In addition, peritoneovenous shunt does not reduce mortality during the initial hospitalization and does not improve long-term survival in cirrhotic patients. Therefore, peritoneovenous shunts should be considered in only cirrhotic patients with refractory ascites who are not candidates for liver transplantation or TIPS, and in whom large-volume paracentesis is difficult.

Which patients with cirrhosis and ascites should be considered for TIPS?

TIPS is an interventional radiologic technique that consists of creating a fistula between a hepatic vein and a portal vein and then placing an expandable metal stent in the balloon-dilated fistula to maintain patency. This technique was introduced to treat patients with recurrent variceal hemorrhage by decreasing portal pressure. Initial results show that TIPS could be useful in the treatment of cirrhotic patients with refractory ascites. However, the incidence of shunt dysfunction is still quite high. Two recent trials performed in patients with refractory ascites have demonstrated that TIPS plus medical therapy is superior to medical therapy (diuretics plus total paracentesis when required) alone for the control of ascites, but does not improve survival, length of hospitalization, and quality of life. The incidence of hepatic encephalopathy was higher in the TIPS group, but other complications of cirrhosis, such as variceal hemorrhage or acute renal failure, were similar in both groups. In one study, the cost of the TIPS group was significantly higher than in the medical therapy group. These data suggest that TIPS should be reserved as second-line therapy or a bridge to liver transplantation, especially in those patients with relatively preserved liver function. An additional concern regarding TIPS is the high incidence of TIPS dysfunction that requires frequent ultrasound evaluations and reinterventions. The recent introduction of PTFE-covered stents improves shunt patency and reduces the incidence of TIPS dysfunction and episodes of encephalopathy.

Which patients with cirrhosis and ascites should be evaluated for liver transplantation?

The probability of survival after the first onset of ascites has been estimated at 50% and 20% after 1 and 5 years of follow-up, respectively. The prognosis is even worse in patients with diuretic-resistant ascites; the 1-year survival rate is 25%. Because the 1-year survival rate after liver transplantation is >75% patients with cirrhosis who develop ascites should be considered for liver transplantation. Once the fluid becomes diuretic-resistant, consideration for transplantation becomes even more urgent. However, some alcoholic patients with diuretic-resistant ascites may become diuretic-sensitive after months of alcohol abstinence.

What is the treatment of hepatic hydrothorax?

The initial treatment of hepatic hydrothorax is the same for ascites: salt restriction, diuretics, and large-volume paracentesis, if the patient has ascites. Therapeutic thoracocentesis has a high incidence of complications in cirrhotic patients (10% develop pneumothorax) and should be avoided if it is not necessary to relieve pulmonary symptoms. Patients with recurrent or refractory hepatic hydrothorax should be carefully evaluated. Thoracotomy and pleurodesis is usually ineffective. Thoracotomy and surgical repair of the diaphragmatic defects could be performed by using a videothoracoscope and could be useful for selected patients. Use of TIPS is under evaluation and could be a good option for patients with refractory hepatic hydrothorax, a Child-Pugh score <12, and Model for End-Stage Liver Disease (MELD) score <18.

31. **What is the hepatorenal syndrome?**

The hepatorenal syndrome occurs in patients with advanced liver failure and portal hypertension. It is characterized by impaired renal function caused by arterial vasodilatat reflex activation of the endogenous vasoconstrictive systems. According to clinical outco hepatorenal syndrome can be divided into two types:

Type I is characterized by a rapid and progressive reduction of renal function defined b doubling of the initial serum creatinine to a level >2.5 mg/dL or a 50% reduction of the in 24 hour creatinine clearance to a level <20 mL/min in less than 2 weeks.

In *type II*, renal failure does not have such a rapidly progressive course.

32. **What are the criteria of hepatorenal syndrome?**

- Chronic or acute liver disease with advanced hepatic failure and portal hypertension.
- Low glomerular filtration rate, as indicated by serum creatinine >1.5 mg/dL or 24-hour nine clearance <40 mL/min.
- Absence of shock, ongoing bacterial infection, current or recent treatment with nephro drugs, and absence of gastrointestinal fluid losses by repeated vomiting or intense dia renal fluid losses.
- No sustained improvement in renal function following diuretic withdrawal and expansi plasma volume with 1.5 L of isotonic saline.
- Proteinuria <500 mg/dL and no ultrasonographic evidence of obstructive uropathy or parenchymal disease.

33. **Describe the treatment of patients with hepatorenal syndrome.**

Liver transplantation is currently the treatment of choice in patients with hepatorenal syne Unfortunately, patients with hepatorenal syndrome type I die usually before an organ is available. The mortality rate of patients with hepatorenal syndrome type I is almost 100% than 2 months. Treatments such as hemodialysis, peritoneovenous shunt, albumin infusi dopamine infusion have been evaluated and found to be of only transient benefit or withou benefit. Recent prospective, but uncontrolled, studies have shown that hepatorenal syndr can be reversed by the administration of vasoconstrictive drugs, such as octreotide and midodrine, ornipressin, terlipressin or noradrenaline, with albumin infusion or other volu expanders. Randomized controlled trials are ongoing. These agents allow some patients t survive long enough to undergo liver transplantation. TIPS insertion seems to be another for the temporary treatment of hepatorenal syndrome. More information is required.

WEBSITES

1. http://www.aasld.org

2. http://www.aasld.org/eweb/docs/practiceguidelines/ascites.pdf

3. http://www.aasld.org/eweb/docs/practiceguidelines/tip.pdf

BIBLIOGRAPHY

1. Akriviadis EA, Runyon BA: The value of an algorithm in differentiating spontaneous from secondary bacte peritonitis. Gastroenterology 98:127–133, 1990.

2. Aparicio JR, Such J, Pascual S, et al: Development of quinolone-resistant strains of *Escherichia coli* in sto patients with cirrhosis undergoing norfloxacin prophylaxis: Clinical consequences. J Hepatol 31:277–283

3. Arroyo V, Ginés P, Gerbes AL, et al: Definition and diagnostic criteria of refractory ascites and hepatorenal drome in cirrhosis. Hepatology 23:164–176, 1996.

Bureau C, Garcia-Pagan JC, Otal P, et al: Improved clinical outcome using polytetrafluoroethylene-coated stents for TIPS: results of a randomized study. Gastroenterology 126:469–475, 2004.

Castellote J, Lopez C, Gornals J, et al: Rapid diagnosis of spontaneous bacterial peritonitis by use of reagent strips. Hepatology 37:893–896, 2003.

Chiva M, Guarner C, Peralta C, et al: Intestinal oxidative mucosal damage and bacterial translocation in cirrhotic rats. Eur J Gastroenterol Hepatol 15:145–159, 2003.

Chiva M, Soriano G, Rochat I, et al: Effect of Lactobacillus johnsonii La1 and antioxidants on intestinal flora and bacterial translocation in rats with experimental cirrhosis. J Hepatol 37:456–462, 2002.

Coll S, Vila MC, Molina LL, et al: Mechanisms of early decrease in systemic vascular resistance after total paracentesis: influence of flow rate of ascites extraction. Eur J Gastroenterol Hepatol 16:347–353, 2004.

Duvoux C, Zanditenas D, Hezode C, et al: Effects of noradrenaline and albumin in patients with type I hepatorenal syndrome: A pilot study. Hepatology 36:374–380, 2002.

Evans LT, Kim WR, Poterucha JJ, Kamath PS: Spontaneous bacterial peritonitis in asymptomatic outpatients with cirrhotic ascites. Hepatology 37:897–901, 2003.

Felisart J, Rimola A, Arroyo V, et al: Cefotaxime is more effective than is ampicillin-tobramycin in cirrhotics with severe infections. Hepatology 5:457–462, 1985.

Ginés P, Planas R, Angeli P, et al: Treatment of patients with cirrhosis and refractory ascites using LeVeen shunt with titanium tip: Comparison with therapeutic paracentesis. Hepatology 22:124–131, 1995.

Ginés P, Rimola A, Planas R, et al: Norfloxacin prevents spontaneous bacterial peritonitis recurrence in cirrhosis: Results of a double-blind, placebo-controlled trial. Hepatology 12:716–724, 1990.

Ginés P, Tito L, Arroyo V, et al: Randomized comparative study of therapeutic paracentesis with and without intravenous albumin in cirrhosis. Gastroenterology 94:1493–1502, 1998.

Ginés P, Uriz J, Calahorra B, et al: Transjugular intrahepatic portosystemic shunting versus paracentesis plus albumin for refractory ascites in cirrhosis. Gastroenterology 123:1839–1847, 2002.

Guarner C, Runyon BA, Young S, et al: Intestinal bacterial overgrowth and bacterial translocation in an experimental model of cirrhosis in rats. J Hepatol 26:1372–1378, 1997.

Guarner C, Solá R, Soriano G, et al: Risk of a first community-acquired spontaneous bacterial peritonitis in cirrhotics with low ascitic fluid protein levels. Gastroenterology 117:414–419, 1999.

Guarner C, Soriano G: Spontaneous bacterial peritonitis. Semin Liver Dis 17:203–217, 1997.

McHutchison JG, Runyon BA: Spontaneous bacterial peritonitis. In Surawicz CM, Owen RL (eds): Gastrointestinal and Hepatic Infections. Philadelphia, W.B. Saunders, 1994, pp 455–475.

Moore KP, Wong F, Gines P, et al: The management of ascites in cirrhosis: Report on the consensus conference of the international ascites club. Hepatology 38:258–266, 2003.

Moreau R, Durand F, Poynard T, et al: Terlipressin in patients with cirrhosis and type I hepatorenal syndrome: A retrospective multicenter study. Gastroenterology 123:923–930, 2002.

Mouroux J, Perrin C, Venissac N, et al: Management of pleural effusion of cirrhotic origin. Chest 109:1093–1096, 1996.

Navasa M, Follo A, Llovet JM, et al: Randomized, comparative study of oral ofloxacin versus intravenous cefotaxime in spontaneous bacterial peritonitis. Gastroenterology 111:1011–1017, 1996.

Novella MT, Solá R, Soriano G, et al: Continuous vs inpatient prophylaxis of the first episode of spontaneous bacterial peritonitis with norfloxacin. Hepatology 25:532–536, 1997.

Ortega R, Gines P, Uriz J, et al: Terlipressin therapy with and without albumin for patients with hepatorenal syndrome: Results of a prospective, nonrandomized study. Hepatology 36:941–954, 2002.

Ortiz J, Soriano G, Coll P, et al: Early microbiologic diagnosis of spontaneous bacterial peritonitis with BacT/ALERT. J Hepatol 26:839–844, 1997.

Ortiz J, Vila MC, Soriano G, et al: Infections caused by Escherichia coli resistant to norfloxacin in hospitalized cirrhotic patients. Hepatology 29:1064–1069, 1999.

Ricart E, Soriano G, Novella MT, et al: Amoxicillin-clavulanic acid versus cefotaxime in the therapy of bacterial infections in cirrhotic patients. J Hepatol 32:596–602, 2000.

Rimola A, Garcia-Tsao G, Navasa M, et al: for the International Ascites Club: Diagnosis, treatment and prophylaxis of spontaneous bacterial peritonitis: A consensus document. J Hepatol 32:142–153, 2000.

Rossle M, Ochs A, Gulberg V, et al: A comparison of paracentesis and transjugular intrahepatic portosystemic shunting in patients with ascites. N Engl J Med 342:1701–1707, 2000.

Runyon BA: Ascites. In Schiff E, Schiff L (eds): Diseases of the Liver, 7th ed. Philadelphia, J.B. Lippincott, 1993, pp 990–1015.

32. Runyon BA: Care of patients with ascites. N Engl J Med 330:337–342, 1994.

33. Runyon BA: Low-protein-concentration ascitic fluid is predisposed to spontaneous bacterial peritonitis. Gastroenterology 191:1343–1346, 1986.

34. Runyon BA: Malignancy-related ascites and ascitic fluid humoral tests of malignancy [Editorial]. J Clin Gastroenterol 18:94–98, 1994.

35. Runyon BA: Management of adult patients with ascites caused by cirrhosis. Hepatology 27:264–272, 1998.

36. Runyon BA: Refractory ascites. Semin Liver Dis 13:343–351, 1993.

37. Runyon BA, Canawati HN, Akriviadis EA: Optimization of ascitic fluid culture technique. Gastroenterology 95:1351–1355, 1988.

38. Runyon BA, McHutchison JG, Antillon MR, et al: Short-course vs long-course antibiotic treatment of spontane bacterial peritonitis: A randomized controlled study of 100 patients. Gastroenterology 100:1737–1742, 1991.

39. Runyon BA, Montano AA, Akriviadis EA, et al: The serum-ascites albumin gradient is superior to the exudate-transudate concept in the differential diagnosis of ascites. Ann Intern Med 117:215–220, 1992.

40. Sanyal AJ, Genning CH, Reddy KR, et al: The North American study for the treatment of refractory ascites. Gastroenterology 124:634–641, 2003.

41. Sola-Vera J, Miñana J, Ricart E, et al: Randomized trial comparing albumin and saline in the prevention of pa centesis-induced circulatory dysfunction in cirrhotic patients with ascites. Hepatology 37:1147–1153, 2003.

42. Soriano G, Guarner C, Teixido M, et al: Selective intestinal decontamination prevents spontaneous bacterial peritonitis. Gastroenterology 100:477–481, 1991.

43. Soriano G, Guarner C, Tomas A, et al: Norfloxacin prevents bacterial infection in cirrhotics with gastrointestin hemorrhage. Gastroenterology 103:1267–1272, 1992.

44. Sort P, Navasa M, Arroyo V, et al: Effect of intravenous albumin on renal impairment and mortality in patients with cirrhosis and spontaneous bacterial peritonitis. N Engl J Med 341:403–409, 1999.

45. Stanley MM, Ochi S, Lee KK, et al: Peritoneovenous shunting as compared with medical treatment in patients with alcoholic cirrhosis and massive ascites. N Engl J Med 321:1632–1638, 1989.

46. Such J, Runyon BA: Spontaneous bacterial peritonitis. Clin Infect Dis 27:669–704, 1998.

47. Terg R, Cobas S, Fassio E, et al: Oral ciprofloxacin after a short course of intravenous ciprofloxacin in the trea ment of spontaneous bacterial peritonitis: Results of a multicenter, randomized study. J Hepatol 33:564–569 2000.

48. Wu S, Lin OS, Chen Y, et al: Ascitic fluid carcinoembryonic antigen and alkaline phosphatase levels for the diffe entiation of primary from secondary bacterial peritonitis with intestinal perforation. J Hepatol 34:215–221, 200

49. Xiol X, Guardiola J: Hepatic hydrothorax. Curr Opin Pulm Med 4:239–242, 1998.

CHAPTER 32

LIVER ABSCESS

Jorge L. Herrera, MD, and Jason M. Wilkes, MD

. What are the two major categories of liver abscess?

The two types of liver abscess are pyogenic and amebic. Pyogenic abscesses usually arise from intra-abdominal infections, whereas amebic abscesses arise from colonic infection with invasive *Entamoeba histolytica*. This differentiation is important because diagnostic approach and management differ for the two conditions.

. Describe the clinical features of pyogenic liver abscess.

Most patients are middle-aged or older, with a recent shift in age toward younger patients. The median age is 51 years. The condition is equally prevalent in both sexes, although some series reflect a male predominance. The clinical findings are nonspecific but may include fever, chills, right-upper-quadrant pain, malaise, and weight loss. Fever may be absent in up to 30% of cases. Abdominal pain is present in only 45% of cases. Only 37% present with the classic findings of fever and right-upper-quadrant tenderness, reinforcing the often nonspecific nature of signs and symptoms. In many patients, the clinical presentation may be dominated by the underlying cause, such as appendicitis, diverticulitis, or biliary disease.

Comorbidities are common, including diabetes mellitus, prior liver transplantation, malignancy, alcoholism, cardiovascular disease, and chronic renal failure. The mean duration of symptoms before hospital admission is 26 days, with a range of 1–200 days and a median of 14 days.

. What are the clinical features of amebic liver abscess?

Patients tend to be younger (ages 30–40), are more often male, have more severe right-upper-quadrant pain, and are febrile in 85% of cases. A history of travel to endemic areas is common, although it may be remote. Prior symptoms suggestive of previous colonic amebiasis are present in only 5–15% of patients. Concurrent hepatic abscess and amebic dysentery are unusual. Approximately 80% of patients present with symptoms that develop quickly over 2–4 weeks. Involvement of the diaphragmatic surface of the liver may lead to right-sided pleural pain or referred shoulder pain. Colonic involvement, presenting as right-sided colonic ulcerations are present in 55% of cases, even in the absence of diarrhea.

4. What laboratory features are distinctive in patients with liver abscess?

Results of routine laboratory tests are not diagnostic for pyogenic or amebic liver abscess. Leukocytosis is often present but may be absent in a significant number of patients. Normochromic normocytic anemia is present in over 70% of patients. Eosinophilia is characteristically absent in patients with amebic abscess. The erythrocyte sedimentation rate is invariably raised. Liver test abnormalities are not specific. Over 90% of patients have elevation of alkaline phosphatase (AP), but aspartate aminotransferase (AST) and alanine aminotransferase (ALT) are elevated to lesser degrees. If significant hyperbilirubinemia is present, the biliary tree is the likely source of the abscess; bilirubin levels are lowest in patients with cryptogenic liver abscess. Hypoalbuminemia is described frequently, and a level <2 gm/dL carries a poor prognosis. Blood cultures are positive in 50% of patients with pyogenic abscess, and 75–90% of aspirates from the abscesses are positive for bacteria.

5. **What are the most common sources of pyogenic liver abscess?**
   Biliary tract disease is the most common known source of pyogenic liver abscess, accounting for 35% of cases. In most cases the cause cannot be identified, and the disease is therefore termed *cryptogenic*. Most abscesses related to biliary disease result from cholangitis or acute cholecystitis. Malignant tumors of the pancreas, common bile duct, and ampulla account for 10–20% of hepatic abscesses originating in the biliary tree. Endoscopic or surgical intervention in the biliary tree may also result in hepatic abscess formation. Parasitic invasion of the biliary tree by roundworms or flukes can lead to biliary infection and hepatic abscess.

   Another common source of pyogenic liver abscesses is intra-abdominal infection with bacterial seeding through the portal vein. Diverticulitis, Crohn's disease, ulcerative colitis, and bowel perforation account for 30% of pyogenic liver abscesses. Appendicitis is a rare cause of liver abscess, except in older or immunocompromised patients, in whom the diagnosis of appendicitis may be delayed. About 15% of liver abscesses arise by direct extension from a contiguous source, such as a subphrenic abscess or empyema of the gallbladder. Pyogenic infection may be carried to the liver in hepatic arterial blood flow from distant localized infections, such as endocarditis or severe dental disease.

6. **List the organisms that commonly cause pyogenic liver abscess.**
   Gram-negative organisms are implicated in 50–70% cases. *Escherichia coli* is the most common aerobic gram-negative, cultured organism. Aerobic gram-positive organisms account for approximately 25% of infections, and up to 50% of cases are caused by anaerobes. Recent reports suggest that aerobes are becoming a more common cause of abscess than anaerobes (Table 32-1).

TABLE 32-1. BACTERIOLOGY OF PYOGENIC LIVER ABSCESS		
Gram-Negative Aerobes (50–70%)	**Gram-Positive Aerobes (25%)**	**Anaerobes (40–50%)**
Escherichia coli (35–45%)	*Streptococcus faecalis*	*Fusobacterium nucleatum*
Klebsiella sp.	β Streptococci	*Bacteroides* sp.
Proteus sp.	α Streptococci	*Bacteroides fragilis*
Enterobacter sp.	Staphylococci	*Peptostreptococcus* sp.
Serratia sp.	*Streptococcus milleri*	*Actinomyces* sp.
Morganella sp.		*Clostridium* sp.
Actinobacter sp.		
Pseudomonas sp.		

Adapted from Frey CF, Zhu Y, Suzuki M, Isaji S: Liver abscess. Surg Clin North Am 69:259–271, 1989.

7. **Do negative cultures from an abscess aspirate indicate a nonpyogenic abscess?**
   No. Although most cultures are positive, a negative culture may reflect improper handling of the specimen or prior antibiotic therapy. Proper collection and culture techniques are of critical importance for growing anaerobic organisms. Culture material should be transported to the laboratory immediately in the syringe used for aspiration to avoid exposure to air. Never submit swabs for culture of liver abscess. Anaerobic organisms may require at least several days and up to 1 week or more for sufficient growth to establish a diagnosis. For this reason, a Gram stain of the aspirate is of paramount importance. A Gram stain that demonstrates organisms with no

growth in cultures after 2 or 3 days suggests an anaerobic pathogen. All aspirated material should be cultured for aerobic, anaerobic, and microaerophilic organisms.

8. **What abnormalities can be detected on standard radiologic studies of patients with liver abscess?**

A chest radiograph may be abnormal in 50–80% of patients with liver abscess. Right-lower-lobe atelectasis, right pleural effusion, and an elevated right hemidiaphragm may be clues to the presence of a liver abscess. Perforation of a pyogenic liver abscess into the thoracic cavity may result in empyema. In plain abdominal films, air can be seen in the abscess cavities in 10–20% of cases. Gastric displacement due to enlargement of the liver may also be seen. These features are not sensitive for the diagnosis of liver abscess.

9. **Which imaging studies should be obtained in evaluating a suspected liver abscess?**

Ultrasonography has traditionally been considered the initial procedure of choice. It is noninvasive, readily available, and highly accurate, with a sensitivity of 80–90%. It is the preferred modality to distinguish cystic from solid lesions and, in most patients, is more accurate than computed tomographic (CT) scanning for visualizing the biliary tree. Ultrasonography, however, is operator-dependent, and its accuracy may be affected by the patient's habitus or overlying gas. Currently, with the increasing availability of helical CT with intravenous contrast, some consider it the initial procedure of choice. It is not operator-dependent, it is more sensitive than ultrasound, and it aids in the identification of smaller abscesses that may be missed on ultrasound examination. CT scanning provides an assessment not only of the liver but also of the entire peritoneal cavity, which may provide information about the primary lesions causing the liver abscess.

Magnetic resonance imaging (MRI) does not add much to the sensitivity of CT scanning. Scintigraphy with technetium sulfur colloid is sensitive for detecting lesions >2 cm in diameter. Gallium scanning may add to the sensitivity of technetium scanning, because pyogenic liver abscess avidly takes up gallium. Amebic abscesses, however, tend to concentrate gallium only in the periphery of the abscess cavity. In general, scintigraphy is the least helpful of the scanning modalities.

10. **Which areas of the liver are usually affected by hepatic abscess?**

Right lobe only	60% of patients
Both lobes	20–30%
Left lobe only	5–20%

11. **How can the location, size, and number of liver abscesses help to determine the source?**

Pyogenic liver abscesses, arising from a biliary source, tend to be multiple and of small size and involve both lobes of the liver. Septic emboli from the portal vein may be solitary and tend to be more common in the right lobe of the liver because most of the portal vein flow goes to the right lobe. Abscesses arising from a contiguous source tend to be solitary and localized to one lobe only.

Amebic liver abscesses tend to be solitary and large. Most commonly, they are located in the right lobe of the liver. The right lobe receives a major part of the venous drainage from the cecum and ascending colon, which are the parts of the bowel most commonly affected by amebiasis. Abscesses located in the dome of the liver, or complicated by a bronchopleural fistula, are typically amebic in origin.

12. **When should a hepatic abscess be aspirated?**

Hepatic abscesses should be aspirated if they are thought to be pyogenic and not amebic. Patients with multiple abscesses, coexistent biliary disease, or an intra-abdominal inflammatory process are more likely to have pyogenic abscess. In such patients, aspiration under ultrasound guidance with Gram stain and culture helps to guide antibiotic selection. Aspiration of amebic abscesses should be considered under the following circumstances: (1) when pyogenic abscess or secondary infection of an amebic abscess cannot be excluded; (2) when the patient does not respond to adequate therapy for amebic liver abscess; or (3) when the abscess is very large with risk of rupture and/or causes severe pain.

13. **In what situation should an amebic liver abscess be treated by open surgical drainage?**
When the amebic abscess is located in the left lobe of the liver, and response to therapy is not dramatic within the first 24–48 hours, open surgical drainage should be performed. Complications of left-lobe amebic abscess, such as cardiac tamponade, are associated with high mortality and require prompt intervention to prevent their occurrence.

14. **Does aspiration of an amebic hepatic abscess yield diagnostic material in most patients?**
No. Trophozoites are found in <20% of aspirates. Although, classically, the contents of amebic abscess are described as "anchovy paste" in appearance, in practice most aspirated material does not conform to this description. The contents of an amebic abscess are typically odorless. Foul-smelling aspirates or a positive Gram stain should suggest a pyogenic abscess or secondarily infected amebic abscess.

15. **How often is the biliary tree involved in patients with amebic liver abscess?**
Bile is lethal to amebas; thus, infection of the gallbladder and bile ducts does not occur. In patients with a large amebic or pyogenic abscess, compression of the biliary system may result in jaundice, but cholangitis occurs with secondary bacterial infection only.

16. **How can the diagnosis of an amebic abscess be confirmed?**
Amebic abscesses are best differentiated from pyogenic abscesses by serologic tests:

Hemagglutination (IHA)	Gel diffusion precipitin (GDP)
Indirect immunofluorescence (IF)	Complement fixation (CF)
Counterimmunoelectrophoresis (CIE)	Latex agglutination (LA)
Immunoelectrophoresis (IEP)	Enzyme-linked immunosorbent assay (ELISA)

Serologic tests are positive in patients with invasive amebiasis only, such as hepatic abscess or amebic colitis. They are negative in asymptomatic carriers. With the exception of CF, these tests are highly sensitive (95–99%). The IHA is extremely sensitive, and a negative test excludes the diagnosis; a titer >1:512 is present in almost all patients with invasive disease. IHA, however, remains positive for many years, and a positive titer may indicate prior infection. GDP titers become negative usually 6 months after the infection, and this is the test of choice for patients from endemic areas with prior exposure to amebiasis. A high GDP titer in a patient with hepatic abscess suggests an amebic abscess, even if the patient has a prior history of invasive amebiasis. In general, the choice of serologic tests depends on availability and epidemiologic considerations.

17. **Describe the treatment for pyogenic liver abscess.**
For single abscess or several large abscesses, treatment consists of antibiotics and appropriate drainage. Drainage should be performed percutaneously whenever possible. The combination of percutaneous drainage with intravenous antibiotics results in a 76% cure rate, compared with 65% for antibiotic alone and 61% for surgery alone.
It is not clear whether percutaneous catheter drainage is superior to aspiration without catheter placement. Most centers favor catheter drainage over simple aspiration. Surgical drainage should be performed only if more conservative measures do not result in complete resolution or if surgery is needed to treat a primary intra-abdominal lesion. For multiple microabscesses, antibiotic therapy and correction of the underlying biliary abnormality may suffice.

Antibiotic coverage involves a combination of antibiotics directed against anaerobes, gram-negative aerobes, and enterococci. Thus, the combination of an aminoglycoside or cephalosporin for aerobic gram-negative organisms, clindamycin or metronidazole for anaerobes, and penicillin or ampicillin for enterococci is commonly used. The antibiotic regimen may be altered as needed, depending on culture results or clinical response. Intravenous treatment should be continued for 14 days, or longer if drains are still in place, with a minimum of 4 weeks of therapy.

Describe the treatment for amebic liver abscess.

Metronidazole is the only drug active against the extraintestinal form of amebiasis. A dose of 750 mg three times/day for 10 days is recommended. Even at this dose, metronidazole is somewhat less effective in the intestinal form of the disease; thus, a luminal amebicide (such as iodoquinol (diiodohydroxyquin), paromomycin, or diloxanide furoate) should be prescribed to eradicate the intestinal form and prevent recurrence. Uncomplicated amebic abscess should be managed conservatively with metronidazole. Needle aspiration should be considered for large (>7 cm) abscesses and for patients who fail to respond after 7 days of metronidazole. Operative intervention should be performed only for complications or when conservative therapy fails.

List the potential complications of pyogenic liver abscess.

Untreated, pyogenic liver abscesses have a mortality rate of 100%. Other complications include rupture into the peritoneal cavity, which may form subphrenic, perihepatic, or subhepatic abscess or peritonitis. Rupture into the pleural space may cause empyema. Rupture into the pericardial sac may result in pericarditis and pericardial tamponade. Metastatic septic emboli involving the lungs, brain, or eyes may also occur.

List the potential complications of amebic liver abscess.

The complications of amebic liver abscess are similar to those of pyogenic liver abscess. Rupture into the pleural space results in amebic empyema. Rupture into the lung parenchyma may produce a lung abscess or bronchopleural fistula. Pericardial extension occurs in 1–2% of patients and is associated with amebic abscesses in the left lobe of the liver. A serous pericardial effusion may indicate impending rupture. Constrictive pericarditis occasionally follows suppurative amebic pericarditis. Brain abscess from hematogenous spread of the infection has also been reported.

What is the prognosis for patients with liver abscess?

The prognosis depends on the rapidity of diagnosis and the underlying illness. Patients with amebic liver abscess generally do well with appropriate treatment; morbidity and mortality rates are 4.5% and 2.2%, respectively, in recent series. Response to treatment is prompt and dramatic. Healing of the abscess leads to residual scar tissue associated with subcapsular retraction. Occasionally, in patients with a large abscess, a residual cavity surrounded by fibroconnective tissue may persist.

The mortality rate associated with pyogenic liver abscess has been reduced to 5–10%, with prompt recognition and adequate antibiotic therapy; it is highest in patients with multiple abscesses. Mortality is highly dependent on the underlying disease process. Morbidity remains high at 50%, primarily because of the complexity of therapy and the need for prolonged drainage.

Is a vaccine against amebiasis feasible?

Yes. Although vaccination is not currently available, ongoing research suggests that an effective vaccine may be feasable. Gal/GalNAc-specific lectin is a recombinant antigen that provides protection in animal models to amebiasis. Human immunity is linked to intestinal IgA against the lectin. The clonal population structure of *E. histolytica* and, specifically, the high degree of sequence conservation of the Gal/GalNAc-specific lectin, suggests that a vaccine could be broadly protective.

BIBLIOGRAPHY

1. Akgun Y, Tacyildiz IH, Celik Y: Amebic liver abscess: Changing trends over 20 years. World J Surg 23:102–106 1999.

2. Block MA: Abscesses of the liver (other than amebic). In Haubrich WS, Schaffner F, Berk JE (eds): Bockus Gastroenterology, 5th ed. Philadelphia, W.B. Saunders, 1995, pp 2405–2427.

3. Chou FF, Sheen-Chen SM, Chen YS, Chen MC: Single and multiple pyogenic liver abscesses: Clinical course, e ology and results of treatment. World J Surg 21:384–389, 1997.

4. Chung RT, Friedman LS: Liver abscess and bacterial, parasitic, fungal and granulomatous liver disease. In Sleisenger MH, Fordtran JS (eds): Gastrointestinal Disease: Pathophysiology, Diagnosis, Management, 7th e Philadelphia, W.B. Saunders, 2002, pp 1343–1373.

5. Crippin JS, Wang KK: An unrecognized etiology for pyogenic hepatic abscesses in normal hosts: Dental disea Am J Gastroenterol 87:1740–1742, 1992.

6. DeCock KM, Reynolds TB: Amebic and pyogenic liver abscess. In Schiff L, Schiff ER (eds): Diseases of the Liv 7th ed. Philadelphia, J.B. Lippincott, 1993, pp 1320–1337.

7. Filice C, Di Perri G, Strosselli M, et al: Outcome of hepatic amebic abscesses managed with three different the peutic strategies. Dig Dis Sci 37:240–247, 1992.

8. Frey CF, Zhu Y, Suzuki M, Isaji S: Liver abscesses. Surg Clin North Am 69:259–271, 1989.

9. Haque R, Huston CD, Hughes M, et al: Amebiasis. N Engl J Med 348:1565–1573, 2003.

10. Kandel G, Marcon NE: Pyogenic liver abscess: New concepts of an old disease. Am J Gastroenterol 79:65–71 1984.

11. Kaplan GG, Gregson DB, Laupland KB: Population-based study of the epidemiology and the risk factors for py genic liver abscess. Clin Gastroenterol Hepatol 2:1032–1038, 2004.

12. Knight R: Hepatic amebiasis. Semin Liver Dis 4:277–292, 1984.

13. Misra SP, Misra V, Dwivedi M, et al: Factors influencing colonic involvement in patients with amebic liver abscess. Gastrointest Endosc 59:512–516, 2004.

14. Lederman ER, Crum NF: Pyogenic liver abscess with a focus on *Klebsiella pneumoniae* as a primary pathoge An emerging disease with unique clinical characteristics. Am J Gastroenterol 100:322–331, 2005.

15. Monroe LS: Gastrointestinal parasites. In Haubrich WS, Schaffner F, Berk JE (eds): Bockus Gastroenterology 5th ed. Philadelphia, W.B. Saunders, 1995, pp 3123–3134.

16. Rajak CL, Gupta S, Jain S, et al: Percutaneous treatment of liver abscesses: Needle aspiration versus catheter drainage. AJR Am J Roentgenol 170:1035–1039, 1998.

17. Ralls PW, Barnes PF, Johnson MB, et al: Medical treatment of hepatic amoebic abscess: Rare need for percuta neous drainage. Radiology 165:805–807, 1987.

18. Seeto RK, Rockey DC: Pyogenic liver abscess: Changes in etiology, management and outcome. Medicine 75:99–113, 1996.

19. Teague M, Baddour LM, Wruble LD: Liver abscess: A harbinger of Crohn's disease. Am J Gastroenterol 83:1412–1414, 1988.

20. Vukmir RB: Pyogenic hepatic abscess. Ann Emerg Med 20:421–423, 1991.

CHAPTER 33

INHERITABLE FORMS OF LIVER DISEASE

Bruce R. Bacon, MD

HEMOCHROMATOSIS

1. **How are the various iron-loading disorders in humans classified?**

The usual way to classify iron-overload syndromes is to distinguish among hereditary hemochromatosis, secondary iron overload, and parenteral iron overload. *Hereditary hemochromatosis* (HH) results in increased iron absorption from the gut, with preferential deposition of iron in the parenchymal cells of the liver, heart, pancreas, and other endocrine glands. Most HH is found in patients who are homozygous for the C282Y mutation found in HFE, the gene for hemochromatosis. Over the past several years, however, mutations in other genes have been found that can result in iron overload. These include transferrin receptor-2, ferroportin, hemojuvelin, and hepcidin.

In *secondary iron overload,* some other stimulus causes the gastrointestinal tract to absorb increased amounts of iron. Here, the increased absorption of iron is caused by an underlying disorder rather than by an inherited defect in regulation of iron absorption. Examples include various anemias due to ineffective erythropoiesis (e.g., thalassemia, aplastic anemia, red cell aplasia, and some patients with sickle cell anemia), chronic liver disease, and, rarely, excessive intake of medicinal iron.

In *parenteral iron overload,* patients have received excessive amounts of iron as either red blood cell transfusions or iron-dextran given parenterally. In patients with severe hypoplastic anemias, red blood cell transfusion may be necessary. Over time, patients become significantly iron-loaded. Unfortunately, some physicians give iron-dextran injections to patients with anemia that is not due to iron deficiency; such patients can become iron-loaded. Parenteral iron overload is always iatrogenic and should be avoided or minimized. In patients who truly need repeated red blood cell transfusions (in the absence of blood loss), a chelation program with deferoxamine should be initiated to prevent toxic accumulation of excessive iron.

2. **What are neonatal iron overload and African iron overload?**

Neonatal iron overload is a rare condition that may be related to an intrauterine viral infection. Infants are born with increased amounts of hepatic iron. Many patients do very poorly, and liver transplantation can be lifesaving.

African iron overload, previously called "Bantu hemosiderosis," was thought to be a disorder in which excessive amounts of iron were ingested from alcoholic beverages brewed in iron drums. Recent studies have suggested that this disorder may have a genetic component distinct from the genetic disorder found in HH (i.e., it is not HFE-linked). Some patients have a mutation in ferroportin. Thus, African Americans may be at risk for developing iron overload from a genetic disease.

3. **How much iron is usually absorbed per day?**

A typical Western diet contains approximately 10–20 mg of iron, which is usually found in heme-containing compounds. Normal daily iron absorption is approximately 1–2 mg, representing about a 10% efficiency of absorption. Patients with iron deficiency, HH, or ineffective erythropoiesis absorb increased amounts of iron (up to 3–6 mg/day).

4. **Where is iron normally found in the body?**
The normal male adult contains about 4 gm of total body iron, which is roughly divided between the 2.5 gm of iron in the hemoglobin of circulating red blood cells, 1 gm of iron in storage sites in the reticuloendothelial system of the spleen and bone marrow and the parenchymal and reticuloendothelial system of the liver, and 200–400 mg in the myoglobin of skeletal muscle. In addition, all cells contain some iron because mitochondria contain iron in both heme, which is the central portion of cytochromes involved in electron transport, and iron sulfur clusters, which are also involved in electron transport. Iron is bound to transferrin in both the intravascular and extravascular compartments. Storage iron within cells is found in ferritin and, as this amount increases, in hemosiderin. Serum ferritin is proportional to total body iron stores in patients with iron deficiency or uncomplicated HH and is biochemically different from tissue ferritin.

5. **Discuss the genetic defect in patients with hereditary hemochromatosis.**
In 1996, the gene responsible for hemochromatosis was identified and named *HFE*. HFE codes for a major histocompatibility complex (MHC) type 1-like protein that is membrane-spanning with a short intracytoplasmic tail, a transmembrane region, and three extracellular alpha loops. A single missense mutation results in loss of a cysteine at amino acid position 282, with replacement by a tyrosine (C282Y), which leads to disruption of a disulfide bridge and thus to the lack of a critical fold in the alpha$_1$ loop. As a result, HFE fails to interact with beta$_2$ microglobulin (β_2M), which is necessary to the function of MHC class 1 proteins.
   In 1997, it was demonstrated that the HFE/β_2M complex binds to transferrin receptor and is necessary for transferrin receptor-mediated iron uptake into cells. This observation linked HFE with a protein of iron metabolism. C282Y homozygosity is found in approximately 85–90% of patients with hemochromatosis. A second mutation, whereby a histidine at amino acid position 63 is replaced by an aspartate (H63D), is common but less important in cellular iron homeostasis. Recently, a third mutation has been characterized, whereby a serine is replaced a cysteine at amino acid position 65 (S65C). Like H63D, S65C has little impact on iron loading unless it is present as a compound heterozygote with the C282Y mutation. Cell and molecular biologic studies have demonstrated that when C282Y-mutant HFE is transfected into cells, a decrease in intracellular iron (due to either a decrease in cellular uptake or a decrease in transferrin receptor cycling within the cell) leads to up-regulation of the divalent metal transporter-1 (DMT-1), which is responsible for iron absorption in the villus cells of the intestine, and ferroportin, which is involved in iron egress out of the enterocyte. It is presumed that the crypt cells of the intestine are involved in whole-body iron sensing. If these cells sense iron deficiency because of the C282Y mutation in HFE, up-regulation of DMT-1, as cells mature to migrate up the villus, results in an increase in absorption of iron and the ultimate development of hemochromatosis.

6. **What are the usual toxic manifestations of iron overload?**
In chronic iron overload, an increase in oxidant stress results in lipid peroxidation to lipid-containing components of the cell, such as organelle membranes. This process causes organelle damage. Hepatocellular injury and/or death ensues with phagocytosis by Kupffer cells. Iron-loaded Kupffer cells become activated, producing profibrogenic cytokines, such transforming growth factor beta$_1$ (TGF-β_1), which, in turn, activates hepatic stellate cells. Hepatic stellate cells are responsible for increased collagen synthesis and hepatic fibrogenesis.

7. **What are the most common symptoms in patients with hereditary hemochromatosis?**
Currently, most patients are identified by abnormal iron studies on routine screening chemistry panels or by screening family members of a known patient. When identified in this manner, patients typically have no symptoms or physical findings. Nonetheless, it is useful to be aware the symptoms that patients with more established HH can exhibit. Typically, they are nonspecific and include fatigue, malaise, and lethargy. Other more organ-specific symptoms are arthralgia

and symptoms related to complications of chronic liver disease, diabetes, and congestive heart failure.

8. **Describe the most common physical findings in patients with hereditary hemochromatosis.**

The way in which patients come to medical attention determines whether they have physical findings. Thus, patients identified by screening tests have no abnormal physical findings. In contrast, physical findings in patients with advanced disease may include grayish or "bronzed" skin pigmentation, typically in sun-exposed areas; hepatomegaly with or without cirrhosis; arthropathy with swelling and tenderness over the second and third metacarpophalangeal joints; and other findings related to complications of chronic liver disease.

9. **How is the diagnosis of hemochromatosis established?**

Patients with abnormal iron studies on screening blood work, any of the symptoms and physical findings of hemochromatosis, or a positive family history of hemochromatosis should have blood studies of iron metabolism, either repeated or performed for the first time. These studies include serum iron, total iron-binding capacity (TIBC) or transferrin, and serum ferritin. The transferrin saturation (TS) should be calculated from the ratio of iron to TIBC or transferrin. Blood samples for these studies are drawn in the fasting state to minimize the possibility of false-positive results. If the TS is >45% or if the serum ferritin is elevated, hemochromatosis should be strongly considered, especially in patients without evidence of other liver disease (e.g., chronic viral hepatitis, alcoholic liver disease, nonalcoholic steatohepatitis) known to have abnormal iron studies in the absence of significant iron overload.

If iron studies are abnormal, mutation analysis of HFE should be performed. If patients are homozygous for the C282Y mutation, compound heterozygotes (C282Y/H63D) and under age 40, or have normal liver enzymes (alanine aminotransferase and aspartate aminotransferase), no further evaluation is necessary. Plans for therapeutic phlebotomy can be initiated. In patients over age 40 or those with abnormal liver enzymes or markedly elevated ferritin (>1000 ng/mL), the next step is to perform a percutaneous liver biopsy to obtain tissue for routine histology, including Perls' Prussian blue staining for storage iron and biochemical determination of hepatic iron concentration (HIC). The main purpose for performing a liver biopsy in these individuals is to determine the degree of fibrosis because increased fibrosis has been associated with markedly elevated ferritin levels and elevated liver enzymes.

10. **How commonly do abnormal iron studies occur in other types of liver disease?**

In various studies, approximately 30–50% of patients with chronic viral hepatitis, alcoholic liver disease, and nonalcoholic steatohepatitis have abnormal serum iron studies. Usually, the serum ferritin is abnormal. In general, an elevation in transferrin saturation is much more specific for HH. Thus, if the serum ferritin is elevated and the transferrin saturation is normal, another form of liver disease may be responsible. In contrast, if the serum ferritin is normal and the transferrin saturation is elevated, the likely diagnosis is hemochromatosis, particularly in young patients. Differentiation of HH in the presence of other liver diseases is now much easier with the use of genetic testing (HFE mutation analysis for C282Y and H63D).

11. **Is computed tomography (CT) or magnetic resonance imaging (MRI) useful in diagnosing hemochromatosis?**

In massively iron-loaded patients, CT and MRI show the liver to be white or black, respectively, consistent with the kinds of changes associated with increased iron deposition. In more subtle and earlier cases, overlap is tremendous and imaging studies are not useful.

12. **On liver biopsy, what is the typical cellular and lobular distribution of iron in hereditary hemochromatosis?**

In early HH in young people, iron is found entirely in hepatocytes and a periportal (zone 1) distribution. In heavier iron-loading in older patients, iron is still predominantly hepatocellular, but some iron may be found in Kupffer cells and bile ductular cells. The periportal-to-pericentr[al] (zone 1–to–zone 3) gradient is maintained but may be less distinct in more heavily loaded patients. When patients develop cirrhosis, the pattern is typically micronodular and regenerati[ve] nodules may show less intense iron staining.

13. How useful is hepatic iron concentration?

Since genetic testing has become readily available, liver biopsy and determinations of HIC and HII are less important. Nonetheless, whenever a liver biopsy is performed in a patient with suspected HH, the quantitative HIC should be obtained. In symptomatic patients, HIC is typica[lly] >10,000 µg/gm. The iron concentration threshold for the development of fibrosis is approximately 22,000 µg/gm. Lower iron concentrations can be found in cirrhotic HH with a coexistent toxin, such as alcohol or hepatitis C or B virus. Young people with early HH may ha[ve] only moderate increases in HIC. In the past, discrepancies in HIC concentration with age were clarified by use of the hepatic iron index (HII).

14. How is the hepatic iron index used in diagnosing hereditary hemochromatosi[s]?

The HII, introduced in 1986, is based on the observation that HIC increases progressively with age in patients with homozygous HH. In contrast, in patients with secondary iron overload or i[n] heterozygotes, there is no progressive increase in iron over time. Therefore, the HII was thoug[ht] to distinguish patients with homozygous HH from patients with secondary iron overload and heterozygotes. The HII is calculated by dividing the HIC (in µmol/gm) by the patient's age (in years). A value >1.9 was thought to be consistent with homozygous HH. With the advent of genetic testing, we have learned that many C282Y homozygotes do not have phenotypic expression to the degree that would cause an elevated HII, and they will not have increased iro[n] stores. Thus, the HII is no longer the gold standard for the diagnosis of HH. The HII is not use[d] in patients with parenteral iron overload.

15. How do you treat a patient with hereditary hemochromatosis?

Treatment of HH is relatively straightforward and includes weekly or twice-weekly phlebotomy [of] 1 unit of whole blood. Each unit of blood contains about 200–250 mg of iron, depending on th[e] hemoglobin. Therefore, a patient who presents with symptomatic HH and who has up to 20 g[m] of excessive storage iron requires removal of over 80 units of blood, which takes close to 2 years at a rate of 1 unit of blood per week. Patients need to be aware that this treatment can be tedious and prolonged. Some patients cannot tolerate removal of 1 unit of blood per week and occasionally, schedules are adjusted to remove only one-half unit every other week. In contras[t,] in young patients who are only mildly iron-loaded, iron stores may be depleted quickly with on[ly] 10–20 phlebotomies. The goal of initial phlebotomy treatment is to reduce tissue iron stores, [or] to create iron deficiency. Once the ferritin is <50 ng/mL and the transferrin saturation is <50% the majority of excessive iron stores have been successfully depleted and most patients can g[o] into a maintenance phlebotomy regimen (1 unit of blood removed every 2–3 months).

16. What kind of a response to treatment can you expect?

Many patients feel better after phlebotomy therapy has begun, even if they were asymptomati[c] before treatment. Energy level may improve, with less fatigue and less abdominal pain. Liver enzymes improve typically once iron stores have been depleted. Increased hepatic size diminishes. Cardiac function may improve, and about 50% of patients with glucose intoleranc[e] are more easily managed. Unfortunately, advanced cirrhosis, arthropathy, and hypogonadism [do] not improve with phlebotomy.

17. What is the prognosis for a patient with hemochromatosis?

Patients who are diagnosed and treated before the development of cirrhosis can expect a nor[mal] lifespan. The most common causes of death in hemochromatosis are complications of chroni[c] liver disease and hepatocellular cancer. Patients who are diagnosed and treated early should not experience any of these complications.

Because hemochromatosis is an inherited disorder, what is one's responsibility to family members once a patient has been identified?
Once a patient has been fully identified, all first-degree relatives should be offered screening with genetic testing (HFE mutation analysis for C282Y and H63D) and tests for transferrin saturation and ferritin. If genetic testing shows that the relative is a C282Y homozygote or a compound heterozygote (C282Y/H63D) and has abnormal iron studies, HH is confirmed. A liver biopsy may not be necessary. Human leukocyte antigen (HLA) studies are no longer performed.

Should general population screening be done to evaluate for hemochromatosis?
With the advent of genetic testing, it was suggested that hereditary hemochromatosis may be a good disease for population screening. This was because genetic testing was available, phenotypic expression was easy to determine, there was a long latent period between diagnosis and disease manifestations, and treatment is effective and safe. Several large-scale population studies have been performed and demonstrate that about half of C282Y homozygotes have evidence of phenotypic expression with increased iron stores. Thus, interest in population screening has waned because many people who do not develop iron overload would be identified with a genetic disorder. Thus, population screening is not recommended.

ALPHA$_1$-ANTITRYPSIN DEFICIENCY

What is the function of α_1-antitrypsin in healthy people?
Alpha$_1$-antitrypsin (α_1-AT) is a protease inhibitor synthesized in the liver. It is responsible for inhibiting trypsin, collagenase, elastase, and proteases of polymorphonuclear neutrophils. In patients deficient in α_1-AT, the function of these proteases is unopposed. In the lung, this can lead to a progressive decrease in elastin and development of premature emphysema. The liver fails to secrete α_1-AT, and aggregates of the defective protein are found, leading by unclear means to the development of cirrhosis. Over 75 different protease inhibitor (Pi) alleles have been identified. Pi MM is normal, and Pi ZZ results in the lowest levels of α_1-AT.

How common is α_1-antitrypsin deficiency?
Alpha$_1$-AT deficiency occurs in approximately 1 in 2000 people.

Where is the abnormal gene located?
The gene is located on chromosome 14 and results in a single amino acid substitution (replacement of glutamic acid by lysine at the 342 position), which causes a deficiency in sialic acid.

What is the nature of the defect that causes α_1-antitrypsin deficiency?
Alpha$_1$-AT deficiency is a protein-secretory defect. Normally, this protein is translocated into the lumen of the endoplasmic reticulum, interacts with chaperone proteins, folds properly, is transported to the Golgi complex, and then is exported out of the cell. In patients with α_1-AT deficiency, the protein structure is abnormal because of the deficiency of sialic acid, and the proper folding in the endoplasmic reticulum occurs for only 10–20% of the molecules, with resultant failure to export via the Golgi complex and accumulation within the hepatocyte. In one detailed Swedish study, α_1-AT deficiency of the Pi ZZ type caused cirrhosis in about only 12% of patients. Chronic obstructive pulmonary disease (COPD) was present in 75% of patients, and of these, 59% were classified as having primary emphysema. It is not

known why some patients with low levels of α_1-AT develop liver or lung disease and others do not.

24. **Describe the common symptoms and physical findings of α_1-antitrypsin deficiency.**
    Adults with liver involvement may have no symptoms until they develop signs and symptoms of chronic liver disease. Similarly, children may have no specific problems until they develop complications from chronic liver disease. In adults with lung disease, typical findings include premature emphysema, which can be markedly exacerbated by smoking.

25. **How is the diagnosis of α_1-antitrypsin deficiency established?**
    It is useful to order α_1-AT levels and phenotypes in all patients evaluated for chronic liver disease because no clinical presentation suggests the diagnosis (apart from premature emphysema). Certain heterozygous states can result in chronic liver disease; for example, SZ as well as ZZ patients can develop cirrhosis. MZ heterozygotes do not usually develop disease unless they have some other liver condition, such as alcoholic liver disease or chronic viral hepatitis. There are, however, occasional patients who have significant liver disease, and no other abnormalities are identified other than MZ heterozygosity. Liver disease due to other causes may progress more rapidly.

26. **What histopathologic stain is used to diagnose α_1-antitrypsin deficiency?**
    Periodic acid-Schiff-diastase. Periodic acid-Schiff (PAS) stains both glycogen and α_1-AT globules with a dark reddish-purple, and diastase digests the glycogen. Thus, when a PAS-diastase stain is used, the glycogen has been removed by the diastase, and the only positively staining globules are those due to α_1-AT. In cirrhosis, these globules characteristically occur at the periphery of the nodules and can be seen in multiple sizes within the hepatocyte. Immunohistochemical staining can also be used to detect α_1-AT globules, and electron microscopy can show characteristic globules trapped in the Golgi apparatus.

27. **How is α_1-antitrypsin deficiency treated?**
    The only treatment for α_1-AT–related liver disease is symptomatic management of complications and liver transplantation. With liver transplantation, the phenotype becomes that of the transplanted liver.

28. **What is the prognosis for patients with α_1-antitrypsin deficiency? Should family screening be performed?**
    The prognosis depends entirely on the severity of the underlying lung or liver disease. Typically, patients who have lung disease do not have liver disease, and those who have liver disease do not have lung disease, although in some patients both organs are severely involved. In patients with decompensated cirrhosis, the prognosis relates largely to the availability of organs for liver transplantation. Patients with transplants do typically fine. Family screening should be performed with α_1-AT levels and phenotype. This screening is largely for prognostic information; definitive therapy for liver disease, other than liver transplantation, is not available.

WILSON'S DISEASE

29. **How common is Wilson's disease?**
    Wilson's disease has an estimated prevalence of 1 in 30,000 people.

30. **Where is the Wilson's disease gene located?**
    The abnormal gene responsible for Wilson's disease, an autosomal recessive disorder, is located on chromosome 13 and has been cloned recently. The gene has homology for the Menke's

disease gene, which also results in a disorder of copper metabolism. The Wilson's disease gene (called *ATP7B*) codes for a P-type adenosine triphosphatase, which is a membrane-spanning copper-transport protein. The exact location of this protein within hepatocytes is not definite, but it most likely causes a defect in transfer of hepatocellular lysosomal copper into bile. This defect results in the gradual accumulation of tissue copper with subsequent hepatotoxicity. Unfortunately, there are over 60 mutations in the Wilson's disease gene, and genetic testing has limited usefulness.

31. **What is the usual age of onset of Wilson's disease?**
    Wilson's disease is characteristically a disease of adolescents and young adults. Clinical manifestations have not been seen before age 5. By age 15, almost one half of the patients have some clinical manifestations of the disease. Rare cases of Wilson's disease have been identified in patients in their 40s or 50s.

32. **Which organ systems are involved in Wilson's disease?**
    The liver is uniformly involved. All patients with neurologic abnormalities due to Wilson's disease have liver involvement. Wilson's disease can also affect the eyes, kidneys, joints, and red blood cells. Thus, patients can have cirrhosis, neurologic deficits with tremor and choreic movements, ophthalmologic manifestations such as Kayser-Fleischer ring, psychiatric problems, nephrolithiasis, arthropathy, and hemolytic anemia.

33. **What are the different types of hepatic manifestations in Wilson's disease?**
    The typical patient who presents with symptoms from Wilson's disease already has cirrhosis. However, patients can present with chronic hepatitis, and in all young people with chronic hepatitis, a serum ceruloplasmin level should be performed as a screening test for Wilson's disease. Rarely, patients present with fulminant hepatic failure, which is uniformly fatal without successful liver transplantation. Finally, patients can present early in the disease with hepatic steatosis. As with chronic hepatitis, young patients with fatty liver disease should be screened for Wilson's disease.

34. **How is the diagnosis of Wilson's disease established?**
    Initial evaluation should include measurement of serum ceruloplasmin and, if abnormal, a 24-hour urinary copper level. About 85–90% of patients have depressed serum ceruloplasmin levels, but a normal level does not rule out the disorder. If the ceruloplasmin is decreased or the 24-hour urinary copper level is elevated, a liver biopsy should be performed for histologic interpretation and quantitative copper determination. Histologic changes include hepatic steatosis, chronic hepatitis, or cirrhosis. Histochemical staining for copper with rhodamine is not particularly sensitive. Usually, in established Wilson's disease, hepatic copper concentrations are >250 μg/gm (dry weight) and can be as high as 3000 μg/gm. Although elevated hepatic copper concentrations can occur in other cholestatic liver diseases, the clinical presentation allows an easy differentiation between Wilson's disease and primary biliary cirrhosis, extrahepatic biliary obstruction, and intrahepatic cholestasis of childhood.

35. **What forms of treatment are available for patients with Wilson's disease?**
    The mainstay of treatment has been the copper-chelating drug D-penicillamine. Because D-penicillamine is frequently associated with side effects, trientine has also been used. Trientine is equally efficacious and probably has fewer side effects. Maintenance therapy with dietary zinc supplementation has also been used. Neurologic disorders can improve with therapy. Patients who present with complications of chronic liver disease or with fulminant hepatic failure should be quickly considered for orthotopic liver transplantation.

36. **Is it necessary to perform family screening in Wilson's disease?**
    Wilson's disease is an autosomal recessive disorder, and all first-degree relatives of the patient should be screened. If the ceruloplasmin level is reduced, a 24-hour urinary copper level should

be obtained, followed by a liver biopsy for histology and quantitative copper determination. Genetic testing can be valuable for family screening, if genotyping has been done on the proband and is available to family members.

37. **Compare Wilson's disease and hereditary hemochromatosis.**
Both disorders involve abnormal metal metabolism and are inherited as autosomal recessive disorders. The mechanism of tissue damage is probably related to metal-induced oxidant stress for both disorders. In HH, the gene is on chromosome 6, whereas in Wilson's disease the abnormal gene is on chromosome 13. HH occurs in approximately 1 in 250 people, but Wilson's disease occurs in only about 1 in 30,000. The inherited defect in HH causes an increased absorption of iron by the intestine, with the liver as a passive recipient of the excessive iron; in contrast, the inherited defect in Wilson's disease is in the liver, resulting in decreased hepatic excretion of copper with excessive deposition and subsequent toxicity. Although the liver is affected in both Wilson's disease and HH, the other affected organs are quite variable. In hemochromatosis, the heart, pancreas, joints, skin, and endocrine organs are affected; in Wilson's disease, the brain, eyes, red blood cells, kidneys, and bone are affected. Both disorders are fully treatable, if diagnosis is made promptly before the development of end-stage complications.

WEBSITE

http://www.aasld.org/

See Practice Guidelines (metabolic/genetic/autoimmune)

BIBLIOGRAPHY

1. Bacon BR: Causes of iron overload. N Engl J Med 326:126–127, 1992.
2. Bacon BR, Britton RS: Hemochromatosis and other iron storage disorders. In Schiff ER, Sorrell MF, Maddrey WC (eds): Diseases of the Liver, 9th ed. Philadelphia, Lippincott-Raven, 2003, pp 1187–1205.
3. Bacon BR, Olynyk JK, Brunt EM, et al: *HFE* genotype in patients with hemochromatosis and other liver diseases. Ann Intern Med 130:953–962, 1999.
4. Bacon BR, Powell LW, Adams PC, et al: Molecular medicine and hemochromatosis: At the crossroads. Gastroenterology 116:193–207, 1999.
5. Bassett ML, Halliday JW, Powell LW: Value of hepatic iron measurements in early hemochromatosis and determination of the critical iron level associated with fibrosis. Hepatology 6:24–29, 1986.
6. Crystal RG: α1-Antitrypsin deficiency, emphysema, and liver disease: Genetics and strategies for therapy. J Clin Invest 85:1343–1352, 1990.
7. Edwards CQ, Griffen LM, Goldgar D, et al: Prevalence of hemochromatosis among 11,065 presumably healthy blood donors. N Engl J Med 318:1355–1362, 1988.
8. Eriksson S, Calson J, Veley R: Risk of cirrhosis and primary liver cancer in alpha$_1$-antitrypsin deficiency. N Engl J Med 314:736–739, 1986.
9. Feder JN, Gnirke A, Thomas W: A novel MHC class I-like gene is mutated in patients with hereditary haemochromatosis. Nature Genet 13:399–408, 1996.
10. Hill GM, Brewer GJ, Prasad AS, et al: Treatment of Wilson's disease with zinc. I: Oral zinc therapy regimens. Hepatology 7:522–528, 1987.
11. Hodges JR, Millward-Sadler GH, Barbatis C, Wright R: Heterozygous MZ alpha$_1$-antitrypsin deficiency in adults with chronic active hepatitis and cryptogenic cirrhosis. N Engl J Med 304:557–560, 1981.

. Larsson C: Natural history and life expectancy in severe alpha$_1$-antitrypsin deficiency, Pi Z. Acta Med Scand 204:345–351, 1978.

. Niederau C, Fischer R, Sonnenberg A, et al: Survival and causes of death in cirrhotic and noncirrhotic patients with primary hemochromatosis. N Engl J Med 313:1256–1262, 1985.

. Perlmutter DH: The cellular basis for liver injury in α_1-antitrypsin deficiency. Hepatology 13:172–185, 1991.

. Powell LW, Jazwinska E, Halliday JW: Primary iron overload. In Brock JH, Halliday JW, Powell LW (eds): Iron Metabolism in Health and Disease. London, W.B. Saunders, 1994, pp 227–270.

. Scheinberg IH, Jaffe ME, Sternlieb I: The use of trientine in preventing the effects of interrupting penicillamine therapy in Wilson's disease. N Engl J Med 317:209–213, 1987.

. Schilsky ML: Identification of the Wilson's disease gene: Clues for disease pathogenesis and the potential for molecular diagnosis. Hepatology 20:529–533, 1994.

. Sternlieb I: Perspectives on Wilson's disease. Hepatology 12:1234–1239, 1990.

. Stremmel W, Meyerrose KW, Niederau C, et al: Wilson's disease: Clinical presentation, treatment, and survival. Ann Intern Med 15:720–726, 1991.

CHAPTER 34

LIVER HISTOPATHOLOGY

Janet K. Stephens, MD, PhD, and George H. Warren, MD

LIVER MICROANATOMY AND INJURY PATTERNS

1. **Explain the role of liver biopsy.**
   Liver biopsies play an important role in patient care. They may confirm or advance a diagnosis, guide additional studies, help to evaluate therapeutic efficacy, and gauge prognosis. The liver biopsy must be of adequate size and contain an appropriate number of portal tracts and central veins to allow proper assessment. However, the liver has a limited pattern of pathologic response to injury, especially for inflammatory diseases, and, as in other organs, biopsy represents a static look at an ongoing dynamic process.

2. **Many liver biopsy reports say that the basic architecture is intact and then list a string of abnormalities. What is the basic architecture?**
   Histologically, the liver has three functional components: hepatocytes, central veins and sinusoids, and portal tracts (triads). The basic liver architecture is formed by cords of hepatocytes, which, in adults, are one cell-layer thick. The liver cells are separated by vascular sinusoids lined by endothelial cells and Kupffer cells; the latter are part of the reticuloendothelial system and have macrophage function. Central veins, also called *terminal hepatic venules,* collect the circulating blood after it percolates through the sinusoids and then carry the blood to larger hepatic veins. Distributed at regular intervals are portal tracts, which contain interlobular bile ducts, small hepatic arteries, small portal veins, and fibrous stroma with scant numbers of mononuclear cells. The row of hepatocytes immediately adjacent to the portal tract is termed the *limiting plate.*

3. **What are the geographic differences in pathology between portions of hepatic acini?**
   The functional unit of the liver is represented by hepatic acini, which are three-dimensional units built around a central axis containing a portal tract and its blood vessels. From the portal area, plates of hepatocytes radiate out toward central veins, located at the periphery of the acinus. The acinus can be divided into three zones: zone 1 is closest to the portal tracts, zone 3 is closest to the central veins, and zone 2 lies between. A gradient exists between zone 1 and zone 3; zone 1 is the best supplied with oxygen and various nutrients.

4. **What is meant by distortion of the hepatic architecture?**
   Usually, it indicates fibrosis and perhaps formation of regenerative nodules of hepatocytes. These changes can alter the relationships of central veins, portal tracts, and hepatic cords.

5. **How are degrees of fibrosis designated?**
   The pathologist indicates how generalized scarring is, how much collagen is present, whether anatomic structures, such as portal tracts and central veins, are connected by scar (bridging fibrosis) and whether the scarring has altered the architecture into nodules of hepatocytes (cirrhosis).

6. **What criteria are used to define the presence of cirrhosis?**
   Cirrhosis is the end stage of all chronic liver disease. By definition, it is a process that diffusely involves the liver with progressive fibrosis, resulting in the formation of nodules. Therefore,

focal scarring, even if significant and associated with nodules, is not cirrhosis because the process is not diffuse.

Can the presence of cirrhosis be proved by a needle biopsy specimen?
Not always. *Micronodular cirrhosis* (nodules ≤3 mm), most often caused by ethanol injury (also biliary tract disease, hemochromatosis), is highly uniform throughout the liver, and nodules are usually clearly defined on a needle specimen. *Macronodular cirrhosis* (nodules >3 mm), due most commonly to chronic viral hepatitis, is less uniform. One sometimes sees relatively sparse fibrosis in a needle specimen, with some fairly normal lobules noted, even when cirrhosis is suspected clinically. By nature of the biopsy technique, the softer lobular tissue may come out in the needle more easily than the fibrous tissue, or the needle may pass through large nodules and appear relatively uninvolved. The end result is that scarring can be underrepresented.

What types of liver cell injury are seen on needle specimens? What causes each type?
It may be difficult to determine a specific cause for liver injury seen on needle biopsy, because both hepatocytes and bile ducts have a limited pattern of response. Histopathologic features may overlap in many disease processes (Table 34-1).

TABLE 34-1. TYPES OF LIVER CELL INJURY	
Type	**Causes**
Fatty change	Ethanol, obesity, diabetes, drugs
Councilman bodies (acidophilic bodies)	Viral hepatitis, drugs, nonspecific reaction
Mallory's bodies (hyaline)	Ethanol, obesity, diabetes, drugs, Wilson's disease, biliary tract disease, hepatocellular carcinoma
Hydropic change (ballooning degeneration)	Viral hepatitis, drugs, cholestasis
Cholestasis	Duct obstruction or injury, drugs, viral hepatitis
Interlobular duct injury	Primary biliary cirrhosis, primary sclerosing cholangitis, hepatitis C
Piecemeal necrosis	Viral hepatitis, primary biliary cirrhosis, drugs, Wilson's disease
Increased iron stores	Hemochromatosis, transfusions, hemolysis
Granulomas	Tuberculosis, fungi, drugs

FATTY CHANGE AND STEATOHEPATITIS

Injury from either acute or chronic ethanol ingestion is one of the most common insults to the liver. Describe the major characteristics of mild and severe injury.
Alcoholic liver disease results in a spectrum of changes, including fatty liver, alcoholic hepatitis, and alcoholic cirrhosis. In fatty liver, as the name implies, the hepatocytes contain globules of fat, usually larger than and compressing the hepatocyte nucleus (referred to as macrovesicular

steatosis). Initially, this change occurs around central veins but may extend to involve the enti
acinus. Biopsies from patients with alcoholic hepatitis may also show fatty change. In additio
hepatocytes are swollen, with areas of necrosis, associated with acute inflammation
(polymorphs, polymorphonuclear neutrophils [PMNs]). Hepatocytes may contain perinuclea
Mallory's hyaline. Hyaline represents aggregates of the intermediate filament cytokeratin.
However, hyaline may also be found in a number of other conditions (nonalcoholic
steatohepatitis [NASH], Wilson's disease, hepatocellular carcinoma, primary biliary cirrhosis
Alcoholic cirrhosis, which is micronodular, may have superimposed fatty change and/or
hepatitis (Fig. 34-1).

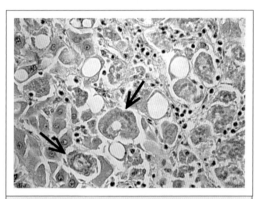

Figure 34-1. Alcoholic hepatitis with prominent hyaline
(hematoxylin-eosin stain).

10. **What is hyaline?**
    Hyaline is composed of irregular, ropelike strings that represent aggregates of microfilaments
    eosinophilic material in the cytoplasm. Although the fat and neutrophils can resolve relatively
    quickly after alcohol abstinence, hyaline can take up to 6 weeks to disappear.

11. **How does scarring progress with alcohol injury?**
    Many patients with ethanol injury show initial scarring around central veins with delicate, spic
    web–like fibrosis along the sinusoids. Eventually, bridging fibrosis connects central veins and
    portal tracts and adjacent portal tracts. When cirrhosis is fully developed, most of the native
    central veins have been obliterated.

12. **Is alcoholic cirrhosis micronodular or macronodular?**
    Micronodular, because the scarring is relatively uniform throughout the liver. These small or
    "micro" nodules have become subdivided by the portal-central bridging fibrosis. With comple
    alcohol abstinence, the nodules can regenerate to a size >3 mm, but the central veins are
    decreased in number and the nodules lack multiple portal tracts. One sees usually central vein
    and portal tracts in some nodules of macronodular cirrhosis (e.g., those from viral hepatitis).

13. **Sometimes a biopsy shows "alcoholic hepatitis," but the patient denies drinki
    ethanol. Is the pathologist's diagnosis incorrect, or is there a differential
    diagnosis for alcoholic hepatitis?**
    Steatohepatitis is the better term to describe the histologic changes. It is clear that similar
    patterns of injury can be seen in nonalcoholics, especially in the setting of diabetes and
    obesity, and is referred to as *nonalcoholic steatohepatitis* (NASH) or, simply, fatty liver

disease. This represents a significant form of chronic liver disease in both adults and children, with a spectrum ranging from indolent to end-stage liver disease. It may be a significant cause of cryptogenic cirrhosis and has been reported to recur in allograft livers. Other conditions associated with NASH include: acute starvation, accelerated weight loss, intestinal bypass, disorders of lipid metabolism (i.e., abetalipoproteinemia, hyperlipidemia, lipodystrophy) and various drugs (i.e., amiodarone, perhexiline, tamoxifen, synthetic estrogens, nifedipine, corticosteroids). Careful clinicopathologic correlation is required to determine the cause.

How are the diseases resembling alcoholic hepatitis differentiated?
Most of these conditions can be detected by history taking. The common ones are obesity and diabetes mellitus. Obese or diabetic patients occasionally show pathologic changes quite similar to alcoholic liver disease, including fat, hyaline, and sinusoidal scarring. In patients younger than 40 years, particularly those under age 30, Wilson's disease should be excluded by multiple laboratory tests and quantitative liver copper analysis. Hyaline can be present in primary biliary cirrhosis (PBC), but it is characteristically limited to the periportal zone. Of the important drugs, the antiarrhythmic amiodarone may have a half-life of up to 3 months, and ongoing injury may lead to death from liver failure. Clinical history of drug and toxin exposure is critical in liver disease. When all choices in the differential are exhausted, one should recognize that many alcoholics are exquisitely good at keeping their drinking a secret. The biopsy may confirm the nature and degree of injury, but the history taker solves the case.

VIRAL HEPATITIS

How can a liver biopsy help in patients with viral hepatitis?
A biopsy is helpful in assessing the amount of inflammatory activity (grade), its chronicity, and the degree of irreversible fibrosis or cirrhosis (stage). It can help to predict and evaluate response to medication. It is also useful in determining the presence of a second process, in addition to viral hepatitis.

When, if ever, is a biopsy ordered for patients with hepatitis A? With hepatitis B and C?
Because hepatitis A does not cause chronic liver disease, biopsy is rarely needed. Biopsies may be ordered to distinguish severe cholestasis in hepatitis A from large duct obstruction or to determine whether bridging necrosis or the rare fulminant necrosis is present. Usually, if a patient is positive for antihepatitis A, IgM type, there is no need for biopsy. Hepatitis B, hepatitis B and D coinfection, and hepatitis C can cause chronic hepatitis leading to cirrhosis, in addition to acute and/or fulminant disease. Liver biopsy helps to determine the severity of liver injury with regard to inflammatory activity and fibrosis. The histologic features may help to determine both treatment and prognosis.

Does chronic hepatitis have unique histopathologic features?
No. Chronic hepatitis is a clinical and pathologic syndrome that may have a variety of causes. It is a chronic necroinflammatory process in which hepatocytes are preferentially injured compared with bile ducts. In addition to viral infection, chronic hepatitis may be autoimmune or drug-related. Histologic features of chronic cholestatic disease, including PBC, primary sclerosing cholangitis (PSC), and autoimmune cholangitis, as well as metabolic diseases including Wilson's disease and alpha$_1$-antitrypsin (α_1-AT) deficiency, may overlap with those of chronic hepatitis.

What features are typical of chronic hepatitis?
Whereas parenchymal inflammation predominates in acute hepatitis, chronic hepatitis is usually associated with varying degrees of portal and periportal inflammation, parenchymal

hepatitis, and fibrosis. The inflammatory cell infiltrate is typically mononuclear and includes lymphocytes, plasma cells, and macrophages. Once the inflammatory infiltrate crosses the limiting plate, it is usually associated with local hepatocyte damage, piecemeal necrosis, and inflammation. Lobular inflammation is accompanied by some hepatocellular necrosis (acidophilic or Councilman bodies). With time, chronic hepatitis leads to progressive fibrosis and, without treatment, to cirrhosis. The fibrosis begins in portal areas, extends to periportal areas, and begins bridging to other portal tracts and central veins (Fig. 34-2).

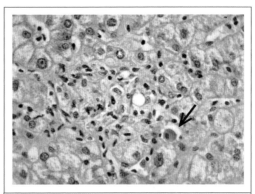

Figure 34-2. Biopsy, ordered to investigate fever of unknown origin, shows hepatitis with disorganized hepatocytes, lymphocytic infiltrate, and Councilman body (*arrow*) (hematoxylin-eosin stain).

19. **How is chronic hepatitis graded and staged?**
Various systems are used to evaluate chronic hepatitis, the simplest of which was proposed by Batts and Ludwig. A four-point grading system is used for both inflammatory activity and degree of fibrosis:

Inflammatory activity
Grade 1: Minimal patchy, piecemeal necrosis, and lobular inflammation/necrosis.
Grade 2: Mild portal inflammation with piecemeal necrosis involving some or all portal tracts with focal hepatocellular damage.
Grade 3: Moderate piecemeal necrosis involving all portal tracts with increased hepatocellular damage.
Grade 4: Severe portal inflammation with piecemeal necrosis; bridging fibrosis and diffuse hepatocellular damage may be present.

Fibrosis
Stage 1: Portal fibrosis (fibrous portal expansion)
Stage 2: Periportal fibrosis (periportal fibrosis with rare portal-portal septa)
Stage 3: Septal fibrosis (fibrous septa with architectural distortion)
Stage 4: Cirrhosis
Example: A liver biopsy from a patient with hepatitis C (Fig. 34-2), which shows mild portal inflammation with piecemeal necrosis in most of the portal tracts and periportal expansion with a few fibrous septa, is characterized as chronic hepatitis C with mild activity (grade 2) and portal and focal bridging fibrosis (stage 2).

What features in the liver biopsy help to predict etiology?
Biopsies from patients with chronic hepatitis B may show some of the changes described previously, as well as a "ground-glass" change to the cell cytoplasm. This change reflects accumulation of hepatitis B surface antigen within the endoplasmic reticulum of the hepatocytes. Chronic hepatitis C may be associated with prominent lymphoid aggregates within portal tracts, sometimes including germinal centers and, occasionally, bile duct damage, although not to the degree seen in primary biliary disorders. In addition, biopsies may show focal, nonzonal macrovesicular steatosis. The inflammatory infiltrate in patients with autoimmune hepatitis shows typically a predominance of plasma cells.

Can chronic viral hepatitis be confused with other injuries?
Autoimmune hepatitis looks quite similar to chronic viral hepatitis, but plasma cells are more prominent in autoimmune injury, and various confirmatory serologic tests are available. Some drug injuries, PBC, PSC, and other disorders can pose difficult diagnostic problems. Some cases of α_1-AT deficiency show piecemeal necrosis, but a periodic acid – Schiff–diastase stain reveals numerous magenta cytoplasmic globules in hepatocytes.

CHOLESTASIS

In patients with acute or chronic cholestasis, can the liver biopsy distinguish among the various differential diagnoses?
Maybe. Diagnosing cholestasis requires evaluation of the many causes in a systematic fashion: increased production of bilirubin, decreased excretion of bilirubin, and liver cell injuries. Hemolysis causes typically only mild hyperbilirubinemia. Extrahepatic obstruction is diagnosed typically by tests other than liver biopsy. Therefore, cases coming to liver biopsy are the difficult ones to solve; clinical and radiologic findings have solved the easy cases. The pathologist must ask whether the specimen shows associated inflammation or noninflammatory, "bland" cholestasis. The pathologist must also look for clues that suggest large duct obstruction or interlobular duct inflammatory injury. Subtle lesions in the head of the pancreas and ampulla of Vater can be missed. A stone may be missed. Other questions include the following: (1) Does the patient have hepatitis? (2) Has viral injury been excluded? (3) What are the patient's toxic exposures at work, home, or play? (4) Has every drug been sought and disclosed? (5) Have granulomatous causes been excluded?

DRUG INJURY

What histologic changes suggest drug- or toxin-related liver injury?
Three findings should make a pathologist press the clinician to "find the drug":
1. Significant fatty change, which most often is related to toxic ethanol injury.
2. A liver biopsy that shows features of a hypersensitivity reaction. Such cases resemble viral hepatitis, with an abundance of eosinophils. Eosinophils may also be present nonspecifically with viral hepatitis, connective tissue disorders, and some neoplasms (usually an infiltrate of Hodgkin's disease), but when eosinophils are a striking feature, the clinician should search for a drug or toxin (Fig. 34-3).
3. A liver that looks like it is recovering from a point-in-time injury, with numerous liver cell mitotic figures. These findings suggest that a single or short episode of drug or toxin exposure may be to blame.

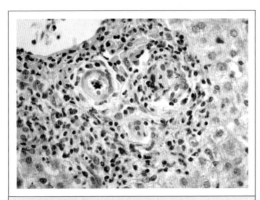

Figure 34-3. Nitrofurantoin hepatitis with prominent eosinophils (hematoxylin-eosin stain).

BILE DUCT DISORDERS

24. **In a patient with large duct obstruction, conjugated hyperbilirubinemia, an ultrasound showing bile duct stones, and clinical cholangitis, what would a biopsy show?**

    In this clinical situation, it is unusual that a liver biopsy would be necessary. If done, such a biopsy would show centrilobular cholestasis, portal tract edema, and neutrophils within portal tract stroma and within bile duct epithelium and lumens. One needs to remember that neutrophils within edematous portal stroma are a feature of large duct obstruction, even when frank cholangitis is not present.

25. **When is primary biliary cirrhosis (PBC) diagnosed?**

    PBC is chronic progressive cholestatic liver disease that occurs in middle-aged patients, usually women, and is often associated with other autoimmune diseases. Patients may present with jaundice and pruritus. Laboratory testing reveals an elevated serum antimitochondrial antibody as well as increased alkaline phosphatase, bilirubin, and GGT.

26. **How is PBC staged?**

    Stage depends on the degree of bile duct damage and fibrosis. *Stage 1* (early changes) consists of damage to septal and larger interlobular bile ducts, characterized by biliary epithelial damage with infiltration of the duct by lymphocytes, plasma cells, eosinophils, and rare polymorphs. The inflammatory infiltrate may include granulomas and lymphoid follicles (florid duct lesion; Fig. 34-4). At this point, the process is confined within the portal tract.

    In *stage 2* disease, the inflammatory process extends beyond the portal tract, and piecemeal necrosis may be seen. Bile ducts begin to disappear. Associated with this scenario may be bile ductular (cholangiolar) proliferation (along the edges of the portal tracts) and evidence of chronic cholestasis, including feathery degeneration within the cytoplasm of hepatocytes, accumulation of bile pigment, periportal accumulation of copper (not generalized as in Wilson disease), and, occasionally, Mallory's bodies.

    Stage 3 is associated with increasing fibrosis and bridging between portal areas, with decreased amounts of inflammation.

    Stage 4 represents "biliary" (micronodular) cirrhosis.

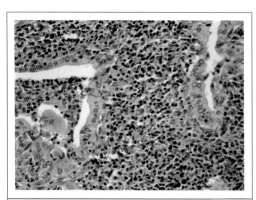

Figure 34-4. Primary biliary cirrhosis, with a florid duct lesion (hematoxylin-eosin stain).

When is primary sclerosing cholangitis (PSC) diagnosed?

PSC shares many clinical biochemical and pathologic features with PBC, although it can affect both intrahepatic and extrahepatic ducts. PSC is strongly associated with inflammatory bowel disease, particularly ulcerative colitis. Patients may present with increased alkaline phosphatase, IgG and/or IgM, and positive perinuclear antineutrophil cytoplasmic antibodies (p-ANCAs). The classic lesion of PSC is "onionskin" or concentric periductular fibrosis, with damage to the ductal epithelium.

How is PSC staged?

Like PBC, PSC is staged according to bile duct changes and fibrosis. *Stage 1* (early disease) is associated with bile duct damage and inflammation and is largely confined within portal tracts. In *stage 2* disease, the fibroinflammatory process is periportal. In *stage 3,* bridging fibrosis is present and bile ducts are decreased in numbers. *Stage 4* represents end-stage disease (cirrhosis).

What are the most common biopsy findings in patients with primary sclerosing cholangitis?

The onionskin lesion is seen *rarely* on percutaneous biopsy. The most common findings on biopsy are nonspecific fibrosis with inflammation of portal tracts and paucity of normal bile ducts. In addition, in patients with extrahepatic disease, it may be hard to separate intrahepatic PSC from the effects of obstruction. Obstruction causes proliferation and dilatation of interlobular ducts and an increased number of periportal PMNs. A major goal of the biopsy interpretation is to consider PSC and then to suggest endoscopic retrograde cholangiopancreatography (ERCP) to confirm the diagnosis.

GRANULOMATOUS INFLAMMATION

What is a granuloma?

A granuloma is a sharply (or fairly sharply) defined aggregate of histiocytes.

How common are granulomas in liver biopsies?

Most systemic granulomatous diseases involve the liver to some extent. Granulomas may be identified in 10% of routine liver biopsies, probably in relation to the liver's large population of phagocytic cells, including Kupffer cells and other macrophages.

32. **What causes granulomas in the liver?**

The differential list is long and varied. Tuberculosis and sarcoidosis are the most common causes. Other infectious agents include viruses (cytomegalovirus, Epstein-Barr virus), bacteria (brucellosis, nocardiosis, tularemia), *Rickettsia* spp. (Q fever *[Coxiella burnetii]*), spirochetes, various fungi, and protozoa. Noninfectious causes, in addition to sarcoidosis, include PBC, drug reaction, extrahepatic inflammatory disease (chronic granulomatous disease of childhood, chronic inflammatory bowel disease, rheumatoid arthritis), neoplasms (Hodgkin's disease), and foreign substances (talc, mineral oil).

33. **In patients with fever of unknown origin, do negative stains for fungi and acid-fast bacilli exclude infection?**

Not at all. Cultures for these organisms are more sensitive than special histologic stains. If infection is a possibility, a core of liver should be submitted with sterile precautions and without fixative to the microbiology laboratory. In addition, tissue in formalin should be sent to the surgical pathology laboratory for microscopic sections. Tissue may also be sent for molecular analysis to determine whether an infectious agent is present.

34. **Are acid-fast bacilli hard to identify on biopsy?**

In *Mycobacterium tuberculosis* infection, few organisms may be detected in the sections. Usually, stains are negative but cultures are positive.

35. **What are the different types of granulomas? Is the distinction of diagnostic use?**

Epithelioid granulomas are nodular aggregates of plump macrophages, often associated with multinucleated giant cells, lymphocytes, and plasma cells. They are typically seen in sarcoidosis and central caseating necrosis or tuberculosis.

Fibrin-ring granulomas are formed by a fibrin band encircling a lipid droplet, with associated inflammation. They were first described with Q fever but may also be seen after infection with cytomegalovirus or Epstein-Barr virus as well as with drug (allopurinol) toxicity and in association with systemic lupus erythematosus.

Lipogranulomas are composed of lipid deposits and vacuolated macrophages. They are formed in the presence of exogenous or endogenous fat accumulation.

Microgranulomas are composed of small, round clusters of plump Kupffer cells. They are a relatively nonspecific finding.

36. **How often are liver granulomas secondary to a drug reaction?**

Perhaps one third of granulomatous liver reactions are caused by drugs, including allopurinol, nitrofurantoin, alpha-methyldopa, phenylbutazone, carbamazepine, procainamide, diphenylhydantoin, quinidine, isoniazid, and sulfanilamide.

INHERITED LIVER DISEASE

37. **If the ratio of serum iron to total iron-binding capacity (TIBC) and serum ferritin levels are significantly elevated, is a liver biopsy indicated?**

Yes. The biopsy can tell you where the iron is stored (hepatocytes versus Kupffer cells), the amount of iron can be graded, the complications of iron storage (fibrosis, cirrhosis, hepatocellular carcinoma) can be assessed, and the biopsy can be sent for quantitative iron determination.

38. **What is hematochromatosis? Can it be diagnosed by histologic findings?**

Hemochromatosis is an autosomal recessive disorder characterized by massive deposits of iron in many organs, including liver, pancreas, heart, joints, and skin. Untreated, it leads to the development of micronodular cirrhosis. In genetic hemochromatosis, hepatocytes and biliary epithelium contain increased stainable iron. The biopsy may be relatively normal or show bridging fibrosis or even micronodular cirrhosis. Hepatocyte iron is deposited in a graded fashion, from periportal areas to central veins, and can be scored on a four-point system.

39. **If the laboratory tests are supported by Fe^{4+} deposition, is this sufficient evidence to diagnose genetic hemochromatosis?**
   The diagnosis of genetic hemochromatosis can be established with liver biopsy, quantitative iron determination performed on liver tissue, and genetic testing for the C282Y or H63D mutation.

40. **What disorders are problematic in the clinical differential diagnosis of hemochromatosis?**
   The list of disorders associated with increased hepatic iron is long. The pattern of distribution of the iron may be of some help in establishing the diagnosis:

   Predominantly hepatocellular distribution
   Genetic hemochromatosis
   Alcoholic liver disease
   Porphyria *cutanea tarda*

   Distributed predominantly in Kupffer cells
   Multiple transfusion
   Hemolytic anemias

   Mixed hepatocellular and Kupffer cell distribution
   Megaloblastic anemia
   Anemia secondary to chronic infection

1. **How does age affect the interpretation of quantitative iron results?**
   Among patients with hemochromatosis, young patients will have accumulated less iron than older patients, and menstruating women will have less iron than men of the same age. The hepatic iron index (HII) takes these factors into account:

$$HII = \text{Hepatic iron concentration (mg/gm liver dry wt)}/\text{age}/55.8$$

   Patients with genetic homozygous hemochromatosis characteristically show an HII >1.9, whereas patients with other causes of iron overload, including chronic alcoholic liver disease, show an HII <1.9.

2. **What is Wilson's disease? Can liver biopsy help to establish the diagnosis?**
   Wilson's disease is an autosomal recessive disorder of copper metabolism, characterized by excessive accumulation of copper in the liver and other organs. The gene for Wilson's disease has been localized to chromosome 13 (13q14-q21). The disease can show a range of appearances on liver biopsy, depending to some extent on the patient's age. In children and young adolescents, the most common appearance may be fatty change. In older adolescents and young adults, a liver biopsy may show chronic hepatitis with piecemeal necrosis. Adults tend to show cirrhosis, and Mallory's hyaline may be part of this change. In either adolescents or adults, confluent necrosis leading to fulminant hepatic failure may follow.

3. **What other tests are helpful in patient's with Wilson's disease?**
   Quantitative copper testing of the liver is useful; in patients with Wilson's disease, levels are typically >250 µg/gm dry weight liver (normal level = 38 µg/gm). The levels may be much higher in the absence of cirrhosis. Conditions associated with chronic cholestasis (PBC, PSC) also have elevated liver copper levels (range = 150–350 µg/gm). Other helpful measurements include serum ceruloplasmin (<20 mg/dL in patients with Wilson's disease; normal levels = 23–50 mg/dL) and 24-hour urinary copper (>100 µg/dL; normal = <30 µg/dL).

44. **What are the features of α_1-AT deficiency on liver biopsy?**

Alpha$_1$-AT is the major circulating inhibitor of serine proteases (Pi). Its primary target is the potent elastase found in PMNs. It thus acts to protect tissues against injury during active, ac inflammation. It is a 52-kd glycoprotein synthesized in the liver under the control of codomir alleles at a locus on the long arm of chromosome 14. These genes are highly polymorphic, v more than 75 known alleles. Many of the Pi variants are associated with fairly normal serum concentration and function and are thus of little clinical significance. However, a few result in low circulating levels of α_1-AT (i.e., PiZZ) and are of pathologic significance. Liver biopsies show classic PAS-positive, diastase-resistant globules with periportal hepatocytes. Portal fibrosis and chronic hepatitis may also be present. Liver cell dysplasia may be seen, and patients older than age 50, especially men, are at risk of developing hepatocellular carcinoma.

45. **Is the presence of PAS-positive, diastase-resistant globules diagnostic for α_1-AT deficiency?**

No. Various inflammatory conditions may be associated with overproduction of the enzyme, may congestion or hypoxia. Clinical correlation with electrophoretic analysis is key.

NEOPLASMS

46. **Discuss the role of liver biopsy in diagnosing metastatic neoplasms.**

First, an adequate sample of the neoplasm must be obtained. Biopsy can confirm metastasis the liver from a known primary tumor. Most metastatic disease is not curable, and it is appropriate to make the diagnosis with the minimally invasive technique of liver needle biops Some biopsies show a tumor that is probably metastatic but for which no primary tumor is known. In such cases, biopsy findings can guide further work-up, but it may not be possible identify the primary tumor from the needle specimen. A needle specimen may be used to diagnose or stage malignant lymphoma.

47. **Discuss the role of biopsy in diagnosing primary liver tumors.**

For vascular tumors, radiologic methods may be used rather than biopsy, but three types of li masses deserve special consideration: hepatocellular carcinoma, liver cell adenoma, and foca nodular hyperplasia. Each of these diagnoses may be suggested by needle biopsy samples, b definitive diagnosis is frequently difficult and, in some cases, impossible without larger samp or complete resection of the mass.

Higher-grade *hepatocellular carcinomas* are usually straightforward, but low-grade hepatocellular carcinomas can be difficult to distinguish from normal tissue or a regenerative nodule in the setting of cirrhosis (Fig. 34-5).

Liver cell adenomas in women taking oral contraceptives may show characteristic features but, occasionally, well-differentiated hepatocellular carcinomas can resemble liver cell adenomas.

Focal nodular hyperplasia is a localized lobulated nodule of hyperplastic liver cells surrounding a central scar. This condition can be confused with macronodular cirrhosis on a needle biopsy specimen (or even a wedge biopsy specimen). Definitive classification may require excision of the nodule.

48. **Can the clinical laboratory help in classifying tumors?**

Marked elevation of serum alpha-fetoprotein levels in hepatocellular carcinomas or similar markers for other tumors can be a great help.

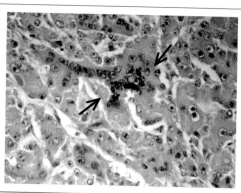

Figure 34-5. Hepatocellular carcinoma with prominent giant cell (*arrows*) (hematoxylin-eosin stain).

TRANSPLANTATION

9. Describe the role of liver biopsy in the evaluation of transplant recipients with abnormal liver function tests in the early postoperative period.

Liver transplantation is a well-accepted treatment for patients with advanced liver disease that is unresponsive to conventional therapy. In the first few weeks and months after transplant, the major causes of abnormal liver function tests (LFTs) include preservation injury, acute rejection, opportunistic infections (e.g., cytomegalovirus, hepatitis), vascular compromise, and/or biliary stricture. Acute allograft rejection is, perhaps, the most common and results from direct alloantigenic stimulation of recipient T cells by donor dendritic cells (antigen-presenting cells). The effector T cells can then preferentially injure biliary epithelial cells of both interlobular and septal bile ducts as well as endothelial cells of intrahepatic arteries and veins. Hepatocytes and sinusoidal lining cells are not prime targets.

0. What are the three main features of acute rejection?

1. Predominantly mononuclear with mixed portal inflammation (lymphocytes, macrophages, plasma cells, PMNs, eosinophils)
2. Subendothelial inflammation (endothelialitis), which may involve both portal and central veins and even the hepatic artery
3. Bile duct infiltration by inflammatory cells with associated damage

. What criteria help to distinguish recurrent hepatitis C after transplantation from allograft rejection?

Hepatitis C recurs in virtually all patients transplanted for that disease. The distinction of recurrent hepatitis from acute allograft rejection can be difficult. In general, however, recurrent hepatitis C is characterized by a mononuclear rather than a mixed portal infiltrate. Bile duct damage, although it may occur, is focal and mild. Hepatitis C is usually associated with a lobular hepatitis and, perhaps, hepatocyte necrosis. These findings are unusual in allograft rejection, unless it is severe. As with any disease process, correlation with clinical findings is key.

. Describe the role of liver biopsy in the evaluation of abnormal liver function tests in the first year after transplantation (and beyond).

Common causes of abnormal LFTs in the first year after transplantation include acute rejection (usually caused by inadequate immunosuppression), opportunistic infection, recurrent viral hepatitis, chronic rejection, steatohepatitis, and various recurrent diseases (e.g., PBC, PSC, autoimmune hepatitis). Chronic rejection is characterized histologically by either loss of small bile ducts ("ductopenic" rejection) or obliterative vasculopathy (affecting hilar structures). The former can be diagnosed by liver biopsy, whereas the latter may require examination of the explanted liver. Chronic rejection on liver biopsy is characterized classically by bile duct loss more than 50% of portal tracts, either in a single biopsy or a series of biopsies. It is probably irreversible. Chronic rejection may first manifest as prominent bile duct abnormalities or damage with some degree of bile duct loss. Unlike acute allograft rejection, the amount of bile duct damage is typically out of proportion to the degree of inflammation.

53. **How can a liver biopsy help in the evaluation of a bone marrow transplant recipient with elevated liver function tests?**

Complications of bone marrow transplantation include veno-occlusive disease (VOD) and graft versus host disease (GVHD). VOD is characterized by liver dysfunction and is due to the use of high-dose cytoreductive therapy. It develops within 1–4 weeks after transplantation. On biopsy it is characterized by occlusion of central veins, sinusoidal fibrosis, and pericentral hepatocyte necrosis. Acute GVHD develops within 6 weeks after transplantation and affects the skin, gastrointestinal tract, and liver. It is characterized by degenerative bile duct lesions with some degree of mononuclear inflammation. Cholestasis may be present. Chronic GVHD is a multiorgan process that develops 80–400 days after transplantation and is often preceded by acute GVHD. The changes in the liver are similar to those in acute disease, but the ducts show more prominent changes and are likely to be reduced in number or destroyed. A prominent periportal mononuclear infiltrate, or even piecemeal necrosis, may be seen.

WEBSITES

1. http://www-medlib.med.utah.edu/WebPath/LIVEHTML/LIVERIDX.html

2. http://www-medlib.med.utah.edu/WebPath/ORGAN.html#2

3. http://www-medlib.med.utah.edu/WebPath/GIHTML/GIIDX.html

4. http://www.afip. org/Departments/HepGastr_dept/index.html

5. http://www. gastroatlas.com

BIBLIOGRAPHY

1. Andrews NC: Disorder of iron metabolism. N Engl J Med 341:1986–1995, 1999.

2. Batts KP, Ludwig J: Chronic hepatitis: An update on terminology and reporting. Am J Surg Pathol 19:1409–1417, 1995.

3. Brunt EM: Nonalcoholic steatohepatitis: Definition and pathology. Semin Liver Dis 21:3–16, 2001.

4. DeMetris AJ, Batts KP, Dhillon AP, et al: Banff schema for grading liver allograft rejection: An international consensus document. Hepatology 25:658–663, 1997.

5. Edwards CQ, Ajoika RS, Kushner JP: Hemochromatosis: A genetic definition. In Barton JC, Edwards CQ (eds): Hemochromatosis: Genetics, Pathophysiology, Diagnosis and Treatment. Cambridge, United Kingdom, Cambridge University Press, 2000, pp 8–11.

6. Gerber JA, Thung SN: Histology of the liver. Am J Surg Pathol 11:709–722, 1987.

7. Kanel GC, Korula J: Developmental, familial and metabolic disorders. In Atlas of Liver Pathology. Philadelphia, W.B. Saunders, 1992, pp 135–174.

8. Krawitt EL: Autoimmune hepatitis. N Engl J Med 334:897–903, 1996.

Lee RG: General principles. In Diagnostic Liver Pathology. St. Louis, Mosby, 1994, pp 1–22.

Olynyk JK, Cullen DJ, Aquillia S, et al: A population-based study of the clinical expression of the hemochromatosis gene. N Engl J Med 341:718–724, 1999.

Scheuer PJ: Pathologic features and evolution of primary biliary cirrhosis and primary sclerosing cholangitis. Mayo Clin Proc 73:179–183, 1998.

Shulman HM, Fisher LB, Schoch HG, et al: Veno-occlusive disease of the liver after marrow transplantation: Histological correlates of clinical signs and symptoms. Hepatology 19:1171–1180, 1994.

Shulman HM, Sharma P, Amos D, et al: A coded histologic study of hepatic graft-versus-host disease after human bone marrow transplantation. Hepatology 8:463–470, 1988.

Snover DC, Freese DK, Sharp HL, et al: Liver allograft rejection: An analysis of the use of biopsy in determining outcome of rejection. Am J Surg Pathol 11:1–10, 1987.

Zimmerman HJ, Maddrey WE: Toxic and drug-induced hepatitis. In Schiff L, Schiff ER (eds): Diseases of the Liver. Philadelphia, J.B. Lippincott, 1993, pp 707–783.

CHAPTER 35

HEPATOBILIARY CYSTIC DISEASE

Randall E. Lee, MD

1. **Describe the five major classes and subtypes of congenital bile duct cysts (Fig. 35-1).**

   Type Ia: cystic extrahepatic bile duct dilation[*]

   Type Ib: segmental extrahepatic bile duct dilation

   Type Ic: fusiform, diffuse, or cylindrical bile duct dilation[*]

   Type II: extrahepatic duct diverticula

   Type III: choledochocele

   Type IVa: multiple intrahepatic and extrahepatic duct cysts[*]

   Type IVb: multiple extrahepatic duct cysts

   Type V: intrahepatic duct cysts

   [*]Usually associated with an anomalous pancreatobiliary junction (APBJ).

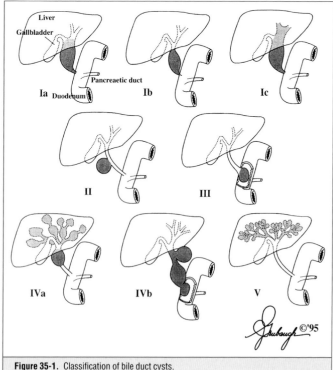

Figure 35-1. Classification of bile duct cysts.

What is the incidence of malignancy within a congenital bile duct cyst?
The reported incidence of malignancy within a congenital bile duct cyst ranges from 10–30%, although this may be an overestimation because the true incidence of choledochal cyst disease is unknown. The risk of malignancy appears to increase with the age of the patient at presentation. Malignancy has been reported in all types of choledochal cysts, including type III (choledochocele).

Describe the typical clinical presentation of a bile duct cyst.
The classic clinical presentation of a bile duct cyst is the triad of abdominal pain, jaundice, and abdominal mass. Infants and children manifest this symptom triad more than adults. Often, only one or two of these symptoms are present at any one time. Other presenting symptoms include cholangitis and pancreatitis. Bile duct cysts may also be incidental findings.

Provide a differential diagnosis for bile duct cyst disease.
- Biliary atresia
- Bile duct stone impaction
- Pancreatic pseudocyst
- Hydatid cyst
- Primary sclerosing cholangitis
- Cholangiocarcinoma

Describe the preferred treatment for patients with bile duct cyst disease.
The preferred treatment is complete surgical excision of the cyst with hepatoenterostomy rather than cystenterostomy and internal drainage. Complete excision significantly reduces, but does not eliminate, the risks of developing bile duct malignancy, strictures, and cholangitis. Patients with symptomatic intrahepatic bile duct cyst disease may have the affected lobe resected, or be considered for liver transplantation.

What is the role of cholangiopancreatography in patients with bile duct cyst disease?
Patients with extrahepatic bile duct cysts have an increased incidence of anomalous pancreaticobiliary junction. Cholangiopancreatography—percutaneously, endoscopically, or intraoperatively—allows definitive identification of the pancreatic duct insertion, which may be important to the planning of excision. In addition, cholangiography can distinguish multiple intrahepatic bile duct cysts from multiple hepatic cysts, which appear similar on computed tomography (CT). Magnetic resonance cholangiopancreatography (MRCP) is not as good as direct cholangiopancreatography for characterizing the pancreatobiliary junction, but it has less risk. Endoscopic retrograde cholangiopancreatography (ERCP) should be performed with caution in patients with suspected Caroli's disease or Caroli's syndrome because of the increased risk of recurrent cholangitis and sepsis. Nevertheless, therapeutic ERCP remains a useful tool for the management of acute cholangitis due to bile duct stones.

Compare the main features of Caroli's disease and Caroli's syndrome.
Initially described by Caroli in 1958, both entities are characterized by congenital dilations of the intrahepatic bile ducts. Patients usually become symptomatic as children or young adults, presenting with abdominal pain and hepatomegaly. Patients with the rare *Caroli's disease* have cystic dilations limited to the larger intrahepatic bile ducts. Some reports of Caroli's disease describe lesions in only one of the hepatic lobes. The cystic dilations of the larger intrahepatic ducts predispose to recurrent intrahepatic calculi and cholangitis. The mode of inheritance is uncertain.

In the more common *Caroli's syndrome,* the cystic dilations are distributed along the portal tract. This distribution is believed to result from a ductal plate malformation that affects the bile ducts at all levels, including the smaller interlobular ducts. Caroli's syndrome is associated with congenital hepatic fibrosis. Consequently, patients often have manifestations of portal hypertension, such as splenomegaly and esophageal varices. The mode of inheritance is autosomal recessive.

KEY POINTS: HEPATOBILIARY DISEASE

1. Patients with any class of congenital bile duct cyst have an increased risk of cholangiocarcinoma.

2. Patients with congenital choledochal cysts have an increased incidence of an anomalous pancreaticobiliary junction.

3. Polycystic liver disease (PLD) is the most common extrarenal manifestation of autosomal dominant polycystic kidney disease (ADPKD). Massive PLD associated with ADPKD has been reported in women only.

4. In the absence of complications, liver cysts do not affect hepatic function.

5. Communities involved in sheep farming have the highest rates of human hepatic cystic echinococcosis.

8. **What disease is commonly associated with polycystic liver disease (PLD)?**

PLD is characterized by numerous cysts scattered throughout the liver parenchyma. Most commonly, it is associated with autosomal dominant polycystic kidney disease (ADPKD). There are also strong associations between ADPKD and intracranial saccular aneurysms (berry aneurysms), mitral valve prolapse, and colonic diverticula. Most families affected by ADPKD have a genetic defect located on chromosome 16 (ADPKD1) or chromosome 4 (ADPKD2). Slightly less than one half of ADPKD patients develop end-stage renal disease.

Polycystic liver disease also exists as a rare autosomal dominant disorder (ADPLD) that is caused by a mutation in the gene encoding for the protein hepatocystin. Patients with ADPLD have no kidney disease but may have an increased risk for intracranial aneurysms.

9. **What are the risk factors for polycystic liver disease in patients with autosomal dominant polycystic kidney disease?**

Polycystic liver disease is the most common extrarenal manifestation of ADPKD. The presence and severity of polycystic liver disease in patients with ADPKD increase with age, female gender, number and frequency of pregnancies, and severity of renal disease. Massive PLD associated with ADPKD has been reported only in women.

10. **Describe the clinical manifestations of complicated polycystic liver disease.**

The common complications of polycystic liver disease include mass effect and cyst infection. Compression of adjacent structures by large cysts or by massive involvement may be manifest by chronic pain, anorexia, or obstructive jaundice. Clinical clues to the presence of a cyst infection include fever, right upper quadrant abdominal pain, and leukocytosis. A definitive diagnosis of cyst infection requires usually percutaneous CT or ultrasound-guided fine-needle aspiration.

11. **How does the presence of liver cysts affect hepatic function?**

Hepatic function is not usually affected by liver cysts. In the absence of complications, the serum aminotransferase, bilirubin, and alkaline phosphatase are typically within normal range only slightly elevated. In patients with ADPKD, serum chemistry abnormalities reflect generally the degree of renal dysfunction.

What are the treatment options for patients with symptomatic polycystic liver disease?

Symptomatic liver cysts may be treated either percutaneously or surgically. Simple ultrasound- or CT-guided percutaneous aspiration results in rapid reaccumulation of the cyst fluid. The rate of cyst recurrence is greatly reduced by instilling a sclerosing agent, such as absolute ethanol, at the time of aspiration. Patients treated in this manner may experience a low-grade fever and transient pain as well as ethanol intoxication. Percutaneous sclerosis of a liver cyst is contraindicated when the cyst communicates with either the biliary system or peritoneal cavity.

Infected cysts do not resolve with systemic antibiotic therapy alone. Administration of antibiotics should be combined with either percutaneous or surgical drainage. Patients with intractable pain or anorexia due to massive polycystic hepatomegaly may be candidates for either isolated orthotopic liver transplantation or combined liver and kidney transplantation (if they are dialysis-dependent).

What is the significance of a simple hepatic cyst?

Simple hepatic cysts (often called *solitary hepatic cysts*) are benign fluid collections surrounded usually by a thin columnar epithelium. They are frequently noted as an incidental finding on hepatic ultrasonography or CT scanning. Simple hepatic cysts are not associated with cystic disease in other organs, and there is no genetic transmission. Many, but not all, simple hepatic cysts are solitary, and most are asymptomatic. Treatment is indicated if symptoms develop. Cyst-related symptoms include abdominal pain, increasing abdominal girth, and obstructive jaundice.

Describe the ultrasonographic characteristics of a simple hepatic cyst.

On ultrasound examinations, a simple hepatic cyst has no internal echoes, a smooth margin with the surrounding parenchyma, and no appreciable wall. The absence of any of these characteristics should make one suspect a complication, such as a cyst infection, or another diagnosis, such as hydatid cyst or biliary cyst disease.

What are the characteristics of a simple hepatic cyst on computed tomography and magnetic resonance imaging (MRI)?

A simple hepatic cyst appears on CT as a thin-walled lesion that does not enhance with iodinated intravenous contrast agents. The density of the lesion is that of water. On MRI, a simple hepatic cyst is a homogeneous, very-low-intensity lesion on T1-weighted scans and a discrete high-intensity lesion on T2-weighted scans.

What is *Echinococcus granulosus*?

E. granulosus is the small tapeworm responsible for unilocular hydatid cyst disease. The adult worm is 2–8 mm long and consists of a bulbous scolex with four suckers and a coronet of hooklets, followed by three or four body segments called *proglottids*. The last proglottid is typically gravid with hundreds of eggs. Each egg measures only about 0.03 mm in diameter.

Describe the life cycle of *Echinococcus granulosus*.

The adult worm lives in the intestinal lumen of the definitive host, usually a predator, such as a dog, fox, or cat. Eggs discharged from the gravid proglottid segment leave the definitive host in the feces. The eggs are ingested through contaminated food or water by intermediate hosts, such as sheep, cattle, goats, rabbits, and horses. Ingested eggs hatch in the duodenum, and the larvae penetrate the intestinal mucosa to be carried by the circulatory system to the capillary beds of distant organs. As a defense mechanism, the intermediate host lays down layers of connective tissue around each larva, thus forming the hydatid cyst. New scolices bud from the inner wall of the cyst. Over time, daughter cysts may form within the original cyst. When infected viscera are eaten by a predator, the scolices develop into adult worms.

18. **Where and how does *Echinococcus granulosus* infect humans?**

Human infection by *E. granulosus* occurs throughout the world. It is a significant public health problem in South and Central Americas, China, Mediterranean countries, and the Russian Federation. Human cystic echinococcosis has been also reported in Alaska, Canada, and the western United States. Infections occur most commonly in sheep- and cattle-raising areas, where dogs assist in herding. Humans are usually infected as intermediate hosts when they ingest egg-contaminated food or water or allow infected dogs to lick them in the mouth. Over one half of all human infections involve the liver. Additional common sites for hydatid cysts are the lungs, spleen, kidneys, heart, bones, and brain (Fig. 35-2).

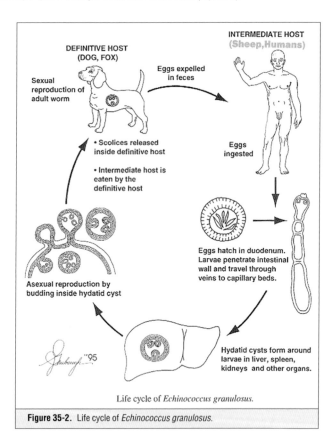

Life cycle of *Echinococcus granulosus*.

Figure 35-2. Life cycle of *Echinococcus granulosus*.

19. **Describe the typical clinical presentation of hepatic hydatid cyst disease.**

Many patients unsuspectingly harbor the infection until they present with a palpable abdominal mass or other symptoms. The symptoms of hydatid cyst disease are related primarily to the mass effect of the slowly enlarging cyst: abdominal pain from the stretching hepatic capsule, jaundice from compression of the bile duct, or portal hypertension from portal vein obstruction. Approximately 20% of patients have cysts that rupture into the biliary tree and may have symptoms similar to those of choledocholithiasis or cholangitis. Rupture of a cyst into the peritoneal cavity may cause an intense antigenic response, resulting in eosinophilia, bronchial spasm, or anaphylactic shock.

. **How is echinococcosis diagnosed?**

Confirming a diagnosis of echinococcosis usually requires a combination of diagnostic imaging and serologic tests. CT scans may show the hydatid cyst as a sharply defined, low-density lesion with spoke-like septations. The presence of a calcified rim of daughter cysts greatly enhances the specificity of the CT findings. When imaged by ultrasound, the hydatid cyst appears as a complex mass with multiple internal echoes from debris and septations. Enzyme-linked immunosorbent assay or indirect hemagglutinin serologic assays for echinococcal antibodies are positive in about 85–90% of patients. Recovery of scolices from a suspected hydatid cyst by percutaneous needle aspiration is diagnostic, but this technique must be used with caution because of the risk of spilling scolices into the peritoneal cavity.

. **What are the treatment options for hepatic hydatid cyst disease?**

Open surgical drainage of the hydatid cysts is, generally, the preferred method of therapy, especially for large or infected cysts. Percutaneous cyst drainage and irrigation with a scolicidal agent (Puncture, Aspiration, Injection, Reaspiration or PAIR) is an accepted alternative, especially in patients who are not surgical candidates. Chemotherapy with albendazole in the peridrainage period reduces the recurrence rate of both techniques. Peridrainage ERCP helps to rule out cyst communication with the biliary or pancreatic duct systems. Persistent postoperative biliary fistulas may be diagnosed and treated by ERCP with endoscopic sphincterotomy.

BLIOGRAPHY

Bernardino ME, Galamobs JT: Computed tomography and magnetic resonance imaging of the liver. Semin Liver Dis 9:32–49, 1998.

Biava MF, Dao A, Fortier B: Laboratory diagnosis of cystic hydatic disease. World J Surg 25:10–14, 2001.

Bilsel Y, Bulut T, Yamaner S, et al: ERCP in the diagnosis and management of complications after surgery for hepatic echinococcosis. Gastrointest Endosc 57:210–213, 2003.

D'Agata ID, Jonas MM, Perez-Atayde AR, Guay-Woodford LM: Combined cystic disease of the liver and kidney. Semin Liver Dis 14:215–227, 1994.

Drenth JP, Tahvanainen E, te Morsche RH, et al: Abnormal hepatocystin caused by truncating PRKCSH mutations leads to autosomal dominant polycystic liver disease. Hepatology 39:924–931, 2004.

Durgun AV, Gorgun E, Kapan M, et al: Choledochal cysts in adults and the importance of differential diagnosis. J Hepatobiliary Pancreat Surg 9:738–741, 2002.

Gabow PA: Autosomal dominant polycystic kidney disease. N Engl J Med 329:332–342, 1993.

Gustafsson BI, Friman S, Mjornstedt L, et al: Liver transplantation for polycystic liver disease?indications and outcome. Transplant Proc 35:813–814, 2003.

Khuroo MS, Wani NA, Javid G, et al: Percutaneous drainage compared with surgery for hepatic hydatid cysts. N Engl J Med 337:881–887, 1997.

Kim MJ, Han SJ, Yoon CS, et al: Using MR cholangiopancreatography to reveal anomalous pancreaticobiliary ductal union in infants and children with choledochal cysts. Am J Roentgenol 179:209–214, 2002.

Larssen TB, Jensen DK, Viste A, Horn A: Single-session alcohol sclerotherapy in symptomatic benign hepatic cysts. Long-term results. Acta Radiol 40:636–638, 1999.

McManus DP, Zhang W, Li J, Bartley PB: Echinococcosis. Lancet 362:1295–1304, 2003.

Mergo PJ, Ros PR: Benign lesions of the liver. Radiol Clin North Am 36:319–331, 1998.

Metcalfe MS, Wemyss-Holden SA, Maddern GJ: Management dilemmas with choledochal cysts. Arch Surg 138:333–339, 2003.

Nisenbaum HL, Rowling SE: Ultrasound of focal hepatic lesions. Semin Roentgenol 30:324–346, 1995.

Polat P, Kantarci M, Alper F, et al: Hydatid disease from head to toe. Radiographics 23:475–494, 2003.

Sayek I, Onat D: Diagnosis and treatment of uncomplicated hydatid cyst of the liver. World J Surg 25:21–27, 2001.

18. Schievink WI, Spetzler RF: Screening for intracranial aneurysms in patients with isolated polycystic liver disease. J Neurosurg 89:719–721, 1998.

19. Todani T, Watanabe Y, Narusue M, et al: Congenital bile duct cysts: Classification, operative procedures, and review of thirty-seven cases including cancer arising from choledochal cyst. Am J Surg 134:263–269, 1977.

20. Ulrich F, Steinmuller T, Settmacher U, et al: Therapy of Caroli's disease by orthotopic liver transplantation. Transplant Proc 34:2279–2280, 2002.

CHAPTER 36

GALLBLADDER: STONES, SLUDGE, AND POLYPS

Cynthia W. Ko, MD, MS, and Sum P. Lee, MD, PhD

How common is gallstone disease in Western populations?
In studies performed in the United States and Italy, about 10–20% of adults have gallstones. Only about 20–30% of persons with gallstones develop symptoms; the risk of developing symptoms or complications is approximately 2–4% per year.

Which populations are at greatest risk for gallstones?
- Gallstones are more common with increasing age and body mass index.
- Women are twice as likely as men to develop gallstones.
- Native Americans and Hispanics are at higher risk for gallstones. Female Pima Indians of the western United States carry the highest risk; about 75% develop gallstones by the fourth decade of life.
- Scandinavian women are also highly predisposed to gallstones (50% by age 50).

What are the symptoms of biliary colic?
Biliary colic is characterized by severe, episodic pain in the epigastrium or right upper quadrant. Pain sometimes occurs following a large meal but may occur without any precipitating events. The interval between attacks of biliary colic is unpredictable. Nonspecific dyspeptic symptoms, such as ill-defined abdominal discomfort, nausea, vomiting, or fatty food intolerance, are not characteristic of biliary tract disease. A cholecystectomy done for nonspecific dyspeptic complaints will not usually relieve these symptoms.

What are the three principal factors involved in gallstone formation?
- Cholesterol supersaturation—the amount of cholesterol exceeds the carrying capacity of bile acids and phospholipids in bile.
- Accelerated nucleation—precipitation of cholesterol crystals from supersaturated bile. Certain proteins, most importantly mucin, may accelerate precipitation of cholesterol crystals.
- Gallbladder hypomotility—gallbladder stasis alters bile composition and allows crystals to precipitate.

Are bacteria involved in gallstone formation?
Yes. Bacteria can be found in gallstones using molecular techniques. Different bacterial species may promote initial precipitation of bilirubin salts, which may serve as a nidus for stone formation. Gallstones may also become colonized with bacteria, resulting in precipitation of bilirubinate salts or remodeling of the existing stones.

Name drugs, medical conditions, and medical therapy associated with gallstone/sludge formation.
- The antibiotic ceftriaxone is excreted into bile. It may precipitate with calcium and form sludge or stones in the gallbladder.
- Biliary sludge and stones form commonly during pregnancy. Gallstones are also more common in patients with diabetes mellitus, ileal Crohn's disease, or spinal cord injury.

- Total parenteral nutrition (TPN) and fasting cause gallbladder stasis and promote sludge and stone formation.
- Progestins, oral contraceptives, and octreotide (somatostatin) impair gallbladder emptying and promote sludge and stone formation.

7. **What is biliary sludge?**
Biliary sludge is composed of microscopic precipitates of cholesterol or calcium bilirubinate. On ultrasonography, sludge appears as low-amplitude echoes without postacoustic shadows that layer with gravity (Fig. 36-1). It can also be diagnosed by microscopic examination of a fresh sample of gallbladder bile. In certain clinical situations, sludge may evolve into gallstones. It may also disappear spontaneously. Sludge is thought to represent the earliest stages of gallstone formation.

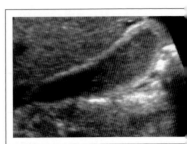

Figure 36-1. Ultrasonography showing biliary sludge. Microscopic crystals in the gallbladder generate low-amplitude echoes without postacoustic shadowing.

8. **Can gallbladder sludge cause symptoms or complications?**
Yes. Passage of sludge out of the gallbladder into the cystic duct and common bile duct can cause symptoms identical to those caused by gallstones. Sludge is associated with biliary colic, pancreatitis, cholangitis, and cholecystitis. Biliary sludge can be found in a large proportion of patients with "idiopathic" pancreatitis.

9. **What is the risk of gallstones in the obese? Why are gallstones more common with obesity?**
The incidence of gallstones in obese women is estimated at 2–3% per year, with approximately two thirds of these stones being asymptomatic. The risk of gallstones relative to nonobese women is increased twofold in women with a body mass index >30 kg/m^2 and sevenfold in women with body mass index >45 kg/m^2. In the obese, there is marked cholesterol supersaturation of bile. Obesity is also associated with gallbladder hypomotility. Both of these factors may predispose to gallstone formation.

10. **Why is rapid weight loss a risk factor for development of gallstones? Can such gallstones be prevented?**
About 25% of obese patients undergoing rapid weight loss develop gallstones. During rapid weight loss through dieting or bariatric surgery, cholesterol is mobilized from adipose tissue and secreted into bile. Prolonged fasting leads to supersaturation of bile with cholesterol, increased mucin production, and decreased gallbladder motility, all of which promote gallstone formation. Both aspirin and ursodeoxycholic acid may prevent stone formation during rapid weight loss. Some experts advocate prophylactic cholecystectomy in obese patients undergoing bariatric surgery. Maintaining some fat intake (>10 gm/day) may help maintain gallbladder motility and prevent gallstone formation.

11. **How do yellow, black, and brown biliary stones differ clinically?**
Yellow stones are almost pure cholesterol monohydrate. They account for over 80% of gallstones in Western populations. *Brown stones* are associated with colonization of bile by bacteria and/or parasites. Brown stones have a soft, clay-like consistency and are found in the intrahepatic and extrahepatic ducts but not the gallbladder. They are more common among Asian populations and may present as acute pyogenic cholangitis. *Black stones* are associated with chronic hemolysis, long-term TPN, and cirrhosis. They form in the gallbladder from

bilirubin precipitation and are usually quite soft; however, they may contain some calcium salts and be radiopaque. They rarely cause obstruction.

Discuss complications from the migration of gallstones.
Large gallstones occasionally erode through the gallbladder into the gastrointestinal tract, where they may cause obstruction. Most frequently, the stones impact in a normal ileum. This *gallstone ileus* is the second most common cause of small bowel obstruction in adults without prior surgery. Stones escaping the small bowel may impact in the colon, if it is narrowed by previous diverticular disease. Rarely, stones may enter the stomach by way of a fistula and obstruct the pylorus *(Bouveret's syndrome)*. Cholecystocolonic fistulas may also occur, leading, in some cases, to diarrhea provoked by the entry of bile salts into the colon. Plain films frequently demonstrate air in the gallbladder or biliary tree. In patients with a bowel obstruction and air in the biliary tree, a gallstone complication should be suspected.

What causes acute cholecystitis in patients with gallstones?
Stones may impact in the neck of the gallbladder or cystic duct, resulting in distention and inflammation of the gallbladder wall (cholecystitis). Cultures of bile during the early phase of the disease are usually sterile. Secondary bacterial infection, and even gangrene, may ensue after prolonged cholecystitis.

KEY POINTS: CLINICAL CHARACTERISTICS AND MANIFESTATIONS OF BILIARY STONES AND SLUDGE

1. Gallbladder stones and sludge are frequent but often asymptomatic.

2. Biliary colic is characterized by intermittent, severe abdominal pain in the epigastrium or right upper quadrant.

3. Nonspecific symptoms, such as nausea, dyspepsia, or fatty food intolerance, are not usually attributable to gallbladder disease.

What are the symptoms of acute cholecystitis? How should patients with acute cholecystitis be treated?
Patients with acute cholecystitis have typically epigastric or right upper quadrant abdominal pain lasting longer than 3 hours. Low grade fevers and vomiting are common. *Murphy's sign,* an inspiratory pause during palpation of the right upper quadrant, may be present. On ultrasound, patients will have a thickened gallbladder wall with pericholecystic fluid. Patients with acute cholecystitis should be hospitalized and given intravenous fluids and antibiotics. The timing of cholecystectomy in these patients is controversial. However, early surgery (<3 days) may be associated with faster recovery and shorter hospital stays, with morbidity rates similar to delayed surgery (4–6 weeks).

Should patients with asymptomatic stones be treated? What is the treatment of choice for patients with symptomatic stones?
The risk of developing gallstone-related symptoms is not great (2–4% per year). In patients with gallbladder stones, complications usually occur after development of uncomplicated biliary colic, so there is no advantage to prophylactic cholecystectomy. Once complications develop, laparoscopic cholecystectomy is the treatment of choice, with a mortality rate of 0.1–0.2%.

Patients with common bile duct stones, even if asymptomatic,
are at higher risk for complications and should be advised to undergo cholecystectomy
and stone extraction. Depending on local expertise, common bile duct stones may be remove
at the time of surgery or with endoscopic retrograde cholangiopancreatography (ERCP).

16. **What treatment options are available for patients who do not want to undergo
    cholecystectomy?**
    In selected patients, stones may be treated with dissolution therapy or with endoscopic or
    extracorporeal shock-wave lithotripsy.

17. **Describe the two types of dissolution therapy.**
    Oral bile acid dissolution therapy, usually with ursodeoxycholic acid, is limited to patients with
    small stones (usually <1 cm), which are composed of cholesterol and are not calcified. The
    cystic duct must be patent. Oral dissolution therapy is slow, costly, and limited by frequent
    recurrence of stones.
       Contact dissolution uses solvents, most commonly methyl tertbutyl ether, administered by
    catheter placed directly into the gallbladder. Complications include those caused by the cathet
    placement and side effects from solvent leakage into the duodenum, such as hemolytic anemi
    erosive or hemorrhagic duodenitis, and aspiration pneumonia. Stone recurrence is also
    common, unless oral therapy is added.

18. **What nonsurgical methods are available for stone removal or destruction?**
    Endoscopic sphincterotomy and *stone extraction* remain the nonsurgical procedures of choic
    for removal of common bile duct stones. Large, common bile duct stones may be crushed wit
    an endoscopically placed mechanical lithotriptor prior to removal. For gallbladder stones,
    extracorporeal shock wave lithotripsy has been used with some success. This procedure is m
    likely to be successful with small, single stones. Lithotripsy is combined frequently with oral b
    acid therapy to maximize dissolution rates. A functioning gallbladder is necessary to expel the
    fragments into the duodenum during the months after therapy, but biliary colic occurs
    frequently with lithotripsy as stone fragments pass.

KEY POINTS: DIAGNOSIS OF BILIARY SLUDGE AND STONES

1. Transabdominal ultrasonography should be the initial imaging modality to diagnose gallbladde
   sludge and stones.

2. Abdominal CT is less sensitive than ultrasonography in diagnosing sludge and stones.

3. Magnetic resonance cholangiopancreatography (MRCP) has high sensitivity and specificity fo
   diagnosing common bile duct stones.

19. **How accurate is ultrasonography for detection of cholecystolithiasis? Of
    choledocholithiasis?**
    Gallbladder stones can be diagnosed by ultrasonography with a sensitivity and specificity
    of over 90%, where they appear as high amplitude echoes with postacoustic shadowing
    (Fig. 36-2). Sludge can be seen usually as movable echogenic material without shadowing.
    Transabdominal sonography is the radiologic procedure of choice for diagnosing gallbladder
    disease. Unfortunately, the sensitivity of transabdominal ultrasound drops to about 30–40%
    for detection of stones within the common duct. Common bile duct stones may be

suspected in appropriate clinical situations, if dilated intrahepatic and common ducts are visualized. Endoscopic ultrasonography can detect over 90% of common bile duct stones.

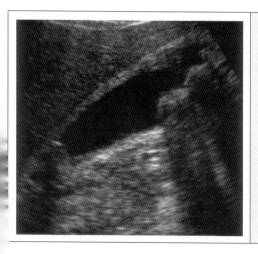

Figure 36-2. Ultrasonography showing gallstones. Stones appear as high-amplitude echoes within the gallbladder with postacoustic shadows.

20. **What is the role of magnetic resonance cholangiopancreatography in diagnosing common bile duct stones?**
Magnetic resonance cholangiopancreatography has high sensitivity (>90%) and specificity (>97%) for diagnosing common bile duct stones, when compared to ERCP. It is a useful test for the noninvasive diagnosis of common bile duct stones and may be the test of choice if the pretest probability of stones is low.

KEY POINTS: MANAGEMENT OF BILIARY SLUDGE AND STONES

1. Asymptomatic sludge or stones may be managed expectantly.

2. The treatment of choice for symptomatic sludge or stones is laparoscopic cholecystectomy.

3. Endoscopic retrograde cholangiopancreatography (ERCP) is useful in the management of common bile duct stones.

4. In selected patients who cannot or do not wish to undergo surgery, nonsurgical therapy with oral bile acid therapy or lithotripsy may be useful.

21. **A 65-year-old woman undergoes transabdominal ultrasonography due to postprandial abdominal pain. A 1-cm polyp is found in the gallbladder. What is the differential diagnosis?**
Polypoid lesions of the gallbladder wall include cholesterol polyps (the most common type), inflammatory polyps, adenomas, adenocarcinoma, and metastatic disease, particularly melanoma. The differentiation of neoplastic and benign lesions is a primary problem. Malignant lesions are more likely to be sessile and larger than 1 cm. Computed tomography (CT) or endoscopic ultrasound (EUS) may help in this differential diagnosis. In appropriate candidates

with polyps >1 cm, cholecystectomy is recommended due to the potential for malignancy. Smaller polyps may be followed by ultrasound, looking for a change in size or the appearance of new polyps.

22. **What is a porcelain gallbladder?**
A porcelain gallbladder is characterized by intramural calcification of the gallbladder wall. The diagnosis can be made by plain abdominal radiographs or abdominal CT. Prophylactic cholecystectomy is recommended to prevent development of carcinoma, which may occur in over 20% of cases.

23. **What is Mirizzi's syndrome?**
Mirizzi's syndrome occurs when a stone becomes impacted in the neck of the gallbladder or cystic duct, causing extrinsic compression of the common bile duct. The diagnosis should be considered in patients with cholecystitis who have higher than usual bilirubin levels (>5 mg/dL) or dilation of the intrahepatic or common hepatic duct (but *not* the common bile duct).

24. **What is the clinical significance of a low gallbladder ejection fraction?**
Gallbladder dysmotility is defined as a gallbladder ejection fraction less than 35%. It may be diagnosed by hepatobiliary scintigraphy with cholecystokinin infusion. Gallbladder dysmotility is often suspected in patients with biliary-type pain who do not have gallstones on ultrasonography. Management of patients with gallbladder dysmotility is controversial. Symptoms of biliary-type pain will resolve in 25–40% without treatment. In patients who undergo cholecystectomy, symptoms do not uniformly resolve. However, symptoms may also improve following treatment for other upper gastrointestinal tract disorders. Thus, the clinical significance of gallbladder dysmotility is not clear.

25. **Describe the clinical manifestations and treatment of acute acalculous cholecystitis.**
Acute acalculous cholecystitis occurs usually in older patients who are critically ill. Symptoms frequently associated with gallstone-related cholecystitis are often absent, and patients may present with fevers only. Complications can develop rapidly, and 50–70% of patients may develop gangrene, empyema, or perforation of the gallbladder. The most useful diagnostic test is transabdominal ultrasound. Hepatobiliary scintigraphy is limited by frequent false-positive results. Management should include supportive treatment with antibiotic coverage of anaerobic and gram-negative bacteria. Gallbladder decompression by percutaneous cholecystostomy tube placement is often effective.

WEBSITE

http://davel.mgh.harvard.edu

BIBLIOGRAPHY

1. Barie PS, Fischer E: Acute acalculous cholecystitis. J Am Coll Surg 180:232–244, 1995.
2. Carr-Locke DL: Therapeutic role of ERCP in the management of suspected common bile duct stones. Gastrointest Endosc 56:S170–S174, 2002.

3. Diehl AK: Epidemiology and natural history of gallstone disease. Gastroenterol Clin North Am 20:1–19, 1991.

4. Everhart JE, Khare M, Hill M, Maurer KR: Prevalence and ethnic differences in gallbladder disease in the United States. Gastroenterology 117:632–639, 1999.

5. Goncalves RM, Harris JA, Rivera DE: Biliary dyskinesia: Natural history and surgical results. Am Surg 64:493–497, 1998.

6. Gracie WA, Ransohoff DF: The natural history of silent gallstones. N Engl J Med 307:798–800, 1982.

7. Ko CW, Sekijima JH, Lee SP: Biliary sludge. Ann Intern Med 130:301–311, 1999.

8. Lai PB, Kwong KJ, Leung KL, et al: Randomized trial of early versus delayed laparoscopic cholecystectomy for acute cholecystitis. Br J Surg 85:764–767, 1998.

9. Lee SP, Nicholls JF, Park HZ: Biliary sludge as a cause of acute pancreatitis. N Engl J Med 326:589–593, 1992.

10. Maclure KM, Hayes KC, Colditz GA: Weight, diet, and the risk of symptomatic gallstones in middle-aged women. N Engl J Med 321:563–569, 1989.

11. Prat F, Amouyal G, Amouyal P, et al: Prospective controlled study of endoscopic ultrasonography and endoscopic retrograde cholangiography in patients with suspected common-bile duct lithiasis. Lancet 347:75–79, 1996.

12. Romagnuolo J, Bardou M, Rahme E, et al: Magnetic resonance cholangiopancreatography: A meta-analysis of test performance in suspected biliary disease. Ann Intern Med 139:547–557, 2003.

13. Shiffman ML, Kaplan GD, Brinkman-Kaplan V, Vickers FF: Prophylaxis against gallstone formation with ursodeoxycholic acid in patients participating in a very-low-calorie diet program. Ann Intern Med 122:899–905, 1995.

14. Shiffman ML, Sugerman HJ, Kellum JM, et al: Gallstone formation after rapid weight loss: A prospective study in patients undergoing gastric bypass surgery of morbid obesity. Am J Gastroenterol 86:1000–1005, 1991.

15. Swidsinski A, Lee SP: The role of bacteria in gallstone pathogenesis. Front Biosci 6:E93–E103, 2001.

16. Terzi C, Sokmen S, Seckin S, et al: Polypoid lesions of the gallbladder: Report of 100 cases with special reference to operative indications. Surgery 127:622–627, 2000.

17. Tint GS, Salen G, Colalillo A, et al: Ursodeoxycholic acid: A safe and effective agent for dissolving gallstones. Ann Intern Med 97:351–356, 1982.

CHAPTER 37

SPHINCTER OF ODDI DYSFUNCTION

Erik W. Springer, MD, and Raj J. Shah, MD

1. What is the sphincter of Oddi?

The sphincter of Oddi is a fibromuscular sheath that encircles the terminal portion of the common bile duct, main pancreatic duct (Wirsung), and common channel in the second portion of the duodenum. It is made up of smooth muscle. Three interconnected sphincters exist: choledochus, pancreaticus, and ampulla (Fig. 37-1). Ruggero Oddi, as a medical student, published the early morphologic observations of the sphincter in 1887.

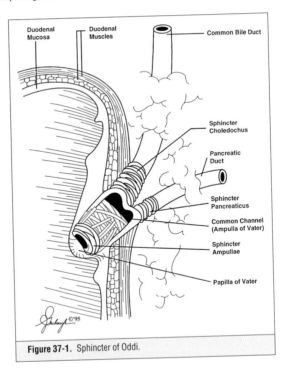

Figure 37-1. Sphincter of Oddi.

2. How does the sphincter of Oddi function?

- Regulates bile and pancreatic juice into the duodenum
- Reduces duodenal reflux into the pancreatic and biliary ducts
- Contracts tonically during the interdigestive period to promote gallbladder filling
- Contracts phasically in the digestive period to promote flow of bile into the duodenum

Its activity is increased by cholinergic stimulation. Endogenous substances also control the sphincter. Motilin increases the intensity of sphincter contractions. Cholecystokinin (CCK) is induced by food intake and stimulates contraction of the gallbladder and relaxation of the sphincter. Vasoactive intestinal peptide (VIP) and nitric oxide promote sphincter relaxation.

3. **What is sphincter of Oddi dysfunction (SOD)?**

Sphincter of Oddi dysfunction is a benign disorder characterized by a functional or structural obstruction at the level of the sphincter of Oddi. It is suspected in patients presenting with upper abdominal pain, suggestive of a biliary or pancreatic origin. Objective measures, such as transient elevations in liver or pancreatic enzymes and ductal dilation on noninvasive imaging, are sought to support the clinical suspicion.

4. **Describe the pathophysiology of sphincter of Oddi dysfunction.**

There seem to be two abnormalities that can lead to SOD, and both may be present in a single patient. One is a primary motor abnormality of the sphincter termed *biliary dyskinesia* or "spasm" (elevated pressure). The other is fibrosis or inflammation, most likely from recurrent passage of biliary stones/microlithiasis. One explanation as to why these patients present postcholecystectomy is that gallbladder distention can accommodate increased biliary pressure. Further, it has been postulated that cholecystectomy may sever neuroinhibitory pathways that normally cause sphincter relaxation in response to increased biliary pressure. However, SOD is also identified in patients with an intact gallbladder.

5. **Name typical symptoms of sphincter of Oddi dysfunction.**

Symptoms can be either biliary or pancreatic in nature. Pain is located in the epigastrium or right upper quadrant with radiation to the back or to the right infrascapular region and may be meal-related. It is episodic or continuous with periodic exacerbations. Symptoms compatible with irritable bowel syndrome (IBS) often coexist, and it can often be difficult to distinguish SOD from patients with non-nuclear dyspepsia. Another manifestation is "idiopathic" acute recurrent pancreatitis as a result of sphincter hypertension. Other structural abnormalities, such as costochondritis, ulcer, gastroesophageal reflux disease, malignancy, stones, and chronic pancreatitis, must be ruled out before the diagnosis of SOD is pursued.

6. **Who is at risk for sphincter of Oddi dysfunction?**

Females in their third through fifth decades of life are at risk. The female predominance is as high as 90%. Symptoms often become apparent after cholecystectomy (hence the older term *postcholecystectomy syndrome*), but, in many cases, patients will have had empiric cholecystectomy for pain that was thought to originate from the gallbladder.

7. **How common is sphincter of Oddi dysfunction?**

The incidence in patients who have undergone cholecystectomy has been estimated to be approximately 1%.

8. **What diagnostic evaluation should be considered in a patient presenting with symptoms suggestive of sphincter of Oddi dysfunction?**

Start with a thorough history and physical exam. The history will often determine which diagnostic testing is required prior to pursuing a diagnosis of SOD. The physical exam during a flare of pain often reveals a nontoxic-appearing patient with tenderness in the epigastrium or right upper quadrant. Hepatic enzymes and pancreatic enzymes should be obtained during or soon after any flare of pain. Imaging with ultrasound or computed tomography (CT) is performed to exclude cholelithiasis, chronic pancreatitis, or other intra-abdominal pathology. If nausea and vomiting is a predominant feature, then gastric emptying studies can be considered. If dyspeptic or reflux-type symptoms are apparent, then a 24-hour esophageal pH study or upper endoscopy is reasonable.

9. **Name noninvasive tests that may be utilized to diagnose sphincter of Oddi dysfunction.**

Provocation studies involve a stimulus with a fatty meal or cholecystokinin (CCK) and ultrasound imaging to assess for an abnormal increase of the bile duct diameter (>2 mm). Secretin is used to evaluate for outflow obstruction in the pancreatic duct by assessing pancreatic duct diameter with transabdominal ultrasound or magnetic resonance cholangiopancreatography (MRCP). In general, if there is a sustained dilation (>30 minutes), the test is considered positiv The Nardi provocation test involves the administration of morphine and neostigmine to increas sphincter pressure and pancreatic secretion, respectively. The test is considered positive if pai or elevation in hepatic or pancreatic enzymes occurs. Hepatobiliary scintigraphy utilizes a tech netium-99m labeled dye that is hepatically excreted and assesses for delayed biliary drainage. Noninvasive tests rarely exclude with certainty stones or strictures as a cause of outflow obstruction and are not commonly used to diagnose SOD.

10. **When should one consider endoscopic retrograde cholangiopancreatography (ERCP) with sphincter of Oddi dysfunction (SOM)?**
    SOM should be considered in those patients with symptoms that cannot be explained by other diagnoses and have failed therapeutic medication trials. Because there often exists an overlap wi dysmotility or IBS-type symptoms, antispasmodics and low-dose antidepressants or selective serotonin reuptake inhibitors should be tried initially. Narcotic-requiring pain may suggest a need for manometric studies; however, these medications interfere with accurate pressure measure- ments. Ideally, manometry should be performed prior to patients becoming narcotic-dependent.

11. **How is sphincter of Oddi manometry performed, and what manometric criteria define sphincter of Oddi dysfunction?**
    Deep cannulation of the biliary or pancreatic duct is required. SOM is most commonly performe using a water perfusion, aspirating catheter introduced through the working channel of the ERCP scope. The catheter is attached to external transducers, and the recordings are displaye and recorded on a computer monitor or paper strip. Prior to performing pull-through measure ments in a stepwise fashion across the sphincter, a duodenal baseline is obtained. The major criterion for SOD is defined as a mean basal pressure increase of >40 mm Hg above the duodenal baseline for a 30-second duration on two separate pull-throughs. Less established criteria assess basal ductal pressure, phasic sphincter contractile frequency and amplitude, and phasic contractile duration.

12. **Which medications can interfere with sphincter of Oddi manometry pressure measurements?**
    Narcotics and smooth muscle relaxants should be held prior to the procedure. During the ERC narcotic analgesia and antimotility agents (i.e., glucagon) should be avoided. Benzodiazepines or propofol are used predominantly. The 1994 study by Elta and Barnett showed, however, tha meperidine had no effect on the basal sphincter pressure. Nevertheless, it is still generally avoided or limited to 1 mg/kg.

13. **What are the possible complications of endoscopic retrograde cholangiopancreatography with sphincter of Oddi manometry?**
    The types of complications are similar to ERCP performed for other indications. These include pancreatitis, cholangitis, perforation, bleeding, and sedation or anesthesia-related adverse events. However, there is an elevated risk of pancreatitis in the patient subgroup that has sus- pected SOD. This is as high as 15–30% and applies to all patients with suspected SOD who undergo ERCP.

14. **Is manometry an independent risk factor for postendoscopic retrograde cholangiopancreatography pancreatitis?**
    Likely, the answer is no. Although previous studies have suggested that manometry carries increased risk, more recent data have shown that the increased risk of pancreatitis in patients with suspected SOD is intrinsic to the patient population and characteristics of the procedure. Examples include difficult cannulation, number of pancreatic duct injections, female gender, a prior episode of pancreatitis. These patients are at an elevated risk for pancreatitis from ERCP,

KEY POINTS: COMMON MANIFESTATIONS OF SPHINCTER OF ODDI DYSFUNCTION ✓

1. Epigastric or right upper quadrant pain

2. Transient elevation in liver enzymes

3. Dilated bile or pancreatic duct

4. Idiopathic acute recurrent pancreatitis

whether or not manometry is performed. However, although the duration of pancreatic manometry has not been specifically assessed, it likely plays a role. Suspected SOD alone is an independent risk factor for the development of post-ERCP pancreatitis (Freeman, et al. 2001).

15. **What is the Milwaukee Classification?**

The standard categorization of SOD is the Milwaukee classification (also known as *Geenen-Hogan*) applied generally in the postcholecystectomy patient. Classification is performed before SOM and is predictive of the frequency of abnormal SOM and symptomatic response to sphincterotomy. Currently, the Modified Milwaukee criteria (less stringent than the original Milwaukee criteria) are used. Laboratory values are during an episode of pain and should normalize in the absence of pain to be consistent with transient outflow obstruction and SOD. The schemes are similar for both biliary and pancreatic types (Tables 37-1 and 37-2).

Table 37-3 displays the results of studies where patients were stratified into SOD types prior to SOM. The right column gives the percentage of those who had biliary sphincter hypertension. In general, it is thought that patients with SOD type I or II are more likely to have a structural outflow obstruction (i.e., stenosis) versus SOD type III patients, who are more likely to have a functional problem with the sphincter.

TABLE 37-1. MODIFIED MILWAUKEE CLASSIFICATION: BILIARY

Type I	Biliary type pain, ALT/AST/Alk Phos >1.1X ULN, bile duct >10 mm
Type II	Biliary type pain and either ALT/AST/Alk Phos >1.1X ULN or bile duct >10 mm
Type III	Biliary type pain only

ALT = alanine aminotransferase, AST = aspartate aminotransferase, Alk Phos = alkaline phosphatase, ULN = upper limit of normal.

TABLE 37-2. MODIFIED MILWAUKEE CLASSIFICATION: PANCREATIC

Type I	Pancreatic-type pain and amylase/lipase >ULN and dilated pancreatic duct[*]
Type II	Pancreatic-type pain and either amylase/lipase >ULN or dilated pancreatic duct[*]
Type III	Pancreatic-type pain only

[*]Pancreatic duct >6 mm in the head and >5 mm in the body of the pancreas.
ULN = upper limit of normal.

TABLE 37-3. SUMMARY OF STUDY RESULTS	
Suspected Biliary SOD Type	Elevated Basal Sphincter Pressure
Type I	>90%
Type II	55–65%
Type III	25–60%

SOD = sphincter of Oddi dysfunction.

16. **Does normal sphincter of Oddi manometry on one occasion rule out sphincter of Oddi dysfunction?**
No, SOD has been documented in patients with persistent symptoms who have previously had normal sphincter pressures.

17. **Are there medicines to treat sphincter of Oddi dysfunction?**
SOD, especially milder cases, can be treated medically. A low-fat diet to decrease pancreaticobiliary stimulation may improve symptoms. The improvement, however, can also related to concomitant upper intestinal tract dysmotility as fat increases gastric emptying time. Pharmacologic therapy has also been investigated. Medications that decrease the pressure of the sphincter (such as calcium channel blockers and nitrates) have been shown to reduce symptoms in some patients. However, treatment is often hampered by side effects. Antispasmodic agents may be useful, as well.

18. **How is sphincter of Oddi dysfunction treated endoscopically?**
The standard endoscopic treatment for SOD is sphincterotomy. Manometry is deferred in patients with type I SOD because of the high clinical response rate. In SOD types II and III patients, manometry should be performed to document either biliary or pancreatic sphincter hypertension. Only those with sphincter hypertension are expected to benefit from sphincterotomy. In patients with suspected biliary SOD type III with an intact gallbladder, it is probably reasonable to first perform cholecystectomy and proceed to ERCP with manometry if there is no response, or for recurrent symptoms.

19. **What is the clinical response rate of sphincterotomy for treatment of sphincter of Oddi dysfunction?**
It is dependent on the initial SOD classification. There is a higher benefit in patients with SOD type I (Table 37-4). If benefit is achieved, improvement is generally long-term (years) in the absence of restenosis of the sphincterotomy.

TABLE 37-4. RESPONSE RATE OF SPHINCTEROTOMY		
SOD Type	Pain Relief from Sphincterotomy if SOM is Abnormal	Pain Relief from Sphincterotomy if SOM is Normal
Type I	>90%	>90%
Type II	85%	35%
Type III	55–65%	<10%

SOD = sphincter of Oddi dysfunction, SOM = sphincter of Oddi manometry.

20. Can pharmacologic agents cause clinical sphincter of Oddi dysfunction?

Yes. Among the most notable substances are opiates. Increased pressure in the biliary duct has been documented following administration of fentanyl and morphine. Some patients will experience biliary-type pain following use of these agents. In addition, SOD has been documented in a series of male opium addicts. It is theorized that long-term opium use leads to sphincter hypertension and sustained dysfunction (Sharma, 2003).

21. In sphincter of Oddi dysfunction patients, when should the pancreatic duct be stented prophylactically?

Prophylactic stenting of the pancreatic duct in patients with pancreatic sphincter hypertension undergoing biliary sphincterotomy reduces the incidence of post-ERCP pancreatitis (26% vs. 7%, according to Tarnasky et al. in 1998). Pancreatic duct stenting should also be performed in patients undergoing pancreatic sphincterotomy and considered in those with a history of post-ERCP pancreatitis. Some experts recommend placing a pancreatic stent in all patients with suspected SOD who undergo ERCP, especially if biliary cannulation was difficult.

22. Why do some patients with documented sphincter of Oddi dysfunction not respond to sphincterotomy?

Abnormal manometry in a symptomatic patient does not prove a cause-effect relationship. It may be a consequence (i.e., chronic narcotic use or chronic pancreatitis) rather than an etiology of disease. Potential reasons for a lack of response or recurrent symptoms following a clinical response include an incomplete sphincterotomy, restenosis, concomitant pancreatic sphincter hypertension, underlying chronic pancreatitis, or a disease unrelated to the biliary or pancreatic system.

WEBSITES

1. http://www.pancreas.org/

2. http://www.ccc.musc.edu/ddc_pub/patientinfo/surgeries/pancreatic/Page16.html

3. http://www.indiana.edu/~engs/hints/oddi.html

4. http://www.ddc.musc.edu/ddc_pub/digestiveProbs/diseases/pancBiliary/sphincterOddi.htm

5. http://www.dave1.mgh.harvard.edu

BLIOGRAPHY

Aymerich RR, Prakash C, Aliperti G: Sphincter of Oddi manometry: Is it necessary to measure both biliary and pancreatic sphincter pressures? Gastrointest Endosc 52(2):183–186, 2000.

Corazziari E, Shaffer EA, Hogan WJ, et al: Functional disorders of the biliary tract and pancreas. Gut 45(S2):II48–II54, 1999.

Coyle WJ, Pinau BC, Tarnasky PR, et al: Evaluation of unexplained acute and acute recurrent pancreatitis using endoscopic retrograde cholangiopancreatography, sphincter of Oddi manometry and endoscopic ultrasound. Endoscopy 34(8):617–623, 2002.

Craig AG, Peter D, Saccone GT, et al: Scintigraphy versus manometry in patients with suspected biliary sphincter of Oddi dysfunction. Gut 52:352–357, 2003.

Elta GH, Barnett JL: Meperidine need not be proscribed during sphincter of Oddi manometry. Gastrointest Endosc 40(1):7–9, 1994.

Eversman D, Fogel EL, Rusche R, et al: Frequency of abnormal pancreatic and biliary sphincter manometry compared with clinical suspicion of sphincter of Oddi dysfunction. Gastrointest Endosc 50(5):637–641, 1999.

7. Fazel A, Quadri A, Catalano MF, et al: Does a pancreatic duct stent prevent post-ERCP pancreatitis? A prospective randomized study. Gastrointest Endosc 57(3):291–294, 2003.

8. Freeman ML, DiSario JA, Nelson DB, et al: Risk factors for post-ERCP pancreatitis: A prospective, multicenter study. Gastrointest Endosc 54(4):425–434, 2001.

9. Kaw M, Brodmerkel GJ: ERCP, biliary crystal analysis, and sphincter of Oddi manometry in idiopathic recurrent pancreatitis. Gastrointest Endosc 55(2):157–162, 2002.

10. Lai K: Sphincter of Oddi and acute pancreatitis: A new treatment option. JOP 3(4):83–85, 2003.

11. Linder JD, Geels W, Wilcox CM: Prevalence of sphincter of Oddi dysfunction: Can results from specialized centers be generalized? Dig Dis Sci 47(11):2411–2415, 2002.

12. Maldonado ME, Brady PG, Mamel JJ, Robinson B: Incidence of pancreatitis in patients undergoing sphincter Oddi manometry (SOM). Am J Gastroenterol 94(2):387–390, 1998.

13. Park S, Watkins JL, Fogel EL, et al: Long-term outcome of endoscopic dual pancreatobiliary sphincterotomy patients with manometry-documented sphincter of Oddi dysfunction and normal pancreatogram. Gastrointest Endosc 57(4):481–491, 2003.

14. Rosenblatt ML, Catalano MF, Alcocer E, Geenen JE: Comparison of sphincter of Oddi manometry, fatty meal sonography, and hepatobiliary scintigraphy in the diagnosis of sphincter of Oddi dysfunction. Gastrointest Endosc 54(6):697–704, 2001.

15. Sharma SS: Sphincter of Oddi dysfunction in patients addicted to opium: An unrecognized entity. Gastrointest Endosc 55(3):427–430, 2003.

16. Sherman S: What is the role of ERCP in the setting of abdominal pain of pancreatic or biliary origin (suspected sphincter of Oddi dysfunction)? Gastrointest Endosc 56(6S):S258–S266, 2002.

17. Sherman S, Lehman GA: Sphincter of Oddi dysfunction: Diagnosis and treatment. Pancreas 2(6):382–400, 2001.

18. Silverman WB, Slivka A, Rabinovitz M, Wilson J: Hybrid classification of sphincter of Oddi dysfunction based simplified Milwaukee criteria. Dig Dis Sci 46(2):278–281, 2001.

19. Tanaka M: Advances in research and clinical practice in motor disorders of the sphincter of Oddi. J Hepatobiliary Pancreat Surg 9:564–568, 2002.

20. Tarnasky PR: Mechanical prevention of post-ERCP pancreatitis by pancreatic stents: Results, techniques, and indications. JOP 4(1):58–67, 2003.

21. Tarnasky PR, Palesch YY, Cunningham JT, et al: Pancreatic stenting prevents pancreatitis after biliary sphincterotomy in patients with sphincter of Oddi dysfunction. Gastroenterology 115:1518–1524, 1998.

22. Toouli J, Roberts-Thomson IC, Kellow J, et al: Manometry based randomized trial of endoscopic sphincterotomy for sphincter of Oddi dysfunction. Gut 46:98–102, 2000.

23. Varadarajulu S, Hawes RH, Cotton PB: Determination of sphincter of Oddi dysfunction in patients with prior normal manometry. Gastrointest Endosc 58(3):341–344, 2003.

IV. PANCREATIC DISORDERS

ACUTE PANCREATITIS

Michael W. Cheng, MD, and Jamie S. Barkin, MD

CHAPTER 38

1. **What are the causes of acute pancreatitis (AP)?**
   - *Mechanical:* gallstones, microlithiasis (biliary sludge), sphincter of Oddi dysfunction, papillary stenosis, duodenal diverticula, pancreas divisum, trauma
   - *Toxins:* alcohol, drugs, scorpion venom
   - *Infectious:* viral, bacterial, parasitic
   - *Metabolic:* hypertriglyceridemia, hypercalcemia
   - *Ischemic:* thromboembolic, vasculitis, hypotension, dehydration
   - *Genetic:* cystic fibrosis, hereditary
   - *Tumors:* ampullary, pancreatic, intraductal papillary mucinous tumors (IPMT)
   - *Other:* idiopathic, postoperative, postendoscopic retrograde cholangiopancreatography (ERCP), pregnancy

2. **What are the most common causes of acute pancreatitis?**
   Gallstones and alcohol abuse are the most common causes of AP in the United States, each accounting for at least 30–35% of cases. The leading etiology depends on the population studied; for instance, alcoholism may predominate in many inner cities.

   Idiopathic AP, in which a source is not identified, ranks as the third leading cause of AP. Recent studies, however, have demonstrated the presence of microlithiasis in up to two thirds of these patients when they undergo further investigation with repeated gallbladder ultrasound or bile crystal analysis. The theory that many cases of idiopathic AP are caused by microlithiasis is supported by a reduction in recurrences of AP in patients who undergo endoscopic sphincterotomy or cholecystectomy when compared with untreated patients (10% vs. 73%, $p<.01$). Chemical dissolution with ursodeoxycholic acid can also prevent recurrences.

3. **Which drugs have been reported to cause acute pancreatitis?**
   The list can be remembered by using the mnemonic **"NO IDEA"**:
   N = *N*SAIDs (sulindac, salicylates)
   O = *O*ther (valproate)
   I = *I*BD drugs (sulfasalazine, 5-aminosalicylic acid)
      = *I*mmunosuppressants (L-asparaginase, azathioprine, 6-mercaptopurine)
   D = *D*iuretics (furosemide, thiazides)
   E = *E*strogens
   A = *A*ntibiotics (metronidazole, sulfonamides, tetracycline, nitrofurantoin, stibogluconate)
      = *A*IDS drugs (didanosine, pentamidine)
   Drug-induced pancreatitis can occur immediately upon initiation of the drug or be delayed by months.

4. **How is pregnancy associated with acute pancreatitis?**
   Coexisting cholelithiasis or microlithiasis is present in about 90% of cases. Other causes include hyperlipidemia and medications. Most episodes occur in the third trimester or postpartum period. The overall prognosis is good.

5. **Which infectious agents have been implicated in causing acute pancreatitis?**
    Viruses (i.e., mumps, coxsackievirus, cytomegalovirus, varicella-zoster, herpes simplex, Epstein-Barr, hepatitis A, hepatitis B); bacteria (i.e., *Mycoplasma, Legionella, Leptospira, Salmonella*, tuberculosis, brucellosis); fungi (i.e., *Aspergillus, Candida albicans*); and parasites (*Toxoplasma, cryptosporidium, ascaris, Clonorchis sinensis*)

6. **How do *Clonorchis sinensis* and *ascaris* cause acute pancreatitis?**
    These parasites cause AP by blocking the main pancreatic duct and obstructing drainage of pancreatic secretions.

7. **Is there an increased incidence of acute pancreatitis in patients with acquired immunodeficiency syndrome (AIDS)?**
    Yes. Up to 10% of patients with AIDS develop AP. The cause is usually multifactorial, with drugs and infections being the most common.

8. **How does trauma cause acute pancreatitis?**
    AP can be caused by either blunt trauma or penetrating trauma. Blunt trauma occurs usually from compression of the pancreatic body against the spine. In adults, this may be seen during an automobile accident with a steering wheel or seat-belt injury. Trauma is the most common cause of AP in children, usually as a result of bicycle handle-bar injury. Less frequently, AP can also be caused by penetrating trauma, for instance, gunshot or stab wounds with damage to the pancreas.

    Traumatic pancreatitis can range from mild contusion to severe crush injury with transection of the gland. Possible sequelae from trauma include acute duct rupture with pancreatic ascites or pancreatic duct strictures that result in recurrent and chronic pancreatitis.

9. **What is pancreas divisum? Is it associated with an increased incidence of recurrent acute pancreatitis?**
    Pancreas divisum is the most common congenital variant of the pancreatic anatomy, occurring in approximately 5–10% of the population. It results when the embryologic dorsal and ventral pancreases fail to fuse, causing most of the pancreatic exocrine secretions to drain through the duct of Santorini (dorsal duct) and through the smaller minor papilla into the duodenum. Normally, pancreatic drainage flows through the duct of Wirsung (ventral duct) and through the larger major papilla into the duodenum. Pancreas divisum is usually diagnosed by endoscopic retrograde pancreatography (ERP) but may also be diagnosed by magnetic resonance cholangiopancreatography (MRCP), with or without secretin and endoscopic ultrasound (EUS).

    Whether pancreas divisum causes recurrent AP is controversial. Ninety-five percent of peop with pancreas divisum are asymptomatic, and their anomaly is discovered incidentally. It is, however, generally accepted that the combination of pancreas divisum along with a stenotic minor papilla leads to dorsal pancreatic duct obstruction and pancreatitis. Therapeutic options for these patients are decompression of the obstructed pancreatic duct with endoscopic sphinc terotomy or surgical sphincteroplasty of the minor papilla. Stenting across the minor papilla may serve as a diagnostic test of sphincter dysfunction, if episodes of AP or pain occur frequently.

10. **What is the relationship between hypertriglyceridemia and acute pancreatitis?**
    Hypertriglyceridemia may cause up to 4% of AP cases. Usually, serum triglyceride levels above 1000 mg/dL are required to induce an attack of AP. Treatment with diet and lipid-lowering ager can reduce recurrence when the initial episode has resolved.

11. **What is the relationship between hypercalcemia and acute pancreatitis?**
    Hypercalcemia from any cause (e.g., hyperparathyroidism, metastatic bone disease, sarcoidosis) may lead to AP. Possible mechanisms include calcium activation of trypsinogen to trypsin within the pancreas, and calcification with possible stone formation in the pancreatic duct.

12. **How is the diagnosis of acute pancreatitis made?**

The diagnosis of AP is based on clinical assessment, biochemical analysis, and radiologic evaluation. In general, AP is clinically characterized by acute onset of epigastric abdominal pain that radiates into the back in a patient with risk factors such as alcohol and biliary disease. Compatible laboratory data include at least a threefold elevation in the serum amylase and/or lipase. Presentation may be mild to severe, depending on the amount of pancreatic inflammation and injury to regional or distant organs. The role of imaging with computed tomography (CT) is twofold, to find pancreatic inflammation and to exclude another source of pathology.

13. **How does serum amylase compare to serum lipase in the diagnosis of acute pancreatitis?**

Serum amylase rises typically within 6–12 hours of AP onset and declines gradually over 3–5 days. Serum lipase is elevated within the first 24 hours of AP and remains elevated for a longer period than serum amylase. Therefore, it may be more valuable than serum amylase in patients with delayed onset of suspected AP. Sensitivity of serum amylase and lipase are similar; however, some feel that specificity is greater with serum lipase given that most lipase stems from the pancreas. Fractionation of elevated total serum amylase into pancreatic-type (p-type) and salivary-type (s-type) isoamylase is available in most laboratories and may help in the diagnosis of AP. Recall that abdominal pathology (i.e., intestinal obstruction) can cause elevation of pancreatic isoamylase (see later).

14. **What are the nonpancreatic sources of hyperamylasemia and hyperlipasemia?**

Hyperamylasemia may be seen in diseases of the salivary glands, lungs, fallopian tubes, ovarian cysts, gallbladder, small bowel, and appendix. Certain malignancies may also be associated with hyperamylasemia, including tumors of the pancreas, colon, lung, and ovary. Elevations in serum amylase may also be seen in macroamylasemia (see later), metabolic acidosis, and anorexia nervosa.

Although most serum lipase originates from the pancreas, other possible sources include the stomach, intestine, liver, and tongue. Serum lipase is also elevated in macrolipasemia. Conditions that increase intestinal permeability (inflammation, perforation, obstruction) or decrease renal clearance can also result in hyperamylasemia or hyperlipasemia.

15. **What are macroamylasemia and macrolipasemia?**

These are entities in which amylase or lipase is bound to a serum immunoglobulin, thus forming a large molecule that does not readily undergo renal clearance. This results in elevation of the serum amylase or lipase level. In macroamylasemia, the serum amylase is high; however, urine amylase and amylase:creatinine clearance ratio (ACR) are low (usually ACR <1%). Associated conditions include celiac disease, inflammatory bowel disease, lymphoma, and connective tissue disease.

16. **What cause of acute pancreatitis should be suspected in patients who present with normal serum amylase levels?**

Hypertriglyceridemia. One possible mechanism is that hypertriglyceridemia interferes with the laboratory measurement of the actual amylase level by preventing the calorimetric reading of the assay endpoint. Diluting the serum allows for true values of serum amylase to be measured. Whether this dilution reduces interference of light transmission by the lactescent plasma or decreases the concentration of a circulating amylase inhibitor associated with triglyceride elevation is unclear.

17. **Does the magnitude of hyperamylasemia or hyperlipasemia correlate with the severity of acute pancreatitis?**

No. The magnitude of elevation in pancreatic enzymes does not generally correlate with the severity of pancreatitis and has no prognostic value.

18. **What is the most reliable marker for diagnosing biliary acute pancreatitis?**
A greater than threefold elevation of *serum alanine aminotransferase (ALT) level* has a positive predictive value of 95% for biliary AP. Bilirubin and alkaline phosphatase levels are not specific for biliary tract origin of AP. Amylase:lipase ratios and the magnitude of their elevation are also not helpful in distinguishing the cause of AP.

19. **How is acute pancreatitis classified?**
The most widely accepted classification system is based on the collaboration of 40 international experts on AP known as the 1992 Atlanta Symposium. AP is divided into mild and severe disease. *Mild AP* is defined as minimal or no organ dysfunction and is usually associated with a self-limited course and an uneventful recovery. *Severe AP* consists of multiorgan failure and/or local complications, including pseudocyst or necrosis with possible superimposed infection. Severe AP may be predicted by clinical criteria, including Ranson's criteria and APACHE-II prognostic scoring systems (see later).
Distinction is also made between *interstitial pancreatitis* and *necrotizing pancreatitis* based on the findings of a contrast-enhanced dynamic CT. Interstitial pancreatitis is characterized by interstitial edema and inflammation, with no macroscopic parenchymal necrosis. Mortality is approximately 1%. This CT finding is usually associated with mild AP. Conversely, necrotizing pancreatitis is characterized by macroscopic focal or diffuse necrosis with nonviable parenchyma. Mortality for sterile necrosis approaches 10–15% and increases to 30–35% if the necrosis becomes infected. Patients with pancreatic necrosis have a 30–50% chance of developing infection of the necrosis.

20. **What prognostic scoring systems are used to assess the severity of acute pancreatitis?**
Clinical prognostic scores include Ranson's criteria, simplified Glasgow criteria, and APACHE-II system. Additionally, a CT severity index can be used.
Ranson's criteria (Table 38-1) consist of 11 indices used to assess the severity of AP. Five indices are measured on admission, and the remaining six indices are measured at 48 hours after admission (*see* Table 38-1). Thus, one of the limitations of this system is that a full 48 hours is required after admission prior to fully assessing disease severity. In addition, since the 1970s when the Ranson system was developed, subsequent studies have suggested that Ranson's criteria are more predictive of ethanol-associated AP and less so for biliary AP. The score calculated from Ranson's criteria correlates with mortality (score <3 = 5%, score 3–5 = 10%, score ≥6 = more than 60%). Ranson score ≥6 is also associated with more complications from AP, including necrosis and infected necrosis.

TABLE 38-1. RANSON'S CRITERIA	
At Admission	**Within 48 Hr of Admission**
Age >55 yr	Hct drop >10%
WBC >16,000/mm^3	BUN rise >5 mg/dL
Glucose >200 mg/dL	Calcium <8 mg/dL
LDH >350 IU/L	PaO$_2$ <60 mmHg
AST >250 U/L	Base deficit >4 mEq/L
	Fluid sequestration >6 L

WBC = white blood cell, LDH = lactate dehydrogenase, AST = aspartate aminotransferase, Hct = hematocrit, BUN = blood urea nitrogen, PaO$_2$ = partial pressure of oxygen in arterial blood.

The *simplified Glasgow criteria* (Table 38-2) consist of eight indices used to assess the severity of AP measured at 48 hours. It was initially developed by Clement Imrie in Glasgow, Scotland, based on Ranson's criteria. It has since undergone several modifications and, subsequently, is more predictive of severity in biliary AP. A score >2 predicts a severe attack.

TABLE 38-2. SIMPLIFIED GLASGOW CRITERIA

During Initial 48 Hr

Age >55
WBC >15,000/mm^3
LDH >600 IU/L
Glucose >180 mg/dL
Albumin <3.2 g/dL
Calcium <8 mg/dL
PaO$_2$ <60 mmHg
BUN >45 mg/dL

WBC = white blood cell, LDH = lactate dehydrogenase, PaO$_2$ = partial pressure of oxygen in arterial blood, BUN = blood urea nitrogen.

The *APACHE-II* (Acute Physiology and Chronic Health Evaluation) score's advantage is that it can be applied at the time of admission and used continuously (Table 38-3). The scoring system assigns points for age, acute physiologic variables, and chronic health status in determining a total score. An APACHE-II score ≥8 is associated with an unfavorable prognosis. Unfortunately, it is a cumbersome scoring system.

TABLE 38-3. APACHE-II SCORING SYSTEM

Age: ≥45 yr assigned ascending points to age 75 (6 points maximum)

Acute physiology score (points assigned for abnormal values; 50 points maximum)
　　Vital signs
　　Arterial blood gases
　　Serum electrolytes
　　Glasgow coma score (15 – actual GCS)

Chronic health score (points assigned for severe organ system dysfunction or immunocompromise)
　　Liver: cirrhosis, portal hypertension, encephalopathy/coma
　　Cardiovascular: New York Heart Association, class IV
　　Respiratory: severe chronic obstructive, restrictive, or vascular disease
　　Renal: chronic dialysis
　　Immunocompromise: leukemia, lymphoma, AIDS, or immunosuppressive therapy

GCS = Glasgow Coma Score.

The *CT Severity Index* (Table 38-4), characterized by Balthazar, assigns points based on presence and extent of pancreatic inflammation, fluid collection, and the degree of necrosis scoring system correlates with Ranson's criteria for assessing severity, morbidity, and mo The presence of pancreatic necrosis increases the likelihood of infection, which portends a favorable prognosis. Morbidity and mortality are low with scores up to 2. A score of 7–10 associated with morbidity of 92% and mortality of 17%.

TABLE 38-4. COMPUTED TOMOGRAPHY SEVERITY INDEX	
	Points
Grade of Acute Pancreatitis	
A Normal pancreas	0
B Pancreatic enlargement	1
C Pancreatic or peripancreatic inflammation	2
D Single peripancreatic fluid collection	3
E Multiple fluid collections	4
Degree of Necrosis	
No necrosis	0
Necrosis in one third of pancreas	2
Necrosis in one half of pancreas	4
Necrosis in more than one half of pancreas	6
AP grade (0–4) + necrosis (0–6) = CT severity index	

21. **What is the role of serum markers in assessing the severity of acute pancreatitis?**
Recent studies suggest that hemoconcentration on admission with a hematocrit ≥44% and ure of hematocrit to decrease at 24 hours may be predictive of necrotizing AP and organ fa

22. **What are the major systemic complications of acute pancreatitis?**
Hypotension secondary to cardiovascular collapse may occur due to significant third-spac fluids, peripheral vasodilatation from circulating vasoactive kinins, and depressed left ventr function.

Acute renal failure due to renal hypoperfusion and shock may lead to acute tubular necre with a mortality rate approaching 50%.

Pleural effusions are usually left-sided (although bilateral and right-sided effusions do o and exudative with a high amylase level. *Early arterial hypoxia* results from microthrombi o pulmonary vasculature with subsequent right-to-left shunt. *Acute respiratory distress synd* (ARDS) occurs in up to 20% of patients with severe AP.

Gastrointestinal (GI) bleeding may result from *stress-induced gastritis* and *ulceration*. Isolated *gastric varices* may form from splenic vein thrombosis. Splenectomy is the treatm choice for bleeding gastric varices. *Pseudoaneurysm* and *hemosuccus pancreaticus* are als causes of GI bleeding in AP. Dynamic contrast-enhanced CT is the most useful initial diagn test, which may show a pseudocyst with contrast within it (so-called target sign). Selective mesenteric arteriography with embolization is the treatment of choice.

Pancreatic encephalopathy manifested by agitation, disorientation, confusion, hallucinat and possible coma may occur.

Fat necrosis affecting subcutaneous tissue, bone, peritoneum, retroperitoneum, mediastinum, pleura, and pericardium may occur. Subcutaneous fat necrosis causes circumscribed, tender, red nodules over the skin, resembling erythema nodosum. Involvement of joints may result in arthritis.

Purtscher's retinopathy, a rare complication of AP, leads to sudden blindness secondary to occlusion of the posterior retinal artery with aggregated granulocytes.

When is infection of pancreatic necrosis suspected?

Suspect infected pancreatic necrosis when the patient is not improving clinically, despite aggressive, supportive care, and there is persistence of systemic toxicity (fever >101°F, leukocytosis >20,000/mm^3) or organ failure. Infection does not occur usually until 5–7 days after the onset of AP; however, it can be its presenting symptom. Infection is diagnosed by CT-guided percutaneous aspiration of the necrotic pancreas with Gram stain and culture of the aspirate for aerobic/anaerobic bacteria and fungi. Visualization of retroperitoneal gas bubbles on CT also suggests infection from gas-forming organisms.

What is the most common organism isolated in infected pancreatic necrosis?

Infected pancreatic necrosis may be due to a single organism (75–80% of the time) or a polymicrobial infection. The organisms probably infect the pancreas by translocation across the bowel wall with subsequent local lymphatic, hematogenous, or biliary spread.

Escherichia coli is isolated in 51% of percutaneous aspirates that are infected. Other organisms include *Enterococcus* spp. (19%), *Staphylococcus* spp. (18%), *Klebsiella* spp. (10%), *Proteus* spp. (10%), *Pseudomonas* spp. (10%), *Streptococcus faecalis* (7%), *Bacteroides* spp. (6%), and, rarely, fungi like *Candida* spp.

How is acute pancreatitis treated?

Treatment of AP depends on the severity of disease and the presence of complications. *Mild AP* is treated with supportive care, which includes intravenous hydration, parenteral analgesics, and nothing by mouth. Nasogastric suction may be used in cases of ileus or intractable nausea and vomiting. There is no indication for prophylactic antibiotics in mild AP.

Severe AP has higher morbidity and mortality as well as risk of developing systemic complications. These patients should be monitored in the Intensive Care Unit. Close attention should be paid to volume status because large amounts of fluid may third-space and accumulate in the injured pancreatic bed. Therefore, fluid resuscitation is a foundation of supportive therapy. If there is *pancreatic necrosis,* prophylactic antibiotics with good pancreatic tissue penetration may be utilized to prevent secondary infection and septic complications. There is no consensus regarding use of antibiotic prophylaxis in patients with severe AP without demonstrable necrosis by CT. Antibiotics with adequate pancreatic penetration include imipenem, third-generation cephalosporins, piperacillin, mezlocillin, fluoroquinolones, and metronidazole. Prophylactic antibiotic use may promote development of fungal infections, therefore use of prophylactic fungal therapy may also be advised. Other possible ways to prevent infection of necrotizing pancreatitis include selective digestive tract decontamination and use of enteral rather than parenteral feeding. Because the gut is the source of bacteria causing pancreatic infection, use of oral nonabsorbable antibiotics (norfloxacin, colistin, and amphotericin) for gut decontamination may reduce secondarily infected pancreatic necrosis. Enteral feeding eliminates complications like line sepsis and thrombophlebitis seen commonly with parenteral nutrition, and reduces bacterial translocation through decreasing gut permeability (*see* question 27).

Patients with *infected pancreatic necrosis* should undergo urgent surgical debridement with continued antibiotic coverage. The surgical techniques vary, and debridement may be done in conjunction with closure of the abdomen with external drainage alone or with local saline lavage, or with open packing of the abdomen and repeated debridement. Because of the prolonged hospitalization associated with surgical debridement, recent advances with endoscopic drainage of

infected pancreatic necrosis, or with catheters placed by interventional radiology, have be
described. Their application presently remains limited.

In patients with persistent *sterile pancreatic necrosis,* there is no clear consensus on t
ment. Most experts advise medical management for 4–6 weeks and monitor for resolutic
studies have clearly shown an advantage for surgical debridement, although some favor 1
approach in severely ill patients with continued organ dysfunction.

26. **When, and by what route, should nutritional support be initiated in patient**
acute pancreatitis?
Oral feeding should be initiated as soon as possible in patients with pancreatitis. Clinicall
translates to when the patient is hungry and is without nausea, vomiting, or evidence of g
trointestinal ileus. It is irrelevant if pain is present or if there is elevation of serum pancrea
enzymes. If oral feedings are not tolerated, then nutritional supplementation should be
considered.

The decision to use parenteral or enteral nutrition is controversial, although there is m
evidence that enteral feeding is more beneficial. *Enteral nutrition,* given via a jejunal feedi
placed beyond the ligament of Treitz, has the advantage over parenteral nutrition of prese
bowel function and integrity. This can reduce bacterial translocation and theoretically dec
the incidence of pancreatic infection. Enteral nutrition is also less expensive than parente
nutrition, has fewer problems with stress-induced hyperglycemia, and has a lower incide
septic complications (i.e., catheter sepsis). A recent study showed that although enteral i
sions of elemental diets did not rest the pancreas in healthy subjects, the enzyme secreto
responses to elemental diets were suppressed in all patients with AP.

27. **When should endoscopic retrograde cholangiopancreatography be perfo**
in biliary acute pancreatitis?
Early ERCP with endoscopic sphincterotomy for stone extraction and biliary decompressior
proved beneficial for patients with biliary pancreatitis and evidence of persistent or progress
iary obstruction with cholangitis or biliary sepsis. Of note, the best clinical predictor of persi
common bile duct stones is an elevated *serum total bilirubin level* (>1.35 mg/dL) on hospita
(sensitivity 90%, specificity 63%). However, the routine use of prelaparoscopic cholecystec
ERCP in all patients with presumed gallstone pancreatitis is not justified. Patients without ev
of ongoing biliary obstruction or sepsis should have intraoperative cholangiogram at time o
laparoscopic cholecystectomy, with bile duct exploration or postoperative ERCP as indicate

28. **Should patients undergo a cholecystectomy after an episode of biliary acu**
pancreatitis?
Yes. There is a 25% risk of recurrent AP, cholecystitis, or cholangitis within 6 weeks of the
episode of biliary AP if cholecystectomy is not done.

29. **How soon should a cholecystectomy be performed after an attack of biliar**
acute pancreatitis?
In patients with mild AP (Ranson's criteria <3), laparoscopic cholecystectomy performed
the first week of admission is generally considered safe. Studies have shown no differenc
mortality or length of postoperative stay when early cholecystectomy is compared with la
scopic cholecystectomy performed later. However, in patients with more severe AP (Rans
criteria ≥3), laparoscopic cholecystectomy should be delayed for more than a week after
admission given that patients tended to have a shorter postoperative stay if operated on la

30. **Should patients with coexisting alcoholism and cholelithiasis undergo**
cholecystectomy to prevent further attacks of acute pancreatitis?
No. Cholecystectomy does not prevent recurrent attacks of AP in patients with coexisting
holism because the disease almost always follows the pattern of alcohol-related pancreat

31. **What are acute fluid collections?**

Acute fluid collections (AFC) occur in more than 50% of patients with moderate-to-severe AP. They are an accumulation of transudative or exudative fluid secondary to the local inflamed pancreatic tissue. They lack a clear wall of granulation tissue and are irregularly shaped. In general, they do not communicate directly with the pancreatic duct, and therefore do not have high pancreatic enzyme concentrations, as do pseudocysts. Acute fluid collections may occur as early as 48 hours after the onset of AP, with most resolving spontaneously by 4–6 weeks. However, 10–15% may develop a capsule and progress to pseudocyst formation.

32. **What are pseudocysts?**

Pancreatic pseudocysts are an accumulation of fluid containing necrotic tissue, debris, blood, and high concentrations of pancreatic enzymes. They develop usually 4 weeks after onset of AP and represent extravasated pancreatic secretions with an inflammatory response, often in communication with the pancreatic duct. They appear round or oval in shape and are surrounded by a capsule of granulation tissue and collagen. Unlike pancreatic cysts, pancreatic pseudocysts lack a true epithelial lining. Approximately 85% are located in the body or tail, with 15% found in the head of the pancreas. They may also occur in the lesser peritoneal sac and can extend into the paracolic gutters, pelvis, mediastinum, and, rarely, to the neck or scrotum.

33. **When should a pseudocyst be suspected?**

A pseudocyst should be suspected in the following scenarios:
- Serum amylase remains persistently high.
- An episode of AP fails to resolve.
- The patient has persistent abdominal pain after clinical resolution of AP.
- An epigastric mass is felt after an episode of AP.

34. **What are the indications for pseudocyst drainage?**

An asymptomatic pseudocyst does not require treatment regardless of size and may be followed every 3–6 months with abdominal ultrasound. Indications for pseudocyst drainage include presence of symptoms, progressive enlargement, presence of complications (i.e., infection, hemorrhage, rupture, obstruction), and suspicion of malignancy.

35. **How are pancreatic pseudocysts drained?**

Pseudocysts may be drained endoscopically, percutaneously under radiologic guidance, or surgically. Endoscopic or percutaneous drainage is successful in 85% of cases. *Endoscopic drainage* can be done when the pseudocyst is adherent to the wall of the stomach or duodenum, creating an endoluminal bulge, in which case an endoscopic cyst-gastrostomy or cyst-duodenostomy is performed. Bleeding is a potential complication, and use of endoscopic ultrasonography is recommended to avoid puncturing large blood vessels in the drainage area. Moreover, if there is continuity between the main pancreatic duct and pseudocyst, endoscopic placement of a transpapillary pancreatic duct stent into the pseudocyst may be done for drainage. *Percutaneous catheter drainage* under radiologic guidance is preferred for high-risk patients, immature pseudocysts with thin walls, and infected pseudocysts. It is not to be used in the presence of a main pancreatic duct obstruction close to the ampulla secondary to the risk of developing a permanent external fistula. *Surgical drainage* still remains the gold standard. It is warranted when: (1) there are complications of bleeding or fistula formation, (2) endoscopic or percutaneous drainage fails, (3) multiple or giant pseudocysts are present, and (4) if malignancy is suspected to obtain excisional histopathology.

What are possible complications of an untreated pancreatic pseudocyst?

Secondary infection occurs in approximately 10% of pseudocysts. CT scan may suggest infection by demonstrating gas bubbles within the pseudocyst. Diagnosis is made by percutaneous aspiration with Gram stain and culture.

Pseudocyst rupture occurs in <3% of patients. Clinical presentation varies widely from an acute abdomen to a silent event producing pancreatic ascites or pleural effusion.

Pancreatic ascites, secondary to leakage from a pseudocyst (70%) or pancreatic duct (10–20%), is characterized by ascitic fluid with a high amylase level (usually >1000 U/dL) and protein (usually >2.5 g/dL). Medical management consists of total parenteral nutrition and octreotide (50–200 µg subcutaneously every 8 hours). ERCP can demonstrate the site of leakage, and endoscopic stenting of the main pancreatic duct may allow resolution of the ascites. Surgical approach remains the gold standard of treatment, if the aforementioned are unsuccessful.

Pancreatic fistulas develop usually from external drainage of a pseudocyst. They may close spontaneously or with the aid of octreotide, which decreases fistula output. Surgery may be necessary for persistent high-output fistulas (>200 mL/day).

Obstruction of the GI tract, urinary system, vena cava, or portal vein by a pseudocyst necessitates drainage.

Jaundice is associated with pseudocyst in approximately 10% of cases. Its causes include hepatic dysfunction, extrahepatic biliary obstruction, and stenosis of the intrapancreatic portion of the distal common bile duct from pancreatitis and choledocholithiasis.

Pseudoaneurysm occurs when the pseudocyst erodes into an adjacent vessel (5–10% of patients). Clinical signs include an expanding pseudocyst with pain, hypotension, and a falling hematocrit. If the pseudocyst communicates with the pancreatic duct, massive GI bleeding with hematemesis or melena occurs secondarily to bleeding directly through the pancreatic duct into the duodenum (*hemosuccus pancreaticus*). Intraperitoneal bleeding results from pseudoaneurysm rupture.

37. **What is a pancreatic abscess?**
A circumscribed collection of pus located usually in or near the pancreas. It is caused by secondary infection of a pancreatic pseudocyst (*see* question 36) or an area of pancreatic necrosis. It is a late event, occurring at least 4 weeks after the onset of AP. The mortality rate associated with pancreatic abscess is generally less than that of infected necrosis. Treatment includes percutaneous catheter or surgical drainage, with possible debridement of necrotic tissue.

BIBLIOGRAPHY

1. Abou-Assi S, Craig K, O'Keefe SJ: Hypocaloric jejunal feeding is better than total parenteral nutrition in acute pancreatitis: Results of a randomized comparative study. Am J Gastroenterol 97:2255–2262, 2002.

2. Balthazar EJ, Robinson DL, Megibow AJ, et al: Acute pancreatitis: Value of CT in establishing prognosis. Radiology 174:331–336, 1990.

3. Banks PA: Predictors of severity in acute pancreatitis. Pancreas 6(Suppl 1):S7–S12, 1991.

4. Banks PA, Gerzof SG, Langevin RE, et al: CT-guided aspiration of suspected pancreatic infection: Bacteriology and clinical outcome. Int J Pancreatol 18:265–270, 1995.

5. Blamey SL, Imrie CW, O'Neill J, et al: Prognostic factors in acute pancreatitis. Gut 25:1340–1346, 1984.

6. Bradley EL III: A clinically based classification system for acute pancreatitis. Summary of the International Symposium on Acute Pancreatitis, Atlanta, GA, September 11–13, 1992. Arch Surg 128:586–590, 1993.

7. Brown A, Orav J, Banks PA: Hemoconcentration is an early marker for organ failure and necrotizing pancreatitis. Pancreas 20:367–372, 2000.

8. Calvo MM, Bujanda L, Calderon A, et al: Role of magnetic resonance cholangiopancreatography in patients with suspected choledocholithiasis. Mayo Clin Proc 77:422–428, 2002.

9. Chang L, Lo SK, Stabile BE, et al: Gallstone pancreatitis: A prospective study on the incidence of cholangitis and clinical predictors of retained common bile duct stones. Am J Gastroenterol 93:527–531, 1998.

10. DiMagno EP, Chari S: Acute pancreatitis. In Feldman M (ed): Sleisenger and Fordtran's Gastrointestinal and Liver Disease, 7th ed. Philadelphia, W.B. Saunders, 2002, pp 913–941.

11. Fan ST, Lai EC, Mok FP, et al: Early treatment of acute biliary pancreatitis by endoscopic papillotomy. N Engl J Med 328:228–232, 1993.

Kalfarentzos F, Kehagias J, Mead N, et al: Enteral nutrition is superior to parenteral nutrition in severe acute pancreatitis: Results of a randomized prospective trial. Br J Surg 84:1665–1669, 1997.

Karimgani I, Porter KA, Langevin RE, et al: Prognostic factors in sterile pancreatic necrosis. Gastroenterology 103:1636–1640, 1992.

Kozarek RA, Ball TJ, Patterson DJ, et al: Endoscopic transpapillary therapy for disrupted pancreatic duct and peripancreatic fluid collections. Gastroenterology 100:1362–1370, 1991.

Lankisch PG, Mahlke R, Blum T, et al: Hemoconcentration: An early marker of severe and/or necrotizing pancreatitis? A critical appraisal. Am J Gastroenterol 96:2081–2085, 2001.

Lans JI, Greenen JE, Johanson JF, et al: Endoscopic therapy in patients with pancreas divisum and acute pancreatitis: A prospective, randomized, controlled clinical trial. Gastrointest Endosc 38:430–434, 1992.

Lee SP, Nicholls JF, Park HZ: Biliary sludge as a cause of acute pancreatitis. N Engl J Med 326:589–593, 1992.

Neoptolemos JP, Carr-Locke DL, London NJ, et al: Controlled trial of urgent endoscopic retrograde cholangiopancreatography and endoscopic sphincterotomy versus conservative treatment for acute pancreatitis due to gallstones. Lancet ii:979–983, 1988.

Neoptolemos JP, Kemppainen EA, Mayer JM, et al: Early prediction of severity in acute pancreatitis by urinary trypsinogen activation peptide: A multicentre study. Lancet 355:1955–1960, 2000.

Pederzoli P, Bassi C, Vesenteni S, et al: A randomized multicenter clinical trial of antibiotic prophylaxis of septic complications in acute necrotizing pancreatitis with imipenem. Surg Gynecol Obstet 176:480–483, 1993.

Pitchumoni CS, Agarwal N: Pancreatic pseudocysts: When and how should drainage be performed? Gastroenterol Clin North Am 28:615–639, 1999.

Powell JJ, Miles R, Siriwardena AK: Antibiotic prophylaxis in the initial management of severe acute pancreatitis. Br J Surg 85:582–587, 1998.

Ranson JH: Etiologic and prognostic factors in human acute pancreatitis: A review. Am J Gastroenterol 77:633–638, 1982.

Ratschko M, Fenner T, Lankisch PG: The role of antibiotic prophylaxis in the treatment of acute pancreatitis. Gastroenterol Clin North Am 28:641–659, 1999.

Steinberg W, Tenner S: Acute pancreatitis. N Engl J Med 330:1198–1210, 1994.

Tandon M, Topazian M: Endoscopic ultrasound in idiopathic acute pancreatitis. Am J Gastroenterol 96:705–709, 2001.

Tenner S, Dubner H, Steinberg W: Predicting gallstone pancreatitis with laboratory parameters: A meta analysis. Am J Gastroenterol 89:1863–1866, 1994.

Venu RP, Brown RD, Marrero JA, et al: Endoscopic transpapillary drainage of pancreatic abscess: Technique and results. Gastrointest Endosc 51:391–395, 2000.

CHAPTER 39

CHRONIC PANCREATITIS

Michael W. Cheng, MD, and Jamie S. Barkin, MD

1. **What classification system is used for chronic pancreatitis (CP)?**
   CP is an inflammatory condition that leads to progressive and irreversible changes in the pancreas, which ultimately results in impairment of exocrine and endocrine function. This differs from acute pancreatitis, which is a nonprogressive event with pancreatic function returning to normal after the attack. The modified Marseilles-Rome classification classifies CP into four groups based on morphology, molecular biology, and epidemiology:

   Lithogenic CP (calcifying CP) is characterized by irregular fibrosis of the pancreas with intraductal protein plugs, intraductal stones, and ductal injury. Most cases of CP belong to this group, and the leading cause is alcohol abuse.

   Obstructive CP demonstrates glandular changes, including uniform fibrosis, ductal changes with dilation, and acinar atrophy, all of which may improve when obstruction of the pancreatic duct is removed. Common causes of obstruction include intraductal tumor or benign ductal stricture.

   Inflammatory CP is characterized histologically by mononuclear cell infiltration with exocrine parenchymal destruction, diffuse fibrosis, and atrophy. Associated disorders include auto-immune diseases, such as Sjögren's syndrome, primary sclerosing cholangitis, and auto-immune pancreatitis.

   Asymptomatic pancreatic fibrosis is characterized by silent, diffuse perilobular fibrosis as seen in so-called idiopathic senile CP.

2. **What is the most common cause of chronic pancreatitis in adults?**
   Chronic alcohol abuse is the most common cause of CP in Western societies. It accounts for 70–80% of all cases. The risk of developing CP appears to be related to the duration and amount of alcohol consumed and not to the type of alcohol or pattern of drinking. Although there is variation in individual sensitivity to alcohol, published reports suggest that at least 5 years of alcohol intake exceeding 150 gm/day is needed prior to developing CP. Because only 5–10% of alcoholics develop CP, other cofactors may be involved. Proposed cofactors include a diet high in fat and protein, deficiency of antioxidants or trace elements, smoking, and, possibly, genetic predisposition.

3. **What are the other causes of chronic pancreatitis?**
   - Genetic (including hereditary pancreatitis and cystic fibrosis)
   - Obstructive (from a benign stricture resulting from trauma or previous episodes of acute pancreatitis or malignant pancreatic duct obstruction)
   - Tropical/nutritional
   - Metabolic (resulting from hypercalcemia or hypertriglyceridemia)
   - Autoimmune
   - Idiopathic

4. **What is hereditary pancreatitis?**
   Hereditary pancreatitis is an autosomal dominant disorder with 80% penetrance and variable expression. It accounts for approximately 1% of all cases of CP and has been described in families throughout the world. Hereditary pancreatitis affects both sexes equally and presents

typically as episodes of acute pancreatitis in childhood by ages 10–12. Recurrent episodes of acute pancreatitis lead to the development of CP. They have a predisposition for development of pancreatic carcinoma, with a 40% incidence by age 70. Genetic testing for trypsinogen gene mutations are specific for hereditary pancreatitis and should be offered to young patients with recurrent pancreatitis and a positive family history of pancreatic disease. The diagnosis is suspected when several family members have pancreatic disease, especially CP without other identifiable causes.

How is cystic fibrosis associated with chronic pancreatitis?

Cystic fibrosis is the most common autosomal recessive defect in Caucasians and is due to mutations in the cystic fibrosis transmembrane conductance regulator (CFTR) gene. Approximately 85% of patients with cystic fibrosis develop exocrine pancreatic insufficiency. The CFTR mutation causes reduced and defective ductular and acinar pancreatic secretions, ultimately resulting in pancreatic duct obstruction and acinar cell destruction with fibrosis. It should be suspected in all young persons with acute pancreatitis in whom another cause is not readily apparent. A clue to its presence is difficulty conceiving in a male.

What is obstructive chronic pancreatitis?

Benign or malignant obstruction of the pancreatic duct can lead to CP. Causes include strictures from trauma, pseudocysts, calcific stones, papillary stenosis, pancreas divisum, and malignant tumors. Relief of the obstruction can reverse some of the pancreatic damage and preserve pancreatic function.

What is tropical pancreatitis?

Tropical or nutritional pancreatitis is seen commonly in residents of Southern India, Indonesia, and sub-Saharan Africa. It presents in young adults who manifest with abdominal pain, severe malnutrition, and exocrine or endocrine insufficiency with diabetes and large pancreatic duct calculi. The cause of tropical pancreatitis is unknown. Proposed theories include tropical pancreatitis being the sequela of prolonged severe protein-calorie malnutrition and, possibly, oxidative injury from consumption of the cassava fruit.

What is autoimmune pancreatitis?

Autoimmune pancreatitis, also known as *sclerosing pancreatitis* or *lymphoplasmacytic pancreatitis,* is the most recently described form of CP. It is characterized by the presence of autoantibodies, increased levels of serum immunoglobulins, elevated serum IgG4 levels, and response to steroid therapy. Anatomically, there is diffuse or focal enlargement of the pancreas with pancreatic duct strictures. Histologic findings are characterized by a dense lymphoplasmacytic infiltrate. In 60% of cases, autoimmune pancreatitis is associated with other autoimmune disorders, such as primary sclerosing cholangitis, primary biliary cirrhosis, autoimmune hepatitis, Sjögren's syndrome, and scleroderma. The serologic and histologic findings are useful in diagnosing autoimmune pancreatitis and in distinguishing it from other forms of CP. It presents most commonly with jaundice secondary to intrapancreatic common bile duct obstruction, and patients respond with amelioration of symptoms to corticosteroids.

What is idiopathic chronic pancreatitis?

Idiopathic CP remains a wastepaper basket of the unknown causes of CP. It accounts for 10–30% of all cases of CP. Misdiagnosis may occur if there is concealed alcohol use, or if genetic studies are not done to rule out cystic fibrosis or trypsinogen gene mutations. There appears to be a bimodal age distribution with two forms: early-onset juvenile form and late-onset senile form. *Early-onset juvenile form* has a median age of 18 years and is characterized by severe pain with delayed development of pancreatic calcifications, exocrine insufficiency, and endocrine insufficiency. Conversely, the *late-onset senile form* has a median age of

56 years and is characterized by exocrine and endocrine insufficiency, albeit in the absence of pain.

10. **What is the most common presenting symptom of chronic pancreatitis?**
Abdominal pain is the most common presenting symptom, occurring in 50–100% of patients with CP. Although the pain associated with CP is highly variable, it is described usually as epigastric, dull, constant, radiating to the back, improvement with sitting or leaning forward worsening after meals. Frequently, there is associated nausea and vomiting. Over time, the of CP may persist, diminish, or resolve completely.

11. **What are the causes of weight loss in patients with chronic pancreatitis?**
   - Decreased caloric intake as a result of fear of aggravating pain (sitophobia)
   - Malassimilation due to pancreatic exocrine insufficiency
   - Uncontrolled diabetes
   - Early satiety secondary to delayed gastric emptying or duodenal obstruction

12. **Is steatorrhea an early symptom of chronic pancreatitis?**
No. Steatorrhea occurs when pancreatic exocrine secretion is insufficient to maintain normal digestion and absorption of lipids. Because 90% of exocrine function must be lost before steatorrhea develops, it signifies advanced disease.

13. **Is diabetes mellitus an early manifestation of chronic pancreatitis?**
Similar to steatorrhea secondary to exocrine insufficiency, diabetes mellitus with endocrine insufficiency occurs late in the course of CP. Up to 70% of patients with CP will eventually develop diabetes, which is caused by the destruction of insulin-producing beta cells. In contrast to type 1 diabetes, CP also destroys glucagon-producing alpha cells, which results in a brittle type of diabetes subject to frequent episodes of hypoglycemia. Diabetic ketoacidosis and nephropathy are uncommon in diabetes caused by CP; however, retinopathy and neuropathy occur at similar frequencies to other forms of diabetes.

14. **Are measurements of serum pancreatic enzymes helpful in the diagnosis of chronic pancreatitis?**
No.

15. **What do elevated levels of bilirubin and alkaline phosphatase suggest in the patient with chronic pancreatitis?**
Elevations in bilirubin and alkaline phosphatase suggest biliary obstruction secondary to compression of the intrapancreatic portion of the bile duct by edema, fibrosis, or pancreatic carcinoma. Elevations can also occur in patients from toxic effects of alcohol intake or other hepatotoxins (i.e., medications). Attempts to document biliary obstruction must be a priority because biliary cirrhosis can result.

16. **What specialized test *directly* measures pancreatic exocrine function?**
The *secretin stimulation test,* with or without concomitant cholecystokinin (CCK) administration measures the volume of secretion and the concentration of bicarbonate output (via aspiration duodenal contents) in response to injection of secretin. Bicarbonate levels <50 mEq/L are consistent with CP; levels >50 mEq/L but below 75 mEq/L, are indeterminate; levels >75 mEq/L normal. The test is invasive, requiring duodenal catheter (Dreiling tube) insertion for collection of secretions, but has a reported sensitivity of 75–95%.

17. **What conditions may be associated with a false-positive secretin stimulation test?**
Primary diabetes mellitus, Billroth II gastrectomy, celiac sprue, cirrhosis, and the recovery phase after an attack of acute pancreatitis.

8. **What *indirect* tests of pancreatic exocrine function are used?**

The bentiromide and pancreolauryl tests are noninvasive methods of assessing pancreatic exocrine function but are no longer available in the United States. Most indirect tests of pancreatic function measure the absorption of a compound that first requires digestion by pancreatic enzymes, thereby assessing indirectly pancreatic function. The *bentiromide test* exploits the lack of the digestive enzyme chymotrypsin, which occurs in patients with CP. This test involves the ingestion of bentiromide, a tripeptide digested by pancreatic chymotrypsin with subsequent release of para-aminobenzoic acid (PABA). Free PABA is absorbed in the small intestine, conjugated in the liver, and is then excreted in the urine. Recovery of ≥50% of the administered dosage in a 6-hour urine collection is considered normal. False-positive results may occur in patients with diabetes mellitus, renal insufficiency, liver disease, or malabsorptive states other than CP. The *pancreolauryl test* exploits the reduced secretion of arylesterases from the pancreas. After ingestion of fluorescein dilaurate (with a standard breakfast), arylesterases release fluorescein from the dilaurate. Free fluorescein is absorbed in the small intestine, conjugated in the liver, then excreted in the urine. False-positive results may be seen in patients with chronic inflammatory bowel disease, severe biliary diseases, and Billroth II gastrectomy. Both tests have sensitivities of 80–100% in patients with advanced CP with steatorrhea.

Another test to indirectly assess pancreatic exocrine function is the measurement of *serum trypsinogen*, which is very low (<20 ng/mL) in patients with CP. Serum trypsinogen levels tend to be low in patients with advanced CP and steatorrhea and are usually normal in patients with less advanced disease. Other causes of low trypsinogen levels include pancreatic ductal obstruction.

Additional indirect tests of pancreatic exocrine function include the *fecal chymotrypsin* and *fecal elastase, [^{14}C] olein test*, and 72-hour quantitative *fecal fat determination*. The limitation of most of these tests is their lack of sensitivity, except in patients with advanced CP, characterized by malassimilation and steatorrhea. Unfortunately, we do not have a serologic or noninvasive test for the diagnosis of mild or moderate CP not characterized by exocrine insufficiency of the magnitude to result in steatorrhea.

9. **Are plain abdominal radiographs helpful in the diagnosis of chronic pancreatitis?**

Yes. The identification of focal or diffuse pancreatic calcifications on plain abdominal radiographs makes the diagnosis of advanced CP almost certain. It is seen in 30–40% of patients with CP. Because calcification is not found in early CP, plain abdominal films cannot be used to exclude the diagnosis. Of note, one must be certain that the calcifications are within the pancreas and do not simply represent vascular calcifications (*see* question 20).

10. **What other imaging modalities are used in the diagnosis of chronic pancreatitis?**

Transabdominal ultrasound (US) findings of CP include pancreatic duct dilation, calcifications, pancreatic ductal stones, pseudocysts, and, in milder disease, reduction in parenchymal echogenicity or irregular gland contour. The sensitivity and specificity of US in the diagnosis of CP are 60–70% and 80–90%, respectively. The major limitation of US is that the pancreas cannot be adequately visualized in many patients secondary to overlying bowel gas.

Computed tomography (CT) findings of CP include pancreatic duct dilation, intraductal filling defects, calcifications, cavitary, and cystic lesions. Other significant findings include heterogeneous density of the pancreatic gland with atrophy or enlargement. CT is 10–20% more sensitive than US, with a similar specificity.

Magnetic resonance imaging (MRI) gives more accurate pancreatic duct evaluation than CT. It may reveal enlargement, stenosis, and pancreatic duct filling defects.

11. **What is the role of endoscopic retrograde cholangiopancreatography (ERCP) in the diagnosis of chronic pancreatitis?**

Abnormalities of the pancreatic duct are visualized by ERCP in patients with moderate to advanced CP. Conversely, patients with early CP may have a normal pancreatogram. Findings on

ERCP include characteristic "chain of lakes" beading of the main pancreatic duct, ectatic side branches, and intraductal filling defects. ERCP is considered the gold standard imaging procedure for the diagnosis of CP, with a 90% sensitivity and 100% specificity.

In general, there is good correlation between the findings seen on ERCP and results of the secretin stimulation test in the diagnosis of CP. ERCP may also be useful in distinguishing CP from pancreatic carcinoma. The presence of a dominant stricture is highly suggestive of pancreatic carcinoma, whereas CP is characterized by ductular changes (with multiple areas of stenosis, dilation, irregular branching ducts, and intraductal calculi).

22. **What is the Cambridge grading system of chronic pancreatitis, based on ERCP findings?**

Normal	Main pancreatic duct normal; side branches normal
Equivocal	Main pancreatic duct normal; <3 abnormal side branches
Mild	Main pancreatic duct normal; ≥3 abnormal side branches
Moderate	Main pancreatic duct abnormal; ≥3 abnormal side branches
Marked	Main pancreatic duct abnormal; ≥3 abnormal side branches

and one or more of the following:
Large cavities (>10 mm)
Intraductal filling defects or calculi
Duct obstruction
Severe duct dilation or irregularities

23. **What is the role of endoscopic ultrasound (EUS) in the diagnosis of chronic pancreatitis?**

EUS allows high-resolution imaging of the pancreas without interference by overlying bowel gas typically encountered with transabdominal ultrasound. The diagnosis of CP by EUS is based on presence of abnormal pancreatic ductal and parenchymal findings (*see* question 24). The diagnosis requires the presence of at least three criteria. CP is unlikely in the absence of any criteria and highly likely if there are ≥5 criteria. A prospective evaluation comparing EUS with ERCP and secretin stimulation test in the diagnosis of CP showed good correlation, especially in patients advanced CP. In mild CP, EUS may show findings not detected by ERCP or functional testing, and remains controversial whether a diagnosis of CP can be made by EUS findings alone.

24. **What are the endoscopic ultrasound criteria for the diagnosis of chronic pancreatitis?**

Ductal findings
Dilated main duct
Dilated side branches
Duct irregularities
Hyperechoic duct margins
Stones/calcification
Parenchymal findings
Hyperechoic foci
Hyperechoic strands
Gland lobularity
Cystic cavities

25. **What is the role of magnetic resonance cholangiopancreatography (MRCP) in the diagnosis of chronic pancreatitis?**

Preliminary studies have shown close correlation of the ductular findings seen on MRCP with ERCP in patients with CP, including the presence of pancreatic ductal dilation, ductal narrowing, and filling defects. Imaging by MRCP is limited in assessing areas where the pancreatic duct is small, for instance, pancreatic tail and side branches. The benefits of MRCP over ERCP include that of being noninvasive and being able to evaluate both pancreatic parenchyma and ducts at the same time. It can visualize the ductular anatomy not seen on ERCP when a stricture is present and visualize cystic lesions not in connection with the ductular system. Thus, it is an excellent initial study in patients with suspected CP. If negative, additional studies can be performed for further evaluation.

6. What is the most common complication of chronic pancreatitis?
The most common complication of CP is pseudocyst formation, occurring in up to 25% of patients. Pseudocysts should be suspected in any patient with stable CP who has worsening abdominal or back pain. Other less common presentations of pseudocysts include a palpable mass on physical exam when they are very large, nausea, vomiting, jaundice, and gastrointestinal (GI) bleeding. In contrast to acute pseudocysts (defined as being present for <6 weeks), chronic pseudocysts, especially those >6 cm, almost never resolve spontaneously. Although most pseudocysts are asymptomatic, problems like pseudoaneurysm and abscess formation can occur. Of note, cystic collections in the pancreas are most often due to pseudocysts, accounting for 70–90% of cases.

7. How are pseudocysts treated?
In general, asymptomatic pseudocysts do not require treatment regardless of size. Initially, they may be followed by abdominal ultrasound at 3 and 6 months. If asymptomatic, there is no need in most patients for further routine evaluation. Indications for pseudocyst treatment include presence of symptoms, progressive enlargement, presence of complications (i.e., infection, hemorrhage, intraperitoneal rupture, intestinal obstruction), and suspicion of malignancy. Effective treatment includes surgical excision for pseudocysts localized to the tail of the pancreas, and internal or external drainage (performed by surgical, endoscopic, or percutaneous means). Surgical or endoscopic *internal drainage* is usually the treatment of choice, especially for mature pseudocysts (i.e., present for longer than 6 weeks with a formed cyst wall). Surgical options include cyst-gastrostomy, cyst-duodenostomy, or cyst-jejunostomy. Endoscopic cyst-gastrostomy or cyst-duodenostomy requires abutment of the pseudocyst onto adjacent viscera. EUS can determine the distance of a pseudocyst from the GI lumen, while assessing cyst contents and avoiding adjacent vasculature during performance of endoscopic drainage. *External drainage* is necessary for immature or infected pseudocysts, and this can be achieved surgically or percutaneously under radiologic guidance. Complications of external drainage include higher recurrence rates, drain track superinfection, and formation of pancreatic-cutaneous fistulas.

8. What are other complications of chronic pancreatitis?
Distal *common bile duct* (CBD) *obstruction* occurs in 5–10% of patients with CP. Compression of the intrapancreatic portion of the CBD by edema, fibrosis, or pseudocyst in the pancreatic head can lead to cholestasis, jaundice, biliary pain, and, potentially, cholangitis. If left untreated, secondary biliary cirrhosis can occur. *Duodenal obstruction* may occur secondary to external compression by edema or fibrosis of the pancreatic head. It affects up to 5% of patients with CP. Presenting symptoms include nausea, vomiting, weight loss, postprandial abdominal pain, and early satiety. *External pancreatic fistulas* are rare, and occur most frequently after surgical or percutaneous drainage of a pseudocyst. *Internal pancreatic fistulas* occur usually spontaneously from main pancreatic duct rupture or pseudocyst leakage, typically in patients with CP secondary to alcohol. This can lead to a collection of pancreatic fluid in the peritoneal cavity or into the pleural space, resulting in pancreatic ascites or pleural effusion, respectively. *Pseudoaneurysms* result from pseudocyst erosion into the splenic vein. If the pseudocyst is in communication with the main pancreatic duct, GI bleeding may occur. Gastric varices result from *splenic vein thrombosis* and may also cause GI bleeding. Patients with CP are also predisposed to developing *pancreatic adenocarcinoma,* with a lifetime risk of approximately 4%.

29. How is distal common bile duct obstruction diagnosed and treated?

Imaging by ERCP or MRCP may demonstrate narrowing of the distal CBD in the form of gra tapering, bird's beak stenosis, or "hourglass" stricture. Complications of biliary obstruction include jaundice, abdominal pain, ascending cholangitis, and secondary biliary cirrhosis. O causes of jaundice, such as intrinsic liver disease, should be ruled out. Treatment options include close observation for a short period of time (<2 months), with serial liver function te (LFTs) or endoscopic or surgical decompression procedures. If abnormal LFTs persist seco ary to obstruction, decompression is advised to prevent secondary biliary cirrhosis. Endos biliary stent placement may provide temporary benefit, especially in the acute setting, but lc term success is low due to the need for multiple stent exchanges, stent blockage, and stent migration. Particularly for younger patients, surgical biliary bypass with cholecystojejunost or choledochojejunostomy is preferred. When associated with concomitant pseudocyst or dilated pancreatic duct, surgical biliary decompression may be combined with lateral pancr cojejunostomy.

30. How is duodenal obstruction diagnosed and treated?

Duodenal obstruction is best diagnosed by upper GI series, given that endoscopy may unde appreciate the degree of duodenal stenosis. Treatment includes supportive medical therapy tially, but with persistent stenosis, surgery is warranted. Usually, a gastrojejunostomy is do and this can be combined with biliary drainage (if there is concomitant CBD obstruction) or lateral pancreaticojejunostomy (if pain results from pancreatic duct obstruction). In nonope tive patients, endoscopic placement of metal stents may provide palliation.

31. How are pancreatic fistulas treated?

General treatment strategies for pancreatic fistulas include reducing pancreatic secretions v long-acting somatostatin analogs (octreotide 50–200 µg subcutaneously every 8 hours) an with total parenteral nutrition and nothing by mouth. Successful treatment may take weeks, time is usually the healer. Endoscopic stenting of the main pancreatic duct may facilitate hea if ERCP identifies the site of ductal disruption or leak. For internal pancreatic fistulas, additic treatment options include large volume paracentesis for pancreatic ascites, thoracentesis fo pancreatic pleural effusion, and diuretics. Surgical decompression or resection may be requ if ERCP cannot visualize the source of ductal disruption or leak or there is persistence of the tula after medical therapy.

32. How is pancreatic ascites or pancreatic pleural effusion diagnosed?

The diagnosis is made by examining the fluid obtained from paracentesis or thoracentesis, which has typically a very high amylase concentration (>1000 IU/L).

33. Why does the presence of gastric varices in the absence of esophageal vari suggest chronic pancreatitis?

Anatomically, the splenic vein is in close proximity to the pancreas, and chronic inflammatio seen in CP, may lead to splenic vein thrombosis. Thrombosis of the splenic vein leads to intrasplenic venous hypertension, splenomegaly, and collateral formation through the short gastric veins, resulting in gastric varices. Isolated gastric varices occur in approximately 5% patients with CP. Massive gastrointestinal hemorrhage may occur. Splenectomy is curative. Treatment is not required in the absence of bleeding.

34. Are signs of fat-soluble vitamin deficiencies highly suggestive of chronic pancreatitis?

No. Although absorption of fat-soluble vitamins (A, D, E, K) is decreased in CP, clinical mani tations of vitamin deficiencies, like easy bruisability, bone pain, and poor night vision, are uncommon.

Are patients with chronic pancreatitis predisposed to nephrolithiasis?

Yes. Steatorrhea from CP may lead to hyperoxaluria and subsequent oxalate kidney stone formation. Patients with untreated steatorrhea have high concentrations of long-chain fatty acids in the colon, which bind intraluminal calcium by formation of insoluble calcium soaps. With less calcium in the intestinal lumen to bind oxalate, more intestinal oxalate is absorbed, which results in hyperoxaluria and nephrolithiasis.

How should hyperoxaluria be treated in patients with chronic pancreatitis?

Treatment options include pancreatic enzyme replacement, low dietary oxalate intake, low dietary long-chain triglyceride intake, and increased intake of calcium (3 g/day) or aluminum in the form of antacids (3.5 gm/day).

Can patients with chronic pancreatitis develop vitamin B_{12} malabsorption?

Yes. Vitamin B_{12} (cobalamin) malabsorption occurs in up to 40% of patients with advanced CP. The probable mechanism is competitive binding of cobalamin by cobalamin-binding proteins instead of by intrinsic factor. Cobalamin-binding proteins are destroyed usually by pancreatic proteases, and treatment with pancreatic enzyme replacement may correct the condition.

How is steatorrhea in chronic pancreatitis treated?

The primary therapeutic modality for patients with steatorrhea is *pancreatic enzyme replacement*. These consist of lipase, which is necessary to prevent fat malabsorption that occurs when lipase secretion is <10% of normal levels. The usual dose of lipase is at least 30,000 units with each meal, given as 10,000 units before eating and 20,000 units during the meal to ensure adequate mixing. Pancreatic enzymes are available in enteric and nonenteric-coated formulations. The major advantage of enteric-coated compounds is that they do not dissolve in the stomach and thus are less susceptible to acid pepsin inactivation of pancreatic enzymes, which limits effectiveness of therapy. With nonenteric-coated pancreatic enzymes, the addition of an H_2-receptor antagonist or proton pump inhibitor is suggested to prevent acid inactivation of lipase and improve efficacy. Pancreatic enzyme replacements differ in their dissolution qualities and therefore their effectiveness. This decreased physiologic availability is most often found with generic substitutions. In patients with weight loss and poor response to pancreatic enzyme replacement, *medium chain triglycerides* (MCT) may provide much needed nutritional support given that they are more easily degraded and absorbed. *Restricting fat intake,* usually to <20 gm/day, may also help with steatorrhea. However, this is inappropriate in cachectic patients who need optimal caloric intake for support of nutritional status.

What are nonsurgical modalities of pain control in chronic pancreatitis?

Abdominal pain is the most common symptom of CP that requires medical care. *Alcohol cessation, small low-fat meals,* and *nonnarcotic analgesics* may provide some initial relief.

If abdominal pain persists, other nonsurgical therapeutic options include pancreatic enzyme supplements, narcotic analgesics, somatostatin, and celiac plexus block. *Pancreatic enzyme supplements* should be the first measure used in patients with persistent, severe abdominal pain. They may decrease pain by reducing the abdominal distention and diarrhea associated with malassimilation, as well as by possibly limiting pancreatic stimulation. Treatment of chronic pain in CP is usually facilitated by pancreatic enzyme supplements with high protease content and nonenteric-coating, which differ from the high lipase, enteric-coated supplements preferred in the treatment of steatorrhea. *Somatostatin* at a dose of 200 µg subcutaneously every 8 hours may also reduce the pain of CP. In patients with inadequate pain control from these measures, *narcotic analgesics* may be needed, realizing that secondary addiction is a significant risk if pain persists. Antidepressants may be added as an adjunctive agent. *Celiac plexus block,* with alcohol or steroids, has limited results in alleviating pain due to CP because of its short benefits. The occasional benefits last usually between 2 and 6 months, with less effective pain relief with repeat sessions. Other potential medical therapies that are being studied for pain control in CP include the use of antioxidants.

40. **Does endoscopy have a role in pain control in chronic pancreatitis?**
The role of endoscopy in the management of pain in patients with CP is evolving, especially in patients with a dominant stricture. Numerous reports suggest that endoscopic sphincterotomy with pancreatic stricture dilation and pancreatic duct stent placement relieves recurrent or persistent pain associated with CP. Several studies have also reported marked improvement in pain after endoscopic removal of intraductal pancreatic stones with extracorporeal lithotripsy and pancreatic duct sphincterotomy with stone extraction. Although endoscopic techniques show promise for pain management in CP, substantiation is needed in the form of randomized, blinded, prospective studies.

41. **What is the role of surgery in pain control in chronic pancreatitis?**
Surgery is reserved generally for patients who have continued, persistent pain, despite the aforementioned medical therapies. They are difficult technically but may provide longer-lasting pain control. Surgical treatments include ductal decompression with a lateral pancreaticojejunostomy (modified Puestow's procedure) or partial resection of the pancreas. Lateral pancreaticojejunostomy is preferred in patients with ductal obstruction in the head of the pancreas and distal duct obstruction, whereas partial pancreatic resection is most appropriate in patients without ductal dilation, so-called small duct disease, or localized distal (tail) disease. Pain relief can be achieved with surgery in up to 80% of patients with CP. Other surgical techniques for the treatment of chronic pain in CP include total pancreatectomy followed by autologous islet cell transplantation, which is presently experimental and being studied.

WEBSITES

1. http://www.pancreas.org/assets/patients/HPTesting_FAQ_1201.pdf

2. http://www.pancreas.org/physicians/physicians_diseaseinfo.html

3. http://usagicdu.com/articles/pancpath/pancpath.pdf

4. http://www.dave1.mgh.harvard.edu/

BIBLIOGRAPHY

1. Applebaum SE, O'Connell JA, Aston CE, et al: Motivations and concerns of patients with access to genetic testing for hereditary pancreatitis. Am J Gastroenterol 96:1610–1617, 2001.

2. Barkin JS, Reiner DK, Deutch E: Sandostatin for control of catheter drainage of pancreatic pseudocyst. Pancreas 16:245–248, 1991.

3. Bhatia E, Choudhuri G, Sikora SS, et al: Tropical calcific pancreatitis: Strong association with SPINK1 trypsin inhibitor mutations. Gastroenterology 123:1020–1025, 2002.

4. Bhutani M: Endoscopic ultrasound in pancreatic diseases: Indications, limitations, and the future. Gastroenterol Clin North Am 28:747–770, 1999.

5. Brown A, Hughes M, Tenner S, et al: Does pancreatic enzyme supplementation reduce pain in patients with chronic pancreatitis: A meta-analysis. Am J Gastroenterol 92:2032–2035, 1997.

Catalano MF, Lahoti S, Geenen JE, et al: Prospective evaluation of endoscopic ultrasonography, endoscopic retrograde pancreatography, and secretin test in the diagnosis of chronic pancreatitis. Gastrointest Endosc 48:11–17, 1998.

Choudari CP, Lehman GA, Sherman S: Pancreatitis and cystic fibrosis gene mutations. Gastroenterol Clin North Am 28:543–549, 1999.

Cohn JA, Friedman KJ, Noone PG, et al: Relation between mutations of the cystic fibrosis gene and idiopathic pancreatitis. N Engl J Med 339:653–658, 1998.

Creighton J, Lyall R, Wilson DI, et al: Mutations in the cationic trypsinogen gene in patients with chronic pancreatitis. Lancet 354:42–43, 1999.

Greenberger NJ: Enzymatic therapy in patients with chronic pancreatitis. Gastroenterol Clin North Am 28:687–693, 1999.

Gress F, Schmitt C, Sherman S, et al: Endoscopic ultrasound-guided celiac plexus block for managing abdominal pain associated with chronic pancreatitis: A prospective single center experience. Am J Gastroenterol 96:409–416, 2001.

Hamano H, Kawa S, Horiuchi A, et al: High serum IgG concentrations in patients with sclerosing pancreatitis. N Engl J Med 344:732–738, 2001.

Kozarek RA, Ball TJ, Patterson DJ, et al: Endoscopic pancreatic duct sphincterotomy: Indications, technique, and analysis of results. Gastrointest Endosc 40:592–598, 1994.

Kozarek RA, Jiranek GC, Traverso LW: Endoscopic treatment of pancreatic ascites. Am J Surg 168:223–226, 1994.

Layer P, Yamamoto H, Kalthoff L, et al: The different courses of early- and late-onset idiopathic and alcoholic pancreatitis. Gastroenterology 107:1481–1487, 1994.

Lehman GA, Sherman S: Pancreas divisum. Diagnosis, clinical significance, and management alternatives. Gastrointest Endosc Clin N Am 5:145–170, 1995.

Lowenfels AB, Maisonneuve P, Lankisch PG: Chronic pancreatitis and other risk factors for pancreatic cancer. Gastroenterol Clin North Am 28:673–685, 1999.

Saeed ZA, Ramirez FC, Hepps KS: Endoscopic stent placement for internal and external pancreatic fistulas. Gastroenterology 105:1213–1217, 1993.

Scolapio JS, Malhi-Chowla N, Ukleja A: Nutritional supplementation in patients with acute and chronic pancreatitis. Gastroenterol Clin North Am 28:695–707, 1999.

Shea JC, Bishop MD, Parker EM, et al: An enteral therapy containing medium-chain triglycerides and hydrolyzed peptides reduces postprandial pain associated with chronic pancreatitis. Pancreatology 3:36–40, 2003.

Smits ME, Badiga SM, Rauws EA, et al: Long-term results of pancreatic stents in chronic pancreatitis. Gastrointest Endosc 42:461–467, 1995.

Sossenheimer MJ, Aston CE, Preston RA, et al: Clinical characteristics of hereditary pancreatitis in a large family, based on high risk haplotype. Am J Gastroenterol 92:1113–1116, 1997.

Steer ML, Waxman I, Freedman S: Chronic pancreatitis. N Engl J Med 32:1482–1490, 1995.

Uden S, Bilton D, Nathan L, et al: Antioxidant therapy for recurrent pancreatitis: Placebo-controlled trial. Aliment Pharmacol Ther 4:357–371, 1990.

Warshaw AL, Popp JW Jr, Schapiro RH: Long-term patency, pancreatic function, and pain relief after lateral pancreaticojejunostomy for chronic pancreatitis. Gastroenterology 79:289–293, 1980.

Whitcomb DC: The spectrum of complications of hereditary pancreatitis: Is this model for future gene therapy? Gastroenterol Clin North Am 28:525–541, 1999.

Yoshida K, Toki F, Takeuchi T, et al: Chronic pancreatitis caused by an autoimmune abnormality: Proposal of the concept of autoimmune pancreatitis. Dig Dis Sci 40:1561–1568, 1995.

CHAPTER 40

PANCREATIC CANCER

Sergey V. Kantsevoy, MD, PhD, and Anthony N. Kalloo, MD

1. **What are the most common histologic forms of malignant tumors of the pancreas?**

   Almost 90% of pancreatic cancers are moderately well-differentiated adenocarcinomas, deriv from the pancreatic ductal epithelium. About 5% of pancreatic cancers originate from the pancreatic islet cells. Other rare types of pancreatic cancer include sarcomas, lymphomas, and cy tadenocarcinomas.

2. **Define intraductal papillary-mucinous tumors of the pancreas.**

   Intraductal papillary-mucinous tumors (IPMT) of the pancreas (also called *mucinous ductal ectasia, mucin-producing tumors, ductectatic mucinous cystadenomas, intraductal cystaden mas, intraductal papillary tumors*) are characterized by intraductal papillary growth and produ tion of mucin. These tumors usually grow slowly and cause dilatation of the main pancreatic duct and its branches with potential development of cellular hyperplasia, atypia, and malignan

3. **What is the most common location of the pancreatic adenocarcinoma?**

   Eighty percent of pancreatic adenocarcinomas are located in the head of the pancreas. This lo tion may lead to obstruction of the distal common bile duct with development of obstructive jaundice.

4. **What is Courvoisier's sign?**

   A palpable, distended gallbladder in the right upper quadrant in a patient with jaundice is calle *Courvoisier's sign*. Usually, it results from a malignant bile duct obstruction, such as pancreat cancer with complete obstruction of the distal common bile duct and accumulation of bile in t gallbladder. This finding is not specific for pancreatic cancer. Patients with distal cholangiocar noma or an ampullary mass may also present with Courvoisier's sign.

5. **What is the survival rate for patients with pancreatic cancer?**

   Less than 20% of patients with pancreatic cancer are alive 1 year after diagnosis, and less tha 3% survive longer than 5 years. Surgical resection of the tumor is the only curative treatment. the time of diagnosis, 40% of patients already have locally advanced disease, and more than 40% have visceral metastasis. The stage of the disease at presentation and the surgeon's abili to remove the tumor completely are the most important determinants of treatment outcome a long-term survival.

6. **What are the risk factors for development of pancreatic cancer?**

   Smokers are twice as likely to develop pancreatic cancer as nonsmokers. Pancreatic cancer is more common in countries where the diet contains a large amount of fat and meat products. I contrast, high intake of dietary fiber appears to be protective. Extensive studies have failed to prove a definitive link between coffee intake and development of pancreatic cancer. Recent stu ies indicated that diabetes mellitus (especially recent onset of diabetes in an older patient) ma be a risk factor. Chronic pancreatitis increases the risk. Some patients may have a genetic (familial) predisposition. Patients with pernicious anemia, and patients who have undergone partial gastrectomy, have an elevated risk. Predisposing environmental hazards include oil refining, paper manufacturing, and chemical manufacturing.

7. What is the estimated risk for pancreatic cancer among persons with hereditary pancreatitis (HP)?

Hereditary pancreatitis is an autosomal dominant trait with high phenotypic penetrance. International study groups have calculated a 50- to 70-fold increased risk of pancreatic cancer among patients with HP, with a 40% cumulative risk at age 70. Ideally, screening for pancreatic cancer should be offered to patients of ages 35–40. Optimally, screening should be conducted at expert medical centers with state-of-the-art imaging in conjunction with standardized collection of blood/serum and pancreatic juice for scientific study.

8. Is alcohol consumption an important risk factor for development of pancreatic cancer?

Many epidemiologic studies in Europe and the United States have failed to find a consistent, direct association between alcohol intake and development of pancreatic cancer.

9. What are the most common symptoms in patients with pancreatic cancer?

Patients with pancreatic cancer present usually with abdominal pain, radiating frequently to the back; weight loss; nausea; anorexia; generalized weakness; and easy fatigability. Obstructive jaundice may develop early in the disease in patients with a mass in the head of the pancreas. Jaundice may never develop or develop late in patients with a tumor in the body or tail of the pancreas; in such patients, jaundice indicates the presence of liver metastases.

0. What imaging modalities are used to diagnose pancreatic cancer?

Transabdominal ultrasound is usually the first diagnostic test. Its sensitivity in the detection of pancreatic tumors is around 70%. CT and MRI are more sensitive than transabdominal ultrasound, especially for detection of regional and distal metastases. Endoscopic ultrasonography is the most accurate (sensitivity: 77–100%) diagnostic modality to detect small tumors and to evaluate the local spread of tumor into surrounding organs and blood vessels. Endoscopic retrograde cholangiopancreatography (ERCP) is sensitive (78–95%) and specific (88–95%) for pancreatic cancer and is frequently used to perform palliative drainage of the biliary ducts.

KEY POINTS: PANCREATIC CANCER

1. Most patients with pancreatic carcinoma develop symptoms late in the course of the disease.

2. The lack of early warning symptoms leads to a delay in diagnosis, and less than 20% of patients present with resectable disease.

. What is the "double-duct sign" in patients with pancreatic cancer?

The double-duct sign, noted on ERCP, demonstrates the presence of stenosis of the common bile duct and pancreatic duct in the head of the pancreas. In patients with obstructive jaundice or a pancreatic mass, the double-duct sign has a specificity of 85% in predicting pancreatic cancer.

. Can serum markers diagnose pancreatic cancer?

Many potential serum markers are currently under evaluation to facilitate the early detection of pancreatic cancer. The carbohydrate antigen CA19-9 is highly sensitive (>90%) in diagnosing pancreatic cancer but has low specificity (75%) and is often normal in early stages of the disease (tumor <1 cm in diameter). Many conditions can lead to elevation of CA19-9: chronic pancreatitis, biliary diseases, and other types of gastrointestinal (GI) cancer. After complete resection of pancreatic cancer, the serum level of CA19-9 usually falls. Persistently elevated serum levels of CA19-9 after surgery may indicate inadequate resection or metastatic lesions. Recurrence of pancreatic cancer can manifest with elevation of CA19-9 levels following a declin after surgical resection.

13. **What are the common biochemical abnormalities in patients with pancreatic cancer?**
Patients with biliary tract obstruction can present with elevated serum bilirubin and alkaline phosphatase (obstructive pattern). Serum amylase is elevated in only 5% of patients.

14. **Is chemotherapy effective for patients with advanced pancreatic cancer?**
Traditional chemotherapy with 5-fluorouracil has an overall response rate below 10%, with no effect on quality of life or survival. Gemcitabine, which in one study demonstrated improvemen in disease-related symptoms and survival in advanced pancreatic cancer, is now under clinical evaluation as a single agent and in combination with 5-fluorouracil and cisplatin.

15. **What is the median survival after the diagnosis of advanced pancreatic cancer**
Pancreatic cancer has the poorest prognosis among other GI tumors. It is the fifth leading caus of death in the United States. The median survival of patients with advanced pancreatic carcinoma is approximately 4 months.

16. **Describe the role of celiac blockade in patients with pancreatic cancer.**
Celiac blockade (chemical splanchnicectomy) is injection of 50% alcohol on each side of the aorta at the level of celiac axis. This procedure has been shown, prospectively, to improve pree isting pain significantly and to delay onset of pain in asymptomatic patients. Celiac blockade ca be done at laparotomy, under radiologic guidance, or at the time of endoscopic ultrasound.

17. **What is a Whipple's resection?**
Whipple's resection (pancreaticoduodenectomy) is the most common surgical procedure for resectable cancer located in the head of the pancreas. It involves a partial gastrectomy (resection of the antrum), cholecystectomy, and removal of the distal common bile duct, duodenum, head of the pancreas, proximal jejunum and regional lymphatic nodes. The procedure includes usually pancreaticojejunostomy, hepaticojejunostomy, and gastrojejunostomy.

18. **What surgical procedures are used for cancer in the body and tail of the pancreas?**
Surgical resection consists usually of distal pancreatectomy and splenectomy. This operation technically easier than Whipple's procedure.

19. **When do patients with pancreatic cancer need palliative procedures?**
Patients with unresectable cancer in the head of the pancreas can develop obstructive jaundice pruritus, or cholangitis. These conditions can be palliated by endoscopic placement of plastic self-expending metal stents (Wallstent). If endoscopic stent placement is not possible, transhepatic transcutaneous stents can be inserted by an interventional radiologist. When placement of stents by an endoscopist or radiologist fails, bypass surgical procedure (cholecystojejunostomy or hepaticojejunostomy) may be indicated. In patients with duodenal obstruction by a large pancreatic mass, endoscopy with palliative placement of an expandable stent into the duodenum is indicated to relieve the obstruction. If endoscopy is not possible, surgical bypass procedure (gastrojejunostomy) may be performed.

WEBSITES

1. http://www.path.jhu.edu/pancreas

2. http://www.dave1.mgh.harvard.edu

3. http://www.vhjoe.com

BIBLIOGRAPHY

Alonso Casado O, Hernandez Gallardo D, Moreno Gonzalez E, et al: Intraductal papillary-mucinous tumors: An entity which is infrequent and difficult to diagnose. Hepatogastroenterology 47:275–284, 2000.

Cello JP: Pancreatic cancer. In Feldman M, Scharschmidt BF, Sleisenger MH (eds): Sleisenger & Fordtran's Gastrointestinal and Liver Disease: Pathophysiology/Diagnosis/Management, vol 1. Philadelphia, W.B. Saunders, 1998, pp 863–870.

Lee JH, Whittington R, Williams NN, et al: Outcome of pancreaticoduodenectomy and impact of adjuvant therapy for ampullary carcinomas. Int J Radiat Oncol Biol Phys 47:945–953, 2000.

Lillemoe KD: Current management of pancreatic carcinoma. Ann Surg 221:133–148, 1995.

Lorenz M, Heinrich S, Staib-Sebler E, et al: Regional chemotherapy in the treatment of advanced pancreatic cancer—is it relevant? Eur J Cancer 36:957–965, 2000.

Menges M, Lerch MM, Zeitz M: The double duct sign in patients with malignant and benign pancreatic lesions. Gastrointest Endosc 52:74–77, 2000.

Parker SL, Tong T, Bolden S, Wingo PA: Cancer statistics, 1997. CA Cancer J Clin 47:5–27, 1997.

Parks RW, Garden OJ: Ensuring early diagnosis in pancreatic cancer. Practitioner 244:336–338, 340–341, 343, 2000.

Rice D, Geller A, Bender CE, et al: Surgical and interventional palliative treatment of upper gastrointestinal malignancies. Eur J Gastroenterol Hepatol 12:403–408, 2000.

Todd KE, Gloor B, Reber HA: Pancreatic adenocarcinoma. In Yamada T (ed): Textbook of Gastroenterology, vol 2. Philadelphia, Lippincott Williams & Wilkins, 1999, pp 2178–2192.

Urlich CD: Pancreatic cancer in hereditary pancreatitis, consensus guidelines for prevention, screening and treatment. Pancreatology 1:416–422, 2001.

van Riel JM, van Groeningen CJ: Palliative chemotherapy in advanced gastrointestinal cancer. Eur J Gastroenterol Hepatol 12:391–396, 2000.

Watanapa P, Williamson RC: Surgical palliation for pancreatic cancer: Developments during the past two decades. Br J Surg 79:8–20, 1992.

CHAPTER 41

CYSTIC DISEASE OF THE PANCREAS

Randall E. Lee, MD

1. **Provide a differential diagnosis for a cystic pancreatic lesion.**
   - *Pancreatic pseudocyst* (about 75–90% of cystic pancreatic lesions)
   - *Cystic neoplasm* (about 10% of cystic pancreatic lesions)
     - Primary cystic neoplasms
       - Serous cystadenoma
       - Mucinous cystic neoplasm (MCN)
       - Intraductal papillary mucinous neoplasm (IPMN)
       - Pseudopapillary-solid epithelial neoplasm (PSEN)
       - Mesenchymal neoplasm (lymphangioma, teratoma)
     - Solid neoplasms with cystic degeneration
       - Pancreatic ductal adenocarcinoma
       - Pancreatic metastasis (ovarian adenocarcinoma, most common)
       - Islet cell neoplasms
   - *Retention cyst*

RETENTION CYST

2. **What is the difference between a true pancreatic cyst and a pancreatic pseudocyst?**
   A true pancreatic cyst has an epithelial cell lining. A pancreatic pseudocyst is lined only by inflammatory tissue; it has no epithelium. True pancreatic cysts account for only 10–15% of a cystic lesions of the pancreas.

3. **Define an acute fluid collection.**
   An acute fluid collection is a collection of enzyme-rich pancreatic juice occurring within 48 ho in the course of acute pancreatitis. It is located in or near the pancreas and does not have a w defined wall.

4. **Define an acute pancreatic pseudocyst.**
   An acute pancreatic pseudocyst is a collection of pancreatic juice enclosed by a wall of non-epithelialized granulation tissue that arises due to acute pancreatitis. It requires at least 4 wee to form and contains no significant solid debris.

5. **Define a chronic pancreatic pseudocyst.**
   A chronic pancreatic pseudocyst is a collection of pancreatic juice enclosed by a wall of fibrou or granulation tissue. It arises from pancreatic duct leaks due to pancreatic duct stones or strictures associated with chronic pancreatitis.

6. **Describe the typical clinical presentation of a pancreatic pseudocyst.**
   Formation of a pancreatic pseudocyst should be suspected if a patient with acute pancreatitis develops any of the following:

- Failure of acute pancreatitis symptoms to resolve after about 7–10 days
- Recurrence of acute pancreatitis symptoms after initial improvement
- Epigastric abdominal mass
- Persistently elevated serum amylase
- Obstructive jaundice

7. What criteria suggest that a pseudocyst will not resolve spontaneously?
A pancreatic pseudocyst has a low probability of spontaneous resolution if there is concurrent evidence of chronic pancreatitis, such as pancreatic calcifications, or if the pseudocyst is a consequence of traumatic pancreatitis.

8. When should a pseudocyst be drained?
A pseudocyst should be drained if it causes symptoms, increases in size, shows evidence of infection, causes critical compression of an adjacent structure such as the bile duct, or is complicated by internal hemorrhage. Asymptomatic pseudocysts may be observed carefully, regardless of size or duration. The strict criteria of pseudocyst diameter >6 cm or persistence for >6 weeks are no longer accepted as absolute indications for drainage.

9. List three methods for draining a pancreatic pseudocyst.
1. Surgical drainage
2. Computed tomography (CT)- or ultrasound-guided percutaneous catheter drainage
3. Transpapillary, transgastric, or transduodenal endoscopic drainage

10. Compare the three methods for draining a pancreatic pseudocyst.
Surgical drainage is the procedure of choice for patients in whom a cystic neoplasm cannot be ruled out. An intraoperative biopsy of the cyst wall can confirm the presence or absence of a malignant epithelial cell lining. Surgical drainage is also indicated for patients who have multiple or recurrent pseudocysts or concurrent pancreatic duct stricture. Surgical drainage of a thin walled pseudocyst should be delayed for 4–6 weeks. This delay allows thickening and maturation of the pseudocyst wall, thus increasing the holding power of sutures. The surgical mortality rate is about 3% and the recurrence rate is about 8%.

Percutaneous catheter drainage is preferred for high-risk patients with symptomatic thin-walled or expanding pseudocysts or infected pseudocysts. This method should not be used in patients who have a main pancreatic duct stricture because of the high risk of creating a pancreaticocutaneous fistula. The reported mortality rate is about 2%; the recurrence rate is about 7%.

Endoscopic drainage may be considered for selected patients. The reported mortality rate is about 1% and the recurrence rate is about 16%. The outcome of endoscopic drainage is highly dependent on the skill and expertise of the endoscopist. In one series by a highly skilled endoscopist, the complication rate for endoscopic drainage was about 24%.

11. What criteria suggest that a pancreatic pseudocyst may undergo successful endoscopic drainage?
- Endoscopic retrograde cholangiopancreatography (ERCP) demonstrates a communication between the pseudocyst and the main pancreatic duct.
- The pseudocyst impinges on and is adherent to the wall of the stomach or duodenum, creating an endoluminal bulge. Imaging with endoscopic ultrasound (EUS) and CT is recommended to confirm close contact between the pseudocyst and adjacent gastric or duodenal wall, to avoid puncturing large submucosal blood vessels, to rule out the presence of a pseudoaneurysm, and to help distinguish a true pseudocyst from a cystic neoplasm.
- Endoscopic drainage is more likely to be successful with chronic pseudocysts (aboout 90%) compared with acute pseudocysts (about 70%). A pseudocyst with a wall >1 cm thick is a poor candidate for endoscopic drainage because of the difficulty in puncturing the pseudocyst wall.

12. **Describe a pancreatic abscess.**
   A pancreatic abscess is a circumscribed intra-abdominal collection of pus containing little or no pancreatic necrosis, which is due to acute pancreatitis or pancreatic trauma. A pancreatic abscess may appear as an ill-defined, nonenhancing fluid collection of mixed densities. Unfortunately, this CT appearance may be confused with a noninfected pseudocyst. The presence of gas within the cystic area strongly suggests infection by gas-forming organisms.

13. **What clinical criteria suggest the development of a pancreatic abscess?**
   A pancreatic abscess typically develops from secondary bacterial infection of necrotic pancreatic tissue during an episode of acute pancreatitis. The abscess often causes tempera-tures >38.5°C, leukocytosis >10,000 cells/mm³, and increasing abdominal pain. All of these signs may also be found in noninfected patients with severe pancreatitis. Percutaneous need-le aspiration of the area and Gram stain of the fluid may help to confirm the diagnosis of pancreatic abscess.

14. **Define *hemosuccus pancreaticus.***
   Hemosuccus pancreaticus describes the rare phenomenon of major bleeding into the main pancreatic duct from a pseudoaneurysm. Massive gastrointestinal or intra-abdominal bleeding from pseudocyst erosion into a pancreatic or peripancreatic blood vessel occurs in about 5–10% of patients with pseudocysts. Patients with *hemosuccus pancreaticus* form a subset of this group. Clinical signs suggestive of pseudoaneurysm hemorrhage include an enlarging pulsatile abdominal mass with or without a bruit, recurrent gastrointestinal bleeding, and increasing abdominal pain. For patients suspected of having pseudoaneurysm hemorrhage, obtain a bolus contrast helical CT scan to confirm the diagnosis, followed by angiography for further localization and embolization or immediate surgical exploration.

15. **What is a serous cystadenoma?**
   A serous cystadenoma (SCA) is an uncommon pancreatic neoplasm characterized by numerous cysts filled with a glycogen-rich, low-viscosity serous fluid and lined by flat or cuboidal epithe-lium. Imaging by CT, EUS, or magnetic resonance imaging (MRI) classically shows a honey-comb of small cysts with a sunburst calcification in a central scar. SCAs grow slowly, and more than 99% of reported cases are benign. Conservative observation may be appropriate for an elderly or high-surgical risk patient. Complete surgical resection is indicated if the patient is symptomatic or if the diagnosis is uncertain.

16. **Describe the clinical characteristics of a serous cystadenoma.**
   The usual presenting symptoms of SCAs are nonspecific gastrointestinal complaints, such as nausea, vomiting, abdominal pain, weight loss, or an abdominal mass. Up to one third may be discovered incidentally during autopsy or abdominal imaging. SCAs have been described in adults only.

KEY POINTS: CYSTIC DISEASES OF THE PANCREAS

1. Pancreatic pseudocysts are the most common cystic pancreatic lesion.

2. A pancreatic pseudocyst does not have an epithelial lining.

3. If a patient with acute pancreatitis improves initially then has a relapse of symptoms, or is not improving at all, one should suspect the development of a pseudocyst.

4. Cystic pancreatic neoplasms that produce mucin are considered malignant or premalignant. With very rare exceptions, cystic pancreatic neoplasms that produce serous fluid are considered benign. Both types grow slowly.

17. **What disease commonly manifests by retinal angiomatosis, central nervous system (CNS) hemangioblastomas, and pancreatic serous cystadenomas?**

Retinal angiomatosis and CNS hemangioblastomas in association with multiple pancreatic serous cystadenomas are the common manifestations of von Hippel-Lindau disease (VHL). VHL is also associated with renal cell carcinoma, islet cell tumors, pheochromocytomas, and benign cysts of the liver, lung, spleen, adrenal gland, and kidney. VHL is caused by a mutation of a tumor suppressor gene on chromosome 3p25. The mode of inheritance is autosomal dominant with variable penetrance. The pancreatic cysts may precede other manifestations of the disease by several years and may be the only abdominal manifestation. An evaluation for VHL is recommended for patients who have both pancreatic cysts and cysts in other organ systems.

18. **Describe the characteristics of a mucinous cystic neoplasm (MCN).**

MCN is an uncommon pancreatic tumor characterized by large cysts filled with mucin and lined by a columnar epithelium. Many MCNs have an ovarian-like stroma surrounding the epithelial cells. MCNs form typically in the pancreas tail or body and are much more common in women than in men. The most frequent presenting symptoms are epigastric pain and an enlarging abdominal mass. Obstructive jaundice is rare. Radiologic images usually show larger and less numerous cysts compared with serous cystadenomas. ERCP generally shows no communication between the pancreatic ducts and the neoplasm.

Although MCNs may be subclassified as benign mucinous cystadenomas, borderline mucinous cystic neoplasms, and malignant mucinous cystadenocarcinomas, a single MCN may contain both benign and malignant epithelium. Most clinicians consider all MCNs as potentially malignant. The treatment of choice is complete surgical resection with highly detailed histologic examination. The 2- and 5-year survival rate for patients with invasive mucinous cystadenocarcinoma is about 65% and 30%, respectively, which is much higher than for patients with pancreatic ductal adenocarcinoma.

19. **What is an intraductal papillary mucinous neoplasm (IPMN)? How does it differ from a mucinous cystic neoplasm?**

An intraductal papillary mucinous neoplasm is a pancreatic neoplasm that originates within the duct system and may appear cystic because of duct dilations. IPMN encompasses the pancreatic neoplasms known previously as villous adenoma, papillary carcinoma, and ductectatic mucinous cystadenoma. Unlike mucinous cystic neoplasms, IPMNs afflict both genders equally and tend to arise in the head of the pancreas. An ovarian-like stroma is not found around the epithelial cells. Obstructive jaundice, abdominal pain, and weight loss are common presenting symptoms. ERCP demonstrates direct communication between the pancreatic ducts and the neoplasm. The finding of mucin extruding from the ampulla of Vater is considered highly specific for an IPMN.

20. **How does the surgical management of an intraductal papillary mucinous neoplasm differ from that of a mucinous cystic neoplasm?**

The cystic areas of an MCN usually define the margins of the neoplasm. Careful preoperative imaging studies can usually localize a mucinous cystic neoplasm and allow for a segmental pancreatic resection. In contrast, the cystic areas surrounding an IPMN may extend beyond the margins of the actual neoplasm, resulting in imprecise preoperative localization. Adding to the localization difficulty is the tendency of IPMNs to spread microscopically along the pancreatic duct. Hence, an initial partial pancreatectomy may require extension to total pancreatectomy, based upon the intraoperative frozen section and pancreatoscopy findings.

21. **What is the utility of endoscopic ultrasound imaging in the evaluation of a cystic pancreatic lesion?**

EUS imaging alone may add some incremental diagnostic information to the usual battery of transabdominal ultrasound, contrast-enhanced CT, and MRI. EUS-guided fine-needle aspiration and microbiopsy of cystic pancreatic lesions appear to have very high positive and negative predictive values for determining malignant and nonmalignant characteristics.

22. **What conditions are most commonly associated with a pancreatic retention cyst?**
Pancreatic retention cysts are dilated areas of the pancreatic duct that result from an obstruction of the duct. Retention cysts are usually <1 cm in diameter and are commonly associated with chronic pancreatitis, advanced cystic fibrosis, or a duct-obstructing carcinoma.

WEBSITES

1. http://www.gastroatlas.com (Volume 8: Pancreas)

2. http://www.pancreas.com

BIBLIOGRAPHY

1. Adsay NV, Longnecker DS, Klimstra DS: Pancreatic tumors with cystic dilatation of the ducts: Intraductal papillary mucinous neoplasms and intraductal oncocytic papillary neoplasms. Semin Diagn Pathol 17:16–30, 2000.
2. Baron TH, Harewood GC, Morgan DE, Yates MR: Outcome differences after endoscopic drainage of pancreatic necrosis, acute pancreatic pseudocysts, and chronic pancreatic pseudocysts. Gastrointest Endosc 56:7–17, 2002.
3. Bradley EL III: A clinically based classification system for acute pancreatitis. Summary of the International Symposium on Acute Pancreatitis, Atlanta, GA, September 11–13, 1992. Arch Surg 128:586–590, 1993.
4. Castillo CF: Surgery of cystic neoplasms. Gastrointest Endosc Clin N Am 12:803–812, 2002.
5. Compton CC: Histology of cystic tumors of the pancreas. Gastrointest Endosc Clin N Am 12:673–696, 2002.
6. Fockens P: EUS in drainage of pancreatic pseudocysts. Gastrointest Endosc 56:S93–S97, 2002.
7. Frossard JL, Amouyal P, Amouyal G, et al: Performance of endosonography-guided fine needle aspiration and biopsy in the diagnosis of pancreatic cystic lesions. Am J Gastroenterol 98:1516–1524, 2003.
8. Hammel PR, Vilgrain V, Terris B, et al: Pancreatic involvement in von Hippel-Lindau disease. Gastroenterology 119:1087–1095, 2000.
9. Howell DA, Elton E, Parsons WG: Endoscopic management of pseudocysts of the pancreas. Gastrointest Endosc Clin N Am 8:143–162, 1998.
10. Kloppel G: Pseudocysts and other non-neoplastic cysts of the pancreas. Semin Diagn Pathol 17:7–15, 2000.
11. Pitchumoni CS, Agarwal N: Pancreatic pseudocysts: When and how should drainage be performed? Gastroenterol Clin North Am 28:615–639, 1999.
12. Sahani D, Prasad S, Saini S, Mueller P: Cystic pancreatic neoplasms, evaluation by CT and magnetic resonance cholangiopancreatography. Gastrointest Endosc Clin N Am 12:657–672, 2002.
13. Wilentz RE, Albores-Saavedra J, Hruban RH: Mucinous cystic neoplasms of the pancreas. Semin Diagn Pathol 17:31–42, 2000.

CELIAC DISEASE, TROPICAL SPRUE, WHIPPLE'S DISEASE, LYMPHANGIECTASIA, IMMUNOPROLIFERATIVE SMALL INTESTINAL DISEASE, AND NONSTEROIDAL ANTI–INFLAMMATORY DRUGS

David J. Kaufman, DO, and Ingram M. Roberts, MD

CHAPTER 42

1. What is the best screening test for fat malabsorption?

Microscopic examination of stool using Sudan stain to detect fat is the best screening test for fat malabsorption. This test has a 100% sensitivity and 96% specificity. A stool sample is smeared on a microscope slide and mixed with ethanolic Sudan III and glacial acetic acid. The slide is covered, heated just until boiling, and then examined for the presence of fatty acid globules. The presence of more than 100 globules >6 μm in diameter per high-powered field ($\times$430) indicates a definite increase in fecal fat excretion. The number of globules correlates well with the quantitative amount of fecal fat present.

2. What is the best quantitative test for fat malabsorption?

The 72-hour stool fat collection. The patient is given a diet consisting of 100 gm of fat per day. Stool is collected, usually for 72 hours. The normal coefficient for absorption is approximately 93% of ingested fat. Consequently, if 100 gm of fat is digested, 7 gm or less of fat should appear in stool over a 24-hour period. If >7 gm of fecal fat is present, steatorrhea secondary to malabsorption is confirmed.

3. Under what physiologic conditions is fecal fat excretion increased?

- Diet high in fiber (>100 gm/day)
- Ingestion of solid-form dietary fat (e.g., whole peanuts)
- In the neonatal period, when intraluminal levels of pancreatic lipase and bile salts are low
- When olestra is consumed

4. What is the best test to differentiate malabsorption caused by small bowel enteropathy versus pancreatic insufficiency?

D-Xylose is one of the best tests to differentiate mucosal disease from pancreatic insufficiency as the cause of malabsorption. Normally, D-xylose is absorbed completely in the small bowel and excreted unchanged in the urine.

5. How is the D-xylose test performed?

A 25-gm dose of D-xylose is given orally after an overnight fast, and urine is collected for 5 hours. Normal urine excretion should be >5 gm of D-xylose. One-hour serum collection is also helpful but not as sensitive as urine collection. Normal serum levels 1 hour after ingestion are >20 mg/dL.

6. **What conditions may cause a false-positive D-xylose test?**
   - Delayed gastric emptying
   - Myxedema
   - Vomiting
   - Ascites
   - Renal insufficiency

7. **What is the gluten-sensitive enteropathy panel?**
   A panel of serologic tests used to detect celiac disease or gluten-sensitive enteropathy (GSE). Three antibodies are directed against the connective tissue (reticulin-like structures) or surface component of smooth muscle fibrils:

A-EmA	Antiendomysial antibody (IgA)
AGA	Antigliadin antibody (IgG or pooled Ig)
R1-ARA	Antireticulin antibody (IgA)

   A-EmA has 100% specificity for celiac disease, whereas its sensitivity is 85% and 90%, respectively, for untreated adult and childhood celiac disease. It can persist in low titers in 10–25% of patients on a gluten-free diet, despite normal histology. AGA has fairly good sensitivity (68–76%), but it may also be found in 10–20% of patients with other diseases that affect the small intestinal mucosa. AGA is a helpful test in monitoring GSE, because it always becomes negative with the regrowth of jejunal villi in celiac patients after a gluten-free diet. R1-ARA has a higher specificity than AGA in celiac children but a relatively low sensitivity (<40–50%).

8. **What is tissue transglutaminase?**
   Recently, tissue transglutaminase has been touted as the most sensitive and specific marker for celiac disease. Tissue transglutaminase is believed to be the autoantigen to which the endomysial antibodies react. Studies have shown that specificity for antitransglutaminase is comparable to that for antiendomysial antibodies; however, some investigators have observed that the antibody to transglutaminase is a more sensitive test, detecting 98–100% of patients with celiac sprue.

9. **Name the conditions to consider in previously responsive patients with celiac sprue who begin to deteriorate.**
   Noncompliance with gluten-free diet is the most common cause of deterioration in a previously responsive patient.
   Lymphoma is the most common malignancy complicating celiac disease, especially that of mucosal T-cell origin. Diagnosis of lymphoma requires a high index of suspicion because onset can be insidious or abrupt, and the histologic appearance can be indistinguishable from that of celiac sprue. A careful search for lymphoma is needed in patients with celiac sprue who do not respond to gluten withdrawal and patients with recurrent weight loss and malabsorption, despite strict adherence to a gluten-free diet. Computed tomography (CT) scan and exploratory laparotomy may be necessary to establish the diagnosis.
   Refractory sprue has clinical features and mucosal lesions indistinguishable from celiac sprue, but patients do not respond to a gluten-free diet, either at the onset of diagnosis or after becoming refractory to dietary therapy. Some patients may respond to corticosteroids or other immunosuppressive drugs, such as azathioprine, cyclophosphamide, or cyclosporine. Other patients do not respond to any treatment and face a dismal prognosis. The absence of Paneth cells on small bowel biopsy is a poor prognostic sign.

Collagenous sprue is a subset of refractory sprue characterized by the progressive development of a thick band of collagen-like material beneath the basement membrane of epithelial cells. It is usually refractory to all forms of treatment other than parenteral alimentation.

10. **What are the hepatic manifestations of celiac sprue, and how are they managed?**

Asymptomatic elevation of liver function tests, predominantly aminotransferases, can be seen in up to 42% of celiac patients. Strict adherence to a gluten-free diet will lead to a reduction in aminotransferase levels in the majority of individuals. Failure of liver function test improvement, despite treatment with a gluten-free diet, should prompt consideration of coexistent forms of autoimmune liver disease, such as autoimmune hepatitis, primary biliary cirrhosis, or primary sclerosing cholangitis.

11. **Describe the manifestations of Whipple's disease.**

Whipple's disease is a chronic systemic illness with various potential manifestations. The most common presentation includes weight loss (90%), diarrhea (>70%), and arthralgia (>70%). Arthralgia may exist for many years before the diagnosis of Whipple's disease. Cardiac involvement includes congestive heart failure, pericarditis, and valvular heart disease (30%). Lymphadenopathy and hyperpigmentation are frequent findings on physical examination. Hematochezia is rare, but occult bleeding has been detected in up to 80% of patients with Whipple's disease. The most common central nervous system manifestations (5%) are dementia, ocular disturbances, meningoencephalitis, and cerebellar symptoms, including ataxia and mild clonus.

12. **What is the differential diagnosis of a macrophage infiltrate of the small bowel lamina propria?**

Whipple's disease: inclusions are rounded or sickle-shaped.

Mycobacterium avium-intracellulare: inclusions contain acid-fast bacilli. This condition is seen commonly in AIDS patients with small bowel involvement.

Histoplasmosis or *cryptococcosis:* inclusions contain large, round, encapsulated organisms.

Macroglobulinemia: no inclusions are seen, and there are only faintly staining, homogeneously periodic acid–Schiff (PAS)-positive macrophages.

Miscellaneous disease: PAS-positive macrophages are frequently present in the normal gastric and rectal mucosa and may contain lipids or mucin, respectively.

13. **What causes Whipple's disease?**

Tropheryma whippelii causes the disease in humans but has been cultured only recently. The organism was identified by direct amplification of a 16S-rRNA sequence from a microbial pathogen in tissue. According to phylogenetic analysis, this bacterium is a gram-positive actinomycete that is not closely related to any known genus. Prolonged treatment with antibiotics (up to 6 months) is often required to eradicate the organism. Measurements of *T. whippelii* DNA concentration in tissue by polymerase chain reaction is the most sensitive marker of patient response to antibiotic therapy. Of interest, *T. whippelii* DNA has been found in the small intestine of asymptomatic patients, suggesting that host factors play a role in disease penetration, just as in *Helicobacter pylori* infection.

. **What are the complications of the enteropathy induced by nonsteroidal anti-inflammatory drugs (NSAIDs)?**

NSAID-induced enteropathy is associated with intestinal bleeding, protein loss, ileal dysfunction, and malabsorption. There is no close relationship between upper endoscopic findings and evidence of intestinal bleeding among NSAID-treated patients, even when blood loss has led to iron-deficiency anemia. Chronic blood loss and protein loss seem to occur from the inflammatory site. Protein loss can result in significant hypoalbuminemia. Ileal dysfunctic can lead to bile acid malabsorption and, in rare cases, mild vitamin B_{12} malabsorption. Mefenamic acid (Postel) and sulindac (Clinoril) have been implicated as causes of severe malabsorption with subtotal villus atrophy that resembles celiac disease.

15. **Does scleroderma produce any manifestations in the small bowel?**
Patients with scleroderma may have small bowel dysfunction caused by absent cycling of the normal contractile pattern, known as the migrating motor complex. Small bowel motility stuc reveal markedly diminished amplitude in all phasic pressure waves. This finding may manifes clinically as intestinal pseudo-obstruction and bacterial overgrowth. Patients may suffer from nausea, vomiting, abdominal pain, diarrhea, and malabsorption. Small bowel radiographic series may show megaduodenum and dilated loops of jejunum.

16. **How does octreotide affect intestinal motility and bacterial overgrowth in scleroderma?**
Octreotide evokes alternating phase-1 and phase-3 activities in normal people and patients with scleroderma. In patients with scleroderma, these complexes propagate at the same velocity and have two-thirds the amplitude of spontaneous complexes in normal people. This effect is independent of motilin because octreotide inhibits motilin release. Octreotide may retard gastric antral motility—unlike erythromycin, which markedly stimulates gastric antral motor activity.

17. **Describe the different forms of lymphangiectasia.**
Congenital intestinal lymphangiectasia (Milroy's disease) results from a malformation of the lymphatic system. Many areas in the body can be affected. Patients with congenital disease m present at any time from childhood to adulthood and have usually asymmetric lymphedema. *Secondary lymphangiectasia* results from a disease that blocks intestinal lymph drainage. Causes of secondary lymphangiectasia include extensive abdominal or retroperitoneal carci- noma, lymphoma, retroperitoneal fibrosis, chronic pancreatitis, mesenteric tuberculosis or sarcoidosis, Crohn's disease, chronic congestive heart failure, and even constrictive pericard

KEY POINTS: SMALL BOWEL ENTEROPATHIES

1. Small bowel enteropathies may present with vague symptoms of bloating, intestinal gas, loos bowel movements.

2. Clinicians should be alert to the subtle presenting symptoms of these disorders to avoid missing the diagnosis.

18. **What are the clinical manifestations of abetalipoproteinemia?**
Abetalipoproteinemia is an autosomal recessive condition characterized by the inability to for chylomicrons and very low density lipoprotein particles by the enterocytes because of abnorr apoprotein B. Most patients suffer severe fat malabsorption and retardation and rarely surviv the third decade. The largest series of patients has been studied at the National Institutes of Health.

19. **What are the different clinical presentations of eosinophilic gastroenteritis?**
Eosinophilic gastroenteritis is characterized by eosinophilic infiltration in the gastrointestinal tract. Clinical features and severity depend on the layer and location of involvement. Mucosal involvement leads to protein-losing enteropathy, fecal blood loss, and malabsorption.

Involvement of the muscle layer often causes obstruction of gastric or small bowel. Subserosal involvement causes ascites, pleural effusion, or, on occasion, pericarditis.

20. **How are patients with eosinophilic gastroenteritis treated?**
The mainstay of treatment for eosinophilic gastroenteritis is corticosteroids, even though no controlled trials have been performed. The recommended dosage of prednisone is usually 20–40 mg/day for treatment of the initial episode and relapses, with 5–10 mg/day for maintenance. Some patients respond to a short course of treatment but may suffer relapse. Others may require long-term maintenance therapy. The course of disease may wax and wane in severity but is rarely life threatening. The therapeutic effect of oral sodium cromoglycate is controversial. Trial elimination diets have, occasionally, been successful, but relapse is common.

21. **What are the common causes of diarrhea in a patient with Crohn's disease and ileal resection?**
Ileal resection <100 cm: bile salt diarrhea. Normally, conjugated bile acids are reabsorbed in the ileum. When <100 cm ileum is resected, bile acids pass into the colon, causing direct irritation of the colonic epithelium and net water secretion by the colon. Bile-salt diarrhea is typically watery, may not start until a normal diet is resumed after surgery, is precipitated by a meal (typically after breakfast when a large amount of bile is stored in the gallbladder), and does not lead to weight loss. Patients benefit from an empiric trial of cholestyramine, a bile acid-binding agent.
Ileal resection >100 cm: steatorrhea. When >100 cm of ileum is lost to surgical resection or disease, the daily loss of bile acids exceeds the ability of the liver to synthesize new bile acids; hence, the total circulation bile acid pool is diminished. Bile acid deficiency leads to impaired intraluminal micellar fat absorption or steatorrhea. Patients benefit from a low-fat diet or supplement of medium-chain triglycerides. The diminished circulating pool of bile acids also promotes formation of cholesterol gallstones.

22. **Where are the endemic areas for tropical sprue?**
Tropical sprue is endemic in Puerto Rico, Cuba, the Dominican Republic, and Haiti but not in Jamaica or the other West Indies islands. It is found in Central America, Venezuela, and Columbia. Sprue is common in the Indian subcontinent and Far East, although little information is available from China. Sprue has been reported among several visitors to countries in the Middle East. It is rare in Africa, although the occurrence of sprue among populations living in the central and southern parts is now well established.

23. **How is tropical sprue treated?**
The most effective therapy for tropical sprue in returning travelers or expatriates is a combination of folic acid and tetracycline. Folic acid should be given in a dosage of 5 mg/day orally and tetracycline in a dosage of 250 mg four times/day. Vitamin B_{12} should be given parenterally, in addition to the previously mentioned combination, if a deficiency of this vitamin is discovered. Treatment should be continued for at least several months or until intestinal unction returns to normal. Treatment with folic acid alone may be effective in reversing small bowel abnormalities or even in curing the acute illness, but not in curing the chronic form. On the other hand, long-term treatment with tetracycline alone may result in cure of both acute and chronic forms of sprue.

24. **How is bacterial overgrowth diagnosed?**
The gold standard for the diagnosis of bacterial overgrowth is demonstration of increased concentrations of bacteria (>10^5 colony-forming units/mL) in fluid obtained from the intestine during duodenal intubation. If quantitative culture of the small bowel aspirate is not possible, the diagnosis can be made with various breath tests. With the lactulose-hydrogen breath test, a rise in breath hydrogen level of 12 ppm from baseline values is taken as diagnostic of bacterial

overgrowth. The 14C-glycocholate and 14C-D-xylose breath tests detect the release of the radi labeled carbon dioxide as the result of bacterial deconjugation of bile acid and metabolism of xylose. Normalization of the Schilling's test after treatment with antibiotics is highly suggestiv of bacterial overgrowth.

25. **What is the mechanism of hyperoxaluria in short bowel syndrome?**
Normally, intraluminal calcium binds to oxalate and prevents intestinal absorption of oxalate. With short bowel syndrome, malabsorption of fat leads to excessive luminal free fatty acids, which bind to calcium, allowing oxalate to pass unbound and become available for absorption. Excessive luminal free fatty acids and bile acids appear to increase colonic permeability to oxalate, further increasing its absorption. Therefore, hyperoxaluria appears to depend on the presence of an intact colon. To prevent calcium oxalate nephrolithiasis in patients with bowel disease, a low-oxalate and low-fat diet should be recommended.

26. **What is immunoproliferative small intestinal disease (IPSID)?**
Also known as alpha heavy-chain disease, IPSID is a type of lymphoma composed of dense lymphoplasmacytic mucosal infiltrate that secretes an abnormal alpha-heavy chain protein. The disease usually affects the small intestine from the second part of the duodenum distally into the jejunum. It presents in young adults and is usually associated with poor socioeconom conditions in the Mediterranean region and many developing nations.

27. **What causes immunoproliferative small intestinal disease?**
Although its exact etiology is unclear, early stage IPSID has been linked to a bacterial origin. Recently, investigators have established an association between IPSID and *Campylobacter jejuni* with use of polymerase chain reaction and DNA sequencing techniques.

28. **What are the most common clinical manifestations of immunoproliferative small intestinal disease?**
   - Abdominal pain
   - Diarrhea
   - Malabsorption
   - Weight loss
   - Growth retardation
   - Paraproteinemia with overproduction of heavy chain of IgA

29. **How is immunoproliferative small intestinal disease treated?**
Early stage disease responds frequently to tetracycline or to other broad-spectrum antibiotic treatment and may result in complete remission. IPSID that has progressed to high-grade lymphoma may respond to systemic combination chemotherapy.

WEBSITES

1. http://www.celiac.org/

2. http://www.consensus.nih.gov
(Search "celiac disease")

3. http://www.vhjoe.com

LIOGRAPHY

Akbulut H, Soykan I, Yakaryilmaz F, et al: Five-year results of the treatment of 23 patients with immunoproliferative small intestinal disease: a Turkish experience. Cancer 80:8–14, 1997.

Balasekaran R, Porter JL, Santa Ana CA, Fordtran JS: Positive results on tests for steatorrhea in persons consuming olestra potato chips. Ann Intern Med 132:279–282, 2000.

Bardella MT, Fraquelli M, Quatrini M, et al: Prevalence of hypertransaminasemia in adult celiac patients and effect of gluten-free diet. Hepatology 22:833–836, 1995.

Bjarnason I, Hayllar J, Macpherson AJ, Russell AS: Side effects of nonsteroidal antiinflammatory drugs on the small and large intestine in humans. Gastroenterology 104:1832–1847, 1993.

Fleming JL, Wiesner RH, Shorter RG: Whipple's disease: Clinical, biochemical, and histopathologic features and assessment of treatment in 29 patients. Mayo Clin Proc 63:539–551, 1988.

Hofmann AF, Poley R: Role of bile acid malabsorption in pathogenesis of diarrhea and steatorrhea in patients with ileal resection: I. Response to cholestyramine or replacement of dietary long chain triglyceride by medium chain triglyceride. Gastroenterology 62:918–934, 1972.

Klipstein FA: Tropical sprue in travelers and expatriates living abroad. Gastroenterology 80:590–600, 1981.

Lecuit M, Abachin E, Martin A, et al: Immunoproliferative small intestinal disease associated with *Campylobacter jejuni*. N Engl J Med 350:239–248, 2004.

Ramzan NN, Loftus E Jr, Burgart LJ: Diagnosis and monitoring of Whipple disease by polymerase chain reaction. Ann Intern Med 126:520–527, 1997.

Raoult D, Birg ML, La Scola B: Cultivation of the bacillus of Whipple's disease. N Engl J Med 342:620–625, 2000.

Relman DA, Schmidt TM, MacDermott RP, Falkow S: Identification of the uncultured bacillus of Whipple's disease. N Engl J Med 327:293–301, 1992.

Roberts IM: Workup of the patient with malabsorption. Postgrad Med 81:32–42, 1987.

Sblattero D, Berti I, Trevisiol C, et al: Human recombinant tissue transglutaminase ELISA: An innovative diagnostic test for celiac disease. Am J Gastroenterol 95:1253–1257, 2000.

Seissler J, Boms S, Wohlrab U, et al: Antibodies to human recombinant tissue transglutaminase measured by radioligand assay: Evidence for high diagnostic sensitivity for celiac disease. Horm Metab Res 31:375–379, 1999.

Sollid LM: Molecular basis of celiac disease. Annu Rev Immunol 18:53–81, 2000.

Soudah HC, Hasler WL, Owyang C: Effect of octreotide on intestinal motility and bacterial overgrowth in scleroderma. N Engl J Med 325:1461–1467, 1991.

Street S, Donoghue HD, Neild GH: Tropheryma whippelii DNA in saliva of healthy people [Letter]. Lancet 354:1178–1179, 1999.

Talley NJ, Shorter RG, Phillips SF, Zinsmeister AR: Eosinophilic gastroenteritis: A clinicopathological study of patients with disease of the mucosa, muscle layer, and subserosal tissues. Gut 31:54–58, 1990.

Trier JS: Celiac sprue. N Engl J Med 325:1709–1719, 1991.

Volta U, Molinaro N, Fusconi M, et al: IgA antiendomysial antibody test: A step forward in celiac disease screening. Dig Dis Sci 36:752–756, 1991.

Yamada T, Alpers DH, Owyang C, et al (eds): Textbook of Gastroenterology, 2nd ed. Philadelphia, J.B. Lippincott, 1995.

CHAPTER 43

CROHN'S DISEASE

Aaron Brzezinski, MD, and Bret A. Lashner, MD

DIAGNOSIS

1. **What are the usual symptoms and signs suggestive of Crohn's disease?**

   The symptoms of Crohn's disease are determined by the site and type of involvement, that is, inflammatory, stenotic, or fistulizing. The most common site of involvement is ileocolitis. These patients present with diarrhea; abdominal pain that is usually insidious in the right lower quadrant, triggered or aggravated frequently after meals; weight loss; and an association with tender, inflammatory mass in the right lower quadrant. The diarrhea is usually nonbloody, and this may be one of the clues in clinical history that helps differentiate Crohn's disease from ulcerative colitis, where bloody diarrhea is almost universal. Patients frequently have fever, weight loss, perianal fistulas and/or fissures, and extra-intestinal manifestations, such as aphthous stomatitis, arthritis, and erythema nodosum. Patients with isolated colonic disease present usually with diarrhea, abdominal pain, and weight loss.

   Perianal skin tags are very common and, at times, mistaken for external hemorrhoids; it is not until these are excised and the course is complicated by a nonhealing wound that the diagnosis of Crohn's disease is entertained. At times the main symptoms are related to perianal fistulas and/or abscess, even though most of these patients have other areas of involvement by Crohn's disease. Gastroduodenal Crohn's disease is less common and can mimic complicated peptic ulcer disease with abdominal pain, early gastric satiety, or symptoms of duodenal obstruction.

   Patients can present with mild, moderate, or severe disease. This is a clinical judgment based on factors such as the severity of diarrhea, abdominal pain, the presence or absence of dehydration, anemia, malnutrition, and tachycardia. For clinical trials, the Crohn's Disease Activity Index (CDAI) has been developed (Table 43-1). Calculation of the CDAI combines

TABLE 43-1. CALCULATION OF THE CROHN'S DISEASE ACTIVITY INDEX (CDAI)		
Variable	Range of Values	Weight
1. Liquid or soft stools summed over 7 days	0–70	2
2. Daily abdominal pain ratings summed over 7 days	0–21	6
3. General well-being ratings summed over 7 days	0–28	6
4. Number of extraintestinal manifestations	0–3	30
5. Use of opiates for diarrhea	0–1	4
6. Abdominal mass	0–5	10
7. 47-Hematocrit (males) 42-Hematocrit (females)	—	6
8. Percent of body weight below standard	—	1

CDAI = the sum of each variable multiplied by its weight.

weighted scores of clinical and laboratory variables. CDAI scores less than 150 indicate a clinical remission, and scores over 450 indicate severely active disease. Even though the CDAI is subjective and cumbersome, it is currently the standard measure of disease activity for all clinical trials.

2. **How is the diagnosis of Crohn's disease established?**
The diagnosis of Crohn's disease is established by history, physical examination, endoscopy, biopsies, x-rays, and laboratory tests. Crohn's disease presents more commonly between ages 15 and 25 years. The diagnosis should be suspected in patients with chronic diarrhea, finding characteristic intestinal ulcerations and excluding alternative diagnoses. The ulcerations of Crohn's disease may be aphthoid (Fig. 43-1) but could be deep and serpiginous along the longitudinal axis of the bowel (Fig. 43-2). Skip areas, cobblestoning, and rectal sparing are characteristic findings. Air contrast barium enema, small bowel series with or without a per-oral pneumocolon, or colonoscopy each may demonstrate these typical lesions. On a small bowel series, Crohn's disease often leads to separation of bowel loops, a narrowed and ulcerated terminal ileum and, in advanced cases, the so-called string sign (Fig. 43-3). The biopsies of involved areas have architectural distortion and a chronic inflammatory infiltrate, and in about 10–30% of cases of Crohn's colitis there are noncaseating granulomas that are usually diagnostic. Typical lesions of Crohn's disease may also be seen in the upper gastrointestinal tract. The inflammation is localized to the ileocecal region in approximately 50% of cases, the small bowel in approximately 25% of cases, the colon in 20% of cases, and the upper gastrointestinal tract or perirectum in 5%.

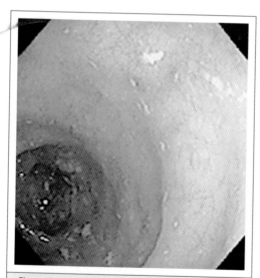

Figure 43-1. Aphthoid ulcers in a patient with Crohn's colitis.

3. **Which diseases can mimic the symptoms and signs of Crohn's disease?**
The differential diagnosis of Crohn's disease is long. The most common mimics of Crohn's colitis are ulcerative colitis, ischemic colitis, diverticulitis, or colorectal cancer. For Crohn's ileitis, infection with *Yersinia enterocolitica* or *Mycobacterium tuberculosis* may mimic disease. In immunosuppressed patients, viral infections such as cytomegalovirus (CMV) can mimic Crohn's disease. Other important diseases in the differential diagnosis of Crohn's disease

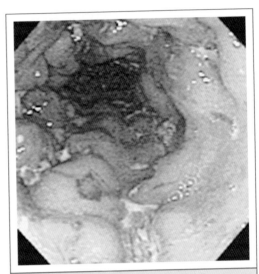

Figure 43-2. Deep, serpiginous ulcers of Crohn's disease.

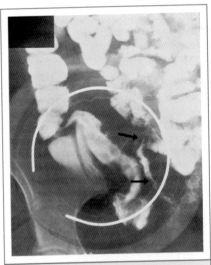

Figure 43-3. "String sign" from a small bowel series in a patient with Crohn's disease

include the irritable bowel syndrome, intestinal lymphoma, celiac sprue, radiation enteropa[??] and nonsteroidal anti-inflammatory drug-induced enteropathy.

4. **What serologic tests can help establish the diagnosis?**
Clinical, endoscopic, and histologic findings can establish the diagnosis and differentiate between Crohn's disease and ulcerative colitis in 85–90% of patients (Table 43-2). Still, in t[??] 10–15% of patients with indeterminate colitis, where the diagnosis is important to determi[??]

optimal medical or surgical therapy, serologic testing may be helpful. Anti-*Saccharomyces cerevisiae* antibody (ASCA) is seen in over 60% of patients with Crohn's disease (sensitivity) and in less than 10% of patients with other gastrointestinal diseases, such as ulcerative colitis and irritable bowel syndrome. *Saccharomyces cerevisiae*, or baker's yeast, becomes antigenic when there is increased intestinal permeability, as there is in Crohn's disease patients. When coupled with the perinuclear antineutrophil cytoplasmic antibody (pANCA), a test with a 70% sensitivity for ulcerative colitis and a 10% sensitivity for Crohn's disease, ASCA and pANCA, testing together, have a sensitivity and specificity of over 90%.

TABLE 43-2. SOME DISTINGUISHING CHARACTERISTICS OF ULCERATIVE COLITIS AND CROHN'S DISEASE

Characteristics	Ulcerative Colitis	Crohn's Disease
Rectal bleeding	Usual	Sometimes
Abdominal mass	Rare	Often
Abdominal pain	Sometimes	Often
Perianal disease	Extremely rare	5–10%
Upper GI symptoms	Never	Occasional
Cigarette smoking	Very rare	Common
Malnutrition	Sometimes	Common
Low-grade fever	Sometimes	Often
Rectal disease	Usual	Sometimes
Continuous disease	Usual	Rare
Granulomas	Never	10–30%
Crypt abscesses	Common	Rare
Discrete ulcers	Rare	Common
Aphthoid ulcers	Rare	Common
Cobblestone lesions	Never	Common
Skip lesions	No, except rarely in treated patients	Common
Ileal involvement	Rare, backwash ileitis	Usual
Fistulas	Never	Common
Cancer	Rare	Very rare
Microscopic skip lesions	No, except rarely in treated patients	Common
Transmural inflammation	Only in fulminant disease	Common

GI = gastrointestinal.

CAUSES

Is cigarette smoking associated with Crohn's disease?
Yes. Crohn's disease is a heterogeneous disease, and a single etiologic agent has not been identified. Cigarette smokers are much more likely than nonsmokers to develop Crohn's disease and, particularly in women, it has a more aggressive behavior. There is evidence that cigarette

smokers with Crohn's disease have a worse prognosis than nonsmokers. Early recurrence, m
severe complications, and a higher likelihood for repeat surgery are all associated with cigare
smoking. Although it has not been shown that quitters can favorably change the course of the
disease, it is reasonable to assume that quitters will have less severe complications and requi
surgery less often than smokers. For reasons related to their disease, the increased risk of
vascular events due to hypercoagulability, as well as related to their cardiovascular health anc
cancer risk, Crohn's disease patients *must quit smoking!*

Over half of Crohn's disease patients are cigarette smokers compared to about one third of
the U.S. adult population. Furthermore, Crohn's disease patients are less likely to quit than co
trols. This finding is in direct contradistinction to the protective effect of cigarette smoking fo
ulcerative colitis. Although nicotine has been used to treat ulcerative colitis patients, it should
only be used in Crohn's disease patients as a means to quit smoking.

6. **What infectious agents might be responsible for Crohn's disease?**
   Mycobacterium paratuberculosis causes Johne's disease, a granulomatous inflammation of t
   terminal ileum and other parts of the intestine in cows. In a small number of Crohn's disease
   patients, *in situ* hybridization and culture of resected specimens has found *M. paratuberculos*
   and other atypical mycobacterium. However, a causal relationship has not been determined; a
   treatment of such infections is effective in a few patients only. Other infectious agents, such a
   the measles virus or the measles vaccine, have been proposed, but the evidence is inconclusi
   and an etiologic association has not been established. It is possible that an infectious agent o
   cellular material from an infectious agent triggers an abnormal immune response by the inna
   intestinal immune system.

7. **Is there a genetic predisposition for developing Crohn's disease?**
   Yes. The principal theory on the pathogenesis of Crohn's disease is that in a genetically predis
   posed individual, an environmental agent (e.g., infection, dietary substance that enters the
   bloodstream through a permeable intestine, or nicotine) triggers an uncontrolled inflammato
   response. The incidence of Crohn's disease ranges between 2 and 10 per 100,000 in the popu
   tion. Crohn's disease occurs in more than one first- or second-degree family member in appro
   mately 20% of cases. Children of a parent with Crohn's disease have a lifetime risk of less tha
   3% of developing Crohn's disease. Spouses of Crohn's disease patients rarely develop Crohn'
   disease. The genetic predisposition occurs from a number of important genetic mutations in l
   regulatory proteins of intestinal inflammation. Studies of genetic linkages among kindreds wi
   inflammatory bowel disease led to the discovery of the NOD 2/CARD 15 mutation in chromosome 16 (IBD-1). Depending on the population studied, this mutation can be seen in as many
   30% of Crohn's disease patients; however, it is also seen in non-Crohn's disease patients, and
   Japan this mutation is rarely seen only in Crohn's disease patients. In the European and
   American Caucasian population, the presence of this mutation appears to predict stenotic
   disease involving the terminal ileum.

NATURAL HISTORY

8. **Is mortality increased in patients with Crohn's disease?**
   Yes. Patients with Crohn's disease, in general, do not have an increased mortality when
   compared with age- and sex-matched controls. Some complications of Crohn's disease,
   such as malignancy, short bowel syndrome, hypercoagulable state, and primary sclerosing
   cholangitis, do have an increased mortality. Fortunately, these complications are rare.

9. **Are there factors that predict a flare of Crohn's disease activity?**
   Yes. Cigarette smoking is the most important clinical risk factor for symptomatic recurrence.
   Smokers have a recurrence at least twice as high as nonsmokers. The effect of oral contracep

tive use on recurrence rate is controversial. Although oral contraceptive use is not associated with an increased recurrence rate, there is a synergistic effect between smoking and oral contraceptive use: the combined effects are greater than the sum of the individual effects. Other important risk factors for symptomatic recurrence are intestinal infections or nonsteroidal anti-inflammatory drug use.

10. **Does behavior of disease predict its natural history?**

Yes. According to its behavior, Crohn's disease has been classified as either inflammatory, stricturing, or fistulizing disease. Inflammatory-type disease is characterized by intestinal ulcerations, and the main symptoms are diarrhea, abdominal pain, an inflammatory mass, and, when it is severely active, fever and weight loss. Inflammatory-type disease responds best to anti-inflammatory therapy, particularly corticosteroids and infliximab, but recurrence is the rule rather than the exception. The natural history of inflammatory-type disease is aggressive with early recurrence. Stricturing-type disease, on the other hand, has a more indolent course that does not respond well to anti-inflammatory therapy. Although all Crohn's disease begin as inflammation, the predominant pathology in patients with stricturing disease is extensive fibrosis in the lamina propria. Surgery is the best therapeutic option in patients with symptomatic stricturing disease, and the need for a second surgery is lower than with other types of Crohn's disease. Fistulizing-type disease is characterized by enterocutaneous and/or entero-enteric fistulas. Fistulas occur in areas of inflammation and often originate in a segment of bowel proximal to a stricture. Following successful medical or surgical therapy for fistulas, recurrence is common. Most patients with inflammatory or fistulizing disease will benefit from maintenance medical therapy to minimize the risk for recurrence.

11. **Do patients with Crohn's disease have an excess cancer risk?**

Yes. Small bowel cancer in Crohn's disease is a rarely reported phenomenon; less than 100 cases have been reported in the literature. Epidemiologic studies, though, have suggested that the relative risk of small bowel cancer in Crohn's disease is greatly elevated. Small bowel cancer in Crohn's disease follows the same distribution as Crohn's disease (ileum > jejunum > duodenum), which is exactly opposite to the distribution of sporadic small bowel cancer. Excluded loops and chronic fistulas are also risk factors for small bowel cancer in Crohn's disease. Like in ulcerative colitis, colorectal cancer is increased in patients with extensive colonic Crohn's disease. Colorectal cancer in Crohn's disease occurs near areas of inflammation. However, because the premalignant lesion of dysplasia is not as widespread when present in the colon of Crohn's disease patients as it is in ulcerative colitis patients, cancer surveillance colonoscopy is less effective in decreasing mortality.

12. **What are the extraintestinal manifestations of Crohn's disease?**

The extraintestinal manifestations of Crohn's disease are similar to those seen in ulcerative colitis. A polyarticular nondeforming arthritis is the most common extraintestinal manifestation, occurring in about 20% of patients; the arthritis responds to treatment of bowel symptoms. Primary sclerosing cholangitis is less common in Crohn's disease patients than in ulcerative colitis patients; it follows a course independent of disease activity and does not respond to anti-inflammatory therapy directed to the bowel, including surgery. Erythema nodosum, pyoderma gangrenosum, iritis, uveitis, pancreatitis, nephrolithiasis, cholelithiasis, amyloidosis, osteoporosis, and ankylosing spondylitis are all extraintestinal manifestations of Crohn's disease. Nephrolithiasis most often is from oxalate stones. Crohn's disease patients with fat malabsorption have preferential binding of luminal calcium to fatty acids rather than oxalate and the subsequent increased absorption of dietary oxalate with stone formation.

TREATMENT

13. **Which 5-aminosalicylic acid preparations are effective in treating Crohn's disease patients?**

    5-Aminosalicylic acid (5-ASA) agents have been used for many years to treat inflammatory bowel disease, mostly in ulcerative colitis patients. The response to 5-ASA in Crohn's disease in induction and maintenance of remission is less than in ulcerative colitis. 5-ASA is a topical agent and not a systemic medication; therefore, it needs to be delivered to the site of inflammation. Sulfasalazine requires bacterial cleavage of the diazo bond between sulfapyridine and 5-ASA for the 5-ASA to have a local anti-inflammatory effect. Because bacteria in sufficient numbers are only present in the large bowel, sulfasalazine is effective only in patients with colitis. Other oral 5-ASA compounds that are used for colonic disease include Asacol that is 5-ASA coated with a compound that dissolves at pH 7 (terminal ileum), Dipentum that is two molecules of 5-ASA bound by a diazo bond, and Colazal that is 5-ASA delivered in pro-form by a carrier. Pentasa is 5-ASA coated with ethylcellulose beads that dissolve and release 5-ASA throughout the small and large bowels. Theoretically, Pentasa should be most effective in patients with extensive small bowel disease. 5-ASA is also available in the form of suppositories or enemas for patients with proctitis or involvement of the sigmoid colon. 5-ASA agents are used only in patients with mildly to moderately active disease; their role in maintenance of remission is debatable.

14. **Should steroids be used in Crohn's disease?**

    Yes. Steroids are effective in treating inflammatory-type Crohn's disease. Long-term use is not recommended, however, due to the many serious adverse effects such as osteoporosis, diabetes, and cataracts, just to name a few. Steroids are not effective in stricturing Crohn's disease and may actually worsen patients with fistulas, especially if localized infection is not drained adequately.

    Budesonide is a very potent steroid with a very high rate first-pass metabolism, 85–90%. Given this, the systemic side effects are diminished greatly but not entirely eliminated. The preparation available in the United States delivers the medication in the distal ileum and cecum in patients who have not had small bowel resection. In Canada, budesonide is also available as an enema. Budesonide has been effective for induction of remission in patients with moderately active Crohn's disease and has some effect in maintenance of remission. It is advisable to prescribe supplemental calcium and vitamin D to patients taking steroids, regardless of the route of administration.

15. **What is the role for immunosuppressive therapy in Crohn's disease?**

    Both azathioprine and 6-mercaptopurine are used commonly in Crohn's disease patients. Both are purine analogs that interfere with DNA synthesis of rapidly dividing cells, such as lymphocytes and macrophages. Because these drugs do not have a clinical effect for 2–3 months or longer, they are used primarily in maintaining remission in inflammatory-type and fistulizing-type Crohn's disease and can be given for 4 years or longer. Important adverse effects include pancreatitis, allergy, hepatitis, and leukopenia. White blood cell counts and liver function tests need to be checked on a periodic basis. There are two main strategies to start these medications: traditionally the medication was started at a low dose and the dose was increased, according to the speed at which the white blood cells (WBCs) decreased. Because the thiopurine methyltransferase (TPMT) enzyme activity can be measured, the preferred option is to start the dose predicted, according to body weight for those patients with a normal enzyme level activity, at a reduced dose for patients with intermediate TPMT enzyme activity, and to explore alternative therapies in patients with low or absent TPMT activity. Whichever regimen one chooses, it is very important to monitor liver tests and the WBC on a regular basis. Nonresponders can have levels of the active metabolite, 6-thioguanine (6-TG), measured to see whether the lack of response is due to lack of adherence to a medical regimen (6-TG level of 0), under dosing (6-TG level of <230 pmol/8×10^8 red blood cells [RBCs]), or true lack of response (6-TG level >230 pmol/8×10^8 RBCs).

16. **Which biologic therapies are effective for Crohn's disease patients?**

Infliximab is an IgG_1 chimeric mouse-human antibody to tumor necrosis factor (TNF) that, when infused intravenously, binds to soluble TNF and to the TNF on surface membranes of inflammatory cells causing cell lysis. It has been approved for use in inflammatory-type Crohn's disease and fistulizing Crohn's disease. In randomized clinical trials, 48% of patients with inflammatory-type disease and 55% of patients with fistulizing disease achieved complete remission, figures significantly higher than placebo-treated patients. Side effects during the infusion, such as nausea, headache, and pharyngitis, can be attenuated with slowing the infusion. Since its approval by the Food and Drug Administration (FDA) in 1998, there has been a great deal of experience gained with the use of infliximab. We have learned that the response rate is 60–70%, and that with continued use every 8 weeks patients maintain remission. Tuberculosis and opportunistic infections have been the main complications of its use, and the analysis of 500 patients at the Mayo Clinic revealed a 1% mortality rate among patients receiving infliximab (but this mortality rate has not been reported in other series). With chronic use, patients form anti-infliximab antibodies that may decrease its effectiveness, in which case higher doses or more frequent infusions are required. When a long period of time elapses between infusions, there is a higher risk of immediate or delayed infusion reactions that precludes its subsequent use.

17. **Which medications are effective in maintaining remission?**

Patients who have a high risk of recurrence following a medically or surgically induced remission should be considered for maintenance medications. Smokers, patients who have had more than one surgery, and patients with inflammatory-type or fistulizing disease, have the highest risk of recurrence. Long-term therapy with azathioprine or 6-mercaptopurine has the best maintenance effects. Methotrexate is effective in some patients and can be used in patients who fail treatment with either azathioprine or 6-mercaptopurine, or in those who have side effects precluding the use of these agents. 5-ASA agents are rarely effective for maintenance. Infliximab infusions every 8 weeks have been approved for maintenance therapy of inflammatory-type Crohn's disease.

18. **What are the indications for surgery in Crohn's disease?**

The adage "a chance to cut is a chance to cure" does not apply to Crohn's disease. Surgery is not a cure for Crohn's disease. The main goal of surgery is to treat the most important problem while preserving as much bowel as possible. Wide resection margins are not associated with decreased recurrence and should be avoided. The indications for surgery include active inflammatory-type disease refractory to medical therapy, prednisone dependence, intestinal strictures, fistulas, abscesses, growth retardation, bleeding, perforation, severe anorectal disease, dysplasia, and cancer. Besides resection and abscess drainage, there is considerable experience with strictureplasty (opening a stricture without removing bowel) and advancement flap surgery (removing a perirectal fistula by advancing normal mucosa over the internal os). A close working relationship between the internist/gastroenterologist and colorectal surgeon is extremely important for controlling disease and decreasing morbidity.

19. **What therapeutic regimen is most often effective for stricturing-type Crohn's disease?**

Usually, stricturing-type Crohn's disease will require surgery. Anti-inflammatory therapy is not likely to relieve symptoms. The goals of surgery are to relieve symptoms and preserve bowel length. The surgery offered need not be a resection, though. Strictureplasties of strictured segments of small bowel or anastomosis can provide long-term relief of obstructive symptoms. In the most common type of strictureplasty, an incision is made on the longitudinal axis of a short stricture that is sutured along a perpendicular. Prior to performing a strictureplasty, the surgeon will send a frozen section to rule out carcinoma at the site of the stricture. In some patients, endoscopic balloon dilatation at the site of an ileocolic anastomosis relieves symptoms, delaying the need for surgery.

KEY POINTS: CROHN'S DISEASE

1. Synonyms include regional enteritis, regional ileitis, granulomatous colitis, or granulomatous enteritis.

2. Intestinal lesions range from erythema and blunted vessel pattern to aphthous ulcers and deep and serpiginous ulcers.

3. The eponym for the disease is taken from the first author of the paper, Burrill B. Crohn, with the first description in the U.S. literature in 1932. The other authors of the paper, Ginzburg and Oppenheimer, have fallen in historic importance since authorship order was determined alphabetically.

4. Crohn's disease is characterized by nonspecific inflammation of any segment of the gastrointestinal tract in a discontinuous fashion with skip areas of ulceration, fissuring, or transmural inflammation.

5. Noncaseating granulomas are characteristic of the disease; however, they are seen in only 10–30% of biopsies.

20. **What therapeutic regimen is most often effective for inflammatory-type Crohn disease?**

Inflammatory-type Crohn's disease should respond to anti-inflammatory agents. In mild disease, 5-ASA agents are usually tried first due to the limited toxicity; however, their efficacy is limited. Antibiotics such as ciprofloxacin or Metronidazole are effective, particularly in patients with colonic and perianal disease. Steroids or infliximab are tried next due to the relatively rapid onset of action. Azathioprine/6-mercaptopurine and methotrexate are reserved usually for steroid-dependent inflammatory disease and for maintenance of remission.

21. **What therapeutic regimen is most often effective for fistulizing Crohn's disease?**

An assessment of the degree of mucosal activity is an important determinant of therapy for fistulizing Crohn's disease. When active disease is present, anti-inflammatory therapy with azathioprine, 6-mercaptopurine, or infliximab can be extremely helpful. In perianal fistulas, combined medical and surgical treatment is usually required. Sepsis should be adequately drained, and placement of noncutting seton sutures can facilitate continued drainage and promote healing (Fig. 43-4). Antibiotics, azathioprine, 6-mercaptopurine, or infliximab are usually beneficial. If the mucosal disease is quiescent, then surgical therapy with an advancement flap procedure may be appropriate.

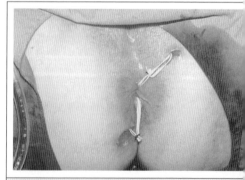

Figure 43-4. Seton sutures placed in the perineum.

When should nutritional support be used in Crohn's disease patients?

Nutritional support can be used as primary or adjuvant therapy for Crohn's disease. Interestingly, bowel rest and total parenteral nutrition (TPN) will greatly improve symptoms in most patients with inflammatory-type or fistulizing-type disease. Enteral nutrition is almost as effective as steroids in inducing remission in inflammatory-type Crohn's disease; it has much fewer side effects, but it takes longer to induce remission. Unfortunately, when food is introduced, symptoms and signs of active disease return quickly. Nutritional support is also effective to promote growth in children with Crohn's disease and growth retardation. Because of the expense and morbidity of TPN, long-term TPN should be reserved for patients with a short bowel syndrome, extensive small bowel disease, or in patients who need nutritional support, when enteral nutrition is not tolerated.

BLIOGRAPHY

Abreu MT, Taylor KD, Lin YC, et al: Mutations in NOD2 are associated with fibrostenosing disease in patients with Crohn's disease. Gastroenterology 123:679–688, 2002.

Belluzzi A, Brignola C, Campieri M, et al: Effect of an enteric-coated fish-oil preparation on relapses in Crohn's disease. N Engl J Med 334:1557–1560, 1996.

Best WR, Becktel JM, Singleton JW: Rederived values of the eight coefficients of the Crohn's disease activity index (CDAI). Gastroenterology 77:843–846, 1979.

Brant SR, Picco MF, Achkar JP, et al: Defining complex contributions of NOD2/CARD15 gene mutations, age at onset, and tobacco use in Crohn's disease phenotypes. Inflamm Bowel Dis 9:281–289, 2003.

Columbel JF, Loftus EV, Tremaine WJ, et al: The safety profile of infliximab in patients with Crohn's disease: The Mayo Clinic experience in 500 patients. Gastroenterology 126:19–31, 2004.

Crohn BB, Ginzburg L, Oppenheimer GD: Regional enteritis: A pathological and clinical entity. JAMA 99:1323–1329, 1932.

Cuthbert AP, Fisher SA, Mirza MM, et al: The contribution of NOD2 gene mutations to the risk and site of disease in inflammatory bowel disease. Gastroenterology 122:867–874, 2002.

Dubinsky MC, Lamothe S, Yang HY, et al: Pharmacogenomics and metabolite measurement for 6-mercaptopurine therapy in inflammatory bowel disease. Gastroenterology 118:705–713, 2000.

Fazio VW, Marchetti F, Church JM, et al: Effect of resection margins on recurrence of Crohn's disease of the small bowel: A randomized controlled trial. Ann Surg 224:563–571, 1996.

Feagan BG, Rochon J, Fedorak RN, et al: Methotrexate for the treatment of Crohn's disease. N Engl J Med 332:292–297, 1995.

Fiocchi C: Inflammatory bowel disease: Etiology and pathogenesis. Gastroenterology 115:182–205, 1998.

Hugot JP, Chamaillard M, Zouali H, et al: Association of NOD2 leucine-rich repeat variants with susceptibility to Crohn's disease. Nature 411:599–603, 2001.

Lichtiger S, Present DH, Kornbluth A, et al: Cyclosporine in severe ulcerative colitis refractory to steroid therapy. N Engl J Med 330:1841–1845, 1994.

Munkholm P, Langholz E, Davidsen M, Binder V: Intestinal cancer risk and mortality in patients with Crohn's disease. Gastroenterology 105:1716–1723, 1993.

Ogura Y, Bonen DK, Inohara N, et al: A frameshift mutation in NOD2 is associated with susceptibility to Crohn's disease. Nature 411:603–606, 2001.

Parsi MA, Achkar JP, Richardson S, et al: Predictors of response to infliximab in patients with Crohn's disease. Gastroenterology 123:707–713, 2002.

Present DH, Rutgeerts P, Targan S, et al: Infliximab for the treatment of fistulas in patients with Crohn's disease. N Engl J Med 340:1398–1405, 1999.

Ruemmele FM, Targan SR, Levy G, et al: Diagnostic accuracy of serological assays in pediatric inflammatory bowel disease. Gastroenterology 115:822–829, 1998.

Silverstein MD, Loftus EV, Sandborn WJ, et al: Clinical course and costs of care for Crohn's disease: Markov model analysis of a population-based cohort. Gastroenterology 117:49–57, 1999.

Singleton JW, Law DH, Delly ML, et al: National Cooperative Crohn's Disease Study: Results of drug treatment. Gastroenterology 77:847–869, 1979.

21. Targan SR, Hoenir SB, Van Deventer SJ, et al: A short-term study of chimeric monoclonal antibody cA2 to TNF alpha for Crohn's disease. N Engl J Med 337:1029–1035, 1997.

22. Timmer A, Sutherland LR, Martin F, et al: Oral contraceptive use and smoking are risk factors for relapse in Crohn's disease. Gastroenterology 114:1143–1150, 1998.

23. Valentine JF, Sninsky CA: Prevention and treatment of osteoporosis in patients with inflammatory bowel disea Am J Gastroenterol 94:878–883, 1999.

CHAPTER 44

ULCERATIVE COLITIS

Ramona O. Rajapakse, MD, and Burton I. Korelitz, MD

1. **What is ulcerative colitis?**

   Ulcerative colitis (UC) is a chronic inflammatory disease of the colon. It is distinct from Crohn's disease (CD) of the colon in that the inflammation is restricted mostly to the mucosa and involves only the colon. *The rectal segment is almost always involved, whereas in CD of the colon the rectum is usually spared.*

2. **Define *backwash ileitis.***

   Backwash ileitis refers to unusual cases of ulcerative colitis that involve the terminal ileum. The endoscopic, *histologic,* and radiologic appearances of backwash ileitis is the same as those of ulcerative colitis. When deep linear ulcers and strictures are seen in the ileum, Crohn's ileitis is the more likely diagnosis.

3. **What is indeterminate colitis?**

   As more information is gathered about the pathogenesis of ulcerative colitis and CD, the distinction between them at times can be unclear. In about 7% of patients, *when the inflammatory process is limited to the colon (no ileal involvement), the endoscopic, histologic, or radiologic findings are insufficiently distinct to separate the two diseases.* The colitis is then referred to as "indeterminate." Other patients carry the diagnosis of UC for many years until a change in signs and symptoms, consistent with CD, influences a change in diagnosis. In some patients, the diagnosis of CD of the colon is recognized only after colectomy and the development of recurrent ileitis in the ileostomy or ileoanal pouch performed for what was thought to be UC.

4. **Why is it important to distinguish between ulcerative colitis and Crohn's disease?**

   Medical treatment of the two diseases overlaps, but ulcerative colitis is "curable" by total colectomy, *whereas CD can never be considered cured by resection.* Therefore, the correct diagnosis is of the utmost importance.

5. **What causes ulcerative colitis?**

   The cause is unknown. The greatest risk factor is a positive family history. Approximately 15% of patients with inflammatory bowel disease (IBD) have a first-degree relative with the disease, but the familial association is less in UC than in CD. Similarly, the incidence of IBD in first-degree relatives of patients with IBD is 30–100 times higher than in the general population. The cause remains technically unknown, although research has clarified that there are genetic, environmental, and immunologic contributions. The exact genetic link for UC has not been identified. Dietary antigens and bacteria have been proposed as possible triggers, but no evidence supports these theories. The incidence of UC is significantly higher in nonsmokers than in smokers and higher still in ex-smokers than in nonsmokers, supporting a protective effect of smoking. Whether this protective effect is secondary to nicotine or other constituents of cigarettes has not been fully established.

6. **Who gets ulcerative colitis?**

In most patients, UC has its onset in the second or third decades of life. However, there may be a second peak in the fifth or sixth decades, although this peak may be false because of other types of colitis that mimic UC. The disease has been described in all nationalities and ethnic groups but is more common in whites than in nonwhites. It is also more common in Jews than non-Jews. The hereditary link is supported by population-based studies.

7. **What are the signs and symptoms of ulcerative colitis?**

The predominant symptom at onset of UC is diarrhea, with or without blood in the stool. If inflammation is confined to the rectum *(proctitis)*, blood may be seen on the surface of the stool; other symptoms include tenesmus, urgency, rectal pain, and passage of mucus, without diarrhea.

Other distributions of UC are proctosigmoiditis; left-sided disease, which extends more proximal to the descending colon, splenic flexure, or distal transverse colon; and universal colitis, which involves any length proximal to the mid-transverse colon and often the entire colon. The inflammation is almost always confluent in distribution and almost always involves the rectum, when it is untreated with medication by enema.

More extensive colitis may be accompanied by systemic symptoms, such as weight loss and malaise, in addition to bloody diarrhea. Although pain is not a dominant feature, patients may complain of crampy abdominal discomfort relieved by a bowel movement and may have abdominal tenderness, localized usually to the left lower quadrant. Occasionally, patients may present with "constipation" secondary to rectal spasm. Although patients may present with extraintestinal manifestations before bowel symptoms, more often they parallel the severity of the primary bowel disease.

8. **Is there a diagnostic blood test for UC?**

Two antibodies have been helpful in differentiating UC from Crohn's colitis. Patients with ulcerative colitis have higher levels of peripheral anti-neutrophil cytoplasmic antibody (p-ANCA) and lower levels of anti-saccharomyces antibody (ASCA) than patients with Crohn's disease. However, these tests lack sufficient sensitivity and specificity to be used alone for diagnostic purposes. The combination of both tests may be helpful in a select group of patients with indeterminate colitis, together with other parameters such as clinical, endoscopic, pathologic, and radiologic features.

9. **How are patients with ulcerative colitis classified?**

Truelove and Witts divided patients into those with severe, moderate, and mild disease based on symptoms, physical findings, and laboratory values. We add to this list the severity of endoscopic and radiologic appearances. A plain film of the abdomen showing any degree of dilation of the colon or ulceration and edema of the mucosa outlined by air (even if not dilated) i indicative of a severe attack. Although endoscopic appearance does not always correlate well with clinical symptoms, the presence of severe mucosal disease indicates the need for more aggressive management. The clinical guide for severity of UC is as follows:

- *Mild:* fewer than four stools daily, with or without blood, with no systemic disturbance and a normal erythrocyte sedimentation rate (ESR).
- *Moderate:* more than four stools daily but with minimal systemic disturbance.
- *Severe:* more than six stools daily with blood and systemic disturbance as shown by fever, tachycardia, anemia, or ESR >30.

10. **How are the extraintestinal manifestations of ulcerative colitis classified?**

Although UC involves primarily the bowel, it may be associated with manifestations in other organs. These manifestations are divided into those that coincide with the activity of bowel disease and those that occur independently of bowel disease.

Extra Colonic Manifestation	Coincides with Colitis Activity
Colitic arthritis	Yes
Ankylosing spondylitis	No
Pyoderma gangrenosum	Yes
Erythema nodosum	Yes
Primary sclerosing cholangitis	No
Uveitis	Often but not always
Episcleritis	Often but not always

11. **What is colitic arthritis?**

Colitic arthritis is a migratory arthritis affecting the knees, hips, ankles, wrists, and elbows. *Usually, the joint involvement is asymmetric not bilateral.* It responds well to corticosteroids.

12. **Describe the association between ulcerative colitis and ankylosing spondylitis.**

Although ankylosing spondylitis is associated more commonly with CD than UC, patients with ulcerative colitis have a 30-fold increased risk of developing ankylosing spondylitis, which does not parallel disease activity. Many patients with early sacroiliitis alone are asymptomatic, and the diagnosis is made on radiographs. See Chapter 65, Rheumatologic Manifestations of GI Diseases.

13. **Discuss the hepatic complications of ulcerative colitis.**

Hepatic complications include fatty liver, pericholangitis, chronic active hepatitis, cirrhosis, and primary sclerosing cholangitis. Although most patients with sclerosing cholangitis have UC, only a minority of patients with UC develop sclerosing cholangitis. It is usually suspected with the finding of an abnormally elevated alkaline phosphatase or gamma glutamyl transferase (GGTP) enzyme. Sclerosing cholangitis is sometimes improved with ursodeoxycholic acid therapy (Actigal). Patients with sclerosing cholangitis and UC have a higher risk of developing colon cancer than those without. In addition, they are also at risk of developing cholangiocarcinoma. Cholestyramine may help in alleviating the pruritus associated with the disease, but the only cure is liver transplantation.

14. **What are the ocular complications of ulcerative colitis?**

Ocular complications include uveitis and episcleritis. Uveitis causes eye pain, photophobia, and blurred vision and requires prompt intervention to prevent permanent visual impairment. It usually responds to topical steroids, but, sometimes, systemic steroids are required.

15. **Describe the association between ulcerative colitis and thromboembolic events.**

Patients with IBD are at increased risk of thromboembolic events, most commonly deep venous thrombosis of the lower extremities. After a search for other causes of a hypercoagulable state, patients should receive standard therapy for the thrombosis.

16. **How do I evaluate a patient with ulcerative colitis?**

The management of UC depends on the severity and location of disease activity, which are best assessed by a careful clinical history with emphasis on the duration and severity of symptoms and physical examination, followed by endoscopic evaluation to determine the extent and severity of mucosal involvement. Although flexible sigmoidoscopy may indicate the severity of the disease, full colonoscopy is essential to determine the extent as well as the full severity. A plain radiograph of the abdomen should also be performed in flat and upright positions to recognize depth of ulceration and early or advanced toxic megacolon, which may be suspected by the presence of tympany in any of the segments of the abdomen (Fig. 44-1).

17. **What are 5-ASA products?**

Sulfasalazine, the first 5-ASA product, has been used successfully for many years in the treatment of mild-to-moderate UC. It is linked to sulfapyridine by a diazo bond that is cleaved by

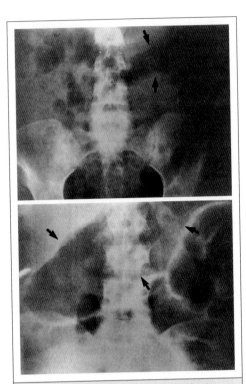

Figure 44-1. Toxic megacolon is a clue to imminent bowel perforation or worsening colitis. The condition is obvious when the width of the colon reaches 9 cm. (A) Early toxic dilation of the transverse colon with scalloped mucosa *(arrows)*. The width of the colon was <6 cm. In addition, a diseased segment of the sigmoid colon is outlined by air. (B) Late toxic megacolon involving primarily the transverse and descending colon *(arrows)*. Inflammation has resulted in thickening of the bowel wall.

colonic bacteria. The active moiety is the 5-ASA. The side effects caused most commonly by s fasalazine include nausea, vomiting, fever, and a rash, all of which are attributable primarily to the sulfapyridine, which is a carrier only. It may also cause agranulocytosis, autoimmune hemolytic anemia, folic acid deficiency, and infertility secondary to changes in sperm count a morphology. Newer preparations that contain only 5-ASA (mesalamine) are carried through c released in the small bowel. Mesalamine is currently available as a 4-gm enema (Rowasa), as suppository, and in oral formulations (Asacol, Pentasa, Dipentum, Colazal) (Table 44-1).

18. **How do I treat proctitis and proctosigmoiditis?**
For mild-to-moderate ulcerative proctitis, topical therapy may suffice. If disease is limited to anorectal region, a *Canasa* suppository can be used once or twice daily. Hydrocortisone foam (cortifoam) or hydrocortisone enemas (Cortenema) may also be used either alone or in alternation with the 5-ASA product. For proctosigmoiditis, the Rowasa enema, used alone or alternation with a hydrocortisone enema, is effective. Only the Rowasa enema—not the Cortenema— has maintenance value. The patient must lie on the left side for at least 20 min

TABLE 44-1. 5-ASA PRODUCTS

5-ASA	Carrier Molecule	Release	Site of Activity
Asacol (mesalamine)	Eudragit-S	pH >7.0	Terminal ileum and colon
Pentasa (mesalamine)	Ethylcellulose beads, time release	pH >6.0	Small bowel and colon
Dipentum (olsalazine)	Azo bond	Bacteria	Colon (ileum with bacterial overgrowth)
Azulfidine (sulfasalazine)	Sulfapyridine	Bacteria	Colon (ileum with bacterial overgrowth)
Colazal (balsalazide)	Dimer	Colon	Colon

after introducing the enema to ensure adequate delivery to the affected area. In some instances when tenesmus is severe, the enema is better introduced in the knee-chest position, taking advantage of the downhill gravity. Occasionally, oral therapy may work better than *enemas* or *suppositories;* in other cases, a combination is required.

19. **How do I treat an exacerbation of ulcerative colitis?**

When the disease extends more proximally, oral therapies are required in addition to, or instead of, topical therapy. Choice of oral 5-ASA product is determined by the extent of involvement. Pentasa (4 gm), Asacol (3.2 gm) or Colazal (6.75 gm) can be used for universal colitis and Dipentum (1 gm) for left-sided colitis. The dose of Asacol may be titrated within the limits of tolerability to a maximum of 4.8 gm/day. It is not yet known whether still higher doses of any of the three would have increased efficacy. If the disease fails to resolve with 5-ASA therapy or is moderately severe at presentation, a short course of oral corticosteroids should be prescribed to bring the disease under control. The maximal effective oral dose of prednisone is 60 mg daily. The dose may be tapered to 40 mg/day after 2–7 days, if the disease is brought under control. The formula for further tapering of prednisone is individualized. The 5-ASA drugs should be given concurrently with prednisone. Prednisone and other corticosteroids are not maintenance drugs.

20. **What should I do if the disease is severe?**

Severe disease requires admission to hospital for intravenous corticosteroids and fluids. Patients should be monitored carefully by serial physical examination, lab tests, and plain radiographs of the abdomen. Severe UC may progress to toxic megacolon and/or perforation. It is treated with intravenous corticosteroids, antibiotics, a small bowel tube attached to suction, "log rolling" from side to side and to the supine and prone positions, and sometimes by rectal tube. If these maneuvers are not successful, subtotal colectomy should be considered, preferably before a perforation occurs. If the colon is dilated and the mucosal surface is ragged on abdominal films, a surgical colleague should be involved in management decisions.

If there is no response to intravenous corticosteroids, intravenous cyclosporine should be considered. Rapid deterioration in clinical condition warrants early surgical intervention with ileostomy and subtotal colectomy. If there is time for a trial of cyclosporine, it should be administered only by physicians with extensive experience in its use. It is administered at a dose of 4 mg/kg/day intravenously by continuous infusion, with close monitoring of blood pressure, renal function, electrolytes, and drug blood levels. Cyclosporine should not be initiated if the serum cholesterol is low because it increases the risk of seizures. Bactrim is administered concurrently to prevent *Pneumocystis carinii* pneumonia. Failure to respond within 3 days portends a poor prognosis for medical therapy. Early medical intervention in expert hands can significantly reduce the number of severely ill patients who go to surgery. Severe UC sometimes responds to intravenous infliximab, even though more frequent success has been confirmed by trials in CD.

21. **Define *toxic megacolon.***

Toxic megacolon is defined as a severe attack of colitis with total or segmental dilation of the colon (diameter of transverse colon usually >5–6 cm). It can be recognized by plain x-rays showing the colon to be outlined by air (not after endoscopy) even with a diameter less than 5 cm. Megacolon is considered toxic if two or more of the following criteria are positive, in addition to the colon persistently outlined by air:

- Tachycardia with a pulse rate >100 beats/min
- Temperature >101.5°F
- Leukocytosis >10,000 cells/mm^3
- Hypoalbuminemia <3.0 gm/dL

22. **How do I prevent a relapse?**

Maintenance therapy should be initiated at the same time or soon after acute-phase therapy. For mild-to-moderate disease, a 5-ASA product may be all that is necessary. For more severe or recurrent disease, an immunosuppressive medication such as 6-mercaptopurine (6-MP) or azathioprine is more effective. 6-MP should be started at a dose of 50 mg/day, and the patient should be followed carefully with weekly blood counts for the first 3 weeks and less often thereafter. If the initial dose is tolerated well and the white cell count is normal, the dose may be increased gradually, if clinically warranted. Early toxic reactions to these medications include pancreatitis (3%), hepatitis, rash, fever, and leukopenia. The occurrence of pancreatitis or hepatitis precludes usually further use of the same drug. Patients with allergic-type reactions may be carefully desensitized to the same or the other immunosuppressive drug. High levels of the 6-MP metabolites 6-MMP (6-methyl mercaptopurine) and 6-TG (6-thioguanine) may predict which patients will develop toxicity. Anti-tumor necrosis factor is an established therapy for CD. There is evidence that it might also be effective in the treatment of UC.

23. **How often should patients have surveillance colonoscopy?**

The current recommendations are as follows: for patients with left-sided colitis, surveillance should begin after 15 years of colitis. For patients with universal colitis, surveillance should begin after 8 years of colitis. Three biopsy specimens should be obtained every 10 cm throughout the colon. In addition, any strictured, raised, polypoid areas, or those with unusual shapes textures, should be biopsied. Surveillance colonoscopy should be repeated annually for universal disease, perhaps less often for left-sided disease.

24. **What should be done if a polyp or dysplasia is found?**

Obvious polyps should be removed and the area surrounding the polyp biopsied. If the area is free of premalignant changes, nothing further need be done except for the usual surveillance. However, if dysplasia is found, colectomy is the treatment of choice. Dysplasia is a premalignant lesion classified as high-grade, low-grade, or indefinite. Although everyone agrees that high-grade dysplasia anywhere in the colon warrants proctocolectomy, there is less consensus about management of low-grade dysplasia. The diagnosis of low-grade dysplasia can be challenged when the biopsies are taken from areas of marked inflammation. Intensive treatment of the disease may lead to the recognition that the diagnosis of dysplasia was not accurate. Biopsies should be taken preferably from flat mucosa without inflammation. If a recommendation of colectomy depends on the diagnosis of dysplasia, a second expert gastrointestinal pathologist should review the biopsy slides before the final decision is made.

25. **Define *dysplasia-associated lesion or mass* (DALM).**

DALM is a dysplasia-associated lesion or mass and is an indication for total colectomy. If, however, the mass is a polyp and no dysplasia is present elsewhere in the colon, a simple polypectomy can be performed without colectomy and the surveillance routine continued.

26. **Is surveillance effective?**

Yes. Studies have shown that as many as 42% of patients with UC who are found to have high-grade dysplasia either already have cancer or develop it within a short time. The presence of low-grade dysplasia is also predictive of cancer: 19% of patients develop cancer of the colon or may even have cancer at the time of diagnosis. The finding of no dysplasia is predictive of a good short-term outcome. Outcome and case-controlled studies have shown that cancer in patients in a surveillance program is detected at an earlier and therefore more favorable stage. Patients who undergo screening have improved survival rates and lower cancer-related mortality rates.

27. **Is diet important in the management of ulcerative colitis?**

No evidence suggests that any one diet is beneficial in patients with UC. Apart from the advice that patients with lactose intolerance should avoid lactose-containing food, no dietary restrictions are necessary. Because chronically ill patients may be in a consistently negative caloric balance, maintaining a balanced diet is of the utmost importance.

28. **Does stress exacerbate ulcerative colitis?**

No studies to date support any role for psychological stresses, personality types, or overt psychiatric illness in the causation or exacerbation of UC. However, many physicians believe that psychosocial stress plays an important role not only in precipitating illness but also in preventing healing. This belief is validated by the fact that many patients experience exacerbations during times of emotional stress. When a patient remains ill, despite maximal medical therapy, consideration should be given to psychological factors. A psychopharmacologist can be invaluable in this setting. Sometimes, the addition of an anxiolytic agent or an antidepressant may be the final step required to bring UC under control.

As with any chronic illness, the approach to management should be multifaceted with expert medical and surgical teams, a psychopharmacologist, and knowledgeable ancillary staff.

29. **How does menstruation affect ulcerative colitis?**

Scattered information supplements our experience that the symptoms of both UC and Crohn's disease are aggravated or provoked coincidentally with the premenstrual period and, in some cases, throughout menstruation. Occasionally, a 2- to 3-day course of steroids is warranted.

30. **Do patients with ulcerative colitis have problems with fertility and pregnancy?**

In considering the effects of UC on pregnancy and vice versa, two aspects are important: the effect of the disease itself and the effect of the medications used to treat the disease. Well-controlled disease appears to have no deleterious effects on fertility or pregnancy. However, if the disease is active at any time during pregnancy, the incidence of fetal loss may be increased. It is therefore important to maintain control of the disease before and during pregnancy.

Mesalamine (5-ASA) has a long record of safety in pregnancy. Corticosteroids have also proven to be safe during pregnancy. With regard to the immunosuppressants 6-MP and azathioprine, data from the transplant literature suggest safety during pregnancy. One study concerning UC and CD treated with immunosuppressives concluded that they are safe and need not be discontinued for pregnancy. In our experience, however, these medications may cause fetal loss when used by women before pregnancy and an increased incidence of congenital abnormalities and spontaneous abortions when used by men within 3 months of conception. We therefore suggest that patients should discontinue these drugs, if clinically feasible, at least 3 months before planned conception. If a woman is in remission, immunosuppressives may be stopped without expectation of early recurrence. If the disease is active, pregnancy should be postponed.

Sulfasalazine causes defects in sperm morphology and motility. It should be replaced with one of the newer 5-ASA products in male patients who are contemplating starting a family.

31. **What medications are contraindicated in patients with ulcerative colitis?**
Evidence suggests that nonsteroidal anti-inflammatory drugs may precipitate exacerbations of the disease and, in some cases, may even be implicated in the onset of disease. These drugs, including aspirin, should be avoided in patients with UC.

Anticoagulant therapy, with warfarin, may lead to increased bleeding in patients with active disease and bloody diarrhea. Ironically, heparin therapy has been reported to improve disease activity in some patients. Although heparin therapy is not the standard of care, it may be useful when anticoagulation is required for patients with active UC. Opioid derivatives should be avoided, if possible, in patients with any type of colitis because of their propensity to cause toxic dilatation of the colon.

32. **What new treatments are available for UC?**
Probiotics are indigenous nonpathogenic microorganisms that are being used in mainstream medical therapy. Currently proposed mechanisms of action in IBD include (1) competition with microbial pathogens for cell surface receptors, (2) immunomodulation, (3) suppression of pathogens via release of antimicrobial factors, and (4) induction of T cell apoptosis in the lamina propria. Several open label studies have shown encouraging results with the use of combinations of lactobacilli in pouchitis and mild to moderate UC. These results have to be confirmed with randomized controlled trials.

Infliximab (anti-tumor necrosis factor) is well established as an effective therapy for Crohn disease. Several open label studies have demonstrated an approximately 50% clinical response rate in UC. Although at the time of writing, infliximab is not an FDA-approved treatment for UC, is a useful therapy for this condition and will likely receive approval in the near future.

Natalizumab is a monoclonal anti-alpha$_4$-integrin antibody that has emerged from recent trials as a promising new agent for the treatment of UC. Further trials are underway.

33. **What are the surgical options for management of ulcerative colitis?**
When medical management fails, or complications such as perforation or dysplasia occur, subtotal colectomy with ileostomy or ileoanal pouch is the procedure of choice. Many patients are frightened by the prospect of having an ileostomy, but education can do much to alleviate their fears. Fortunately, a large number of patients with ileostomies become accustomed to them and continue to lead normal lives.

The ileoanal pouch is a possible alternative. It consists of a double loop of ileum that is fashioned into a pouch and stapled to the rectal stump and stripped of its mucosa, thereby preserving the anal sphincter. Disadvantages of the pouch include recurrent inflammation or "pouchitis," frequent bowel movements, nocturnal incontinence, and the continued need for surveillance endoscopy. Pouchitis responds well to metronidazole, Cipro or Bismuth, alone or combination. These drugs can be used to treat the acute illness and also as maintenance therapy to prevent recurrence. Some patients with refractory pouchitis may require excision of the pouch and substitution of an ileostomy at a later date.

WEBSITES

1. http://www.niddk.nih.gov
2. http://www.ccfa.org/

BLIOGRAPHY

Adler DJ, Korelitz BI: The therapeutic efficacy of 6-mercaptopurine in refractory ulcerative colitis. Am J Gastroenterol 85:717–722, 1990.

Francella A, Dyan A, Bodian C, et al: The safety of 6-mercaptopurine for childbearing patients with inflammatory bowel disease: A retrospective cohort study. Gastroenterology 124:9–17, 2003.

Lichtiger S, Present DH, Kornbluth A, et al: Cyclosporine in severe ulcerative colitis refractory to steroid therapy. N Engl J Med 330:1841–1845, 1994.

Marshall JK, Irvine EJ: Rectal aminosalicylate therapy for distal ulcerative colitis: A meta-analysis. Aliment Pharmacol Ther 9:293–300, 1995.

Orholm M, Munkholm P, Langholz E, et al: Familial occurrence of inflammatory bowel disease. N Engl J Med 324:84–88, 1991.

Pemberton JH, Kelly KA, Beart RW, et al: Ileal pouch-anal anastomosis for chronic ulcerative colitis: Long-term results. Ann Surg 206:504–513, 1987.

Rajapakse RO, Korelitz BI, Zlatanic J, et al: Outcome of pregnancies when fathers are treated with 6-mercaptopurine for inflammatory bowel disease. Am J Gastroenterol 95:684–688, 2000.

Sandborn WJ: Pouchitis following ileal pouch-anal anastomosis: Definition, pathogenesis and treatment. Gastroenterology 107:1856–1860, 1994.

Sutherland LR, May GR, Shaffer EA: Sulfasalazine revisited: A meta-analysis of 5-aminosalicylic acid in the treatment of ulcerative colitis. Ann Intern Med 118:340–349, 1993.

Truelove SC, Witts LJ: Cortisone in ulcerative colitis: Final report on a therapeutic trial. BMJ 2:1041–1048, 1955.

Winawer SJ, Fletcher RH, Miller L, et al: Colorectal cancer screening: Clinical guidelines and rationale. Gastroenterology 112:594–642, 1997.

Woolrich AJ, DaSilva MD, Korelitz BI: Surveillance in the routine management of ulcerative colitis: Predictive value of low-grade dysplasia. Gastroenterology 103:431–438, 1992.

Zlatanic J, Korelitz BI, Rajapakse R, et al: Complications of pregnancy and child development after cessation of treatment with 6-mercaptopurine for inflammatory bowel disease. J Clin Gastroenterol 36:303–309, 2003.

CHAPTER 45

EOSINOPHILIC GASTROENTERITIS

Christian Jost, MD, and Michael B. Wallace, MD, MPH

1. **How is the entity eosinophilic gastroenteritis defined?**
   Eosinophilic gastroenteritis is a rare, nonparasitic inflammatory disease of the gastrointestinal tract with various degrees of eosinophilic infiltration anywhere in the tubular intestinal tract and the biliary tree in the absence of vasculitis or significant extraintestinal tissue eosinophilia. Peripheral blood eosinophilia is present in up to 80%.

2. **Why should one know features of this rare disease?**
   Although it is a rare disease, it is a treatable condition mimicking several gastrointestinal diseases. It presents most often with abdominal pain, diarrhea, nausea, vomiting, dysphagia, and gastric outlet obstruction.

3. **What is the differential diagnosis of eosinophilic gastroenteritis?**
   Patients with eosinophils on intestinal biopsy or any form of inflammation with peripheral eosinophilia should be evaluated for the possibility of eosinophilic gastroenteritis. Many other diseases, however, can produce similar findings (Table 45-1).

4. **How is irritable bowel syndrome (IBS) differentiated from eosinophilic gastroenteritis?**
   Peripheral eosinophilia is *absent* in 20% of the patients with eosinophilic gastroenteritis, reinforcing the need to examine mucosa with biopsies. Careful review of the colonic histology can usually distinguish IBS by its lack of mucosal eosinophils.

5. **How is gastroesophageal reflux disease (GERD) distinguished from eosinophilic gastroenteritis?**
   Solid food dysphagia without a history of heartburn among persons with allergic disorders should raise a red flag and suggest the diagnosis of eosinophilic esophagitis. Endoscopy is remarkable for an absence of typical esophagitis seen with GERD and the presence of subtle granularity with furrows or rings seen frequently with eosinophilic esophagitis. Deep biopsies normal and abnormal mucosal sites in the esophagus, stomach, and duodenum are recommended. In gastroesophageal reflux esophagitis, intraepithelial eosinophils are present (<5 per high power field, but the eosinophilic cell count depends on the absolute thickness of the microscopic sample slice) and vanish usually under acid suppression therapy.

6. **How is intestinal parasitic infestation or extraintestinal disease diagnosed?**
   Ancylostoma (hookworm), *Anisakis, Ascaris, Capillaria, Isospora belli* (immunocompromised patients), *Strongyloides, Toxocara, Trichuris trichiura,* and *Trichinella* are diagnosed by using concentration methods in several fresh stool samples (sedimentation methods, after fixation with ethyl-acetate formalin for ova and cysts, or polyvinyl alcohol fixatives for protozoan trophozoites).

7. **Explain the relationship between inflammatory bowel diseases and eosinophilic gastroenteritis.**
   Collagenous colitis can be associated with eosinophilic infiltration of the colon but has a characteristic collagen band in the submucosa. Classic ulcerative colitis and Crohn's disease are associated rarely with peripheral eosinophilia.

TABLE 45-1.	CLINICAL DIFFERENTIAL DIAGNOSIS OF EOSINOPHILIC GASTROENTERITIS

Irritable bowel syndrome

Reflux esophagitis

Parasitic intestinal or extraintestinal disease: *ancylostoma* (hookworm), *Anisakis, Ascaris, Capillaria, Isospora belli* (immunocompromised patients), *Strongyloides, Toxocara, Trichuris trichiura,* and *Trichinella*

Inflammatory bowel disease (collagenous colitis, ulcerative colitis, Crohn's disease)

Allergies (food, dust, medication), celiac disease, cow's milk protein sensitivity, soybean protein sensitivity, medications (gemfibrozil, clofazimine, gold salt, azathioprine, sulfamethoxazole, carbamazepine, L-tryptophan, enalapril)

Eosinophilia-myalgia syndrome (L-tryptophan)

Idiopathic hypereosinophilic syndrome (overlap with chronic myelogenous leukemia)

Systemic vasculitis syndromes (Churg-Strauss granulomatous vasculitis, polyarteritis nodosa, dermatomyositis/polymyositis, scleroderma, eosinophilic fasciitis)

Eosinophilic granuloma or histiocytosis X

Inflammatory fibroid gastrointestinal polyps

Bowel obstruction warrants the following differential diagnosis:

- Intestinal primary tumors: gastric, colonic, extraintestinal malignancies
- Intussusception
- Extraintestinal tumors and inflammatory diseases
- With peripheral blood eosinophilia: Hodgkin's lymphoma, mycosis fungoides, chronic myelogenous leukemia, and adenocarcinomas of the lung, stomach, pancreas, ovary, or uterus

8. **How do you distinguish between allergies and eosinophilic gastroenteritis?**
Allergies to food (e.g., cow's milk, gliadin), dusts, or medications (e.g., gemfibrozil, clofazimine, gold salt, azathioprine, sulfamethoxazole, carbamazepine, L-tryptophan, enalapril) can imitate eosinophilic gastroenteritis and are often suggested as the pathogenetic mechanism in the pediatric literature. A thorough history and removal of the inciting agent can elucidate the cause.

9. **What is eosinophilia-myalgia syndrome?**
This L-tryptophan–induced syndrome is associated with cutaneous, hematologic, and visceral inflammation with infiltration of eosinophils as well as macrophages and lymphocytes. Immediate withdrawal of L-tryptophan can be lifesaving.

10. **Describe the idiopathic hypereosinophilic syndrome.**
This rare, often lethal multisystemic eosinophilic organ infiltration affects the lungs, heart, kidneys, brain, and gut, with peripheral blood eosinophilia (eosinophils above 1.5 K); persists for at least 6 months; and is associated with gastroenteritis in 14% of cases. The tyrosine kinase inhibitor imatinib offers a new therapeutic option in 90% of patients.

11. **Describe the systemic vasculitis syndromes.**
- Scleroderma, dermatomyositis, and polymyositis can be found with mucosal and muscular eosinophilic/basophilic infiltration accompanied by peripheral blood eosinophilia. Serologic tests for autoantibodies and biopsies will lead to the diagnosis.

- Churg-Strauss syndrome is a granulomatous vasculitic asthma syndrome with eosinophilia. Other organs, such as the kidneys, heart, and colon, can be involved. Asthma as the cardinal feature often precedes vasculitis up to 10 years.
- Polyarteritis nodosa (PAN) has a tremendous variability of manifestations because of the varying involvement of kidneys, lungs, skin, joints, gut, and nervous system. There is a perivascular infiltration with a variable eosinophilic component.
- Eosinophilic fasciitis as part of a paraneoplastic syndrome.
- Eosinophilic granuloma and histiocytosis X are rare and present typically with multisystem involvement (liver, spleen, lung, bone marrow, lymph nodes, brain) in older kids. Rarely, there is isolated involvement of the intestinal tract. Biopsies from the liver, involved bones, or lymph nodes can help to differentiate it from eosinophilic gastroenteritis by the characteristic staining pattern of Langerhans cells (cholesterol accumulation).

12. **How are gastrointestinal inflammatory fibroid polyps diagnosed?**
Most often they are found in the gastric antrum (70%, and 20% in the small bowel) and are not accompanied by peripheral eosinophilia. They present with symptoms of gut obstruction. The typical histopathology allows the differentiation from eosinophilic gastroenteritis: arborizing capillaries are concentrically surrounded by spindle cells (fibroblasts or endothelial cells) and a variable eosinophilic infiltrate.

KEY POINTS: EOSINOPHILIC GASTROENTERITIS

1. Although eosinophilic gastroenteritis is a rare disorder, it is a treatable condition, responsive usually to corticosteroid therapy.
2. The manifestations of eosinophilic gastroenteritis are protean and should always be considered by the astute clinician.
3. The etiology of eosinophilic gastroenteritis is not known. There is no known direct correlation to a distinct allergen. However, it is likely to be a primary regulatory dysfunction of the immune system involving the eosinophilic granulocytes.

13. **How is malignant bowel obstruction similar to eosinophilic gastroenteritis?**
It can present with peripheral blood eosinophilia. Examples are gastric, colonic, and pancreatic tumors, further hematologic malignancies as Hodgkin's lymphoma, mycosis fungoides, chronic myelogenous leukemia, or extraintestinal adenocarcinomas of the lung, ovary, or uterus.

14. **What is the etiology of eosinophilic gastroenteritis? Describe the pathophysiologic background of eosinophilic gastroenteritis.**
This immune-mediated disease is most likely the result of several different factors affecting the immunologic regulation (i.e., allergic, autoimmune). A single etiologic factor is not yet known.

15. **Why does eosinophilic gastroenteritis have so many different clinical faces?**
The anatomic location of the affected organs and the depth of the inflammatory infiltration of the intestinal wall layers and of the surrounding visceral structures determine the clinical manifestation. Examples include:
- Mucosal eosinophilic infiltration without muscular involvement
- Inflammation of the intestinal muscle layer (muscularis propria)
- Subserosal/serosal inflammation (present in 10%)

5. Describe mucosal eosinophilic infiltration without muscular involvement.

Intestinal eosinophilic mucositis presents as abdominal pain, vomiting, nausea, and diarrhea. This can be complicated by malabsorption with weight loss, protein-losing enteropathy, chronic intestinal blood loss (iron deficiency), recurrent gastroduodenal ulcer disease, eosinophilic colitis, or acute intestinal bleeding. Endoscopic biopsy facilitates the diagnosis (Fig. 45-1).

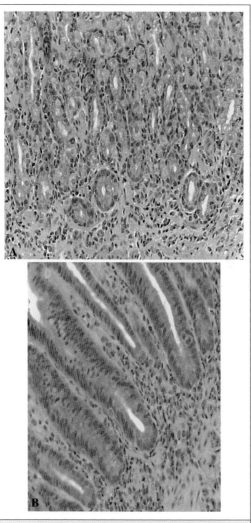

Figure 45-1. *A,* Endoscopic biopsy (H&E, 20×) from the gastric antrum: Histopathology shows the eosinophilic mucosal and submucosal infiltration. *B,* Endoscopic biopsy (H&E, 20×) from the duodenum: Histopathology shows the typical eosinophilic inflammatory infiltration of the mucosa and submucosa.

17. **Describe inflammation of the intestinal muscle layer (muscularis propria).**
    Muscle layer inflammation results in a rigid gut with symptoms of dysmotility, such as dysphagia with esophageal stricture or pseudoachalasia; vomiting and pain with obstruction of the gastric outlet, small intestine, or colon; or bacterial overgrowth. Recurrent acute cholangitis or pancreatitis can present in patients with ampullary infiltration, presumably due to ampullary stenosis. Barium double-contrast study facilitates the diagnosis (Fig. 45-2).

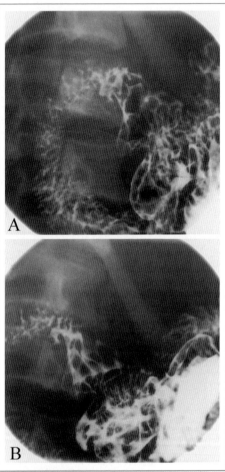

Figure 45-2. *A,* Barium double contrast: Cobblestone pattern is a typical sign of thickened mucosal folds. This patient has gastric and duodenal eosinophilic gastroenteritis. *B,* Barium double contrast of the gastric antrum and duodenum: Roughened mucosal folds are typical in eosinophilic gastroenteritis.

18. **Describe subserosal/serosal inflammation.**
    Subserosal/serosal inflammation (seen in 10% of patients) presents as eosinophilic peritonitis, ascites, rarely pleural effusions, or as an inflammatory tumor with bowel obstruction. Ascitic eosinophil counts can reach more than 80%. The subserosal involvement is often accompanie

by muscular infiltration, what can be visualized by abdominal ultrasound, computed tomography (CT) scan, or magnetic resonance imaging (MRI) (Fig. 45-3).

19. What symptoms and signs suggest a probable diagnosis of eosinophilic gastroenteritis?

Dependent on the involved anatomic structures, eosinophilic gastroenteritis presents as dyspepsia, dysphagia/chest pain, gastric outlet obstruction, duodenal obstruction, gastroduodenal ulcer disease, diarrhea, malabsorption syndrome, protein-losing enteropathy, intestinal blood loss, enteritis syndrome, obstruction of the small or large intestine, intestinal perforation, peritoneal disease with ascites, biliary obstruction, periampullary tumor, or pancreatitis. Peripheral eosinophilia is present in most (80%) but not all patients with eosinophilic gastroenteritis.

20. What are possible x-ray features of eosinophilic gastroenteritis?

Gastric retention, small intestinal hypomotility, or obstruction can be demonstrated by barium studies. Double contrast barium enema or enteroclysis can show mucosal thickening with a cobble-stoned or saw-tooth silhouette, nodular filling defects, or coarse folds in the small intestine (*see* Fig. 45-2). It can mimic regional enteritis (Crohn's disease). Eosinophilic esophagitis presents with circumferential rings or feline esophagus. Muscle layer disease presents with stiffened and narrowed tubular gut structures, complicated by obstruction of the esophagus, gastric outlet, duodenum, jejunum, ileum, or colon. Computer tomography or MRI imaging can reveal duodenal, jejuno-ileal, or colonic wall thickening, inflammatory tumors, or ascites.

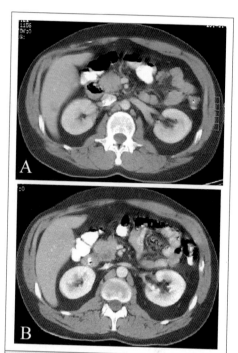

Figure 45-3. *A,* Early pancreatitis in duodenal eosinophilic gastroenteritis. *B,* Early pancreatitis in eosinophilic gastroenteritis. Duodenal wall thickening.

1. What are rational steps to diagnose eosinophilic gastroenteritis?

- Check the medical history for atopic diseases (present in 50%).
- Exclude parasitic intestinal disease by history and three stool samples.
- Obtain tissue samples.
- Perform eosinophil counts (Table 45-2).

When *endoscopic biopsies* are taken, it is recommended to retrieve large, deep biopsies (caused by inflammation sparing the mucosal layer) at up to 10 different locations, including the stomach and the small bowel (patchy distribution with sampling error leads to nondiagnostic biopsies in up to 20%). It is also recommended that endoscopic biopsies be taken from mucosa with abnormal and normal appearance. Although not often involved, colonic or ileal biopsies can prove the diagnosis. In deep muscular or peritoneal disease, the diagnosis is sometimes only found in the surgical resection specimen or in the *full-thickness surgical biopsy* (open or laparoscopic surgery). Eosinophilic duodenitis with involvement of the duodenal papilla (Vater) can manifest as pancreatitis or cholangitis. Then systemic corticosteroid or endoscopic retrograde cholangiopancreatography (ERCP) with sphincterotomy is indicated.

TABLE 45–2.   EOSINOPHIL COUNTS IN EOSINOPHILIC GASTROENTERITIS

Test	Finding Supportive of the Diagnosis
Peripheral blood smear	Eosinophils >0.250 K/CUMM and 5–35%, respectively; normal peripheral blood counts are found in 20%
Stool specimens	>5% eosinophils in differential count of the leucocytes
Ascites	>5% eosinophils in differential count of the leucocytes
Deep mucosal biopsies	>20 eosinophils/high-power (×1000) field of at least three different histopathology slides because the intraepithelial cell count is dependent on the thickness of the cut slices (microtomes cut variable number of micrometers)

22. **What should one exclude in patients with suspected eosinophilic gastroenteritis?**
    - Drug-induced: aspirin, gold therapy, gemfibrozil, clofazimine, L-tryptophan, enalapril
    - Intestinal parasites
    - Inflammatory bowel disease or collagenous colitis
    - Collagen-vascular disease: PAN, SLE, systemic sclerosis, dermatomyositis, Churg-Strauss syndrome
    - Malignant infiltration
    - Lymphoma: Sezary T-cell and intestinal lymphomas, chronic myelogenous leukemia, Hodgkin's disease.

23. **How should one treat eosinophilic gastroenteritis?**
    Traditionally, *glucocorticoid* therapy is recommended. Oral prednisone 0.5 mg/kg/day for a period of 2 weeks will induce remission in 90% of patients, irrespective of the affected gut layer. Most patients do not require maintenance therapy; however, a small number will require 2–3 months of corticosteroid therapy for symptoms to resolve. Severe disease should be treated with parenteral methylprednisolone (bolus of 125 mg followed by 0.5 mg/kg/day b.i.d.). Even in severe duodenal obstruction, a parenteral glucocorticoid therapeutic trial is recommended before surgery is considered.
        Recurrences occur in up to 40% and can be treated with repeat short courses of prednisone. Topical corticosteroids have been reported to be effective. Cases of eosinophilic esophagitis have clinically and histologically responded to *fluticasone propionate MDI* that are *swallowed* NOT *inhaled*. One report documented effectiveness of *nonenteric coated budesonide* (formula of water soluble tablets produced for rectal enema dissolutions) in gastric transmural eosinophilic gastroenteritis with ascites.
    Nonglucocorticoid immune-modulatory therapies may be an alternative in the future:
    - *Montelukast:* a leukotriene$_1$-receptor antagonist
    - *Suplatast tosilate:* a leukotriene inhibitor (not available in the US)
    - *Cromoglycate sodium:* a mast cell stabilizer
    - *Ketotifen:* a mast cell stabilizer
        Elemental diet was used for a period of 1–3 months with some success in pediatric patients. In suspected food allergy a *trial elimination diet* can rarely elucidate the individual

pathogenesis and resolve the disease in a few patients. *Symptomatic treatment* includes adequate pain relief, loperamide for diarrhea, and supplementation of deficiencies acquired by malabsorption.

WEBSITES

. http://www.vhjoe.com

. http://www.dave1.mgh.harvard.edu/

BIBLIOGRAPHY

Babb RR: Cromolyn sodium in the treatment of ulcerative colitis. J Clin Gastroenterol 2(3):229–231, 1980.

Cello JP: Eosinophilic gastroenteritis?a complex disease entity. Am J Med 67(6):1097–1104, 1979.

Desreumaux P, Bloget F, Seguy D, et al: Interleukin 3, granulocyte-macrophage colony-stimulating factor, and interleukin 5 in eosinophilic gastroenteritis [See comments]. Gastroenterology 110(3):768–774, 1996.

Faubion WA Jr, Perrault J, Burgart LJ, et al: Treatment of eosinophilic esophagitis with inhaled corticosteroids. J Pediatr Gastroenterol Nutr 27:90–93, 1998.

Fenoglio LM, Benedetti V, Rossi C, et al: Eosinophilic gastroenteritis with ascites: A case report and review of the literature. Dig Dis Sci 48(5):1013–1020, 2003.

Gallamini A, Carbone A, Lista P, et al: Intestinal T-cell lymphoma with massive tissue and blood eosinophilia mediated by IL-5. Leuk Lymphoma 17(1-2):155–161, 1995.

Gruber BL, Baeza ML, Marchese MJ, et al: Prevalence and functional role of anti-IgE autoantibodies in urticarial syndromes. J Invest Dermatol 90(2):213–217, 1988.

Hertzman PA, Blevins WL, Mayer J, et al: Association of the eosinophilia-myalgia syndrome with the ingestion of tryptophan [See comments]. N Engl J Med 322(13):869–873, 1990.

Hogan SP, Mishra A, Brandt EB, et al: A critical role for eotoxin in experimental oral antigen-induced eosinophilic gastrointestinal allergy. Proc Natl Acad Sci U S A 97(12):6681–6686, 2000.

Katsinelos P, Pilpilidis I, Xiarchos P, et al: Oral administration of ketotifen in a patient with eosinophilic colitis and severe osteoporosis. Am J Gastroenterol 97(4):1072–1074, 2002.

Kweon MN, Kiyono H: Eosinophilic gastroenteritis: A problem of the mucosal immune system? Curr Allergy Asthma Rep 3(1):79–85, 2003.

Lee CM, Changchien CS, Chen PC, et al: Eosinophilic gastroenteritis: 10 years experience. Am J Gastroenterol 88(1):70–74, 1993.

MacCarty RL, Talley NJ: Barium studies in diffuse eosinophilic gastroenteritis. Gastrointest Radiol 15(3):183–187, 1990.

Markowitz JE, Spergel JM, Ruchelli E, Liacouras CA: Elemental diet is an effective treatment for eosinophilic esophagitis in children and adolescents. Am J Gastroenterol 98(4):777–782, 2003.

Martin DM, Goldman JA, Gilliam J, Nasrallah SM: Gold-induced eosinophilic enterocolitis: Response to oral cromolyn sodium. Gastroenterology 80(6):1567–1570, 1981.

Mishra A, Hogan SP, Brandt EB, Rothenberg ME: IL-5 promotes eosinophil trafficking to the esophagus. J Immunol 168:2464–2469, 2002.

Mishra A, Hogan SP, Brandt EB, Rothenberg ME: Peyer's patch eosinophils: Identification, characterization, and regulation by mucosal allergen exposure, interleukin-5, and eotaxin. Blood 96(4):1538–1544, 2000.

Moots RJ, Prouse P, Gumpel JM: Near fatal eosinophilic gastroenteritis responding to oral sodium chromogly-cate. Gut 29(9):1282–1285, 1988.

Neustrom MR, Friesen C: Treatment of eosinophilic gastroenteritis with montelukast. J Allergy Clin Immunol 104:506, 1999.

Perez-Millan A, Martin-Lorente JL, Lopez-Morante A, et al: Subserosal eosinophilic gastroenteritis treated efficaciously with sodium cromoglycate. Dig Dis Sci 42:342, 1997.

Schoonbroodt D, Horsmans Y, Laka A, et al: Eosinophilic gastroenteritis presenting with colitis and cholangitis. Dig Dis Sci 40(2):308–314, 1995.

22. Schwartz DA, Pardi DS, Murray JA: Use of montelukast as steroid-sparing agent for recurrent eosinophilic gastroenteritis. Dig Dis Sci 46(8):1787–1790, 2001.

23. Shirai T, Hashimoto D, Suzuki K, et al: Successful treatment of eosinophilic gastroenteritis with suplatast tosilate. J Allergy Clin Immunol 107:924, 2001.

24. Talley NJ, Shorter RG, Phillips SF, Zinsmeister AR: Eosinophilic gastroenteritis: A clinicopathological study of patients with disease of the mucosa, muscle layer, and subserosal tissues. Gut 31(1):54–58, 1990.

25. Tan AC, Kruimel JW, Naber TH: Eosinophilic gastroenteritis treated with non-enteric-coated budesonide tablets. Eur J Gastroenterol Hepatol 13(4):425–427, 2001.

26. Teitelbaum JE, Fox VL, Twarog FJ, et al: Eosinophilic esophagitis in children: Immunopathological analysis and response to fluticasone propionate. Gastroenterology 122(5):1216–1225, 2002.

27. Vitellas KM, Bennett WF, Bova JG, et al: Idiopathic eosinophilic esophagitis [See comments]. Radiology 186(3):789–793, 1993.

28. Weltman JK: Cytokines: Regulators of eosinophilic inflammation [In process citation]. Allergy Asthma Proc 21(4):203–207, s

CHAPTER 46

BACTERIAL OVERGROWTH

Jack A. DiPalma, MD

1. **Define *bacterial overgrowth*.**

   Overgrowth is defined by an increased number of bacteria in areas of the gastrointestinal tract that do not usually provide the environment suitable for the colonization and proliferation of bacteria.

2. **What is the usual bacterial presence in the gastrointestinal tract?**
   - Stomach $<10^4$/mL
   - Jejunum $<10^5$/mL
   - Ileum $<10^6$/mL
   - Colon $<10^{10}$/mL

   The type of species that colonize the small intestine is changed in bacterial overgrowth. In health, small bowel bacteria resemble oropharyngeal flora with gram-positive, aerobic organisms. In overgrowth, bacteria are mostly gram-negative, including *Escherichia coli*; anaerobic bacteria, including *Clostridia* and *Bacteroides* species, also predominate.

3. **What factors influence small intestinal bacterial proliferation?**
   - Structural lesions
   - Motility
   - Excessive bacterial load
   - Deficiency in host defenses

4. **What kind of structural lesions predispose to overgrowth?**

   Obstruction to outflow of luminal contents can occur at the site of surgical anastomosis or with webs, adhesions, or strictures. Surgical diversions and blind loops or neoreservoirs, such as the continent ileostomy, predispose to small intestinal bacterial overgrowth. The jejunoileal bypass, once a popular surgical procedure for morbid obesity, created a long segment of diverted bowel and was often complicated by overgrowth. Diverticula and duplications are frequently colonized with colonic-type bacteria, leading to overgrowth.

5. **How do motility disorders cause overgrowth?**

   Delayed transit of intestinal contents results in stasis. Overgrowth complicates intestinal pseudo-obstruction syndromes. The intestinal "housekeeper" migratory motor complex, when disrupted, is associated with bacterial overgrowth. Paralytic ileus results in bacterial proliferation.

6. **How can an excessive bacterial load be delivered to the small bowel?**

   Absence or incompetence of the ileocecal valve and enteric fistula can deliver bacteria to the small bowel in amounts that exceed clearing capacity.

7. **Which impairments of host defenses are important?**
   - Acid suppression by surgery or medications
   - Hypochlorhydric disorders, such as pernicious anemia
   - Immune deficiencies, particularly absence of secretory immunoglobulin A (IgA)
   - Undernutrition, which can decrease gastric acidity and immune function

8. **What conditions are associated with small intestinal bacterial overgrowth?**

   Reduced gastric acid
   - Pernicious anemia

- Atrophic gastritis
- Gastric surgery
- Medications (H_2-receptor antagonists, proton-pump inhibitors)
- Neoreservoirs

Structural abnormalities

- Small bowel diverticula
- Surgical anastomosis and diversions
- Strictures
- Webs
- Adhesions
- Fistulas (colo-enteric, gastrocolic)
- Absent or incompetent ileocecal valves
- Neoreservoirs

Dysmotility syndromes

- Diabetes
- Scleroderma
- Acute enteric infection
- Intestinal pseudo-obstruction syndromes

9. **What are the other risk factors for bacterial overgrowth?**
Evidence indicates that overgrowth with colonic-type bacteria should be considered in patients over age 75 with chronic diarrhea, anorexia, or nausea, even if they have no apparent predisposition. Dysmotility is probably responsible. Additional data suggest that overgrowth may cause diarrhea or abdominal pain in children, especially those younger than age 2. Recent data implicate bacterial overgrowth in some patients with irritable bowel syndrome.

10. **What are the symptoms of overgrowth?**
Clinical manifestations vary. Diarrhea, anorexia, nausea, weight loss, and anemia are cardinal symptoms, but the nature of the small bowel abnormality influences the presentation. Patients obstructed by stricture may have bloating and pain. Overgrowth in small intestinal diverticula may present insidiously with metabolic derangements. The eventual clinical consequence of overgrowth, regardless of cause, is steatorrhea, leading to weight loss. Malabsorption results in hypocalcemic disorders, night blindness, vitamin K deficiency, and osteomalacia. Cobalamin deficiency is common with severe overgrowth.

11. **Why do patients with bacterial overgrowth develop anemia?**
Anemia may be megaloblastic and macrocytic as a result of cobalamin deficiency. Microcytic anemia due to iron deficiency results mainly from blood loss not bacterial overgrowth. Anaerobic bacteria compete for uptake of cobalamin–intrinsic factor complex. Whereas luminal bacteria consume cobalamin, folic acid is a product of bacterial substrate fermentation. Thus, an important clinical observation in small intestinal bacterial overgrowth is the finding of low B_{12} and high folate levels.

12. **What other micronutrient deficiencies are clinically important?**
In addition to iron and cobalamin deficiencies, other micronutrient deficiencies include deficiencies of water-soluble vitamins (e.g., thiamine and nicotinamide) and decreased absorption of fat-soluble vitamins (vitamins A, D, E, and K). Trace element malabsorption has not been studied carefully in overgrowth syndromes.

13. **How is bacterial overgrowth diagnosed?**
Small intestinal bacterial overgrowth is confirmed by the demonstration of elevated numbers of small bowel bacteria colonies and the replacement of oropharyngeal with predominantly colonic organisms. Because small bowel intubation and aspiration for microbial analysis are cumbersome, overgrowth is considered in patients with predisposing factors and appropriate history. Indirect testing may help to substantiate the diagnosis.

14. **What indirect testing can be used?**
See Table 46-1.

TABLE 46–1.	DIAGNOSIS OF BACTERIAL OVERGROWTH
History	Prior surgery, medical conditions (e.g. osteomalacia, night blindness, easy bruisability, tetany)
Examination	Systemic disease: weight loss and malabsorption
Laboratory values	Hemoglobin (decreased), mean corpuscular volume (increased), vitamin B_{12} (decreased), folic acid (increased), fecal fat (increased)
Tests	Schilling's test with intrinsic factor (decreased), ^{14}C-glycocholic acid (increased), ^{14}C-D-xylose (decreased), hydrogen testing with glucose or lactulose, jejunal aspirate for bacterial colony counts and strain identification.

15. **What are the limitations of testing?**

Jejunal intubation for aspiration with bacterial colony counts and stain identification can provide a definitive diagnosis by showing jejunal counts $>10^5$ with colonic organisms. Because the test is cumbersome, some clinicians rely on indirect testing. Jejunal intubation can be performed endoscopically, and protected catheters can be used to obtain reliable aspirates.

Radiolabelled breath tests, using glycocholic acid or xylose, have been used for diagnosis of overgrowth. Glycocholic acid is released by bacterial deconjugation of radiolabelled bile acids. Xylose is catabolized by gram-negative aerobes and is absorbed in the proximal small bowel.

Fasting breath hydrogen is elevated in overgrowth patients, and early rises after glucose or lactulose challenge reflect small bowel fermentation of the substrate by abnormal concentrations of bacteria. In general, *scintigraphic* and *hydrogen breath tests* are attractive alternatives to intubation tests for bacterial overgrowth. Hydrogen testing, although simple, inexpensive, and nonradioactive, does not have sufficient sensitivity or specificity.

16. **What about other testing methods?**

Quantification of urinary excretion of indican, drug metabolites, and conjugated para-aminobenzoic acid does not distinguish overgrowth from other types of malabsorption.

17. **What is the treatment for bacterial overgrowth?**
   I. **Correction of the underlying condition**
      - Surgery
      - Prokinetic agents

   II. **Nutrition**
      - Lactose-free, low-residue diet
      - Increase calories
      - Micronutrient supplementation (B_{12}, fat-soluble vitamins, trace elements)

   III. **Antibiotics**

18. **Do prokinetic agents help?**

Surgery is often impractical or unacceptable, and prokinetic agents are tried to relieve stasis and improve outflow of small intestinal contents. However, standard stimulatory agents are not very effective. The long-acting somatostatin analog, octreotide, has been shown to stimulate motility in normal subjects and patients with scleroderma. It reduces overgrowth and improves symptoms in scleroderma.

19. **Which antibiotics are preferred?**
The optimal choice of antibiotic and dosage regimen has not been determined. Some investigators prefer broad-spectrum antibiotics, such as cephalosporins, tetracyclines, or chloramphenicol. Others recommend narrower-spectrum drugs active against anaerobes, such as metronidazole, or against aeroanaerobes, such as fluoroquinolones. A recent study showed efficacy with either norfloxacin or amoxicillin-clavulanic acid.

20. **How long should overgrowth be treated with antibiotics?**
A single 7- to 10-day course usually suffices, but recurrence is frequent. Some patients require retreatment in weeks or months; others need continuous therapy. Prolonged antibiotic therapy poses significant risk, including resistance and enterocolitis.

21. **What about probiotics?**
Saccharomyces boulardii is a probiotic used in treatment of pseudomembranous colitis that has stated efficacy for bacterial overgrowth in children. Because antibiotics have potential side effects, probiotic therapy is attractive. A recent study in adults, however, showed no efficacy of *Saccharomyces boulardii* in treatment of overgrowth.

BIBLIOGRAPHY

1. Ahar A, Flourie B, Rambaud JC, et al: Antibiotic efficacy in small intestinal bacterial overgrowth-related chronic diarrhea: A cross-over, randomized trial. Gastroenterology 117:794–797, 1999.
2. de Boissieu D, Chaussain M, Badoual J, et al: Small-bowel bacterial overgrowth in children with chronic diarrhea, abdominal pain, or both. J Pediatr 128:203–207, 1996.
3. Pimentel M, Lin HC: Eradication of small bowel bacterial overgrowth reduces symptoms of irritable bowel syndrome. Am J Gastroenterol 95:3503–3506, 2000.
4. Riordan SM, McIver CJ, Wakefield D, et al: Small intestinal bacterial overgrowth in the symptomatic elderly. Am J Gastroenterol 92:47–51, 1997.
5. Riordan SM, McIver CK, Walker BM, et al: The lactulose breath hydrogen test and small intestinal bacterial overgrowth. Am J Gastroenterol 91:1795–1803, 1996.
6. Rose S, Young MA, Reynolds JC: Gastrointestinal manifestations of scleroderma. Gastroenterol Clin North Am 27:563–594, 1998.
7. Sherman PM: Bacterial overgrowth. In Yamada T (ed): Textbook of Gastroenterology. Philadelphia, J.B. Lippincott, 1991, pp 1530–1539.
8. Soudah HC, Hasller WL, Owyang C: Effect of octreotide on intestinal motility and bacterial overgrowth in scleroderma. N Engl J Med 325:1461–1467, 1991.
9. Toskes PP, Kumar A: Enteric bacterial flora and bacterial overgrowth syndrome. In Feldman M (ed): Sleisenger and Fordtran's Gastrointestinal and Liver Disease, 6th ed. Philadelphia, W.B. Saunders, 1998, pp 1523–1535.

CHAPTER 47

COLORECTAL CANCER AND COLON CANCER SCREENING

Stephen P. Laird, MD, MS, and Neil W. Toribara, MD, PhD

What is colorectal cancer?

Colorectal cancer (CRC) includes both colon and rectal cancer. Over 95% of the primary cancers arising in the large bowel are adenocarcinomas; the remainder are lymphomas, malignant carcinoids, leiomyosarcomas, and Kaposi's sarcoma.

How does the pathophysiology of rectal cancer differ from cancer elsewhere in the colon?

The rectum is relatively immobile, lacks a serosal covering, and is located largely behind the peritoneal reflection, surrounded by perirectal fat. As a result, rectal cancers spread, more commonly, contiguously by direct extension into local structures, whereas colon cancer spreads, more commonly, via lymphatics and hematogenously. Thus, rectal cancers that have spread beyond the mucosa are treated with surgery and adjuvant radiation, with or without chemotherapy, whereas colon cancers are treated with surgery and chemotherapy rather than radiation.

How common is CRC?

Cancer is the second leading cause of death in the United States (after cardiovascular disease), and colorectal cancer is the second leading cause of death from malignancies (after lung cancer). The lifetime risk of developing CRC is 1 in 18 (5.5%) in women and 1 in 17 (5.9%) in men and is influenced by hereditary and lifestyle factors. The incidence is estimated at 146,000 new cases per year, with an estimated 56,290 deaths in the year 2005. The incidence of CRC peaked in the mid-1980s and has slowly declined since that time, reflecting the effects of increased availability of colonoscopy, gradual acceptance of CRC screening, and the lag time between polyp formation and malignant transformation.

Do the genetic defects leading to sporadic CRC differ from those in genetic syndromes associated with colon cancer?

Yes. In most sporadic CRC and familial adenomatous polyposis (FAP) syndrome, genetic abnormalities accumulate via loss of large pieces of DNA, known as loss of heterozygosity (LOH). The most common acquisition sequence of genetic abnormalities is thought to be APC, *ras*, p53, and DCC, although the order of allelic deletion is not as important as the cumulative loss of DNA or LOH. The knowledge of these genetic abnormalities has been utilized in developing the current generation of stool-based DNA tests, in which DNA isolated from a stool sample is tested for a panel of mutations in genes involved commonly in colonic carcinogenesis. In hereditary nonpolyposis colorectal cancer (HNPCC) and a small minority of sporadic CRCs, the abnormalities accrue through accumulation of point mutations, which cannot be corrected because of defects in the DNA repair system.

Describe the natural sequence from colon adenoma to colon cancer.

The National Polyp Study showed that removal of colonic adenomas during colonoscopy prevented subsequent development of colorectal cancer, showing that colonic adenomas are a vital step, which can be interrupted, in the carcinogenic progression of sporadic CRC. The prevalence curves for adenomas and colorectal cancers parallel each other, with the adenoma curve shifted 5–10 years earlier than carcinomas. This suggests that the time needed for an adenoma to develop into cancer is 5–10 years, thus giving a significant window of time to discover and remove premalignant lesions.

6. **How prevalent are colonic adenomas among the U.S. population?**
   The prevalence of adenomatous polyps appears to be highly dependent on the population studied. Two colonoscopic studies in asymptomatic populations have reported somewhat low rates of 23–25% prevalence in male and female patients between ages 50 and 82. Two other studies involving only men in Department of Veterans Affairs Medical Centers had prevalence rates of approximately 40%.

7. **Where in the colon are polyps located most commonly?**
   Autopsy series have shown a relatively even distribution of adenomas throughout the colon, although larger polyps have a distal predominance, as expected from the distribution of CRCs.

8. **Give the mean age of onset, and describe the anatomic distribution of CRC.**
   True sporadic CRCs occur at a mean age of 69; approximately 60% are distal to the splenic flexure (thus theoretically within the reach of a flexible sigmoidoscope). However, some studies have suggested that older patients and African Americans appear to have an increased proportion of CRCs in the right colon.

9. **How are malignant polyps defined? How are they managed clinically?**
   Pathologists prefer the term *severe dysplasia* for adenomas with a focus of carcinoma in situ intramucosal carcinoma, because complete endoscopic removal is curative. The term *malignant polyp* is reserved for the approximately 5% of adenomas in which a focus of carcinoma has invaded beyond the muscularis mucosa into the submucosa, where lymphatic spread with metastasis is possible. A malignant polyp has at least one of the following characteristics: (1) poorly differentiated cancer, (2) invasion of veins or lymphatics, (3) extension of the carcinoma to <2 mm of the margin, or (4) invasion of submucosa of the bowel wall. When malignant polyps are found, consideration should be given to early reendoscopy and/or local surgical resection. Endoscopic removal of a malignant polyp is associated with a 10–25% relapse rate.

10. **How is colon cancer staged, and how does this impact prognosis?**
    Although the overall 5-year survival is about 62% in the United States, there are significant differences among ethnic groups. Although histology and syndromes (i.e., HNP colorectal cancers) have a better prognosis stage for stage than sporadic CRCs, the best determinant of prognosis stage at diagnosis. The two most widely used staging methods are the Dukes and TNM (tumor, node, metastasis) systems. Both give essentially equivalent information for prognostic purposes. The Dukes' system (Table 47-1) is simpler and still widely used by gastroenterologists and surgeons, whereas TNM staging is used more widely among oncologists and pathologists.

11. **Describe the work-up for colorectal cancer after initial diagnosis.**
    Surgical removal of the cancer remains the only curative therapy. Before surgery, visualization of the entire bowel, preferably by full colonoscopy, is indicated to exclude synchronous lesions (either adenomas or cancers) that may influence the operation. Preoperative laboratory tests should include complete blood count, blood chemistry panel-20, and carcinoembryonic antigen (CEA). If the CEA level is elevated at the time of diagnosis (approximately 60% of cases), it provides a convenient method for assessing effectiveness of the surgery and detecting early recurrences. Preoperative abdominal CT scan and chest radiograph are useful in looking for metastatic disease. In rectal cancers, preoperative staging with transrectal ultrasound helps determine the utility of adjunct radiation therapy.

TABLE 47-1. DUKES' CLASSIFICATION VERSUS TNM STAGING

Dukes' Classification*	5-Year Survival (%)	TMN Staging[†]		5-Year Survival (%)
		Stage 0		
		Carcinoma in situ	Tis N0 M0	100
Stage A		**Stage I**		
Limited to mucosa	95–100	Tumor invades submucosa	T1 N0 M0	95
		Tumor invades muscularis propria	T2 N0 M0	80
Stage B1		**Stage II**		
Into muscularis propria	80–85	Tumor invades through muscularis propria into serosa or pericolonic/perirectal tissue	T3 N0 M0	
Stage B2		Tumor perforates or	T4 N0 M0	
Through serosa	75	directly invades other organs		
Stage C1		**Stage III**		
1-4 regional nodes positive	65	Any perforation with nodal metastases		
		N1: 1–3 nodes	TX, N1, M0	
Stage C2		N2: ≥4 nodes	TX, N2, M0	
> 4 regional nodes positive	42	N3: Any lymph node along named vascular trunk	TX, N3, M0	
Stage D[‡]		**Stage IV**		
Distant metastases	5	Any invasion of bowel wall with or without lymph node metastases but with evidence of distant metastases	TX, NX, M1	

TNM = tumor, node, metastasis.
* Gastrointestinal Study Group Modification.
[†] American Joint Committee on Cancer.
[‡] Included only in the Turnbull modification of Dukes' classification.

12. **What surgical margins are recommended?**
Most surgeons attempt to include at least 5 cm on either side of the tumor within the resection block, although margins as small as 2 cm may be acceptable in the distal rectum to preserve sphincter function.

13. **Describe the recommended schedule of colonoscopic follow-up after surgery.**
If a preoperative colonoscopy clears the remainder of the colon of polyps or synchronous malignancy and the surgical margins are tumor-free, colonoscopy before 1–3 years after resection is probably not indicated. The risk for developing metachronous neoplasms in a postmalignancy resection patient is about the same as for a patient with an adenoma of unfavorable histology; therefore, intervals between colonoscopic screening exams should be similar, every 3–5 years.

14. **Are there any effective blood tests to screen for CRC?**
Serum tests to diagnose colorectal cancer are limited by the inherent problem that markers produced by malignant cells are hardest to detect in the early, small tumors that have the best prognosis. To date, no putative serum markers of CRC have sufficient sensitivity or specificity to warrant use as primary screening modalities. CEA, the most widely used CRC tumor marker is, therefore, useful only to assess efficacy of surgery or monitoring for recurrences in cancers already known to be CEA-positive. Even this use has been challenged by those who feel that the clinical benefit of diagnosing recurrences is minimal. (*Caveat:* Because CEA is excreted in the bile, elevated levels may be difficult to interpret in the presence of biliary obstruction or hepatic dysfunction.) A reasonable surveillance approach in CEA positive tumors is to check CEA levels every 2 months for the first 6 months, every 4 months for up to 2 years, and then every 6 months for up to 5 years.

15. **List the risk factors for developing CRC.**
Age, diet, environment, personal history of colonic neoplasm, family history of colonic neoplasm, familial colon cancer syndromes, and inflammatory bowel disease.

16. **What is the effect of age on the risk of developing CRC?**
The risk of developing colorectal cancer increases with age, starting at about age 40 and roughly doubling with each decade. Below age 40, the incidence of CRC is less than 6 in 100,000; however, by age 80 the incidence is approximately 500 per 100,000 in men and 400 per 100,000 in women. Because over 90% of colorectal cancers occur after age 50, most screening programs have arbitrarily chosen this as a starting age.

17. **Discuss the effect of diet on the risk for developing CRC.**
Diet is thought to account for the major differences in the incidence rates of CRC worldwide. Although epidemiologic studies and animal models suggest that a high-fat, low-fiber diet (typical of Western nations) increases the risk of developing CRC, prospective trials of low-fat, high-fiber diets have shown no significant effect. Similarly, other micronutrients, such as folate reducing agents (vitamins C and E), and beta-carotene, have shown promise in experimental conditions but failed to yield positive results in controlled trials. Calcium supplementation is the only dietary intervention that has shown a positive, albeit modest, effect in humans, using adenomas as a surrogate marker for the development of CRC.

18. **Do environmental factors increase the risk for developing colorectal cancer?**
The risk of developing CRC is related directly to environmental factors. This effect is evident in comparing the rates of colorectal cancer in populations emigrating from a region with a low rate to a region with a high rate. For example, the incidence of colon cancer in the Japanese (low incidence) immigrating to the United States (high incidence) led to a 10-fold increase in incidence over a single generation, much too fast to be a selection phenomenon. In general,

the United States and Western European nations have a higher rate of CRC than developing nations.

Which adenoma features are associated with a greater malignant potential?
Adenomatous polyps are considered premalignant lesions, but the actual risk of neoplastic transformation is unknown. Large size, villous architecture, and dysplasia are features of adenomas that have a higher risk of developing a carcinoma within a given polyp.

What are the recommendations for CRC screening in people at average risk for CRC?
Men and women at average risk should be offered screening for CRC and adenomatous polyps at age 50. Options for CRC screening include fecal occult blood test (FOBT), flexible sigmoidoscopy, FOBT and flexible sigmoidoscopy, or colonoscopy. Stool DNA testing and CT colonography are two methods that appear to have a great deal of promise, although their utility in everyday clinical practice has yet to be defined. Each approach has its advantages and disadvantages, and each person should make an informed decision regarding his or her preference.

Is colon cancer screening cost-effective?
Yes. All strategies of colon cancer screening are cost-effective compared to no screening and cost less than $20,000 per life-year saved. Twice-lifetime colonoscopy and flexible sigmoidoscopy, combined with fecal occult blood testing, are the two most effective screening strategies. Twice-lifetime colonoscopy is the most cost-effective screening method followed by once-lifetime colonoscopy.

Give the current guidelines for surveillance colonoscopy in patients with a history of adenomatous polyps.
A periodic surveillance program should be customized according to adequacy of the preparation and endoscopic findings.

Colonoscopy Findings	Next Colonoscopy
One-two tubular adenomas	5 years
Large sessile (>2 cm) adenoma	3–6 months
Inadequate colon preparation	Repeat within 3–6 months
Villous histology or dysplasia	3 years

Who is considered to be at increased risk for developing colorectal cancer?
People at increased risk are defined as those individuals who have a personal history of CRC or an adenomatous polyp, a predisposing illness for CRC, such as inflammatory bowel disease, a first-degree relative (parent, sibling, child) with CRC or an adenomatous polyp, or a gene carrier for familial colon cancer syndromes. The risk of developing CRC is increased approximately twofold if a first-degree relative has been diagnosed with CRC over age 65. The younger the age at which the relative was diagnosed, the higher the risk. The risk also rises if more than one first-degree relative has been diagnosed with CRC. Perhaps more significantly, the same risk seems to apply if first-degree relatives were found to have adenomatous polyps. Evidence suggests a slightly increased risk (approximately 1.5-fold) if third-degree relatives (e.g., cousins) have been diagnosed with CRC.

Which method of CRC screening is recommended for individuals at increased risk of developing CRC?
Colonoscopy is the only recommended screening modality in this patient population.

List the familial colon cancer syndromes.
- Familial adenomatous polyposis (FAP) and Gardner's syndrome (FAP with extracolonic manifestations)

- Hamartomatous polyp syndromes: Peutz-Jeghers syndrome (PJS) and juvenile polyposis syndrome (JPS)
- HNPCC

26. **What tests are available for hereditary CRC?**

Diagnosis of an APC germ-line mutation is based on one of several DNA-based tests:
- Sequencing of the entire genome (95% sensitive)
- Combination of confirmation strand gel electrophoresis screening and protein truncation testing (80–90% sensitive)
- Protein truncation alone (80% sensitive)
- Linkage analysis (98% sensitive in most families with the FAP mutation)

There are >228 germ-line mutations and >47 polymorphisms in the seven mismatch repair (MMR) genes associated with HNPCC. These multiple mutations have limited the development of inexpensive diagnostic assays for HNPCC, and diagnosis is now based on direct DNA sequencing. JPS patients and their family members are appropriate candidates for genetic testing for germ-line mutations MAD4 and BMP1A, using direct DNA sequencing. The only clearly identified gene mutation is PJS *STK11/LKB1*, which leads to 40–60% of cases and can be diagnosed by mutation analysis of STK11. Candidate mutations associated with common familial colon cancer have not been characterized well enough to warrant routine genetic testing (Table 47-2).

27. **What is the recommended surveillance for people with a family history of CRC who do not fit the genetic profiles?**

- People with a first-degree relative (FDR) with CRC or adenomatous polyp diagnosed at age <60 or two FDRs with CRC diagnosed at any age should have a screening colonoscopy starting at age 40 or 10 years younger than the earliest diagnosis in the family (whichever is first) and repeated every 5 years.
- People with an FDR with CRC or adenomatous polyp diagnosed at age >60 or two second-degree relatives (grandparent, aunt, or uncle) with CRC should be screened as average risk persons but beginning at age 40.
- People with one second-degree relative with CRC should be screened as average risk.

28. **How do FAP and Gardner's syndrome increase the risk of CRC?**

FAP and Gardner's syndrome are inherited in an autosomal dominant manner. Their fully expressed forms are characterized by the development of hundreds to thousands of colonic adenomas. One hundred percent of patients expressing this phenotype develop CRC without colectomy. Most patients begin developing adenomas in their teens, and screening in families with a known proband should start at that time. One third of FAP cases arise as de novo mutations. The increased risk of CRC is thought to be due to the sheer number of adenomatous polyps; each polyp has the same risk of malignant transformation as an "ordinary" sporadic adenoma.

29. **How are FAP and Gardner's syndrome diagnosed?**

The APC gene is responsible for both FAP and Gardner's syndrome. Most disease-causing mutations result in premature stop codons, which give rise to truncated proteins. Commercial tests are available to detect truncated proteins and to directly sequence the gene. The results can be used for accurate screening of affected kindreds. Members of FAP kindreds who have not developed adenomas by age 40 have not inherited the polyposis phenotype. The position of the mutation gives rise to the phenotype of the FAP. For example, mutations in the extreme beginning or end of the APC gene can cause an attenuated form of FAP, which is characterized by fewer adenomas (1–100) with a right-sided predominance.

30. **In addition to colonoscopy, what other tests should be considered in FAP?**

Patients with FAP are at increased risk of extracolonic tumors, including thyroid cancer, pancreatic cancer, duodenal and ampullary cancer, and gastric cancer; therefore, periodic thyroid function

TABLE 47-2. FEATURES OF COLON CANCER SYNDROMES

Features	Sporadic CRC	HNPCC	FAP	Attenuated FAP	JPS	PJS
Average age of CRC (yr)	69	44	39	49	34	46
Incidence	Lifetime 1/18 (F) 1/17 (M)	1:2000	1:10,000	1:9000	1:100,000	1:200,000
Colon polyps	Few polyps	Few polyps, proximal distribution	>100 polyps in teens	~30 polyps with proximal distribution	~100s in colon, scattered else-where in GI tract	>2 P-J polyps in GI tract
Gene abnormality	Multiple	MLH1, MSH2, MSH6, PMS2, PMS1	APC (>90%), ?MYH (~5%)	APC (>90%), ?MYH (~5%)	MADH4/SMA4, & BMPRIA (53%)	STK11/LKB1 (~55%)
Mode of inheritance	?	Autosomal dominant	Autosomal dominant	Autosomal dominant	Autosomal dominant	Autosomal dominant

CRC = colorectal cancer, HNPCC = hereditary nonpolyposis colorectal cancer, FAP = familial adenomatous polyposis, JPS = juvenile polyposis syndrome, PJS = Peutz-Jeghers syndrome, F = female, M = male, GI = gastrointestinal.

tion tests, liver function tests, and upper gastrointestinal (GI) tract screening with both forwa
and side-viewing endoscopes are recommended.

31. **What is the role of NSAIDs in treating FAP?**

    Both sulindac and celecoxib decrease the number of adenomas in patients with FAP, but neit
    is associated with complete regression. Therefore, chemoprevention cannot replace prophyl
    tic colectomy, although the timing of the colectomy may be delayed.

32. **How do hamartomatous polyp syndromes affect the risk of developing CRC?**

    Along with PJS and JPS, the differential diagnosis includes Cowden's disease and the Banna
    Ruvalcaba-Riley syndrome. Phenotypic features of hamartomatous syndromes display cons
    erable overlap. Emerging understanding of the germ-line mutations may allow and provide n
    accurate distinctions between these. Hamartomatous polyp syndromes appear to be associa
    with a slightly increased risk of developing CRC, although nowhere near the risk associated v
    APC syndromes.

33. **What is HNPCC?**

    HNPCC is an autosomal dominant inherited disease in which colon cancer is caused by inact.
    tion of one of the proteins involved in DNA proofreading (usually hMSH2 or hMLH1) leading
    early onset of colon cancers and extracolonic cancers (e.g., endometrial, ovarian, gastric, uri
    nary tract, renal cell, biliary, and gallbladder). Colon cancer arises from discrete adenomas th
    rapidly accumulate point mutations resulting in a markedly accelerated progression from ade
    noma to carcinoma. Because the term "nonpolyposis" is misleading, there has been a trend
    toward calling this entity by its original designation, the Lynch syndromes I (colon cancer alc
    and II (colon cancer and a spectrum of other malignancies).

34. **How is HNPCC diagnosed?**

    Diagnosis is based on either the Amsterdam criteria, the Amsterdam criteria II, or the Bethes
    guidelines. The more stringent Amsterdam criteria increase the chances of finding a germ-lin
    mutation in either MSH2 or MLH1 to 25–86%. The Bethesda guidelines (Table 47-3) are mor
    sensitive but less specific than the Amsterdam criteria (Table 47-4).

TABLE 47-3.   AMSTERDAM CRITERIA

Amsterdam Criteria*	Amsterdam Criteria II[†]
1. One member diagnosed with CRC before age 50	1. At least three affected relatives with an HNPCC-associated cancer
2. Two affected generations	2. One of whom is an FDR of the other two
3. Three affected relatives, one of them an FDR[2] of the other two	3. At least two successive generations
4. Exclude FAP	4. One member diagnosed with CRC before age 5
5. Pathologic confirmation	5. Exclude FAP
	6. Pathologic confirmation

*All criteria must be met.
[†]First-degree relative.

TABLE 47-4.	BETHESDA GUIDELINES (MEETING ANY LISTED FEATURE IS SUFFICIENT)

1. Individuals in families that meet the Amsterdam criteria
2. Individuals with two HNPCC-related cancers (CRC or associated extracolonic cancers)
3. Individuals with CRC and an FDR with CRC, HNPCC-associated cancer, or colorectal adenoma (cancer diagnosed at younger than age 45, adenoma at younger than age 40)
4. Individuals with CRC or endometrial cancer diagnosed at younger than age 45
5. Individuals with an undifferentiated right-sided CRC diagnosed at younger than age 45
6. Individuals with signet-ring cell-type CRC diagnosed at younger than age 45
7. Individuals with adenomas diagnosed at younger than age 40

HNPCC = hereditary nonpolyposis colorectal cancer, CRC = colorectal cancer, FDR = first-degree relative.

Outline the screening recommendation for patients with HNPCC.
Screening with colonoscopy for all members of the family should begin at ages 20–25, repeated semiannually until age 40, then yearly thereafter. Some individuals with known mutations may elect to have a subtotal colectomy before developing malignancies.

What is MYH-associated polyposis (MAP)?
MYH polyposis is a recently described autosomal recessive polyposis syndrome that is phenotypically similar to attenuated APC (15–500 adenomas) but does not have an APC germ-line mutation. This biallelic germ-line mutation causes nucleotide transversion G:C → T:A in the APC gene. MYH is a protein that acts synergistically with two other proteins OGG1 and MTH1 in the base excision repair pathway to repair DNA replication errors caused by oxidative stress. These mutations have been demonstrated in both adenomas and carcinomas. The percentage of polyposis syndrome patients with this mutation is unknown.

What is microsatellite instability (MSI)?
Microsatellites are short, repeated DNA sequences (5–10 nucleotides) that are susceptible to somatic mutation by misalignment. Ordinarily, this mismatch in the number of repeats is repaired by the DNA proofreading complex (that includes MSH2, MLH1, MSH6, MLH3, PMS1, and PMS2, the so-called mismatch repair genes). When this complex is inactivated, usually by mutations in MSH2 or MLH1 mismatched bases, including the commonly occurring microsatellite, repeat misalignments cannot be repaired, leading to a rapid accumulation of genome wide mutations. MSI is observed in approximately 85% of HNPCC colon cancers and 15% of sporadic colon cancers.

How does inflammatory bowel disease affect the risk of developing CRC?
Patients with chronic inflammatory bowel disease (IBD) have an increased risk of developing colorectal cancer, particularly those with chronic ulcerative colitis (CUC). In patients with CUC, the risk begins to rise approximately 7 years after onset and increases with duration of the disease, as high as 35% by 30 years in tertiary care referral centers (in the community the risk may be much lower). Crohn's disease is also thought to have an increased risk (but lesser than ulcerative colitis) for developing CRC, probably because the noncontiguous nature of the lesions puts less mucosa at risk. It is thought that increased cell turnover due to inflammation is the important factor predisposing the colon to the development of malignancies in patients with IBD.

39. **Describe the recommended screening protocol for patients with IBD.**
The cost-effectiveness of screening for CRC in IBD is controversial. Current screening regimens rely on random biopsies taken during colonoscopies (usually four quadrant biopsies every 10 cm) to identify dysplasia, the premalignant lesion in IBD. Even the most aggressive screening regimens sample <0.1% of the colonic mucosa, thus limiting the probability that a discrete focus of dysplasia or malignancy will be discovered. Because most malignancies in IBD appear to arise within larger fields of dysplasia, the presence of even mild dysplasia, if confirmed, should be a cause for concern, and consideration needs to be given to total colectomy, particularly if the dysplasia is associated with a lesion or mass (DALM). Patients willing to consider colectomy, if dysplasia is found, should begin surveillance 8–10 years after onset of disease and, with negative examinations, probably every 2 years thereafter until 20–25 years, at which time annual examinations should begin. In an IBD clinic in a tertiary care center, annual colonoscopies beginning at 15–20 years of disease duration may be appropriate, with some experts advocating semiannual exams beginning at 30 years of disease duration.

40. **How are high-grade dysplasia and low-grade dysplasia managed?**
High-grade dysplasia carries a 40–45% risk that a malignancy will be found in a resected specimen and therefore proctocolectomy is recommended. Low-grade dysplasia carries an approximately 20% risk of an existing cancer, and an increasing number of clinicians therefore advocate colectomy rather than the traditional program of intensive surveillance (every 3–6 months).

41. **In the setting of chronic ulcerative colitis, does a sporadic adenomatous colon polyp carry an increased risk of cancer?**
No. Although polyps are considered to be premalignant lesions, they do not carry an increased risk of cancer in the remainder of the colon. Therefore, the polyp should be treated the same as in the general population and be removed. The remainder of the colon should be sampled for mucosal dysplasia, as described previously.

42. **Can CRC be prevented?**
Not completely. However, it is possible to reduce mortality by discovering and removing neoplasms at premalignant stages (e.g., polypectomy [secondary prevention]), discovering cancers earlier, more curable stages (tertiary prevention), and using chemoprevention. Colonoscopy with removal of all adenomas is the most effective means of preventing colorectal cancers. Cost-effectiveness depends largely on the interval between screening examinations, cost of the procedures, and prevalence of adenomas and cancers within the target population. Analyses indicate that most strategies fall well below the benchmark figure of $40,000 per year of life saved, comparing favorably with mammography in women over age 50 (approximately $25,000 per year of life saved). The acceptance of colonoscopic screening every 10 years in asymptomatic patients as a Medicare benefit (with most third-party carriers following suit) has made colonoscopy the preferred method of screening. Acceptance by the general population is now the major challenge if the mortality of CRC is to be reduced.

43. **Which two clinical conditions should raise suspicion for the presence of colon cancer?**
An unexplained iron deficiency anemia or sepsis with *Streptococcus bovis* as the pathogen should trigger investigation for colorectal cancer.

44. **What is the sensitivity and specificity of an air contrast barium enema?**
Carefully performed air contrast barium enemas have sensitivities and specificities in the 90% range; however, in most centers the figures are considerably lower, perhaps because modern ultrasound-, CT-, or MRI-based procedures have become more fashionable.

5. How effective is "virtual colonoscopy" as a screening test?

Also known as CT colonography, virtual colonoscopy is an emerging technology for CRC screening. Early studies of virtual colonoscopy showed favorable results but were skewed because only symptomatic patients, or patients at high risk for colonic neoplasm, were selected and thus did not represent a true screening population. One study of average risk patients showed a sensitivity of 28–57% for any polyp between 5–9 mm and 32–73% for any polyp ≥10 mm with high interobserver variability. A more recent study using stool tagging with barium for "digital cleansing" along with a traditional colon preparation as well as three-dimensional endoluminal display reported sensitivities of 93.8% for adenomatous polyps at least 10 mm and 88.7% for polyps at least 6 mm. However, the sensitivity was calculated on 210 adenomas of 6 mm or more and did not include the 134 nonadenomatous polyps of the same size and, therefore, may have resulted in higher estimates of sensitivity. A threshold polyp size of 6 mm would result in approximately 30% of patients being referred for colonoscopy.

6. Can CRC be prevented with medicines (chemoprevention)?

Because we cannot prevent CRCs by elimination of causative factors, the possibility of chemoprevention has generated considerable enthusiasm. Nonsteroidal anti-inflammatory drugs, including sulindac and aspirin, have shown promise in both experimental models and epidemiologic studies. Recent studies have shown protective effects; however, maximum efficacy requires higher doses (>14 tablets/week), which markedly increase the risk of GI tract toxicity and potential bleeding. Aspirin use for adenoma prevention, at present, can only be recommended for those at increased risk for adenoma formation who have no history of ulcer disease or stroke. Sulindac decreases the number and size of adenomas in patients with FAP but does not completely prevent progression to cancer. Its efficacy in sporadic adenomas is unclear. Selective cyclo-oxygenase-2 inhibitors, which have a much lower GI toxicity profile, are effective in animal models and patients with FAP, although they may be somewhat less effective than sulindac for FAP. Ongoing trials have shown benefits in reducing adenoma recurrence, but significant questions regarding cardiovascular safety must be resolved before their use can be recommended.

BIBLIOGRAPHY

1. Baron JA, Cole BF, Sandler RS, et al: A randomized trial of aspirin to prevent colorectal adenomas. N Engl J Med 348(10):891–899, 2003.
2. Boland CR: Malignant tumors of the colon. In Yamada T, Alpers DH, Laine L, et al (eds): Textbook of Gastroenterology. Philadelphia, Lippincott Williams & Wilkins, 2003, pp 1940–1989.
3. Bresalier RS: Malignant neoplasms of the large intestine. In Feldman M, Friedman LS, Sleisenger MH (eds): Gastrointestinal and Liver Disease. Philadelphia, W.B. Saunders, 2002, pp 2215–2256.
4. Burt R: Colon cancer screening. Gastroenterology 119:837–853, 2000.
5. Chan AT, Giovannucci EL, Schernhammer ES, et al: A prospective study of aspirin use and the risk for colorectal adenoma. Ann Intern Med 140:157–166, 2004.
6. Fearon ER, Vogelstein B: A genetic model for colorectal tumorigenesis. Cell 61:759–767, 1990.
7. Giardiello FM, Hamilton SR, Krush AJ, et al: Treatment of colonic and rectal adenomas with sulindac in familial adenomatous polyposis. N Engl J Med 328:1313–1316, 1993.
8. Grady WM: Genetic testing for high-risk colon cancer patients. Gastroenterology 124:1574–1594, 2003.
9. Imperiale TF: Aspirin and the prevention of colorectal cancer. N Engl J Med 348(10):879–880, 2003.
10. Jemal A, Tiwari RC, Murray T, et al: Cancer statistics, 2004. CA Cancer J Clin 54:8–29, 2004.
11. Johnson CD, Harmsen WS, Wilson LA, et al: Prospective blinded evaluation of computed tomographic colonoscopy for screen detection of colorectal polyps. Gastroenterology 125:311–319, 2003.
12. Lieberman DA, Weiss DG, Bond JH, et al: Use of colonoscopy to screen asymptomatic adults for colorectal cancer. Veterans Affairs Cooperative Study Group 380. N Engl J Med 343:162–168, 2000.

13. Lynch HT, de la Chapelle A: Hereditary colorectal cancer. N Engl J Med 348(10):919–932, 2003.

14. Morrin MM, LaMont TL: Screening virtual colonoscopy: Ready for prime time? N Engl J Med 349(23):2261–2264, 2003.

15. Pickhardt PJ, Choi JR, Hwang I, et al: Computed tomographic virtual colonoscopy to screen for colorectal neoplasia in asymptomatic adults. N Engl J Med 349(23):2191–2200, 2003.

16. Pineau BC, Paskett ED, Chen GJ, et al: Virtual colonoscopy using oral contrast compared with colonoscopy for the detection of patients with colorectal polyps. Gastroenterology 125:304–310, 2003.

17. Ransohoff DF, Sandler RS: Screening for colorectal cancer. N Engl J Med 346(1):40–44, 2002.

18. Rustgi A: Hereditary gastrointestinal polyposis and non polyposis syndromes. N Engl J Med 331:1694–1702, 1994.

19. Sandler RS, Halabi S, Baron JA, et al: A randomized trial of aspirin to prevent colorectal adenomas in patients with previous colorectal cancer. N Engl J Med 348(10):883–890, 2003.

20. Selby JV, Friedman GD, Quesenberry CP, Weiss NS: A case-control study of screening sigmoidoscopy and mortality from colorectal cancer. N Engl J Med 326:653–657, 1992.

21. Steinbach G, Lynch PM, Phillips RK, et al: The effect of celecoxib, a cyclooxygenase-2 inhibitor, in familial adenomatous polyposis. N Engl J Med 342:1946–1952, 2000.

22. Toribara NW, Sleisenger MH: Screening for colorectal cancer. N Engl J Med 332:861–867, 1995.

23. Vasen HF, Watson P, Mecklin JP, Lynch HT: New clinical criteria for hereditary nonpolyposis colorectal cancer (HNPCC, Lynch syndrome) proposed by the International Collaborative group on HNPCC. Gastroenterology 116:1453–1456, 1999.

24. Vijan S, Hwang EW, Hofer TP, Hayward RA: Which colon cancer screening test? A comparison of costs, effectiveness, and compliance. Am J Med 111:593–601, 2001.

25. Winawer S, Fletcher R, Rex D, et al: Colorectal cancer screening and surveillance: Clinical guidelines and rationale—update based on new evidence. Gastroenterology 124:544–560, 2003.

26. Winawer SJ, Zauber AG, Gerdes H, et al: Risk of colorectal cancer in the families of patients with adenomatous polyps. N Engl J Med 334:82–87, 1996.

27. Winawer SJ, Zauber AG, Ho MN, et al: Prevention of colorectal cancer by colonoscopic polypectomy. N Engl J Med 329:1977–1981, 1993.

CHAPTER 48

CONSTIPATION AND FECAL INCONTINENCE

Peter E. Legnani, MD, and Suzanne Rose, MD, MSEd

. What is constipation?

Infrequent bowel movements, painful passage of stool, hard consistency of stool, or difficulty in evacuating stool may be considered constipation by the patient, usually defined as fewer than three bowel movements per week.

. Describe the normal mechanism of stool passage.

The first step is sensing that material is in the rectum. Stretch receptors in the muscularis propria of the rectum initiate a spinal reflex arc (rectoanal inhibitory reflex), stimulating inhibitory nerves that lead to relaxation of the internal anal sphincter. Next, the striated muscles of the pelvic floor (puborectalis and pubococcygeus) relax, resulting in perineal descent. The rectoanal angle is opened further from 90 to 130 degrees, and the anal canal is stretched in the anteroposterior direction by flexure of the hips, when the person assumes a sitting or squatting position. When the external anal sphincter relaxes, the final resistance to passage of stool is removed. Finally, rectal smooth muscle contraction, often with concomitant diaphragmatic and abdominal muscular contraction, results in expulsion of the rectal contents, followed by restoration of tone in the internal anal sphincter.

. What are the major causes of constipation?

See Table 48-1.

TABLE 48-1. MAJOR CAUSES OF CONSTIPATION	
Causes	**Examples**
Metabolic disorders	Hypothyroidism, diabetes mellitus
Collagen vascular diseases	Scleroderma
Inherited muscular disorders	Familial visceral myopathy
Colonic disorders	Colonic inertia
Enteric neurologic disorders	Hirschsprung's disease, chronic intestinal pseudo-obstruction
Nonenteric neurologic disorders	Parkinson's disease, spinal cord injury, multiple sclerosis
Anorectal disorders	Anal stricture, rectocele
Medications	Opiates, antacids (calcium and aluminum), anticholinergics, anticonvulsants, antidepressants, parkinsonian agents, diuretics, iron, antihypertensive agents, calcium channel blockers

4. **Describe the work-up for constipation.**
   A thorough history should focus on duration of constipation, presence of danger signs, such as blood per rectum and weight loss, risk factors for colonic malignancy, signs of systemic illnesses, and direct questioning about medical history, diet and exercise, prescription and over-the-counter medications. Physical exam, including a detailed digital rectal exam and neurologic assessment, is supplemented by a limited laboratory analysis of thyroid-stimulating hormone and calcium to exclude metabolic disorders. Colonoscopy or flexible sigmoidoscopy should be considered in all patients. If this work-up is unrevealing, the patient is considered to have chronic idiopathic constipation.

5. **What tests are used in the evaluation of chronic constipation?**
   Colonic marker studies with radiopaque plastic rings are used to measure gut transit time. This safe, effective technique involves swallowing inert rings in a capsule, followed by plain abdominal radiography on subsequent days. In normal patients, more than 80% of the rings should be passed by 5 days, and all of the markers should be passed by 1 week. Another method uses capsules with easily viewed markers of different shapes, which are swallowed on days 1, 2, and 3, followed by a plain abdominal film on day 5. Other protocols have been described using differing numbers of markers with x-rays at various intervals. Four patterns are generally observed: (1) normal transit (majority of rings passed); (2) colonic inertia, in which the markers remain and are evenly distributed throughout the colon (Fig. 48-1); (3) hindgut delay, in which the markers leave the right colon and progress to the left side but are not evacuated; and (4) functional outlet obstructions, which may reflect transit time delay or suggest pelvic floor dysfunction. The markers can be commercially purchased (Sitzmarks, Konsyl Pharmaceuticals, Inc., Edison, NJ) or made in the office/hospital by sectioning a nasogastric tube into small rings.

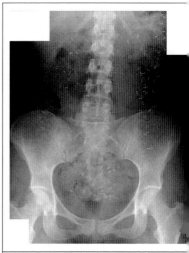

Figure 48-1. Plain radiograph of the abdomen showing Sitzmarks evenly distributed throughout the colon, consistent with finding of colonic inertia.

   Anorectal manometry involves passing a pressure-recording catheter across the anal sphincter. Through techniques involving balloon distention within the rectum, rectal sensory thresholds and internal anal sphincter relaxation can be assessed directly. Manometry can be combined with surface electromyography (EMG) studies of the pelvic floor musculature and external anal sphincter to diagnose entities, such as anorectal dyssynergia or anismus (see later text).

   Defecography involves the placement of barium paste into the rectum, with radiography taken before and during evacuation of rectal contents. In addition to assessing the completeness of rectal expulsion, this test is also used to demonstrate anatomic abnormalities of the rectum (rectocele), prolapse, or pelvic floor dysfunction. New modalities using MRI to evaluate the function of the pelvic floor may also be considered, if available.

6. **What are the subsets of chronic idiopathic constipation?**
   Based on assessment of colonic and anorectal function, chronic idiopathic constipation can be separated into the four major classes: (1) impaired colonic transit, (2) isolated anal

sphincter dysfunction caused by impaired rectoanal inhibitory reflex, (3) anorectal dysfunction caused by physiologic abnormalities, and (4) constipation-predominant irritable bowel syndrome.

7. What causes impaired rectoanal inhibitory reflex? How is it diagnosed?

An impaired rectoanal inhibitory reflex is found in 8–10% of adults with severe idiopathic constipation. In children, it is often seen in conjunction with aganglionosis of the colon (*Hirschsprung's disease*). Adults may have a similar condition called *short-segment Hirschsprung's disease*. Aganglionosis occurs within a very short segment of the distal colon, but ganglia are present in full-thickness biopsies of the remaining colon. The diagnostic finding on anal manometry is failure of the internal anal sphincter to relax with balloon distention (also known as a loss of the rectoanal inhibitory reflex [RAIR]). It is important to consider this syndrome, especially in young adults with long-standing severe constipation, because surgical posterior sphincterotomy often provides good symptomatic response.

8. What physiologic abnormalities may lead to anorectal dysfunction? How are they diagnosed?

Various physiologic abnormalities may lead to *dyschezia* (difficulty in defecating). Functional rectal obstruction may result from dysfunction of the pelvic musculature, also termed *anismus, spastic pelvic floor syndrome,* or *anorectal dyssynergia.* Impaired relaxation during a defecatory effort secondary to spasticity of the levator ani, failure of perineal descent, an abnormally angulated rectoanal axis, or a combination of these factors leads to functional obstruction of the anal outlet, terminating defecation. Measurement of the rectoanal angle and the change in the angle during defecography is necessary to make the diagnosis. Occasionally, biofeedback ameliorates this condition.

Impaired rectal sensation leads to a decreased motor response and a decrease in the urge to defecate, as determined by balloon distention studies of the rectum. *Megarectum* occurs usually in the setting of fecal impaction and is seen most often in children and physically or mentally impaired elderly patients. Occasionally, megarectum is associated with neurologic disease, such as lumbosacral spinal cord lesions, but most often it is associated with long-standing fecal impaction. Increased rectal compliance, diminished rectal sensation, and impaired internal anal sphincter relaxation are noted on manometry. Finally, rectal contents can be directed away from the anal canal into a *rectocele* during increased abdominal pressure, leading to incomplete evacuation and retention of feces in the pouch. Endoscopy and barium enema often fail to diagnose a rectocele. Defecography remains the test of choice for diagnosing a rectocele. Clinically, the patient may report a need to insert a finger in the vagina to facilitate defecation. The finding of a rectocele is not uncommon but the rectocele may be clinically insignificant.

9. What other symptoms may be associated with fecal impaction?

- Constipation
- Abdominal pain
- Rectal discomfort
- Paradoxical diarrhea
- Anorexia
- Fecal incontinence
- Nausea
- Urinary frequency
- Vomiting
- Urinary overflow incontinence

10. How is constipation caused by irritable bowel syndrome diagnosed?

Constipation-predominant irritable bowel syndrome is diagnosed clinically. Usually, it is seen in young or middle-aged adults, predominantly women. Constipation is noted along with abdominal pain, bloating, flatulence, straining, or incomplete evacuation.

11. **Describe the general management of constipation.**

    Primary care physicians manage most patients who complain of constipation. Reassurance is beneficial to those who are concerned with less than daily stool patterns or weekly irregularitie and may alleviate fears of severe disease. Dietary modifications, such as increasing fiber and daily fluid intake, may increase weekly bowel movements. In addition, increased exercise acce erates colonic transit time and may lead to an improvement in general well-being. Changes or substitutions of medications that alter colonic function may allow resumption of normal bowel pattern.

12. **What medical agents can be used for treatment of chronic constipation?**

    Therapeutic agents fall into five major categories:
    1. Bulk-forming agents and dietary fiber
    2. Enemas
    3. Laxatives and cathartics
    4. 5-HT$_4$ agonists
    5. Prokinetic agents

13. **Describe the proper use of bulk-forming laxatives and dietary fiber.**

    Bulk-forming laxatives and dietary fiber often benefit patients with mild constipation and should be initiated in every patient with chronic constipation once fecal impaction and obstruction have been ruled out. All patients should be encouraged to increase daily con- sumption of dietary fiber. A goal of 20–35 gm/day of cereals, fruits and vegetables, and bran is desirable but often requires specific dietary suggestions and relies on patient motivation. Over-the-counter supplements include psyllium, wheat fiber, and methylcellulose. When any kind of bulk laxative is initiated, the starting dose should be low and gradually increased ove 2–3 weeks to minimize the bloating and increased gas that often develop. Patients should be counseled to drink adequate fluids.

14. **Describe the role of enemas.**

    Retention enemas provide direct and reliable results in fecal impaction and are the mainstay of therapy for keeping the rectal vault clean in the setting of megarectum. Agents delivered via enema, including lukewarm tap water and water with soap suds, mineral oil, or phosphate sulfates, can be given on a daily or as-needed basis. In megarectum, prevention of recurrent impaction in conjunction with scheduled bowel training may allow resumption of a more norm bowel pattern. In this clinical setting, a low residue diet may be of benefit.

15. **What are 5-HT$_4$ agonists?**

    A new class of agents targeting the 5-HT$_4$ receptor has been under investigation. 5-HT$_4$ agonists stimulate GI transit and, in animal studies, have accelerated colonic and whole gut transit. Tegaserod, a 5-HT$_4$ partial agonist, was approved in 2002 for the treatment of constipation- predominant irritable bowel syndrome female patients. Tegaserod has been shown to relieve pai and constipation in this population of constipation-predominant irritable bowel syndrome patien

16. **Outline the approach to evaluation of patients with constipation.**

    See Figure 48-2.

17. **What is fecal incontinence? Who is generally affected?**

    Fecal incontinence in adults is the involuntary loss of stool. In population-based studies involv ing all ages, the prevalence of incontinence ranges from 2–14%. In geriatric patients, the preva lence is even higher: 10–17% of nursing home residents and 13–47% of hospitalized elderly patients report incontinence. Women develop incontinence more often than men (in some stu ies up to eight times more frequently).

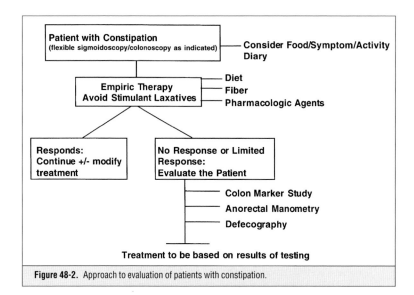

Figure 48-2. Approach to evaluation of patients with constipation.

8. Describe the pathophysiology of fecal incontinence.

Normal functioning requires an intact neuromuscular system; the ability to sense impending defecation and to differentiate between gas, liquid, and solid; and the motivation to maintain continence. The major abnormalities of continence mechanisms involve impairments in rectal sensation, abnormal rectal compliance, and anal sphincter dysfunction secondary to muscle dysfunction or interruption and nerve damage.

Impaired proprioception in the levator ani, puborectalis, and sphincters can decrease the ability to sense rectal filling, leading to loss of the normal warning of imminent defecation. Because autonomic pathways remain intact, the IAS relaxes before the patient senses rectal distention, leading to incontinence. Long-standing patients with diabetes may develop sensory abnormalities from neuropathy with similar consequences.

Changes in *rectal compliance* can lead to incontinence. The rectum has elastic properties that allow it to maintain low intraluminal pressure in response to increasing volumes. If compliance is diminished, smaller volumes may lead to increased intraluminal pressures and incontinence, often associated with urgency and frequency. A reduced compliance may result from inflammation or fibrosis, such as that seen in radiation proctitis or inflammatory bowel disease. Conversely, incontinence may also result from increased rectal compliance and diminished sensation, as in fecal impaction and megarectum. In this setting, intact involuntary pathways relax the internal anal sphincter before the patient senses rectal distention, with resultant incontinence from "overflow" diarrhea.

Myopathic damage from disruption of the anal sphincters and sacral neuropathic disorders can diminish the high-pressure zone necessary to maintain continence, leading to soiling. A functional component may also lead to early muscle fatigue and incontinence. Rarely, massive diarrhea may overwhelm the normal continence mechanism.

9. What are the major causes of incontinence?

Anatomic defects	Obstetric injury (high birthweight infants, forceps-assisted deliveries)
	Surgical injury (fistula repair, hemorrhoidectomy)
	Trauma

Collagen vascular disease	Scleroderma
Congenital disorders	Spina bifida
Diarrheal conditions	Inflammatory bowel disease
	Infection
	Irritable bowel syndrome
	Laxatives
	Malabsorption
Neurologic disorders	Cerebrovascular accident
	Dementia
	Diabetes
	Multiple sclerosis
Overflow incontinence	Fecal impaction
Aging	May be multifactorial

20. **Describe the work-up of incontinence.**

A good history and physical exam are vital. The *history* should include general information about frequency, duration, and pattern of soilage; symptoms of diarrhea, constipation, urgency, or straining; and dietary intake. Prior anorectal surgery or trauma, diabetes mellitus or thyroid disease, neurologic events or illness, and progressive dementia may contribute to incontinence. A thorough obstetric history includes information about all deliveries, use of forceps for delivery, length of second stage of labor, history of episiotomy, or significant perineal lacerations that may have affected the perineal floor. Finally, a comprehensive medication history must be obtained, including direct inquiry about over-the-counter medications, laxatives, and dietary substitutes, such as sorbitol.

The *physical exam* must include careful inspection of the perineum, looking for scars, obvious lacerations, fissures, and hemorrhoids. Digital rectal exam detects distal rectal masses and fecal impaction. The resting tone and squeeze pressures of the anal sphincter should be noted and the strength of puborectalis contraction assessed. Neurologic evaluation should include a mental status examination, assessment of sacral reflexes (anal wink), checking the integrity of the spinal pathway, and evaluation of perineal sensation. Visualization of the anus with anoscopy, and flexible sigmoidoscopy or colonoscopy, as indicated, completes the exam. (See Fig. 48-3.)

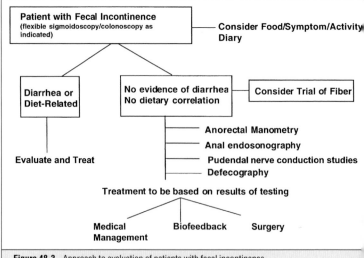

Figure 48-3. Approach to evaluation of patients with fecal incontinence.

1. **What specialized tests are available for the evaluation of incontinence?**

   Anorectal manometry, which is performed with balloon catheters to test the function of the sphincters, enables measurement of the resting tone of the IAS, squeeze pressure of the EAS, and functional length of the high-pressure zone created by the sphincters. Certain manometric devices are also capable of measuring rectal sensation and rectal compliance.

   Electromyography of the sphincters and puborectalis, performed with surface electrodes or needles, allows detection of denervation, conduction defects, and abnormalities in striated muscle function. This test may serve as both a diagnostic and therapeutic function.

   Pudendal nerve terminal motor assessment (PNTML) is performed by stimulating the right and/or left pudendal nerves at the ischial tuberosities and measuring the time to detect a muscular response (latency). This test is most useful in patients with obstetric injury, neurogenic incontinence, and rectal prolapse, all of which may have prolonged PNTML.

   Defecography (described earlier) evaluates the anatomy and change in pelvic floor muscle position with defecation. Abnormalities often missed in endoscopic evaluation of the rectum, such as prolapse, perineal descent, and intussusception, are often detected with defecography.

   Endoscopic ultrasound is a safe method for quick and easy evaluation of the structural integrity of the IAS and EAS.

2. **How is incontinence treated?**

   The initial step is *correction of all modifiable factors.* Dietary changes, such as limiting sorbitol, lactose, and fructose ingestion and increasing dietary fiber, may firm the stool, allowing better rectal sensation and enhancing sphincter function. Over-the-counter medications that may cause diarrhea (e.g., magnesium-containing antacids) should be eliminated. Loperamide or diphenoxylate may be helpful in reducing the gastrocolic reflex and limiting rectal filling.

   Biofeedback requires a patient who is able to understand the process, is sufficiently motivated, has some rectal sensation, and can generate a squeeze pressure through voluntary control of the EAS. Patients can be taught to recognize rectal distention and to increase the EAS pressure in response to balloon distention. In well-selected patients, good results may be noted after a single session.

   Other nonsurgical options have focused on mechanisms to tighten the anal canal and include encirclement with nonabsorbable mesh and perianal injections of fat, collagen, or synthetic gel. There are reports of success of using radiofrequency electrical energy to accomplish this tightening effect. Finally, several studies show improvement in symptoms of incontinence in patients who have been treated with sacral nerve stimulation.

   Various surgical techniques have been used. Operative resuspension of rectal prolapse restores continence in up to two thirds of patients. Repair of sphincter defects, with removal of scar tissue and direct apposition of the sphincters, successfully relieves incontinence in approximately 50% of patients. Anterior plication of the levator ani, puborectalis, and EAS with restoration of the anorectal angle and tightening of the anal canal improves symptoms in approximately 62% of patients with idiopathic incontinence. Other techniques, such as anal encirclement with a wire or a silastic ring to tighten the anal canal mechanically, have been used, but frequent complications occur. Newer techniques using artificial sphincters are currently under study. Colostomy has been used for immobile patients suffering from recurrent bacteremia secondary to skin breakdown with fecal contamination of decubitus ulcers.

3. **List the indications and contraindications for use of biofeedback.**

   See Table 48-2.

TABLE 48-2. INDICATIONS AND CONTRAINDICATIONS FOR USE OF BIOFEEDBACK	
Indications	**Contraindications**
Anal sphincter weakness	Dementia
Anal sphincter muscle fatigue	Spinal cord injuries
Obstetric damage	Absent rectal sensation
Idiopathic fecal incontinence	Lack of motivation
Diabetes mellitus	Impaired rectal storage capacity
Meningomyelocele	

BIBLIOGRAPHY

1. Bishoff JT, Garrick M, Optenberg SA, et al: Incidence of fecal and urinary incontinence following radical perineal and retropubic prostatectomy in a national population. J Urol 160:454–458, 1998.

2. Burkitt DP, Walker AR, Painter NS: Effect of dietary fiber on stools and transit times, and its role in the causation of disease. Lancet 2:1408, 1972.

3. Camilleri M, Thompson WG, Fleshman JW, et al: Clinical management of intractable constipation. Ann Intern Med 121:520–528, 1994.

4. Caruana BJ, Wald A, Hinds JP, et al: Anorectal sensory and motor function in neurogenic fecal incontinence. Gastroenterology 100:465–470, 1991.

5. Cooper ZR, Rose S: Fecal incontinence: A clinical approach. Mount Sinai J Med 67:96–105, 2000.

6. De Lillo AR, Rose S: Functional bowel disorders in the geriatric patient: Constipation, fecal impaction, and incontinence. Am J Gastroenterol 9:901–905, 2000.

7. Enck P: Biofeedback training in disordered defecation: A critical review. Dig Dis Sci 38:1953–1960, 1993.

8. Freckner B, Von Euler C: Influence of pudendal block on the anal sphincters. Gut 16:482–489, 1975.

9. Gattuso JM, Kamm MA: Clinical features of idiopathic megarectum and idiopathic megacolon. Gut 41:93–99, 1997.

10. Goei R: Anorectal function in patients with defecation disorders and asymptomatic subjects: Evaluation with defecography. Radiology 174:121, 1990.

11. Ho YH, Tan M, Goh HS: Clinical and physiologic effects of biofeedback in outlet obstruction constipation. Dis Colon Rectum 39:520–524, 1996.

12. Jost WH, Schrank B, Herold A, Leiss O: Functional outlet obstruction: Anismus, spastic pelvic floor syndrome, and dyscoordination of the voluntary sphincter muscles. Definition, diagnosis, and treatment from the neurologic point of view. Scand J Gastroenterol 34:449–453, 1999.

13. Kelvin FM, Maglinte DD, Benson JT: Evacuation proctography (defecography): An aid to investigation of pelvic floor disorders. Obstet Gynecol 83:307–314, 1994.

14. Kumar D, Benson MJ, Bland JE: Glutaraldehyde cross-linked collagen in the treatment of faecal incontinence. Br J Surg 85:978–979, 1998.

15. Metcalfe AM, Phillips SF, Zinmeister AR, et al: Simplified assessment of segmental colonic transit. Gastroenterology 92:40, 1987.

16. Miller R, Orrom WJ, Cornes H, et al: Anterior sphincter plication and levatorplasty in the treatment of fecal incontinence. Br J Surg 76:1058–1060, 1989.

17. Muller-Lissner SA, Fumagalli I, Bardhan KD, et al: Tegaserod, a 5-HT4 receptor partial agonist, relieves symptoms in irritable bowel syndrome patients with abdominal pain, bloating and constipation. Aliment Pharmacol Ther 15:1655–1666, 2001.

18. Nelson R, Norton N, Cautley E, Furner S: Community based prevalence of anal incontinence. JAMA 274:559–561, 1995.

19. Prather CM, Camilleri M, Zinsmeister AR, et al: Tegaserod accelerates orocecal transit in patients with constipation predominant irritable bowel syndrome. Gastroenterology 118:463–468, 2000.

20. Rose S, Reynolds JC: Motility disorders of the colon. In Anuras S: Motility Disorders of the Gastrointestinal Tract: Principles and Practice. New York, Raven Press, 1992.

1. Sultan AH, Kamm MA, Hudson CN, et al: Anal sphincter disruption during vaginal delivery. N Engl J Med 329:1905–1911, 1993.

2. Sun WM, Read NW, Miner PB: Relation between rectal sensation and anal function in normal subjects and patients with fecal incontinence. Gut 1056–1061, 1990.

3. Takahashi T, Garcia-Osogobio S, Valdovinos MA, et al: Radiofrequency energy delivery to the muscle of the anal canal for the treatment of fecal incontinence. Dis Colon Rectum 45:915–922, 2002.

4. Vaizey CJ, Kamm MA, Roy AJ, et al: Double-blind crossover study of sacral nerve stimulation for fecal incontinence 43:298–302, 2000.

5. Wald A: Colonic transit and anorectal manometry in chronic idiopathic constipation. Arch Intern Med 146:1713, 1986.

6. Wong WD, Jensen LL, Bartolo DC, et al: Artificial anal sphincter. Dis Colon Rectum 39:1345–1351, 1996.

7. You YT, Wang JY, Changchien CR: Segmental colectomy in the management of colonic inertia. Am Surg 64:775–777, 1998.

CHAPTER 49

DIVERTICULITIS

Erik J. Pieramici, MD, JD, and Stephen R. Freeman, MD

1. **What is a diverticulum? Which types are colonic diverticula?**
   A diverticulum is a circumscribed pouch or sac that either occurs naturally or is created by herniation of a lining mucous membrane through a muscular defect of a tubular organ. Typical colonic diverticula are false or pulsion diverticulum, with only the mucosa and submucosa herniating through the muscle layers of the colon. True diverticula containing all layers of the bowel wall do occur in the colon and are congenital.

2. **How common is diverticular disease? What are the most frequent complications?**
   Diverticulosis is known to increase with age, with prevalence rates of 5% by age 40, 30% by age 60, and 65% by age 85 in Western societies. However, there are no recent population-based studies in the last 30 years in the United States. Most (70%) remain asymptomatic, 15–25% develop diverticulitis, and 5–15% develop bleeding.

3. **How do diverticula develop?**
   Although the specific cause is unknown, development of diverticula likely involves mechanical, environmental, and lifestyle factors. Etiologic factors include increased luminal pressure, lack of dietary fiber, age-related factors, and hypersegmentation. Decreased dietary fiber in the colonic lumen leads to decreased stool volume and increasing segmentation during peristalsis.

4. **What is hypersegmentation?**
   Segmentation is the motility process in which proximal and distal segmental muscular contractions separate the lumen into isolated chambers. In diverticulosis, this process is believed to be exaggerated, leading to herniation of the mucosa at four constant points of weakness in the colonic wall, where the vasa recta penetrate the circular muscle layer. The diverticula, therefore, tend to develop in rows between the mesenteric and lateral teniae coli. This concept is based, partly, on the principles of the law of LaPlace. This law states that colonic wall pressure is proportional to wall tension and inversely proportional to the radius of the colon. This helps explain, in part, why the sigmoid colon, with its smaller diameter, is at higher risk of developing diverticula.

5. **What is myochosis?**
   Myochosis is thickening of the circular and longitudinal (teniae) muscular layers of the colon, shortening of the teniae and luminal narrowing, and is usually seen grossly in people with sigmoid diverticulosis. The thickening shortens the teniae leading to a narrowing of the sigmoid colon, allowing obliteration of the lumen and segmentation of the colon. This thickening occurs without hypertrophy or hyperplasia of the smooth muscle. Histologically, the teniae have excess elastin deposition.

6. **Where are diverticula located?**
   In Western societies, 95% of diverticula are located in the sigmoid and distal descending colon. Sixty-five percent are isolated to sigmoid colon, 24% involve other areas to a lesser degree, and 7% are equally dispersed throughout the colon. Only 3–4% of cases spare the sigmoid colon. In Asian populations, diverticula are more common in the right colon, demonstrating that other

factors (genetic and environmental) must be important in this site-specific pathogenesis. As these cultures adopt Western diets, the incidence of diverticulosis and left-sided diverticula increases.

7. **How should symptomatic diverticulosis be managed?**
   Most clinicians emphasize the benefits of a high-fiber diet, regardless of the presence or absence of symptoms. Abdominal pain is thought to be related to spasm or distention of the colon, probably a factor in the pathogenesis of diverticulosis. Although no therapy has been proven to be effective, high-fiber diet and antispasmodics are often recommended. Advice to avoid foods containing seeds and nuts has no scientific foundation and eliminates many nutritious and high-fiber foods. A recent survey of colorectal surgeons concluded that a high-fiber diet without concern for avoiding nuts and seeds is probably the most appropriate advice.

KEY POINTS: DIVERTICULOSIS

1. Acquired colonic diverticula are false or pulsion diverticula.

2. Diverticulosis affects one third of people by age 60, and two thirds by age 80 in Western societies and is associated with low dietary fiber intake.

3. The majority of patients remain asymptomatic with complications of bleeding or diverticulitis occurring in 20–30%.

4. Myochosis is the gross appearance of the sigmoid colon exhibited in most patients with diverticulosis.

8. **What are the common signs and symptoms of early diverticulitis?**
   The most common symptoms are abrupt onset of abdominal pain and an alteration in bowel pattern. Early acute diverticulitis is characterized by circumscribed abdominal pain and tenderness. The usual location of the pain is the left lower quadrant, but because diverticula, and hence diverticulitis, can develop at any site, inflammation may mimic other conditions. For example, transverse colon diverticulitis may mimic peptic ulcer disease, and right colon diverticulitis may mimic acute appendicitis. Signs of inflammation, such as fever and elevated white blood cell count, help to distinguish diverticulitis from the spasm of irritable bowel syndrome.

9. **What are the signs and symptoms of severe diverticulitis?**
   As the disease progresses in severity, localized abscess and phlegmonous reaction may develop. In addition to pain and tenderness, a mass may develop. Systemic signs of infection become more pronounced (i.e., fever and leukocytosis). In elderly patients and patients taking corticosteroids, abdominal exam and usual signs are unreliable. Therefore, a high index of suspicion and use of imaging studies, such as CT scan, are important to avoid significant delay in diagnosis and increased operative mortality.
   Obstipation has long been taught as a symptom of diverticulitis, but, in fact, diarrhea is not uncommon. Rectal bleeding is not a symptom of diverticulitis.
   Table 49-1 summarizes the diagnostic approach to diverticulitis.

10. **What is the natural history of diverticulitis?**
    Most initial presentations of diverticulitis are uncomplicated (75%). Of these cases, 85% are effectively managed medically. After successful medical management of first episode:
    - About one third remain asymptomatic.
    - About one third have episodic discomfort without frank diverticulitis.
    - About one third have a second episode.

TABLE 49-1. DIAGNOSTIC APPROACH FOR ACUTE DIVERTICULITIS

History and Physical Examination
Usually >age 60
Left lower quadrant tenderness and unremitting abdominal pain
Fever
Leukocytosis

Differential Diagnosis

Elderly patients	*Middle-aged and young patients*	*Other*
Ischemia	Appendicitis	Amebiasis
Carcinoma	Salpingitis	Collagen vascular disease
Volvulus	Inflammatory bowel disease	Infectious colitis
Obstruction	Penetrating ulcer	Post-irradiation
Penetrating ulcer	Urosepsis	proctosigmoiditis
Nephrolithiasis/urosepsis	Pancreatitis	Prostatitis
		Irritable bowel syndrome

Qualifiers
Extremes of age (more virulent)
Asian ancestry (right-sided symptoms)
Corticosteroids
Immunosuppression
Chronic renal failure (abdominal examination insensitive)

Evaluations
Plain x-rays: good initial first step. May show ileus, obstruction, mass effect, ischemia, perforation
CT scan: very helpful in staging the degree of complications and evaluating for other diseases. Should be considered in all cases of diverticulitis with a palpable mass or clinical toxicity, failure of medical therapy, orthopedic complications, and corticosteroid use.
Ultrasound: can be a safe and helpful noninvasive test to evaluate acute diverticulitis. Over 20% of exams are suboptimal because of intestinal gas; highly operator-dependent.
Contrast enema: for mild-to-moderate cases when the diagnosis is in doubt, water-soluble contrast exam is safe and helpful; otherwise, delay the exam for 6–8 weeks.
Endoscopy: acute diverticulitis is a relative contraindication to endoscopy; must first exclude perforation. Examine only when the diagnosis is in doubt (rectal bleeding, anemia) to exclude ischemic bowel, Crohn's disease, carcinoma, and other possibilities.

Adapted from Freeman SR, McNally PR: Diverticulitis. Med Clin North Am 77:1152, 1993.

With a second attack of diverticulitis, the morbidity increases from 25–50% and mortality from 1.3–5% to 5–10%.

Initial presentations of diverticulitis complicated by abscess usually require surgery (90–95%). A recurrence of diverticulitis after surgery is seen in 2–11% of cases.

1. **List the common complications of diverticulitis.**
Fistula, abscess, obstruction, and peritonitis from perforation.

2. **Between which organs do fistulous communications develop?**
Bowel, urinary bladder, skin, pelvic floor, and vagina may be involved in fistulous disease associated with diverticulitis. The most common is *colovesicular fistula* (colon to urinary bladder), which is seen almost exclusively in men or in women after a hysterectomy. Pneumaturia is a pathognomonic sign of this fistula. Another clue is recurrent urinary tract infections, especially involving multiple organisms. *Colovaginal fistula* occurs almost exclusively in women with prior hysterectomies. The differential diagnosis includes Crohn's disease, previous pelvic irradiation, gynecologic surgery, and pelvic abscess from any cause. The diagnosis is suspected in the proper setting (recent diverticulitis) with the presence of vaginal symptoms: vaginal discharge, severe vaginitis, flatus vaginalis, and feculent discharge.

3. **What techniques are used to diagnose and localize fistulas?**
Demonstration of a colovesical fistula is often difficult. Reflux of contrast through the fistula via contrast enema or cystogram confirms the diagnosis, but such reflux is seen in a minority of patients. Cystoscopy and endoscopy are not very sensitive means of demonstrating the fistula. Identification of a colovaginal fistula can also be difficult. Barium enema, oral charcoal, vaginography, methylene blue installation into the vagina and/or colon, and combined vaginoscopy and colonoscopy are various means of attempting to localize the fistula. Treatment is surgical resection of the diseased section of bowel.

4. **How is a diverticular stricture differentiated from strictures of other causes?**
The signs favoring a diverticular stricture are the presence of diverticula in the region of the colonic stricture, the suggestion of an extraluminal mass contributing to the stricture, and intramural or extraluminal extravasation of contrast. The length of the stricture is helpful. *Malignant strictures* are usually <3 cm in length and associated with abrupt shoulders at either end. *Diverticular strictures* are longer (3–6 cm) with smoother contours. Strictures between 6–10 cm are more likely to be due to *Crohn's disease* or *ischemia*. Location of the stricture may be helpful. For example, the splenic flexure is an uncommon site for diverticulitis but a common site for ischemia.

5. **Which drugs are known to exacerbate diverticulitis?**
Corticosteroids in high doses have been associated with development of acute diverticulitis. A cause-and-effect relationship is debatable, but inhibition of epithelial cell renewal has been hypothesized. Clearly, high-dose steroids may mask the usual signs and symptoms of diverticulitis, leading to a delay in diagnosis and more serious disease.

Nonsteroidal anti-inflammatory drugs have also been associated with more severe diverticulitis. The masking of early signs and symptoms has been hypothesized as the most likely reason.

6. **What imaging modalities are available to diagnose diverticulitis? What is the role of each?**
CT is the test of choice for the diagnosis of simple and complicated diverticulitis, with a sensitivity of 90–95% and a specificity of 72% for diverticulitis. CT offers the added advantage of providing extraluminal information and helps identify patients with nondiverticular causes for their symptoms, including ischemic colitis, mesenteric thrombosis, tubo-ovarian abscess, and

pancreatitis. *Ultrasonography* of the abdomen and pelvis has a sensitivity and specificity of 84 and 80%, respectively. *Contrast enema* and *colonoscopy* are generally discouraged when diverticulitis is severe or abscess is suspected (*see* Table 49-1).

17. **How is mild diverticulitis defined and treated?**
    Mild diverticulitis should be suspected in patients with appropriately localized abdominal pain (usually in the left lower quadrant) with associated fever and/or leukocytosis. Patients with mild diverticulitis are nontoxic and able to take food and fluids orally without vomiting. Keep in mind qualifying factors (*see* Table 49-1). Treatment of mild disease is generally performed on an outpatient basis. Diet is commonly modified to include clear liquids only. After complete resolution of the acute event, the entire colon should be evaluated to determine the extent of disease and exclude other diagnostic considerations, that is, colon carcinoma. Colonoscopy is the preferred method of evaluation. However, barium enema with flexible sigmoidoscopy or virtual colonoscopy are reasonable alternatives.

18. **What antibiotic regimen is appropriate for moderately severe disease? How is treatment otherwise different?**
    Antibiotics are given usually intravenously, most often on an inpatient basis. If present, abscess drainage is required and can be performed percutaneously under CT guidance. Many antibiotic regimens are appropriate (Table 49-2). One goal for more severe disease is adequate coverage of *Pseudomonas aeruginosa*. Resistance of *Bacteroides fragilis* group microorganisms to cefoxitin or cefotetan precludes their selection as a single antibiotic choice. Aminoglycoside-based regimens have fallen out of favor because of their associated toxicity profile (ototoxicity and nephrotoxicity) and the availability of less toxic alternatives that have demonstrated equal efficacy.

19. **How is the management of severely ill patients different?**
    Severely ill patients are usually toxic with signs of peritonitis. The main difference in treatment compared with patients with less serious disease is the threshold for surgery. In toxic patients an imaging study, such as CT scan, may be helpful in directing treatment, but early surgery is most likely to result in a favorable outcome and rarely necessitates prior diagnostic studies. Mortality is high in patients with peritonitis from perforated diverticulitis, with a rate of 6% for purulent peritonitis and 35% for fecal peritonitis.

KEY POINTS: DIVERTICULITIS

1. Constant, noncolicky left lower quadrant abdominal pain, obstipation, and, occasionally, diarrhea are common symptoms of diverticulitis, whereas hematochezia is not.

2. Fistula, abscess, obstruction, and peritonitis from perforation are the common complications of diverticulitis and may be indications for surgery.

3. Bowel, urinary bladder, skin, pelvic floor, and vagina are the most common areas involved in the fistulous disease of diverticulitis, the most common being colovesical fistula (colon to urinary bladder).

4. Simple diverticulitis is treated medically in the majority of cases. Complicated diverticulitis requires usually surgical management.

20. **What are the indications and goals for surgery?**
    Surgery is indicated for complications such as sepsis, fistula formation, and obstruction. Patients with recurrent episodes of diverticulitis are candidates for surgery, as are those who fa

TABLE 49-2. A GUIDE TO ANTIMICROBIAL THERAPY IN ACUTE DIVERTICULITIS

Modifying Circumstances	Cause	First Choice	Alternative	Comments
Mild, nonperforating, with no high-risk factors	Aerobes; *Escherichia coli*; *Klebsiella* spp.; Streptococci; *Proteus* spp.; *Enterobacter* spp.; Anaerobes; *Bacteroides fragilis*; Peptostreptococci; Peptococci; *Clostridium* spp.	TMP/SMX + metronidazole *or* Ciprofloxacin + metronidazole	Cephalexin for TMP-SMX or Cipro clindamycin for metronidazole *or* amoxicillin-clavulanic acid	Outpatient, oral
Moderately ill, possible local abscess ± high-risk factors	Same, including *Pseudomonas aeruginosa*	Ampicillin-sulbactam Ticarcillin-clavulanate Imipenem-cilastatin Ertapenem	Ciprofloxacin + metronidazole 2nd gen ceph* + metronidazole	Inpatient, IV + CT (catheter drainage of abscess), consider surgery
Severely ill, toxic, peritonitis	Same, including *Pseudomonas aeruginosa*	Same	Same + 3rd or 4th gen ceph† + metronidazole	Inpatient, IV + CT, consider early surgery

Modified from Freeman SR, McNally PR: Diverticulitis. Med Clin North Am 77:1161, 1993.
TMP-SMX = trimethoprim-sulfamethoxazole.
*Cefazolin or cerfuroxime.
†Cefotaime, cettriaxone, cettizoxime, ceftazidime, cefepime.

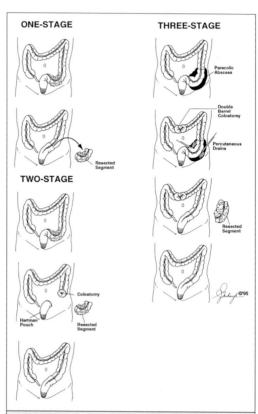

Figure 49-1. Surgical options for treating complicated diverticulitis. *One-stage surgery* includes resection of diseased bowel and reanastomosis to reestablish normal bowel continuity. *Two-stage surgery* for more complicated disease involves fecal diversion via a proximal colostomy and resection of the diseased segment. The distal segment of the colon can be oversewn (Hartman's pouch) or brought out as a mucous fistula. This is currently the most frequently performed operation for diverticulitis complicated by abscess. The first step in *three-stage surgery* involves fecal diversion and simple drainage of the involved area. Later, the involved area is resected at a second operation and a reanastomosis of the segment is performed, leaving the suture line protected by the diverting colostomy. At a third surgery, the colostomy is taken down and bowel continuity is reestablished. (From Freeman SR, McNally PR: Diverticulitis. Med Clin North Am 77:1161, 1993, with permission.)

medical therapy or deteriorate during initial treatment. Occasionally, patients with colonic stric tures that cannot convincingly be shown to be nonmalignant are candidates for resection. The goals of surgical management are to remove the septic focus with resection of the diseased colon, to treat complications including obstruction and fistula, and to restore bowel continuity The threshold for surgery is modified by the presence of high-risk factors: extremes of age, us of steroids, immunocompromised state, and right-sided diverticulitis.

1. **What operations are available in the management of diverticulitis?**

   Surgery requiring abscess drainage and fecal diversion may be done in one, two, or, in rare cases, three stages (Fig. 49-1) and is based on a classification that assesses the degree of peritoneal contamination and determines the advisability of performing a primary anastomosis.

   In the past decade, laparoscopic surgery has become applicable to an increasingly wider range of problems. This attractive technique has been used successfully for complicated diverticulitis. Several series demonstrate equal safety and effectiveness with laparoscopic surgery compared to the conventional approach of open laparotomy. The advantages of the laparoscopic approach include decreased morbidity and lower costs of hospitalization.

2. **What are the available and preferred operations for diverticulitis?**

   Single operation—ideal; thorough preoperative bowel preparation allowed; surgery is elective; diseased bowel is resected, and the remaining colon is anastomosed to maintain normal continuity. Examples of appropriate clinical scenarios include chronic obstruction, intractable pain, or recurrent episodes of medically responsive diverticulitis.

   Two-stage procedure—bowel preparation cannot be performed beforehand; usually for medically unresponsive disease. A diverting colostomy is created, and the diseased bowel segment is removed. Later (3–6 months), a second operation is performed to reestablish bowel continuity. The two-stage procedure is the procedure of choice for perforated diverticulitis.

   Three-stage procedure—outdated and rarely, if ever, indicated; has a higher mortality rate of 12–32% versus 1–12% compared to the two-stage procedure, as well as higher morbidity. The initial operation is simple drainage of the pericolonic abscess and creation of a diverting colostomy. A second operation in 2–8 weeks is performed for resection of the diseased bowel with reanastomosis to maintain bowel continuity and preservation of the colostomy to protect the anastomosis. A third surgery is performed in 2–4 weeks to take down the colostomy.

BIBLIOGRAPHY

1. Almy TP, Howell DA: Medical progress: Diverticular disease of the colon. N Engl J Med 302:324–331, 1980.
2. Chautems RC, Ambrosetti P, Ludwig A, et al: Long term follow-up after first acute episode of sigmoid diverticulitis: Is surgery mandatory?: A prospective study of 118 patients. Dis Colon Rectum 45:962–966, 2002.
3. Dwivedi A, Chahin F, Agrawal S, et al: Laparoscopic colectomy vs. open colectomy for sigmoid diverticular disease. Dis Colon Rectum 45:1309–1314, 2002.
4. Ferzoco LB, Raptopoulos V, Silen W: Acute diverticulitis (a clinical review). N Engl J Med 338:1521–1526, 1998.
5. Freeman SR, McNally PR: Diverticulitis: Med Clin North Am 77:1149–1167, 1993.
6. Greenall MJ, Levine AW, Nolan DT: Complications of diverticular disease: A review of the barium enema findings. Gastrointest Radiol 8:353–358, 1983.
7. Klein S, Mayer L, Present DH, et al: Extraintestinal manifestations in patients with diverticulitis. Ann Intern Med 108:700–702, 1988.
8. Ludeman L, Shepard NA: What is diverticular colitis? Pathology 34:568–572, 2002.
9. Mendeloff AI: Dietary fiber and gastrointestinal disease. Med Clin North Am 62:165–171, 1978.
10. Mendeloff AI: Thoughts on the epidemiology of diverticular disease. Clin Gastroenterol 15:855–877, 1986.
11. Painter NS, Burkitt DP: Diverticular disease on the colon: A deficiency disease of western civilization. Br Med J 2:450–454, 1971.
12. Reve RV, Nahrwold DL: Diverticular disease. Curr Prob Surg 26:136, 1989.
13. Schechter S, Mulvey J, Eisenstat TE: Management of uncomplicated acute diverticulitis: Results of a survey. Dis Colon Rectum 42:470–475; discussion, 475–476, 1999.
14. Smith TR, Cho KC, Morehouse HT, et al: Comparison of computed tomography and contrast enema evaluation of diverticulitis. Dis Colon Rectum 33:1–6, 1990.
15. Solomkin JS, Mazuski JE, Baron EJ, et al: Guidelines for the selection of anti-infective agents for complicated intra-abdominal infections. CID 37:997–1005, 2003.

16. Wong WD, Wexner SD, Lowry A, et al: Practice parameters for the treatment of sigmoid diverticulitis—supporting documentation. The Standards Task Force, American Society of Colon and Rectal Surgeons. Dis Colon Rectum 43:290–297, 2000.

17. Woods RJ, Lavery IC, Fazio VW, et al: Internal fistulas in diverticular disease. Dis Colon Rectum 31:591–596, 1988.

18. Young-Fadok TM, Sarr MG: Diverticular disease of the colon. In Yamada T (ed): The Textbook of Gastroenterology, 4th ed. Philadelphia, Lippincott, 2003, pp 1843–1863.

CHAPTER 50

DISEASES OF THE APPENDIX

Jonathan A. Schoen, MD, and Frank H. Chae, MD

1. **Describe the anatomy and function of the human appendix.**
   The appendix is usually 6–9 cm in length situated on the end of the cecum, where the three taenia coli converge. It is now considered an immunologic organ that participates actively in the secretion of immunoglobulins, particularly IgA.

2. **What is the etiology of appendicitis?**
   Fecaliths or hypertrophied lymphoid tissue, causing obstruction of the lumen, are the dominant etiologic factors. Fecaliths are found in about 90% of cases of gangrenous, ruptured appendicitis. The luminal obstruction causes distention of the appendix from both continued mucosal secretion and resident bacterial overgrowth. Ultimately, venous pressure is exceeded and areas of wall infarction with bacterial invasion occur.

3. **What are the signs and symptoms of appendicitis?**
   The acute appendiceal distention initially stimulates visceral afferent pain fibers, producing vague, dull, diffuse pain in the mid-abdomen (peri-umbilical) or lower epigastrium. Low-grade fever, anorexia, nausea, and vomiting may occur after the onset of pain. The inflammatory process soon involves the serosa of the appendix and, in turn, the parietal peritoneum, producing the characteristic shift in pain to the right lower quadrant.

4. **What are the laboratory findings?**
   Mild leukocytosis, ranging from 10,000–18,000/mm^3, is usually present with acute, uncomplicated appendicitis. C-reactive protein is elevated as well, with a sensitivity of 93% and specificity of 80%.

5. **Where and what is McBurney's point?**
   The point of maximal tenderness elicited in the right lower quadrant during a physical exam indicates an inflammation in the area. It is a point located two thirds distally from the umbilicus along an axis drawn from the umbilicus to the anterior superior iliac spine.

6. **What are the psoas and obturator signs?**
   Irritation of the retroperitoneal psoas muscle (pain on right hip extension) or internal obturator muscle (pain on internal rotation of the flexed right hip) by an inflamed retrocecal appendix.

7. **What is Rovsing's sign?**
   Palpation of the left lower quadrant leads commonly to right lower quadrant pain in acute appendicitis.

8. **Peak incidence of acute appendicitis occurs in what age group?**
   Ages 15–19.

9. **The risk of perforation of the appendix is highest in what age groups?**
   Children (<age 5) and elderly people (as high as 75%). Those with diabetes and immunosuppressed patients are also at risk.

10. **What is the surgery mortality rate for nonperforated appendicitis? Perforated?**
    Less than 0.1% for nonperforated and as high as 3% for perforated appendicitis. In the elderly the mortality rate of perforated appendicitis is about 15%!

11. **List the differential diagnoses for right lower quadrant pain.**
    Ectopic pregnancy, tubo-ovarian abscess, pelvic inflammatory disease, Mittelschmerz, torsion of ovary, incarcerated hernia, Crohn's disease, ulcerative colitis, diverticulitis, Meckel's diverticulitis, carcinoid tumor, infectious colitis/ileitis, cholecystitis, and peptic ulcer disease.

12. **How may acute cholecystitis and peptic ulcer disease present with right lower quadrant pain?**
    Perforation of gangrenous gallbladder or duodenal/gastric ulcer leads to collection of biliary and/or gastric fluid in the right lower quadrant (Valentino's sign).

13. **What is a Meckel's diverticulum?**
    A congenital omphalomesenteric mucosal remnant that may contain ectopic gastric mucosa. Located on the antimesenteric side of the ileum, usually 2 feet from the ileocecal valve, it is found in 2% of the population, and 2% will develop diverticulitis. The gastric mucosa, if present, may lead to ileal ulcer and cause a small intestinal bleed.

14. **In children, what two other conditions mimic acute appendicitis?**
    Gastroenteritis and mesenteric lymphadenitis. This is usually viral in etiology; however, infection with *Yersinia enterocolitica* may lead to terminal ileitis.

15. **What is an acceptable incidence rate for false-positive diagnosis of appendicitis?**
    A false-positive rate of 10–15% on appendectomy is within acceptable standards of surgical care. Lower false-positive rates may imply decreased vigilance for the diagnosis of appendicitis.

16. **In older patients (age >50), what condition may be indistinguishable from acute appendicitis?**
    Acute diverticulitis of either a redundant sigmoid colon or the cecum may present with right lower quadrant pain, fever, and leukocytosis. It is also important to rule out perforated cecal cancer in this setting.

17. **List the differentiating features of pelvic inflammatory disease (PID).**
    High fever, cervical motion tenderness, cervical discharge, and pain related to menses with tendency for bilateral onset.

18. **Define *mittelschmerz*.**
    From the German "mittel" for middle and "schmerz" for pain, it is used to describe pain accompanying the rupture of ovarian follicle at mid-menstrual cycle. Although it is a common nonsurgical ailment, appendicitis should be ruled out.

19. **How does appendicitis lead to Charcot's triad and gas in the portal vein?**
    Charcot's triad (fever/chills, right upper quadrant pain, and jaundice) and gas in the portal venous system may result from suppurative thrombosis of the portal vein resulting from appendiceal abscess. It should be seen rarely in the current setting of effective antibiotic coverage with early surgical removal of the infected appendix.

What is the most common tumor of the appendix? Describe its management.
Carcinoid. Malignant potential is related to size, and appendectomy is usually all that is required, provided that the tumor is less than 2 cm. If the tumor is greater than 2 cm, or there is extension into the mesoappendix, right hemicolectomy is required. If metastatic disease is present, the tumor should still be removed for palliation.

How is an appendiceal abscess best treated?
An established abscess, as imaged by a CT scan, may be drained via CT-guided catheter placement, provided that the patient has no evidence of diffuse peritonitis or sepsis while taking antibiotics. An appendectomy is required after about 6–8 weeks of recovery because the rate of recurrent appendicitis may approach 20%.

2. What is the most common complication after appendectomy?
Subcutaneous wound infection. For perforated appendix or abscess, the fascia is closed and the skin is usually left open for delayed closure.

3. Does ultrasound help in the diagnosis of acute appendicitis?
An ultrasound may help when an examination is equivocal, especially in pediatric and pregnant patients, when a CT scan is preferably avoided. It is also very helpful when a gynecologic etiology needs to be ruled out. A noncompressible, distended (>6 mm), tubular structure that is tender with focal compression predicts acute appendicitis. The reported sensitivity is 84–94% and specificity is 92%.

4. What other imaging modality is often used (and abused)?
CT scanning has become popular with a quoted sensitivity of 90–100% and a 95–97% specificity (in the best of hands). Although it appears to be a very accurate test, CT scanning has never been conclusively proven to reduce the negative (or normal) appendectomy rate or reduce the rate of perforated appendicitis. This means that nothing can or should replace the clinical decision-making of the examining surgeon. The examining surgeon should decide whether further imaging studies in a patient with right lower quadrant pain is necessary.

5. When is laparoscopic appendectomy appropriate?
Laparoscopy helps as a minimally invasive evaluation tool when the diagnosis is uncertain, especially in young women or morbidly obese patients. If the appendix appears normal, it should be removed via laparoscope to narrow the differential diagnosis, in the event of recurrent symptoms. Improved cosmesis, less wound infection, decreased pain, and earlier return to normal activity are the potential benefits of laparoscopy. There is some concern over an increased intra-abdominal abscess rate with laparoscopic appendectomy, although this remains unproven. It is an appropriate procedure in the hands of a skilled surgeon.

6. During an abdominal exploration for right lower quadrant pain, is removal of a normal appendix appropriate in patients with Crohn's disease?
Yes. If the base of the appendix and the surrounding area of the cecum are free of inflammation, despite active terminal ileal disease, an appendectomy should still be performed. If an enterocutaneous fistula develops postoperatively, it almost always results from the diseased ileum and not from the surgical site on the cecum.

7. Is an appendectomy during pregnancy a safe procedure?
Acute appendicitis is the most frequently encountered extrauterine disease requiring surgery during pregnancy. The appendix shifts superiorly above the right iliac crest by the fourth month of pregnancy. Abdominal tenderness is less localized because the inflamed appendix is no

longer near the parietal peritoneum. These factors along with the nausea, vomiting, and leukocytosis of pregnancy makes the clinical diagnosis of appendicitis more difficult. Fetal mortality increases from 5% in simple appendicitis to 28% if there is perforation. Therefore, early intervention is the rule. Excision of a normal or nonperforated appendix poses little risk t mother of fetus, as opposed to the significant correlation of fetal demise with perforation.

28. **Ovarian tumor is discovered during laparoscopic or open exploration. What steps should be taken?**

The normal appendix should be removed after obtaining peritoneal washings with saline irrigation in the abdominal cavity. The washing is collected to look for free tumor cells. The ovarian mass should not be touched or biopsied. A strictly followed, elaborate ritual is performed for staging ovarian cancer. Patients should be brought back at a later time for surgical staging.

29. **Does nonoperative therapy have any role in treating acute appendicitis?**

In general, treating acute appendicitis with antibiotic therapy alone is not recommended in No America. The British have been known to treat uncomplicated acute appendicitis with antibioti however, their claims of success have been offset by high recurrence rates (40%) and high costs of delivery. This mode of therapy is controversial and not universally accepted. On the other hand, delayed appendectomy is appropriate after resolution of contained abscess or inflammation by antibiotic therapy (with or without catheter drainage) in patients with a perforated appendix—provided that the abscess does not cause systemic toxicity and is well contained.

BIBLIOGRAPHY

1. Affleck DG, Handrahan DL, Egger MJ, Price RR: The laparoscopic management of appendicitis and cholelithias in pregnancy. Am J Surg 178:523–529, 1999.
2. Carr NJ: The pathology of acute appendicitis. Ann Diagn Pathol 4:46–58, 2000.
3. Khalili TM, Hiatt JR, Savar A, et al: Perforated appendicitis is not a contraindication to laparoscopy. Am Surg 65:965–967, 1999.
4. Lane JS, Sarkar R, Schmidt PJ, et al: Surgical approach to cecal diverticulitis. J Am Coll Surg 188:629–634, 1999.
5. Martin JP, Connor PD, Charles K: Meckel's diverticulum. Am Fam Physician 61:1037–1042, 2000.
6. McKellar DP, Reiling RB, Eiseman B: Prognosis and Outcomes in Surgical Disease. St. Louis, Quality Medical Publishing, 1999.
7. Meakins JL: Appendectomy and appendicitis. Can J Surg 42:90, 1999.
8. Norton LW, Stiegmann GV, Eiseman B: Surgical Decision Making. Philadelphia, W.B. Saunders, 2000.
9. Schumpelick V, Dreuw B, Ophoff K, Prescher A: Appendix and cecum: Embryology, anatomy, and surgical approach. Surg Clin North Am 80:295–318, 2000.
10. Temple LK, Litwin DE, McLeod RS: A meta-analysis of laparoscopic versus open appendectomy in patients suspected of having acute appendicitis. Can J Surg 42:377–383, 1999.

CHAPTER 51

COLITIS: PSEUDOMEMBRANOUS, MICROSCOPIC, AND RADIATION

Jill M. Watanabe, MD, MPH, and Christina M. Surawicz, MD

PSEUDOMEMBRANOUS COLITIS

1. **How common is *Clostridium difficile* disease?**

   Although 20–30% of persons who take antibiotics develop diarrhea, only 10–20% of antibiotic-associated diarrhea is caused by *C. difficile*. The frequency of *C. difficile* disease is not known, but it is estimated at 12 in 100,000 outpatients and 21 in 100 inpatients. As many as two thirds of infected, hospitalized patients are asymptomatic carriers. The clinical course of patients with *C. difficile* disease is quite variable, ranging from mild self-limited diarrhea to more severe and prolonged diarrhea that can progress to pseudomembranous colitis (PMC). During a hospital outbreak, 60% of patients with *C. difficile* disease had mild-to-moderate symptoms that resolved within 10 days, 32% had prolonged symptoms, and 8% had severe colitis. In general, the most severe complication, PMC, occurs in about 5–8% of all cases of *C. difficile* infection.

2. **What causes PMC?**

   Pseudomembranous colitis is caused by overgrowth of the anaerobic gram-positive bacteria *C. difficile*, which causes disease by production of two toxins, A and B. *C. difficile* strains that do not produce toxins are not pathogenic. In turn, these toxins cause mucosal damage and inflammation of the colon. Susceptibility to the overgrowth of *C. difficile* occurs most often after antibiotic exposure, which disrupts the normal colonic flora and allows *C. difficile* to grow. Cases of *C. difficile* can also develop sporadically as well as in association with chemotherapy. The key factor appears to be an alteration in colon flora that allows the organism to grow and produce its toxins.

3. **Which antibiotics are implicated most commonly?**

   Clindamycin, cephalosporins (especially third-generation), and broad spectrum penicillins. *C. difficile* disease can occur with any antibiotic, even single-dose preoperative antibiotics.

4. **What are the risk factors for *C. difficile* disease?**

   Hospitalization (especially surgical, ICU, and posttransplant patients), advanced age, and antibiotic exposure. Other risk factors include invasive procedures (especially gastrointestinal procedures), renal failure, cancer chemotherapy, residence in nursing home, and enteral feeding. Hospital settings remain an important reservoir for exposure, in part, because the spores of the anaerobic bacillus, *C. difficile*, can survive for many years. As many as 20–30% of hospitalized patients become colonized with *C. difficile*.

5. **Why do some people develop *C. difficile* diarrhea, whereas others are simply colonized?**

   Studies of patients with *C. difficile* colonization have shown that serum levels of IgG antibody against toxin A have been associated with protection from disease expression and prevention of recurrences. Further studies are underway to determine vaccine feasibility in susceptible patients.

6. **How is the diagnosis of *C. difficile* colitis made?**
   See Table 51-1.

TABLE 51-1. DIAGNOSIS OF *CLOSTRIDIUM DIFFICILE* COLITIS		
Diagnostic Test	**Accuracy**	**Comments**
Cytotoxin B assay	Good sensitivity and specificity	Gold standard: detects up to 10 pg toxin B, but expensive
		Results unavailable for 24–48 hr
Enzyme immunoassays to detect toxin A or B	Good specificity	EIAs are quick (hours) and less expensive
	Sensitivity varies	Test detects up to 100 to 1000 pg toxin
		1–2% of *C. difficile* strains that cause disease produce toxin B with a variant of toxin A that is undetectable
Stool cultures	Sensitive	Carriers test positive, results unavailable for 3–4 days
	Poor specificity	

KEY POINTS: IMPORTANT RISK FACTORS FOR *CLOSTRIDIUM DIFFICILE* DISEASE

1. Recent use of antibiotics—virtually all antibiotics, even in single doses—has been implicated.

2. Hospitalization, especially in the ICU setting.

3. Advanced age.

4. The ability of the host to mount an IgG response to toxin A may be protective from expression of disease and from its recurrence.

7. **What are the typical findings on colonoscopy?**
   Colonoscopy may be normal or show nonspecific colitis. With severe disease, the colon mucos
   has creamy white-yellow plaques (pseudomembranes). Histologic studies show that the
   pseudomembrane arises usually from a point of superficial ulceration, accompanied by acute
   and chronic inflammation of the lamina propria. (*See* Figs. 51-1 and 51-2.)

8. **When is treatment indicated? Which antibiotics are used?**
   The first step is to discontinue antibiotics, if possible. About 20% of cases, which are mild,
   resolve spontaneously. Treatment to eradicate *C. difficile* should be given in all but the mildest
   cases. The two most common antibiotics used to treat PMC are metronidazole and vancomycin
   (Table 51-2).

9. **What should be the first-line choice of antibiotic?**
   Metronidazole is the first choice because it is less expensive and does not promote the developmen
   of vancomycin-resistant organisms. However, vancomycin is indicated when metronidazole cannot

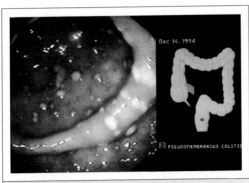

Figure 51-1. Endoscopic photograph of the white-yellow raised exudates seen in pseudomembranous colitis.

be used (i.e., first-trimester pregnancy, intolerable side effects, or when the patients fail to respond to metronidazole).

When should you expect a response to treatment?
Usually within 2–4 days, with resolution of diarrhea by 2 weeks.

When should you consult a surgeon?
When severe PMC is associated with toxic megacolon, increased abdominal pain, or development of subserosal air in the colon on abdominal flat-plate radiographs.

What should you do if symptoms recur after therapy?
Although most patients respond to therapy, about 20% have recurrent symptoms after stopping the antibiotics, probably because continued abnormal fecal flora allows C. difficile to persist and, perhaps, spores germinate. One recurrence makes further recurrences even more likely (up to 40%). Patients with recurrent C. difficile disease

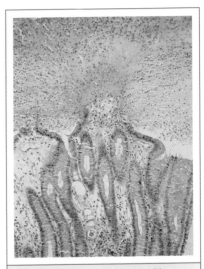

Figure 51-2. Pseudomembranous colitis. Microscopic section of colonic mucosa illustrates the pseudomembrane, composed of fibrin, polymorphonuclear cells, and debris, that emanates in a volcano-like fashion from the colon mucosa.

need retreatment, with either metronidazole or vancomycin in standard doses. Pulsed treatment with lower doses of antibiotic will decrease recurrences. Management of repeated relapses include courses of metronidazole or pulsed vancomycin and the use of probiotic agents, such as the nonpathogenic yeast, *Saccharomyces boulardii* (Table 51-3).

How can C. difficile epidemics be controlled in hospitals?
Control mechanisms include handwashing, use of disposable equipment and vinyl gloves, judicious use of antibiotics, and education/infection control programs. Active or passive immunization against C. difficile may have a role in preventing future nosocomial C. difficile infection in the most vulnerable patients.

TABLE 51-2.   TREATMENT FOR *CLOSTRIDIUM DIFFICILE* DISEASE

Drug	Dose	Comment
Metronidazole	250–500 mg orally 4 times/day for 7–10 days	First line Avoid in first-trimester pregnancy Inexpensive IV metronidazole may also be effective when oral medication cannot be given
Vancomycin	125–500 mg orally 4 times/day for 7–10 days	Expensive ($600/10-day course), recently in limited supply in the United States Use if severely ill or no response to metronidazole
Bacitracin	25,000 U orally 4 times/day for 7–10 days	Expensive Does not taste good
Fusidic acid		Not available in the United States

TABLE 51-3.   TREATMENT OF RECURRENT *CLOSTRIDIUM DIFFICILE* DISEASE

1. Retreat with antibiotic for 10–14 days.
2. Reduce antibiotic to half dose and pulse or taper pulsed therapy to once daily, once every other day, and once every third day, with lengthening intervals.
3. Add probiotic agent, if available.

MICROSCOPIC COLITIS

14. **What is microscopic colitis?**
    Microscopic colitis (MC) is a clinical syndrome characterized by chronic watery diarrhea, grossly normal-appearing colonic mucosa, and well-defined histologic features. There are two forms of MC, each named for their characteristic histologic findings: collagenous colitis (CC) and lymphocytic colitis (LC). Microscopic colitis may account for 10% of patients examined for chronic diarrhea in referral centers.

15. **Describe the clinical features of microscopic colitis.**
    The clinical manifestations of MC include at least a 1-month history of watery, nonbloody diarrhea. Patients have an average of six bowel movements a day, but as many as 20 is not uncommon. The clinical course can be chronic and continuous or intermittent and recurrent. The diarrhea can be associated with abdominal cramping, loss of appetite, and mild weight loss. Nocturnal stools are typical in this disease entity and help distinguish MC from irritable bowel syndrome.

16. **What are the histologic features of microscopic colitis?**
    Patients with microscopic colitis have normal radiographic studies and a grossly normal colonoscopy, though mild nonspecific findings of erythema, edema, or superficial tears have been noted. The histologic criteria of MC are:

- Increased chronic inflammatory infiltrate in the lamina propria
- Increased number of intraepithelial lymphocytes (>15–20 lymphocytes per 1000 epithelial cells)
- Damage of the surface epithelium, with flattening of epithelial cells.

The additional presence of a subepithelial collagenous band (>10 microns) is a specific feature of CC and distinguishes CC from cases of LC.

How common is microscopic colitis?
The occurrence rates of CC and LC are similar. The incidence for MC is 1–3 cases/100,000, and the prevalence is about 10–16 cases/100,000. There are reports that LC is as much as three times more common than CC, but both are less common than inflammatory bowel disease.

How are collagenous colitis and lymphocytic colitis different?
Differences include the female preponderance of CC (as high as 3–9:1) that is not seen as prominently in LC. Lymphocytic colitis is thought to be more limited in its course. The onset of both conditions occurs at approximately the same age (50–60), and both have been reported rarely in children. Clinically, these conditions cannot be distinguished, and the treatment approach is the same for both.

Which parts of the colon are affected most commonly?
CC can be patchy, and multiple studies report a decrease in the density of the intraepithelial lymphocytes from the right to the left colon; sparing of the rectum is also not uncommon. In one study the highest diagnostic yield was from biopsies from the transverse colon (83%) and the right colon (70%); the lowest diagnostic yield was found in the rectosigmoid colon (66%). Nonetheless, most cases can be diagnosed by biopsies taken within the range of flexible sigmoidoscopy; left-sided biopsies are thought to miss less than 5% of the cases. Colonoscopy with biopsy of the right colon may be necessary when left-sided biopsies are negative, and there is a high clinical suspicion for MC. Histologic changes consistent with CC and LC are typically limited to the colon but have also been seen in the terminal ileum and stomach.

What is the role of nonsteroidal anti-inflammatory agents and other medications in the pathogenesis of microscopic colitis?
Nonsteroidal anti-inflammatory drugs (NSAIDs) have been long associated with the potential to cause diarrhea syndromes. Collagenous colitis has been associated with the use of NSAIDs, and resolution of symptoms has been reported when NSAIDs were stopped. In addition to NSAIDs, ranitidine, lansoprazole, ticlopidine, and simvastatin have been associated with the development of MC.

What are the associated conditions?
A wide variety of associated conditions is found in case reports, including rheumatologic conditions (e.g., rheumatoid arthritis, polyarthritis), thyroid disease, diabetes mellitus, systemic lupus erythematosus, sicca syndrome, atrophic gastritis, and primary biliary cirrhosis.

What are the treatment options?
There are limited data to guide the treatment of CC and LC. The natural history of MC may be chronic and relapsing, but spontaneous resolution can also occur. MC is thought to be a benign condition without premalignant potential, and surveillance colonoscopies are not necessary. Small, double-blinded placebo-controlled trials have demonstrated the efficacy of bismuth subsalicylate and budesonide. The goals of therapy are directed at symptom management while minimizing the side effects of the interventions. This can often be accomplished by discontinuing the NSAIDs along with any other agents that might worsen the diarrhea (e.g., dairy and caffeine). Some patients do well on antidiarrheals or cholestyramine alone. Retrospective studies have demonstrated the efficacy of sulfasalazine, mesalamine, and 5-ASA. Steroids can also be effective, but their use is often limited by recurrent symptoms once the

steroids are discontinued. These steroid-dependent patients may require stronger immunosuppressants, such as methotrexate or azathioprine.

RADIATION COLITIS

23. **What is radiation colitis?**
Radiation injury to the colon occurs following treatment of rectal, cervical, uterine, prostate, urinary bladder, and testicular cancer. The peristaltic movement of intestine in and out of the field of radiation decreases the degree of injury to the small bowel. The colon, especially the rectosigmoid, is highly susceptible to radiation injury because it is immobile. In general, implant radiation therapy causes less severe damage than external beam radiation because the field of radiation is smaller. Tumors in the pelvic area often require high dosages of radiation and result in greater risk of radiation injury to the colon. Coadministration of chemotherapeutic agents enhances the damaging effects of radiation.

24. **What can be done to prevent radiation damage?**
Radiation damage can be prevented, in part, by limiting the dosage and area of exposure and shielding adjacent tissues. Amifostine, misoprostol, and sulfasalazine have shown some protective benefit in small clinical trials.

25. **What symptoms are associated with irradiation?**
Total-body irradiation can induce nausea and vomiting. Diarrhea develops typically 5 days later. Loss of mucosal defenses increases the patient's chance of developing sepsis. Acute radiation injury to the colon occurs typically within 6 weeks and is manifested by diarrhea and tenesmus. Chronic symptoms of radiation colitis and proctitis can occur late within the first year following radiation therapy but have also been seen decades following the initial radiation exposure. The primary symptoms associated with chronic injury to the colon and rectum include: diarrhea, rectal pain, and rectal bleeding.

KEY POINTS: MICROSCOPIC COLITIS

1. Biopsy is warranted in patients with chronic diarrhea, even when the colonic mucosa appears normal.

2. Histologically, two variations of microscopic colitis (MC) have been identified: collagenous colitis (CC) and lymphocytic colitis (LC). Debate continues as to whether CC and LC represent a clinical spectrum of the same disease or distinct clinical entities.

3. NSAIDs and/or other medicines may play a causal role in the development of MC.

4. Despite the histologic and epidemiologic differences between CC and LC, the treatment approach is currently the same.

5. There are only a few randomized, controlled clinical trials to guide therapy of MC.

26. **What are the effects of localized radiation to the colon?**
Colonoscopy may be normal or may show telangiectasias or friable mucosa. Early or acute changes include microscopic damage to mucosal and vascular epithelial cells. One typical histologic feature is the presence of atypical fibroblasts. Late changes commonly involve fibrosis with obliterative endarteritis resulting in chronic ischemia, stricture formation, and bleeding.

7. How can radiation colitis and proctitis be managed?
There are limited data on the appropriate treatment for radiation colitis and proctitis. Treatment should be directed by the severity of symptoms. Various medications have been tried, including oral and topical sucralfate, oral and topical steroids, 5-ASA compounds, sulfasalazine, hyperbaric oxygen, pentosan polysulfate, and antibiotics.

8. What are the endoscopic therapies for chronic bleeding?
Argon laser photocoagulation, heater probe, and bipolar cautery have been used to treat localized bleeding from telangiectasias. Multiple treatment sessions are often needed. Patients should be transfused with blood, as needed, and take oral iron.

9. How are chronic radiation-induced bowel strictures managed?
Endoscopic dilation may be helpful, but surgery is occasionally needed.

KEY POINTS: RADIATION COLITIS

1. Acutely, diarrhea can be induced by radiation therapy to the abdomen and pelvis approximately 5 days after radiation therapy begins because the cell turnover rate in the GI tract is 5 days.

2. The typical manifestations of acute radiation colitis include diarrhea and tenesmus.

3. Rectal bleeding is seen more often with chronic radiation colitis and proctitis rather than in the acute setting.

4. Treatment and interventions should be guided by the severity of symptoms.

BIBLIOGRAPHY

. Aboudola S, Kotloff KL, Kyne L, et al: *Clostridium difficile* vaccine and serum immunoglobulin G antibody response to toxin A. Infect Immun 71:1608–1610, 2003.

. Alfa JM, Kabani A, Lyerly D, et al: Characterization of a toxin A-negative, toxin B-positive strain of *Clostridium difficile* responsible for a nosocomial outbreak of *Clostridium difficile*-associated diarrhea. J Clin Microbiol 38:2706–2714, 2000.

3. Babb, RR: Radiation proctitis: A review. Am J Gastroenterol 91:1309–1311, 1996.

4. Bartlett JG: Antibiotic-associated diarrhea. N Engl J Med 346:334–339, 2003.

5. Brar HS, Surawicz CM: Pseudomembranous colitis: An update. Can J Gastroenterol 14:51–56, 2000.

6. Cleary RK: *Clostridium difficile*-associated diarrhea and colitis: Clinical manifestations, diagnosis, and treatment. Dis Colon Rectum 41:1435–1449, 1998.

7. Fernandez-Banares F, Salas A, Eteve M, et al: Collagenous and lymphocytic colitis: Evaluation of clinical and histological features, response to treatment and long-term follow-up. Am J Gastroenterol 98:340–347, 2003.

8. Goff JS, Barnett JL, Pelke T, Appleman HD: Collagenous colitis: Histopathology and clinical course. Am J Gastroenterol 92:57–60, 1997.

9. Jackson BK: Collagenous and lymphocytic colitis: Diagnosis and treatment. Clin Perspect Gastroenterol May/June:173–180, 1999.

10. Kochhar R, Sriram PV, Sharma SC, et al: Natural history of late radiation proctosigmoiditis treated with topical sucralfate suspension. Dig Dis Sci 44:973–978, 1999.

11. Kyne L, Warny M, Qamar A, Kelly C: Asymptomatic carriage of *Clostridium difficile* and serum levels of IgG antibody against toxin A. N Engl J Med 342:390–397, 2000.

12. Kyne L, Warny M, Qamar A, Kelly CP: Association between antibody response to toxin A and protection against recurrent *Clostridium difficile* diarrhoea. Lancet 357:189–193, 2001.

13. Miehlke S, Heymer P, Bethke B, et al: Budesonide treatment for collagenous colitis: A randomized, double-blind, placebo-controlled, multicenter trial. Gastroenterology 123(4):978–984, 2002.

14. Nair S, Yadav D, Corpuz M, Pitchumoni CS: *Clostridium difficile* colitis: Factors influencing treatment failure and relapse—a prospective evaluation. Am J Gastroenterol 93:1873–1876, 1998.

15. Pardi DS: Microscopic colitis. Mayo Clin Proc 78:614–617, 2003.

16. Pardi DS, Ramnath VR, Loftus EV Jr, et al: Lymphocytic colitis: Clinical features, treatment, and outcomes. Am J Gastroenterol 97(11):2829–2833, 2002.

17. Shiraishi M, Hiroyasu S, Ishimine T, et al: Radiation enterocolitis: Overview of the past 15 years. World J Surg 22:491–493, 1998.

18. Surawicz CM, McFarland LV: Pseudomembranous colitis: Causes and cures. Digestion 60:91–100, 1999.

19. Surawicz CM, McFarland LV: Recurrent *Clostridium difficile* disease. Clin Perspect Gastroenterol March/April:24–26, 1999.

20. Tagkalidis P, Bhathal P, Gibson P: Microscopic colitis. J Gastroenterol Hepatol 17:236–248, 2002.

CHAPTER 52

UPPER GASTROINTESTINAL TRACT HEMORRHAGE

John S. Goff, MD

. **What are the signs and symptoms of upper gastrointestinal (UGI) bleeding?**
Hematemesis can vary from material that looks like coffee grounds (blood darkened from acid exposure) to massive amounts of bright red blood. Melena (black, tarry) stool is usually found in patients with an upper source but may be seen in patients with a right colon bleed and slow transit. Brisker UGI bleeding will result in maroon to bloody red stool.

. **What historic facts will help with determining the source of UGI bleeding?**
Use of aspirin, other nonsteroidal anti-inflammatory drugs (NSAIDs), alcohol, or cigarettes are risk factors for gastric and duodenal lesions. Physical stress (i.e., trauma, CNS injury, burns, etc.) is seen commonly in patients with UGI bleeding sources. A history of heartburn and abdominal pain prior to onset of the bleeding strongly suggests a peptic source. A history of liver disease or suspected liver disease because of heavy alcohol use should alert one to the possibility of bleeding from varices or portal hypertensive gastropathy. Vomiting prior to bleeding suggests a Mallory-Weiss tear as the possible cause. Inquiring about previous bleeding episodes is often useful.

. **How can the amount of acute blood lost be estimated clinically?**
The acute loss of 500 mL of blood will not result in detectable physiologic changes; however, loss of 1000 mL will produce orthostatic changes of 10–20 mmHg in systolic blood pressure and a pulse rise of 20 beats/min or more. Loss of >2000 mL of blood will produce shock.

. **How might one distinguish a UGI bleed from a lower GI bleed in a patient who presents with blood per rectum?**
The most obvious factor that points to a UGI source is finding a positive gastric aspirate for blood. Melena suggests UGI bleeding, but it can also be seen in some patients with bleeding from the right colon. Red blood per rectum is not likely to be from an upper source if there is no associated syncope or orthostatic blood pressure changes. The presence of risk factors for UGI bleeding may be of some help (alcohol use, smoking, NSAID use, prior UGI bleed, UGI symptoms).

. **What are the first steps in managing a patient with UGI bleeding?**
The first step in management is to establish intravenous access with at least one 18-G or larger catheter. Volume replacement should be initiated (*see* question 8) and vasopressors are to be used if the patient is hypotensive and does not respond promptly to fluid resuscitation. Complete blood count (CBC), prothrombin time, and partial thromboplastin time are run on blood obtained at the time of achieving intravenous access. A nasogastric (NG) tube, preferably of moderate to larger size, is placed next followed by consultation with the Gastroenterology and Surgery services.

6. **How does one interpret the hematocrit values in a patient with acute UGI bleeding?**

The hematocrit (Hct) will fall over time as there is replacement of lost volume from extravascu- fluid. In about 2 hours, approximately 25% of the final fall will be achieved and approximately 50% will be seen in 8 hours. The final Hct value will be seen at 72 hours after the initial acute loss of blood. Obviously, this timetable will be accelerated if the patient is given intravenous fluid.

7. **Why place an NG tube?**

The major reasons for placing an NG tube are to determine source of bleeding and whether the patient is still bleeding. The finding of red blood from the NG tube is associated with increased mortality rates, increased number of complications, and higher blood transfusion requirement A secondary benefit is the clearing of blood from the stomach to aid in performing an urgent upper endoscopy (EGD). There should be no worry about causing increased bleeding in patient with known liver disease when passing an NG tube.

8. **What types of fluid should be used for resuscitation and when?**

The fluid of choice for initial resuscitation is crystalloid (normal saline or Ringer's lactate). Packed red blood cells are the blood product of choice. Type-specific or universal donor blood can be given if the patient needs urgent replacement due to massive and ongoing losses. In elderly patients, the Hct should be kept in the 30 range to help avoid cardiac complications. Fresh frozen plasma (FFP) is to be considered if the patient is still bleeding and the internationa normalized ratio [INR] is >1.5. Platelets are to be used if the count is <50,000 and there is ongoing bleeding.

9. **Does every UGI bleeding patient need to be hospitalized in the intensive care unit or even hospitalized?**

Patients are best treated by triaging them according to their risk factors for further bleeding. This can mean that some can go home the same day as they present, and others will need to g to the intensive care unit. The Rockall Score (Lancet, 1996) has been successfully used to achieve such triage. Risk factors for increased mortality associated with an acute UGI bleed are age >65, comorbid illness, shock, and continued bleeding in the hospital. Patients with none of these risk factors and a clean-based, nonbleeding ulcer, mild gastritis, or low-grade esophagiti can be considered for discharge to home from the emergency room or the GI lab.

10. **What are the common causes, and uncommon causes, of UGI bleeding?**

Duodenal ulcers are the most common cause of acute UGI bleeding (30%) followed by gastric erosions (27%), gastric ulcers (22%), esophagitis (11%), duodenitis (10%), varices (5%), and Mallory-Weiss tears (5%). More unusual causes include (in no particular order): Dieulafoy's ulcers, GAVE (gastric antral vascular ectasia), cancer, portal hypertensive gastropathy, angiodysplasia, aortoenteric fistula, and hemobilia.

11. **What is the role of NSAIDs in UGI bleeding?**

There is an overall 2.74 increase in the relative risk for any GI complication associated with the use of NSAIDs. If the patient is >age 50, the risk increase is 5.57. If the patient has a history of prior GI bleed, the relative risk increase is 4.76, which is similar to the increase related to concomitant corticosteroid use. The increased relative risk is 12.7 for patients using NSAIDs and anticoagulants. There is a sixfold increased risk of GI bleeding in patients taking NSAIDs a who also have *Helicobacter pylori*.

12. **How can one prevent bleeding in patients taking NSAIDs?**

Misoprostol given along with the NSAIDs will prevent bleeding complication, whereas H_2RA drugs will not. Proton pump inhibitors have been shown to decrease the ulcer/bleed risk by fourfold. The new COX-2 selective prostaglandin inhibitors are associated with significantly fewer ulcers than the traditional NSAIDs.

3. What are the possible sources of bleeding in a patient with cirrhosis who presents with UGI bleeding?

One must remember that having cirrhosis means there is only a 50% chance that the patient is bleeding from varices. The most common nonvariceal source of bleeding in such patients is gastric erosions (approximately 50%), followed by Mallory-Weiss tears (15%), duodenal and gastric ulcers (13.8% each), and esophagitis (11%). Portal hypertensive gastropathy (PHG) is also a nonvariceal source of bleeding in cirrhotic patients but is related to portal pressure, unlike the other cited sources.

4. How does one diagnose bleeding to be from a varix?

The easiest way to confirm that varices are the source of bleeding is to see active bleeding coming from a varix. The next best criterion is seeing a fibrin/platelet plug on a varix. The weakest criterion is finding no other identifiable source in the setting of a moderate-to-large volume bleed. Endoscopic ultrasound (EUS) may be helpful in differentiating large gastric folds from gastric varices.

5. Which patients need endoscopy and when?

Ideally, all patients with UGI bleeding need an upper endoscopy (EGD), but this is only beneficial if the results of the EGD will impact on patient management. Management changes include endoscopic therapy and triage that would result in shorter or no hospital stay. Patients over age 60, patients with liver disease, those with active bleeding, and those who rebleed are in clinical situations that have been shown to benefit from EGD because they often lead to therapeutic interventions that positively impact on the patient's outcome.

6. What techniques are available to the endoscopist for controlling active bleeding?

Modalities available include monopolar probes, bipolar probes, heater probes, the argon plasma coagulator, and Nd-YAG lasers. They are all effective in controlling bleeding and preventing rebleeding, except the monopolar technique. Frequently, epinephrine (1:10,000) is used before cautery to slow or to stop the bleeding, which allows for more directed cautery treatment. Epinephrine alone is not as effective. Sclerosants (alcohol, ethanolamine, and others) injected into the bleeding site have been used alone with some success. A newer technique is to use endoscopically placed clips to clamp off small bleeding vessels.

7. What nonendoscopic therapies can be used to stop variceal bleeding?

The addition of intravenous infusions of octreotide will lower portal pressure and can thus prevent rebleeding during the initial hospitalization. Vasopressin can be used to decrease portal pressure, but significant side effects are common. The Sengstaken-Blakemore tube, preferably with the Minnesota modification (a suction port above the esophageal balloon), is still a reasonable method for gaining control of a patient with massive bleeding from varices. If medical or endoscopic therapy is ineffective, shunt surgery and a transjugular intrahepatic portosystemic shunt (TIPS) procedure will need to be considered.

8. What endoscopic therapy is available to control variceal hemorrhage?

Endoscopic sclerotherapy (ES) and endoscopic variceal ligation (EVL) are the main methods for controlling variceal bleeding via an endoscope. Both are reported to control active bleeding in up to 90% of cases. Rebleeding is less with EVL than ES (26% vs. 44%). Patient mortality is reduced with use of endoscopic methods for treating varices. Mortality is less with EVL than ES (24% vs. 31%). There are fewer complications with EVL (11% vs. 25%), and it takes fewer sessions to obliterate a patient's varices with EVL (3.7 vs. 4.9 sessions).

19. **What are the special considerations that need to be addressed in patients with cirrhosis who have acute UGI bleeding?**

There is a higher likelihood of the patient having a serious coagulopathy that will need to be corrected. The patient is more prone to mental confusion from encephalopathy or alcohol withdrawal, which increases the risk of aspiration with its associated increase in mortality. Encephalopathy-related complications can be prevented by early endotracheal intubation and aggressive use of lactulose. Prophylactic antibiotics will prevent complications and reduce mortality. Norfloxacin and ciprofloxacin alone or in combination with Augmentin (amoxicillin and clavulanate) have been used successfully.

20. **What is a visible vessel? What is its significance?**

A visible vessel is the exposed side of a small vessel at the base of an ulcer. It may contain a fibrin/platelet plug or have an adherent clot over it. The finding is significant because of the increased risk for rebleeding. Those with an associated adherent clot have a rebleed rate of 20–30%, whereas true visible vessels have rebleeding rates of approximately 50%. If the vessel is seen to be spurting at the time of endoscopy, there is a 90% chance it will rebleed. If the ulcer has only a red dot in its base, the rebleeding rate is around 10%. The rebleeding rate for an ulcer with a clean base is <5%. Endoscopic intervention will lower these rebleeding rates.

21. **Is there a role for other diagnostic tests when evaluating UGI bleeding patients?**

Radiolabeled red blood cell scans are not usually helpful for defining a UGI bleeding source, unless it is beyond the reach of an endoscope. Barium studies have no place in the diagnosis of acute UGI bleeding. Angiography can be used to define an active bleeding site (the site needs to be bleeding at a rate of at least 0.5 mL/min) and to possibly treat it with either a selective vasopressin infusion or embolization of the feeding blood vessel. Patients with ulcerative lesions in the stomach or duodenum need to be tested for *H. pylori*.

22. **Which medications, if any, can be used to reduce rebleeding from UGI tract ulcers?**

The use of intravenous H_2-receptor antagonists for prevention of rebleeding has only marginal, if any, benefit. Intravenous omeprazole has been shown to reduce rebleeding in several studies but is not available in the United States. Intravenous pantoprazole 80 mg IV bolus, then 8 mg/hr continuous infusion for 72 hr, can be substituted for omeprazole. There is some evidence that intravenous octreotide can reduce the rebleeding rate of nonportal hypertensive sources of UGI tract bleeding. Factor replacement therapy may be needed for patients with specific clotting deficiencies. Fresh frozen plasma, recombinant factor VIIa (Novo-Seven), and desmopressin (DDAVP) can be useful in various situations.

23. **When and who should be treated with surgery for continued nonvariceal UGI bleeding?**

Patients more than 60 years old and patients with significant comorbid illness need to be considered for surgery earlier due to the increased likelihood of a poor outcome with prolonged bleeding and multiple transfusions. Patients who have failed at least one (and certainly after two) attempt(s) at endoscopic therapy need to go to surgery for rebleeding. Giant ulcers (>2 cm) are unlikely to be manageable with endoscopic methods, as are ulcers with bleeding from major arteries.

24. **What medications are used for patients who go home after a bleeding episode?**

The main treatment after bleeding is acid suppression. Thus, patients need H_2-receptor antagonists or proton pump inhibitors. The latter are generally better at healing because of greater acid suppression. Antibiotics are added if the patient was found to be positive for *H. pylori*. Iron supplementation orally is indicated for replacement if the patient had a major bleed. Beta blockers possibly in conjunction with long-acting nitrates, should be considered for maintenance therapy in patients with bleeding due to portal hypertension. The selective COX-2 inhibitors should be substituted for standard NSAIDs in patients who need therapy for arthritic conditions.

5. When and what should patients receive by mouth after a UGI bleed?
Traditionally, patients are started on clear liquids once they have had an endoscopic evaluation or after several hours of observation, during which there seems to be no more signs and symptoms of further bleeding. Solid food is reintroduced in 24–48 hours. If there is a substantial risk of rebleeding, it would be best that there was no solid food in the stomach to deal with at the time of endoscopic or surgical intervention.

6. When should patients be sent home after a UGI bleed?
There is little need for prolonged hospital observation after a mild-to-moderate UGI bleed. Elderly patients who have required blood transfusions need to be observed for 1 or 2 days after their last sign of bleeding or transfusion.

7. What should patients avoid once they have had a UGI bleed?
Patients need to be instructed to avoid all alcohol, tobacco, aspirin, and NSAIDs.

8. How and when should patients be followed after their episode of UGI bleeding?
An office visit is scheduled in 2–4 weeks to reinforce use of treatment medications and to make long-term plans. Patients need to be seen promptly if there are any signs of bleeding or return of their peptic symptoms. Endoscopy is repeated in only patients with major GI bleeding and no antecedent symptoms of peptic disease to confirm healing at 1–2 months after their bleed. Gastric ulcers need to be followed to complete endoscopic healing to be sure there is no cancer present. Patients with varices are seen for repeat ES or EVL within 7–10 days of their first treatment and then every 2 weeks until the varices are eradicated.

BLIOGRAPHY

1. Bjorkman DJ, Kimmey MD: Non-steroidal anti-inflammatory drugs and gastrointestinal disease: Pathophysiology, treatment and prevention. Dig Dis 13:19–29, 1995.
2. Corley DA, Stefan AM, Wolf M, et al: Early indicators of prognosis in upper gastrointestinal hemorrhage. Am J Gastroenterol 93:336, 1998.
3. D'Amico G, Pagliaro L, Bosch J: Pharmacological treatment of portal hypertension: An evidence-based approach. Semin Liver Dis 39:475–505, 1999.
4. Huang JQ, Sridhan S, Hunt RH: Role of *H. pylori* infection and non-steroidal anti-inflammatory drugs in peptic ulcer disease: A meta-analysis. Lancet 359:14–22, 2002.
5. Katshinski B, Logan R, Davis J, et al: Prognostic factors in upper GI bleeding. Dig Dis Sci 39:706–712, 1994.
6. Khuroo MS, Yattoo GN, Javid G, et al: A comparison of omeprazole and placebo for bleeding peptic ulcers. N Engl J Med 336:1054–1058, 1997.
7. Lau JY, Sung JJ, Lam YH, et al: Endoscopic retreatment compared with surgery in patients with recurrent bleeding after initial endoscopic control of bleeding ulcers. N Engl J Med 340:751–756, 1999.
8. Lee JG, Turnipseed S, Romano PS, et al: Endoscopy-based triage significantly reduces hospitalization rates and costs of treating upper gastrointestinal bleeding. A randomized controlled trial. Gastrointest Endosc 50:755–761, 1999.
9. Levine JE, Leontiadis GI, Sharma VK, Howden CW: Meta-analysis: The efficacy of intravenous H_2-receptor antagonists in bleeding peptic ulcer disease. Aliment Pharmacol Ther 16:1137–1142, 2002.
10. Lin HJ, Lo WC, Lee FY, et al: A prospective randomized comparative trial showing that omeprazole prevents rebleeding in patients with bleeding peptic ulcer after successful endoscopic therapy. Arch Int Med 158:54–59, 1998.

11. Nevens F, Bustami K, Scheys I, et al: Variceal pressure is a factor predicting the risk of first variceal bleeding. A prospective cohort study in cirrhotic patients. Hepatology 27:15–19, 1998.

12. Rockall TA, Logan RF, Devlin HB, et al: Selection of patients for early discharge or outpatient care after acute upper gastrointestinal haemorrhage. National audit of acute upper gastrointestinal haemorrhage. Lancet 347:1138–1140, 1996.

13. Stiegmann GV, Goff JS, Michalitz-Onody PA, et al: Endoscopic sclerotherapy as compared with endoscopic variceal ligation for bleeding esophageal varices. N Engl J Med 326:1527–1532, 1992.

LOWER GASTROINTESTINAL TRACT BLEEDING

Peter R. McNally, DO

CHAPTER 53

1. **Define lower gastrointestinal (LGI) bleeding.**
   Bleeding distal to the ligament of Treitz.

2. **How common is LGI bleeding?**
   The annual incidence of LGI bleeding is estimated to be 20–27 cases/100,000 adult population.

3. **Is LGI bleeding seen more commonly in men?**
   Yes. LGI tract bleeding is more common in men. The incidence increases with age with a 200-fold increased incidence between the third to ninth decades of life.

4. **What is the overall mortality rate of LGI bleeding?**
   3.6%, which is similar to the mortality rate for UGI hemorrhage.

5. **What is the likelihood that LGI bleeding will stop spontaneously?**
   About 80%.

6. **How is history important in assessing a patient with lower GI bleeding?**
   - *Onset:* Did symptoms start months ago with associated diarrhea or that day with a difficult to pass, hard, and constipated bowel movement?
   - *Volume and consistency of bleeding:* Clots of blood on formed stool suggest an anorectal source. Squirts of blood with defecation suggest internal hemorrhoids as the source bleeding, whereas repeated rectal bleeding of large volumes over a short time suggest arterial bleeding, as can be seen with a diverticular or angiodysplastic cause.
   - *Symptoms:* Associated abdominal pain is uncommon with diverticular and vascular ectasia LGI bleeding and may suggest UGI bleeding from ulcer or intestinal ischemia. Acute or chronic diarrhea may suggest Crohn's disease, infectious, or ulcerative colitis. Chronic abdominal pain with large meals may be a sign of intestinal ischemia.
   - *Medical history:* Prior history of ulcer disease, cirrhosis, use/prescription of aspirin, nonsteroidal anti-inflammatory drugs (NSAIDs), or blood thinners. History of aortic aneurysm may suggest aortoenteric fistula. Recent colonoscopy may indicate post-polypectomy bleeding. Prior radiation therapy for cervical or prostate carcinoma suggests angiodysplasia.

7. **What are the first steps taken in the management of a patient with significant LGI bleeding?**
   1. Stabilize and resuscitate.
   2. Place at least one large-bore IV line (lactated Ringer's or normal saline).
   3. Evaluate hemodynamic status: blood pressure, pulse, orthostatic vital signs, if stable.
   4. Give supplemental oxygen by nasal cannula.
   5. Order lab tests: complete blood count (CBC), electrolytes, international normalized ratio (INR), and type and screen for packed RBCs.
   6. Get electrocardiogram for those with known arteriosclerotic heart disease (ASHD) or older than age 50.

7. Perform physical examination:
   - Ear, nose and throat (ENT) examination for telangiectasias or pigmented macules may indicate Osler-Weber-Rendu disease, Peutz-Jeghers syndrome, or vascular ectasia in the gut.
   - Cardiac auscultation for aortic stenosis, perhaps associated with vascular ectasia of the GI tract.
   - Abdominal examination should assess for bowel sounds, abdominal bruit, tenderness, masses, and surgical scars. Hepatosplenomegaly, ascites, and/or caput medusae may indicate chronic liver disease with portal hypertension, suggesting an esophageal, gastric, or colonic variceal bleed.
   - Cutaneous purpura or petechiae suggest a coagulopathy, and spider angiomata or jaundice may be another indicator of chronic liver disease.
   - Joint hypermobility, swelling, or deformity may indicate a connective tissue disorder and possible use of aspirin or NSAIDs.
   - Digital rectal exam is *mandatory* for all patients with LGI bleeding to evaluate for prolapsed internal hemorrhoids or masses and to characterize color and consistency of blood/stool in the rectal vault.

8. **How often are experienced clinicians wrong in their estimation of source of LGI bleeding?**
   Several studies have shown that significant rectal bleeding suspected to be of an LGI source was from a UGI etiology. Placement of a nasogastric tube can confirm upper GI source of bleeding, but an aspirate negative for blood does not entirely exclude the possibility of a UGI source. Unless bile is confirmed on the nasogastric (NG) aspirate, one cannot exclude the possibility of bleeding beyond the level of the pylorus.

9. **How can one determine whether rectal bleeding is caused by a UGI versus an LGI source?**
   Suggestion of UGI source
   - History: ulcer disease, chronic liver disease, use of ASA or NSAIDs
   - Symptoms: nausea, vomiting, or hematemesis
   - NG aspirate: identification of blood or "coffee ground" material

   Suggestion of LGI source
   - Absence of UGI symptoms or risk factors
   - NG aspirate positive for bile but negative for blood

10. **Name three methods for localization of LGI bleeding.**
    - Technetium (Tc) 99m-pertechnetate-labeled RBC scan
    - Mesenteric arteriogram
    - Urgent colonoscopy
    Of importance is that recent studies have questioned the accuracy of RBC scanning to localize LGI bleeding. One study showed that 42% of patients who underwent surgery, based on only positive RBC scan, had recurrent bleeding. Some have relegated the RBC scan to identify active GI bleeding and candidate for emergent arteriography.

11. **What are the bleeding rates needed for localization of LGI source?**
    Tc 99m-pertechnetate-labeled RBC scan: 0.1–0.5 mL/min
    Mesenteric arteriogram: 0.5–1.0 mL/min

12. **What are some of the advantages of mesenteric arteriogram for the evaluation of LGI bleeding?**
    When bleeding is active, arteriogram may localize the source, and treatment can be instituted with selective arterial embolization with polyvinyl alcohol particles or microcoils. Selective

intra-arterial infusion of vasopressin is effective in 70–90%, but rebleeding is frequent and precipitation of angina and cardiovascular complications in the elderly can be devastating.

3. What is the role of urgent colonoscopy in the evaluation of LGI bleeding?
Jensen and others have shown that administration of a "rapid bowel prep" followed by urgent colonoscopy (12–24 hr) can identify the source of LGI bleeding in 74–90% of patients.

4. List the most common causes of LGI bleeding.

Etiology	Percentage
Diverticulosis	30
Colitis	15
Cancer/polyp	13
Angiodysplasia	10
Anorectal	11
Other	6
No site	8
UGI source	8

5. What is the role of urgent colonoscopy in the treatment of LGI bleeding?
Active bleeding from diverticulosis and angiodysplasia can be successfully treated with injection of dilute epinephrine (1:10,000) and or thermal techniques. Nonbleeding, visible vessels may be treated with monopolar cautery probes at 10–15 watts, 1 second, and moderate coaptive pressure. This is considerably less aggressive than hemostatic techniques used to treat bleeding ulcers in the UGI tract.

6. Are bleeding colonic diverticula inflamed or infected?
No. Clinical evidence of diverticulitis or inflammation is not present with bleeding diverticula, and the vessel rupture is believed to be the result of pressure erosion. LGI bleeding from diverticulosis is painless, usually of a maroon to bright red in color and large in volume.

7. What is the natural history of LGI bleeding from diverticulosis?
- About 80% of patients stop bleeding spontaneously.
- 70% will not rebleed and not require further treatment.
- 30% will rebleed and require treatment.

8. What types of colitis are associated with LGI bleeding?
Ischemia, Crohn's disease, and ulcerative colitis. LGI bleeding caused by segmental colitis usually indicates an ischemia etiology.

9. Do all colonic vascular ectasias or angiodysplasia cause LGI bleeding?
No. Angiodysplasia are found commonly in the colon during cancer screening examinations. They are more common among the elderly. Most (75%) of the bleeding vascular ectasias are found in the right colon. Endoscopic treatment of bleeding ectasias with injection, laser, or thermal techniques have been shown to be effective. One should be cautious with any endoscopic treatment of these lesions, especially in the thin-walled right colon.

10. How is postpolypectomy LGI bleeding best managed?
Postpolypectomy bleeding is the cause of 2–5% of all acute LGI bleeding. Most bleeding occurs at a mean of 5 days after polypectomy. The majority of patients have been on NSAIDs/aspirin or anticoagulants. Endoscopic treatment has been shown to be successful in 95% of the cases.

21. **When is surgery considered in patients with LGI bleeding?**
First, it is *always* advisable to make the surgeon part of the initial management team, rather tha waiting until the patient is in dire circumstances. Severe hematochezia with hemodynamic instability or blood transfusion greater than 6 units over 24 hours or recurrent LGI bleeding is typical indication for surgery. Accurate preoperative localization of the bleeding site, with eithe arteriography or colonoscopy, decreases postoperative rebleeding rates and allows for segmental colonic resections. When right- or left-sided localization of LGI bleeding is not possible, subtotal colectomy is recommended. Surgical mortality for acute LGI hemorrhage is 5–10%.

BIBLIOGRAPHY

1. Debarros J, Rosas L, Coen J, et al: The changing paradigm for the treatment of colonic hemorrhage: Superselective angiographic embolization. Dis Colon Rectum 45:802, 2002.

2. Dennison AR, Wherry DC, Morris DL: Hemorrhoids: Nonoperative management. Surg Clin North Am 68:1401 1988.

3. Eisen GM, Dominitz JA, Faigel DO, et al: An annotated algorithmic approach to acute lower gastrointestinal bleeding. Gastrointest Endosc 53:859–863, 2001.

4. Elta GH: Urgent colonoscopy for acute lower-GI bleeding. Gastrointest Endosc 59:402, 2004.

5. Jensen DM, Machicado GA: Colonoscopy for diagnosis and treatment of severe lower gastrointestinal bleedin Routine outcomes and cost analysis. Gastrointest Endosc Clin North Am 7:477–498, 1997.

6. Jensen DM, Machicado GA: Diagnosis and treatment of severe hematochezia: The role of urgent colonoscopy after purge. Gastroenterology 95:1569, 1988.

7. Jensen DM, Machicado GA, Jutabha R, Kovacs TO: Urgent colonoscopy for the diagnosis and treatment of severe diverticular hemorrhage. N Engl J Med 342:78–82, 2000.

8. Longstreth GF: Epidemiology and outcome of patients hospitalized with acute lower gastrointestinal hemorrhage: A population-based study. Am J Gastroenterol 92:419, 1997.

9. Miller LS, Barbarevech C, Friedman LS: Less frequent causes of lower gastrointestinal bleeding. Gastroentero Clin North Am 23:21, 1994.

10. Reinus JF, Brandt LJ: Vascular ectasias and diverticulosis: Common causes of lower intestinal bleeding. Gastroenterol Clin North Am 23:1, 1994.

11. Savides TJ, Jensen DM: Colonoscopic hemostasis for recurrent diverticular hemorrhage associated with a vis ble vessel: A report of three cases. Gastrointest Endosc 40:70, 1994.

12. Sorbi D, Norton I, Conio M, et al: Polypectomy lower GI bleeding: Descriptive analysis. Gastrointest Endosc 51:690–696, 2000.

13. Zuckerman DA, Bocchini TP, Birnbaum EH: Massive hemorrhage in the lower gastrointestinal tract in adults: Diagnostic imaging and intervention. AJR Am J Roentgenol 161:703, 1993.

CHAPTER 54

OCCULT AND OBSCURE GASTROINTESTINAL BLEEDING

John S. Goff, MD

1. **What is occult gastrointestinal (GI) bleeding?**
   Bleeding that is not visible or hidden and is manifested by positive fecal occult blood (FOB) testing or iron deficiency anemia.

2. **What physical examination findings might provide a clue about the source of bleeding?**
   Facial or oral telangiectasia can suggest hereditary telangiectasia (Osler-Weber-Rendu disease). Acanthosis nigricans in the axilla suggest possible malignancy. Perioral pigment spots are associated with Peutz-Jeghers syndrome (hereditary hamartomatous polyposis; see Fig. 54-1). Purpura or ecchymosis implies a possible bleeding disorder.

   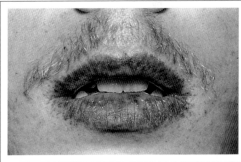

   Figure 54-1. Perioral hyperpigmentation seen with Peutz-Jeghers syndrome.

3. **What tests are used to identify patients with occult GI bleeding, and which are the best?**
   Hemoccult, Hemoccult II Sensa, HemeSelect, FECA, and HemoQuant are techniques for identifying nonvisible blood in a patient's stool. Hemoccult and Hemoccult II Sensa cards are made of guaiac-impregnated paper that is developed by dropping on it a solution of hydrogen peroxide and denatured alcohol. If blood is present, the spot will turn blue. HemeSelect and FECA are immunologic tests for hemoglobin in stool samples, whereas HemoQuant uses a fluorometric method to quantitatively measure heme and heme-derived porphyrin in stool. The sensitivity and specificity of Hemoccult testing is 0.67 and 0.90, respectively, whereas they are 0.97 and 0.94, respectively, for HemoQuant. However, the HemoQuant is not a bedside test and is about 10-fold more expensive.

4. **What are the factors that influence the results of fecal occult blood (FOB) testing besides bleeding from the GI tract?**
   Pseudoperoxidase in various foods can result in a false-positive FOB test. The foods that can produce this unwanted situation are rare red meat, raw broccoli, turnips, cauliflower, radishes, cantaloupe, and parsnips. Rehydrating Hemoccult cards will also produce more false-positive results. A false-negative result can be caused by vitamin C ingestion and delayed development of the card (>6 days). Iron ingestion probably does not cause false-positive results. There is some controversy over whether a stool specimen collected at digital rectal examination is more prone to produce false-positive results. Published studies seem to support the validity of a specimen collected at rectal examination.

5. **What is the proper procedure for doing FOB testing?**
For about 3 days before testing, the patient should avoid the items listed in the previous question. The patient should also avoid aspirin and nonsteroidal anti-inflammatory drugs (NSAIDs). A sample of stool from three separate movements should be collected. The cards need to be developed in <7 days and should not be rehydrated.

6. **How much blood is needed to cause a positive FOB test?**
As little as 2 mL of blood in the GI tract can produce a positive FOB test.

7. **Who should be electively tested for occult blood, and how often?**
All patients age 50 or greater should have annual FOB testing, unless they have already had a normal colonoscopic examination within the past 5–10 years. Colonoscopy is now considered the preferred screening test for colon polyps and cancer.

8. **What can be expected to be found at colonoscopy in a patient over age 50 and who is FOB-negative? Who is FOB-positive?**
Those who are FOB-negative have a cancer find rate at colonoscopy of 0.5–3%, with a polyp find rate of 7–35%. These numbers change to 7–17% for cancer and 20–43% for polyps in those who are FOB-positive.

9. **How should a patient with a positive FOB test be evaluated?**
The patient needs a full colonoscopy and, if negative, should be considered for evaluation of the upper GI tract with endoscopy (EGD). The yield for EGD is increased by approximately 50% (13% vs. 27%) if the patient is also iron deficient. Barium x-rays can be substituted, but the sensitivity for detecting causes of the positive FOB will be less.

10. **What are some of the signs and symptoms of iron deficiency anemia?**
Symptoms of iron deficiency include fatigue, tachycardia (anemia), pica (eating clay and other objects), and pagophagia (ice eating). Physical signs of iron deficiency are rare; they include cheilitis, glossitis, and koilonychia. Laboratory findings include high platelet counts, microcytosis, elevated total iron binding capacity, and low ferritin values. Microcytosis can also be seen with thalassemia, anemia of chronic disease, and sideroblastic anemia.

11. **How should a patient with a positive FOB and iron deficiency anemia be initially evaluated?**
If the patient has no GI symptoms, which is most common, the evaluation should start with a colonoscopy. If the colon is normal, an upper endoscopy (EGD) with biopsies of the proximal small bowel (duodenum) to look for sprue (celiac disease) is the next test. If both endoscopies are negative and the patient does not have sprue, a small bowel x-ray should be performed.

12. **What tests would you do in a patient with iron deficiency (microcytic) anemia, who does not respond to iron nor has recurrence after an initial negative evaluation?**
The first thing to consider would be repeat upper and lower endoscopies. Small bowel endoscopy would be the next step in evaluating these patients. The choices are push enteroscopy, Sonde enteroscopy, and capsule or wireless endoscopy (CE). Of these it would appear that CE is the most accurate, but it has no ability to provide any therapeutic intervention. Consultation with a hematologist to consider bone marrow production problems might also be considered.

13. **How would the evaluation be different if the patient was only iron deficient?**
The initial emphasis would be on diagnosing sprue (celiac disease), non-GI tract sources of blood loss (e.g., menstrual bleeding, urinary tract), nutritional factors, and an evaluation for

infectious causes (hookworm, strongyloidosis, ascariasis), if the patient is <age 50. If they are >age 50, they will need a full GI tract evaluation.

4. **What is the yield for combined colonoscopy and EGD in patients who are FOB positive with or without iron deficiency?**
    Lesions can be found in 48–71% of such patients. Colonoscopy will be positive in 20–30% with 5–11% having cancer. EGD will be positive in 29–56% of cases. Synchronous lesions are found in 1–10% of patients.

5. **What is meant by obscure GI bleeding?**
    Clinically observable bleeding with a negative standard evaluation, including such tests as an upper GI series, barium enema, upper endoscopy (EGD), and colonoscopy, defines obscure GI bleeding.

6. **What endoscopic tests are available for evaluating a patient with obscure GI bleeding, and how useful are they?**
    Repeat standard upper and lower endoscopy has a total yield of about 35% (29% upper, 6% lower). Enteroscopy with a long scope (Sonde versus push), which has yields of 30–75%, is also helpful in evaluating the small bowel. CE is a relatively new noninvasive method for evaluating the entire small bowel. The yield for a source of obscure or occult bleeding with CE is 5–70%. Intraoperative endoscopy is moderately risky and highly invasive. The yield is high for finding a bleeding site (70–100%), and any lesion found can then be easily handled.

7. **What radiologic tests are available for evaluating a patient with obscure GI bleeding, and how useful are they?**
    Small bowel evaluation with enteroclysis is preferred over a small bowel follow through because of the increased yield (0–20% vs. 0–6%). Radiolabeled-RBC scanning should be used for instances when it is felt that the patient might be actively bleeding. If confirmed, the radiologist can then proceed to an urgent angiogram. Elective angiography may have yields up to 40%, but the data in this area are limited. Pharmacologically altering the patient's coagulation system to enhance angiography is not to be encouraged because of the high risk and poor yield. Meckel scans are useful in the young, but are rarely useful in the middle-aged to elderly patient.

8. **How would you sequence an evaluation of a patient with obscure GI bleeding?**
    The first step is to try to catch the patient in the act of bleeding. When there are obvious findings of hematemesis or hematochezia, one should try to obtain a radiolabeled-RBC scan to confirm continued active bleeding. A positive scan may help localize the bleeding to a specific part of the GI tract and will indicate that it would be a good time to perform an angiogram to better define the type and site of bleeding. If the patient does not have such acute bleeding episodes, the sequence for evaluation would start with repeating the upper and lower endoscopies, followed by small bowel enteroclysis, small bowel endoscopy, CE, and then elective angiography. A last resort, but best diagnostic and therapeutic procedure, would be to do intraoperative endoscopy.

9. **Angiodysplasia (vascular malformations) are a common cause of obscure GI bleeding. How are these treated?**
    Endoscopic cautery (laser, bipolar, heater probe) is effective for reducing the blood requirements in these patients, if the lesions can be reached with the endoscope. Angiographic embolization is useful if a feeding vessel can be selectively cannulated. Surgery may be useful for a localized lesion that is not otherwise accessible. Treatment for multiple vascular malformations—hereditary (Osler-Weber-Rendu syndrome) or nonhereditary—is use of estrogen-progesterone combinations or, in difficult cases, octreotide may be helpful but is clearly more difficult to administer. Patients need to avoid NSAIDs and anticoagulants.

20.   **What other lesions are found to be a cause of obscure GI bleeding?**
      Cameron's erosions (associated with large hiatal hernias; Fig. 54-2), portal hypertensive
      gastropathy (Fig. 54-3), GAVE (gastric antral vascular ectasia—watermelon stomach; Fig. 54-4
      Crohn's disease, nonesophageal varices, tumors (lymphoma, leiomyoma, carcinoid, others),
      diverticula (particularly a Meckel's diverticulum in younger patients), small bowel or colonic
      ulcers, Dieulafoy's ulcers, amyloidosis, and hemorrhoids.

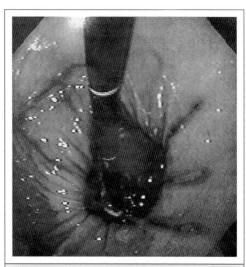

Figure 54-2. Endoscopic photograph of Cameron's (riding)
erosions associated with large hiatal hernia. Here linear
erosions can be seen running perpendicular to the
impression of the diaphragmatic hiatus on the proximal
stomach. (Courtesy of Peter McNally, DO.)

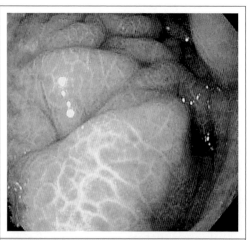

Figure 54-3. Endoscopic photograph of portal hypertensive
gastropathy. (Courtesy of Mark Powis, MD.)

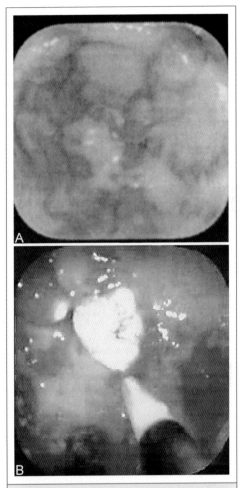

Figure 54-4. (A) Endoscopic photograph of gastric antral vascular ectasia (GAVE) or watermelon stomach. (B) Endoscopic photograph of GAVE after BICAP therapy. (Courtesy of Mark Powis, MD.)

WEBSITES

1. http://www.givenimaging.com/

2. http://www.gastroatlas.com/

3. http://www.vhjoe.com/volume3Issue4/3-4-3.htm./

BIBLIOGRAPHY

1. Ackerman Z, Eliakin R, Stalnikowicz R, Rachmilowitz D: Role of small bowel biopsy in the endoscopic evaluation of adults with iron deficiency anemia. Am J Gastroenterol 91:2099–2102, 1996.

2. Allison JE, Tekawa IS, Ranson CJ, Adrian AL: A comparison of fecal occult-blood tests for colorectal cancer. N Engl J Med 334:155–159, 1996.

3. Cave DR, Cooley JS: Intraoperative enteroscopy. Indications and techniques. Gastrointest Endosc Clin North A 6:793–802, 1996.

4. Chen YK, Gladden DR, Kestenbaum DJ, Collen MJ: Is there a role of upper gastrointestinal endoscopy in the evaluation of patients with occult-positive stool and negative colonoscopy? Am J Gastroenterol 88:2026–2029, 199■

5. Costamagna G, Shah SK, Riccioni ME, et al: A prospective trial comparing small bowel radiographs and video capsule endoscopy for suspected small bowel disease. Gastroenterol 123:994–1005, 2002.

6. Ell C, Remke S, May A, et al: The first prospective controlled trial comparing wireless capsule endoscopy to pu enteroscopy in chronic gastrointestinal bleeding. Endoscopy 43:685–689, 2002.

7. Kepczyk T, Cremins JE, Long BD, et al: A prospective, multidisciplinary evaluation of premenopausal women with iron-deficiency anemia. Am J Gastroenterol 94:109–115, 1999.

8. Kepczyk T, Kadakia SC: Prospective evaluation of the gastrointestinal tract in patients with iron deficiency anemia. Dig Dis Sci 40:1283–1289, 1995.

9. Lewis BS, Waye JD: Chronic gastrointestinal bleeding of obscure origin: Role of small bowel enteroscopy. Gastroenterology 94:1117–1120, 1998.

10. Lieberman DA, Weiss DG, Bond JH, et al: Use of colonoscopy to screen asymptomatic adults for colorectal car cer. Veterans Affairs Cooperative Study Group 380. N Engl J Med 343:162–168, 2000.

11. Pignone M, Saha S, Hoergert T, Mandelblatt J: Cost effectiveness analysis of colorectal cancer screening: A systematic review for the U. S. Prevention Service Task Force. Ann Intern Med 16:96–104, 2002.

12. Ransohoff DF, Lang CA: Screening for colorectal cancer with fecal occult blood testing: A background paper. American College of Physicians. Ann Intern Med 126:811–822, 1997.

13. Rex DR, Lehman GA, Ulbright TM, et al: Colonic neoplasms in asymptomatic persons with negative fecal occu blood tests: Influence of age, gender, and family history. Am J Gastroenterol 88:825–831, 1993.

14. Rockey DC, Koch J, Cello JP, et al: Relative frequency of upper gastrointestinal and colonic lesions in patients with positive fecal occult-blood tests. N Engl J Med 339:153–159, 1998.

15. Rossini FP, Arrigoni A, Pennazio M: Octreotide in the management of bleeding due to angiodysplasia of the sm intestine. Am J Gastroenterol 88:1424–1428, 1993.

16. Winawer SJ, Stewart ET, Zauber AG, et al: A comparison of colonoscopy and double-contrast barium enema fc surveillance after polypectomy. N Engl J Med 342:1766–1772, 2000.

17. Zuckerman GR, Prakash C, Askin MP, Lewis BS: AGA technical review on the evaluation and management of occult and obscure gastrointestinal bleeding. Gastroenterology 118:201–204, 2000.

CHAPTER 55

EVALUATION OF ACUTE ABDOMINAL PAIN

Peter R. McNally, DO, and James E. Cremins, MD

Provide a useful clinical definition of an acute abdomen.
This clinical scenario is characterized by severe pain, often of rapid onset, that prevents bodily movement. When patients experience symptoms of pain for more than 6 hours, surgical intervention is usually necessary.

What are the four types of stimuli for abdominal pain?
1. Stretching or tension   3. Ischemia
2. Inflammation   4. Neoplasms

What are the three categories of abdominal pain?
1. *Visceral pain* occurs when noxious stimuli affect an abdominal viscus. The pain is usually dull (cramping, gnawing, or burning) and poorly localized to the ventral midline because the innervation to most viscera is multisegmental. Secondary autonomic effects, such as diaphoresis, restlessness, nausea, vomiting, and pallor, are common (*see* Fig. 55-1).
2. *Parietal pain* occurs when noxious stimuli irritate the parietal peritoneum. The pain is more intense and localized more precisely to the site of the lesion. Parietal pain is likely to be aggravated by coughing or movement.
3. *Referred pain* is experienced in areas remote from the site of injury. The remote site of pain referral is supplied by the same neurosegment as the involved organ; for example, gallbladder pain may be referred to the right scapula, and pancreatic pain may radiate to the mid back.

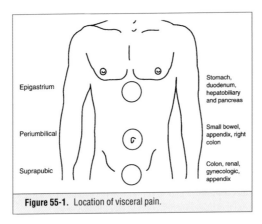

Figure 55-1. Location of visceral pain.

How does the character of the abdominal pain help in the evaluation?
See Table 55-1.

TABLE 55-1. CLASSIFICATION OF PAIN BY THE RATE OF DEVELOPMENT	
Explosive and excruciating (instantaneous)	Myocardial infarction
	Perforated ulcer
	Ruptured aneurysm
	Biliary or renal colic (passage of a stone)
Rapid, severe, and constant (over minutes)	Acute pancreatitis
	Complete bowel obstruction
	Mesenteric thrombus
Gradual and steady pain (over hours)	Acute cholecystitis
	Diverticulitis
	Acute appendicitis
Intermittent and colicky pain (over hours)	Early subacute pancreatitis
	Mechanical small bowel obstruction

5. **What are the important components of the physical examination for patients with acute abdominal pain?**
    - *General status:* Is the patient hemodynamically unstable? Does he or she need immediate hemodynamic resuscitation and emergent laparotomy (e.g., ruptured spleen, hepatic tumo aneurysm, ectopic pregnancy, or mesenteric apoplexy)?
    - *Inspection:* Visually evaluate for distention, hernias, scars, and hyperperistalsis.
    - *Auscultation:* Hyperperistalsis suggests obstruction; absence of peristalsis >3 minutes sug gests peritonitis (silent abdomen); bruits suggest presence of an aneurysm.
    - *Percussion:* Tympany suggests either intraluminal or free abdominal air.
    - *Palpation:* Start the examination away from the area of tenderness and be gentle. Abdomina pain with voluntary coughing suggests peritoneal signs. Deeply palpating the abdomen onl diminishes patient trust and cooperation. The enlarged gallbladder will be missed on deep palpation. Inspiratory arrest during light palpation of the right hypochondrium suggests ga bladder pain (Murphy's sign). Localized pain suggests localized peritonitis (e.g., appendicit cholecystitis, diverticulitis). Findings on the abdominal examination of visceral ischemia or infarction are characteristically disproportionate to the degree of abdominal pain.
    - *Pelvic and rectal exams:* These exams should be done in any patient with abdominal pain. A painful examination may be the only sign of pelvic appendicitis, diverticulitis, or tubo-ova ian pathology. Bimanual examination is critical to exclude an obstetric or gynecologic cause
    - *Iliopsoas test:* With the legs fully extended in a supine position, the patient is requested to raise the legs. Pain occurs when the psoas muscle is inflamed (e.g., appendicitis).
    - *Obturator test:* This test is performed by flexing the patient's thigh at right angles to the trur and then rotating the leg externally. Inflammation of the obturator internus muscle causes pain (e.g., tubo-ovarian abscess or pelvic appendicitis).

6. **Which laboratory tests should be obtained in patients with acute abdominal pain?**
    Although laboratory tests are helpful in confirming the evolution of a disease process, they are frequently not helpful in localizing the cause of abdominal pain.
    - *Complete blood count (CBC):* Elevation of the white blood cell count suggests inflammation however, absence of leukocytosis may be unhelpful early in the course of disease. A low hematocrit with a normal mean corpuscular volume (MCV) suggests acute blood loss, whereas a low hematocrit with a low MCV suggests iron deficiency from chronic gastro-intestinal (GI) blood loss or malabsorption.

- *Amylase elevations* (>500 IU) suggest pancreatitis but are not specific. Lipase enzyme elevations are more specific for pancreatic origin.
- *Liver enzyme elevations* may be suggestive of hepatobiliary causes of pain. Elevations of aspartate or alanine aminotransferase suggest hepatocyte injury. Alkaline phosphatase or gamma glutamine transferase (GGT) elevations suggest canalicular or biliary injury. Total bilirubin elevations >3 mg/dL suggest common bile duct obstruction or associated intrahepatic cholestasis.
- *Evidence of pyuria* on urinalysis suggests urinary tract infection, but it may also be seen in nephrolithiasis or even pelvic appendicitis.
- *Chemistry analysis* can be helpful in the global assessment of patient health, hyperglycemia, acidosis, and electrolyte disturbances.
- *Pregnancy tests* (beta human chorionic gonadotropin) should be ordered for all premenopausal women.
- *Stool examination* for occult blood is necessary.
- *Electrocardiography* is performed for all patients with possible myocardial infarction or those >age 50.

7. **Which radiologic tests should be ordered to evaluate the patient with acute abdominal pain?**

The selection of tests depends on the likelihood of the pretest clinical diagnosis and the ability of the radiologic test to confirm clinical suspicion.

- *Plain radiographs* of the abdomen are quick and readily available and can be done at the bedside. They reliably detect bowel obstruction and viscus perforation. Occasionally, they may suggest stone disease (one third of gallbladder and two thirds of renal stones are calcified) or ruptured aortic aneurysm (separation of aortic wall calcium and mass effect). Free intraabdominal air is best detected with the patient in the left lateral decubitus position for 10 minutes (see Chapter 68, Radiography and Radiographic/Fluoroscopic Contrast Studies).
- *Ultrasound* of the abdomen is quick and noninvasive and can be performed at the bedside. The disadvantages of ultrasound include variable operator expertise and suboptimal examination in the obese or gaseous abdomen. Ultrasound is excellent for evaluating the gallbladder, bile ducts, liver, kidneys, and appendix (see Chapter 71, Interventional Radiology: Fluoroscopic and Angiographic Procedures).
- *Computed tomography (CT)* of the abdomen provides a detailed view of the anatomy. It is expensive, requires transportation of the patient, and is not always readily available. Oral and intravenous contrast agents are usually required. CT provides the best evaluation of the pancreas (see Chapter 71, Noninvasive Gastrointestinal Imaging: Ultrasound, Computed Tomography, and Magnetic Resonance Imaging).
- *Hepatoiminodiacetic (HIDA) scan* is the most accurate test for acute cholecystitis (see Chapter 72, Nuclear Medicine Studies).

8. **Pain referred to the abdomen can be confusing. What are the common extraabdominal causes of referred abdominal pain?**

- *Thoracic:* pneumonia, pulmonary embolism, pneumothorax, myocardial infarction or ischemia, esophageal spasm, or perforation
- *Neurogenic:* tabes dorsalis, radicular pain (spinal cord compression from tumor, abscess, compression, or varicella zoster infection)
- *Metabolic:* uremia, porphyria, acute adrenal insufficiency
- *Hematologic:* sickle cell anemia, hemolytic anemia, Henoch-Schönlein purpura
- *Toxins:* insect bites (scorpion bite–induced pancreatitis), lead poisoning

9. **List the common causes of acute abdominal pain in gravid women.**

- Appendicitis
- Ovarian cysts complicated by torsion, rupture, and hemorrhage

- Ectopic pregnancy
- Gallbladder problems

10. **When the appendix is found to be entirely normal during a laparotomy performed for presumed appendicitis in a gravid woman, should the appendix be removed?**
No. Removal of the normal appendix triples the risk of fetal loss.

11. **What is the most common cause of acute abdominal pain in elderly patients?**
Biliary tract disease is responsible for 25% of all cases of acute abdominal pain in elderly patients requiring hospitalization. Bowel obstruction and incarcerated hernia are the next most common, followed by appendicitis.

12. **What symptoms are helpful in evaluating for appendicitis?**
It is decidedly uncommon for acute appendicitis to present with nausea, vomiting, or diarrhea before abdominal pain. Usually, acute appendicitis is heralded by pain and is often followed by anorexia, nausea, and, sometimes, single-episode vomiting. Acute appendicitis should be first on the differential diagnosis list in any patient with acute abdominal pain without a prior history of appendectomy. The diagnosis of typical appendicitis requires careful history and physical examination only. Laboratory tests and radiographic studies are ancillary.

13. **Discuss atypical forms of appendicitis.**
When the appendix is retrocecal or retroileal in location, the inflamed appendix is often shielded from the anterior abdomen. The pain is often less pronounced, and localizing signs on physical examination are uncommon. Symptoms and signs of appendicitis in elderly patients are subtle. Pain is often minimal, fever mild only, and leukocytosis unreliable. A high index of suspicion is essential.

14. **Describe the ultrasound findings of acute appendicitis.**
The appendix appears as a round target with an anechoic lumen, surrounded by a hypoechoic and thickened (>2 mm) appendiceal wall. This finding with reproduction of pain under the transducer has a diagnostic accuracy of 95% and a negative predictive value of 97%.

15. **When laparotomy is performed for presumed appendicitis, what is the acceptable false-negative rate? How often is another cause identified in this setting?**
A false-negative laparotomy rate of 10–20% is reported. In roughly 30% of these cases some other cause of abdominal pain is identified, such as mesenteric lymphadenitis, Meckel's diverticulum, cecal diverticulitis, pelvic inflammatory disease, ectopic pregnancy, or ileitis.

16. **What is the single best test to evaluate patients who, infected with human immunodeficiency virus (HIV), complain of acute abdominal pain?**
Because of the variety of causes of abdominal pain in such patients, it has been argued that CT scan is the single best test.

17. **What are the cardinal features of a ruptured tubal pregnancy?**
- Amenorrhea (missed period or scant menses)
- Abdominal and pelvic pain
- Unilateral, tender adnexal mass
- Signs of blood loss

8. **What are the characteristics of acute intestinal obstruction?**
   - Nausea and vomiting
   - Failure to expel flatus
   - Prior abdominal surgery or presence of hernia
   - Peristaltic pain (colicky pain—every 10 minutes for jejunal obstruction and every 30 minutes for ileal obstruction)

9. **List the clinical characteristics of large bowel obstruction.**
   - Most patients are over age 50.
   - Lower abdominal cramping pain is gradual in onset.
   - Abdominal distention is a prominent feature.
   - Dilated loops of bowel with haustra distinguish the colon from the small bowel.
   - Sigmoidoscopy or single-column barium enema is important.
   - Causes include obstructing neoplasm and cecal or sigmoid volvulus.

10. **List the clinical characteristics of diverticulitis.**
    - Age >50
    - Localized left lower abdominal pain
    - Palpable mass in the left lower quadrant

11. **List the clinical hallmarks of acute cholecystitis.**
    - Patients often give a history of prior episodes of milder abdominal pain.
    - Abdominal pain arises usually after a meal, especially in the evening after a large meal.
    - Pain crescendos typically over 20–30 minutes and then plateaus.
    - Pain lasting >1–2 hours is accompanied usually by gallbladder wall inflammation.
    - Associated nausea occurs in 90% of patients; vomiting may follow onset of pain in 50–80%.
    - Radiation of pain to the back is common; pain radiates to the right scapula in 10% of cases.
    - Low-grade fever is common.
    - Right hypochondrium tenderness is generally present. Inspiratory arrest during gentle palpation of the right upper quadrant (Murphy's sign) suggests acute cholecystitis.
    - Diagnostic tests include HIDA scan or ultrasound.

12. **What is the differential diagnosis of acute cholecystitis?**
    - *Liver:* alcoholic hepatitis, liver metastasis, Fitz-Hugh and Curtis syndrome, congestive hepatopathy
    - *Pancreas:* pancreatitis, pseudocyst
    - *GI tract:* peptic ulcer disease with or without perforation, acute appendicitis (retrocecal)
    - *Kidney:* pyelonephritis, renal colic
    - *Lung:* pneumonia, pulmonary embolism, emphysema
    - *Heart:* myocardial infarction, pericarditis
    - Pre-eruptive varicella zoster

13. **When should a patient undergo surgery for an acute abdomen?**
    When, in the judgment of the surgeon, a problem will be identifiable or treatable by surgical intervention. There is no substitute for good surgical judgment and intuition.

14. **What conditions can result in an acute abdomen in HIV-infected patients?**
    Patients with HIV can have any of the usual causes of an acute abdomen; all non–HIV-specific diagnoses must be considered. Perforation is most often due to cytomegalovirus (CMV) infection in the distal small bowel or colon; this is the most common cause of the acute abdomen in late-stage HIV infection. CMV infection of the vascular endothelial cells leads to mucosal ischemic ulceration and perforation. HIV-associated lymphoma and Kaposi's sarcoma can also

lead to perforation, but this finding is rare. AIDS cholangiopathy, papillitis, and drug-induced pancreatitis (e.g., pentamidine, bactrim, didanosine, ritonavir) are unique causes of abdominal pain in HIV-infected patients.

25. **Are patients with systemic lupus erythematosus (SLE) at increased risk for intra-abdominal catastrophe?**

    Approximately 2% of patients with SLE develop lupus vasculitis, one of the most devastating complications of SLE. The fatality rate is >50%. Small vessels of the bowel wall are affected, leading to ulceration, hemorrhage, perforation, and infarction.

26. **How common are severe GI manifestations of polyarteritis nodosa (PAN)?**

    PAN is a vasculitis that may have visceral involvement. GI bleeding from intestinal ischemia is seen in 6% of cases, bowel perforation in 5%, and bowel infarction in 1.4%. Acalculous cholecystitis occurs in up to 17% because of direct vasculitic involvement of the gallbladder.

27. **What causes of acute abdominal pain should be considered in illicit drug users?**

    Intravenous and smoked cocaine has been reported to cause acute mesenteric ischemia, or "crack belly." Endocarditis in parenteral drug abusers may be associated with mesenteric emboli and bowel infarction.

BIBLIOGRAPHY

1. Brandt CP, Priebe PP, Eckhauser ML: Diagnostic laparoscopy in the intensive care patient: Avoiding the nontherapeutic laparotomy. Surg Endosc 7:168–172, 1993.
2. Clement DJ: Evaluation of the acute abdomen with CT: Is image everything? Am J Gastroenterol 88:1282–1283, 1993.
3. Connor TJ, Garcha IS, Ramshaw BJ, et al: Diagnostic laparoscopy for suspected appendicitis. Am Surg 61:187–189, 1995.
4. de Dombal FT: Acute abdominal pain in the elderly. J Clin Gastroenterol 19:331–335, 1994.
5. Epstein FB: Acute abdominal pain in pregnancy. Emerg Med Clin North Am 12:151–165, 1994.
6. Haubrich WS: Abdominal pain. In Haubrich WS, Schaffner F, Berk JE (eds): Bockus Gastroenterology, 5th ed. Philadelphia, W.B. Saunders, 1995, pp 11–29.
7. Klein KB: Approach to the patient with abdominal pain. In Yamada T (ed): Textbook of Gastroenterology, 2nd ed. Philadelphia, J.B. Lippincott, 1995, pp 750–771.
8. Kovachev LS: "Cough sign": A reliable test in the diagnosis of intra-abdominal inflammation. Br J Surg 81:1542 1994.
9. Linder JD, Monkemuller KE, Raijman I, et al: Cocaine-associated ischemic colitis. South Med J 93:909–913, 2000.
10. Mulholland MW: Approach to the patient with acute abdomen and fever of abdominal origin. In Yamada T (ed): Textbook of Gastroenterology, 2nd ed. Philadelphia, J.B. Lippincott, 1995, pp 783–796.
11. Nusair S, Nahir M, Almogy G, et al: Pancreatitis and chronic abdominal pain in patients with AIDS. Postgrad Med J 75:371–373, 1999.
12. Ridge JA, Way LW: Abdominal pain. In Sleisenger MH, Fordtran JS (eds): Gastrointestinal Disease: Pathophysiology, Diagnosis, Management, 5th ed. Philadelphia, W.B. Saunders, 1993, pp 150–162.
13. Sheikh RA, Prindiville TP, Yeramandra S, et al: Microsporidial AIDS cholangiopathy due to encephalitozoon intestinalis: Case report and review. Am J Gastroenterol 95:2364–2371, 2000.
14. Silen W: Cope's Early Diagnosis of the Abdomen. New York, Oxford University Press, 1979.
15. Taourel P, Baron MP, Pradel J, et al: Acute abdomen of unknown origin: Impact of CT on diagnosis and management. Gastrointest Radiol 17:287–291, 1992.
16. Wyatt SH, Fishman EK: The acute abdomen in individuals with AIDS. Radiol Clin North Am 32:1032–1043, 199
17. Wattoo MA, Osundeko O: Cocaine-induced intestinal ischemia. West J Med 170:47–49, 2000.

CHAPTER 56

EVALUATION OF ACUTE DIARRHEA

Col. Kent C. Holtzmuller, MD

1. **What is the definition of acute diarrhea?**
   Diarrhea is defined as the passage of an increased number of stools of less-than-normal form and consistency. Acute diarrhea refers to acute onset of symptoms of <14–30 days' duration. Diarrhea lasting longer than 1 month is considered chronic. The severity of acute diarrhea can be defined as mild, where no change in daily activities is noted; moderate, where a change in daily activities is required but the patient is able to function; and severe, where the patient is disabled by the symptoms.

2. **What is the impact of acute diarrhea in the United States and worldwide?**
   American adults average about one episode of acute diarrhea annually. Acute diarrhea is one of the most common medical conditions seen by primary care practitioners. In the United States, approximately 1 million hospital admissions and 6000 deaths per year are attributed to acute diarrhea. Worldwide, diarrheal-related diseases are the single greatest cause of morbidity and mortality and, for children under age 4, the most common cause of death.

3. **Who should undergo medical evaluation for acute diarrhea?**
   Most cases of acute diarrhea are self-limited and require no medical evaluation. Nearly half of the cases last for less than 1 day. Evaluation should be reserved for patients with evidence of systemic toxicity (dehydration, bloody diarrhea, fever, severe abdominal pain), diarrhea of >48 hours' duration, and elderly or immunocompromised patients.

4. **What are the most common causes of acute bloody diarrhea?**
   Infectious dysentery, inflammatory bowel disease (ulcerative colitis and Crohn's disease), and ischemic colitis.

5. **What is dysentery?**
   Dysentery is a disease process characterized by diarrhea that contains blood and polymorphonuclear cells. Dysentery results when an organism causes an inflammatory reaction, either by direct invasion of the colonic/ileal epithelium or by producing a toxin that causes cellular death and tissue damage. Symptoms associated with dysentery may include abdominal pain and cramping, tenesmus (painful urgency to evacuate stool), fever, and dehydration.

6. **Name the common causes of infectious dysentery in the United States.**
   Campylobacter and *Salmonella* species are the principal causes of dysentery in the United States. *Shigella* species and certain strains of *Escherichia coli* (specifically O157H) are less common. Rarer causes include *Yersinia, Entamoeba, Aeromonas,* and *Plesiomonas* species.

7. **What is the significance of stool leukocytes (white blood cells)?**
   The presence of fecal leukocytes helps to distinguish inflammatory from noninflammatory diarrhea. Normally, leukocytes are not present in stool. Fecal leukocytes are found usually in infectious diarrhea caused by *Campylobacter, Salmonella, Shigella,* and *Yersinia* species, *Clostridium difficile*, enterohemorrhagic and enteroinvasive strains of *E. coli*, and *Aeromonas*

species. In cases of ischemic colitis and inflammatory bowel disease, fecal leukocytes are the result of mucosal bleeding. Diarrhea secondary to toxigenic bacteria (e.g., Enterotoxigenic *E. coli* [ETEC], *Vibrio cholerae*), viruses, and small bowel protozoa (e.g., *Giardia* sp.) do not contain stool leukocytes.

8. **How does one evaluate a stool specimen for leukocytes?**
   The presence of white blood cells (WBCs) in the stool can be assayed by microscopic exam of the stool or by means of an immunoassay for the neutrophil marker lactoferrin. The sensitivity fecal lactoferrin and microscopy for fecal WBCs is 92% and 72%, respectively. Microscopy is best performed on liquid stool or mucus:
   1. Place a drop of liquid stool or mucus on a glass microscope slide.
   2. Add several drops of methylene blue or Gram stain.
   3. Mix the material thoroughly.
   4. Place a coverslip over the mixture.
   5. Wait several minutes to allow nuclear staining.
   6. Scan the slide under high power to observe for leukocytes and red blood cells (positive result ≥3 leukocytes in four or more fields).

9. **If 100 random patients with acute diarrhea underwent evaluation with stool cultures, how many would be positive? Which patients with acute diarrhea should be evaluated with a stool culture?**
   Published studies show the diagnostic yield of stool cultures to be 1.5–5.6%. This percentage range can be increased if tested patients are selected carefully. A stool culture should be obtained from patients with dysentery symptoms, persistent diarrhea (beyond 3–5 days), or from patients who are immunocompromised. Patients with dysentery symptoms are much more likely than the other two groups to have a positive stool culture. The rate of positive stool culture in patients hospitalized with dysentery is 40–60%.

10. **Which patients with acute diarrhea should be evaluated with an endoscopic exam?**
    Generally, a flexible sigmoidoscopy or colonoscopy is not needed for the evaluation of acute diarrhea. Most cases of acute diarrhea are self-limited, and endoscopic exam findings add usually little information to the history, physical exam, and stool tests. However, patients with prolonged symptoms or those suspected to have pseudomembranous colitis, ischemic colitis, or inflammatory bowel disease should be considered for endoscopic evaluation.

11. **By what mechanisms do toxigenic organisms produce diarrhea?**
    The toxins produced by organisms can be classified into two categories: cytotonic and cytotoxic. Cytotonic toxins cause a watery diarrhea by activation of intracellular enzymes, which cause net fluid secretion into the intestinal lumen. Examples of cytotonic toxins include those produced by *V. cholerae* and enterotoxigenic strains of *E. coli*. Cytotoxic toxins cause structural injury to the intestinal mucosa, which, in turn, causes inflammation and mucosal bleeding. Enterohemorrhagic *E. coli* produces a cytotoxic toxin (Shiga-like toxin).

12. **Which *Campylobacter* species are implicated as causes of dysentery? How is *Campylobacter* transmitted?**
    C. jejuni accounts for 98% of reported *Campylobacter* isolates. The less common isolates are *C. fetus* and *C. fecalis*. Direct contact with fecal matter from infected persons or animals and ingestion of contaminated food or water have been implicated in the transmission of *Campylobacter* infection.

13. **Describe the clinical and endoscopic features of *Campylobacter* diarrhea.**
    The incubation period from ingestion until onset of symptoms is 1–7 days. Symptoms include diarrhea (often bloody), abdominal pain, malaise, headache, and fever (sometimes high). With

or without antibiotic therapy, most patients recover within 7 days. Relapse may occur. The rectosigmoidoscopic findings of *Campylobacter* diarrhea may be indistinguishable from those of ulcerative colitis or Crohn's disease. The identification of comma-shaped, gram-negative bacteria on stool Gram stain suggests the diagnosis of *Campylobacter* infection. A rare, extraintestinal complication of *Campylobacter* infection is Guillain-Barré syndrome. Up to a third of Guillain-Barré cases in the United States are caused by *Campylobacter* infection.

4. **How are *Salmonella* organisms classified?**
Salmonella species are gram-negative, aerobic, and facultative anaerobic bacteria of the *Enterobacteriaceae* family. Using O and H antigens, 2200 different serotypes have been identified. The term *nontyphoidal salmonellosis* is used to denote disease caused by serotypes other than *S. typhi*.

5. **List the types of illnesses that can be caused by *Salmonella*.**
   - Acute gastroenteritis (The degree of colonic involvement determines the extent of the dysentery-like symptoms.)
   - Bacteremia (with or without gastrointestinal [GI] involvement)
   - Localized infection (Bacteremia can result in localized nonintestinal infections—e.g., bone, joints, meninges. Predisposing conditions for localized infection include abdominal aortic aneurysm, prosthetic heart valve, vascular grafts, and orthopedic hardware.)
   - Typhoidal or enteric fever
   - Asymptomatic carrier states (more common in older age, in women [3:1], and in people with biliary disease)

6. **What is typhoid fever?**
Typhoid fever is a clinical syndrome characterized by marked hectic fever, persistent bacteremia, hepatosplenomegaly, and abdominal pain. The illness can be caused by any serotype of *Salmonella* but results most commonly from *S. typhi* and less commonly from *S. paratyphi*. Because humans are the only known reservoir of *S. typhi*, transmission is primarily by the fecal-oral route. The illness usually lasts for 3–5 weeks. Up to 90% of patients experience a "rose spot" rash on the upper anterior trunk within the first or second week of illness. Although diarrhea is unusual, ulceration of Peyer's patches in the intestinal wall may cause hemorrhage or perforation. A number of vaccines are successful against typhoid.

7. **How is *Salmonella* infection treated?**
Healthy patients with mild symptoms do not require antibiotic therapy. In fact, antibiotic therapy may prolong intestinal life and shedding of the organism. Antibiotic therapy is appropriate for patients at the extremes of age (the very young or elderly), patients who are immunosuppressed, patients with evidence of bacteremia, and patients with severe cases of intestinal salmonellosis. A quinolone antibiotic is the treatment of choice, or, if susceptible, trimethoprim-sulfamethoxazole.

8. **Describe the characteristics of *Shigella* infection. How is it treated?**
Shigella species is a gram-negative rod and member of the *Enterobacteriaceae*. Most (90–95%) infections are caused by four species: *S. sonnei, S. flexneri, S. dysenteriae,* and *S. boydii*. The organism is highly infectious, having a fecal-oral route of transmission. Infection can occur with the ingestion of as few as 10–100 organisms. Intestinal damage results primarily from direct invasion of the organism into the colonic epithelium and, to a lesser extent, from the production of an enterotoxin. The *Shigella* toxin is composed of an A subunit, which is catalytic, and a B subunit, which is responsible for binding. The endoscopic appearance of shigellosis shows intense involvement of the rectosigmoid with variable proximal involvement. Approximately 15% of cases present with pancolitis. In children, *Shigella* infection has been associated with seizures. Antimicrobial therapy is recommended for all cases of shigellosis: a fluoroquinolone may be used, or, if susceptible, trimethoprim-sulfamethoxazole.

19. **What diarrheogenic illnesses are caused by *Escherichia coli*?**

    E. coli belongs to the family Enterobacteriaceae, a facultative anaerobic, gram-negative bacter
    The organisms are common inhabitants of the human GI tract, and most strains do not have th
    virulence factors necessary to cause disease. The four primary pathogenic strains of *E. coli* an
    the syndromes that they cause are listed below.

    ETEC accounts for most cases of traveler's diarrhea but is relatively rare in the United States.
    Fecal-oral transmission through the ingestion of contaminated food or water is the primary mean
    of spread. Disease is produced by the adherence of ETEC to the mucosa, followed by the produc-
    tion of toxins (heat-labile "cholera-like" toxins). Invasion of the mucosa does not occur. The illne
    is usually self-limited, lasting 3–5 days. Symptoms include watery diarrhea and abdominal cram
    ing. Occasionally associated with this illness is low-grade fever and, rarely, bloody diarrhea.

    Enteropathogenic E. coli (EPEC) lacks invasive properties. Disease results from its entero-
    adherent properties. Illness caused by EPEC affects primarily young children (<age 3) and mu
    be considered as a probable cause of nursery and pediatric outbreaks of diarrhea. Profuse
    watery diarrhea, which may become chronic, is the usual presentation. As with ETEC-caused il
    nesses, those caused by EPEC rarely result in bloody diarrhea.

    Enteroinvasive E. coli (EIEC) can invade the intestinal mucosa and cause acute dysente
    EIEC strains share characteristics with *Shigella* species and are not commonly found in th
    United States. Infants under age 1 are most susceptible to EIEC strains in developed
    countries.

    Enterohemorrhagic E. coli (EHEC) has a number of serotypes, but *E. coli* O157:H7 is the mo
    important. *E. coli* O157:H7 is acquired primarily from the ingestion of contaminated beef,
    although outbreaks have also been associated with contaminated water, raw milk, unpasteuriz
    juices, and person-to-person transmission among household members. Drinking water contai
    inated with farm waste has been implicated in several recent large outbreaks. The typical clinic
    presentation begins with severe abdominal cramps and watery diarrhea followed by rapid pro-
    gression to bloody diarrhea. The organism is not invasive but produces a Shiga-like toxin, whi
    is cytotoxic to vascular endothelium. The disease can cause hemolytic uremic syndrome and
    thrombotic thrombocytopenia purpura (<10% of cases). The very young and very old are the
    most susceptible to fatal complications. The most common cause of acute renal failure in Nort
    American children is O157:H7 infection.

20. **What is the therapy for O157:H7–induced diarrhea?**

    Antibiotic therapy for O157:H7 is controversial. Early therapy with antibiotics may encourage
    development of hemolytic uremia syndrome. Supportive care, correction of fluid and electrolyt
    disturbances, and hemodialysis for acute renal failure are the mainstays of therapy. Antimotilit
    agents should be avoided.

21. **Describe the clinical presentation of infection with *Yersinia enterocolitica*.**

    The most common presentation includes diarrhea, abdominal pain, and low-grade fever.
    Microscopic examination of the stool usually shows red and white blood cells. Approximately 25
    of the cases are grossly bloody. The clinical presentation of children and young adults may
    resemble that of appendicitis (right lower quadrant abdominal pain and tenderness, fever, and
    leukocytosis). Findings at surgery show mesenteric lymphadenitis and terminal ileitis. On rare
    occasions, a patient may progress to fulminant enterocolitis with intestinal perforation, peritonitis
    and hemorrhage. Pharyngitis is common in children with *Y. enterocolitica* infection and is seen in
    up to 10% of adult cases. Patients with iron overload (hemochromatosis) are more susceptible to
    yersinial sepsis. Postinfectious manifestations of reactive arthritis, erythema nodosum, Reiter's
    syndrome, thyroiditis, myocarditis, and glomerulonephritis have been reported.

22. **How is infection with *Y. enterocolitica* treated?**

    Most cases are self-limited and do not require antibiotic therapy. Severe cases can be treated
    with ceftriaxone, trimethoprim-sulfamethoxazole, fluoroquinolone, or the combination of
    doxycycline and aminoglycoside.

3. **Which organisms are associated with seafood-induced dysentery?**
Vibrio parahaemolyticus, a member of the *Vibrionaceae* family, is a halophilic organism (i.e., it grows only in media containing salt) that has been isolated in fish, crustaceans, and shellfish. The diarrhea is characteristically watery, but bloody diarrhea may be seen in up to 15% of patients. Other causes of seafood-induced dysentery include *Plesiomonas shigelloides* and *Campylobacter* species.

4. **What parasites cause bloody diarrhea?**
Entamoeba histolytica, Balantidium coli, Dientamoeba fragilis, and *Schistosoma* species. The most common cause of parasitic dysentery in the United States is amebiasis (*E. histolytica*). Although parasitic diarrhea is uncommon in the United States, it is a significant cause of morbidity and mortality worldwide.

5. **Who is at risk for amebiasis? What are the potential complications of amebic dysentery?**
Travelers to and immigrants from endemic areas, institutionalized patients, and homosexual men. Complications include toxic megacolon, intestinal perforation, peritonitis, ameboma, and liver abscess.

6. **What is an ameboma?**
An ameboma is a mass of granulation tissue and mucosal/submucosal inflammation in the cecum or right colon. The inflammatory process clinically manifests itself as a tender mass in the right lower abdomen. Approximately 0.5–1.5% of patients with amebic colitis have an ameboma. Barium enema may show an "apple-core" appearance. Diagnosis is confirmed with colonoscopy, and biopsy is necessary to rule out carcinoma or tuberculosis. Amebomas respond to antiamebic therapy; surgery is not generally required.

7. **Which laboratory studies are useful in the diagnosis of amebic dysentery?**
Microscopic examination of the stool for cysts and/or trophozoites or detection of circulating antibodies to *E. histolytica* by the indirect hemagglutination (IHAA) test. Approximately 80–90% of patients with amebic dysentery have a positive IHAA serology. A positive IHAA test in a patient with presumptive inflammatory bowel disease should raise the possibility of amebiasis.

8. **Describe the treatment of amebic dysentery. What are the potential side effects?**
Acute amebic dysentery is treated with metronidazole, 500–750 mg three times/day for 5–10 days, plus either treatment with iodoquinol 650 mg three times/day for 20 days or paromomycin 500 mg three times/day for 7 days. Consumption of alcohol during metronidazole therapy may induce an Antabuse effect (e.g., abdominal cramps, nausea, emesis, headache, flushing). Peripheral neuropathy is a potentially severe and chronic side effect of metronidazole. Other possible symptoms include a metallic taste and GI distress manifested by nausea, flatus, and diarrhea. Metronidazole is teratogenic and should not be taken during the first trimester of pregnancy.

9. **Which parasites typically cause nonbloody diarrhea? What are the risks for acquisition?**
Giardia, Cryptosporidiosis, and *Cyclospora* species typically cause nonbloody diarrhea. Contaminated water is the primary source for community outbreaks. *Giardia* species is a frequent culprit after consumption of water from mountainous lakes and streams. *Cyclospora* species should be considered in travelers from Nepal. *Cryptosporidiosis* is a significant cause of HIV-related diarrhea.

10. **How do you obtain a stool specimen for ova and parasites exam?**
An inverted, hat-like container is a convenient receptacle for collection of stool. The specimen should be free of contamination from urine and toilet water. Protozoan trophozoites degenerate

rapidly with drying. The specimen should be fresh and processed expeditiously or preserved with a two-vial preservation technique. One vial contains a buffered formalin mixture; the other a polyvinyl alcohol fixative. Erratic shedding of parasites requires stool collection for 3 consecutive days. Barium, antibiotics, mineral oil, antacids, bismuth, and enemas may interfere with parasite identification. Newer enzyme immunoassay (EIA) and immunofluorescence methods are available for the detection of *E. hystolytica, Giardia,* and *Cryptosporidiosis.*

31. What is the most common cause of hospital-acquired diarrhea?

Diarrhea starting during or shortly after hospitalization is most commonly due to *C. difficile* infection. It is rare that another bacterial agent is the cause of diarrhea in patients who develop diarrhea after being hospitalized for more than 3 days. Other causes of hospital-acquired diarrhea include enteral nutrition and hyperosmolar liquid medications (which commonly contain sorbitol). Other medications that can cause diarrhea include antacids, magnesium supplements, antibiotics, antineoplastics, cholinergics, theophylline, and prostaglandins.

32. Describe the treatment of pseudomembranous colitis.

Antibiotic discontinuation results in complete cessation of symptoms in many patients. Consider drug therapy with oral metronidazole, vancomycin, or Bacitracin in patients with moderate-to-severe symptoms. Vancomycin is expensive (up to $500 for a 5- to 10-day course). Intravenous *metronidazole* can be used in patients who cannot tolerate oral intake. Symptomatic relapse is seen in 15–20% of cases, regardless of which antibiotic is used.

An alternative to antibiotic therapy is oral *cholestyramine.* The cholestyramine resin binds *C. difficile* toxin while the colonic flora reconstitutes itself. Resin therapy has been advocated for use in mild cases and relapses.

Fecal enemas have been used experimentally to reestablish bacterial flora. The theoretic value of fecal enemas in clinical practice is diminished by limited patient acceptance.

33. Outline the differential diagnosis of a patient with AIDS who presents with bloody diarrhea.

1. As with nonimmunosuppressed patients, colitis secondary to invasive bacteria (*Salmonella, Shigella, Campylobacter,* and *Yersinia* species), bacteria that produce cytotoxins (EHEC), and amebiasis must be considered.
2. Infections that can result in proctitis and bloody diarrhea include rectal gonorrhea, lymphogranuloma venereum (*Chlamydia trachomatis*), primary anorectal syphilis, and herpes simplex. The hallmark of herpes proctitis is severe rectal pain and tenesmus. In addition, a purulent rectal discharge is frequently present, and difficulty with urination, inguinal lymphadenopathy, and perianal ulcerations may also be noted.
3. Colitis characterized by abdominal pain, diarrhea, hematochezia, and fever is a common manifestation of cytomegalovirus (CMV) infection. Patchy involvement of the colonic mucosa is often seen on colonoscopy with CMV infection, and the diagnosis is aided by the identification of amphophilic intranuclear inclusion bodies.
4. Pseudomembranous colitis should be considered in AIDS patients with diarrhea, because they are often prescribed antibiotics.
5. Rarer causes of bloody diarrhea in AIDS are *Mycobacterium tuberculosis* and histoplasmosis. It should be noted that multiple concurrent causes of diarrhea can be present in this population.
6. *Cryptosporidium* species, *Isospora belli, Cyclospora* spp., *Microsporidia* spp., *Giardia* spp., *Mycobacterium avium-intracellulare,* and lymphoma can affect the small bowel and cause nonbloody diarrhea.
7. AIDS patients with inflammatory bowel disease often exhibit amelioration of symptoms as the immune suppression worsens.

4. List the risk factors and therapy for infectious dysentery.
   See Table 56-1.

TABLE 56–1. RISK FACTORS AND THERAPY FOR INFECTIOUS DYSENTERY

Organism	Risk Factors/Reservoirs	Therapy
Campylobacter spp.*	Contaminated food, water, raw milk, infected animals and humans	Erythromycin Fluoroquinolone
Salmonella spp.* (nontyphoidal)	Food (milk, eggs, poultry, meats), water, infected humans	Fluoroquinolone TMP-SMX, ceftriaxone
Shigella spp.*	Food, water, infected humans	Fluoroquinolone TMP-SMX
Escherichia coli	Beef, raw milk, untreated water, direct contact	Supportive care
Aeromonas spp.*	Untreated water, shellfish	TMP-SMX
Plesiomonas spp.	Water, seafood, chicken	TMP-SMX
Yersinia spp.*	Food (milk products, tofu), water	TMP-SMX Ceftriaxone (severe)
Entamoeba histolytica	Travel to endemic areas (food, water, fruit)	Metronidazole
Clostridium difficile	Antibiotic use, hospitalization, chemotherapy	Metronidazole Vancomycin Cholestyramine

TMP-SMX = trimethoprim-sulfamethoxazole.
*Mild-to-moderate symptoms do not require antibiotic therapy.

5. The use of empiric antibiotics in the treatment of acute diarrhea is potentially detrimental in what ways?
   Antibiotic therapy in patients with O157:H7 can precipitate the hemolytic uremia syndrome and, in patients with *Salmonella,* can prolong the chronic carrier state and increase relapse. Most patients with acute diarrhea do not require antibiotic therapy. Bacterial resistance is a significant problem in treating the bacterial organisms that cause diarrhea. Many of the diarrhea-causative bacterial organisms are resistant to the penicillins, tetracycline, and TMP/SMX. On the average, significant resistance is noted approximately 10 years following the introduction of an antibiotic.

6. What is loperamide?
   Loperamide is an antimotility agent that also has antisecretory properties. It is a peripherally acting opioid that does not cross the blood-brain barrier. Antimotility agents slow intestinal transit and increase intraluminal fluid and ion absorption.

7. Are antimotility agents contraindicated in patients with dysentery?
   Historically, treatment of dysentery with antimotility agents, such as diphenoxylate-atropine (Lomotil) and loperamide (Imodium), has been contraindicated. It was believed that reduced intestinal motility would worsen dysentery by slowing pathogen clearance. Recent studies of

patients with shigellosis dysentery who were given a combination of loperamide and antibiotic therapy had a shortened duration of diarrhea without adverse effects. Antimotility agents contin to be contraindicated in children with dysentery because of recurrent adverse case reports.

38. **Several members of a family develop nausea, emesis, and watery diarrhea 2–(hours after a picnic. Food at the picnic included ham, rice, and custard pie. What type of bacteria is likely to be the cause?**

   Enterotoxin-producing bacteria must be considered because the symptoms began soon after ingestion of the food. Two enterotoxin-producing bacteria that cause symptoms with such a she incubation are *Staphylococcus aureus* and *Bacillus cereus*. Coagulase-positive strains of *S. aureus* are responsible for many cases of food poisoning in the United States. *S. aureus* enterotoxin is heat-stable. The incubation period from ingestion to symptoms is approximately 3 hours (range = 1–6 hours). *S. aureus* favors growth in foods with high sugar content (e.g., custard) and high salt intake (e.g., ham). Recovery is generally complete in 24–48 hours. *B. cereus* is a spore-forming, gram-positive rod that produces a diarrheogenic, heat-labile enterotoxin. Vomiting can occur within 2 hours of ingestion of contaminated food. Almost all cases of *B. cereus* develop diarrhea. Meat and rice are the most common food vehicles for infection.

39. **What are the common causes of traveler's diarrhea?**

   More than 80% of these cases are secondary to a bacterial pathogen. *E. coli* (ETEC strains mos common), *Campylobacter, Salmonella*, and *Shigella* species account for most traveler's diarrhea.

40. **How can one avoid traveler's diarrhea?**

   "Safe" foods include steaming hot food and beverages, acidic foods such as citrus, dry foods, foods with high sugar content such as syrups and jellies, and carbonated drinks. Bottled, uncarbonated water is not always safe. Avoid uncooked vegetables and unpeeled fruits. Also consume only safe foods on airplanes that are departing from high-risk areas.
   Chemoprophylaxis with bismuth salicylate (2 tablets with meals and at bedtime) is effective in reducing diarrhea. Chemoprophylaxis should be given to persons with prior gastric surgery, those taking acid blocking medicines (H_2 blockers and proton pump inhibitors), or those debilitated and immunosuppressed. Travelers who cannot risk or afford a short illness while traveling may opt for chemoprophylaxis.

41. **Describe the treatment of traveler's diarrhea.**

   Patients with moderate-to-severe illness (e.g., daily activities restricted by diarrhea symptoms, fever, or bloody diarrhea) should be empirically treated with a fluoroquinolone antibiotic or TMP/SMX for 3–5 days to shorten the duration of symptoms. Bismuth subsalicylate is effective for mild-to-moderate diarrhea. Antimotility drugs can be used alone or with antibiotic therapy i adults but acute be avoided in children.

42. **What is cholera?**

   Cholera is a severe diarrheal disorder caused by *V. cholerae*, a gram-negative, comma-shaped bacteria. The illness is characterized by massive watery stool output, at times in excess of 1 L/h Dehydration, hypovolemic shock, and death occur rapidly if fluid replacement is not provided. The cholera organisms colonize the upper small bowel and release an enterotoxin that binds to and activates mucosal cyclic adenosine monophosphate (cAMP), which, in turn, activates chloride channels in mucosal crypts and leads to the massive secretory diarrhea. A second toxin, called the *zonula occludens toxin* (ZOT), increases intestinal permeability. The intestinal mucosa is not altered by the organism.

3. **How is cholera treated?**
Fluid replacement with either intravenous fluids or oral rehydration solution is the mainstay of therapy. A 2-day course of tetracycline is also beneficial.

4. **What is oral rehydration solution? How does it work?**
Oral rehydration solution (ORS) is composed primarily of water, salt, and glucose (1 liter of purified water combined with 20 gm of glucose, 3.5 gm of sodium chloride, 2.5 gm of sodium bicarbonate, and 1.5 gm of potassium chloride). Glucose enhances sodium and water absorption across the small bowel villi, even in the presence of cholera enterotoxin. Rice starch can be substituted for glucose.

5. **What is a BRAT diet?**
BRAT stands for bananas, rice, applesauce, and toast. This diet, with its avoidance of dairy products, because a transient lactase deficiency may occur, is often recommended to patients with gastroenteritis and diarrhea.

6. **What viruses cause acute diarrhea?**
Acute viral gastroenteritis can be caused by caliciviruses (includes Norwalk-like viruses), Rotavirus, enteric adenoviruses, coronavirus, and astrovirus. Rotavirus is a common cause of acute diarrhea in patients <age 2. The Norwalk-like virus can cause widespread community outbreaks that affect persons of all ages. Fecal-oral transmission has been implicated as the transmission route for viral gastroenteritis. Raw shellfish has been implicated in outbreaks of Norwalk infection.

7. **What are the clinical features of Rotavirus gastroenteritis? What tests are available for diagnosis?**
The clinical presentation of Rotavirus can range from an asymptomatic carrier state to severe dehydration that can lead to death. Children under age 2 are at greatest risk for infection. Following a 1- to 3-day incubation period, the Rotavirus illness is characterized by vomiting and diarrhea for 5–7 days. Rotavirus accounts for 25% of acute diarrhea among U.S. children. Rotavirus is more prevalent during cooler months. Adults can develop mild infection with Rotavirus. Commercial immunoassays are available to detect rotavirus in the stool.

8. **You are on your honeymoon cruise, and 25% (300 people) of the ship's occupants are afflicted with acute gastroenteritis. What is the most likely causative agent?**
The most likely agent is a Norwalk-like virus. Norwalk-like viruses are single-stranded RNA viruses in the family of *Caliciviridae*. Most nonbacterial gastroenteritic illnesses are caused by Norwalk-like viruses.

9. **What are the factors that contribute to high attack rates of Norwalk-like viruses?**
- The virus can survive at varying temperatures.
- The infection dose is <100 viral particles.
- Viral shedding can be prolonged.
- There is a lack of long-term immunity following infection.
- The virus can be spread through fecal-oral, airborne, and fomite contact routes.

10. **What is Reiter's syndrome? Which enteric infections are associated with its development?**
Reiter's syndrome is a triad of arthritis, urethritis, and conjunctivitis. Infections with *Salmonella* spp., *Shigella* spp., *Campylobacter jejuni*, and *Yersinia enterocolitica* have been associated with

this syndrome. Approximately 80% of patients affected by Reiter's syndrome are HLA-B27 antigen-positive. The male-to-female ratio is 9:1.

INFLAMMATORY BOWEL DISEASE

51. **How does one differentiate between acute infectious dysentery and acute onset of inflammatory bowel disease as the cause of bloody diarrhea?**

The clinical symptoms and endoscopic findings of the colon are often similar in the two diagnoses. When evaluating a patient with bloody diarrhea, the clinician must use historic data, assess the patient's potential risk factors and associated symptoms, and evaluate endoscopic appearance, radiologic findings, and laboratory data to narrow the differential. Many of the infectious dysentery illnesses are self-limited in nature. Dysenteric illnesses that do not spontaneously resolve and are culture-negative should undergo investigation for inflammatory bowel disease. Inflammatory bowel disease should be considered in patients with any additional findings, such as oral apthous ulcers, sacroileitis, spinal or peripheral arthropathy, perianal or cutaneous fistulas, a palpable abdominal mass, erythema nodosum, or erythema gangrenosum.

52. **Can a mucosal biopsy obtained on flexible sigmoidoscopy assist in differentiating among acute bacterial dysentery, ulcerative colitis, and Crohn's disease?**

Yes. Biopsy findings are not 100% specific; however, there are distinguishing features among the three diseases:

- *Bacterial infection:* mucosal edema, neutrophilic infiltration of the superficial lamina propria, absence of plasmacytosis of the deep lamina propria, and preservation of the crypt architecture.
- *Ulcerative colitis:* crypt abscesses (clumps of neutrophils in the crypt lumen), chronic inflammation limited to the mucosa and submucosa, atrophy, and, possibly, dysplasia.
- *Crohn's disease:* the presence of granulomas is a hallmark finding; however, the absence of granulomas does not exclude Crohn's disease, because up to 50% of patients do not show granulomas on biopsy. Submucosal inflammation, focal ulceration, and patchy involvement in the biopsy specimen are also suggestive.

53. **What is toxic megacolon? What are its risk factors?**

Toxic megacolon is a complication of colitis manifested by acute dilatation of the colon, with associated fever, tachycardia, leukocytosis, anemia, and postural hypotension. Transmural inflammation interferes with colonic motility, leading to colonic dilation and risk for perforation. Severe idiopathic panulcerative colitis carries the highest risk for toxic megacolon, but it may occur with any severe colitis (e.g., amebiasis, shigellosis, EHEC, *C. difficile*, and *Campylobacter* spp.). Performance of barium enema or colonoscopy or the administration of antimotility agents (loperamide, diphenoxylate, anticholinergics, or opiates) in patients with severe colitis may precipitate toxic megacolon.

ISCHEMIC COLITIS

54. **How is acute bacterial dysentery differentiated from acute onset of ischemic colitis?**

The degree of bloody diarrhea is variable in patients with ischemic colitis, and it may be difficult to distinguish between the two diseases. Clinically, the patient with ischemic colitis complains of sudden-onset abdominal pain, and an acute abdominal series may show "thumbprinting" of the colonic mucosa.

Flexible sigmoidoscopy is the mainstay of diagnosis for ischemic colitis. The rectum is usually spared because of its collateral blood flow. Above the rectum, the mucosa becomes friable and edematous, and there may be hemorrhagic areas and ulcerations resembling those of Crohn's disease. Angiography is not generally helpful in the evaluation of ischemic colitis; ischemic colitis is a small-vessel disease (nonocclusive), as compared to mesenteric midgut ischemia of the small bowel, which involves thrombosis or embolism in the superior mesenteric artery (occlusive). A barium enema is contraindicated in patients with suspected ischemic colitis, because colonic expansion during barium instillation may promote further ischemia.

5. Name the segment of colon most commonly affected by ischemia.
The left colon is the segment most commonly affected (75%). The next most common segments are the transverse colon (15%) and right colon (5%). Although any area of the colon can be affected by ischemia, the rectum is rarely involved because of its rich blood supply.

6. What are the predisposing factors for ischemic colitis?
Most patients with ischemic colitis are middle-aged or elderly and have a history of atherosclerotic heart disease and/or peripheral vascular disease. Medications implicated in causing colonic ischemia include digitalis, nonsteroidal anti-inflammatory drugs, diuretics, vasopressin, gold compounds, and some cancer chemotherapeutic agents. Colonic ischemia is a common complication of surgical repair of an abdominal aortic aneurysm. During surgery, mucosal ischemia results from the prolonged low blood flow to the colon or from disruption of blood flow in the inferior mesenteric artery.

BIBLIOGRAPHY

1. Ali SA, Hill DR: Giardia intestinalis. Curr Opin Infect Dis 16:453–460, 2003.
2. Allos BM: Campylobacter jejuni infections: Update on emerging issues and trends. Clin Infect Dis 32:1201–1206, 2002.
3. American Academy of Pediatrics: Practice parameter: The management of acute gastroenteritis in young children. Pediatrics 97:424–435, 1996.
4. Bottone EJ: Yersinia enterocolitica: Overview and epidemiologic correlates. Microbes Infect 4:323–333, 1999.
5. Cohen J: Infectious diarrhea in human immunodeficiency virus. Gastroenterol Clin North Am 30:637–664, 2001.
6. Diagnosis and management of foodborne illnesses: A primer for physicians. MMWR Recomm Rep 50:1–69, 2001.
7. DuPont HL: Guidelines on acute infectious diarrhea in adults. Am J Gastroenterol 92:1962–1975, 1997.
8. Edwards BH: Salmonella and Shigella species. Clin Lab Med 19:469–487, 1999.
9. Eisen GM, Dominitz JA, Faigel DO, et al: Use of endoscopy in diarrheal illnesses. Gastrointest Endosc 54:821–823, 2001.
10. Farmer RG: Infectious causes of diarrhea in the differential diagnosis of inflammatory bowel disease. Med Clin North Am 74:29–38, 1990.
11. Greenberg SB: Serious waterborne and wilderness infections. Crit Care Clin 15:387–414, 1999.
12. Guerrant RL, Van Gilder T, Steiner TS, et al: Practice guidelines for the management of infectious diarrhea. Clin Infect Dis 32:331–351, 2001.
13. Haque R, Huston CD, Hughes M, et al: Amebiasis. N Engl J Med 348:1565–1573, 2003.
14. Lew EA, Poles MA, Dieterich DT: Diarrheal diseases associated with HIV infections. Gastroenterol Clin 26:259–290, 1997.
15. Ochoa TJ, Cleary TG: Epidemiology and spectrum of disease of Escherichia coli O157. Curr Opin Infect Dis 16:259–263, 2003.
16. Thielman NM, Guerrant RL: Acute infectious diarrhea. N Engl J Med 350:38–47, 2004.
17. Turgeon DK, Fritsche TR: Laboratory approaches to infectious diarrhea. Gastroenterol Clin North Am 30:693–707, 2001.
18. Wilhelmi I, Roman E, Sanchez-Fauquier A: Viruses causing gastroenteritis. Clin Microbiol Infect 9:247–262, 2003.

CHAPTER 57

CHRONIC DIARRHEA

Lawrence R. Schiller, MD

1. **Define *chronic diarrhea*.**

   Diarrhea is defined as an increase in the frequency and fluidity of stools. For most patients, diarrhea means the passage of loose stools. Although loose stool is often accompanied by an increase in the frequency of bowel movements, most patients do not classify the frequent passage of formed stools as diarrhea. Because stool consistency is difficult to quantitate, many investigators use frequency of defecation as a quantitative criterion for diarrhea. By this standard, passage of more than two bowel movements per day is considered abnormal. Some authors also incorporate stool weight in the definition of diarrhea. Normal stool weight averages approximately 80 gm/day in women and 100 gm/day in men. The upper limit of normal stool weight (calculated as the mean plus two standard deviations) is approximately 200 gm/day. Normal stool weight depends on dietary intake, and some patients on high-fiber diets exceed 200 gm/day without reporting diarrhea. Thus, stool weight by itself is an imperfect criterion.

2. **Summarize the criteria for diagnosis of diarrhea.**

   See Table 57-1.

TABLE 57-1. CRITERIA FOR DIAGNOSIS OF DIARRHEA

Criterion	Normal Range	Diarrhea, If
Increased stool frequency	2–14 stools per week	>2 stools per day
More liquid stool consistency	Soft–formed stools	Loose–unformed
Increased stool weight		
Men	0–240 gm/24 hr	>240 gm/24 hr
Women	0–180 gm/24 hr	>180 gm/24 hr

3. **What other disorder may be described as "diarrhea"?**

   Occasionally, patients with fecal incontinence describe the problem as "diarrhea," even when stools are formed. Physicians must be careful to distinguish fecal incontinence from diarrhea, because incontinence is usually due to problems with the muscles and nerves regulating continence.

4. **What is the basic mechanism of all diarrheal diseases?**

   Diarrhea is due to the incomplete absorption of fluid from luminal contents. Normal stools are approximately 75% water and 25% solids. Normal fecal water output is approximately 60–80 mL/day. An increase in fecal water output of 50–100 mL is sufficient to cause loosening of the stool. This volume represents approximately 1% of the fluid load entering the upper intestine each day; thus, malabsorption of only 1% or 2% of fluid entering the intestine may be sufficient to cause diarrhea (Fig. 57-1).

5. **What pathologic processes can cause diarrhea?**

   Excessive stool water is due to the presence of some solute that osmotically obligates water retention within the lumen. This solute may be a poorly absorbed, osmotically active

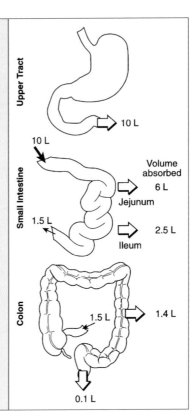

Figure 57-1. Fluid loads through the intestine. Each day approximately 9–10 L of fluid pass into the jejunum. This fluid consists of approximately 2 L of ingested food and drink, 1.5 L of saliva, 2.5 L of gastric juice, 1.5 L of bile, and 2.5 L of pancreatic juice. The jejunum absorbs most of this load as nutrients are taken up, and the ileum absorbs most of the rest. The colon absorbs more than 90% of the fluid load reaching it, leaving only 1% of the original fluid entering the jejunum to be excreted in stool. Substantial fluid malabsorption in the small bowel can overwhelm colonic absorptive capacity and may result in diarrhea. Less severe disruption of colonic absorption can lead to diarrhea because of the lack of a more distal absorbing segment. A reduction of absorptive efficiency of only 1% for the total intestine can result in diarrhea.

substance, such as magnesium ions, or an accumulation of ordinary electrolytes, such as sodium or potassium, that are normally absorbed easily by the intestine. When excessive stool water is due to ingestion of a poorly absorbed substance, the diarrhea is called *osmotic diarrhea*. Examples include lactose malabsorption and diarrhea induced by osmotic laxatives. When the excessive stool water results from the presence of excessive electrolytes due to reduction of electrolyte absorption or stimulation of electrolyte secretion, the diarrhea is known as *secretory diarrhea*. Causes of secretory diarrhea include infection, particularly infections that produce toxins that reduce intestinal fluid electrolyte absorption; reduction of mucosal surface area due to disease or surgery; absence of an ion transport mechanism; inflammation of the mucosa; ingestion of drugs or poisons; endogenous secretagogues, such as bile acids; dysfunction due to abnormal regulation by nerves and hormones; and tumors producing circulating secretagogues.

6. **List three classifications of diarrheal diseases.**
   Several schemes have been proposed, three of which can be useful clinically:
   1. Differentiate between acute and chronic diarrheal diseases. Most cases of acute diarrhea are due to infections that are self-limited and run their courses over a few weeks. Diarrheas that last longer are probably due to some other mechanism. For practical purposes, a duration of 4 weeks can be used to differentiate acute and chronic diarrheas.
   2. Categorize the diarrhea by epidemiologic characteristics (*see* question 7).
   3. Divide diarrheal diseases by the characteristics of the stools produced. In this scheme diarrheas are classified as watery, fatty, or inflammatory (*see* questions 8–11). These

distinctions are based on the gross characteristics of the stool and laboratory testing when appropriate. Watery stools are typically runny and lack blood, pus, or fat. Watery diarrhea is subdivided into secretory or osmotic, depending on stool electrolyte concentrations. Fatty stools have an excess of fat, which can be shown by qualitative testing with the Sudan stain or by quantitative analysis of a timed stool collection for fat. Inflammatory diarrheas contain typically blood or pus. If not grossly evident, these characteristics can be detected by a fecal occult blood test or by staining the stool for neutrophils. Classifying diarrheas by stool characteristics enables the physician to sort quickly through more likely and less likely diagnoses. This scheme is thus quite useful in chronic diarrheas in which construction of a reasonable differential diagnosis can lead to more appropriate testing and more rapid diagnosis.

7. **What are the likely causes of diarrhea, according to epidemiologic characteristics?**

Travelers
- Bacterial infection (mostly acute)
- Protozoal infections (e.g., amebiasis, giardiasis)
- Tropical sprue

Epidemics/Outbreaks
- Bacterial infection
- Viral infection (e.g., Rotavirus)
- Protozoal infections (e.g., cryptosporidiosis)
- Brainerd diarrhea (epidemic idiopathic secretory diarrhea)

Patients with AIDS
- Opportunistic infections (e.g., cryptosporidiosis, cytomegalovirus, herpes, *Mycobacterium avium* complex)
- Drug side effect
- Lymphoma

Institutionalized Patients
- *Clostridium difficile* toxin-mediated colitis
- Food poisoning
- Fecal impaction with overflow diarrhea
- Tube feeding
- Drug side effect

8. **What are the likely causes of osmotic watery diarrhea?**
Osmotic laxatives (e.g., Mg^{2+}, PO_4^{-3}, SO_4^{-2}) and carbohydrate malabsorption.

9. **List the likely causes of secretory watery diarrhea.**
- Congenital syndromes (e.g., congenital chloridorrhea)
- Bacterial toxins
- Ileal bile acid malabsorption
- Inflammatory bowel disease (ulcerative colitis, Crohn's disease, microscopic colitis [lymphocytic and collagenous], diverticulitis)
- Vasculitis
- Drugs and poisons
- Laxative abuse (stimulant laxatives)
- Disordered motility/regulation (postvagotomy diarrhea, postsympathectomy diarrhea, diabetic autonomic neuropathy, irritable bowel syndrome)
- Endocrine diarrhea (hyperthyroidism, Addison's disease, gastrinoma, vipoma, somatostatinoma, carcinoid syndrome, medullary carcinoma of the thyroid, mastocytosis)
- Other tumors (colon carcinoma, lymphoma, villous adenoma)
- Idiopathic secretory diarrhea (epidemic secretory [Brainerd] diarrhea, sporadic idiopathic secretory diarrhea)

0. List the likely causes of inflammatory diarrhea.
- Inflammatory bowel disease (ulcerative colitis, Crohn's disease, diverticulitis, ulcerative jejunoileitis)
- Infectious diseases (pseudomembranous colitis, invasive bacterial infections [e.g., tuberculosis, yersiniosis], ulcerating viral infections [e.g., cytomegalovirus, herpes simplex], invasive parasitic infections [e.g., amebiasis, strongyloides])
- Ischemic colitis
- Radiation colitis
- Neoplasia: colon cancer, lymphoma

1. List the likely causes of fatty diarrhea.
Malabsorption Syndromes
- Mucosal diseases (e.g., celiac disease, Whipple's disease)
- Small bowel bacterial overgrowth
- Mesenteric ischemia
- Short bowel syndrome

Maldigestion
- Pancreatic exocrine insufficiency
- Inadequate luminal bile acid concentration

2. Summarize the initial diagnostic scheme for patients with chronic diarrhea.
The scheme in Figure 57-2 is based on a careful history, looking for specific physical findings, and simple laboratory data to help classify the diarrhea as watery, fatty, or inflammatory. The value of obtaining a quantitative (as opposed to a spot) stool collection is debated among experts. A quantitative collection over 48 or 72 hours permits a better estimation of fluid, electrolyte, and fat excretion but is not absolutely necessary to the appropriate classification of diarrhea.

3. How do you distinguish secretory and osmotic watery diarrhea?
The most useful way to differentiate secretory and osmotic types of watery diarrhea is to measure fecal electrolytes and calculate the fecal osmotic gap. In many diarrheal conditions, sodium and potassium, with their accompanying anions, are the dominant electrolytes in stool water. Secretory diarrhea is characterized by failure to absorb electrolytes completely or actual electrolyte secretion by the intestine. Sodium, potassium, and their accompanying anions are responsible for the bulk of osmotic activity in stool water and the retention of water within the gut lumen. In contrast, in osmotic diarrhea, ingestion of poorly absorbed osmotically active substances is responsible for holding water within the gut lumen. Electrolyte absorption is normal; thus, sodium and potassium concentrations may become quite low (Fig. 57-3). The fecal osmotic gap calculation takes advantage of these distinctions to differentiate the two conditions.

4. How is the fecal osmotic gap calculated?
First, measure sodium and potassium in stool water. The sum of the concentrations of these two ions is multiplied by 2 to account for the anions that are also present. The product is then subtracted from 290 mOsm/kg, the approximate osmolality of luminal contents within the intestine. This number is a constant because the relatively high permeability of the intestinal mucosa beyond the stomach means that osmotic equilibration has taken place by the time luminal contents reach the rectum. As an example, let us assume that a patient with watery diarrhea has a sodium concentration of 75 mmol/L and a potassium concentration of 65 mmol/L in stool water. Adding the two values yields a concentration of 140 mmol/L. Doubling this value to account for anions means that electrolytes account for 280 mOsm/kg of stool water osmolality. Subtracting this value from 290 mOsm/kg yields an osmotic gap of 10 mOsm/kg.

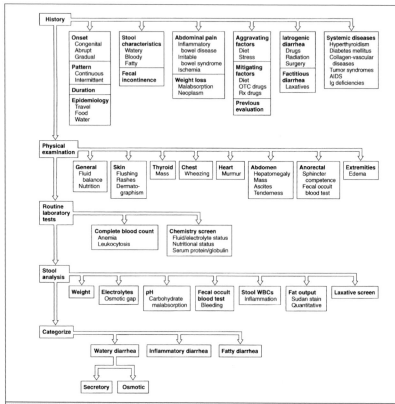

Figure 57-2. The initial evaluation plan for patients with chronic diarrhea is aimed at assessing the severity of the problem, looking for clues to etiology, and classifying the diarrhea as watery (with subtypes of osmotic and secretory diarrhea), inflammatory, or fatty. (From Fine KD, Schiller LR: AGA technical review on the evaluation and management of chronic diarrhea. Gastroenterology 116:1464–1486, 1999, with permission.)

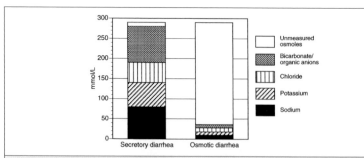

Figure 57-3. Electrolyte patterns differ between osmotic and secretory diarrhea. In secretory diarrhea, electrolytes account for the bulk of the osmotic activity of stool water. In contrast, in osmotic diarrhea, electrolyte absorption is normal; therefore, electrolyte concentrations are very low. Most of the osmotic activity is due to unmeasured osmoles. (Bicarbonate concentrations are "virtual" and are not measurable directly in most circumstances because of reaction with organic acids generated by fermentation by colonic bacteria.)

5. **How is the fecal osmotic gap interpreted?**

   Fecal osmotic gaps <50 mOsm/kg correlate well with diarrheas due to electrolyte secretion (or poor absorption). In contrast, if stool sodium is 10 mmol/L and potassium concentration is 20 mmol/L, the combined contribution of cations and anions in stool water is only 60 mOsm/kg, yielding a fecal osmotic gap of 230 mOsm/kg. This value represents the amount of some unmeasured substance that is contributing to fecal osmolality, presumably some poorly absorbed substance that is ingested but not absorbed. Fecal osmotic gaps >50 mOsm/kg are associated with osmotic diarrheas.

6. **What precaution is necessary in measuring fecal osmotic gap?**

   Be certain that the stool has not been contaminated with either water or urine. Dilution by water or hypotonic urine falsely lowers fecal electrolyte concentrations and elevates the calculated osmotic gap. This problem can be detected by actually measuring fecal osmolality; values that are substantially less than 290 mOsm/kg indicate dilution. Contamination with hypertonic urine may also affect fecal electrolyte concentrations, but it is harder to detect unless the sum of measured cations and assumed anions is much greater than 290 mmol/L.

7. **How does one evaluate osmotic diarrhea?**

   Osmotic diarrheas are typically due to ingestion of poorly absorbed cations, such as magnesium, or anions, such as sulfate. In addition, carbohydrate malabsorption, such as that due to ingestion of lactose in patients with lactase deficiency and ingestion of poorly absorbable sugar alcohols (e.g., sorbitol), can lead to osmotic diarrhea. Measuring stool pH can help distinguish between osmotic diarrheas due to poorly absorbed cations and anions and those due to ingestion of poorly absorbed carbohydrates and sugar alcohols. Carbohydrates and sugar alcohols are fermented by colonic bacteria, reducing fecal pH to <5 due to production of short chain fatty acids. In contrast, ingestion of poorly absorbed cations and anions does not have a significant effect on stool pH, which is typically 7. Once acidic stools have been discovered, check the diet and inquire about food additives and osmotic laxative ingestion. Specific testing for magnesium and other ions in stool is readily available to confirm any suspicions (Fig. 57-4).

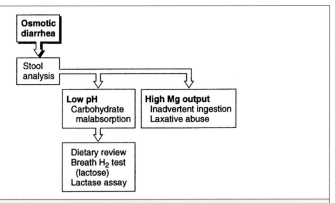

Figure 57-4. Once a diagnosis of osmotic diarrhea is made, evaluation is fairly straightforward. Only a few etiologies are possible. (From Fine KD, Schiller LR: AGA technical review on the evaluation and management of chronic diarrhea. Gastroenterology 116:1464–1486, 1999, with permission.)

8. **Describe the evaluation of chronic secretory diarrhea.**

   Because there are many causes of chronic secretory diarrhea, an extensive evaluation is possible (Fig. 57-5). Rare cases of infection should be excluded by bacterial culture and examination of stool for parasites. Stimulant laxative abuse is best excluded by looking for

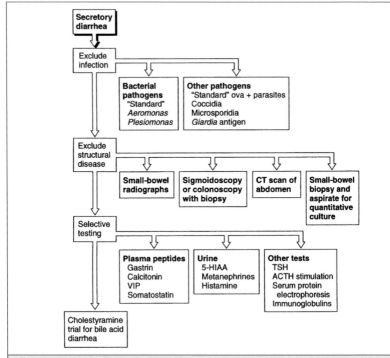

Figure 57-5. Evaluation of secretory diarrhea can be quite complex. This "mind map" can be used to guide the evaluation, depending on the specifics of each case. Not every test needs to be done in every patient. (From Fine KD, Schiller LR: AGA technical review on the evaluation and management of chronic diarrhea. Gastroenterology 116:1464–1486, 1999, with permission.)

laxatives in the urine or stool. Structural disease and internal fistulas can be evaluated with small bowel radiography and CT scanning of the abdomen and pelvis. Endoscopic examination of the upper gastrointestinal tract and colon is occasionally helpful and should include biopsy of even normal-appearing mucosa, looking for microscopic evidence of disease. Systemic diseases, such as hyperthyroidism, adrenal insufficiency, and defective immunity, can be evaluated with appropriate tests (*see* question 19).

19. **Summarize the tests for evaluation of systemic diseases associated with chronic secretory diarrhea.**
   See Table 57-2.

20. **When should neuroendocrine tumors be suspected as a cause of chronic secretory diarrhea?**
   Neuroendocrine tumors are an uncommon cause of chronic secretory diarrhea. For example, one vipoma may be expected per 10 million people per year. Table 57-3 lists these tumors and their markers. Because of their rarity as a cause for chronic diarrhea, other causes should first be considered. If tumor is visualized by CT scan, or if systemic symptoms (e.g., flushing) are present, evaluation for neuroendocrine tumors may have a better yield. Blanket testing for tumor-associated peptides is likely to yield many more false-positives than true-positives and can therefore be quite misleading.

TABLE 57–2. TESTS FOR EVALUATION OF SYSTEMIC DISEASES ASSOCIATED WITH CHRONIC SECRETORY DIARRHEA

Condition	Diagnostic Tests
Endocrine diseases	
Hyperthyroidism	Thyroid-stimulating hormone, T_4
Addison's disease	ACTH-stimulation test, cortisol
Panhypopituitarism	ACTH-stimulation test, TSH
Diabetes mellitus	Blood glucose, glycosylated hemoglobin
Endocrine tumor syndromes	
MEN-1 (Werner's syndrome)	
Hyperparathyroidism	Parathormone
Pancreatic endocrine tumors	Gastrin, VIP, insulin, glucagon
Pituitary tumors	Prolactin, growth hormone, ACTH
(may also have adrenal cortical tumors, thyroid adenomas)	
MEN-2a (Sipple's syndrome)	
Medullary thyroid cancer	Calcitonin
Pheochromocytoma	Urine metanephrine
Hyperparathyroidism	Parathormone
MEN-2b (same as MEN-2a + neuromas, marfanoid phenotype)	
Hematologic diseases	
Leukemia, lymphoma	Complete blood count
Multiple myeloma	Serum protein electrophoresis
Immune system disorders	
AIDS	HIV serology
Amyloidosis	Mucosal biopsy
Common variable immunodeficiency, IgA deficiency	Immunoglobulin levels
Heavy metal poisoning	Heavy metal screen

T_4 = thyroxine, ACTH = adrenocorticotropic hormone, TSH = thyroid-stimulating hormone, MEN= multiple endocrine neoplasia, VIP = vasoactive intestinal polypeptide, AIDS = acquired immunodeficiency syndrome, HIV= human immunodeficiency virus.

1. **What is Bayes' theorem? How does it relate to peptide-secreting tumors?**
   Bayes' theorem links the prevalence of the diagnosis to the positive predictive value of a diagnostic test. The positive predictive value of a test depends on the likelihood of the condition in the population to be screened, not only on the accuracy of the test. For example, peptide-secreting tumors are a rare cause of chronic diarrhea, with a prevalence of 1/5000 to 1/500,000 patients with chronic diarrhea, depending on tumor type. The following is a simplified formula for Bayes' theorem:

$$\text{Posttest odds} = \text{pretest odds} \times \text{likelihood ratio}$$

TABLE 57-3. NEUROENDOCRINE TUMORS CAUSING CHRONIC DIARRHEA AND THEIR MARKERS

Tumor	Typical Symptoms	Mediator/ Tumor Marker
Gastrinoma	Zollinger-Ellison syndrome: pancreatic or duodenal tumor, peptic ulcer, steatorrhea, diarrhea	Gastrin
Vipoma	Verner-Morrison syndrome: watery diarrhea, hypokalemia, achlorhydria, flushing	Vasoactive intestinal polypeptide
Medullary thyroid carcinoma	Thyroid mass, hypermotility	Calcitonin, prostaglandins
Pheochromocytoma	Adrenal mass, hypertension	Vasoactive intestinal polypeptide, norepinephrine, epinephrine
Carcinoid	Flushing, wheezing, right-sided cardiac valvular disease	Serotonin, kinins
Somatostatinoma	Nonketotic diabetes mellitus, steatorrhea, diabetes, gallstones	Somatostatin
Glucagonoma	Skin rash (migratory necrotizing erythema), mild diabetes	Glucagon
Mastocytosis	Flushing, dermatographism, nausea, vomiting, abdominal pain	Histamine

where the likelihood ratio = true-positive/true-negative result. Because the pretest odds of a peptide-secreting tumor are so long, and the false-positive rate of serum peptide assays for peptide-secreting tumors is so high (approximately 45%), the positive predictive value for serum peptide assays is substantially less than 1%. An abnormal result would be misleading more than 99% of the time.

22. **What is the likely outcome in patients with chronic secretory diarrhea in whom a diagnosis cannot be reached?**
Diagnostic testing may fail to reveal a cause for chronic diarrhea in up to 25% of patients with chronic diarrhea, depending on referral bias and extent of evaluation. Patients with continuous idiopathic secretory diarrhea have remarkably similar courses. In most cases, diarrhea begins suddenly, is associated with some initial weight loss, and resolves in 1–2 years without recurrence. It is therefore preferable to treat patients symptomatically rather than to repeat diagnostic testing once a thorough evaluation has been concluded.

23. **Describe the evaluation of chronic fatty diarrhea.**
Chronic fatty diarrhea is due to either maldigestion or malabsorption. Maldigestion can occur with pancreatic exocrine insufficiency or a bile acid deficiency that reduces fat emulsification. Malabsorption is typically due to mucosal diseases such as celiac disease, bacterial overgrowth, or small bowel fistula or resection.

Pancreatic exocrine insufficiency can be evaluated with a secretin test, or stool chymotrypsin or elastase measurement. Because these tests are not widely available or have poor specificity and sensitivity, clinicians often resort to a therapeutic trial of pancreatic enzymes. The patient should be treated with a high dose of enzymes, and the effect of treatment on stool fat excretion as well as symptoms should be assessed.

Bile acid deficiency, a rare cause of maldigestion, is best assessed by measuring postprandially the bile acid concentration in duodenal contents. Tests showing excessive bile acid excretion in stool (radiolabeled bile acid excretion or total bile acid excretion tests) do not directly assess duodenal bile acid concentration, but if fecal bile acid excretion is high, reduced duodenal bile acid concentration can be inferred. Mucosal disease can be evaluated with small bowel biopsy, and bacterial overgrowth can be assessed by breath hydrogen testing after an oral glucose load or by quantitative culture of intestinal contents (Fig. 57-6).

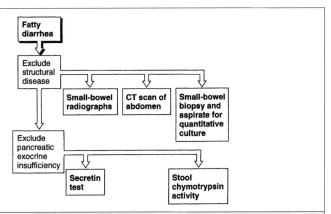

Figure 57-6. Evaluation of chronic fatty diarrhea is designed to determine whether malabsorption or maldigestion is the cause of excessive fecal fat excretion. (From Fine KD, Schiller LR: AGA technical review on the evaluation and management of chronic diarrhea. Gastroenterology 116:1464–1486, 1999, with permission.)

24. How does one make a diagnosis of celiac disease?

Celiac disease is a common cause of chronic fatty diarrhea but may be present without causing diarrhea. Serologic testing for immunoglobulin (Ig)A antibodies to tissue transglutaminase is the preferred indirect test, but mucosal biopsy remains the gold standard for diagnosis. Antigluten antibodies are less specific and sensitive but can be used to follow adherence to a gluten-free diet (the titer should decrease with adherence to the diet). Patients with IgA deficiency (approximately 10% of the population with celiac disease) will not have IgA antibodies against tissue transglutaminase or gluten, so a negative serologic test does not exclude the diagnosis of celiac disease.

25. Describe the further evaluation of chronic inflammatory diarrhea.

Inflammatory diarrheas can be due to idiopathic inflammatory bowel diseases, such as ulcerative colitis or Crohn's disease; invasive chronic infectious diseases, such as tuberculosis or yersiniosis; ischemic colitis; radiation colitis; or some tumors. To sort through these diagnoses, the most appropriate tests include sigmoidoscopy or colonoscopy to visually inspect the colonic mucosa, colonic biopsy to look for microscopic evidence of inflammation, small bowel radiography or CT scanning of the abdomen, and special cultures for chronic infections, such as tuberculosis or yersiniosis. In most cases the diagnosis becomes apparent after these tests are completed (Fig. 57-7).

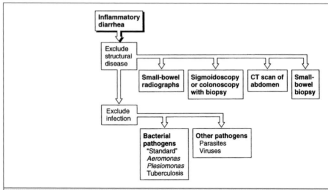

Figure 57-7. Chronic inflammatory diarrhea has a diverse differential diagnosis. Structural evaluation with endoscopic or radiographic techniques often yields a diagnosis. Mucosal biopsy may be needed to confirm the diagnosis. (From Fine KD, Schiller LR: AGA technical review on the evaluation and management of chronic diarrhea. Gastroenterology 116:1464–1486, 1999, with permission.)

26. **How does one distinguish irritable bowel syndrome from chronic diarrhea?**
    The diagnosis of irritable bowel syndrome should be based on the presence of abdominal pain associated with defecation and abnormal bowel habits. Chronic continuous diarrhea in the absence of pain is not irritable bowel syndrome, although it may be functional in nature. The diagnosis of irritable bowel syndrome can be based on symptomatic criteria, the Rome criteria. The most recent iteration of these criteria ("Rome II") includes the presence of abdominal pain or discomfort for at least 12 of the preceding 12 months that is characterized by at least two of the following three features: (1) relieved by defecation, (2) onset associated with a change in stool frequency, or (3) onset associated with a change in stool form or consistency.

27. **What causes of chronic diarrhea may be difficult to diagnose?**
    - Fecal incontinence
    - Iatrogenic diarrhea (drugs, surgery, radiation)
    - Surreptitious laxative ingestion
    - Microscopic colitis syndrome
    - Bile acid-induced diarrhea
    - Small bowel bacterial overgrowth
    - Pancreatic exocrine insufficiency
    - Carbohydrate malabsorption
    - Peptide-secreting tumors
    - Chronic idiopathic secretory diarrhea

    These conditions are seen in referral centers after routine evaluation has not disclosed a diagnosis. In general, the necessary tests are not difficult but have not been done because physicians have not considered these disorders in the differential diagnosis of chronic diarrhea.

28. **What are common causes of iatrogenic diarrhea?**
    Most iatrogenic diarrheas are due to ingestion of drugs, some of which may not commonly cause diarrhea. About two thirds of the drugs listed in the *Physician's Desk Reference* mention diarrhea as a possible side effect. Therefore, the physician should obtain a history of all ingested drugs, including prescription medications, over-the-counter drugs, and herbal remedies (Table 57-4). Other causes of iatrogenic diarrhea include operations, such as vagotomy, gastrectomy, and cholecystectomy, and radiation therapy during which the intestine is exposed to high doses of ionizing radiation.

29. **What features should suggest surreptitious laxative ingestion?**
    Some patients who present with chronic diarrhea have diarrhea due to laxative abuse. In general, four groups of patients have this diagnosis:

TABLE 57-4. DRUGS ASSOCIATED WITH DIARRHEA	
Antibiotics (most)	Antacids (e.g., containing magnesium)
Antineoplastic agents (many)	Acid-reducing agents (e.g., H_2-receptor antagonists, proton pump inhibitors)
Anti-inflammatory agents (e.g., NSAIDs, gold, 5-aminosalicylates)	Prostaglandin (e.g., misoprostol)
Antiarrhythmics (e.g., quinidine)	Vitamin/mineral supplements
Antihypertensives (e.g., beta-receptor blocking drugs)	Herbal products

- Patients with bulimia: usually adolescent to young adult women concerned about weight or manifesting an eating disorder.
- Secondary gain: pending disability claim, induction of concern or caring behavior in others.
- Munchausen's syndrome: peripatetic patients who relish being diagnostic challenges; may undergo extensive testing repeatedly.
- Polle's syndrome (Munchausen's syndrome by proxy): dependent child or adult poisoned with laxatives by parent or caregiver to show effectiveness as caregiver; may have history of sibling who died with chronic diarrhea.

  Laxatives can be detected by chemical testing of stool or urine. The diagnosis should be confirmed before confronting the patient, and psychiatric consultation should be available to help with further management.

30. **What is microscopic colitis syndrome?**
Microscopic colitis is a syndrome characterized by chronic secretory diarrhea, a normal gross appearance of the colonic mucosa, and a typical pattern of inflammation in colon biopsy specimens. This pattern includes changes of the surface epithelium (flattening and irregularity), intraepithelial lymphocytosis, and an increased density of inflammatory cells in the lamina propria. There are two varieties: (1) collagenous colitis, in which the subepithelial collagen layer is thickened, and (2) lymphocytic colitis, in which the subepithelial collagen layer is of normal thickness. Microscopic colitis occurs frequently in older patients and is often associated with fecal incontinence. In many cases an actual or suspected rheumatologic disease is present. Treatment is variably effective, but budesonide, bile-acid-binding resins, and bismuth subsalicylate (Pepto-Bismol) have the greatest reported response rates in controlled trials.

31. **Define *bile acid diarrhea*.**
In patients with ileal resection or disease, the part of the small intestine with high-affinity bile acid transporters has been removed or is dysfunctional. Thus, excessive bile acid finds its way into the colon. If the bile acid concentration in colonic contents reaches a critical level of approximately 3–5 mmol/L, salt and water absorption by the colonic mucosa is inhibited and diarrhea results. Patients who have had extensive small bowel resections (>100 cm) often have so much fluid entering the colon that this critical bile acid level is not reached (Fig. 57-8).

  In addition to this classic form of diarrhea due to bile acid malabsorption, some investigators have speculated that in many patients with an intact ileum, bile acid malabsorption drives chronic diarrhea. Although tests of bile acid absorption are frequently abnormal in patients with idiopathic diarrhea, treatment with bile acid-sequestering resins, such as cholestyramine, is not often as effective in this group of patients as in those who have had surgical resection of the ileum.

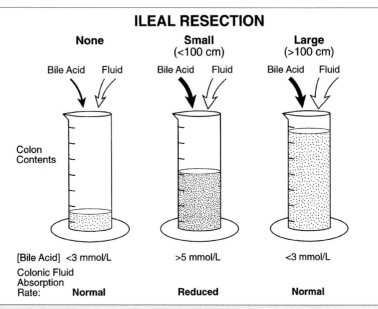

Figure 57-8. Bile acid diarrhea occurs when bile acid malabsorption in the ileum is linked with relatively low fluid flows into the colon. As a result, the concentration of bile acid in colon contents is greater than the cathartic threshold of 3–5 mmol/L. If fluid flows are high (as with substantial small bowel resection), bile acid malabsorption may be just as severe, but bile acid concentrations are not high enough to impair absorption by the colon.

32. **What is the likely outcome in idiopathic secretory diarrhea?**
    Patients with chronic secretory diarrhea that evades a serious diagnostic evaluation may have a similar history of previous good health with sudden onset of diarrhea, often accompanied by acute but not progressive, weight loss. Although acute onset suggests an acute infectious process, patients have negative microbiologic studies and do not respond to empiric antibiotics. Diarrhea persists usually for 12–30 months and then gradually subsides. This condition can be sporadic or occur in epidemics. The epidemic form (Brainerd diarrhea) seems to be associated with ingestion of potentially contaminated food or drink, but no organism has been implicated. Management consists of the effective use of nonspecific antidiarrheals until the process subsides.

33. **What is the best nonspecific therapy for chronic diarrhea?**
    Because the evaluation of chronic diarrhea may extend over several weeks and the diagnosis is not always forthcoming, patients may need symptomatic therapy. The most effective agents are opiates. Traditional antidiarrheal agents, such as diphenoxylate and loperamide, work well in many patients but should be given on a routine schedule in patients with chronic diarrhea rather than on an as-needed basis. Typical doses of 1–2 tablets or capsules before meals and at bedtime improve symptoms in most people. When this therapy is ineffective, more potent opiates, such as codeine, opium, or morphine, can be used. With the stronger agents, doses should be low at first, and increased gradually so that tolerance to the central nervous system effects can develop. Fortunately, the gut does not become tolerant to these agents; thus, one can usually find a dose that controls symptoms without producing severe side effects. Other agents sometimes used to manage chronic diarrhea include clonidine, octreotide, and cholestyramine, but they tend to be less effective than opiates and are often less well tolerated by patients, making them second-line agents in most circumstances (Table 57-5).

TABLE 57-5. NONSPECIFIC THERAPY FOR CHRONIC DIARRHEA

Agent	Dose
Opiates	
μ-opiate receptor selective	
Diphenoxylate	2.5–5 mg 4 times/day
Loperamide	2–4 mg 4 times/day
Codeine	15–60 mg 4 times/day
Morphine	2–20 mg 4 times/day
Opium tincture	2–20 drops 4 times/day
δ-opiate receptor selective	
Racecadotril (acetorphan)	1.5 mg/kg 3 times/day*
Adrenergic agonist	
Clonidine	0.1–0.3 mg 3 times/day
Somatostatin analog	
Octreotide	50–250 μg 3 times/day (subcutaneously)
Bile acid-binding resin	
Cholestyramine	4 gm 1–4 times/day

*Not yet approved in the United States.

WEBSITE

http://www.guideline.gov/

Search "diarrhea"

BIBLIOGRAPHY

1. Afzalpurkar RG, Schiller LR, Little KH, et al: The self-limited nature of chronic idiopathic diarrhea. N Engl J Med 327:1849–1852, 1992.

2. Arrambide KA, Santa Ana CA, Schiller LR, et al: Loss of absorptive capacity for sodium chloride as a cause of diarrhea following partial ileal and right colon resection. Dig Dis Sci 34:193–201, 1989.

3. Bernstein CN, Riddell RH: Colonoscopy plus biopsy in the inflammatory bowel diseases. Gastrointest Endosc Clin North Am 10:755–774, 2000.

4. Bini EJ, Weinshel EH: Endoscopic evaluation of chronic human immunodeficiency virus-related diarrhea: Is colonoscopy superior to flexible sigmoidoscopy? Am J Gastroenterol 93:56–60, 1998.

5. Brandt LJ, Greenwald D (eds): Acute and Chronic Diarrhea: A Primer on Diagnosis and Treatment. Arlington, VA, American College of Gastroenterology, 1997.

6. Camilleri M: Chronic diarrhea: A review on pathophysiology and management for the clinical gastroenterologist. Clin Gastroenterol Hepatol 2:198–206, 2004.

7. Chande N, McDonald JW, MacDonald JK: Interventions for treating collagenous colitis. Cochrane Database Syst Rev 3:CD003575, 2003.

8. Donowitz M, Kokke FT, Saidi R: Evaluation of patients with chronic diarrhea. N Engl J Med 332:725–729, 1995.

9. Eherer AJ, Fordtran JS: Fecal osmotic gap and pH in experimental diarrhea of various causes. Gastroenterology 103:545–551, 1992.

10. Farthing MJ: Oral rehydration therapy: An evolving solution. J Pediatr Gastroenterol Nutr 34(Suppl 1):S64–S67 2002.

11. Field M: Intestinal ion transport and the pathophysiology of diarrhea. J Clin Invest 111:931–943, 2003.

12. Fine KD, Schiller LR: AGA technical review on the evaluation and management of chronic diarrhea. Gastroenterology 116:1464–1486, 1999.

13. Freeman HJ: Small intestinal mucosal biopsy for investigation of diarrhea and malabsorption in adults. Gastrointest Endosc Clin North Am 10:739–753, 2000.

14. Giannella RA: Infections of the intestine. In Feldman M, Schiller LR (eds): Gastroenterology and Hepatology: The Comprehensive Visual Reference, vol 7, Small Intestine. Philadelphia, Current Medicine, 1997, pp 12.1–12.19.

15. Green PH, Jabri B: Coeliac disease. Lancet 362:383–391, 2003.

16. Loftus EV: Microscopic colitis: Epidemiology and treatment. Am J Gastroenterol 98(Suppl 12):S31–S36, 2003.

17. Powell DW: Approach to the patient with diarrhea. In Textbook of Gastroenterology, 4th ed. Philadelphia, Lippincott Williams & Wilkins, 2003, pp 844–894.

18. Schiller LR: Review article: Anti-diarrhoeal pharmacology and therapeutics. Aliment Pharmacol Ther 9:87–106 1995.

19. Schiller LR, Hogan RB, Morawski SG, et al: Studies of the prevalence and significance of radiolabeled bile acid malabsorption in a group of patients with idiopathic chronic diarrhea. Gastroenterology 92:151–160, 1987.

20. Schiller LR, Rivera LM, Santangelo WC, et al: Diagnostic value of fasting plasma peptide concentrations in patients with chronic diarrhea. Dig Dis Sci 39:2216–2222, 1994.

21. Schiller LR, Santa Ana CA, Morawski SG, et al: Studies of the antidiarrheal action of clonidine: Effects on motility and intestinal absorption. Gastroenterology 89:982–988, 1985.

22. Schiller LR, Sellin JH: Diarrhea. In Feldman M, Friedman L, Sleisenger MH (eds): Sleisenger and Fordtran's Gastrointestinal and Liver Disease: Pathophysiology, Diagnosis, Management, 7th ed. Philadelphia, W.B. Saunders, 2003, pp 131–153.

23. Thillainayagam AV, Hunt JB, Farthing MJ: Enhancing clinical efficacy of oral rehydration therapy: Is low osmolarity the key? Gastroenterology 114:197–210, 1998.

24. Thompson WG, Longstreth GF, Drossman DA, et al: Functional bowel disorders and functional abdominal pain. Gut 45(Suppl 2):II43–II47, 1999.

25. Wenzl HH, Fine KD, Schiller LR, Fordtran JS: Determinants of decreased fecal consistency in patients with diarrhea. Gastroenterology 108:1729–1738, 1995.

CHAPTER 58

AIDS AND THE GASTROINTESTINAL TRACT

C. Mel Wilcox, MD

1. What is the role of barium esophagram for patients with AIDS and esophageal symptoms?

Infections are the most common cause of esophageal disease in patients with AIDS. Although many of these infections have a characteristic appearance on barium x-ray, overlap is frequent, thus mandating a definitive diagnosis before long-term antimicrobial therapy is given. In addition, some therapies for these disorders (e.g., corticosteroids) may be associated with significant toxicity, further emphasizing the importance of a histologic diagnosis. Last, in patients with severe odynophagia, the barium study may be inadequate because severe pain on swallowing will limit the amount of barium that can be swallowed, thus limiting the quality of the study.

2. What is the role of empiric antifungal therapy for new-onset esophageal symptoms in patients with AIDS?

Candida esophagitis is the most common cause of esophageal disease in patients with AIDS (Fig. 58-1). Because of this high prevalence, an empiric approach to new-onset esophageal symptoms with potent antifungal therapy is commonly undertaken. A randomized study has shown the efficacy and cost-effectiveness of such an approach, using a loading dose of 200 mg of fluconazole followed by 100 mg/day for 7 days. Because *Candida* responds very rapidly to fluconazole, in the patient who doesn't symptomatically improve within the first few days of treatment, endoscopic evaluation to exclude other causes of disease (viral esophagitis) should be performed.

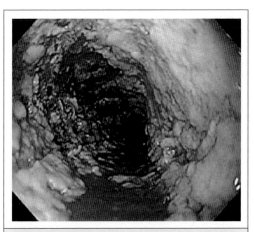

Figure 58-1. Candidal esophagitis. Yellow plaques coating the esophageal wall are typical for *Candida*. Note that on one portion of the wall, the material has been removed and the underlying mucosa is normal.

3. **What are the most common causes of esophageal ulceration in AIDS?**

The most common causes are cytomegalovirus (CMV) and idiopathic esophageal ulcer (IEU). O endoscopy, CMV and IEU appear most often as large, well-circumscribed solitary ulcerations, with normal-appearing surrounding mucosa. Multiple ulcers may also be observed. Antiretrovir medications, such as didanosine (ddl) and zidovudine (AZT) have also been associated with pill induced esophagitis. Like most pill-induced esophageal ulcers, these lesions are typically solitar but multiple small, well-circumscribed ulcerations are more characteristic and seen in the mid and proximal esophagus. Herpes simplex virus (HSV) is usually associated with multiple small, shallow esophageal ulcerations, often raised with a "volcano crater" appearance.

Gastroesophageal reflux disease (GERD) can also present with ulcerations of the distal esophagus generally involving the gastroesophageal junction; these lesions are generally linear and superficial. Neoplasms (e.g., lymphoma), parasites (e.g., leishmania), and fungal infections (e.g., histoplasmosis and *Candida* spp.) are rare causes of esophageal ulcers (Table 58-1).

TABLE 58-1.   REPORTED CAUSES OF ESOPHAGEAL ULCERS IN AIDS

Viruses: cytomegalovirus, herpes simplex virus type II, Epstein-Barr virus, papovavirus, human herpes virus-6

Fungi: Candida spp., *Histoplasma capsulatum, Cryptococcus neoformans*, mucormycosis, aspergillosis, *Penicillium chrysogenum, Exophiala jeanselmei*

Bacteria: Mycobacterium avium-complex, *M. tuberculosis, Bartonella henselae, Nocardia asteroides, Actinomyces israelii*

Protozoa: cryptosporidia, *Leishmania donovani, Pneumocystis carinii*

Tumors: non-Hodgkin's lymphoma, Kaposi's sarcoma, cancer (squamous cell and adenocarcinoma), lymphoma

Pill-induced: zalcitabine, zidovudine, other

Gastroesophageal Disease
Idiopathic: idiopathic esophageal ulcer

---

4. **What biopsy technique should be used to sample an esophageal ulcer?**

The exact number of biopsies required for maximal sensitivity is not clearly established, but several studies suggest the range of 8–10. It is important to obtain biopsies from the ulcer margin to investigate for HSV and from the ulcer base to investigate for CMV. Biopsy of the ulcer edge is important to exclude HSV because the viral cytopathic effect is present in squamous epithelium; conversely, CMV resides in granulation tissue in the ulcer base. The role of culture and cytology for esophageal ulcers is not settled. If all biopsies are negative for viral bacterial, fungal, and parasitic infections, a diagnosis of idiopathic esophageal ulcer can be made.

5. **What is AIDS-cholangiopathy? How do patients present?**

AIDS-cholangiopathy is a spectrum of biliary tract abnormalities resembling sclerosing cholangitis that can be caused by a wide array of microorganisms and neoplasms, usually in patients with advanced immunodeficiency. Patients generally present with epigastric or right upper quadrant pain, fever, and malaise. Although AIDS-cholangiopathy is a cholestatic diseas jaundice and pruritus are uncommon. The most common laboratory finding in this syndrome i a markedly elevated alkaline phosphatase, usually more than three times the upper limits of normal. Bilirubin rarely exceeds 3 mg/dL, and transaminases are only mildly elevated. General these patients have a dilated bile duct that is identifiable on abdominal ultrasonography. The diagnosis is best established by endoscopic retrograde cholangiopancreatography (ERCP). Several cholangiographic patterns have been described, including papillary stenosis, sclerosing cholangitis, combined papillary stenosis and sclerosing cholangitis, isolated intrahepatic disease, and long extrahepatic bile duct strictures. The most common pattern is papillary stenosis with intrahepatic sclerosing cholangitis. Endoscopic sphincterotomy is appropriate only for the relief of pain in patients with papillary stenosis. Unfortunately, the disease is progressive and medical therapy has no influence on its outcome.

6. What are the most common causes of AIDS-cholangiopathy? How are they diagnosed?

1. *Cryptosporidium parvum*
2. Microsporidia
   Enterocytozoon bieneusi
   Encephalitozoon intestinalis
   Encephalocytozoon cuniculi
3. Cytomegalovirus
4. *Mycobacterium avium*-complex (MAC)
5. *Cyclospora cayetanensis*
6. Non-Hodgkin's lymphoma
7. Kaposi's sarcoma

The diagnosis is usually established by obtaining biopsy specimens of the ampulla or duodenal mucosa, aspirated bile specimens, or biliary epithelial brush cytology. Despite its infectious origin, medical therapies aiming at the eradication of these organisms have not produced marked improvement in AIDS-cholangiopathy, which is a gradually progressive disease.

7. What are the most common causes of pancreatitis in HIV-infected patients?

Several studies have documented chronic and/or recurrent elevations of serum amylase and lipase in up to 50% of patients with AIDS. Pancreatograms at the time of ERCP have shown abnormalities of the pancreatic ducts consistent with chronic pancreatitis. These findings have led many investigators to hypothesize that pancreatic insufficiency from chronic pancreatitis is an important cause of chronic diarrhea in AIDS; however, most cases of chronic pancreatitis are attributable to conditions, such as alcohol abuse. The most common medications associated with pancreatitis in AIDS are pentamidine, ddI, and zalcitabine (ddC). Reported infectious causes of pancreatitis include CMV, HSV, MAC, and tuberculosis. An infectious cause of pancreatitis is difficult to establish and would require pancreatic biopsy.

8. Describe the work-up for abdominal pain in AIDS.

As in any patient, the differential diagnosis and diagnostic evaluation of abdominal pain is broad, especially in those with AIDS. Like any patient, the diagnostic evaluation should be targeted to the primary symptom(s). Patients with esophageal complaints or epigastric pain may benefit from upper endoscopy, whereas patients with lower abdominal pain associated with diarrhea may benefit from colonoscopic examination. When pain is more severe, abdominal CT scan is appropriate to evaluate for small bowel cancer, pancreatitis, and colitis (Fig. 58-2).

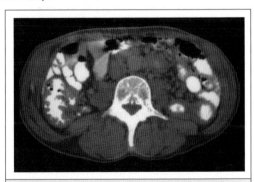

Figure 58-2. Cytomegalovirus colitis. Abdominal CT scan shows colonic wall thickening most pronounced in the right colon.

9. **How has highly active antiretroviral therapy (HAART) affected the incidence of opportunistic gastrointestinal (GI) disorders?**
    Since the introduction of protease inhibitors and HAART in 1996, there has been a constant and dramatic decline of GI opportunistic disorders in AIDS. It is postulated that improvement in the immune status, as reflected by an increase in CD4 cells, prevents the development of opportunistic disorders. In several reports, symptoms resolved even before any changes in the total CD4 cell count were apparent, suggesting that the antiretroviral medications promote elimination of the offending GI infection, probably secondary to immune-boosting mechanisms independent of the CD4 cell count and intrinsic antimicrobial activity.

10. **Describe the clinical features and causes of enterocolitis in AIDS.**
    In evaluating an AIDS patient with diarrhea, careful attention should be directed to the history and physical exam. Enteritis (small bowel diarrhea) is associated with voluminous, watery bowel movements, abdominal bloating, cramping, borborygmi, and nausea. Abdominal pain, if present, tends to be periumbilical or diffuse. Abdominal exam reveals an increase in number and frequency of bowel sounds, which may be high-pitched. Conversely, colitis (large bowel diarrhea) is characterized by frequent, small bowel movements, with the presence of mucus, pus, and/or blood ("dysentery"). Patients with prominent involvement of the distal colon also have "proctitis" symptoms, such as tenesmus, dyschezia (pain on defecation), and proctalgia (rectal pain). The most common causes of enteritis include cryptosporidiosis, microsporidiosis, giardiasis, cyclosporiasis, and viral infections. Colitis is generally secondary to CMV or bacteria such as *Shigella* spp., *Salmonella* spp., *Campylobacter jejuni*, and *Clostridium difficile*. *C. difficile* has become increasingly common because of the frequent use of antimicrobial medications.

11. **Describe the clinical features of HSV proctitis in AIDS.**
    HSV proctitis is the most common cause of nongonococcal proctitis in sexually active homosexual men. HSV proctitis classically presents with tenesmus, purulent rectal discharge, severe proctalgia, fever, constipation, and anorectal bleeding. Painful inguinal lymphadenopathy is an almost universal finding. The pain tends to distribute in the region of the sacral roots (i.e., buttocks, perineal region, and posterior thigh). Because of the neural involvement by HSV and the presence of severe pain, patients also have impotence and difficulty in initiating micturition. Visual inspection and anoscopy commonly reveal the following lesions: vesicles, pustular rectal lesions, or diffuse ulcerations. HSV is a pathogen of the squamous mucosa; therefore, diffuse proctitis involving the entire rectum is rare. In severe cases, the columnar rectal and sigmoid mucosa has been involved. The differential diagnoses of HSV proctitis include lymphogranuloma venereum (*Chlamydia trachomatis*), *Entamoeba histolytica*, *Salmonella* spp. and *Campylobacter jejuni*.

12. **What is the recommended work-up for diarrhea in AIDS?**
    In general, a stepwise approach should be followed. A thorough history and physical examination are essential first steps. It is also important to consider geographic location. For example, rotavirus is a common cause of diarrhea in Australian patients, microsporidiosis is uncommon in the south of the United States, and *Cyclospora cayetanensis* is a common cause of diarrhea in South America. A recent visit to a farm, contact with farm animals, or use of public swimming pools should raise the suspicion of cryptosporidiosis or microsporidiosis. Giardia is also associated with certain epidemiologic settings. Knowledge of the patient's immune status, as reflected by CD4 cell count, is also essential, because patients with more severe immunocompromise are predisposed to a wider array of opportunistic disorders. History of new medications or an alteration in a current regimen, such as antiretrovirals or antibacterials, is important because many protease inhibitors are associated with diarrhea, and antibacterials are associated with *C. difficile* colitis.

The first step in the evaluation of diarrhea is to obtain at least three stool samples to investigate for ova and parasites and to culture for common bacteria, such as *Shigella*, *Salmonella*, and *Campylobacter* spp. Stool samples should also be submitted for *C. difficile* toxin. A more urgent work-up may be necessary in the patient with acute severe symptoms, and the diagnosis of acute diarrhea differs from chronic diarrhea in this setting. In febrile patients, blood cultures should be obtained for common bacteria. If the CD4 count is below 50 cells/μL, blood cultures for *Mycobacterium avium*-complex should be obtained. If stool and blood culture studies are negative, the next step is endoscopic evaluation. In the presence of "colitis" symptoms, flexible sigmoidoscopy or colonoscopy is recommended. Because CMV colitis may be isolated to the right colon, some suggest the performance of a full colonoscopy. Ileal biopsies at the time of colonoscopy should be performed. In the presence of "enteritis" symptoms or long-standing diarrhea, an EGD with duodenal biopsies can evaluate for cryptosporidia, microsporidia, and giardiasis. Table 58-2 summarizes the studies and laboratory tests used in the evaluation of diarrhea in AIDS. Table 58-3 lists the most common infectious causes of diarrhea in AIDS.

3. **How useful is endoscopy for the evaluation of diarrhea in AIDS?**
The advantage of endoscopy is that it permits direct visualization and retrieval of tissue for histologic examination. The diagnostic yield of colonoscopy in HIV-infected patients with chronic diarrhea and negative stool studies ranges from 27–37%; CMV is the most common etiology identified. Because CMV colitis is usually present in the distal colon, sigmoidoscopy with biopsy may be sufficient work-up, but in 13–39% of cases of CMV enterocolitis, the virus can be detected in the right colon only. Therefore, if CMV is suspected as the cause of diarrhea, a full colonoscopy is warranted, especially if sigmoidoscopy is negative. However, it is still not clear whether colonoscopy has a higher yield than flexible sigmoidoscopy for the detection of organisms other than CMV. Evaluation with colonoscopy would be prudent if sigmoidoscopy is negative and right-sided abdominal complaints are reported. The value of upper endoscopy and small bowel biopsy in the evaluation of chronic diarrhea has also been demonstrated, although specific treatment options for most small bowel pathogens are limited. Some would obtain ileal biopsy at the time of colonoscopy rather than proceed with upper endoscopy and biopsy. The most commonly detected organisms involving the small bowel are cryptosporidia and microsporidia.

4. **What is the most common cause of viral diarrhea in AIDS?**
CMV is one of the most common opportunistic infections in patients with AIDS, occurring late in the course of HIV infection when immunodeficiency is severe (CD4 lymphocyte count <100/mm^3). CMV has been identified in mucosal biopsies in as many as 45% of patients with AIDS and diarrhea, especially in those patients with negative stool studies. CMV causes both enteritis and colitis. A number of other viral pathogens have been reported to involve the GI tract in patients with AIDS, but their clinical importance remains to be determined. Examples include adenovirus, rotavirus, astrovirus, picobirnavirus, and coronavirus. There are also reports that HIV itself can be isolated from enterocytes and colonic cells, but its role in causing disease is uncertain. HSV can cause proctitis that mimics diarrhea because of the rectal mucous discharge. However, HSV does not cause enterocolitis because it invades the squamous mucosa, not the columnar epithelium, such as the one lining the colonic and small bowel mucosa.

5. **What are the treatment options for CMV enterocolitis?**
The natural history of CMV colitis is variable. In untreated patients, it usually has a chronic course characterized by progressive diarrhea and weight loss, although occasionally symptoms and histologic abnormalities remit spontaneously. Unlike CMV retinitis, for which strong evidence supports induction therapy followed by lifelong maintenance therapy, the optimal duration of therapy and the need for maintenance therapy in CMV colitis are undefined. Two

TABLE 58-2.   STUDIES AND LABORATORY TESTS USED IN THE EVALUATION OF DIARRHEA IN AIDS

Stool
Cultures (*Salmonella, Shigella, Campylobacter* spp.)
Toxin (*Clostridium difficile*)
Ova and parasites (*Giardia lamblia, Entamoeba histolytica, Cryptosporidium* spp.)
Modified Kinyoun acid-fast (*Cryptosporidium* spp., *Isospora belli*)
Concentrated stool (zinc sulfate, Shether sucrose flotation) (microsporidia)

Blood
Cultures (*Mycobacterium avium*-complex, *Salmonella, Campylobacter* spp.)
Antibodies (*Entamoeba histolytica*, cytomegalovirus [CMV])

Gastrointestinal fluids
Duodenal aspirate (*Giardia lamblia*, microsporidia)
Electron microscopy (*Cryptosporidium* spp., adenovirus)

Biopsy stains
Hematoxylin-eosin
Giemsa or methenamine silver (fungi)
Methylene blue-azure II-basic fuchsin (microsporidia)
Fite (mycobacteria)

Immunohistochemical stains (CMV)

Immunologic methods
In situ hybridization (CMV)
DNA amplification (CMV)

Culture of tissue
CMV
Herpes simplex virus
Mycobacteria

antivirals (foscarnet and ganciclovir) have been studied extensively in the therapy of CMV colitis and/or enteritis. Cidofovir, the newest intravenous agent, has been used primarily in patients with retinal disease, but in our experience it is effective for GI disease as well. The newest agent is valganciclovir. This drug can be given orally and achieves serum levels similar to intravenous ganciclovir. Studies for GI disease are limited. Fundoscopic examination at the time of diagnosis of CMV enterocolitis is mandatory, because duration of therapy is considerably longer for disseminated diseases than for disease limited to the GI tract.

A number of open-label trials of ganciclovir for HIV-infected patients with CMV GI disease have demonstrated clinical improvement in approximately 75% of patients. Open-label trials of

TABLE 58-3. INFECTIOUS CAUSES OF DIARRHEA IN AIDS

Viruses	Bacteria	Parasites	Fungi
Cytomegalovirus	Salmonella spp.	Giardia lamblia	Histoplasma capsulatum
Astrovirus	Shigella spp.	Entamoeba histolytica	Candida albicans
Picornavirus	Campylobacter jejuni	Microsporidia	
Coronavirus	Clostridium difficile	Enterocytozoon bieneusi	
Rotavirus	Mycobacterium avium-	Encephalitozoon intestinalis	
Herpesvirus	complex	(formerly Septata)	
Adenovirus	Treponema pallidum		
Small round virus	Spirochetes	Cyclospora cayetanensis	
HIV	Neisseria gonorrhoeae	Cryptosporidium spp.	
	Vibrio cholerae	Isospora belli	
	Aeromonas spp.	Blastocystis hominis (?)	
	Pseudomonas spp. (?)		
	Staphylococcus aureus		

HIV = human immunodeficiency virus.

foscarnet have yielded comparable results. The only placebo-controlled trial of ganciclovir in AIDS-associated CMV colitis found no clinically significant differences, probably because the treatment period was only 2 weeks. A randomized trial comparing ganciclovir with foscarnet in 48 AIDS patients with CMV GI disease found similar clinical efficacy (73%), regardless of the location of disease (esophagus vs. colon). Endoscopic improvement was documented in over 80% of patients. For all patients, institution of HAART is important and, if there is an immunologic response, long-term maintenance therapy can be discontinued.

6. **Name the parasites that cause diarrhea in AIDS.**
Among the protozoa, *Cryptosporidium parvum* is the most common parasite causing diarrhea in AIDS and has been identified in up to 11% of symptomatic patients. Although a cause of acute diarrhea, cryptosporidiosis is found most commonly in HIV-infected patients with chronic diarrhea. In some studies of HIV-infected patients with chronic diarrhea, microsporidia (*Enterocytozoon bieneusi* and *Encephalitozoon intestinalis*) are the most commonly identified pathogens. Giardia is also a consideration in patients with diarrhea, especially when chronic and associated with the upper gastrointestinal symptoms of nausea and bloating. *Isospora belli* is a rare GI pathogen in HIV-infected patients in North America, whereas it is endemic in many developing countries, such as Haiti.

7. **Describe the clinical features and therapy for microsporidiosis.**
Gastrointestinal microsporidial infection is generally attributed to two species, *E. bieneusi* and *E. intestinalis*. In general, intestinal disease is relatively mild in contrast to the severe diarrhea typical for cryptosporidiosis. Loose stool is most common, and colonic symptoms are typically absent. Mild weight loss is frequent. Gastrointestinal bleeding suggests another diagnosis

KEY POINTS: AIDS AND THE GASTROINTESTINAL TRACT

1. Opportunistic infections are the most common cause of gastrointestinal symptoms in patients with AIDS.

2. The likelihood of an opportunistic process as a cause of gastrointestinal symptoms in an HIV-infected patient is directly proportional to the degree of immunodeficiency as reflected by the CD4 lymphocyte count.

3. *Candida* is the most common cause of esophageal disease in patients with AIDS.

4. A variety of infections, which involve both the upper and lower gastrointestinal tract, may cause diarrhea in patients with AIDS, and infections are oftentimes multiple.

5. Endoscopy has a high yield of identifying intestinal and colonic infections in AIDS patients with chronic diarrhea and negative stool studies.

because this infection does not cause mucosal ulceration. Although stool studies can establish the diagnosis, small bowel biopsies, either of the duodenum or ileum, are more sensitive if the appropriate stains are performed. Although there is no effective antimicrobial therapy for *E. bieneusi*, albendazole is highly effective for *E. intestinalis*. As with all opportunistic infection in AIDS, HAART may result in clinical remission.

18. **Describe the epidemiologic and clinical features of cryptosporidiosis.**
Cryptosporidia are a common cause of chronic diarrhea in HIV-infected patients with severe immunodeficiency. There are at least 40 species of cryptosporidia, but the most common caus of human disease is *C. muri*. Cryptosporidia infect and then reproduce within the columnar small intestinal cells. Infection can occur from person-to-person, animal-to-person, or from waterborne transmission (e.g., swimming pools, lakes). Therefore, a severely immunodeficien patient with AIDS who is not taking HAART is advised to avoid from contact with farm animals public pools, and lakes. The life cycle is completed in a single host. Autoinfectious cycles follow ingestion of a few oocysts, leading to severe disease and persistent infection in severely immunodeficient hosts. The diarrhea is generally voluminous, watery, and yellow-green. Dehydration and weight loss are common in patients with advanced immunodeficiency. The disease tends to be most severe in those with the most compromised immune function. The stool may contain mucus but rarely contains blood or leukocytes. The disease may wax and wane, but persistent and/or progressive disease may be manifested by dehydration and electrolyte imbalances. Constitutional symptoms are prominent, including low-grade fever, malaise, anorexia, nausea, and vomiting.

19. **Which bacteria most commonly cause diarrhea in AIDS?**
Campylobacter, Salmonella, and *Shigella* spp. and *C. difficile. Yersinia enterocolitica, Staphylococcus aureus,* and *Aeromonas hydrophila* have also been associated with severe enterocolitis in HIV-infected patients. *C. difficile* colitis is a frequent cause of diarrhea in HIV-infected patients, perhaps because of frequent exposure to antimicrobials and requirement for hospitalization. *Mycobacterium avium*-complex is a common pathogen in patients with advanced immunosuppression (i.e., CD4 count <50/μL). An incidence of 39% has been described when the CD4 count remains <10/mm^3. Tuberculosis is most frequent in developing countries and is less likely to present with diarrhea alone.

20. **What is bacillary peliosis hepatis (BPH)?**
BPH produces multiple cystic blood-filled spaces in the liver. BPH is caused by an infection with the bacteria *Bartonella henselae* (formerly *Rochalimae*) and occurs in patients with advanced AID

Patients present with generalized and nonspecific symptoms, such as fever, weight loss, and malaise. Abdominal pain, nausea, vomiting, and diarrhea may be prominent. Skin manifestations include reddish vascular papules that can be confused with Kaposi's sarcoma. On abdominal exam hepatosplenomegaly and lymphadenopathy are the most prominent features. Histopathology of the liver lesions shows multiple cystic blood-filled spaces within fibromyoid areas. The treatment of choice is erythromycin for at least 4–6 weeks, but doxycycline is a safe alternative.

BLIOGRAPHY

. Blanshard C, Francis N, Gazzard BG: Investigation of chronic diarrhoea in acquired immunodeficiency syndrome: A prospective study in 155 patients. Gut 39:824–832, 1996.

. Bonacini M, Young T, Laine L: The causes of esophageal symptoms in human immunodeficiency virus infection: A prospective study of 110 patients. Arch Intern Med 151:1567–1572, 1991.

. Bush ZM, Kosmiski LA: Acute pancreatitis in HIV-infected patients: Are etiologies changing since the introduction of protease inhibitor therapy? Pancreas 27:E1–E5, 2003.

. Call SA, Heudebert G, Saag M, Wilcox CM: The changing etiology of chronic diarrhea in HIV-infected patients with CD4 cell counts less than 200 cells/mm^3. Am J Gastroenterol 95:3142–3146, 2000.

. Carr A, Marriott D, Field A, et al: Treatment of HIV-1-associated microsporidiosis and cryptosporidiosis with combination antiretroviral therapy. Lancet 351:256–261, 1998.

. Cello JP: Acquired immunodeficiency syndrome cholangiopathy: Spectrum of disease. Am J Med 86:539, 1989.

. Chen XM, LaRusso NF: Cryptosporidiosis and the pathogenesis of AIDS-cholangiopathy. Semin Liver Dis 22:277–289, 2002.

. Dieterich DT, Wilcox CM: Diagnosis and treatment of esophageal diseases associated with HIV-infection. Am J Gastroenterol 91:2265–2268, 1996.

. Dore GJ, Marriott DJ, Hing MC, et al: Disseminated microsporidiosis due to *Septata intestinalis* in nine patients infected with the human immunodeficiency virus: Response to therapy with albendazole. Clin Infect Dis 21:70–76, 1995.

. Goodgame RW: Understanding intestinal spore-forming protozoa: Cryptosporidia, microsporidia, isospora, and cyclospora. Ann Intern Med 124:429–441, 1996.

. Kearney DJ, Steuerwald M, Koch J, Cello JP: A prospective study of endoscopy in HIV-associated diarrhea. Am J Gastroenterol 94:556–559, 1999.

. Mohle-Boetani JC, Koehler JE, Berger TG, et al: Bacillary angiomatosis and bacillary peliosis in patients infected with human immunodeficiency virus: Clinical characteristics in a case-control study. Clin Infect Dis 22:794–800, 1996.

. Mönkemüller KE, Call SA, Lazenby AJ, Wilcox CM: Decline in the prevalence of opportunistic gastrointestinal disorders in the era of HAART. Am J Gastroenterol 95:457–462, 2000.

. Mönkemüller KE, Wilcox CM: Diagnosis and treatment of colonic disease in AIDS. Gastrointest Endosc Clin North Am 8:889, 1998.

. Mönkemüller KE, Wilcox CM: Diagnosis and treatment of esophageal ulcers in AIDS. Semin Gastroenterol 10:1, 1999.

. Mönkemüller KE, Wilcox CM: Therapy of gastrointestinal infections in AIDS. Aliment Pharmacol Ther 11:425–443, 1997.

. Schwartz DA, Straub RA, Wilcox CM: Prospective endoscopic characterization of cytomegalovirus esophagitis in patients with AIDS. Gastrointest Endosc 40:481–484, 1994.

. Weber R, Bryan RT, Schwartz DA, Owen RL: Human microsporidial infections. Clin Microbiol Rev 7:426–461, 1994.

. Wilcox CM: Etiology and evaluation of diarrhea in AIDS: A global perspective at the millennium. World J Gastroenterol 6:177–186, 2000.

. Wilcox CM, Clark WS, Thompson SE: Fluconazole compared with endoscopy for human immunodeficiency virus-infected patients with esophageal symptoms. Gastroenterology 110:1803–1808, 1996.

. Wilcox CM, Schwartz DA, Clark WS: Causes, response to therapy, and long-term outcome of esophageal ulcer in patients with human immunodeficiency virus infection. Ann Intern Med 122:143–149, 1995.

CHAPTER 59

INTESTINAL ISCHEMIA

Arvey I. Rogers, MD, and David S. Estores, MD

1. **What is ischemic bowel disease?**
   It is a disorder that results from impairment of gut perfusion by oxygen-carrying blood distributed via the mesenteric arterial circulation. A sustained reduction in blood flow or reduce oxygen content of red blood cells results in tissue hypoxia and ischemic injury. This injury principally affects the small and/or large intestine and is clinically manifested as acute or chron abdominal pain, vomiting, sitophobia (fear of eating), weight loss, diarrhea, ileus, gastrointestinal (GI) bleeding, gut infarction, peritonitis, and fibrotic strictures.

2. **What are the main anatomic components of the mesenteric circulation?**
   The mesenteric circulation consists of three major arteries (celiac axis, superior mesenteric, ar inferior mesenteric) as inflow vessels and two major veins (superior and inferior mesenteric) a outflow vessels. This vascular system is referred to as the splanchnic circulation. Both arteries and veins course through the mesentery, providing blood to and draining it from the digestive organs and spleen (Fig. 59-1). The veins empty, ultimately, into the portal and hepatic veins. Th celiac axis provides blood to the stomach, duodenum, spleen, liver, and gallbladder. A portion c

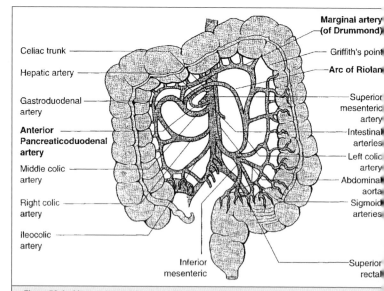

Figure 59-1. Mesenteric arterial anatomy. Three unpaired arterial branches of the aorta (celiac, superior mesenteric, and inferior mesenteric arteries) provide oxygenated blood to the small and large intestines. In most instances, veins parallel arteries. The superior mesenteric vein joins the splenic vein to form the portal vein, which enters the liver at its hilum. The inferior mesenteric vein joins the splenic vein near the juncture of the superior mesenteric and splenic veins. (Adapted from Rogers AI, Rosen CM: Mesenteric vascular insufficiency. In Schiller LR [ed]: Small Intestine. Philadelphia, Current Medicine, 1997, with permission.)

the duodenum, the entire small intestine, and half of the large intestine receives arterial blood via the superior mesenteric artery (SMA). The inferior mesenteric artery provides blood to the left colon and the rectum. The rectum is also perfused by branches of the internal iliac arteries.

3. **An extensive collateral circulatory system exists between the systemic and splanchnic vascular networks. Describe this system.**

The three major systemic-splanchnic and intersplanchnic collateral channels, which anastomose with the three unpaired major mesenteric arteries and their branches, are the *pancreaticoduodenal arcade*, *marginal artery of Drummond*, and *arc of Riolan* (Fig. 59-2). The pancreaticoduodenal arcade provides collateral channels between the celiac axis and SMA. The marginal artery of Drummond, composed of branches of the superior and inferior mesenteric arteries (IMA), is the continuous arterial pathway that runs parallel to the long axis of the colon. The middle colic branch of the SMA and the left colic branch of the IMA are anastomosed through the arc of Riolan.

Slowly developing occlusion of the mesenteric arteries via atherosclerosis promotes the opening of these collateral channels to assure the maintenance of arterial flow to and oxygenation of the small and/or large intestine. As a result, chronic mesenteric arterial insufficiency (that is, abdominal angina) is distinctly unusual unless there is occlusion of two of the three major mesenteric arteries.

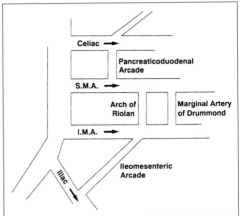

Figure 59-2. Schematic representation of collateral channels between the three major mesenteric arteries. The development of alternative anastomoses and collateral flow makes it theoretically possible that any single artery could supply all of the abdominal viscera with arterial blood given sufficient time and opportunity, that is, gradual occlusion of one or two of the other major arterial vessels. One major anastomosis exists between the left branch of the middle colic artery (from the superior mesenteric artery [SMA]) and the left colic artery from the inferior mesenteric artery (IMA), forming the meandering mesenteric artery or the arc of Riolan. Its demonstration by angiography indicates occlusion of the SMA or IMA. The marginal artery of Drummond is an arterial connection that provides a continuous channel of collateral flow via the vasa recta to the small and large intestines. The ileomesenteric arcade establishes an important anastomosis between the mesenteric and systemic circulation between the superior hemorrhoidal artery, a branch of the IMA and the hypogastric artery, a branch of the iliac artery. (Adapted from Rogers AI, Rosen CM: Mesenteric vascular insufficiency. In Schiller LR [ed]: Small Intestine. Philadelphia, Current Medicine, 1997, with permission.)

4. **A unique microcirculation functions to maintain oxygen delivery to the gut. Describe its components, and discuss how they respond to alterations in gut blood flow.**

The microcirculation consists of arterioles, capillaries, and venules, all lined by endothelial cells. Arterioles resist and therefore regulate the flow of blood through the tissues. A steep gradient of pressure exists between the artery and terminal portion of the arteriole. The arterioles dilate when arterial perfusion pressure is reduced. Capillaries allow the exchange of materials between gut wall cells and blood vessels. When tissue hypoxia occurs, underperfused capillaries are recruited, increasing the density of perfused capillaries and thereby compensating for the steep gradient in tissue oxygen levels. The venules store blood for short periods before it is returned to the heart after meals or in response to exercise. In the face of systemic hypotension, the tone of venous capacitance vessels is increased, enhancing venous return to the heart to ensure maintenance of cardiac output (Fig. 59-3).

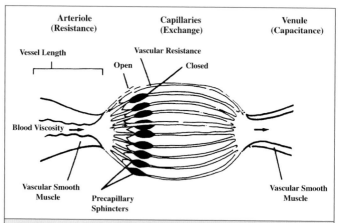

Figure 59-3. Intramural vascular anatomy. The assured delivery of oxygen-rich arterial blood to the various layers of the small and large intestinal wall during basal, meal-stimulated, and stress states depends on the interplay between various anatomic and physiologic factors, that is, blood viscosity, red blood cell oxygen saturation, arteriole length and resistance to flow, tone of precapillary sphincters, tone of vascular smooth muscle, and venous capacitance. See question 5 to gain a better understanding of the various factors influencing the regulation of blood flow. (Adapted from Rogers AI, Rosen CM: Mesenteric vascular insufficiency. In Schiller LR [ed]: Small Intestine. Philadelphia, Current Medicine, 1997, with permission.)

5. **What factors contribute to the regulation of gut blood flow?**
   Maintenance of gut blood flow, adequate to assure effective tissue oxygenation, includes cardiac output, net arterial, arteriole and capillary perfusion pressures, oxygen content of red blood cells, volume status, red cell and platelet mass, diameter and patency of arteries and arterioles, and neural and neuroendocrine elements, as outlined in the following:
   1. Cardiovascular factors (cardiac output, blood pressure, blood volume)
   2. Autonomic nervous system
      - Sympathetic nerves constrict, whereas parasympathetic nerves dilate vessels.
      - Nonadrenergic, noncholinergic (NANC) nerves dilate, whereas the intrinsic enteric nervous system both constricts and dilates vessels.
   3. Circulating hormones: norepinephrine, angiotensin II, and vasopressin constrict, whereas hormones elaborated locally by gut mucosa dilate vessels.
   4. Tissue substances released in response to ischemia, inflammation, or increased tissue metabolism (elaborated by endothelial cells lining the vessels of the microcirculation and by immunocytes, such as mast cells and leukocytes).
   5. Physical forces (transmural pressure and streaming velocity).

6. **What are the different varieties of ischemic bowel disease?**
   Arterial and venous, acute and chronic, occlusive and nonocclusive. Ischemic bowel disease can also be divided into three clinical entities: acute mesenteric ischemia (AMI) from emboli, arterial or venous thrombi, or vasoconstriction; chronic mesenteric ischemia (CMI); and colonic ischemia (CI) (Fig. 59-4).

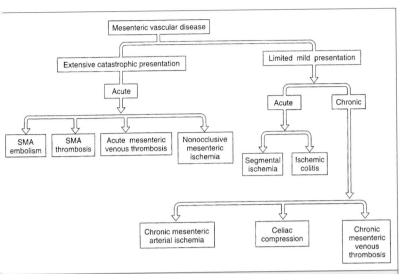

Figure 59-4. Classification of mesenteric vascular disease based on the extent of resulting ischemia. This particular classification, proposed by Williams et al. (1988) may facilitate more effective evaluation and management by focusing on extent of gut involvement.

7. **What clinical circumstances predispose to ischemic bowel disease?**

   Arterial:
   - Embolus: cardiac arrhythmias, valvular heart disease (atrial fibrillation), myocardial infarction, mural thrombus, atrial myxoma, angiography.
   - Thrombosis: atherosclerosis, hypercoagulable states (pregnancy, protein C or S deficiency, factor V Leiden deficiency, hyperhomocysteinemia, antithrombin deficiency, phospholipid syndromes, birth control pills, neoplasms, polycythemia vera, thrombocytosis), vascular aneurysms or dissections, vasculitides.

   Nonocclusive mesenteric ischemia: cardiac arrhythmias, cardiogenic shock, pulmonary edema, hypovolemia, sepsis, vasoconstricting drugs.

   Venous: hypercoagulable states (see Arterial), congestive heart failure, shock, portal hypertension, Budd-Chiari syndrome, carcinoma, trauma, sclerotherapy, peritonitis, diverticulitis, pancreatitis, inflammatory bowel disease, intestinal obstruction, postoperative states, trauma.

8. **Describe the pathophysiology and precipitating events leading to occlusive intestinal ischemia.**

   Intestinal ischemia results from tissue hypoxia. Hypoxia ensues when blood volume, its physical characteristics (red cell mass), flow rate, or oxygen content is altered in the mesenteric arterial or venous circulation. Decreased flow affecting the arterial vasculature can result from an obstruction caused by a thrombus (acute or chronic), embolus (acute), or vasoconstriction. Thrombosis is usually secondary to rupture of an atherosclerotic plaque. The most common location for thrombotic or embolic occlusion is at the origin of the superior mesenteric artery; its angular branching off the aorta is a predisposing factor.

   Patients can develop a syndrome of chronic, recurrent abdominal pain when the thrombosis or arterial wall thickening is complete enough to compromise luminal diameter by <50%. With insufficient development of collateral circulation to provide compensated arterial flow to fulfill physiologic demands for increased delivery of oxygen to tissues (i.e., 30–90 minutes after a meal), ischemia and resulting tissue hypoxia lead to gut spasm and abdominal pain.

9. **Describe the pathophysiology of nonocclusive mesenteric ischemia.**
   Shock, profound hypovolemia, impaired cardiac output, or major thoracic or abdominal surge are risk factors for gut hypoperfusion as a consequence of vasoconstriction of the mesenteric vasculature. This condition is known as nonocclusive mesenteric ischemia (NOMI). These patients have decreased perfusion of the mesenteric arteries due to vasoconstriction precipitated by an event or events resulting in hypoperfusion (i.e., hypovolemia or cardiac failure). No occluding thrombus or embolus is present. NOMI is encountered most commonly patients who have undergone major abdominal or thoracic surgery complicated by pulmonary edema, cardiac arrhythmias, or shock. Digitalis preparations can aggravate mesenteric vasoconstriction. Affected patients manifest the same symptoms and signs as patients with occlusive disease. Angiography reveals intense vasoconstriction and spasm that may persist, even if the precipitating event is remedied. Selective (intra-arterial) papaverine infusion may relieve the vasoconstriction.

10. **What is focal (short segment) segmental ischemia?**
    The same pathophysiologic processes (embolus, thrombosis, venous occlusion, NOMI) capab of causing extensive bowel ischemia can also lead to a form of ischemia that is limited to a sho segment of bowel. It is the result of the involvement of a few small arteries (or, more rarely, veins) and is known as focal segmental ischemia.

11. **What should one know about mesenteric venous occlusion as a cause of ischemic bowel disease?**
    Mesenteric venous occlusion is a rare cause of ischemic bowel disease. Just as in mesenteric ischemia complicating arterial occlusion (or nonocclusion), most patients present with mid-abdominal pain that is severe and disproportionate to the minimal findings on physical examination of the abdomen. However, patients with venous occlusion can present acutely or subacutely (weeks to months). Accurate diagnosis requires a high index of suspicion. Abdominal computed tomography (CT) with contrast enhancement is the diagnostic test of choice, revealing findings consistent with venous occlusion in more than 90% of patients: thickening and contrast enhancement of the bowel wall, enlarged SMV, thrombosis in the lumen of the SMV, and collateral vessels. If there are no signs of intestinal infarction, patients should treated with anticoagulation and thrombolytics; otherwise, they should be operated on immediately.

12. **What are the common presenting complaints in patients with suspected gut ischemia?**
    Presenting complaints vary with the etiology of the ischemia. Most patients with intestinal ischemia complicating acute embolic or thrombotic occlusion of the SMA present with the abrupt onset of acute, severe abdominal pain, usually mid-abdominal in location and of colicky character. Simultaneously, involuntary evacuation of bowel contents may occur because of the intense tonic contractions of gut smooth muscle provoked by ischemia. Abdominal pain resulting from smooth muscle spasm presents few abdominal physical findings. Abdominal distention and a Hemoccult-positive stool *(late findings)* may be the only presenting signs in th intensive or coronary care unit patient who develops NOMI and is incapable of complaining of abdominal pain.

    Patients with acute mesenteric ischemia secondary to thrombotic occlusion may provide a history consistent with mesenteric angina, that is, recurring postprandial mid or diffuse abdominal pain, sometimes with a back-radiation component. Weight loss usually ensues because of sitophobia. Pain radiating to the back (possibly due to duodenal or pancreatic ischemia) and weight loss suggest pancreatic carcinoma. A negative abdominal CT mitigates against this consideration. Diarrhea, steatorrhea, and/or protein-losing enteropathy may complicate ischemia-induced atrophy of the small intestinal mucosa.

Venous occlusive disease may have a more insidious onset characterized by vague abdominal pain, diarrhea, and vomiting. Acute occlusion may result in profound fluid sequestration and shock. It should be suspected in the appropriate clinical setting.

3. What are the physical findings in a patient with gut ischemia?

These vary with the etiology and duration of the ischemia. In the appropriate clinical setting, acute occlusion of the SMA via embolus or thrombosis should be suspected when a striking disparity exists between the subjective complaint of severe, diffuse abdominal pain and the minimal findings on abdominal examination. Early in the course of disease, only mild distention and normal or hyperactive bowel sounds are likely to be encountered. Abdominal arterial bruits are too nonspecific to be of value. Stools may be Hemoccult-positive. As the ischemic injury progresses, ileus develops, bowel sounds diminish, and abdominal distention ensues. Bloody diarrhea may occur. Hypotension and tachycardia signal volume sequestration, whereas fever and peritoneal signs indicate transmural injury and probable infarction.

Nonocclusive ischemia should be considered in the appropriate setting (see question 9). Subjective complaints are less dramatic than with acute arterial occlusion. Physical findings vary with the duration of the arterial occlusion and may be similar to those described for acute arterial occlusion. Chronic, recurring abdominal pain on the basis of compromised flow through the SMA (i.e., mesenteric abdominal angina) is not associated with specific physical findings. Most patients have evidence of peripheral vascular disease; they may also exhibit findings associated with weight loss.

Physical findings in venous occlusive disease depend on its etiology and severity (e.g., congestive heart failure, stigmata of chronic liver disease and portal hypertension, hepatomegaly, splenomegaly, evidence of hypercoagulability, abdominal mass). Tachycardia and hypotension are present if splanchnic volume has been sequestered.

4. When should you suspect mesenteric ischemia, and what is a realistic differential diagnosis?

Acute mesenteric ischemia should be suspected in patients complaining of severe abdominal pain out of proportion to findings on physical examination and when pain is present for more than 2 hours.

The differential diagnosis is broad and should include any cause of acute abdominal pain, unexplained ileus in the appropriate setting, and hypotension. Conditions usually considered include perforated viscus, small bowel obstruction, cecal volvulus, incarcerated hernia, dissecting aortic aneurysm, acute pancreatitis, and cholecystitis.

5. Do laboratory findings help at all?

Not much. Laboratory findings in gut ischemia are usually nonspecific and probably vary with the etiology, duration, severity, potential for reversing precipitating and complicating events, and extent of ischemic injury (i.e., which organs are involved). Early stages are associated with no abnormalities (other than those associated with a preexisting illness that may or may not have predisposed to gut ischemia). Abnormalities seen with gut ischemia and/or infarction are the consequence of volume sequestration and tissue hypoxia, inflammation, and necrosis (i.e., hemoconcentration, leukocytosis, and lactic acidosis). Increased levels of amylase, alkaline phosphatase, and creatine phosphokinase (CPK) are nonspecific findings. Laboratory test results may help to exclude mimicking etiologies, such as pancreatitis (increased levels of amylase and lipase) and choledocholithiasis (increased levels of alkaline phosphatase, alanine aminotransferase [ALT], aspartate aminotransferase [AST], and bilirubin). Increased levels of CPK and alkaline phosphatase are nonspecific consequences of gut injury. The more abnormal the laboratory findings, the more advanced the injury.

16. **What radiographic studies are available to confirm a suspected diagnosis of gut ischemia? To exclude differential diagnostic considerations?**

Conventional radiography, contrast-enhanced CT, Doppler ultrasound of mesenteric vessels, mesenteric angiography (magnetic resonance or invasive arteriography), laparoscopy, and enteroscopy are among the diagnostic techniques applied most frequently. The clinical circumstances and findings dictate choices and sequence. Unless dictated otherwise by clinical circumstances that point clearly to gut ischemia and/or infarction and away from mimicking etiologies, abdominal plain films (flat and upright) should first be obtained. Helpful clues to diagnose the cause of abdominal pain (ischemic bowel disease or other causes) that may be seen on the plain radiographs of the abdomen are listed in Table 59-1.

The administration of barium for a small bowel study should be avoided in anticipation that an abdominal CT or angiogram may be undertaken; the oral contrast interferes with the ability to perform and/or interpret findings on these studies. As mentioned earlier (*see* question 11), a dynamic, contrast-enhanced abdominal CT can be very valuable in diagnosing venous occlusive disease. Both plain abdominal x-rays and CT scans show only nonspecific abnormalities in 35% of patients with infarcted bowel. Angiography is superior to CT for the identification of mesenteric arterial branch occlusions or NOMI.

TABLE 59-1. RADIOGRAPHIC CLUES TO DIAGNOSIS	
Disorder	**Finding on Plain Abdominal Radiographs**
Small bowel obstruction	Dilated loops of bowel with or without air-fluid levels
	Stair-step overlapping of loops of small bowel
	May see termination of luminal small bowel air at lead point of obstruction
Pancreatitis	Sentinel loop of jejunum or colon cutoff sign
Volvulus	Characteristic jejunual, sigmoid, or cecal bowel dilation
Pneumobilia	Air in the biliary tree, seen in emphysematous cholangitis or intra-abdominal sepsis, caused by gas-forming bacteria
Pylephlebitis	Air in the hepatic/portal venous system suggests severe gut injury, infarction, advanced intra-abdominal sepsis
Perforation	Free air under the diaphragm or air dissecting between loops of bowel or retroperitoneally along solus muscles
Bowel ischemia	Bowel wall thickening, loop separation, or thumbprinting
Pneumatosis intestinalis	Air in the bowel wall indicates usually pre- or actual bowel infarction

17. **What is the role of magnetic resonance angiography (MRA) in patients with abdominal angina?**

MRA may be useful in the patient with suspected chronic mesenteric ischemia who has severe iodine allergies. Three dimensional reconstruction may also be feasible with MRA.

18. **Describe the role of Doppler ultrasound studies in diagnosis.**

Fasting and meal-stimulated Duplex ultrasound is a noninvasive test that can be used to assess the patency of and blood flow through the major mesenteric vessels. Its greatest use is in diagnosing multivessel stenosis in cases of suspected mesenteric angina; findings include narrowing or occlusion at vessel origin and excessively turbulent flow. Its major limitations for diagnosing acute mesenteric arterial or venous occlusion include visualization limited to the proximal segment of the vessels and compromised visualization, when ileus is present or the patient is obese. Overlying bowel gas may also prevent adequate visualization of mesenteric vasculature. For these reasons, Duplex ultrasonographic scanning cannot be recommended in acutely ill patients. As with CT scans, angiography is superior to duplex sonography to visualize mesenteric arterial branch occlusions or NOMI.

9. **What are the roles of endoscopy (sigmoidoscopy, colonoscopy, enteroscopy) and laparoscopy?**

Conventional enteroscopy should not be undertaken for purposes of diagnosing small bowel ischemic disease. Despite the fact that scattered case reports describe diagnostic findings in selected clinical settings, the technique using available endoscopic instruments and scope passage through the small intestine can be dangerous. Smaller scope diameter and improved technology to facilitate intestinal intubation may modify conventional wisdom. However, lower endoscopy (sigmoidoscopy or colonoscopy) is relatively safe and may be highly informative in patients with suspected ischemic colitis (*see* questions 27–32).

Laparoscopy has been considered as a technique to diagnose and assess severity of ischemic injury to the gut. Despite the observation by Liolios et al. (1999) that this invasive but relatively safe technique can diagnose full-thickness mesenteric injury (late finding), its limitation is that it will miss earlier stages of potentially reversible ischemia. Brandt and Boley (2000) emphasize that although the serosa can appear completely benign, the mucosal surface may be undergoing necrosis. They also emphasize that when intraperitoneal pressure exceeds 20 mmHg (a level reached possibly during laparoscopy), blood flow decreases through the superior mesenteric artery.

20. **When should one undertake mesenteric arteriographic studies?**

Early diagnosis and definitive nonsurgical or surgical therapy are important in patients with suspected ischemic bowel disease. The mortality rate is quite high when diagnosis and therapy are delayed and when peritoneal signs and acidosis ensue. Angiography is the gold standard for the diagnosis of mesenteric arterial occlusion and sometimes differentiates an embolic from a thrombotic event. The angiographic demonstration of an abrupt cutoff of a nonatherosclerotic) artery in the absence of collateral vessel enlargement suggests embolic occlusion, whereas associated vessel narrowing by atherosclerosis in association with the development of prominent collaterals is more consistent with thrombosis. The venous phase of the arteriogram may demonstrate venous occlusive disease. The angiographic findings in nonocclusive mesenteric ischemia include vessel narrowing, arterial beading, and lack of arterial blush in the intestinal wall.

On occasion, angiography can also be therapeutic, allowing the selective infusion of vasodilating drugs or thrombolytic agents, respectively, to the spastic or acutely occluded artery(ies) or by facilitating the performance of therapeutic angioplasty, balloon embolectomy, or stent placement. The infusion of thrombolytic agents is considered experimental at present, but may have a limited applicability in tertiary medical centers with technical expertise, in patients considered poor surgical candidates without peritoneal signs, and in patients in whom the ischemic event is considered to be of short duration. Angiography is not a benign procedure and carries definite risk, inasmuch as many affected patients have considerable atherosclerotic changes in femoral and mesenteric arteries. Infused contrast in association with hypovolemia, impaired cardiac output, and reduced renal blood flow increases the likelihood of renal damage, especially if the patient is diabetic. Nonetheless, angiography is the only definitive technique, short of exploratory surgery, to establish the diagnosis of mesenteric ischemia early in the disease when there is still a chance for survival.

21. **When should a patient with ischemic bowel disease be sent to the operating room?**

A clinical picture compatible with acute ischemic bowel disease, in which other diagnoses have been excluded, should prompt angiography. If the findings are amenable to nonoperative management (i.e., NOMI treated with papaverine infusion, embolectomy), and there is no indication of bowel necrosis, the patient should be treated conservatively. Otherwise, patients should be taken to the operating room to: (1) assess the degree and extent of gut injury, (2) identify the site of and to relieve arterial obstruction, (3) resect irreversibly damaged bowel, and (4) possibly undergo revascularization. Bowel viability may be assessed by the injection of fluorescein dye.

22. **Is there ever an indication for a "second-look" operation?**

At the time of surgery, there may be some doubt about the viability of a segment of bowel left intact, whether or not revascularization has been attempted. Under such circumstances, the patient may undergo a second operation 24–48 hours later to assess bowel viability. This is an area of ongoing, active controversy.

23. **What is meant by reperfusion injury?**

Reestablishing normal blood flow to the ischemic bowel does not always arrest injury to the bowel. Reperfusion of ischemic tissue can lead to paradoxical exaggeration of the injury. One of the prevailing theories to account for this observation is that reperfusion increases the number of active oxidants (free oxygen, H_2O_2, hydroxy radicals) that further injure the cells. The membranes of the enterocytes are initially damaged by the ischemic process, thereby making the intracellular components more vulnerable to injury. The enzyme xanthine dehydrogenase is abundantly present in cell cytoplasm and, when exposed to the pancreatic enzyme trypsin, undergoes conversion to xanthine oxidase. This enzyme is responsible for the formation of active oxidants during reperfusion. Some experimental data suggest that allopurinol, an inhibitor of xanthine oxidase, may reduce the risk of reperfusion injury.

24. **What is abdominal angina? What is its clinical significance?**

Abdominal angina refers to chronic, recurring abdominal pain caused by diminished arterial flow through the mesenteric arteries. Affected patients are often hyperlipidemic, diabetic, or chronic tobacco users and have associated peripheral vascular (arterial) disease. Abdominal angina can be viewed as claudication of the gut. Most often, the equivalent exercise stimulus is a meal; the pain is experienced 30–90 minutes postprandially and can last up to 4 hours. Some authorities believe that as food enters the stomach and the demand for oxygen increases, the flow of blood to the small intestine diminishes ("stealing blood"). Although minimal at first, postprandial abdominal pain progressively increases in severity over weeks to months. Profound and prolonged hypoxia of small intestinal mucosa may result in villous atrophy and diarrhea as well as protein-losing enteropathy and steatorrhea.

25. **What is the role of angioplasty and stenting in the management of abdominal angina?**

Angioplasty with or without stent placement may have a role in some patients with intestinal angina. Lesions located at the aortic orifices of the mesenteric arteries are not readily amenable to angioplasty because of their fixed diameter, but more distal lesions can be dilated without the morbidity and mortality of surgical intervention.

26. **Which patients with abdominal angina should undergo surgical revascularization?**

Surgical revascularization should probably be limited to a few patients. Indications include typical disabling symptoms of abdominal angina (chronic postprandial abdominal pain, sitophobia, weight loss), angiographic evidence of occlusion of at least two major mesenteric arteries, inclusive of the SMA, and acceptable risk for surgery. Whether multiple vessels or only the SMA should be revascularized is controversial. Most recent studies report a mortality rate of <16%, success rate of >90%, and recurrence rate of <10%.

7. **Can ischemia be isolated to the colon?**
Yes. Ischemic colitis is the most common form of intestinal ischemia. Most patients are older than age 60 and have experienced nonoperative or postoperative reduction in blood flow to the large intestine, but the condition can be encountered in younger patients with risk factors (vasculitides, coagulopathies, sickle cell disease, cocaine use, long-distance runners). Psychotropic drugs, danazol, and estrogen have been implicated.

8. **What are the most common symptoms of ischemic colitis?**
The most common symptoms are the sudden onset of crampy, mild left lower abdominal pain and urgency to defecate. In the postoperative state, mild symptoms are often dismissed. Bright red blood per rectum or hematochezia may be seen. Tenderness can be elicited over the involved segment of bowel. Inflammatory bowel disease is the most frequently confused diagnosis.

9. **How does one confirm a suspected diagnosis of ischemic colitis?**
Abdominal plain films may demonstrate "thumbprint" abnormalities along the wall of a colonic segment (often the splenic flexure) filled with air. These changes are the result of submucosal edema or hemorrhage. If ischemic colitis is suspected and there are no clinical features to suggest peritoneal irritation, a colonoscopy should be undertaken to confirm the diagnosis. Any region of the colon may be affected, but the key endoscopic feature of ischemic colitis is the tendency for segmental distribution. The rectosigmoid (20%), descending colon (20%), splenic flexure (11%), and all three in combination (14%) are affected most commonly. Changes may be isolated to the rectum (6%) or right colon (8%). Flexible sigmoidoscopy may not disclose changes consistent with ischemic colitis isolated to the splenic flexure. When the rectosigmoid region is involved with sparing of the rectum, the diagnosis is strongly suspected. The rectum is involved infrequently because of its dual blood supply derived from the inferior mesenteric and internal iliac arterial branches. Barium enemas are less sensitive than colonoscopy for detecting mucosal changes but may reveal thumbprinting changes because of submucosal edema and hemorrhage. Angiography is not indicated in ischemic colitis, because the predisposing nonocclusive vascular factors are not demonstrable by angiography once ischemic injury has occurred.

10. **Can endoscopic findings or histologic features establish a definitive diagnosis?**
Neither endoscopic findings (edema, submucosal hemorrhage, friability, and/or ulcerations) nor histologic findings (nonspecific inflammation, epithelial sloughing, subepithelial hemorrhage, cell dropout and hemosiderin deposition in muscle layers) are specific enough to make a definitive diagnosis. But in the right clinical setting (i.e., acute systemic hypotension, aortic bypass surgery), the diagnosis can be made with a high degree of certainty on clinical grounds. Infectious colitis and inflammatory bowel disease should be considered in the differential diagnosis.

11. **What are the sequelae of ischemic colitis? Can anything be done to modify the course of the disease?**
Ischemic colitis is reversible in up to 50% of patients whose symptoms abate within 24–48 hours; in these patients, healing occurs without stricture in 1–2 weeks. The severely injured colon may require 1–6 months to heal completely. Irreversible damage occurs in the remaining 50% and includes the following courses: gangrene and perforation, segmental colitis, fulminant colitis, and ischemic stricture. The course cannot be predicted at the time of initial presentation.

Optimizing cardiac function is imperative; impaired cardiac output and cardiac arrhythmias should be corrected. Factors predisposing to vasoconstriction, digitalis therapy, vasopressor agents, and hypovolemia should be avoided when possible. Vasodilating agents are ineffective because low colonic blood flow has already returned to normal by the time the ischemia has occurred. The bowel should be placed at rest, broad-spectrum antibiotics should be administered, and a distended colon should be decompressed colonoscopically or by placement of a rectal tube. Rolling the patient from a supine posture alternating with right and left lateral decubitus positions may facilitate movement of air and its rectal passage. Urgent surgery is necessary only in rare cases of rapid progression of ischemic injury to gangrene and infarction.

32. **When is surgery indicated in patients with ischemic colitis?**
Surgery is indicated in patients who present with or develop peritoneal signs, massive bleeding or evidence of fulminant colitis. Surgery should be considered even with apparent healing in patients who have recurrent bouts of sepsis and in patients who fail to respond to conservative measures over 2–3 weeks. Symptomatic colon strictures may also warrant surgical correction.

BIBLIOGRAPHY

1. Brandt LJ, Boley SJ: AGA technical review on intestinal ischemia. Gastroenterology 118:954–968, 2000.
2. Brandt LJ, Boley SJ: Intestinal ischemia. In Feldman M, Friedman LS, Sleisenger MH (eds): Gastrointestinal and Liver Diseases, 7th ed. Philadelphia, W.B. Saunders, 2000, pp 2321–2339.
3. Jacobson E: Intestinal ischemia. In McNally PR (ed):GI/Liver Secrets. Philadelphia, Hanley & Belfus, 1996, pp 403–414.
4. Kim AY, Ha HK: Evaluation of suspected mesenteric ischemia: Efficacy of radiologic studies. Radiol Clin North Am 41:327–342, 2003.
5. Lefkovitz Z, Cappell MS, Lookstein R, et al: Radiologic diagnosis and treatment of gastrointestinal hemorrhage and ischemia. Med Clin North Am 86:1357–1399, 2002.
6. Liolios A, Oropello JM, Benjamin E: Gastrointestinal complications in the intensive care unit. Clin Chest Med 20:329–345, 1999.
7. Marston A: Vascular Disease of the Gastrointestinal Tract. Baltimore, Williams & Wilkins, 1986, pp 1–15.
8. Nicoloff AD, Williamson WK, Moneta GL, et al: Duplex ultrasonography in evaluation of splanchnic artery stenosis. Surg Clin North Am 77:339–356, 1997.
9. Shanley CJ, Ozaki K, Zelenock GB: Bypass grafting for chronic mesenteric ischemia. Surg Clin North Am 77:381–396, 1997.
10. Smithline AE, Brandt LJ, Boley SJ: Acute and chronic mesenteric ischemia. In Brandt LJ (ed): Clinical Practice Gastroenterology, vol 1. Philadelphia, Current Medicine, 1999, pp 574–586.
11. Williams LF Jr.: Mesenteric ischemia. Surg Clin North Am 68:331–353, 1988.

CHAPTER 60

NUTRITION AND MALNUTRITION

Peter R. McNally, DO, and Jonathan P. Kushner, MD

1. **What is meant by nutritional status?**

   Nutritional status reflects how well nutrient intake contributes to body composition and function in the face of the existing metabolic needs. The four major body compartments are water, protein, mineral, and fat. The first three compose the lean body mass (LBM); functional capacity resides in a portion of the LBM called the *body-cell mass.* Nutritionists concentrate their efforts on preservation or restoration of this vital component.

2. **Define *malnutrition.***

   Malnutrition refers to states of overnutrition (obesity) or undernutrition relative to body requirements, resulting in dysfunction.

3. **How do different types of malnutrition affect function and outcome?**

   Marasmus is protein-calorie undernutrition associated with significant physical wasting of energy stores (adipose tissue and somatic muscle protein) but preservation of visceral and serum proteins. Patients are not edematous and may have mild immune dysfunction. Hypoalbuminemic malnutrition occurs with stressed metabolism and is common in hospitalized patients. They may have adequate energy stores and body weight but have expanded extracellular space, depleted intracellular mass, edema, altered serum protein levels, and immune dysfunction. A similar state of relative protein deficiency occurs in classic kwashiorkor, in which caloric provision is adequate but quantity and quality of protein are not.

4. **How does one perform a simple nutritional assessment?**

   Simple bedside assessment may be as valuable for predicting nutrition-associated outcomes as sophisticated composition and function tests. One popular method, the Subjective Global Assessment, incorporates basic questions about weight history, intake, gastrointestinal (GI) symptoms, disease state, functional level, and a physical examination to classify patients as well-nourished, mildly to moderately malnourished, or severely malnourished.

   A weight history, estimate of recent intake, brief physical exam, consideration of disease stress/medications, and assessments of functional status and wound healing allow a good estimate of nutritional status. They predict the risk for malnutrition-associated complications as well as, or better than, laboratory data. Poor intake for longer than 1–2 weeks, a weight loss of more than 10%, or a weight less than 80% of desirable weight guidelines warrants closer nutritional assessment and follow-up.

5. **List desirable weights for men and women, according to the Metropolitan Life Tables.**

   Men: 135 lb for the first 5 feet, 3 inches of height plus 3 lb per additional inch (±10%)
   Women: 119 lb for the first 5 feet, 0 inches of height plus 3 lb per additional inch (±10%).

6. **Describe the types of commonly prescribed oral diets.**

   The clear liquid diet supplies fluid and calories in a form that requires minimal digestion, stimulation, and elimination by the GI tract. It provides about 600 calories and 150 gm carbohydrate but inadequate protein, vitamins, and minerals. Clear liquids are hyperosmolar;

diluting the beverages and eating slower may minimize GI symptoms. If clear liquids are needed for >3 days, a dietitian can assist with supplementation.

The full liquid diet is used often in progressing from clear liquids to solid foods. It may also be used in patients with chewing problems, gastric stasis, or partial ileus. Typically, the diet provides >2000 calories and 70 gm protein. It may be adequate in all nutrients (except fiber), especially if a high-protein supplement is added. Patients with lactose intolerance need special substitutions. Progression to solid foods should be accomplished with modifications or supplementation, as needed.

7. **What is a "hidden" source of calories in the ICU?**
   Watch out for significant amounts of lipid calories from propofol, a sedative in 10% lipid emulsion (1.1 kcal/mL).

8. **Summarize the typical findings in deficiency or excess of various micronutrients.**
   See Table 60-1.

9. **What are the nutritional concerns in patients with short bowel syndrome?**
   Loss of bowel surface puts the patient at great risk for dehydration and malnutrition. The small bowel averages 600 cm in length and absorbs about 10 L/day of ingested and secreted fluids. A patient may tolerate substantial loss of small bowel, although preservation of more than 2 ft with an intact colon and ileocecal valve or more than 5 ft in the absence of the colon and ileocecal valve may make survival impossible with enteral use alone. In addition, the loss of the distal ileum precludes absorption of bile acids and vitamin B_{12}. Remaining bowel, especially ileum, may adapt its absorptive ability over several years, but underlying disease may hamper this process.

10. **Describe the management of nutritional problems in patients with short bowel syndrome.**
    Therapy in the acute postsurgical phase is aimed at intravenous fluid and electrolyte restoration. Parenteral nutrition may be required while the remaining gut function is assessed and adaptation takes place. Attempts at oral feeding should include frequent, small meals with initial limitations in fluid and fat consumption. Osmolar sugars (e.g., sorbitol), lactose, and high-oxalate foods are best avoided. In patients with small bowel-colon continuity, increased use of complex carbohydrates may allow the salvage of a few hundred calories from colonic production and absorption of short-chain fatty acids. Antimotility drugs and gastric acid suppression should be used if stool output remains high. Oral rehydration with glucose- and sodium-containing fluids (e.g., sports drinks) may help to prevent dehydration. Pancreatic enzymes, bile acid-binding resins (if bile acids are irritating the colon), and octreotide injections may play a role in selected cases. If oral diets fail, the use of elemental feedings may enhance absorption and nutritional state. Studies of gut rehabilitation with growth hormone and glutamine, as well as intestinal or combined intestinal-liver transplantation, are available at selected centers.

11. **Describe the approach to nutritional support in patients with acute pancreatitis**
    Pancreatitis can resemble other cases of stressed metabolism. If severe pancreatitis precludes the resumption of food intake beyond 4–5 days, consideration should be given to nutrition support. The route of feeding remains controversial; neither bowel/pancreatic rest nor nutritional support has been shown conclusively to alter the clinical course beyond improvement of the nutritional state. Several recent randomized trials suggest that distal (jejunal) enteral feeding may be tolerated as well as bowel rest/total parenteral nutrition (TPN), with fewer complications. The enteral route may be tried in the absence of GI dysfunction (e.g., ileus). Energy expenditure is variable, but most likely only 20–30% above basal. Use partial or total parenteral nutrition if the enteral approach fails. Experiments suggest that parenteral

TABLE 60-1. VITAMIN AND MINERAL DEFICIENCIES AND TOXICITIES

Micronutrient	Deficiency	Toxicity
Vitamin A	Follicular hyperkeratosis, night blindness, corneal drying, keratomalacia	Dermatitis, xerosis, hair loss, joint pain, hyperostosis, edema, hypercalcemia, hepatomegaly, pseudotumor
Vitamin D	Rickets, osteomalacia, hypophosphatemia, muscle weakness	Fatigue, headache, hypercalcemia, bone decalcification
Vitamin E	Hemolytic anemia, myopathy, ataxia, ophthalmoplegia, retinopathy, areflexia	Rare: possible interference with vitamin K, arachidonic acid metabolism; headache, myopathy
Vitamin K	Bruisability, prolonged prothrombin time	Rapid IV infusion: possible flushing, cardiovascular collapse
Vitamin C	Scurvy: poor wound healing, perifollicular hemorrhage, gingivitis, dental defects, anemia, joint pain	Diarrhea; possible hyperoxaluria, uricosuria; interference with glucose, occult blood tests; dry mouth, dental erosion
Vitamin B_1 (thiamine)	Dry beriberi (polyneuropathy): anorexia, low temperature Wet beriberi (high-output congestive heart failure): lactic acidosis Wernicke-Korsakoff syndrome: ataxia, nystagmus, memory loss, confabulation, ophthalmoplegia	Large dose IV: anorexia, ataxia, ileus, headache, irritability
Vitamin B_2 (riboflavin)	Seborrheic dermatitis, stomatitis, cheilosis, geographic tongue, burning eyes, anemia	None
Vitamin B_3 (niacin)	Anorexia, lethargy, burning sensations, glossitis, headache, stupor, seizures Pellagra: diarrhea, pigmented dermatitis, dementia	Hyperglycemia, hyperuricemia, GI symptoms, peptic ulcer, flushing, liver dysfunction
Vitamin B_6 (pyridoxine)	Peripheral neuritis, seborrhea, glossitis, stomatitis, anemia, CNS/EEG changes, seizures	Metabolic dependency, sensory neuropathy

Continued

TABLE 60-1. VITAMIN AND MINERAL DEFICIENCIES AND TOXICITIES—CONT'D

Micronutrient	Deficiency	Toxicity
Vitamin B$_{12}$	Glossitis, paresthesias, CNS changes, megaloblastic anemia, depression, diarrhea	None
Folic acid	Glossitis, intestinal mucosal dysfunction, megaloblastic anemia	Antagonizes antiepileptic drugs, decreases zinc absorption
Biotin	Scaly dermatitis, hair loss, papillae atrophy, myalgia, paresthesias, hypercholesterolemia	None
Pantothenic acid	Malaise, GI symptoms, cramps, paresthesias	Diarrhea
Calcium	Paresthesias, tetany, seizures, osteopenia, arrhythmia	Hypercalciuria, GI symptoms, lethargy
Phosphorus	Hemolysis, muscle weakness, ophthalmoplegia, osteomalacia	Diarrhea
Magnesium	Paresthesias, tetany, seizures, arrhythmia	Diarrhea, muscle weakness, arrhythmia
Iron	Fatigue, dyspnea, glossitis, anemia, koilonychia	Iron overload (hepatic, cardiac), possible oxidation damage
Iodine	Goiter, hypothyroidism	Goiter, hypo/hyperthyroidism
Zinc	Lethargy, anorexia, loss of taste/smell, rash, hypogonadism, poor wound healing, immunosuppression	Impaired copper, iron metabolism, reduced HDL, immunosuppression
Copper	Anemia, neutropenia, lethargy, depigmentation, connective tissue weakness	GI symptoms, hepatic damage
Chromium	Glucose intolerance, neuropathy, hyperlipidemia	None
Selenium	Keshan's cardiomyopathy, muscle weakness	GI symptoms
Manganese	Possible weight loss, dermatitis, hair disturbances	Inhalation injury only
Molybdenum	Possible headache, vomiting, CNS changes	Interferes with copper metabolism, possible gout
Fluorine	Increased dental caries	Teeth mottling, possible bone integrity/fluorosis

nutrition, including intravenous fat, elicits little significant pancreatic secretion; however, all patients with pancreatitis should be monitored to exclude severe hypertriglyceridemia.

2. **What adverse GI effects may be encountered in a patient using herbal supplements?**

It is estimated that one third to one half of the U.S. population uses herbal products in supplementary form and that 60–75% do not inform health care providers. Because herbal products are not regulated and their composition not standardized, toxicity data are less clear than with regulated pharmaceuticals. However, popular products that may cause adverse GI effects include saw palmetto, Ginkgo biloba (nonspecific GI upset), garlic (nausea, diarrhea), ginseng (nausea, diarrhea), aloe (diarrhea, abdominal pain), and guar gum (obstruction). In addition, hepatotoxicity (ranging from asymptomatic enzyme elevation to fulminant necrosis) has been documented with germander, chapparal, senna, atractylis, and callilepsis. Hepatotoxicity associated with the use of valerian, mistletoe, skullcap, and various Chinese herbal mixtures has been noted but awaits a cause-and-effect confirmation. The pyrrolizidine alkaloids in crotalaria, senecio, heliotropium, and comfrey have long been implicated in cases of veno-occlusive disease.

3. **How is obesity defined, and how common is it among Americans?**

Body mass index (BMI) has become the standard of measurement for obesity:

BMI = weight (kg) / body surface area (m^2)

BMI >30 kg/m^2 is defined as obese.

Body Mass Index Category	BMI kg/m^2
Normal	18.5–24.9
Overweight	25–29.9
Obesity	30–39.9
Morbid/extreme	40–49.9
Super obesity	>50

Adults	1988–1994	1999–2000
Obese	22.9%	30.5%
Overweight	55.9%	64.5%
Extremely obese	2.9%	4.7%

Although the number of adults has doubled since 1980, the number of obese adults has quadrupled: approximately 97 million adults in the United States are obese.

4. **Does obesity carry a significant risk for death?**

Yes; 300,000 persons in the United States die annually from obesity-related diseases:

Cardiomyopathy	Degenerative joint disease
Coronary artery disease	Immobility
Dyslipidemia	Depression
Hypertension	Malignancies
Diabetes	Dyspnea
Infertility	Obstructive sleep apnea
Fatty liver	Obesity hypoventilation
Gastroesophageal reflux disease (GERD)	Deep vein thrombosis
Gallstones	Pulmonary embolus
Chronic fatigue	Venous stasis
Urinary stress incontinence	

5. **What are the medical therapies for obesity?**

Dietary restriction of calories (while maintaining adequate protein, fluid electrolyte) in mineral and vitamin intake is the key. A sensible weight reduction program targets gradual weight reduction by behavior modification, including diet and activity changes. Numerous fad diets claim success, but key to the weight loss is patient commitment and total lifestyle modification.

16. **What are the surgical options for obesity?**
Bariatric surgery dates back to the 1950s when intestinal bypass was first performed. The total weight lost correlates with the total length of bowel bypassed. Gastric bypass (GBP) is the most common weight loss surgery performed in the United States. (See Chapter 79, Obesity and Surgical Weight Loss.)

17. **What are the National Institutes of Health consensus criteria felt to be viable indications for bariatric surgery?**

Failure of a major weight-loss program	plus	morbid obesity BMI >40 kg/m^2

or

Failure of a major weight-loss program	plus	BMI >35 kg/m^2 and obesity-related comorbidities*

*Hypertension, type-2 diabetes mellitus, degenerative joint and disc disease, GERD, sleep apnea, obesity hypoventilation, severe venous stasis, abdominal wall hernias, and pseudotumor cerebri.

18. **What is the operative mortality of GBP surgery?**
Operative mortality ranges from 0.3–1.6%, and perioperative complications occur in 10% of patients:

Splenic injury	Pulmonary failure
Pneumonia	Cardiac events
Wound infection	Wound dehiscence
Thrombotic events	Thrombocytopenia
Anastomotic leaks	Intra-abdominal sepsis
Hemorrhage	Death

19. **What are medical benefits of bariatric surgery?**
Diabetes: 83% of NIDDM and 99% of those with glucose intolerance maintained normal levels of plasma glucose, glycosylated hemoglobin and insulin. 88% with diabetes no longer required medication.
Cardiovascular: 15% decrease in cholesterol, 50% decrease in triglyceride HTN 58% rx treated to 14%
Pulmonary: 14% preoperative have obstructive or hypoventilation syndrome with most improved

20. **What nutritional deficiencies are seen with bariatric surgery?**
- Fat malabsorption
- B_{12} deficiency: 37% develop B_{12} deficiency
- Folate deficiency
- Fat-soluble vitamin deficiency
- Iron deficiency and anemia seen in 33% and 30%, respectively

Recommended supplements: iron, 325 mg b.i.d.; B_{12} as part of a multivitamin; folate as part of multivitamin; calcium, 1200–1500 mg in divided doses over the day. Calcium citrate is better absorbed in a low-acid environment.

WEBSITES

1. http://www.asbs.org

2. http://www.niddk.nih.gov/health/nutrition.htm

3. http://www.obesitylaw.com

4. http://www.weightlosssurgeryinfo.com/

5. www.mypyramid.gov/

BIBLIOGRAPHY

1. Buddeberg-Fischer B, Klaghofer R, Sigrist S, Buddeberg C: Impact of psychosocial stress and symptoms on indication for bariatric surgery and outcome in morbidly obese patients. Obes Surg 14(3):361–369, 2004.

2. Byrne TK: Complications of surgery for obesity. Surg Clin North Am 81:1181–1193, 2001.

3. Detsky A, McGlaughlin J, Baker J, et al: What is subjective global assessment of nutritional status? J Parent Ent Nutr 11:8–13, 1987.

4. Heyland D, MacDonald S, Keefe L, et al: Total parenteral nutrition in the critically ill patient: A meta-analysis. JAMA 280:2013–2019, 1998.

5. Heys S, Walker L, Smith I, et al: Enteral nutritional supplementation with key nutrients in patients with critical illness and cancer: A meta-analysis of randomized controlled clinical trials. Ann Surg 229:467–477, 1999.

6. Hunter D, Jaksic T, Lewis D, et al: Resting energy expenditure in the critically ill: Estimation vs. measurement. Br J Surg 75:875–878, 1988.

7. Institute of Medicine: Dietary reference intakes for calcium, phosphorous, magnesium, vitamin D, and fluoride. Washington, DC, National Academy Press, 1997.

8. Institute of Medicine: Dietary reference intakes for thiamin, riboflavin, niacin, vitamin B6, folate, vitamin B12, pantothenic acid, biotin, and choline. Washington, DC, National Academy Press, 1998.

9. Institute of Medicine: Dietary reference intakes for vitamin C, vitamin E, selenium, and carotenoids. Washington, DC, National Academy Press, 2000.

10. Klein S, Kinney J, Jeejeebhoy K, et al: Nutrition support in clinical practice: Review of published data and recommendations for future research directions. J Parent Ent Nutr 21:133–156, 1997.

11. Lee WJ, Wang W, Chen TC, et al: Clinical significance of central obesity in laparoscopic bariatric surgery. Obes Surg 13(6):921–925, 2003.

12. Moore F, Feliciano D, Andrassy R, et al: Early enteral feeding compared with parenteral reduces postoperative septic complications: Results of meta-analysis. Ann Surg 216:172–183, 1992.

13. Pinkney J, Kerrigan D: Current status of bariatric surgery in the treatment of type 2 diabetes. J Obes Rev 5:69–78, 2004.

14. Rombeau J, Caldwell M (eds): Parenteral Nutrition, 3rd ed. Philadelphia, WB Saunders, 2000.

15. Tripp F: The use of dietary supplements in the elderly: Current issues and recommendations. J Am Diet Assoc 97(10 Suppl 2):S181–S183, 1997.

16. Ukleja A, Stone RL: Medical and gastroenterologic management of the post-bariatric surgery patient. J Clin Gastroenterol 38(4):312–321, 2004.

POTPOURRI: NAUSEA AND VOMITING, HICCUPS, BULIMIA/ANOREXIA, AND RUMINATION

Steven S. Shay, MD

NAUSEA AND VOMITING

1. **How is vomiting distinguished from regurgitation, and what disorders present with regurgitation?**

   Vomiting is characterized by the presence of nausea and autonomic symptoms, such as salivation, followed by the forceful abdominal and thoracic muscle contractions associated with retching. In contrast, regurgitation is the sudden, effortless return of small volumes of gastric or esophageal contents into the pharynx and implies cricopharyngeal relaxation or insufficiency.

   Chronic regurgitation may result from oropharyngeal or esophageal disorders or gastroesophageal reflux. Patients with Zenker's diverticulum may accumulate secretions and food that empty into the pharynx, especially at night. Structural lesions, such as esophageal cancer, may obstruct the esophagus. Esophageal diverticula may cause accumulation of food particles and secretions and result in regurgitation when the contents are discharged into the esophageal lumen. Esophageal motility disorders, such as achalasia and primary esophageal spasm, may also be responsible for regurgitation.

2. **What disorders must be considered in acute nausea and vomiting?**

   See Table 61-1.

3. **What specific symptoms or characteristics of acute nausea and vomiting should be sought to narrow the differential diagnosis?**

   The presence of abdominal pain strongly suggests an intra-abdominal process as the cause of acute nausea and vomiting, and the character of the pain, physical findings, and initial routine diagnostic laboratory tests (e.g., amylase, liver tests, complete blood count) direct the subsequent diagnostic evaluation. Suspicion of peritonitis requires recumbent and upright abdominal radiographs, including the diaphragm, to exclude the presence of free air under the diaphragm. In contrast, the abdominal radiograph in patients with colicky pain may confirm the presence of obstruction (mechanical or pseudo-obstruction). Suspicion of biliary colic or acute cholecystitis requires ultrasound and/or hepato-iminodiacetic acid (HIDA) scan, whereas pancreatitis is typically first suspected because of an increased amylase level.

   The presence of systemic symptoms, such as fever or diarrhea, suggests the possibility of food poisoning with one of several toxins or an infection. Other systemic symptoms, such as polyuria and polydipsia, suggest a metabolic disorder. A chemistry screen should be obtained to exclude such disorders.

   The presence of abnormal mental status, headache, meningismus, or a preceding head injury suggests the possibility of a central nervous system (CNS) etiology and should prompt appropriate investigation. A history of vertigo or the presence of nystagmus suggests a motion disorder rather than CNS disease.

   If there are no systemic symptoms, abdominal complaints, or CNS symptoms or signs, several other considerations should be entertained. The possibility of pregnancy should be

TABLE 61-1.	DISORDERS COMMONLY ASSOCIATED WITH ACUTE NAUSEA AND VOMITING	
Intra-Abdominal Disorders	**Metabolic Disorders**
Mechanical obstruction	Renal failure
Stomach	Ketoacidosis (e.g., diabetes)
Small bowel	Addison's disease
Pseudo-obstruction	
Peritonitis	**Central Nervous System Disorders**
Acute pancreatitis	
Acute cholecystitis	**Vestibular Disorders**
Infections or Toxins	**Pregnancy**
Infection	
Epidemic (e.g., Norwalk agent)	**Drugs**
Viral hepatitis	Narcotics
Toxins	Digitalis
Staphylococcus aureus	Aminophylline
Bacillus cereus	Chemotherapeutic drugs
Clostridium perfringens	

considered early in any evaluation of nausea and vomiting. Serum and/or urine human chorionic gonadotropin levels should be obtained to avoid tests using radiation. All medications should be reviewed to exclude the possibility of drug-associated nausea and vomiting. Finally, Addison's disease needs to be considered.

4. **What are the major etiologic considerations for chronic nausea and vomiting, and how are they evaluated?**
   Disorders that typically present with chronic nausea and vomiting are: (1) gastroparesis, (2) small bowel dysmotility, and (3) psychogenic vomiting. One historic clue is that all of these disorders typically present with repeated postprandial vomiting.

5. **What is gastroparesis, and how is it diagnosed?**
   Gastroparesis is defined as an impairment in gastric emptying in the absence of mechanical obstruction in the stomach or small bowel. It may be seen with certain drugs (e.g., narcotics), after gastrectomy, in patients with diabetes, scleroderma, or amyloidosis, or for no apparent reason (idiopathic). It is often difficult to distinguish idiopathic gastroparesis from psychogenic vomiting. Radionuclide solid-food gastric emptying, most commonly using a radiolabeled fried-egg sandwich, is the most helpful test in making the diagnosis.

6. **What disorders cause small bowel dysmotility, and how should they be evaluated?**
   In patients with intestinal pseudo-obstruction, no obstruction is found with appropriate diagnostic tests (especially small bowel follow-through) performed during recovery from an episode. Other signs, such as abdominal distention, pain, changes in bowel habits, orthostatic hypotension, or bladder symptoms, may be present. Intestinal pseudo-obstruction may be seen with certain medications or systemic disorders, most commonly scleroderma, diabetes, and

amyloidosis. These systemic disorders, as well as jejunal diverticulosis, must be specifically excluded with appropriate diagnostic studies. When these diagnoses have been excluded, primary small bowel myopathy or neuropathy may be present. Esophageal motility may suggest the diagnosis when aperistalsis is found. If these disorders are suspected and esophageal motility is normal, consideration of small bowel motility and/or small bowel biopsy at laparotomy will need to be made on an individual basis. This is best done in a referral center with expertise in such disorders.

7. **How is psychogenic vomiting diagnosed?**
   Psychogenic vomiting is a cause of recurring vomiting in patients, especially young women, with an underlying emotional disturbance. However, it is occasionally a manifestation of major depression or conversion reaction. Although psychogenic vomiting is a diagnosis of exclusion, certain characteristics suggest its presence, including vomiting that has been present for a long time, especially during emotional strain. Moreover, vomiting is typically seen after the meal rather than delayed, and it can be suppressed if necessary. Finally, the vomiting may be of surprisingly little concern to the patient and of more concern to family members. Abdominal pain may be a major associated symptom. The diagnosis needs to be considered to avoid extensive diagnostic procedures or abdominal surgery that may worsen and complicate the issue.

8. **What consequences of vomiting should be anticipated and treated?**
   Be vigilant for metabolic derangements or dehydration that may require hospitalization. Because of the loss of hydrogen ions in vomitus and contraction of extracellular fluid volume, alkalosis commonly develops. Second, potassium deficiency is common due to the loss of potassium in vomitus and wasting from the kidneys. Therefore, the clinical features of potassium deficiency, including muscle weakness, and cardiac arrhythmias may be present.
   Another major consequence of vomiting is an emetogenic injury. With protracted or forceful vomiting, a Mallory-Weiss laceration or, rarely, Boerhaave's syndrome (transmural tear of the esophagus) may occur. These complications need to be considered in patients with vomiting who develop a gastrointestinal bleed, odynophagia, or catastrophic chest pain.

9. **What drugs are used to treat nausea and vomiting?**
   See Table 61-2.

TABLE 61–2.   DRUGS USED TO TREAT NAUSEA AND VOMITING

Antihistamines (H_1-antagonist)	Trimethobenzamide (Tigan)
Dimenhydrinate (Dramamine)	Dopaminergic antagonists
Promethazine (Phenergan)	Metoclopramide (Reglan)
Meclizine (Antivert)	Domperidone
Cyclizine (Marezine)	Octreotide
Anticholinergic drugs	Erythromycin
Scopolamine	Serotonin receptor antagonists
Phenothiazine	Ondansetron (Zofran)
Prochlorperazine (Compazine)	Dolasetron (Anzemet)
Chlorpromazine (Thorazine)	
Butyrophenone	
Haloperidol (Haldol)	

0. **When should these drugs be used in patients with nausea and vomiting?**

The antihistamines (H_1-antagonists) and anticholinergics (scopolamine) are used primarily for patients with nausea and vomiting secondary to vestibular disorders or motion sickness. The phenothiazine, haloperidol, and serotonin receptor antagonists are the most commonly prescribed antiemetics and are useful for a wide variety of disorders.

Metoclopramide has a central dopamine antagonist effect; however, the peripheral dopamine antagonist effect is responsible for prokinetic activity. It has been used in gastroparesis and, in much larger doses, for prophylaxis against chemotherapy-associated nausea and vomiting. Common side effects include anxiety, lethargy, and increased prolactin levels. Rare side effects include depression and dystonia, particularly in older patients. Domperidone has a prokinetic effect, but because it does not readily cross the blood-brain barrier, it has less CNS effect. Side effects are uncommon. Domperidone is not yet available in the United States.

Erythromycin interacts with motilin receptors on gastrointestinal smooth muscle membranes in an action independent of its antibiotic effect. It is effective acutely in gastroparesis, though less evidence exists that it is effective on a prolonged basis.

Octreotide has been found to improve small bowel motility in patients with scleroderma and, in combination with erythromycin, often improves symptoms in patients with either idiopathic or scleroderma-associated pseudo-obstruction.

The newest agents for the treatment of nausea and vomiting are the serotonin antagonists. Ondansetron is an antagonist to the $5-HT_3$ receptor, which is one of three serotonin receptors that have been identified. They are the most common antiemetics now used with chemotherapy-induced emesis and are given frequently for other causes of nausea and vomiting as well. They appear to have only rare adverse effects.

1. **What is the role of gastric pacing in gastroparesis?**

Gastric pacing via electrodes implanted in gastric serosa has been shown to improve gastric emptying and decrease symptoms. Only open-label trials have been reported to date, and controlled studies with more patients are needed. A gastric neurostimulator has been approved for humanitarian use by the FDA, which allows restricted marketing and implantation in centers where Institutional Review Board approval has been granted. Controlled studies, with more patients and longer follow-up, are needed.

HICCUPS

2. **What are hiccups? When are they pathologic?**

Hiccups are spasmodic, involuntary contractions of the muscles of inspiration (not just the diaphragm) almost simultaneously with closure of the glottis. Closure of the glottis is responsible for the audible sound. Hiccups are usually short-lived, typically occur after meals or alcohol ingestion, and subside without treatment or with simple measures, such as breath-holding, water ingestion, or Valsalva's maneuvers.

An episode of hiccups lasting 48 hours, or recurring episodes of protracted hiccups, is defined as chronic. Some unfortunate people have prolonged episodes of hiccups or constant hiccups for years. Chronic hiccups can be disabling, resulting in chronic fatigue, sleep deprivation, interference with normal eating, and depression. Thus, chronic hiccups, which occur predominantly in men, require diagnostic evaluation and prompt treatment. However, even acute hiccups can be devastating and require prompt treatment in certain settings, such as postoperatively or in the early period after myocardial infarction.

3. **What causes chronic hiccups, and what is the diagnostic evaluation?**

Because the afferent limb of the hiccup reflex includes the vagus and phrenic nerves as well as sympathetic fibers T6–T12, a wide variety of intra-abdominal and intrathoracic disorders have been associated with hiccups. In contrast, because hiccups result in physiologic changes (such as a decrease in lower esophageal sphincter pressure), some abnormalities, such as reflux esophagitis, are usually a result of hiccups rather than the cause. A variety of CNS disorders have also been found to cause chronic hiccups. Last, metabolic diseases such as chronic renal failure and, especially, diabetes mellitus are associated with chronic hiccups.

Fluoroscopy of the diaphragm should be performed. If the diaphragm shows unilateral involvement only (usually the left hemidiaphragm), the diagnostic evaluation should focus on the course of the phrenic nerve of the affected side. Bilateral diaphragmatic motion suggests an afferent or central origin. Because a wide variety of intra-abdominal and intrathoracic disorders are associated with the chronic hiccups, unless symptoms point toward a specific organ system, one should begin with laboratory tests (complete blood count, chemistry screen), abdominal flat plate (mechanical obstruction), endoscopy (peptic ulcer disease, gastric cancer, infiltrating diseases), and chest radiograph. If these tests are negative, consider computed tomography (CT) scans of the abdomen and chest and magnetic resonance imaging (MRI) of the brain.

Unfortunately, a thorough evaluation may be negative or find only an abnormal condition that may be coexisting (gastritis) or secondary to the hiccups (esophagitis, for example).

14. **What therapies are available for chronic hiccups?**
The best therapy is directed toward the cause. Unfortunately, the diagnostic evaluation is often negative, and therapy may have to be directed toward the hiccups themselves. Simple measures, such as breath-holding, swallowing water, Valsalva's maneuvers, or rebreathing into a bag, are rarely helpful for protracted hiccups. Instead, more vigorous mechanical approaches or drug therapy are usually necessary, and, occasionally, phrenic nerve ablation should be considered. In my experience, the best way to stop an episode of hiccups is firm digital stimulation of the posterior pharynx, occasionally with a nasogastric tube in place. This technique is unpleasant for patients and is primarily useful for patients with long intervals between isolated episodes of hiccups. For those whose hiccups recur a short time after cessation, this approach is not feasible.

Various drugs have been proposed as effective therapy for hiccups, but experience with each is limited usually to a few cases. Chlorpromazine, metoclopramide, and nifedipine have advocates who proclaim their efficacy in chronic hiccups. In my experience and that of others, the single most effective medication is baclofen, a derivative of gamma aminobutyric acid used as an antispasticity agent in patients with tics or dystonias. Complete cessation of hiccups occurs, but most patients experience a variable decrease in the frequency of episodes. Nevertheless, for some unfortunate patients who suffer near-daily hiccups for a large proportion of their day, this partial response can be gratifying. Dosage begins at 5 mg three times/day and is increased in a stepwise fashion to a maximum dose of 20 mg three times/day. Side effects include somnolence and fatigue. Do not suddenly discontinue the medication, but taper it over time. For postoperative patients with hiccups, nefopam (10 mg IV) has recently been found to be effective.

When unilateral involvement is demonstrated at fluoroscopy and other measures have been exhausted, phrenic nerve intervention should be considered. Because respiratory function may be significantly impaired after diaphragmatic paralysis, pulmonary function tests should be obtained before intervention. Temporary diaphragmatic paralysis confirmed by fluoroscopy and concomitant cessation of hiccups should be demonstrated before permanent ablation of the phrenic nerve is considered. Initial results of phrenic nerve stimulation by surgical placement of electrodes on the phrenic nerve in the neck is a promising new approach but has been reported in only a few patients.

EATING DISORDERS

15. **If eating disorders are psychiatric illnesses, why should an internist be aware of them?**
Anorexia nervosa and bulimia nervosa, the two major well-defined eating disorders, are relatively common. The American Psychiatric Association cited a lifetime prevalence rate of

0.5–1% in women. The internist or gastroenterologist needs to be aware of these disorders, because the family may bring the patient to the physician with concerns that profound weight loss, vomiting, or associated symptoms (e.g., constipation, abdominal pain, dyspepsia) suggest a gastrointestinal disorder. Successful management requires: (1) early suspicion that an eating disorder is present; (2) evaluation for complications; (3) exclusion of a gastrointestinal (e.g., achalasia or Crohn's disease) or systemic (e.g., AIDS) disorder; and (4) prompt referral to a clinician experienced in treating eating disorders.

6. What criteria are required to diagnose anorexia nervosa in Diagnostic and Statistical Manual of Mental Disorders (DSM-IV-TR), and what are typical characteristics?

1. Refusal to maintain body weight at a minimally normal weight for age and height.
2. Intense fear of gaining weight or becoming fat, even though underweight.
3. Disturbance in the way in which body weight or shape is experienced, undue influence of body weight or shape on self-evaluation, or denial of the seriousness of the current low body weight.
4. In postmenarcheal women, amenorrhea (i.e., absence of at least three consecutive menstrual cycles).

Women are overwhelmingly affected; only 5–10% of patients are men. The onset in most patients is in late adolescence and early adulthood, at a mean age of 17 years. The onset is often associated with a stressful life event, such as going to college. There is a high incidence of sexual abuse among these patients. Associated symptoms include depressed mood, obsessive-compulsive acts (such as a preoccupation with food or food hoarding), and overcontrolling behavior, resulting in a typically inflexible attitude in most life situations. Physical examination is dominated by the patient's emaciated state. Other clues include increased size of the salivary glands (especially the parotid gland) and signs of recurring vomiting, such as decreased dental enamel and calluses on the dorsum of the hand (Russell's sign).

7. What complications should be anticipated in patients with anorexia nervosa?

Patients have findings related to degree of starvation. They may have mild leukopenia and normocytic anemia; moreover, endocrine evaluation may reveal regression of the hypothalamic-pituitary-gonadal axis to a prepubertal pattern. Osteoporosis and poor bone growth may occur. Cardiac arrhythmias are the most common cause of death after suicide. Vomiting and purging have sequelae. Repeated vomiting may cause an emetogenic injury. Dehydration and electrolyte disturbances, especially hypokalemia, may be particularly profound in patients using large amounts of laxatives for purging. Rare patients who use ipecac may have a cardiac and skeletal myopathy. Last, amylase may be elevated, although it is typically of the salivary isoamylase type.

8. What is the differential diagnosis for patients with suspected anorexia nervosa?

When the patient has many of the characteristic findings of an eating disorder, it should be the working diagnosis. Only a few disorders need to be considered and expeditiously excluded, including achalasia, inflammatory bowel disease (especially Crohn's disease), celiac sprue, pancreatic insufficiency, or recurring mechanical obstruction. Nongastrointestinal problems include endocrine disorders (especially panhypopituitarism, Addison's disease, or hyperthyroidism), occult neoplasm, and AIDS.

9. How are patients with anorexia nervosa managed, and what is their natural history?

Because of the variable and serious nature of anorexia nervosa, treatment requires an experienced primary physician who can integrate a multiphasic treatment regimen. Medical management is required to restore weight and correct metabolic problems. In general, patients with moderate (65–80% of ideal body weight) and severe (<65% of ideal body weight) weight loss or low prognostic nutritional index scores require nutrition supplementation.

Hospitalization is required for the severely malnourished. Psychological approaches use one or a combination of the following:

1. Behavioral therapies, such as operant conditioning
2. Cognitive therapy, such as assessing and examining distortions in thought processes
3. Family counseling
4. Pharmacotherapy

The course of anorexia nervosa varies markedly, and the spectrum ranges from people with one episode and subsequent recovery to patients who have repeated relapses or an unremitting course leading to death. The early mortality rate is estimated at 5%; the late mortality rate is over 10% because of suicide, arrhythmia, or emaciation. Rates for full recovery are widely variable, ranging from 32–71% after 20 years.

20. **What are the DSM-IV-TR diagnostic criteria for bulimia nervosa?**
   1. Recurrent episodes of binge eating, characterized by both of the following:
      - Eating an amount of food that is definitely larger than most people would eat during a similar period and under similar circumstances.
      - A sense of lack of control over eating during the episode.
   2. Recurrent inappropriate compensatory behavior to prevent weight gain, such as self-induced vomiting; misuse of laxatives, diuretics, enemas, or other medications; fasting; or excessive exercise.
   3. Binge eating and compensatory behaviors both occur, on average, at least twice a week for 3 months.
   4. Body shape and weight unduly influence self-evaluation.
   5. The disturbance does not occur exclusively during episodes of anorexia nervosa.

   Although some argue that bulimic patients are too similar to patients with anorexia nervosa to be differentiated, bulimic patients have less body-image distortion and are more accepting of therapy.

21. **What are other characteristics that may aid in the diagnosis of bulimia nervosa**
   The vast predominance of women and age of onset mirror anorexia nervosa. However, bulimia nervosa is more common and, in various studies, has been reported in 1–3% of the adolescent and young adult female population.

   Characteristically, patients try to conceal their binging or purging behavior, which tends to occur during periods of stress. Vomiting rarely occurs in public, as patients can control their vomiting until they are in a private location. Although vomiting is the most common compensatory behavior (80–90% of cases), approximately one third of patients uses laxatives. The vomiting may be initially forceful but later in the disease becomes nearly effortless. Rare patients use ipecac.

   Bulimic patients characteristically have difficulty in developing personal relationships and may have chemical dependencies, especially alcohol. One third have personality disorders.

   Physical findings are not obvious. Because they are not malnourished, bulimics appear generally healthy, and other people who know the patient well, even family members, may not be aware of the disorder. The physical findings characteristic of patients with repeat vomiting may be present, as noted for anorexia nervosa. Complications are related to the compensatory vomiting and purging behavior and are the same as those for anorexia nervosa.

22. **What therapy is available for bulimic patients, and what is their natural history?**
   Bulimia nervosa can be managed on an outpatient basis. A program that includes both cognitive recognition of the patient's abnormal behavior and therapy directed at the abnormal behavior is the approach of choice. Antidepressants are useful in some.

The course of bulimia nervosa is variable. In one large study, after 6 years after successful therapy, good, intermediate, and poor outcomes were noted in 60%, 29%, and 10%, respectively; 1% had died. Fatalities are most commonly from cardiac arrhythmias.

RUMINATION

3. **What is rumination? Can complications occur?**
   Rumination is the regurgitation of mouthfuls of recently ingested food, with subsequent remastication and reswallowing, in the absence of apparent organic disease. Usually, rumination begins 15–20 minutes after a meal and continues until the stomach contents become sour as a result of acid (20–60 minutes later). As many as 20 episodes per meal are not uncommon. Patients do not describe it as distressful and are often embarrassed and attempt to hide the symptom. Eating large volumes of food quickly, and with a lot of liquids, facilitates rumination.

   Rumination is uncommon in adults, although it is underreported because patients are unlikely to discuss a symptom that they consider embarrassing. Men predominate, and although no consistent intellectual or social characteristics are present, physicians and scientists are highly represented in various reviews.

   Heartburn may start many years after the onset of rumination, suggesting that an acid-sensitive esophagus develops from repeated acid contact during ruminating. Rare reports of gastrointestinal bleeding and hemorrhagic esophagitis at endoscopy have been published.

4. **What is the mechanism of rumination?**
   On observation, most people with rumination have abdominal and thoracic movements that precede and accompany the process. Gastroesophageal manometry performed postprandially has found that Valsalva's maneuvers occur simultaneously with regurgitation. In one report, the Valsalva's maneuver occurred repeatedly over a lower esophageal sphincter and with a pharyngeal maneuver that preceded the upper esophageal sphincter relaxation. Thus, a voluntary component is involved and has led to behavioral therapy and biofeedback as the therapy of choice. No case has been reported in which rumination was accompanied by reverse peristalsis, as described in ruminant animals.

5. **What should be the therapeutic approach?**
   Behavioral therapy is the treatment of choice for adults. Changing the composition of food, slowing the speed of eating, and giving less water with the meal have been effective approaches in some reports. Biofeedback directed against the increased intra-abdominal pressure that always precedes regurgitation episodes has also been effective. Aversive therapies, such as ingesting foods that are distasteful if regurgitated, should be avoided.

BLIOGRAPHY

1. Abell T, Van Cutsam E, Abrahamsson H, et al: Gastric electrical stimulation in intractable symptomatic gastroparesis. Digestion 66:204–212, 2002.
2. American Psychiatric Association: Eating disorders. In Diagnostic and Statistical Manual of Mental Disorders, 4th ed. Washington, DC, American Psychiatric Association, 2000, pp 583–594.
3. Becker A, Grinspoon S, Kubanski A, et al: Eating disorders. NEJM 340:1092–1098, 1999.
4. Bilotta F, Pietropaoli P, Rosa G: Nefopam for refractory postoperative hiccups. Anesth Analg 93:1358–1360, 2001.
5. Cymet T: Retrospective analysis of hiccups in patients at a community hospital from 1995–2000. J Natl Med Assoc 94:480–483, 2002.
6. Dobelle H: Use of breathing pacemakers to suppress intractable hiccups of up to thirteen years duration. ASAIO 45:524–525, 1999.

7. Hasler W: Approach to the patient with nausea and vomiting. In Yamada T (ed): Gastroenterology. Philadelphia, Lippincott Williams & Wilkins, 2003, pp 760–780.

8. Launois S, Bizec JL, Whitelaw WA, et al: Hiccup in adults: An overview. Eur Respir J 6:563–575, 1993.

9. Malcolm MB, Thumshirn MB, Camilleri M, et al: Rumination syndrome. Mayo Clin Proc 72:646–652, 1997.

10. Practice guideline for the treatment of patients with eating disorders. Am J Psychiatry 157(Suppl):1–39, 2000.

11. Ramirez FC, Graham DY: Treatment of intractable hiccup with Baclofen. Am J Gastroenterol 87:1789–1791, 1992.

12. Shay SS: Regurgitation and rumination. In Castell DO (ed): The Esophagus. Philadelphia, Lippincott Williams & Wilkins, 1999, pp 505–509.

FOREIGN BODIES AND THE GASTROINTESTINAL TRACT

George Triadafilopoulos, MD

1. **How common are foreign bodies in the gastrointestinal (GI) tract?**
   Every year, millions of foreign bodies enter the GI tract through the mouth or anus, and about 1500 to 3000 people die every year from ingestion of foreign objects. However, only about 10–20% of foreign bodies require removal through some form of therapeutic intervention; the rest pass through the GI tract without incident.

2. **Which populations are at risk for foreign-body ingestion?**
   Eighty percent of foreign-body ingestions occur in children, whereas almost all foreign bodies inserted into the rectum are described in adults. Other groups at increased risk for foreign-body ingestion include psychiatric patients, inmates, and people who frequently use alcohol or sedative-hypnotic medications. Also at risk are elderly subjects, who may have poorly fitting dentures, impaired cognitive function due to medications, or dementia and/or dysphagia after stroke. Intentional ingestion of foreign objects is well described in smugglers of illicit drugs, jewels, or other valuable items.

3. **Which areas of the GI tract lead to problems in the passage of foreign bodies?**
   Several areas of anatomic or physiologic narrowing exist along the GI lumen and may compromise the spontaneous passage of foreign bodies: cricopharyngeal muscle, extrinsic compression of the middle esophagus from the aortic arch, lower esophageal sphincter, pylorus, ileocecal valve, rectal valves of Houston, and anal sphincters. In addition, numerous pathologic abnormalities, such as strictures or tumors, may impair spontaneous passage of foreign bodies (*see* question 12).

4. **What objects are commonly ingested?**
   The object ingested most commonly by children is a coin. Meat boluses impacted above an esophageal stricture or ring account for most adult cases. Accidental loss of sex stimulant devices account for over one half of foreign objects introduced through the anus.

5. **Describe the typical clinical presentation of foreign-body ingestion.**
   Adults trace the onset of symptoms to the ingestion of a specific meal or foreign body. Mentally retarded, psychiatric patients, or children may remain asymptomatic for months after ingestion, or they may not volunteer the history. Patients with impacted anorectal foreign bodies may relate a wide variety of medical histories to account for their predicament, ranging from accidents or assault to medical remedies.

6. **What is suggested by respiratory symptoms related to foreign-body ingestion?**
   Patients with wheezing, stridor, cough, or dyspnea after foreign-body ingestion may have foreign body entrapment in the hypopharynx, trachea, pyriform sinus, or Zenker's diverticulum.

7. **Do ingested sharp objects perforate the intestine?**
   On rare occasions, sharp objects, such as pins, needles, nails, and toothpicks, may perforate the intestine, but in 70–90% of cases they pass through the alimentary tract without complication. Two phenomena in the intestine allow safe passage: (1) foreign bodies pass with axial flow down

the lumen, and (2) reflex relaxation and slowing of peristalsis cause sharp objects to turn around in the lumen so that the sharp end trails down the intestine. In the colon, the foreign object is centered in the fecal bolus, which further protects the bowel wall.

8. **Why is it important to identify the type of foreign body ingested?**
Although most foreign bodies traverse the GI tract without complication, specific exceptions require special attention. Button alkaline batteries may cause coagulation necrosis in the esophagus, but once they reach the stomach, gastric acid neutralizes their risk. Sharp objects can perforate any part of the alimentary tract. Objects longer than 6 cm may become lodged in the C-loop of the duodenum.

9. **How urgent is removal of a foreign body after ingestion?**
Button batteries, ingested typically by small children, need to be removed urgently because of the severe trauma that they may cause in the esophagus. Any sharp object that carries a high risk for perforation should be removed as soon as possible before it passes to a level that is beyond the reach of an endoscope. For the same reasons, long objects (>6 cm) should be removed when identified. Finally, objects lodged in the esophagus that compromise ability to handle oral secretions should be removed urgently to reduce the risk of aspiration.

KEY POINTS: FOREIGN BODIES IN THE GASTROINTESTINAL TRACT ✔

1. Eighty to ninety percent of ingested foreign bodies pass spontaneously without requiring intervention.

2. Mentally retarded, psychiatric patients, or children may remain asymptomatic for months after foreign body ingestion, or they may not volunteer the history.

3. Ingestion of alkaline batteries, sharp or long (>6 cm) objects, or objects lodged in the esophagus should be removed urgently.

10. **Describe the signs and symptoms of a complication related to foreign-body ingestion.**
Respiratory symptoms suggest entrapment of the foreign body in the hypopharynx, trachea, pyriform sinus, or Zenker's diverticulum (see question 6). Sharp objects may penetrate, obstruct, or perforate the esophagus or intestine, presenting with chest, neck, or abdominal pain that varies from mild discomfort to symptoms and signs of acute abdomen. Injury to the esophagus can lead to hematemesis, fever, tachycardia, neck swelling, and crepitus. Excessive drooling and inability to swallow saliva suggest esophageal obstruction. Abdominal distention, vomiting, and hyperactive bowel sounds suggest intestinal obstruction. Hypoactive or absent bowel sounds, guarding, rebound, and abdominal pain are seen with wall penetration or free perforation. Aortoenteric fistula due to ingestion of a sharp foreign body may cause massive hematemesis.

11. **How should foreign bodies be removed?**
Once identified, nearly all objects can be removed endoscopically. Other modalities have been used with variable success, although major complications have been reported. Consultation with a surgeon is appropriate for cases in which perforation or other major complications are probable. Minimally invasive surgery alone or combined with endoscopy is used increasingly.

12. **Which anatomic/functional defects of the GI tract contribute to foreign-body obstruction?**
See Table 62-1.

TABLE 62-1. ANATOMIC/FUNCTIONAL DEFECTS OF THE GASTROINTESTINAL TRACT THAT CONTRIBUTE TO FOREIGN-BODY OBSTRUCTION

Intestinal Site	Anatomic Defect	Functional Defect
Esophagus	Stenosis, atresia, rings, webs, benign/malignant stricture, diverticula, vascular anomalies	Scleroderma, achalasia, Chagas' disease
Stomach	Pyloric stenosis (congenital, malignancy, postoperative, gastroduodenal ulcer disease)	Gastroparesis (uremia, diabetes, hypothyroidism)
Intestine	Postoperative adhesion, Meckel's diverticulum, strictures (ischemic, anastomotic, Crohn's disease), malignancy	Idiopathic intestinal pseudostruction, scleroderma
Colon	Strictures (ischemic, anastomotic, ulcerative colitis, Crohn's disease, radiation, trauma, infection, surgery), diverticular disease, malignancy	Cathartic colon, idiopathic constipation, familial megacolon, idiopathic intestinal pseudoobstruction
Anus	Stenosis (Crohn's disease, trauma, radiation, infection, surgery)	Hirschsprung's disease

WEBSITE

http://www.guideline.gov/

Search "foreign bodies"

BIBLIOGRAPHY

1. Arana A, Hauser B, Hachimi-Idrissi S, Vandenplas Y: Management of ingested foreign bodies in childhood and review of the literature. Eur J Pediatr 160:468–472, 2001.
2. Barone JE, Yee J, Nealon TF Jr: Management of foreign bodies and trauma of the rectum. Surg Gynecol Obstet 156:453–457, 1983.
3. Busch DB, Starling JR: Rectal foreign bodies: Case reports and a comprehensive review of the world's literature. Surgery 100:512–519, 1986.
4. Caratozzolo E, Massani M, Antoniutti M, et al: Combined endoscopic and laparoscopic removal of ingested large foreign bodies: Case report and decisional algorithm. Surg Endosc 15:1226, 2001.
5. Cheng W, Tam PK: Foreign-body ingestion in children: Experience with 1,265 cases. J Pediatr Surg 34:1472–1476, 1999.

6. Lyons MF, Tsuchida AM: Foreign bodies of the gastrointestinal tract. Med Clin North Am 77:1101–1114, 1993.
7. Mehta D, Attia M, Quintana E, Cronan K: Glucagon use for esophageal coin dislodgment in children: A prospective, double-blind, placebo-controlled trial. Acad Emerg Med 8:200–203, 2001.
8. Mosca S, Manes G, Martino R, et al: Endoscopic management of foreign bodies in the upper gastrointestinal tract: Report on a series of 414 adult patients. Endoscopy 33:692–696, 2001.

CHAPTER 63

IRRITABLE BOWEL SYNDROME

Ashok K. Tuteja, MD, MRCP, MPH

1. **What is irritable bowel syndrome (IBS)?**
   Irritable bowel syndrome comprises a group of functional bowel disorders in which abdominal discomfort or pain is associated with defecation or a change in bowel habits, and with features of disordered defecation.

2. **How does one diagnose IBS?**
   The diagnosis of IBS is based on identifying positive symptoms consistent with the disorder, as described in the Rome Criteria (Table 63-1) and with the exclusion of other conditions (either organic or functional) with similar clinical presentation.

TABLE 63-1. ROME II DIAGNOSTIC CRITERIA FOR IRRITABLE BOWEL SYNDROME

At least 12 weeks or more, which need not be consecutive, in the preceding 12 months of abdominal discomfort or pain that has two out of three features:
   1. Relieved with defecation; and/or
   2. Onset associated with change in frequency of stool; and/or
   3. Onset associated with a change in form (appearance) of stool.

Symptoms that cumulatively support the diagnosis of irritable bowel syndrome:
   1. Abnormal stool frequency (> 3 bowel movements/day or < 3 bowel movements/week);
   2. Abnormal stool form (lumpy/hard or loose/watery stool);
   3. Abnormal stool passage (straining; urgency; feeling of incomplete evacuation)
   4. Passage of mucus
   5. Bloating or feeling of abdominal distension

Adapted from Thompson WG, et al. Functional Bowel Disorders. In Drossman DA, Corazziari E, Talley NJ, Thompson WG, Whitehead WE (eds): Rome II: The Functional Gastrointestinal Disorders. McLean, VA: Degnon Associates, 2000, pp 351-432.

---

3. **What is the Rome Committee?**
   The Rome Committee consists of a group of multinational experts in functional bowel disorders. The working team first met in Rome in 1988 to develop criteria for the diagnosis of functional gastrointestinal disorders (Rome Criteria). In 1998 the working team proposed changes and modifications, which were published in 1999 and are known as Rome II Criteria. A further update, Rome III Criteria, is expected in 2006.

4. **Is there any specific biologic and pathophysiologic marker to diagnose IBS?**
   No. There is no specific discriminatory finding or diagnostic test for IBS.

5. **Describe the supporting symptoms of IBS.**
   1. Fewer than three bowel movements a week
   2. More than three bowel movements a day
   3. Hard or lumpy stools
   4. Loose (mushy) or watery stools
   5. Straining during a bowel movement
   6. Urgency (having to rush to have a bowel movement)
   7. Feeling of incomplete evacuation
   8. Passing mucus (white material) during a bowel movement
   9. Abdominal fullness, bloating, or swelling

6. **What is the importance of the supportive symptoms of IBS?**
   The supportive symptoms help in the classification of IBS as either diarrhea predominant or constipation predominant.

7. **Define diarrhea-predominant and constipation-predominant IBS.**
   Based on supporting symptoms (*see* question 5), these disorders are defined as follows:
   - Diarrhea-predominant (>three bowel movements per day): One or more of supporting systems 2, 4, or 6 and none of 1, 3, or 5; or two or more of 2, 4, or 6 and one of 1 or 5 (3, hard lumpy stools do not qualify).
   - Constipation-predominant (<three bowel movements per week): One or more of 1, 3, or 5 and none of 2, 4, or 6; or two or more of 1, 3, or 5 and one of 2, 4, or 6.
   Subclassification of IBS into constipation-predominant or diarrhea-predominant and mixed patterns has limited value in understanding the pathophysiology of IBS.

8. **Discuss the epidemiology of irritable bowel syndrome.**
   Most estimates indicate that the prevalence is approximately 10%, and this estimate is consistent with multiple non-U.S. studies. Constipation-predominant IBS is more common in women. Functional dyspepsia and IBS appear to overlap in this population.

9. **What is the economic impact of IBS in the United States?**
   IBS is a distressing condition that impairs the quality of life and therefore requires treatment. Most persons with IBS do not consult physicians. Fewer than one quarter of individuals with IBS symptoms present for the evaluation and treatment of their symptoms. Patients with IBS are more likely to undergo surgical procedures, including hysterectomy and appendectomy.

   The cost to society in terms of direct medical expenses and indirect costs, such as absenteeism, is considerable. There are between 2.4 and 3.5 million physician visits annually for IBS in the United States, during which 2.2 million prescriptions are written. IBS is associated with more than $8 billion (U.S.) a year in direct healthcare costs.

KEY POINTS: IRRITABLE BOWEL SYNDROME DIAGNOSTIC STRATEGIES

1. Identify symptoms consistent with IBS.

2. Do physical examination and a limited series of initial laboratory tests to exclude structural, metabolic, or infectious diseases.

3. Eliminate alarm symptoms and signs.

4. Make a confident diagnosis.

10. **Describe the pathophysiology of IBS.**

Initial observations suggest that abnormal motility underlies IBS symptoms. Accelerated small bowel and colon transit has been demonstrated in patients with diarrhea predominant IBS. More than 50% of IBS patients report exacerbation of symptoms after eating, suggesting a prominent gastrocolonic response. Furthermore, high amplitude-propagated contractions in the postprandial period are seen in diarrhea-predominant IBS and a lack of these contractions are seen in severe constipation.

Later observations showed that visceral hypersensitivity is important in explaining the clinical manifestations of IBS. IBS patients have lower visceral pain thresholds than healthy patients. As knowledge increased about the interrelatedness of the brain and gut, it was recognized that the abnormal motility and visceral hypersensitivity in IBS are determined by reciprocal interactions between brain and gut. 5-HT is a neurotransmitter in both the central and enteric nervous systems and is a key mediator of visceral hypersensitivity and heightened bowel motility in patients with IBS.

11. **What is postinfectious irritable bowel syndrome?**

Patients who report an acute onset of IBS symptoms after a bout of gastroenteritis are defined as postinfectious IBS (PI-IBS). These patients have previously normal bowel habits. Up to 30% of IBS patients describe an acute onset of bowel disturbances following an acute infective enteritis. PI-IBS is associated with a modest increase in mucosal T-lymphocytes and serotonin containing enteroendocrine cells. Patients with PI-IBS have the same prognosis as noninfective IBS, with fewer than half recovering after 6 years.

12. **What symptoms are not typical of IBS and should prompt an evaluation for organic disease?**
   - Acute onset of symptoms
   - Fever
   - Rectal bleeding or anemia
   - Weight loss
   - Persistent diarrhea
   - Severe constipation
   - Nocturnal symptoms
   - New onset of symptoms in patients >age 50.
   - Abnormal colonoscopy/sigmoidoscopy
   - Family history of GI cancer, inflammatory bowel disease (IBD), or celiac disease

13. **What diagnostic tests are appropriate in a patient suspected of IBS?**

To rule out anatomic disorders, the following screening tests are normally recommended: complete blood count, sedimentation rate, serum chemistries, thyroid stimulating hormone (TSH), stool, occult blood, stool for ova and parasites, and flexible sigmoidoscopy or colonoscopy (with mucosal biopsy), depending upon age and other associated symptoms (e.g., diarrhea). Serologic testing for celiac disease (tissue transglutaminase) should be performed on all patients suspected to have IBS-diarrhea predominant.

Additional studies should be based on presenting symptoms (diarrhea, constipation, or abdominal pain). The use of diagnostic studies to exclude organic disease should be prudent and cost-effective and made in the context of the entire clinical history, including psychological issues (Fig. 63-1).

14. **What is the role of stress and psychological factors in IBS?**

Stress is widely believed to play a major role in the pathophysiology and clinical presentation of IBS. The effect of stress on gut function is universal, and patients with IBS appear to have greater reactivity to stress compared with healthy individuals.

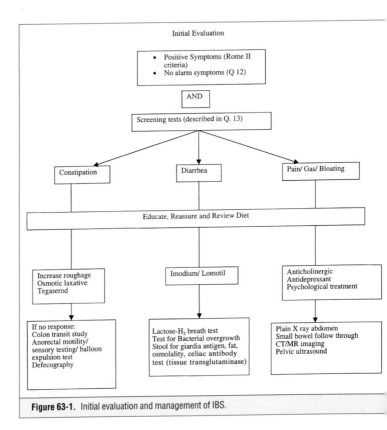

Figure 63-1. Initial evaluation and management of IBS.

Psychological factors include anxiety disorders, depression, somatization, a history of sexual or physical abuse, stressful lifetime events, chronic social stress, or maladaptive coping styles. Psychological symptoms are more prevalent in patients who have severe symptoms and who are seen in tertiary care centers. Furthermore, stress is associated with symptom onset, exacerbations, and severity.

15. **What are essential elements in the management of a patient with IBS?**
    Treatment of IBS patients is indicated when the patient and physician believe that the IBS symptoms diminish the quality of life of the patient. The algorithm for management of IBS based on symptom predominance is described in Figure 63-1.

    It is important to emphasize to the patient the negative results of tests to exclude organic disease and to reassure the patient. Patients should be asked about psychological factors, stress, and history of physical and sexual abuse because these factors may require specific treatment.

    There is evidence to suggest that the outcomes in IBS patients can be improved when physicians: (1) actively listen to patient concerns; (2) provide an adequate explanation of disorder; (3) set realistic goals; (4) establish a long-term relationship; (5) respond to patient concerns and expectations; and (6) identify behavior stressors that exacerbate symptoms.

16. **What is the role of fiber in management of IBS?**
    As a group, patients with IBS do not consume less fiber than control subjects. Fiber has a role in treating constipation; its value for IBS, pain, and diarrhea is controversial.

Many patients with IBS complain of bloating with higher doses of natural fiber. Short chain fatty acids are produced by bacterial fermentation of dietary fiber, resulting in gas formation. Short chain fatty acids can also stimulate rectal contractions and produce pain.

17. **Are anticholinergic and antispasmodic agents useful in IBS?**

The evidence-based position statement on the management of IBS produced by the American College of Gastroenterology states that there is insufficient evidence to make any recommendation about the effectiveness of antispasmodic agents available in the United States. Antispasmodic and anticholinergic agents are sometimes used on an as-needed basis for acute attacks of pain, distention, and bloating.

18. **Discuss the role of psychotropic agents in treating patients with IBS.**

Antidepressants have utility in IBS because many patients present with associated psychological symptoms. Antidepressants have neuromodulatory and analgesic properties, and there is also potential benefit even in the absence of psychiatric comorbidity. Neuromodulatory effects may occur sooner and with lower doses in IBS patients than the dose used in the treatment of depression (e.g., 10–25 mg amitriptyline or 50 mg desipramine). Recent studies suggest that selective serotonin reuptake inhibitors (SSRIs) may offer benefit in some patients with IBS. Tricyclic antidepressants (TCAs), offer benefit for abdominal pain and diarrhea; SSRIs cause diarrhea and may be helpful in patients with constipation-predominant IBS.

KEY POINTS: IRRITABLE BOWEL SYNDROME TREATMENT STRATEGIES

1. Educate and reassure the patient.

2. In diarrhea-predominant IBS, tricyclic antidepressants relieve diarrhea and associated pain.

3. Opioids are useful in relief of diarrhea but may precipitate constipation.

4. Smooth muscle relaxants are indicated in patients with predominant pain/bloating. Their effectiveness is controversial.

5. 5-HT_4-agonists are effective in treating constipation-predominant IBS.

19. **Describe various types of psychological treatments used in patients with IBS.**

- Cognitive behavioral therapy: This attempts to change the way patients perceive and react to their symptoms; uses diaries and exercises to reframe maladaptive thoughts and increase control over symptoms.
- Interpersonal psychotherapy: Identifies and addresses difficulties in relationships. Several studies suggest benefit compared with standard medical therapy.
- Hypnosis: Suggestions are used to reduce gut sensation. This is the best-evaluated psychological treatment. Improvements noted 1 year later.
- Relaxation training: Uses imagery and relaxation techniques to reduce autonomic arousal and stimulate muscular relaxation; improves gut motility.

20. **What is the association between serotonin (5-HT) and IBS?**

A fundamental observation in IBS is the presence of enhanced visceral perception. Serotonin has a role in mediating visceral hypersensitivity and the peristaltic reflex. Ninety-five percent of serotonin is found in the gut, with 90% localized within enterochromaffin cells and 10% in the enteric neurons. Of the various types of serotonin, 5-HT$_3$ and 5-HT$_4$ are involved in sensory and motor functions of the gut and are targets for pharmacotherapy in IBS.

21. **What are the roles for 5-HT$_3$ antagonist and 5-HT$_4$ agonist in management of IBS?**

The indications, mechanism of actions, and major side effects of common 5-HT$_4$ agonist and 5-HT$_3$-receptor antagonist are described in Table 63-2. Alosetron is effective in inducing adequate relief of abdominal pain and discomfort, improvement in bowel frequency, consistency, and urgency in women with diarrhea-predominant IBS. A significant adverse effect is acute ischemic colitis. Because of adverse effects, alosetron was withdrawn from the market in November 2000. As a consequence of vigorous public outcry following withdrawal, the Food and Drug Administration (FDA) approved the restricted use of alosetron in June 2002. Another medication in this class, cilansetron, is undergoing phase III studies for treatment of diarrhea-predominant IBS.

Tegaserod is partial 5-HT$_4$ agonist, which is indicated in women with constipation-predominant IBS. It is the only FDA-approved agent for the short-term treatment of IBS patients with constipation. It improves global assessment and individual symptoms of IBS, including abdominal pain, stool frequency, and bloating.

TABLE 63-2. COMPARISON OF 5–HT$_4$ AGONIST AND 5–HT$_3$ ANTAGONIST DRUGS		
	5-HT$_4$ Agonist (Tegaserod)	**5-HT$_3$ Antagonist (Alosetron)**
Indication	Women with IBS/constipation	Women with IBS/diarrhea
Mechanisms	Increases peristalsis	Delays small bowel and colon transit
	Increases small bowel secretion	Inhibits small bowel secretion
	Antinociceptive/helps bloating	Blunts gastrocolic response; helps urgency
Side effects	Diarrhea/headache	Constipation/ischemic colitis

IBS = irritable bowel syndrome.

WEBSITES

1. http://www.digestive.niddk.nih.gov/

   (Search "IBS")

2. http://www.aboutibs.org/

BIBLIOGRAPHY

1. American College of Gastroenterology Functional Gastrointestinal Disorders Task Force: Evidence-based position statement on the management of irritable bowel syndrome in North America. Am J Gastroenterol 97(11 Suppl):S1–S5, 2002.

2. Camilleri M, Chey WY, Mayer EA, et al: A randomized controlled clinical trial of the serotonin type 3 receptor antagonist alosetron in women with diarrhea-predominant irritable bowel syndrome. Arch Intern Med 161:1733–1740, 2001.

3. Cash BD, Schoenfeld P, Chey WD: The utility of diagnostic tests in irritable bowel syndrome patients: A systematic review. Am J Gastroenterol 97:2812–2819, 2002.

4. Creed F, Fernandes L, Guthrie E, et al: The cost-effectiveness of psychotherapy and paroxetine for severe irritable bowel syndrome. Gastroenterology 124:303–317, 2003.

5. Drossman DA, Camilleri M, Mayer EA, Whitehead WE: AGA technical review on irritable bowel syndrome. Gastroenterology 123:2108–2131, 2002.

6. Drossman DA, Toner BB, Whitehead WE, et al: Cognitive-behavioral therapy versus education and desipramine versus placebo for moderate to severe functional bowel disorders. Gastroenterology 125:19–31, 2003.

7. Hamm LR, Sorrells SC, Harding JP, et al: Additional investigations fail to alter the diagnosis of irritable bowel syndrome in subjects fulfilling the Rome criteria. Am J Gastroenterol 94:1279–1282, 1999.

8. Mayer EA, Raybould HE: Role of visceral afferent mechanisms in functional bowel disorders. Gastroenterology 99:1688–1704, 1990.

9. Mertz H, Naliboff B, Munakata J, et al: Altered rectal perception is a biological marker of patients with irritable bowel syndrome. Gastroenterology 109:40–52, 1995.

10. Muller-Lissner SA, Fumagalli I, Bardhan KD, et al: Tegaserod, a 5-HT(4) receptor partial agonist, relieves symptoms in irritable bowel syndrome patients with abdominal pain, bloating and constipation. Aliment Pharmacol Ther 15:1655–1666, 2001.

11. Rogers J, Henry MM, Misiewicz JJ: Increased segmental activity and intraluminal pressures in the sigmoid colon of patients with the irritable bowel syndrome. Gut 30:634–641, 1989.

12. Saito YA, Schoenfeld P, Locke GR III: The epidemiology of irritable bowel syndrome in North America: A systematic review. Am J Gastroenterol 97:1910–1915, 2002.

13. Sanders DS, Carter MJ, Hurlstone DP, et al: Association of adult coeliac disease with irritable bowel syndrome: A case-control study in patients fulfilling ROME II criteria referred to secondary care. Lancet 358:1504–1508, 2001.

14. Spiller RC: Postinfectious irritable bowel syndrome. Gastroenterology 124:1662–1671, 2003.

15. Talley NJ, Gabriel SE, Harmsen WS, et al: Medical costs in community subjects with irritable bowel syndrome. Gastroenterology 109:1736–1741, 1995.

16. Thompson WG, Longstreth G, Drossman DA, et al: Functional bowel disorders. In Drossman DA, Corazziari E, Talley NJ, et al (eds): Rome II The Functional Gastrointestinal Disorders. McLean, VA, Degnon Associates, 2000, pp 351–432.

CHAPTER 64

ENDOSCOPIC CANCER SCREENING AND SURVEILLANCE

Peter R. McNally, DO, and Scot M. Lewey, DO

1. **What is the difference between endoscopic cancer screening and surveillance**
   - *Screening* is the one-time application of a test in an asymptomatic person. Cancer screening is the search for cancer and precancerous lesions in asymptomatic persons.
   - *Surveillance* is repeated application of such tests over time. Cancer surveillance is the follow up of persons with a known history of cancer or precancerous lesions.

   Recommendations for cancer screening and surveillance are not based solely on medical data but also on patient expectations, state of medical technology, and prevailing medical-legal environment.

ESOPHAGUS

(See Chapter 5, Achalasia; Chapter 6, Esophageal Cancer; and Chapter 8, Barrett's Esophagus.)

2. **What is the risk of esophageal cancer in patients with achalasia?**
   The risk is 2–7%. The pathogenesis is unknown, but chronic stasis is believed to play a role. Th mean interval between diagnosis of achalasia and development of cancer is 17 years. Most cancers are of the squamous cell type. The risk for malignancy is increased among achalasia patients who had unsatisfactory, long delayed, or no treatment. Esophageal cancer is usually fa advanced before the dilated esophagus becomes obstructed and symptoms manifest; hence, th 5-year survival rate is poor (<5%).

3. **Can endoscopic surveillance detect early esophageal cancer among patients with long-standing achalasia?**
   Yes. There are examples of long-term survival after surgery. Periodic endoscopic surveillance for all patients with achalasia is unlikely to be cost-effective.

4. **What are the surveillance recommendations for patients with esophageal achalasia?**
   None. There is no nationally recognized endoscopic surveillance program. A suggested schedul for endoscopic surveillance begins 15–20 years after initial symptoms or 10–15 years after medical or surgical treatment. The esophagus should be cleaned of debris before endoscopic examination. All surface abnormalities of the esophagus should be biopsied. The appropriate frequency of endoscopic surveillance has yet to be determined.

5. **What is the malignant potential of Barrett's esophagus?**
   Barrett's esophagus is a premalignant condition with a reported cancer prevalence of 10–40%. Endoscopic surveillance studies suggest an incidence of 1 in 52–175 patient years. Surgical and medical treatment of gastroesophageal reflux has not been shown to reduce the incidence of cancer

6. **Should every patient with chronic gastroesophageal reflux disease (GERD) be screened for Barrett's esophagus?**
   No. A recent population-based study identified a clear association between chronic reflux symptoms and adenocarcinoma of the esophagus, which continues to exhibit a rising incidence

Because patients with GERD are at increased risk for Barrett's esophagus, some have suggested endoscopic screening for Barrett's esophagus among patients older than age 50 with long-standing GERD. Evidence-based studies are needed to determine whether this recommendation is worthwhile.

7. **What factors seem to increase the risk for Barrett's and esophageal cancer?**
   - Duration of reflux symptoms

Symptoms in Years	Endoscopic Prevalence of Barrett's
<1	4%
1.5	11%
5–10	17%
>10	21%

   - Gender: men > women
   - Ethnicity: Caucasian > African-American
   - Obesity

8. **What are the recommendations for endoscopic screening for Barrett's among patients with GERD?**
   None. Unsedated upper endoscopy with "ultrathin" endoscopes or tethered capsule endoscopy may be cost-effective. In clinical practice, however, the movement has been toward the concept of once-in-a-lifetime endoscopy for patients with chronic gastroesophageal reflux to detect Barrett's esophagus. Chronic symptoms of GERD >5 years and age >40 are commonly used benchmarks.

9. **What is the first step in endoscopic surveillance of patients with Barrett's esophagus?**
   Index endoscopy. Aggressive antireflux therapy should be initiated before a surveillance program is begun because of the difficulty in distinguishing inflammatory dysplasia from neoplasia. Extensive sampling of the entire Barrett's segment should be performed, particularly of any areas with macroscopic abnormalities. A proven method involves quadrant biopsies with large-particle forceps at 1- to 2-cm intervals, starting 1 cm below the esophagogastric junction and extending to 1 cm above the squamocolumnar junction. Further management should be guided by the histologic findings.

10. **What is the appropriate surveillance of patients with Barrett's esophagus?**
    Surveillance intervals are based on the detection of dysplasia with the goal of early intervention to improve the survival rates associated with adenocarcinoma.

    - No Barrett's — No further screening for Barrett's. Additional EGD only to investigate new symptoms
    - Barrett's with no dysplasia (ND) — Every year × 2; if ND, every 3 yrs
    - Barrett's with low-grade dysplasia (LGD) — Every year until ND found, then every 2 yrs
    - Barrett's with high-grade dysplasia — Expert pathologist peer review (for options, see question 11 below)

11. **Describe the management of high-grade dysplasia.**
    Management of high-grade dysplasia is one of the most controversial issues in the treatment of Barrett's esophagus. Current alternatives include more frequent surveillance (every 3 months) until cancer is detected, experimental endoscopic reversal therapy, and esophagectomy. The problems with conventional esophagectomy include operative mortality rate, especially in low-volume centers, the high frequency of morbidity, and the permanent impact on eating and nutrition. Many patients are elderly and are not good surgical candidates because of

comorbidity. It is also not uncommon for patients to refuse surgery even after consulting with a surgeon.

12. **What steps are recommended if cancer is found?**
Review biopsies with an experienced pathologist. If the histologic diagnosis is confirmed and the patient is a surgical candidate, recommend operation after complete staging. If the histologic diagnosis is uncertain, urgent repeat biopsy is required.

13. **Should patients with short segment Barrett's esophagus (SSBE) undergo the same endoscopic surveillance?**
Overall, the risk of cancer appears to be less in SSBE than in long segment Barrett's. Although periodic surveillance of SSBE is probably necessary, no guidelines are available.

14. **Discuss the role of endoscopically applied vital staining of the esophagus for detection of dysplasia and cancer in patients with Barrett's esophagus.**
Specialized columnar mucosa of Barrett's esophagus avidly stains with endoscopically applied methylene blue (MB). Barrett's segments with high-grade dysplasia or adenocarcinoma tend to exhibit a heterogeneous MB-staining pattern marked by variability of stain intensity. Some researchers suggest that MB-directed biopsies of Barrett's esophagus are a more accurate and cost-effective technique than random biopsies for detection of Barrett's dysplasia and cancer.

15. **What is the risk of esophageal cancer in patients with a history of caustic ingestion?**
A thousand times greater than the risk in the general population. The cumulative results of four series have characterized the findings associated with lye-related esophageal cancer:
- Mean age at onset of cancer: 47 years
- Interval from caustic ingestion to development of cancer: 14–47 years (mean = 40 years)
- Location of cancers: mostly in the mid-esophagus
  Malignancy appears to develop after a shorter interval if the corrosive injury occurs later in life. Because the periesophageal fibrosis caused by the corrosive injury decreases esophageal compliance, cancer presents usually at an earlier stage. The resectability rate and 5-year survival rate for lye-associated esophageal carcinoma are 85% and 33%, respectively.

16. **How often is endoscopic surveillance needed in patients with a history of caustic ingestion?**
Begin endoscopic surveillance 15–20 years after the caustic ingestion. Generally, endoscopic examination should not be conducted more frequently than every 1–3 years. The threshold to evaluate swallowing problems with endoscopy should be low.

17. **Define *tylosis*. What is the risk for esophageal malignancy?**
Tylosis is an uncommon genetic disorder characterized by hyperkeratosis of the palms and soles. It is transmitted in an autosomal dominant pattern and associated with a predisposition for development of esophageal cancer. The prevalence of esophageal cancer in patients with tylosis can be >90% by age 65. Death from esophageal cancer has been reported in patients as young as age 30. A prospective endoscopic surveillance program has been initiated for a large family cohort in England.

18. **Outline the recommendations for endoscopic surveillance in patients with tylosis.**
Start surveillance endoscopy at age 30. Symptoms of dysphagia or swallowing difficulties should be evaluated promptly. Generally, endoscopic examination should not be conducted more frequently than every 1–3 years.

STOMACH AND SMALL BOWEL

(See Chapter 11, Gastric Cancer; Chapter 12, Peptic Ulcer Disease and *Helicobacter pylori*; and Chapter 13, Gastric Polyps and Thickened Gastric Folds.)

19. **What is the risk for malignancy among patients with gastric polyps?**
In the United States, gastric polyps are uncommon. The risk of malignant transformation of a gastric polyp depends on histology. Most gastric polyps (70–90%) are hyperplastic, and the risk for malignant transformation is low (<4%). Adenomatous gastric polyps are a true neoplasm, and their risk for malignant transformation is as high as 75%, especially when polyps are large (≥2 cm). Fundic gland polyps have no malignant potential but may suggest the diagnosis of familial adenomatous polyposis syndrome (FAP) and the need for ampullary and lower gastrointestinal (GI) endoscopic surveillance.

20. **What are the recommendations for endoscopic surveillance in patients with adenomatous gastric polyps?**
Begin surveillance endoscopy 1 year after removing all gastric polyps, evaluating for recurrence and new or previously missed polyps. If this exam is negative, surveillance endoscopy should be repeated no more frequently than every 3–5 years for patients with adenomatous polyps. The recurrence rate for gastric adenomas is 16%. When *Helicobacter pylori* gastritis is identified, eradication may inhibit progression of gastric adenoma to carcinoma.

21. **Who is at risk for ampullary and small bowel adenomas and frank malignancy?**
In patients with FAP, the relative risk of duodenal adenocarcinoma and ampullary carcinoma is increased. Adenomatous changes and carcinoma have been reported in the ampulla and lower pancreatic and bile ducts. Such changes may not be readily apparent at endoscopy. Periampullary adenomas have a high risk of dysplasia. Chemoprevention of ampullary adenomas with sulindac has been disappointing. Investigation of the new COX-2 inhibitors and combination chemotherapy with sulindac and HMG-CoA reductase inhibitors (lovastatin) to inhibit apoptosis is underway.

22. **What endoscopic surveillance of the upper GI tract is necessary in patients with FAP?**
Once FAP is diagnosed, periodic surveillance endoscopy should be initiated with both end-viewing and side-viewing instruments. Antral and duodenal polyps should be biopsied. Endoscopic retrograde cholangiopancreatography should be performed when the ampulla appears deformed or abnormal. Recognition of high-grade dysplasia necessitates further therapy, although the type of therapy is not yet fully defined. Studies are needed to ascertain the effectiveness of chemoprevention, endoscopic ampullectomy/polypectomy, and, possibly, more extensive surgical procedures.

23. **What is the risk for malignancy in the gastric remnant after gastrectomy (gastric stump carcinoma)?**
Gastric stump carcinoma is carcinoma arising from the gastric remnant at least 5 years after surgery for benign disease. Cumulative analysis of over 50 studies indicates a twofold to fourfold increased incidence of gastric carcinoma beginning 15 years after the original surgery. Endoscopic surveillance studies have detected gastric stump carcinoma in 4–6% of patients, and the progression from dysplasia to cancer has been documented. Symptoms are an unreliable predictor of early gastric cancer, and multiple random biopsies are necessary to identify dysplasia because the macroscopic abnormalities may not be apparent. The mean interval between gastric surgery and cancer is about 20 years. Variations in the reporting of gastric cancer risk among patients with pernicious anemia may be due to differences in dietary

nitrosamines, genetics, *H. pylori* infection, and/or alcohol and tobacco use. Billroth II procedures are more commonly associated with gastric remnant carcinoma than Billroth I procedures, and dysplastic epithelium is found most commonly near and within the gastroenteric stoma.

24. **How often should patients undergo endoscopic surveillance for stump carcinoma?**
Initiate surveillance endoscopy 15–20 years after gastric surgery. Multiple biopsies should be taken and examined for dysplasia. Periodic endoscopic surveillance is reasonable, but the cost-effective frequency has not been determined. When mucosal dysplasia is identified, more frequent surveillance is indicated.

25. **Are patients with pernicious anemia (PA) at risk for gastric carcinoma?**
Yes. PA is associated with type A gastritis and is thought to arise from chronic autoimmune injury to the gastric mucosa. The reported incidence of gastric cancer in patients with PA ranges from 2–10%. The coincidence of gastric polyps and PA is common. A study of 152 Minnesota residents with PA documented only a single case of gastric cancer during a 30-year period and tempered the enthusiasm for surveillance endoscopy; however, a recent large population-based cohort study in Sweden and a retrospective study of over 30,000 veterans identified the subsequent risk of gastric malignancy after the diagnosis of PA to be increased by at least twofold. The gastric malignancy occurred usually within 1–2 years after initial diagnosis of PA.

26. **Give the recommendations for endoscopic surveillance in patients with pernicious anemia.**
Surveillance endoscopy is not currently recommended. However, index endoscopy at the time of the diagnosis of PA to evaluate other risk factors for gastric cancer (e.g., gastric polyps) seems reasonable.

COLON

(See Chapter 47, Colorectal Cancer and Colon Cancer Screening.)

27. **What are the current guidelines for colorectal cancer screening in U.S. adults at "average" risk?**
   - Screening begins at age 50.
   - Annual fecal occult blood test (FOBT)
   - Annual FOBT plus flexible sigmoidoscopy every 5 years
   - Double-contrast barium enema every 5–10 years
   - Colonoscopy every 10 years

28. **Give the current guidelines for surveillance colonoscopy in patients with a history of adenomatous polyps.**
A periodic surveillance program should be customized according to adequacy of colon preparation and endoscopic findings.

Colonoscopy Findings	*Next Colonoscopy*
Single tubular adenoma	5–10 years
Numerous adenomas (≥5)	1–2 years
Large sessile (>2 cm) adenoma, especially if it was removed piecemeal	3–6 months
Inadequate colon preparation	Repeat within 3–6 months

29. **Does a single first-degree relative with colon cancer increase the risk for colorectal cancer?**

Yes. A positive family history for colon cancer approximately doubles the risk.

30. **Outline the recommended surveillance for people with a family history of colon cancer.**

- Single first-degree relative with colorectal cancer diagnosed at age >60: Begin surveillance at age 40. The preferred surveillance is colonoscopy every 10 years.
- Single first-degree relative with colorectal cancer diagnosed at age <60 or multiple first-degree relatives with colorectal cancer: Begin surveillance at age 40 or 10 years younger than the youngest affected relative (whichever is younger). The preferred surveillance is colonoscopy every 3–5 years.

31. **What is hereditary nonpolyposis colorectal cancer (HNPCC)?**

HNPCC is a disease of autosomal dominant inheritance in which colon cancer arises in discrete adenomas, but polyposis does not occur. The Amsterdam criteria are used for diagnosis (*see* Chapter 47 Colorectal Cancer and Colon Cancer Screening):

1. At least three relatives with colorectal cancer (one must be a first-degree relative of the other two)
2. Colorectal cancer involving at least two generations
3. One or more cases of colorectal cancer before age 50

32. **Outline the recommendation for colonoscopic surveillance in patients who have undergone resection of colorectal cancer.**

Before resection, the yields for synchronous colorectal cancer and adenomatous polyps at initial clearing colonoscopy are about 2% and 25%, respectively. If a well-prepared clearing colonoscopy was performed preoperatively, the yield of surveillance colonoscopy performed 6–24 months after resection is 2–3% for anastomotic recurrence, 3–4% for metachronous cancer, and 25–33% for adenomas (similar to postadenoma removal). If preoperative clearing colonoscopy was not done, or if the results were inadequate because of obstruction or bowel preparation, surveillance should be done 2–3 months postoperatively.

33. **Are patients with long-standing ulcerative colitis at increased risk for colorectal cancer?**

Yes. Their risk is increased by sixfold to 15-fold compared with the general population. The risk increases significantly after 8–10 years of pancolitis or >14 years of left-sided colitis.

34. **What are the current recommendations for colonoscopic surveillance of such patients?**

The yield for cancer or high-grade dysplasia on initial colonoscopic surveillance in long-standing ulcerative colitis may be as high as 12% and 8%, respectively. Surveillance is recommended after 8–10 years of pancolitis and 15 years of left-sided colitis; colonoscopy should be performed every 1–2 years. Because neoplasia and dysplasia are not often evident endoscopically, random biopsies should be taken from the cecum to the rectum (greater than four biopsies for every 10-cm segment) and examined histologically. Any abnormal mucosa or mass lesions should also be biopsied. Approximately 64 biopsies are needed to detect the highest grade of dysplasia with a 95% probability. Some experts recommend four biopsies every 10 cm to the sigmoid, then every 5 cm to the rectum.

35. **Describe management strategy if cancer is found.**

Review biopsies with an experienced pathologist. If the histologic diagnosis is confirmed and the patient is a surgical candidate, recommend proctocolectomy after complete staging. If the histologic diagnosis is uncertain, urgent repeat biopsy is required.

36. **What strategy is recommended for high-grade dysplasia?**
Review biopsies with an expert pathologist. If the diagnosis is confirmed, the likelihood that cancer will be identified in the resected specimen is 42%. Surgery is recommended.

37. **Describe the recommended strategies for dysplasia-associated lesions and low-grade dysplasia.**
For dysplasia-associated lesions, proctocolectomy is recommended because the risk for malignancy is estimated at >50%. For low-grade dysplasia or indefinite results, review biopsies with an expert pathologist. If the histologic diagnosis is confirmed and no endoscopic colitis or histologic inflammatory atypia is present, consider colectomy or more intensive surveillance biopsies every 3–6 months. Low-grade dysplasia carries a 19% likelihood of existing cancer.

38. **What strategy is recommended if no dysplasia is found?**
Serial endoscopy with surveillance biopsies every 12 months.

39. **When a sporadic adenomatous colon polyp is identified in a patient with chronic ulcerative colitis (CUC), should colectomy be performed?**
No. Although all adenomatous polyps of the colon are considered "dysplasia," the polyp itself does not connote the same risk as detecting mucosal dysplasia elsewhere in persons with CUC. The polyp should be removed endoscopically and the remainder of the colon sampled for mucosal dysplasia, as described previously.

40. **What is the risk of colorectal cancer in patients with Crohn's disease?**
When Crohn's disease involves the colon, the risk of colorectal cancer is six times higher than in the general population. When Crohn's disease is confined to the ileum, the risk for colorectal cancer appears to be similar to that in the general population. Screening recommendations are less firmly established than for ulcerative colitis.

41. **What surveillance schedule is appropriate for patients with Crohn's disease?**
Biannual colonoscopy with multiple biopsies after 10 years of colitis is reasonable.

WEBSITE

http://www.guideline.gov

(Search "GI cancer")

BIBLIOGRAPHY

1. Agarwal B, Rao CV, Bhendwal S, et al: Lovastatin augments sulindac-induced apoptosis in colon cancer cells and potentiates chemopreventive effects of sulindac. Gastroenterology 117:838–847, 1999.

2. Aggestrup S, Holm JC, Sorensen HR: Does achalasia predispose to cancer of the esophagus? Chest 102:1013–1016, 1992.

3. Appleqvist P, Salmo M: Lye corrosion carcinoma of the esophagus. Cancer 45:2655, 1980.

4. Armbrecht U, Stockbrugger RW, Rode J, et al: Development of gastric dysplasia in pernicious anemia: A clinical endoscopic follow-up study of 80 patients. Gut 31:1105–1109, 1990.

5. Burt RW: Colon cancer screening. Gastroenterology 119:837–853, 2000.

6. Cooper GS, Yuang Z, Chak A, Rimm AA: Patterns of endoscopic follow-up after surgery for nonmetastatic colorectal cancer. Gastrointest Endosc 52:33–38, 2000.

7. Dunaway CP, Wong CR: Risk and surveillance intervals for squamous cell carcinoma in achalasia. Gastrointest Endosc North Am 11:425, 2001.

8. el Khoury J: Endoscopy in Barrett's esophagus. Surveillance during reflux management and new advances in the diagnosis and early detection of dysplasia. Chest Surg Clin N Am 12:47–58, 2002.

9. Gerson LB, Triadafilopoulos G: Screening for esophageal adenocarcinoma: An evidence-based approach. Am J Med 113:499–505, 2002.

10. Ginsberg G, Al-kawas F, Fleischer D, et al: Should all gastric polyps be removed? Am J Gastroenterol 87:1268, 1992.

11. Katz J, Reynolds JC: The early diagnosis and prevention of gastrointestinal cancer: Problems and promises. Gastroenterol Clin North Am 31(2):369–378, 2002.

12. Lagergren J, Bergstrom R, Lindgren A, et al: Symptomatic gastroesophageal reflux as a risk factor for esophageal adenocarcinoma. N Engl J Med 340:825–831, 1999.

13. Leape LL, Ashcraft KW, Scarpelli DG, et al: Hazard to health—liquid lye. N Engl J Med 248:232–235, 1971.

14. Lieberman D, et al: Impact of GERD: Duration and prevalence of Barrett's (GORE). Am J Gastroenterol 92:1293–129, 1997.

15. Marger RS, Marger D: Carcinoma of the esophagus and tylosis: A lethal genetic combination. Cancer 72:17–79, 1993.

16. Rex DK, Johnson DA, Lieberman DA, et al: Colorectal cancer prevention 2000: Screening recommendations of the American College of Gastroenterology. Am J Gastroenterol 95:868–877, 2000.

17. Rubin PH, Friedman S, Harpaz N, et al: Colonoscopic polypectomy in chronic colitis: Conservative management after endoscopic resection of dysplastic polyps. Gastroenterology 117:1295–1300, 1999.

18. Saito K, Arai K, Mori M, et al: Effect of *Helicobacter pylori* eradication on malignant transformation of gastric adenoma. Gastrointest Endosc 52:27–32, 2000.

19. Schnell T, Sontag SJ, Cheifec G, et al: High grade dysplasia is still not an indication for surgery in patients with Barrett's esophagus: An update. Gastroenterology 14:1149, 1998.

20. Steinbach G, Lynch PM, Phillips RK, et al: The effect of Celecoxib, a cyclooxygenase-2 inhibitor, in familial adenomatous polyposis. N Engl J Med 342:1946–1952, 2000.

21. Trowbridge B, Burt RW: Colorectal cancer screening. Surg Clin North Am 82:943–957, 2002.

22. Winawer SJ, Zauber AG, O'Brien MJ, et al: Randomized comparison of surveillance intervals after colonoscopic removal of newly diagnosed adenomatous polyps. N Engl J Med 328:901–906, 1993.

RHEUMATOLOGIC MANIFESTATIONS OF GASTROINTESTINAL DISEASE

Sterling G. West, MD

CHAPTER 65

ENTEROPATHIC ARTHRITIS

1. **How often does an inflammatory peripheral or spinal arthritis occur in patients with idiopathic inflammatory bowel disease?**
   See Table 65-1.

TABLE 65-1.	FREQUENCY OF PERIPHERAL OR SPINAL ARTHRITIS IN INFLAMMATORY BOWEL DISEASE	
	Ulcerative Colitis	**Crohn's Disease**
Peripheral arthritis	10%	20%
Sacroiliitis	15%	15%
Sacroiliitis/spondylitis*	5%	5%

*Some studies report that ankylosing spondylitis occurs more commonly in Crohn's disease than ulcerative colitis.

2. **What are the most common joints involved in ulcerative colitis and Crohn's disease in patients with an inflammatory peripheral arthritis?**
   Upper extremity and small joint involvement is more common in ulcerative colitis than Crohn's disease. Both ulcerative colitis and Crohn's-related arthritis affect the knee and ankle predominantly. (*See* Fig. 65-1.)

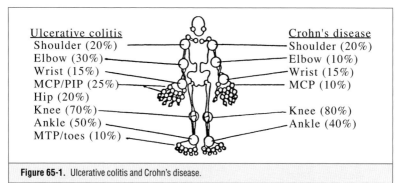

Figure 65-1. Ulcerative colitis and Crohn's disease.

3. **Describe the clinical characteristics of the inflammatory peripheral arthritis associated with idiopathic inflammatory bowel disease (IBD).**
   The most common type of arthritis (type 1) occurs equally in men and women, and children are affected as often as adults. The arthritis is typically acute in onset, migratory, and asymmetric,

and it usually involves less than five joints (i.e., pauciarticular). It is strongly associated with flares of IBD and extra-articular manifestations of IBD. Synovial fluid analysis reveals an inflammatory fluid with up to 50,000 WBC/mm^3 (predominantly neutrophils) and negative findings on crystal examination and cultures. There is an increased prevalence of human leukocyte antigen (HLA)-B27 (26%) in this type of arthritis. Most arthritic episodes resolve in 1–2 months and do not result in radiographic changes or deformities.

A second type of arthritis (type 2) is less common but tends to be polyarticular, runs a course independent of the activity of IBD, does not coincide with extra-articular manifestations, and usually causes symptoms for months to years. This type of arthritis can cause erosions and deformities. There is no association of this arthritis with HLA-B27.

4. **What other extraintestinal manifestations commonly occur in patients with idiopathic IBD and inflammatory peripheral arthritis?**
   P = Pyoderma gangrenosum (<5%)
   A = Aphthous stomatitis (<10%)
   I = Inflammatory eye disease (acute anterior uveitis) (5–15%)
   N = Nodosum (erythema) (<10%)

5. **Do the extent and activity of IBD correlate with the activity of the peripheral inflammatory arthritis?**
   Patients with ulcerative colitis and Crohn's disease are more likely to develop a peripheral arthritis, if the colon is extensively involved. Most arthritic attacks occur during the first few years following onset of the bowel disease, but late occurrences also occur. The episodes coincide with flares of bowel disease in 60–70% of patients. Occasionally, the arthritis may precede symptoms of IBD, especially in children with Crohn's disease. Consequently, lack of gastrointestinal (GI) symptoms and even a negative stool guaiac test does not exclude the possibility of occult Crohn's disease in a patient who presents with a characteristic arthritis.

6. **Which points in the history and physical examination are helpful in separating inflammatory spinal arthritis from mechanical low back pain in an IBD patient?**
   On the basis of history and physical examination, 95% of patients with inflammatory spinal arthritis can be differentiated from patients with mechanical low back pain (Table 65-2).

TABLE 65-2. CLINICAL DIFFERENTIATION OF INFLAMMATORY SPINAL ARTHRITIS (SA) AND MECHANICAL LOW BACK PAIN (LBP)		
	Inflammatory SA	**Mechanical LBP**
Onset of pain	Insidious	Acute
Duration of morning stiffness	>60 min	<30 min
Nighttime pain	Yes	Infrequent
Exercise effect on pain	Improvement	Worsen
Sacroiliac joint tenderness	Usually	No
Range of back motion	Global loss of motion	Abnormal flexion
Reduced chest expansion	Sometimes	No
Neurologic deficits	No	Possible
Duration of symptoms	>3 mo	<4 wk

SA = spinal arthritis, LBP = low back pain.

7. **Does the activity of inflammatory spinal arthritis correlate with the activity of the IBD?**

    No. The onset of sacroiliitis or spondylitis can precede by years, occur concurrently, or follow by years the onset of the inflammatory bowel disease. Furthermore, the course of the spinal arthritis is completely independent of the course of IBD.

8. **What HLA occurs more commonly than expected with inflammatory arthritis as a result of IBD?**

    Eight percent of normal healthy Caucasians have the HLA-B27 gene. Thus, a patient with IBD who possesses the HLA-B27 gene has a 7–10 times increased risk of developing inflammatory sacroiliitis with/without spondylitis compared to IBD patients who are HLA-B27-negative. (See Table 65-3.)

TABLE 65-3.   FREQUENCY OF HLA-B27 IN INFLAMMATORY BOWEL DISEASE

	Crohn's Disease	Ulcerative Colitis
Sacroiliitis/spondylitis	55%	70%
Peripheral arthritis*	26%	26%

*The peripheral arthritis associated with HLA-B27 is the type-1 pauciarticular arthritis.

9. **What serologic abnormalities are seen in patients with inflammatory bowel disease?**
    - Erythrocyte sedimentation rate (ESR) is elevated, whereas rheumatoid factor and anti-nuclear antibody (ANA) are negative.
    - Antineutrophil cytoplasmic antibody (ANCA)—up to 50–60% of ulcerative colitis patients can have pANCA, which is directed against bactericidal permeability increasing protein (BPI), cathepsin G, lactoferrin, lysozyme, or elastase but not myeloperoxidase (MPO).
    - Up to 50% of Crohn's disease patients can have antibodies against *Saccharomyces cerevisiae*.

10. **Describe the typical radiographic features of inflammatory sacroiliitis and spondylitis in IBD patients.**

    The radiographic abnormalities in IBD patients with inflammatory spinal arthritis are similar to those seen in ankylosing spondylitis. Patients with early inflammatory sacroiliitis have frequently normal plain radiographs. In these patients, magnetic resonance (MR) imaging of the sacroiliac joints demonstrates inflammation and edema (Fig. 65-2, *A*). Over several months to years, patients develop sclerosis and erosions in the lower two thirds of the sacroiliac joint (Fig. 65-2, *B*). Some patients may completely fuse these joints.

    Patients with early spondylitis may also have normal radiographs. Later, radiographs may show "shiny corners" at the insertion of the annulus fibrosis, anterior squaring of the vertebrae, and syndesmophyte formation (Fig. 65-3, *A*). Syndesmophytes (calcification of annulus fibrosis) are thin, marginal, and bilateral. A bamboo spine (bilateral syndesmophytes traversing the entire spine from lumbar to cervical) (Fig. 65-3, *B*) occurs in 10% of patients. Patients who develop inflammatory hip disease may be at increased risk for subsequently developing a bamboo spine.

11. **What other rheumatic problems occur with increased frequency in IBD patients?**
    - Achilles tendinitis/plantar fasciitis (enthesopathy)
    - Clubbing of fingernails (5%)

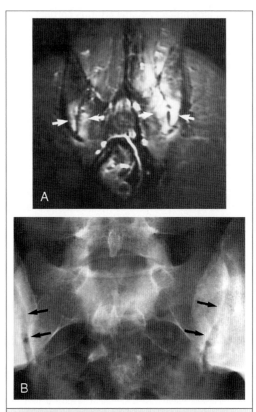

Figure 65-2. (A) MR image of the sacroiliac joints showing inflammation *(arrows)* (T$_2$-weighted image, TE50, TR2500). (B) Radiograph showing early bilateral sacroiliitis *(arrows)*.

- Hypertrophic osteoarthropathy (periostitis)
- Psoas abscess or septic hip from fistula formation (Crohn's disease)
- Osteoporosis secondary to medications (i.e., prednisone)
- Granulomatous lesions of bone and joints
- Vasculitis
- Amyloidosis

12. **Can treatment alleviate the symptoms of inflammatory peripheral arthritis and/or spinal arthritis in IBD patients?**
See Table 65-4.

13. **What rheumatic disorders are associated with pouchitis, microscopic (lymphocytic) colitis (MC), and/or collagenous colitis (CC)?**
See Table 65-5.

14. **Why are patients with IBD more prone to develop an inflammatory arthritis?**
Environmental antigens capable of inciting rheumatic disorders enter the body's circulation b
traversing the respiratory mucosa, skin, or GI mucosa. The human GI tract has an estimated

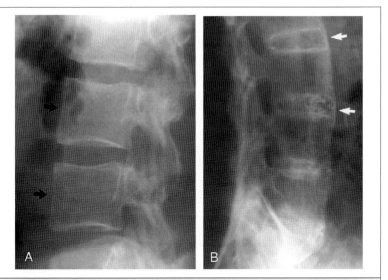

Figure 65-3. *A,* Radiograph showing anterior squaring of the vertebrae in a patient with early inflammatory spondylitis. *B,* Radiograph showing thin, marginal syndesmophytes *(arrows)* causing bamboo spine in a patient with Crohn's disease with advanced inflammatory spondylitis.

TABLE 65-4. ALLEVIATION OF ARTHRITIC SYMPTOMS IN INFLAMMATORY BOWEL DISEASE

	Peripheral Arthritis	Sacroiliitis/Spondylitis
NSAIDs*	Yes	Yes
Intra-articular corticosteroids	Yes	Yes (sacroiliitis)
Sulfasalazine	Yes	No
Immunosuppressives	Yes	No
Antitumor necrosis factor α	Yes	Yes
Bowel resection		
Ulcerative colitis (UC)	Yes	No
Crohn's disease	No	No

*Nonsteroidal anti-inflammatory drugs (NSAIDs) may exacerbate IBD. Sulfasalazine helps the peripheral arthritis in UC patients more than Crohn's disease patients.

surface area of 1000 m² and functions not only to absorb nutrients but also to exclude potentially harmful antigens. The gut-associated lymphoid tissue (GALT), which includes Peyer's patches, the lamina propria, and intraepithelial T cells, constitutes 25% of the GI mucosa and helps exclude entry of bacteria and other foreign antigens. Although the upper GI tract is not normally exposed to microbes, the lower GI tract is constantly in contact with millions of bacteria (up to 10^{12}/gm of feces).

TABLE 65-5.   RHEUMATIC DISORDERS ASSOCIATED WITH POUCHITIS, MICROSCOPIC (LYMPHOCYTIC) COLITIS (MC), AND/OR COLLAGENOUS COLITIS (CC)

	Pouchitis	MC	CC
IBD-like peripheral inflammatory arthritis	Yes	Yes	Yes (10%)
Rheumatoid arthritis	No	Yes	Yes
Ankylosing spondylitis	No	Yes*	No
Thyroiditis/other autoimmune disease	No	Yes	Yes

*Up to 50% of patients with ankylosing spondylitis have asymptomatic MC/Crohn's-like lesions on right-sided colon biopsies.
IBD = inflammatory bowel disease.

Inflammation, whether from idiopathic inflammatory bowel disease or from infection with pathogenic microorganisms, can disrupt the normal integrity and function of the bowel, leading to increased gut permeability. This increased permeability may allow nonviable bacterial antigens in the gut lumen to enter the circulation more easily. These microbial antigens could either deposit directly in the joint synovia, leading to a local inflammatory reaction, or cause a systemic immune response, resulting in immune complexes that then deposit in joints and other tissues.

KEY POINTS: INFLAMMATORY BOWEL DISEASE AND RHEUMATOLOGIC MANIFESTATIONS

1. Inflammatory arthritis is most likely to occur in IBD patients with extensive colonic involvement.

2. Episodes of peripheral arthritis coincide with flares of bowel disease, whereas spinal arthritis occurs independently of bowel disease severity.

3. HLA-B27 increases the risk of developing ankylosing spondylitis 10 times in patients with IBD.

4. Sulfasalazine can help the peripheral arthritis, whereas antitumor necrosis alpha agents help both peripheral and spinal arthritis in IBD patients.

5. All patients with IBD should be screened for osteoporosis.

REACTIVE ARTHRITIS

15. **What is reactive arthritis, and what are the most common GI pathogens causing it?**
A reactive arthritis is a sterile inflammatory arthritis that occurs within 1–3 weeks following an infection by an organism that infects mucosal surfaces, especially the urethra or large bowel. The most common GI pathogens causing reactive arthritis are:
- *Yersinia enterocolitica* or *Y. pseudotuberculosis*
- *Salmonella enteritidis* or *S. typhimurium*
- *Shigella dysenteriae* or *S. flexneri*
- *Campylobacter jejuni*

Approximately 1–3% of patients who get an infectious gastroenteritis during an epidemic subsequently develop a reactive arthritis. It may be as high as 20% in *Yersinia*-infected individuals.

16. **Which joints are involved most commonly in a reactive arthritis following a bowel infection (i.e., postenteric reactive arthritis)?**
See Figure 65-4.

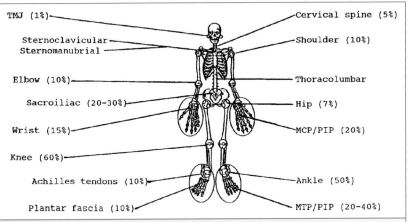

TMJ (1%)

Cervical spine (5%)

Sternoclavicular
Sternomanubrial

Shoulder (10%)

Elbow (10%)

Thoracolumbar

Sacroiliac (20-30%)

Hip (7%)

Wrist (15%)

MCP/PIP (20%)

Knee (60%)

Achilles tendons (10%)

Ankle (50%)

Plantar fascia (10%)

MTP/PIP (20-40%)

Figure 65-4. Joints commonly involved in reactive arthritis after bowel infection.

17. **Describe the clinical characteristics of postenteric reactive arthritis.**
    - Demographics—men > women; average age = 30
    - Onset of arthritis—abrupt, acute
    - Distribution of joints—asymmetric, pauciarticular; lower extremity involved in 80–90%, sacroiliitis in 30%
    - Synovial fluid analysis—inflammatory fluid (usually 10,000–50,000 WBC/mm^3), no crystals, negative cultures
    - Course and prognosis—80% resolve in 1–6 mo; 20% have chronic arthritis with x-ray changes of peripheral and/or sacroiliac joints

18. **What extra-articular manifestations occur in postenteric reactive arthritis?**
    - Sterile urethritis (15–70%)
    - Conjunctivitis
    - Acute anterior uveitis (iritis)
    - Oral ulcers (painless or painful)
    - Erythema nodosum (5% of *Yersinia* infections)
    - Circinate balanitis (25% of *Shigella* infections)
    - Keratoderma blennorrhagicum

19. **How commonly do patients with postenteric reactive arthritis have the clinical features of Reiter's syndrome?**
    The inflammatory arthritis, urethritis, conjunctivitis/uveitis, and mucocutaneous lesions that characterize Reiter's syndrome may develop 2–4 weeks after an acute urethritis or diarrheal illness. The frequency varies with the causative enteric organism:
    - *Shigella* 85%
    - *Salmonella* 10–15%
    - *Yersinia* 10%
    - *Campylobacter* 10%

20. **How do the radiographic features of inflammatory sacroiliitis and spondylitis due to postenteric reactive arthritis differ from those in IBD patients?**
See Table 65-6 and Figure 65-5.

TABLE 65-6.	RADIOLOGIC COMPARISON OF SPINAL ARTHRITIS IN POSTENTERIC REACTIVE ARTHRITIS VERSUS INFLAMMATORY BOWEL DISEASE (IBD)	
	Reactive Arthritis	**IBD**
Sacroiliitis	Unilateral, asymmetric	Bilateral, sacroiliac involvement
Spondylitis	Asymmetric, nonmarginal, jug-handle syndesmophytes	Bilateral, thin, marginal syndesmophytes

21. **Discuss the relationship of HLA-B27 positivity in patients with postenteric reactive arthritis compared to a normal, healthy population.**
    - Reactive arthritis patients, 70–80% HLA-B27–positive; normal healthy controls, 4–8% HLA-B27–positive.
    - Caucasians and patients with radiographic sacroiliitis and/or uveitis are more likely to be HLA-B27–positive.
    - A person who is HLA-B27–positive has a 30–50 times increased risk of developing a reactive arthritis following an episode of infectious gastroenteritis compared to a person who does not have the HLA-B27 gene.
    - Only 20–25% of all HLA-B27–positive individuals who get an infectious gastroenteritis from *Shigella*, *Salmonella*, or *Yersinia* go on to develop a postenteric reactive arthritis.

22. **Explain the current theory for the pathogenesis of a postenteric reactive arthritis.**
Bacterial lipopolysaccharide antigens from the pathogens (*Yersinia, Shigella, Salmonella*) causing the infectious gastroenteritis are deposited in the joints of patients who

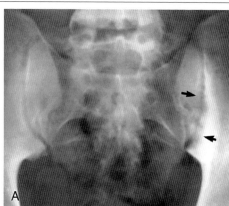
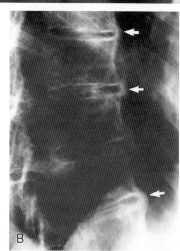

Figure 65-5. *A,* Radiograph showing unilateral sacroiliitis *(arrows)* in a patient with reactive arthritis. *B,* Radiograph showing large, nonmarginal syndesmophytes *(arrows)* of the spine in a patient with reactive arthritis.

develop a postenteric reactive arthritis. These bacterial cell wall components are felt to incite inflammation in the joint. The role that HLA-B27 plays in the pathogenesis is debated. One possibility is that the HLA-B27 molecule presents these bacterial antigens to the immune system in a unique way, leading to inflammation. Another postulate is that there is molecular mimicry between the HLA-B27 molecule and the bacterial antigens, causing an aberrant immune response. It is important to note that intact viable organisms cannot be cultured from the joint of a patient with reactive arthritis. However, chronic persistence of bacterial antigen is an important part of the pathogenesis of reactive arthritis.

23. **Is any therapy beneficial for postenteric reactive arthritis?**
    See Table 65-7.

TABLE 65-7. TREATMENT OF POSTENTERIC REACTIVE ARTHRITIS

	Peripheral Arthritis		
Treatment	Acute	Chronic	Sacroiliitis
NSAIDs	Yes	Yes	Yes
Corticosteroids			
Intra-articular	Yes	Yes	Yes
Oral	Only in high doses	No	No
Antibiotics			
2-week course	No	No	No
3-month course	NA	No	No
Sulfasalazine	NA	Yes	No
Methotrexate	NA	Yes	No
Anti TNF-α	NA	Yes	Yes

NA = not applicable, NSAIDs = nonsteroidal anti-inflammatory drugs, TNF = tumor necrosis factor.

WHIPPLE'S DISEASE

24. **Who was Whipple?**
    George Hoyt Whipple, M.D., in 1907, reported the case of a 36-year-old medical missionary with diarrhea, malabsorption with weight loss, mesenteric lymphadenopathy, and migratory polyarthritis. He named this disease "intestinal lipodystrophy," but it is now known as Whipple's disease. Dr. Whipple also became a Nobel Laureate in Physiology in 1934 and founder of the University of Rochester Medical School.

25. **What are the multisystem manifestations of Whipple's disease?**
    W = Wasting/weight loss   D = Diarrhea
    H = Hyperpigmentation (skin)   I = Interstitial nephritis
    I = Intestinal pain   S = Skin rashes
    P = Pleurisy   E = Eye inflammation
    P = Pneumonitis   A = Arthritis
    L = Lymphadenopathy   S = Subcutaneous nodules
    E = Encephalopathy   E = Endocarditis
    S = Steatorrhea

26. **Describe the clinical characteristics of the arthritis associated with Whipple's disease.**
Whipple's disease occurs most commonly in middle-aged white men. Seronegative oligoarthritis or polyarthritis (knees, ankles, wrists) is the presenting symptom in 60% of patients and may precede the intestinal symptoms by years. Over 70% of patients will develop an arthritis at some time during their disease course. Arthritis is inflammatory, often migratory, and does not correlate with intestinal symptoms. Sacroiliitis or spondylitis occurs in 5–10% of patients, especially in those who are HLA-B27–positive (33% of patients). Synovial fluid analysis shows an inflammatory fluid with 5000–100,000 cells/mm^3. Radiographs remain usually unremarkable.

27. **What is the etiology of Whipple's disease?**
Multiple tissues show deposits in macrophages that stain with periodic acid-Schiff (PAS). These deposits contain rod-shaped free bacilli seen by electron microscopy. Recently, these bacilli have been shown to be a new organism, a gram-positive actinomycete called *Tropheryma whippelii*. The diagnosis is usually made by demonstrating PAS-positive inclusions in macrophages in small bowel or lymph node biopsies. Recently, a more accurate diagnosis can be made by polymerase chain reaction of the DNA sequence of the 16S-ribosomal RNA gene sequence of *T. whippelii* in synovial fluid, cerebrospinal fluid, or small bowel biopsy samples.

28. **How is Whipple's disease best treated?**
Tetracycline, penicillin, erythromycin, or trimethoprim-sulfamethoxazole (TMP-SMX) for >1 year. Relapses can occur (particularly in patients with central nervous system [CNS] involvement) (30%). Chloramphenicol or TMP-SMX is recommended if the CNS is involved.

KEY POINTS: OTHER ENTEROPATHIES WITH RHEUMATOLOGIC MANIFESTATIONS

1. Postinfectious reactive arthritis following an episode of infectious gastroenteritis with *Salmonella, Shigella, Yersinia,* or *Campylobacter* is most likely to occur in HLA-B27–positive individuals.

2. Chronic enteropathic reactive arthritis may respond to sulfasalazine and antitumor necrosis alpha agents but not to prolonged antibiotics.

3. Inflammatory arthritis may be the initial manifestation of Whipple's disease and celiac disease.

4. Whipple's disease is caused by *Tropheryma whippelii,* which can be detected by polymerase chain reaction in synovial/cerebrospinal fluid or biopsied tissue.

5. Pancreatic cancer can release enzymes that cause fat necrosis, resulting in a triad of lower extremity arthritis, tender nodules, and eosinophilia (Schmidt's triad).

OTHER RHEUMATIC DISEASES

29. **What rheumatic manifestations have been described in patients with celiac disease (gluten-sensitive enteropathy)?**
Celiac disease is an enteropathy resulting from an autoimmune reaction to wheat gliadins. It is seen primarily in Caucasians and is associated with HLA-DR3 in 95% of patients compared

to 12% of the general Caucasian population. The most frequent rheumatic manifestations include:

- Arthritis (4–26%): symmetric polyarthritis involving predominantly large joints (knees and ankles > hips and shoulders); may precede enteropathic symptoms in 50% of cases. Oligoarthritis and sacroiliitis can also occur.
- Osteomalacia: due to steatorrhea from severe enteropathy causing vitamin D deficiency
- *Dermatitis herpetiformis*

These rheumatic manifestations can respond dramatically to a gluten-free diet, but not always.

30. Describe the intestinal bypass arthritis-dermatitis syndrome.

This syndrome occurs in 20–80% of patients who have undergone intestinal bypass (jejunoileal or jejunocolic) surgery for morbid obesity. The arthritis is inflammatory, polyarticular, symmetric, and frequently migratory, and it affects both upper- and lower-extremity small and large joints. Radiographic findings usually remain normal, despite 25% of patients having chronic recurring episodes of arthritis. Up to 80% develop dermatologic abnormalities, the most characteristic of which is a maculopapular or vesiculopustular rash.

The pathogenesis involves bacterial overgrowth in the blind loop, resulting in antigenic stimulation that purportedly causes immune complex formation (frequently, cryoprecipitates containing secretory IgA and bacterial antigens) in the serum that deposits in the joints and skin. Treatment includes nonsteroidal anti-inflammatory drugs (NSAIDs) and oral antibiotics, which usually improve symptoms. Only surgical reanastomosis of the blind loop can result in complete elimination of symptoms.

31. What types of arthritis can be associated with carcinomas of the esophagus and colon?

Carcinomatous polyarthritis can be the presenting feature of an occult malignancy of the GI tract. The arthritis is typically acute in onset, asymmetric, and predominantly involves lower extremity joints while sparing the small joints of the hands and wrists. Patients have an elevated erythrocyte sedimentation rate and a negative rheumatoid factor. Another type of arthritis associated with colorectal malignancy is septic arthritis due to *Streptococcus bovis.*

32. What are the clinical features of the pancreatic panniculitis syndrome?

Pancreatic panniculitis is a systemic syndrome occurring in some patients with pancreatitis or pancreatic acinar cell carcinoma. Its clinical manifestations can be remembered by the following mnemonic:

P = Pancreatitis

A = Arthritis (60%) and arthralgia, usually of the ankles and knees. Synovial fluid is typically noninflammatory and creamy in color due to lipid droplets that stain with Sudan black or oil red O.

N = Nodules that are tender, red, and usually on extremities. These are frequently misdiagnosed as erythema nodosum but are really areas of lobular panniculitis with fat necrosis.

C = Cancer of the pancreas more commonly causes this syndrome than does pancreatitis.

R = Radiologic abnormalities caused by osteolytic bone lesions from bone marrow necrosis (10%).

E = Eosinophilia.

A = Amylase, lipase, and trypsin released by the diseased pancreas cause fat necrosis in skin, synovium, and bone marrow.

S = Serositis, including pleuropericarditis frequently with fever.

33. What musculoskeletal problem can occur with pancreatic insufficiency?

Osteomalacia due to fat-soluble vitamin D malabsorption.

BIBLIOGRAPHY

1. Abibotol V, Roux C, Chaussade S, et al: Metabolic bone assessment in patients with inflammatory bowel disease. Gastroenterology 108:417–422, 1995.

2. Bruhlmann P, Michel BA, Altwegg M: Diagnosis and therapy monitoring of Whipple's arthritis by polymerase chain reaction. Rheumatology 39:1427–1428, 2000.

3. Dahl PR, Su WP, Cullimore KC, Dicken CH: Pancreatic panniculitis. J Am Acad Dermatol 33:413–417, 1995.

4. Durand DV, Lecomte C, Cathebras P, et al: Whipple's disease. Medicine 26:170–184, 1997.

5. Farrell RJ, Kelly CP: Celiac sprue. N Engl J Med 346:180–188, 2002.

6. Flores D, Marquez J, Garza M, Espinoza LR: Reactive arthritis: Newer developments. Rheum Dis Clin N Am 29:37–59, 2003.

7. Holden W, Orchard T, Wordsworth P: Enteropathic arthritis. Rheum Dis Clin N Am 29:513–530, 2003.

8. Lubrano E, Cicacci C, Amers PR, et al: The arthritis of coeliac disease: Prevalence and pattern in 200 adult patients. Br J Rheumatol 35:1314–1318, 1996.

9. Naschitz JE, Rosner I, Rozenbaum M, et al: Cancer associated rheumatoid disorders: Clues to occult neoplasia. Semin Arthritis Rheum 24:231–241, 1995.

10. Orchard TR, Wordsworth BP, Jewell DP: Peripheral arthropathies in inflammatory bowel disease: Their articular distribution and natural history. Gut 42:387–391, 1998.

11. Roubenoff R, Ratain J, Giardiello I, et al: Collagenous colitis, enteropathic arthritis, and autoimmune diseases: Results of a patient survey. J Rheumatol 16:1229–1232, 1989.

12. Utsinger PD, Weiner SR, Utsinger JH: Human models: Whipple's disease, coeliac disease, and jejunoileal bypass. Baillieres Clin Rheumatol 10:77–103, 1996.

13. Veloso FT, Carvalho J, Magro F: Immune-related systemic manifestations of inflammatory bowel disease: A prospective study of 792 patients. J Clin Gastroenterol 23:29–34, 1996.

14. Yu D, Kuipers JG: Role of bacteria and HLA-B27 in the pathogenesis of reactive arthritis. Rheum Dis Clin N Am 29:21–36, 2003.

CHAPTER 66

DERMATOLOGIC MANIFESTATIONS OF GASTROINTESTINAL DISEASE

James E. Fitzpatrick, MD

1. **List the most common skin manifestations of hepatobiliary disease.**
   - Dilated abdominal wall veins
   - Hyperpigmentation
   - Jaundice
   - Palmar erythema (liver palms)
   - Peripheral edema
   - Pruritus
   - Purpura
   - Spider hemangiomas

2. **At what serum level of bilirubin do adults and infants develop clinically noticeable jaundice?**
   Adults develop clinically detectable jaundice when the serum levels of bilirubin reach 2.5–3.0 mg/dL in adults, whereas infants may not demonstrate visually detectable jaundice until serum levels reach 6.0–8.0 mg/dL. Hyperbilirubinemia precedes jaundice by several days because the bilirubin has not yet bound to tissue. After serum levels of bilirubin normalize, patients may remain visually jaundiced because it takes several days for tissue-bound bilirubin to be released.

3. **Why is jaundice first noticeable in the sclera of the eyes?**
   Bilirubin has a strong affinity for elastin, which accounts for its early appearance in the sclera of the eye.

4. **What other conditions produce yellowish discoloration of the skin?**
   Jaundice, carotenoderma due to excessive ingestion of carotene (e.g., yellow and orange vegetables, such as carrots and squash), lycopene dermatosis caused by excessive ingestion of lycopene (e.g., red vegetables, such as tomatoes and rose hips), and systemic administration of quinacrine. The skin may also demonstrate a sallow, subtle yellowish hue in patients with profound hypothyroidism.

5. **What are spider angiomas? Why are they associated with liver disease?**
   Spider angiomas (nevus araneus) are vascular lesions characterized by a central arteriole and horizontal radiating thin-walled vessels that produce the "legs" of the vascular spider (Fig. 66-1). The pulsation of the central vertically-oriented arteriole in larger lesions can be visualized

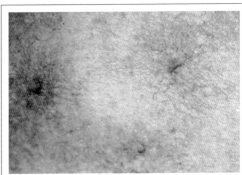

Figure 66-1. Three spider angiomas demonstrating central arteriole and radiating dilated blood vessels.

with diascopy (observing the lesion through a glass slide pressed firmly on the lesion). The mechanism is not proven, but the high incidence of spider angiomas in alcohol-associated hepatitis and pregnancy suggests that elevated levels of estrogens due to higher production or decreased metabolism are responsible. A recent study has shown that patients with liver cirrhosis and spider angiomas have elevated plasma levels of vascular endothelial growth factor and this may play a role in the development of spider angiomas.

6. **Do the number of spider angiomas correlate with the severity of alcohol-induced liver disease?**
Yes, although there is some degree of individual susceptibility to spider angiomas. However, the correlation is high enough that there is report that barmaids in New York used to guess the degree of severity of liver cirrhosis based on the number of spider angiomas visible! The number of spider angiomas also correlates with the presence of esophageal varices. One study demonstrated that the presence of more than 20 spider angiomas correlated with a 50% chance of esophageal bleeding.

7. **Why do many patients with hepatobiliary disease itch?**
Approximately 40% of patients with hepatic cirrhosis demonstrate at least moderate-to-severe pruritus. The mechanism of pruritus associated with hepatobiliary disease has not been firmly established, but it is believed to be due to elevated levels of bile acids secondary to cholestasis. Serum bile acids are frequently but not always elevated in patients with hepatobiliary disease and pruritus. Other mechanisms or chemical mediators may be involved because not all patients demonstrate this finding. Support for elevated bile acids comes from the observation that bile acid-binding resins relieve the pruritus. Studies on purified bile salts placed on blister bases have shown that all bile salts produced pruritus, but unconjugated chenodeoxycholate is the most potent.

8. **A 25-year-old woman presents with painful, tender, red-to-violaceous subcutaneous nodules of the pretibial skin associated with diarrhea. What is the skin lesion?**
The patient most likely has erythema nodosum, although the differential diagnosis includes other types of panniculitis (e.g., erythema induratum, pancreatitis-associated panniculitis), infection, and deep vasculitis (e.g., periarteritis nodosum). Erythema nodosum is a form of hypersensitivity panniculitis that preferentially affect the fibrous septae between the fat lobules. Clinically, erythema nodosum presents most commonly on the anterior surface of the legs, less commonly on the forearms as painful red to violaceous subcutaneous nodules without overlying scale (Fig. 66-2). They

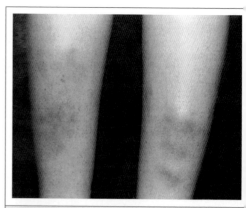

Figure 66-2. Typical lesions of erythema nodosum demonstrating bilateral, red, tender subcutaneous nodules on the anterior lower legs.

are typically bilateral, but unilateral and even annular variants exist. Typical lesions resolve over a period of 3–6 weeks, but atypical lesions may persist for months. The diagnosis is usually made clinically, but occasional cases require biopsy, which is usually diagnostic. The pathogenesis is not understood.

9. **List the three most common gastrointestinal (GI) disorders associated with erythema nodosum.**
   Ulcerative colitis, Crohn's disease, and infectious colitis (e.g., *Salmonella* and *Yersinia enterocolitis*). In patients with inflammatory bowel disease, erythema nodosum is associated most commonly with ulcerative colitis (up to 7% of patients) and less commonly with Crohn's disease. The disease activity of erythema nodosum often parallels the disease activity of the bowel disease.

0. **A 22-year-old woman presents with low-grade fever and an expanding, oozing ulcer of the hand that is rapidly increasing in size, despite aggressive surgical debridement and intravenous antibiotics. What does this patient have?**
   The patient most likely has pyoderma gangrenosum, which usually affects the lower legs, but it can affect any cutaneous surface as well as mucosal surfaces of the eye and oral cavity. The lesions begin as a tender, red papule or pustule that increases rapidly in size to form an ulcer with an undermined border (Fig. 66-3). Lesions of pyoderma gangrenosum may remain fixed or may expand rapidly at a rate of more than 1 cm per day. Pyoderma gangrenosum often demonstrates *pathergy,* which is the development of skin lesions at the site of trauma. Pyoderma gangrenosum, mistaken for bacterial pyodermas, may be treated with surgical debridement, which often makes the lesion worse. The pathogenesis of pyoderma gangrenosum is controversial. Histologically, the predominant effector cells are neutrophils, and some authorities have even considered it to be a form of vasculitis. More recent evidence suggests that it is probably lymphocyte-mediated, which accounts for the marked response to cyclosporine.

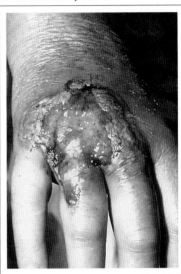

Figure 66-3. Typical lesion of pyoderma gangrenosum demonstrating tender, rapidly expanding ulcer with undermined edge.

1. **List the GI diseases associated most commonly with pyoderma gangrenosum.**
   Ulcerative colitis (most common), Crohn's disease, and chronic infectious hepatitis. One study reported that 50% of all cases of pyoderma gangrenosum are associated with ulcerative colitis, but less than 10% of all patients with ulcerative colitis will develop pyoderma gangrenosum. A separate study reported that one third of patients with pyoderma gangrenosum had inflammatory bowel disease; ulcerative colitis and Crohn's disease were equally represented.

2. **What are the cutaneous manifestations of pancreatitis?**
   Cutaneous manifestations of pancreatitis include Cullen's sign, Grey Turner's sign, and pancreatic fat necrosis. Cullen's sign is a hemorrhagic discoloration of the umbilical area due to intraperitoneal hemorrhage from any cause; one of the more frequent causes is acute hemorrhagic panniculitis. Grey Turner's sign is a discoloration of the left flank associated with acute hemorrhagic pancreatitis. Acute and chronic pancreatitis and pancreatic carcinoma may also produce pancreatic fat necrosis, which presents as very tender, erythematous nodules of the subcutaneous fat that may spontaneously drain necrotic material (Fig. 66-4). Patients have also often associated acute arthritis that may be crippling. Histologically,

pancreatic fat necrosis demonstrates diagnostic changes manifesting as necrosis and saponification of the fat associated with acute inflammation. The fat necrosis is thought to be due to release of lipase and amylase, which have been demonstrated to be elevated within lesions.

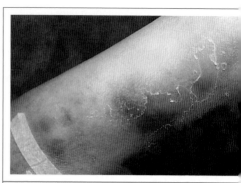

Figure 66-4. Pancreatic fat necrosis in a patient with alcohol-associated pancreatitis. Unlike erythema nodosum, epidermal changes (note scale) and ulceration are common.

13. **A 32-year-old woman presents with recurrent blisters, primarily located over the dorsum aspects of her hands. She reports a history of two episodes of severe abdominal pain, with one episode being associated with stupor. What disease does she have?**
She has most likely variegated porphyria, which is inherited in an autosomal dominant fashion A mutation in the protogen oxidase gene results in a reduction in the enzyme, protogen oxidase Patients clinically resemble a cross between porphyria cutanea tarda (PCT) and acute intermittent porphyria (AIP). The skin lesions consist mainly of tense blisters, erosions, or scars primarily localized to the dorsum of the hands. As in the case of PCT, the patients may als demonstrate increased skin fragility, milia (small, white epidermoid cysts), hyperpigmentation and hypertrichosis. As in the case of AIP, patients demonstrate intermittent abdominal pain tha is often precipitated by certain drugs, such as barbiturates or sulfonamides. The skin findings do not necessarily correlate with the abdominal attacks.

14. **A 32-year-old man presents with a 2-year history of recurrent blisters that are intensely pruritic and have been recalcitrant to antihistamines and topical corticosteroids. They are located primarily on the elbows, knees, and buttocks. What does this patient most likely have?**
This patient most likely has dermatitis herpetiformis, which is an autoimmune vesiculobullous disease characterized by intensely pruritic blisters that are often grouped (herpetiform) or, less commonly, plaques studded with vesicles or bullae (Fig. 66-5). Dermatitis herpetiformis has a classic symmetric distribution; the characteristic sites are the elbows, knees, buttocks, and scalp. Because of the intense pruritus, patients often present with excoriations only. The diagnosis is

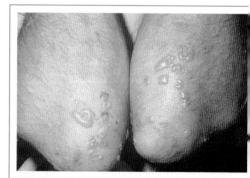

Figure 66-5. Grouped vesicles and bullae on the elbows of a patient with dermatitis herpetiformis.

established usually by demonstrating the presence of IgA autoantibodies along the dermoepidermal junction by direct immunofluorescence.

15. **What GI disease is associated most commonly with dermatitis herpetiformis?**
Celiac disease (gluten-sensitive enteropathy). Although almost all patients demonstrate histologic findings of celiac disease, only one third of patients demonstrate clinical symptoms of celiac disease. Both celiac disease and dermatitis herpetiformis respond to a gluten-free diet.

16. **A 30-year-old man presents with acute GI bleeding. He has yellowish, pebbly papules that coalesce into plaques of the neck, antecubital fossae, and axillae. Similar lesions are also present on his lower lip. What does he have?**
The patient has pseudoxanthoma elasticum (PXE), a disorder characterized by progressive calcification of elastic fibers. It is inherited most commonly in an autosomal dominant fashion, but autosomal recessive variants have also been described. Mutations in the ABCC6 gene have been demonstrated to be the genetic defect, but how this defect produces PXE is not understood. The mucocutaneous manifestations are described as looking like "plucked chicken skin" (Fig. 66-6). The histologic findings are diagnostic and demonstrate fragmentation of abnormal elastic fibers in the dermis associated with calcification. Identical yellowish papules are seen in the GI mucosa, including the mouth, esophagus, and stomach. Involvement of the elastic fibers in gastric arteries may result in acute and sometimes massive hemorrhage. Additional findings associated with PXE include angioid streaks of the retina, claudication, premature angina, and hypertension.

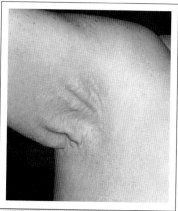

Figure 66-6. Confluent yellowish papules with appearance of "plucked chicken skin" in a patient with pseudoxanthoma elasticum.

17. **A 24-year-old man presents with a history of unexplained melena, nosebleeds, and red macular lesions of his lips and fingers. What does he have?**
This patient most likely has hereditary hemorrhagic telangiectasia (HHT), also known as Osler-Weber-Rendu disease. This uncommon genetic disorder is inherited in an autosomal dominant fashion and is the result of mutations of two genes: ENG (HHT1) and ALK1 (HHT2). The cutaneous lesions typically present at the time of puberty or later and manifest as linear, punctate, or macular lesions that most commonly affect the skin surfaces of the face, fingers, and toes. Similar lesions are also found in many types of mucosal surfaces, including the nasal mucosa, lips, entire GI tract, and urinary tract. Arteriovenous malformations may also develop in the central nervous system, eyes, lungs, and liver. Patients continue to develop new lesions during their lifetime and may experience chronic iron-deficiency anemia due to chronic low-grade blood loss from the GI tract.

18. **During evaluation for GI bleeding, a 25-year-old man is noted to have 2- to 4-mm pigmented macules of the lips and buccal mucosa. What does he most likely have?**
This patient most likely has Peutz-Jeghers syndrome, an autosomal dominant disorder associated with germ-line mutations of the STKII/LKB1 tumor suppressor gene. It is characterized by round to oval pigmented macules that vary from brown to blue-brown in color and small intestine hamartomatous polyps. The pigmented macules are present usually at birth or develop during infancy. The most commonly affected areas are the lips, buccal mucosa, hard palate, gingival, anus, palms, and soles. Because pigmented macular lesions

may be seen in these areas in normal individuals and in association with other syndromes, clinical and historic correlation is necessary to establish a diagnosis of Peutz-Jeghers syndrome.

19. **What is the risk of malignancy developing in the polyps associated with Peutz-Jeghers syndrome?**

The lifetime risk of developing adenocarcinoma is calculated to be between 2% and 13%. Patients with Peutz-Jeghers syndrome also demonstrate an increased incidence of other types of neoplasia—the most common types being breast carcinoma, cervical adenocarcinoma, and both benign and malignant tumors of the ovary and testes.

20. **During evaluation for numerous polyps of the colon, a 19-year-old man is noted to have multiple cysts of the skin and an osteoma. What does he most likely have?**

Gardner's syndrome, which is inherited in an autosomal dominant fashion and due to a mutation in the *APC* gene located at 5q21. This rare disorder occurs in 1 of every 14,000 births. The polyps resemble the polyps of familial adenomatous polyposis. These patients have colonic polyps and 10% have small intestinal polyps. The cutaneous manifestations consist of epidermoid cysts (epidermal inclusion cysts), lipomas, fibromas, desmoid tumors, and, rarely, pilomatrixomas (uncommon hair follicle tumors). Patients often have bone tumors, most of which are osteomas, supernumerary teeth, and congenital hypertrophy of the retinal pigmented epithelium.

21. **What is the risk of development of malignancy in the polyps found in Gardner's syndrome?**

The lifetime risk of colon cancer in Gardner's syndrome approaches 100%. Proctocolectomy is recommended for all patients, followed by periodic monitoring of the rectal mucosal remnant and the upper GI tract. Patients with Gardner's syndrome also have a higher incidence of extracolonic malignancies, including papillary thyroid carcinoma, adrenal carcinoma, hepatoblastoma, periampullary carcinoma, and duodenal carcinoma.

22. **A 44-year-old man presents with multiple hamartomatous polyps of the small and large bowel. Cutaneous examination reveals "cobblestoning" of the oral mucosa and multiple small papules and verrucous papules of his face. What does this patient most likely have?**

Cowden's disease, also known as multiple hamartoma syndrome. This rare syndrome is inherited in an autosomal fashion and is due to mutations in PTEN, a tumor suppressor gene located on chromosome 10q23. The mucocutaneous manifestations include small papules of the oral mucosa that are usually most prominent on the gingival, are often numerous, and have been described as resembling cobblestones; papules and verrucous papules, usually located on the face that are trichilemmomas (benign follicular tumors); hyperkeratotic papules of the extremities; and firm nodules called *sclerotic fibromas*. Sclerotic fibromas are uncommon, benign fibrous tumors that are typically solitary. Multiple sclerotic fibromas are considered to be a specific marker for Cowden's disease; the incidence approaches 100% if two or more are present. Polyps are present in the GI tract in approximately 30% of patients and may be present at any site.

23. **What is the risk of development of malignancy in the polyps associated with Cowden's syndrome?**

The polyps associated with Cowden's syndrome do not demonstrate an increased risk of malignancy. However, patients with Cowden's syndrome demonstrate an increased incidence of thyroid disease—up to two thirds demonstrating goiter and 10% developing thyroid carcinoma.

Seventy-five percent of women demonstrate breast neoplasia manifesting as fibrocystic breast disease, fibroadenomas, and breast carcinoma.

24. What is Trousseau's sign?

Trousseau's sign consists of superficial migratory thrombophlebitis associated with an underlying malignancy. Clinically, it presents as erythematous linear cords that affect the superficial veins of the extremities and trunk. Patients typically continue to develop new lesions at multiple sites and may appear to "migrate." Trousseau's sign may be seen in association with many types of GI malignancies (e.g., gastric carcinoma, pancreatic adenocarcinoma) in addition to lung carcinoma, multiple myeloma, and Hodgkin's disease. The pathogenesis is not understood, and the thrombophlebitis is notoriously resistant to anticoagulant therapy. It was a cruel coincidence that the physician who described this sign, Dr. Armond Trousseau (1801–1867) was himself to develop Trousseau's sign secondary to his underlying gastric carcinoma, which was ultimately fatal.

25. A 50-year-old woman presents with alopecia, unexplained 20-lb weight loss, and very superficial flaccid vesicles and erosions on an erythematous base that preferentially involves the perioral and perianal areas. What does she most likely have?

The cutaneous lesions are consistent with necrolytic migratory erythema, a paraneoplastic cutaneous finding associated with α_2-glucagon-producing islet cell tumors of the pancreas. The cutaneous lesions characteristically start as broad areas of erythema that preferentially affect the face, intertriginous areas, ankles, and feet. The skin often appears to peel or demonstrate superficial vesicles. Patients may also demonstrate stomatitis, glossitis, alopecia, nail dystrophy, weight loss, diabetes mellitus, and anemia. Resection of the glucagon-producing tumor produces prompt resolution of the skin lesions.

26. What is a Sister Mary Joseph's nodule?

Sister Mary Joseph's nodule is an umbilical metastasis of an internal malignancy. In the largest series reported, the most common primary malignancies were stomach (20%), large bowel (14%), ovary (14%), and pancreas (11%). In 20% of cases, the primary could not be established. In 14% of cases, a Sister Mary Joseph's nodule was the initial presentation of the internal malignancy. Umbilical metastases usually indicate advanced disease; the average survival is 10 months.

27. Who was Sister Mary Joseph?

Sister Mary Joseph was the first surgical assistant to Dr. W. J. Mayo. Although it was Dr. Mayo who described the clinical features of nodular umbilical metastases, Sister Mary Joseph is credited with being the first to appreciate that patients with this finding had a poor prognosis. Sister Mary Joseph eventually became the superintendent of St. Mary's Hospital in Rochester, Minnesota.

WEBSITE

http://www.derm.ubc.ca/

BIBLIOGRAPHY

1. Dahl PR, Su WP, Cullimore KC, et al: Pancreatic panniculitis. J Am Acad Dermatol 33:413–417, 1995.
2. Li CP, Lee FY, Hwang SJ, et al: Spider angiomas in patients with liver cirrhosis: Role of vascular endothelial growth factor and basic fibroblast growth factor. World J Gastroenterol 9:2832-2835, 2003.

3. Menachem Y, Gotsman I: Clinical manifestations of pyoderma gangrenosum associated with inflammatory bowel disease. Isr Med Assoc J 6:88–90, 2004.

4. Powell FC, Cooper AJ, Massa MC, et al: Sister Mary Joseph's nodule: A clinical and histologic study. J Am Acad Dermatol 10:610–615, 1984.

5. Reilly PJ, Nostrant TT: Clinical manifestations of hereditary hemorrhagic telangiectasia. Am J Gastroenterol 79:363–367, 1984.

6. Smith KE, Fenske NA: Cutaneous manifestations of alcohol abuse. J Am Acad Dermatol 43:1–16, 2000.

7. Ward SK, Roenigk HH, Gordon KB: Dermatologic manifestations of gastrointestinal disorders. Gastroenterol Clin North Am 27:615–636, 1998.

CHAPTER 67

ENDOCRINE DISORDERS AND THE GASTROINTESTINAL TRACT

John A. Merenich, MD, and William J. Georgitis, MD

1. **Are gastrointestinal (GI) complaints more common in patients with diabetes mellitus?**
   GI complaints are reported by as many as 75% of patients with diabetes mellitus. Most population studies report an increased prevalence of GI symptoms in subjects with type 2 diabetes but not in children with type 1 diabetes, compared to controls. Characteristics of diabetic enteropathy include:
   - Women report symptoms more often than men.
   - Visceral autonomic neuropathy plays a critical role in most GI disorders.
   - Symptoms correlate with glycemic control but *not* with diabetes duration or type of treatment.
   - Manifestations reported most consistently (compared with subjects without diabetes) are nausea, fecal incontinence and urgency, abdominal pain, and diarrhea.

2. **What are the causes and clinical manifestations of gastroparesis in diabetic patients? How should it be treated?**
   Reduced amplitude of fundic contractions, decreased amplitude and frequency of antral contractions, and pylorospasm contribute to a delay in gastric emptying (solids greater than liquids) in patients with diabetes. In addition to worsening nausea/vomiting and early satiety, gastroparesis may contribute to erratic glucose control and weight loss in some individuals. Behavioral, medical, and surgical treatment strategies of gastroparesis are outlined in Table 67-1.

3. **Describe the mechanisms of chronic diarrhea in diabetes mellitus and their treatments.**
   Chronic diarrhea in patients with diabetes mellitus is usually related to either chronic autonomic dysfunction or associated diseases that are more prevalent in the diabetic population. The most common cause of nondiabetic diarrhea in patients with diabetes is drug therapy with metformin. Treatment strategies based on the primary cause of the diabetic diarrhea are depicted in Table 67-2.

4. **What autoimmune GI abnormalities are more prevalent in patients with autoimmune thyroiditis? Do any warrant routine screening?**
   Immune gastritis and pernicious anemia are present in approximately 10%, and antiparietal cell antibodies are detected in up to 33% of patients with autoimmune thyroiditis (Hashimoto's disease). Hypothyroidism occurs in 16%, and thyroid antibody titers are elevated in 26% of patients with primary biliary cirrhosis. Therefore, primary biliary cirrhosis and chronic active hepatitis should be considered if the serum transaminase elevation commonly observed in hypothyroid patients is severe (>2–3 times normal) or persists after thyroid hormone replacement. About 5% of patients with type 1 diabetes have celiac disease. Thus, children with type 1 diabetes and malabsorption, growth failure, unstable diabetes, or even subtle GI upset should be screened for celiac disease.

5. **What are the GI manifestations and their clinical consequences in patients with severe thyrotoxicosis?**
   Patients in thyrotoxic storm almost always manifest some evidence of severe GI dysfunction. Nausea, vomiting, and abdominal pain are common. Hyperdefecation, commonly observed in

TABLE 67–1.   TREATMENT OF GASTROPARESIS IN DIABETES MELLITUS

Maneuver	Comments
Avoid agents that impair gastric emptying	Especially anticholinergics and antidepressants: if needed, use agents with minimal anticholinergic properties, such as desipramine and fluoxetine.
Improve glycemic control	Acute hyperglycemia affects gastric myoelectrical activity and fundic compliance, and slows gastric emptying.
Adjust diet	Decrease fat and fiber intake; avoid uncooked vegetables and fruits with hard-to-digest skins (e.g., apples, grapes, peas); give frequent small meals; increase liquid supplements; antiemetic agents may facilitate oral feeding in certain cases.
Use prokinetic agents	Metoclopramide, 5–20 mg (30 min before meals and at bedtime); erythromycin, 50–250 mg PO t.i.d.–q.i.d.; 2–6 mg/kg every 8 hours, IV
	Domperidone, 20 mg (30 min before meals and at bedtime)
Consider feeding jejunostomy	For refractory patients with severe malnutrition and volume depletion; nasojejunal trial prior to ensure that patients can tolerate minimum 80 mL nutrient/hr

many patients with thyrotoxicosis, may progress to severe diarrhea that can significantly compromise volume status. Hepatic dysfunction characterized by hepatomegaly, abdominal tenderness, and elevated serum transaminase concentrations is frequent; hyperbilirubinemia and jaundice indicate advanced disease and are associated with a high rate of mortality. The combination of increased metabolic demand without compensatory increase in hepatic blood flow results in relative ischemia that may account for some of the clinical and histologic findings.

6. **Name the two metabolic causes of acute pancreatitis.**
    Hypertriglyceridemia and hypercalcemia are the two metabolic disturbances that can cause acute pancreatitis. Triglyceride concentration, almost always in excess of 1000–2000 mg/dL, may account for 4% of acute pancreatitis. Hypertriglyceridemia, because it may resolve with fasting, may be overlooked as a cause unless evaluated early. Although excessive ethanol use may account for both pancreatitis and secondary triglyceride elevation, a direct causative role of severe hypertriglyceridemia in the development of pancreatic inflammation has been postulated. Acute pancreatitis can occur in association with hypercalcemia of any cause, but it is observed most often in patients with hyperparathyroidism. Less than 1% of patients with acute pancreatitis, however, have documented hyperparathyroidism.

TABLE 67-2. CAUSES AND TREATMENT OF DIABETIC DIARRHEA

Cause	Treatment
Metformin induced	Prescribe metformin 250–500 mg with evening meal, and instruct to slowly increase as tolerated to effective dose
Intestinal bacterial overgrowth	Tetracycline, metronidazole, cephalosporins, quinolones, amoxicillin-clavulanic acid (10–14 days each month on rotating basis)
Celiac disease	Gluten-free diet
Use of dietetic foods	Avoid sorbitol products
Pancreatic exocrine deficiency	Pancreatic enzyme
Bile acid malabsorption	Cholestyramine (4–16 gm/day) or aluminum hydroxide
Abnormal colonic motility	Loperamide, diphenoxylate, clonidine (0.1–0.6 mg/day)
Altered intestinal secretion	Octreotide (50–75 μg subcutaneously before meals), clonidine
Anorectal dysfunction	Biofeedback

7. **Define *biochemical hypoglycemia* and *pathologic hypoglycemia*.**
Hypoglycemia signifies a plasma glucose of less than 50 mg/dL (2.7 mmol/L) in most clinical laboratories. Lowering glucose levels, however, provokes measurable physiologic responses (Fig. 67-1) at threshold glucose values much greater than 50 mg/dL. A practical dictum derived from these thresholds is that glucose levels less than 75 mg/dL should be avoided during management of type 1 and type 2 diabetes mellitus to avoid creating hypoglycemic awareness from overzealous glycemic control. Defining the cutoff value for pathologic hypoglycemia is further complicated by the finding that a substantial number of normal young subjects, especially women, exhibit fasting glucose levels less than 50 mg/dL without neuroglycopenic symptoms.

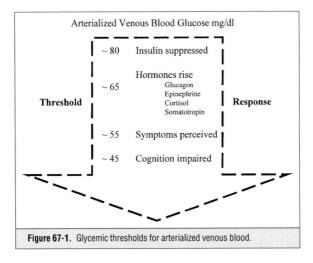

Figure 67-1. Glycemic thresholds for arterialized venous blood.

8. **What is Whipple's triad? Why is it important?**

Whipple described the following triad of findings that should exist before insulin levels are measured and other elaborate testing is performed in the pursuit of rare insulinoma:

1. Presence of neuroglycopenic symptoms* consistent with hypoglycemia
2. Documentation of a low plasma glucose
3. Relief of symptoms after the plasma glucose is normalized

*Neuroglycopenic symptoms due to cerebral glucose deprivation include confusion, difficulty thinking, a sense of increased warmth, weakness, fatigue, bizarre behavior, seizures, and coma, as opposed to reactive adrenergic symptoms like tremulousness, anxiety and palpitations, sweating, and paresthesia.

KEY POINTS: "RULE OF 10s" FOR INSULINOMA

1. 10% are associated with MEN-1 syndrome.

2. 10% are malignant.

3. 10% are bilateral.

4. 10% are <2 cm in size.

5. 10% occur in patients <age 30.

9. **Which GI and hepatic disturbances are associated with hypoglycemia?**

Hypoglycemia (<50 mg/dL) may occur in both the absorptive and postabsorptive state. Postabsorptive (fasting) hypoglycemia includes processes characterized by underproduction or overutilization of glucose; overutilization may be either insulin-dependent or insulin-independent. GI and hepatic disturbances, therefore, may result in or contribute to the development of hypoglycemia, as indicated in Figure 67-2.

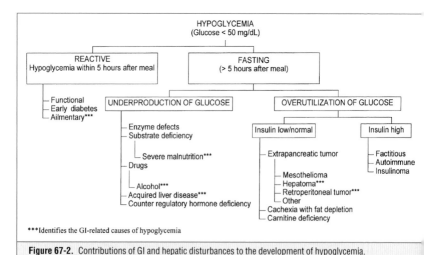

Figure 67-2. Contributions of GI and hepatic disturbances to the development of hypoglycemia.

10. **How does ethanol cause hypoglycemia?**

- Alcohol dampens the normal growth hormone, corticotropin, cortisol, and glucagon responses to induce hypoglycemia.

- Ethanol does *not* impair glycogenolysis.
- Glycogen stores must be depleted for alcohol-induced hypoglycemia to occur.

11. **Should routine screening for polyps and colorectal cancer be performed in patients with acromegaly?**

An increased incidence of tumors (including thyroid, breast, and GI tract types) has been reported in patients with acromegaly. In part, due to improved survival seen in acromegalic patients in the past decade, a 13-fold relative risk of colon cancer in acromegaly has been reported recently. Recommendations regarding the frequency of colorectal screening remain controversial, but it seems prudent to offer screening to all active acromegalic patients >age 40. Frequent surveillance should be conducted in patients with adenoma at first screening, especially when serum IGF-1 levels are elevated. Because up to 25% of adenomas and 50% of carcinomas occur in the ascending or transverse colon, total colonoscopy is recommended.

12. **What GI symptoms may be seen with high serum calcium levels?**

Anorexia, nausea, and vomiting appear early in hypercalcemic crisis. Poor oral intake and accelerated water loss from hypercalcemia-induced nephrogenic diabetes insipidus result in polyuria, dehydration, decreased renal blood flow, and a fall in glomerular filtration rate that leads to increased proximal tubular sodium reabsorption. Enhanced calcium reabsorption linked to the increased sodium uptake further exacerbates the hypercalcemia and can result in stupor, coma, and even death. Additional GI manifestations of hypercalcemia include constipation, pancreatitis, and peptic ulceration stemming from enhanced gastric acid secretion mediated, in part, by calcium-stimulated hypergastrinemia.

13. **When is GI surgery warranted for the treatment of obesity?**

A National Institutes of Health consensus conference concluded that surgical treatment for morbid obesity is acceptable in patients with a body mass index (BMI) >40 or in patients with a BMI >35 who have serious medical problems such as diabetes and cardiopulmonary problems, if nonsurgical attempts at weight reduction have failed. BMI is calculated as weight in kilograms divided by the square of height in meters. All surgical candidates should be screened for endocrine disorders that can cause morbid obesity. They should understand how surgery causes weight loss and that surgery itself does not guarantee good results. Subjects should be psychosocially stable without active drug or alcohol abuse.

14. **How effective are bariatric surgical procedures for long-term control of morbid obesity?**

Currently, bariatric surgery offers the best treatment to produce sustained weight loss in patients who are morbidly obese. Postprocedure weight loss averages from 30–40% of preoperative weight at 6–12 months and is attributable primarily to decreased caloric consumption not malabsorption. Roux-en-Y bypass appears superior to gastric banding and stapled gastroplasty. Surgical treatment of obesity is expensive and associated with some operative morbidity and mortality. Laparoscopic techniques are increasingly utilized for bariatric operations and confer reduced hospitalization, earlier return to normal activity, and fewer postoperative complications. They are technically difficult to perform and are associated with a steep learning curve.

15. **What complications are specific to operations for obesity?**

Jejunoileal bypass eventually achieved about a 1% operative mortality by the end of the 1970s but was fraught with complications, including diarrhea, bile acid malabsorption, fat-soluble vitamin deficiencies, calcium oxalate nephrolithiasis, inflammatory arthritis, and liver disease ranging from steatosis to fibrosis and even frank cirrhosis with hepatic failure. Gastric bypass or plication operations have mortality risks of approximately 1%. Deficiencies in iron, thiamine, and vitamin B_{12} are common.

16. What is multiple endocrine neoplasia syndrome type 1 (MEN-1)?

MEN-1, described by Wermer in 1954, is a disorder characterized by hyperplastic or neoplastic transformation of endocrine glands. Evolution of the syndrome involves the loss of a tumor suppressor gene encoded on the long arm of chromosome 11. A germ cell line mutant allele is inherited. Somatic mutation leads to loss of the gene product menin, which results first in hyperplasia and later in neoplasia. Prevalence is estimated to range from 2–20/100,000.

17. List the MEN-1–associated tumors, in order of frequency.

In Wermer syndrome, the "three P" glands are involved in the following order of decreasing frequency:

- Parathyroid: 80–95% of cases; hyperparathyroidism is also the earliest manifestation to appear. Parathyroid hyperplasia is treated by 3.5 gland parathyroidectomy.
- Pancreas: 80% of cases. Islet cell tumors include gastrinomas (60%) and insulinomas (30%), but they also may be associated with secretion of other peptide hormones (10%) suc as vasoactive intestinal peptide (VIP), somatostatin, and glucagon.
- Pituitary: 50–71% of cases. Prolactinomas are the most prevalent pituitary adenomas, but exces sive secretion of growth hormone, ACTH, and other anterior pituitary tumors can occur.

KEY POINTS: CLINICAL MANIFESTATIONS OF THE PANCREATIC ENDOCRINE TUMORS

1. *Glucagonoma* = hyperglycemia, anorexia, glossitis, anemia, migratory necrolytic erythema

2. *Insulinoma* = hypoglycemia, weight gain, neuroglycopenia, esophagitis, diarrhea

3. *Gastrinoma* = recurrent, refractory peptic ulcer

4. *VIPoma* = watery diarrhea, hypokalemia, hypercalcemia, hypochloremic metabolic alkalosis

5. *Somatostatinoma* = diabetes mellitus, diarrhea, steatorrhea, cholelithiasis

18. Define *carcinoid syndrome*.

Carcinoid syndrome refers to a constellation of symptoms resulting from elaboration of a variety of humoral substances from a carcinoid tumor. Features of the syndrome include flushing, diarrhea, abdominal cramping, eventual development of right-sided valvular heart disease, bronchospasm, and fibrosis of the pleura, peritoneum, or retroperitoneum.

19. How can carcinoid tumors be classified?

Carcinoid tumors can be subdivided by origin into foregut, midgut, hindgut, and other sites (e.g., gonads or thymus). Tumors can also be characterized by the presence or absence of carcinoid syndrome. Secretory products include hormones and biogenic amines (e.g., serotonin, histamine, kallikrein, neurotensin, substance P, corticotropin, prostaglandins). Although the latter are often elaborated, only 5–10% of patients with tumors manifest the syndrome. Small tumors and those with venous drainage into the portal system may be clinically silent because of effective breakdown of tumor products. Large tumors, those with extensive hepatic metastases, or small tumors secreting directly into the systemic venous circulation (e.g., bronchial carcinoid tumors) most often manifest the carcinoid syndrome.

20. Describe the characteristic features of carcinoid tumors by site of origin.

- *Gastric:* Three fourths are associated with chronic atrophic gastritis type A, and one fourth are sporadic with Zollinger-Ellison syndrome. One half of gastric carcinoids are multifocal, but <10% metastasize.

- *Small intestinal:* Frequently located in the distal ileum in patients >age 60 with chronic abdominal pain. Lymph node or hepatic metastases are common. Only 5–7% manifest carcinoid syndrome.
- *Appendiceal:* Present in patients ages 40–50. Less than 10% cause symptoms, and metastases are rare.
- *Colonic:* Present in the seventh decade of life. Less than 5% present with carcinoid syndrome.
- *Rectal:* Usually contain glucagon- and glicentin-related peptides rather than serotonin. One half are asymptomatic. The remainder present with rectal bleeding, pain, or constipation.

21. **How is carcinoid syndrome treated?**
    General treatment measures and agents to ameliorate symptoms associated with carcinoid syndrome are depicted in Table 67-3.

TABLE 67-3. TREATMENT OF CARCINOID SYNDROME	
Carcinoid Symptom/ Problem	**Intervention**
General	Niacin supplementation to compensate for accelerated conversion of tryptophan to serotonin
	High-protein diet
	Avoidance of precipitants for spells, such as sympathomimetics, alcohol, and stress
Flushing	Somatostatin analogs
	H_1 and H_2 blockers (especially for gastric carcinoid)
	Interferon
	Phenoxybenzamine
Diarrhea	Loperamide and diphenoxylate
	Antiserotonin agents (methysergide, cyproheptadine)
	Somatostatin analogs
	Cholestyramine
Asthma and bronchospasm	Methylxanthines and glucocorticoids are the most commonly used agents. Beta agonists and epinephrine should be avoided because they may precipitate attacks.
Excessive tumor burden	Surgery
	Hepatic artery embolization or ligation
	Chemotherapy (streptozocin and fluorouracil; methotrexate and cyclophosphamide; interferon; doxorubicin; cisplatin; etoposide)
	Radiolabeled somatostatin analogs

22. **Weight loss, malaise, nausea, anorexia, vomiting, and skin hyperpigmentation should prompt evaluation for what endocrine disorder suffered by a U.S. president?**
    These signs and symptoms are present in primary adrenal insufficiency (Addison's disease), a malady diagnosed at an early age in former President John F. Kennedy.

23. Which GI symptoms may be present in patients with pheochromocytoma?

Weight loss, anorexia, and abdominal pain due to cholelithiasis are presenting features in some cases of pheochromocytoma.

24. What is the most prominent GI manifestation of medullary cancer of the thyroid?

Diarrhea, sometimes severe, is the most prominent manifestation of medullary cancer of the thyroid. It occurs in 30–50% of patients. Vasoactive intestinal polypeptide, kinins, and prostaglandins (but not calcitonin) account for the diarrhea in most patients. Adrenocorticotropic hormone and serotonin (causing Cushing's syndrome and carcinoid syndrome, respectively) are secreted by the tumor in a few patients.

BIBLIOGRAPHY

1. Arky RA: Hypoglycemia associated with liver disease and ethanol. Endocrinol Metab Clin North Am 18:75, 198●

2. Braverman LE, Utiger RD: The Thyroid, 7th ed. Philadelphia, J.B. Lippincott, 1996.

3. Bravo EL: Evolving concepts in the pathophysiology, diagnosis, and treatment of pheochromocytoma. Endocr Rev 15:356, 1994.

4. Brolin RE: Bariatric surgery and long-term control of morbid obesity. JAMA 288:2793–2796, 2002.

5. Bytzer P, Talley NJ, Leemon M, et al: Prevalence of gastrointestinal symptoms associated with diabetes mellitus A population-based survey of 15,000 adults. Arch Int Med 161:1989–1996, 2001.

6. Chari ST, Vege SS: Etiology of acute pancreatitis. In Rose BD (ed): UpToDate. Wellesley, MA, 1999.

7. Delcore R, Friesen SR: Gastrointestinal neuroendocrine tumors. J Am Coll Surg 178:187, 1994.

8. Gastrointestinal surgery for severe obesity: National Institutes of Health Consensus Development Conference Statement. Am J Clin Nutr 55(Suppl 2):615S–619S, 1992.

9. Greenway FL: Surgery for obesity. Endocrinol Metab Clin North Am 25:1005, 1999.

10. Holmes GK: Screening for coeliac disease in type 1 diabetes. Arch Dis Child 87:495–499, 2002.

11. Jenkins PJ, Fairclough PD: Screening guidelines for colorectal cancer and polyps in patients with acromegaly. Gut 51(Suppl 5):13V–14V, 2002.

12. Kulke MH, Mayer RJ: Carcinoid tumors. N Engl J Med 18:858, 1999.

13. Lauffer JM, Zang T, Modlin IM: Current status of gastrointestinal carcinoids. Aliment Pharmacol Ther 13:271, 1999.

14. Marx SJ: Hyperparathyroid and hypoparathyroid disorders. N Engl J Med 343:1863–1875, 2000.

15. Rensch MJ, Merenich JA, Lieberman M, et al: Gluten-sensitive enteropathy in patients with insulin-dependent diabetes mellitus. Ann Intern Med 124(6):564–567, 1996.

16. Scialpi C, Mosca S, Malguti A: Acromegaly and intestinal neoplasms. Panminerva Med 41:157, 1999.

17. Smith DS, Ferris CD: Current concepts in diabetic gastroparesis. Drugs 63:1339–1358, 2003.

18. Vassilopoulou-Sellin R, Ajani J: Neuroendocrine tumors of the pancreas. Endocrinol Metab Clin North Am 23:5, 1994.

19. Vazeou A, Papadopoulou A, Booth IW, et al: Prevalence of gastrointestinal symptoms in children and adolescents with type 1 diabetes. Diabetes Care 24:962–964, 2001.

20. Veldhuis JD, Norton JA, Wells SA: Surgical versus medical management of multiple endocrine neoplasia (MEN) type 1. J Clin Endocrinol Metab 82:357, 1997.

VII. GASTROINTESTINAL RADIOLOGY

RADIOGRAPHY AND RADIOGRAPHIC/FLUOROSCOPIC CONTRAST EXAMINATIONS

Bernard E. Zeligman, MD

1. **When requesting an imaging examination, what information should a clinician provide for a radiologist?**
   By communicating the following information, a clinician helps ensure that an imaging examination will be conducted and interpreted optimally for each patient.
   1. Known major *diagnoses*.
   2. Pertinent *clinical information*: (a) key findings from history, physical examination, and/or laboratory tests that suggest the diagnoses in question and (b) any surgical alteration of the anatomy to be examined with imaging.
   3. The *purpose* of the examination: possible diagnoses, procedure complications, or an established diagnosis or finding to follow for change.
   4. Using the *precise name* of the requested examination to minimize the possibility that the wrong procedure will be done (i.e., barium swallow, upper gastrointestinal [GI] series, or small bowel follow-through).

ABDOMINAL RADIOGRAPHY

2. **Which radiographs should constitute an acute abdominal series?**
   The optimal series, sometimes called a *three-way abdomen*, includes:
   1. Posteroanterior (PA) upright chest
   2. Supine abdomen
   3. Upright abdomen

   If limited patient mobility precludes upright positioning, the best series is:
   1. Anteroposterior (AP) supine (or semiupright) chest
   2. Supine abdomen
   3. Left lateral decubitus abdomen

   To investigate the cause of an acute abdomen, the entire acute abdominal series should be requested. An upright abdomen radiograph, which is (on average) less sensitive than either an upright chest or left lateral decubitus abdomen for pneumoperitoneum and is also (on average) less diagnostic than a supine abdomen for bowel obstruction, should never be the only radiograph for possible perforation or obstruction of the gut. An upright chest radiograph, though the single most sensitive for pneumoperitoneum, should never be the only image for suspected perforation of the gut. If the patient cannot stand, a radiograph of the entire chest is still important because pneumonia and pulmonary embolism, even if high in the chest, may present as an acute abdomen (Fig. 68-1).

3. **What is the key radiographic finding of bowel obstruction?**
   The hallmark of obstruction (mechanical or functional) is *dilatation* of bowel. If bowel is dilated all the way to the anorectal junction, obstruction is functional (unless from anorectal malformation in a newborn). Alternatively, if bowel is dilated not to the anorectal junction but to

a point of transition to normal or smaller than normal caliber, obstruction is probably mechanical (Figs. 68-2 and 68-3) but may be functional (Fig. 68-4).

Two old axioms are excessively strict: (a) gas in the lumen of duodenal loop, jejunum, or ileum is abnormal and (b) gas-fluid levels in any of those locations or in the colon are abnormal. Gas, with or without fluid levels, can be normal in any part of the intestine.

Abdomen radiographs can be falsely negative for obstruction, even if of high grade.

4. **What are causes of pneumatosis intestinalis?**
The numerous reported causes of pneumatosis (Table 68-1) are difficult to remember, but a logical approach based on pathophysiology will bring the common causes to mind.

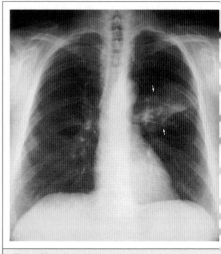

Figure 68-1. Pneumonia presenting as an acute abdomen. The abdomen radiographs were normal, but shown on this PA chest radiograph is fluffy opacification *(arrows)* in the left upper lobe.

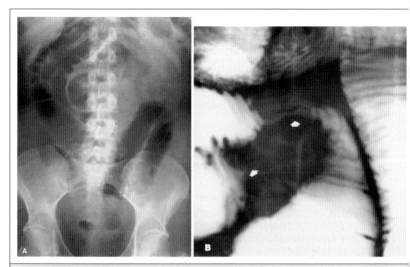

Figure 68-2. Mechanical small bowel obstruction. *A,* Supine abdomen radiograph. Because small bowel dilatation does not reach the right lower quadrant, high-grade mechanical obstruction of upper small bowel (above the lower ileum) is likely. *B,* The appropriate fluoroscopic-radiographic examination, a small bowel follow-through, shows partial obstruction of two nearby foci of jejunum *(arrows)* and strongly suggests the cause: an adhesion.

1. Gas in the bowel wall originates from one of two sites: the lungs or the gut.
2. Gas (or gas-producing bacteria) enters the wall from the lumen by one of two mechanisms: loss of mucosal integrity (bowel ischemia or infection) or increased intraluminal pressure (bowel obstruction or endoscopic procedures).

5. **What distinguishes portal venous gas from pneumobilia?**

Although in both conditions the gas is in a branching, tapering pattern, the location of gas in the liver is usually distinctive. Because portal venous blood normally flows toward the periphery, gas in portal veins tends to accumulate peripherally (Fig. 68-5). Because bile normally flows toward the hilum, biliary gas tends to be near the hilum (Fig. 68-6, *A*). These rules fail occasionally, however, because during the instant a radiograph is exposed, the location of the constantly moving gas may transiently be atypical (Fig. 68-6, *B*).

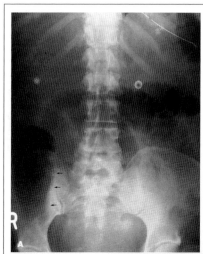

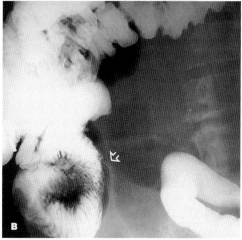

Figure 68-3. Mechanical small bowel obstruction. *A,* Supine abdominal radiograph. Because small bowel is dilated in the right lower quadrant *(arrows)* but colon is not dilated, high-grade mechanical obstruction low in the ileum is likely. *B,* The appropriate fluoroscopic-radiographic examination, a single-contrast barium enema, excluded obstruction of the colon, shows complete obstruction to retrograde flow of barium at a tapered narrowing *(arrow)* of ileum and strongly suggests the cause: an adhesion.

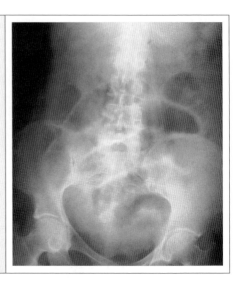

Figure 68-4. Portable supine abdomen radiograph. Because dilatation of small bowel does not reach the right lower quadrant, mechanical obstruction of small bowel well upstream of the terminal ileum is probable. This obstruction, though, was functional, a result of acute pancreatitis.

TABLE 68-1. MAJOR CAUSES OF PNEUMATOSIS INTESTINALIS		
Source of Gas: Lungs	**Source of Gas: Gut Lumen**	
	Mechanism: Increased intraluminal pressure	*Mechanism:* Loss of mucosal integrity
Barotrauma Chronic Obstructive Pulmonary Disease	Air insufflation (endoscopy) Bowel obstruction (mechanical or functional)	Ischemia Inflammation (infectious or noninfectious) Drugs (e.g., glucocorticoids)

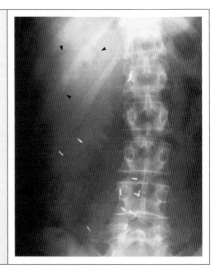

Figure 68-5. Supine abdomen radiograph. These two patterns of pneumatosis intestinalis—linear and bubbly *(arrows)*—are consistent with, but not diagnostic of, bowel ischemia. (A third pattern, not shown here, of pneumatosis—cystic in the colon—is characteristic of pneumatosis cystoids coli and rarely, if ever, from ischemia.) Other gas in an abnormal location—branching and tapering in the liver *(arrowheads)* as its predominantly peripheral location favors—is not in bile ducts but in portal veins.

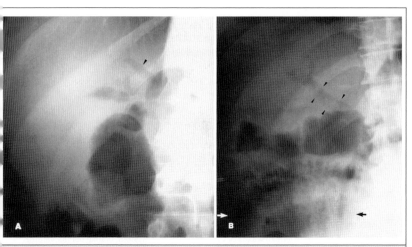

Figure 68-6. A branching and tapering gas pattern in the liver, if predominantly near the hilum *(arrowheads)*, is usually biliary *(A)* but, occasionally, is in portal veins *(B)*. *B,* Bubbly and linear pneumatosis *(arrows)* below the liver is consistent with bowel ischemia.

CONTRAST MEDIA

6. **When is barium preferable to iodinated contrast media to opacify the lumen of the GI tract?**

   Barium contrast media, which consists of barium sulfate particles suspended in water, are generally far superior to iodinated contrast because they produce better images, are less costly, and rarely do harm. Barium is the better choice for examinations for luminal obstruction except for one situation: Because barium may worsen a partial obstruction of the colon, a large volume of barium should be avoided upstream of a mechanical colon obstruction. Adequate assessment of oral and pharyngeal swallowing dysfunction requires barium. The small volumes of barium that enter the larynx during many such examinations and the lungs during a small percentage of examinations do no harm.

7. **What is the role of iodinated (water-soluble) contrast for opacification of the lumen of the GI tract?**

   The major indication for iodinated water-soluble contrast is possible gut perforation. Extravasation of water-soluble contrast into the peritoneum and retroperitoneum is safer than barium. Lower contrast resolution with water-soluble agents is less likely to detect small or walled-off perforations. When no extravasation of water-soluble iodinated contrast is evident, examination with higher resolution barium should follow to avoid missing small or contained perforations.

   To examine the esophagus for perforation, some radiologists begin with water-soluble iodinated contrast. Others prefer to use high-resolution barium because its extravasation into the mediastinum and pleural cavity has not been proven harmful.

8. **Are some iodinated contrast media better than others?**

   Iodinated contrast media are either *high osmolality* or *low osmolality*.
   - High osmolality contrast: aspiration may lead to pulmonary edema; avoid use in proximal GI obstruction.

- Low osmolality contrast: "safer" in proximal gastrointestinal (UGI) tract.
- High osmolality contrast: effective for the "distal intestinal obstructive syndrome" of cystic fibrosis, in which copious viscid intraluminal material accumulates in the colon and lower ileum; an enema (during fluoroscopic monitoring) of high-osmolality contrast may stimulate evacuation when other methods have failed.

SWALLOWING STUDIES

9. **What are barium swallows?**
   Barium swallow is the general term for a fluoroscopic-radiographic examination of oral, pharyngeal, and/or esophageal swallowing. Each examination should be tailored to the patient.
       For symptoms, such as retrosternal dysphagia, that may be of esophageal but not of oral or pharyngeal cause, the examination should be of the esophagus.
       Other symptoms, such as coughing and choking with swallowing and a sensation that swallowed boluses stick in the throat, suggest abnormalities of oral-pharyngeal swallowing. Possible etiologies include diseases of the central nervous system, cranial nerves, neuro-muscular junction (myasthenia gravis), and muscle (dermatomyositis, polymyositis, muscular dystrophy) (see Chapter 1, Swallowing Disorders and Dysphagia). An examination for such symptoms, however, should include not only oral and pharyngeal swallowing but also the esophagus because:
   - A sensation that swallowed boluses stick in the throat is often of esophageal cause with upward referral of symptoms.
   - Chronic esophageal diseases (that is, achalasia) can cause pharyngeal abnormalities.
   - Esophageal abnormalities coexisting with, but unrelated to, oral-pharyngeal swallowing dysfunction may contribute to the dysphagia and tend to be more amenable to treatment than neurogenic oral-pharyngeal dysfunction.
       Examinations limited to oral and pharyngeal swallowing are appropriate to follow known abnormalities or to assess for oral-pharyngeal dysfunction of patients too ill for a complete barium swallow.

10. **What can a barium swallow contribute to an evaluation for dysphagia?**
    Barium swallow is the only single test that can evaluate:
    - The three phases of swallowing: oral, pharyngeal, and esophageal (Fig. 68-7)
    - Both functional and structural abnormalities
    Barium swallow is the preferred first test by many to evaluate dysphagia.

11. **What may a barium swallow contribute to diagnosis and management of gastroesophageal reflux disease (GERD)?**
    A barium swallow is the best examination for the common predisposing condition (hiatus hernia) and for a less common predisposing condition (mechanical gastric outlet obstruction) and may suggest another uncommon predisposing condition (gastric hypomotility). Free gastroesophageal reflux of barium is diagnostic of, but uncommon in, GERD. Minimal reflux of barium is not definitely abnormal, and absence of reflux during the short period of observation provided by a barium swallow is meaningless. A barium swallow may demonstrate esophagitis or Barrett's esophagus but can exclude neither. A barium swallow, therefore, should not be requested to establish or exclude the diagnosis of GERD but may contribute useful information in the setting of GERD:
    - *Dysphagia.* The cause of the dysphagia may be unrelated to GERD. For causes of dysphagia related to GERD, some are functional and others are structural; and, for dysphagia perceived in the throat, the cause may be esophageal and/or pharyngeal. Often more than one cause

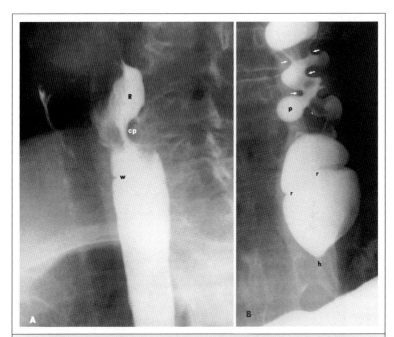

Figure 68-7. This man complained of swallowed boluses stuck in his throat, but abnormalities shown by barium swallow were numerous and widespread. *A,* Occasionally, before initiation of oral swallowing, portions of some boluses leaked from mouth to pharynx and were then aspirated. More limited than normal pharyngeal muscle contraction (and maybe also partial luminal obstruction from incomplete opening of the cricopharyngeus [cp]) contributed to pharyngeal barium residual (R), which became more apparent as his swallow progressed. A cervical esophageal web (w) is small. *B,* Other abnormalities were spasm *(arrows)* and a pulsion diverticulum (p) low in the esophagus; a sliding hiatus hernia (not completely reducible) between a Schatzki's ring (r) and the esophageal hiatus (h); and esophageal barium residual, a result of the spasm and maybe also of weakness and breakup of peristalsis.

affects a given patient. As is true for dysphagia in general, the best first test is a barium swallow.

- *Assessment for surgery.* Useful information about motility and anatomy may be provided: (a) assessment of barium transport by the esophagus is one way to assess for ineffective esophageal motility (a disorder common in GERD) and thereby estimate the possibility that a complete fundoplication will cause dysphagia, and (b) the presence or absence of a hiatus hernia and its size when maximally reduced helps surgeons choose the most appropriate operation.
- *Postoperative symptoms.* A barium swallow can show such possible causes of symptoms, such as excessive esophageal narrowing by a fundoplication, disruption of and "slip" of a fundoplication, and a hiatus hernia (sliding and/or paraesophageal).

2. **What distinguishes achalasia from scleroderma?**
   When the dysmotility is minimal, the barium swallow may be nonspecific, but when the dysmotility is moderate to severe, the radiographic features are usually diagnostic (Table 68-2, Fig. 68-8).

TABLE 68–2.	ACHALASIA VERSUS SCLERODERMA		
	Esophageal Dilatation	Diminished Peristalsis	Esophagogastric Junction
Achalasia	May be marked	Entire esophagus	"Bird beak": smooth, concentric, tapered, flexible No hiatus hernia
Scleroderma	Minimal or moderate	Inferior two thirds	Stricture from esophagitis: cylindrical, rigid, sometimes irregular and/or ulcerated Sliding hiatus hernia

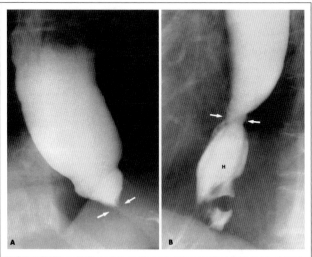

Figure 68-8. Lower esophagus. *A,* Achalasia. Dilatation is marked above a "bird beak" *(arrows)* formed by the closed lower sphincter. *B,* Scleroderma. Dilatation is moderate above a cylindrical reflux esophagitis stricture *(arrows),* below which is a sliding hiatus hernia (H).

13. **What findings help distinguish secondary from primary achalasia?**
Traditionally, achalasia has been thought secondary to cancer only if the "beak," the narrowing at the lower end of the esophagus, resembles malignant strictures elsewhere in the body: eccentric, irregular, and abruptly marginated. However, two other characteristics are more sensitive for secondary achalasia: (a) minimal lumen dilatation above the "beak" (<4.0 cm) and (b) a narrow segment "beak" longer than 3.5 cm.

UPPER GASTROINTESTINAL SERIES

14. **Can benign and malignant gastric ulcers be distinguished?**
Imaging features are best shown with biphasic technique, which includes double-contrast and single-contrast phases. A malignant or possibly malignant appearance warrants endoscopy and biopsy. For unequivocally benign radiographic features, radiologic follow-up is a less costly alternative. If, on follow-up, healing is complete and features of any scar that has developed are unequivocally benign, further assessment for malignancy is unnecessary. If healing is only partial but the appearance remains benign, a second follow-up upper GI is sufficient. If features of or equivocal to malignancy appear during follow-up or, if healing fails despite adequate medical therapy, endoscopy and biopsy are indicated (Table 68-3).

TABLE 68-3.	GASTRIC ULCERS ON UPPER GASTROINTESTINAL SERIES: BENIGN AND MALIGNANT FEATURES	
	Benign	**Malignant**
Location in stomach	Other than upstream half of stomach along greater curvature	Upstream half of stomach along greater curvature
Profile view: relationship of ulcer to lumen	Beyond expected lumen	Within expected lumen
Radiating folds	Regular To margin of ulcer or to ulcer mound (of edema)	Nodular, irregular, fused, clubbed, amputated, or nodular May not reach ulcer margin

If ulcer is within a mass	Ulcer location in mass: central
	Mass:
	  Smooth
	  Junction with wall: obtuse angle
		Ulcer location in mass: eccentric
		Mass:
		  Irregular
		  Junction with wall: acute angle

Surrounding mucosa	Intact	Distorted or obliterated
Ulcer shape	Round, oval, or linear	Angular
Other	Hampton's line	

Healing	Complete	Usually incomplete
		Occasionally complete, but scar:
		  Is nodular
		  Has radiating folds with malignant characteristics

SMALL BOWEL

15. **What are advantages, disadvantages, and indications for enteroclysis (small bowel enema) over small bowel follow-through (SBFT) examination?**
Advantages
■ Enteroclysis provides more anatomic detail than an SBFT.

- Barium can be introduced into the lumen at whatever rate distends the bowel optimally.
- Double contrast examination of the jejunum and much of the ileum is possible by instilling air or methylcellulose through the tube immediately after barium. (Double-contrast examination of downstream ileum—sometimes called a *peroral pneumocolon* because air is introduced per rectum—may accompany either a follow-through or an enteroclysis.)

Disadvantages
- Greater cost
- More patient discomfort
- More radiation exposure
- Nonphysiologic examination

Indications: Opinions vary, but the following guidelines are commonly followed. An SBFT is the routine examination. Enteroclysis is reserved for situations in which the superior anatomic information is especially advantageous:

- The major indication: possible mechanical obstruction of low grade.
- Another indication: gastrointestinal bleeding unexplained by examination of the upper GI tract and colon.

To investigate bleeding, enteroclysis and endoscopy (either push or capsule enteroscopy) are complementary. Unlike endoscopy, enteroclysis cannot show flat vascular lesions. Enteroclysis, unlike push enteroscopy, can examine the entire small bowel. Capsule endoscopy may miss a focal elevated or ulcerated lesion conspicuous by enteroclysis.

For what has been a third indication for enteroclysis—investigating the cause of malabsorption thought not to be from gluten enteropathy—capsule endoscopy is probably now preferable.

16. **How does one choose the best fluoroscopic radiographic examination for evaluation of suspected small bowel obstruction?**
    - For suspected low-grade obstruction, enteroclysis is best to distend the bowel and reveal minimal narrowing.
    - For suspected high-grade obstruction (*see* Fig. 68-2), SBFT is preferred.
    - For suspected distal ileal obstruction, single-contrast barium enema is best for two reasons:
    1. The radiographic bowel gas pattern characteristic of obstruction low in the ileum is sometimes caused by obstruction of the colon, a diagnosis obvious by barium enema.
    2. Barium introduced per rectum may well flow across the ileocolic junction to an obstruction low in the ileum (*see* Fig. 68-3) and, if so, will establish the diagnosis much faster than will barium taken orally.

    Table 68-4 summarizes the previous criteria.

17. **When is computed tomography (CT) preferable to a fluoroscopic-radiographic contrast study for small bowel obstruction?**
    - CT is better for hernias, strangulation, closed-loop obstruction, and abdominal abnormalities outside the gut.
    - Fluoroscopic-radiographic examinations more conclusively show the presence or absence of, and degree of, obstruction.
    - When the right examination is unclear, CT is a better first choice because CT will delay a fluoroscopic examination less than a fluoroscopic procedure will delay CT.

18. **When is a retrograde examination of small bowel indicated?**
    Most small bowel examinations of patients with an ileostomy should be retrograde. It is not only much faster than either enteroclysis or an SBFT, but also shows anatomy as well as single-contrast enteroclysis—with lower cost, less radiation, and, usually, less discomfort.

TABLE 68-4. CHOICE OF FLUOROSCOPIC–RADIOGRAPHIC EXAMINATION FOR SMALL BOWEL OBSTRUCTION		
Setting	Suspected Obstruction	Best Examination
Illness too mild for hospitalization *and* Small bowel dilatation is inconspicuous on radiographs	Low grade	Enteroclysis
Radiographs show dilated small bowel but not in right lower quadrant	High grade Above lower ileum	Small bowel follow-through
Radiographs show dilated small bowel dilatation, including in right lower quadrant	High grade Near terminal ileum	Barium enema: single contrast, no preparation
Illness characteristic of high-grade obstruction, but radiographs show no small bowel dilatation	High grade Anywhere	Small bowel follow-through

COLON

19. **What are indications for single-contrast and double-contrast techniques of barium enema examination?**
    - *Double-contrast:* polyps, cancer, or colitis
    - *Single-contrast:* fistula or sinus track, diverticulitis, or obstruction (requires less patient mobility than double-contrast exam)

20. **What are advantages and disadvantages of screening for colon cancer with a barium enema instead of colonoscopy?**
    Advantages
    - Lower cost
    - Greater safety
    - Greater likelihood that the entire colon will be examined

    Disadvantages
    - Lower sensitivity for detection of polyps (especially diminutive ones)
    - Some false-positive examinations for polyps
    - Positive results (true and false) necessitate a second test: colonoscopy.

21. **What is the role of defecography (evacuation proctography)?**
    Defecography may clarify the cause of anorectal dysfunction responsible for difficult or painful rectal evacuation or fecal incontinence (Fig. 68-9). For this procedure, barium contrast of paste consistency is introduced into the rectum. Barium is also usually given orally and introduced

vaginally so that the location of ileum and vagina will be apparent. Imaging shows the speed and completeness of rectal evacuation and may show one or more of the following: rectocele, intussusception (rectorectal or intra-anal), external rectal prolapse, enterocele, sigmoidocele, peritoneocele, excessive descent of the posterior part of the pelvic floor or perineum, and anismus. For optimal diagnosis and management, defecography findings should be correlated with history, physical examination, nonimaging tests of anorectal function, and often endoanal ultrasound.

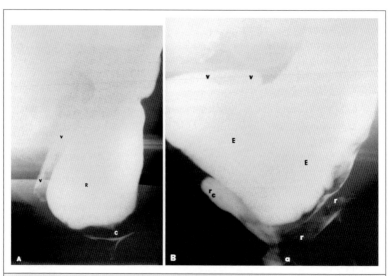

Figure 68-9. Lateral views from a defecogram of a woman who complained of difficult and incomplete rectal evacuation. *A,* The appearance before evacuation was normal. Barium paste opacifies the rectum (R) and anal canal (C). A contrast-impregnated tampon indicates the location of the vagina (v). *B,* Evacuation was slow and incomplete. Intussuscepting rectal tissue (radiolucency demarcated anteriorly and posteriorly by linear barium) has descended into and now obstructs the lower rectum (r) and anal canal (a). A rectocele (rc) retains rectal contents. An enterocele (E) is very large: numerous loops of ileum, opacified by barium swallowed earlier, have descended into the pelvis between the rectum and vagina (v) and widely separate them.

CHOLANGIOPANCREATOGRAPHY

22. **List common causes of obstruction at various locations in the biliary tract.**
    See Figure 68-10 and Table 68-5.

23. **What cholangiopancreatographic features distinguish pancreatitis from ductal adenocarcinoma of the pancreatic head?**
    The characteristics of abnormalities of both ductal systems (Figs. 68-11 and 68-12) are clues to this distinction (Table 68-6).

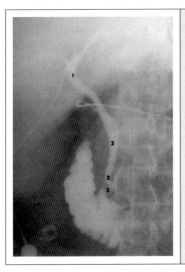

Figure 68-10. Common sites of extrahepatic biliary obstruction are indicated on this operative cholangiogram. (1) Hepatic duct confluence. (2) Intrapancreatic portion of common bile duct. (3) Intraduodenal portion of common bile duct (and/or common channel of individuals whose common bile and pancreatic ducts fuse before reaching the duodenal lumen).

TABLE 68-5.   COMMON CAUSES OF BILIARY OBSTRUCTION BY LOCATION

Liver Hilum-Hepatic Duct Confluence
  Cholangiocarcinoma (Klatskin's tumor)
  Gallbladder cancer
  Porta hepatis lymphadenopathy (usually metastatic cancer)
  Stricture from laparoscopic cholecystectomy injury
  Hepatocellular carcinoma

Intrapancreatic Common Bile Duct
  Cancer of head of pancreas
  Pancreatitis (acute or chronic)

Intraduodenal Common Bile Duct
  Neoplasm of major papilla or peripapillary duodenum
    Adenoma
    Adenocarcinoma
  Nonneoplastic
    Sphincter of Oddi dysfunction
    Stricture (sometimes stenosis of a sphincterotomy)
    Active inflammation
      AIDS
      Acute pancreatitis

Continued

TABLE 68-5. COMMON CAUSES OF BILIARY OBSTRUCTION BY LOCATION—CONT'D

Multiple: Intrahepatic and Extrahepatic
Primary sclerosing cholangitis
Other
    Secondary sclerosing cholangitis
      Include: AIDS cholangiopathy
      Include: oriental cholangiohepatitis
    Cholangiocarcinoma (extensively infiltrating)
    Metastasis

Possible at Most Locations
Stone
Primary sclerosing cholangitis
Cholangiocarcinoma
Other
    Metastasis
    Lymphoma
    Iatrogenic

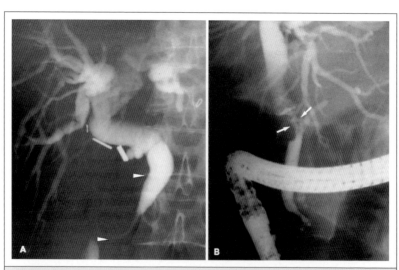

Figure 68-11. Strictures of intrapancreatic common bile duct. *A,* Percutaneous transhepatic cholangiogram. This stricture *(arrowheads),* with all of the characteristics of benignity, is caused by pancreatitis. *B,* Endoscopic retrograde cholangiogram. This stricture *(arrows),* with all of the characteristics of malignancy, is from ductal adenocarcinoma of the pancreatic head.

24. **What is the "double duct sign"?**
A stricture or complete obstruction of the intrapancreatic common bile duct and another stricture or complete obstruction of the main pancreatic duct nearby *(see* Fig. 68-12) constitute the double duct sign. The most common malignant cause is ductal adenocarcinoma of the

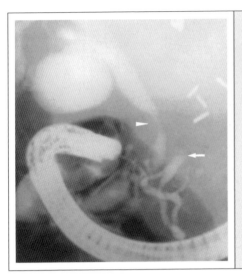

Figure 68-12. Double duct sign. The stricture *(arrowhead)* of the intrapancreatic common bile duct, though smooth and predominantly tapered, is probably malignant because it is short and eccentric. Nearby is a complete obstruction *(arrow)* of the pancreatic duct. No abnormalities of chronic pancreatitis involve the *truncated* opacified part of pancreatic duct. Diagnosis: ductal adenocarcinoma of the pancreatic head.

TABLE 68-6.	PANCREATITIS VERSUS CANCER OF THE PANCREATIC HEAD: CHOLANGIOPANCREATOGRAPHIC FEATURES	
	Pancreatitis	**Carcinoma**
Pancreatogram	If chronic: widespread abnormalities (dilatations, narrowings, calcifications)	Focal abnormality of main duct in pancreatic head (obstruction, stricture, or disruption)
Cholangiogram (stricture of intrapancreatic common bile duct)	Long, smooth, tapered, concentric	Short, irregular, abrupt margins, eccentric

pancreatic head; cholangiocarcinoma, lymphoma, and metastasis are occasional causes. A benign cause of "double duct sign" is chronic pancreatitis.

25. **What pancreatographic features distinguish pancreas divisum from complete obstruction of the main pancreatic duct?**
    Although the main duct opacified via the major papilla is shorter than normal in both conditions, their pancreatographic appearances are generally distinctive.
    - With obstruction (*see* Fig. 68-12), the main duct appears *truncated*. Caliber of the opacified part of main duct and its branches is normal, and upstream termination of the main duct is abrupt. (Two other conditions—traumatic disruption of the main duct and excision of the pancreatic tail and body—can mimic obstruction.)
    - In divisum (Fig. 68-13), the ductal system appears *minified*. Caliber of the main duct and its branches is small, and the main duct terminates upstream not abruptly but by branching and tapering.

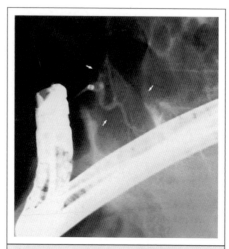

Figure 68-13. Pancreas divisum. This short pancreatic ductal system *(arrows)*, opacified via the major papilla, is *minified*.

OTHER

26. What are advantages of fistulography?

For a suspected fistula between skin and gut lumen, a fistulogram is usually the most informative imaging examination. A fistulagram not only usually provides adequate assessment for obstruction of the gut downstream of a fistula but, compared to barium studies of the gut

- is more likely to show a fistula;
- demonstrates anatomy of a track more completely, and the site of the gut in continuity with the track more precisely; and
- does not delay percutaneous therapy. Immediately after diagnostic fistulography, a catheter may be introduced for drainage or injection of fibrin sealant.

WEBSITES

1. http://www.vhjoe.com

2. http://www.dave1.mgh.harvard.edu/

BIBLIOGRAPHY

1. Levine MS, Creteur V, Kresel HY: Benign gastric ulcers: Diagnosis and follow-up with double-contrast radiography. Radiology 164:9, 1987.

2. Levine MS, Glick SN, Rubesin SE, Laufer I: Double-contrast barium enema examination and colorectal cancer: A plea for radiologic screening. Radiology 222:313–315, 2002.

3. McMahon PM, Bosch JL, Gleason S, et al: Cost-effectiveness of colorectal cancer screening. Radiology 219:44–50, 2001.

4. Woodfield CA, Levine MS, Rubesin SE, et al: Diagnosis of primary versus secondary achalasia: Reassessment of clinical and radiographic criteria. AJR 175:727–731, 2000.

CHAPTER 69

INTERVENTIONAL RADIOLOGY

Paul D. Russ, MD, Stephen W. Subber, MD, Dale L. McCarter, MD, and Keith M. Shonnard, MD

IMAGE–GUIDED INTERVENTIONS

1. What percutaneous procedures are performed using cross-sectional imaging guidance?

The two basic procedures performed in abdominal imaging are biopsies of masses and drainage of fluid collections. Masses and fluid collections of the solid organs, peritoneum, retroperitoneum, vertebras, psoas and paraspinous muscles are usually accessible.

Biopsies can be categorized as fine-needle aspiration (FNA), which yields clusters of cells and occasionally small tissue fragments for cytopathology, or core biopsy, which yields cylinders of tissue, 1–2 cm long, with preserved architecture for histopathologic analysis.

Fluid collections can be needled for Gram stain and culture and aspirated (sometimes repeatedly) for therapeutic decompression. They can be drained with percutaneous catheters for cure or for temporization and medical stabilization before surgery. Some cystic lesions and collections are catheterized for purposes of drainage and subsequent treatment (e.g., sclerotherapy).

2. What materials and equipment are used for FNAs, core biopsies, and percutaneous catheter drainages?

Most FNAs are performed using 21- to 23-G "skinny" needles. The 20-G needles are of intermediate size and should be avoided in cases involving the bowel, bile ducts, or large vessels. *Core biopsies* are usually obtained with 18-G disposable, spring-loaded, automated guns. For most focal pathology, 18-G specimens are as diagnostic as those obtained with 14- to 16-G devices. In most cases, better samples are obtained with 18-G than 20-G guns. An exception is the biopsy of background liver for evaluation of hepatocellular disease. Most advocate the use of 15- or 16-G cores for adequate analysis of hepatic parenchymal architecture.

The vast majority of *fluid collections* can be drained and treated with 8-Fr, self-retaining, pigtail catheters. Except for some percutaneous gallbladder and ascitic fluid drainages, catheters smaller than 8-French offer no advantages, are often more difficult to place, and are dislodged more frequently. The routine use of 10- to 28-Fr catheters is not necessary. However, multiple large catheters are usually required for percutaneous drainage of infected, acute pancreatic necrosis.

3. What steps are taken in preparation for an image-guided procedure?

In all cases, the indications and risks of the procedure are discussed with the referring physician. The necessity for performing the procedure needs to be firmly established and documented. Plans for appropriate medical and surgical backup must be in place, and postprocedure care must be prearranged.

Diagnostic images should be reviewed before the procedure is scheduled. This review allows the interventionalist to establish a presumptive diagnosis, to assess the risks and benefits of the procedure, to decide on the most appropriate procedure, to choose the best imaging modality to guide the procedure, and to plan a safe approach to the lesion.

4. **What four conditions must be satisfied before a percutaneous procedure can be performed?**
   1. The patient or patient representative must provide written, informed consent for both the procedure and anticipated intravenous conscious sedation.
   2. The referring physician must order antibiotic coverage, if there is any possibility that the lesion or fluid collection is infected.
   3. The patient's coagulation profile must be determined.
   4. The patient must be voluntarily cooperative during the procedure.

5. **What coagulation parameters are assessed before a percutaneous procedure?**
   Some literature suggests that the hemostatic evaluation can be stratified according to the patient's history and the predicted risk of the procedure. However, in a referral setting, the preprocedure assessment should be thorough. The patient history should be reviewed for bleeding risks, such as anticoagulant use or hepatocellular disease. At a minimum, prothrombin time (PT), international normalized ratio (INR), partial thromboplastin time (PTT), and platelet count should be assessed in all patients, regardless of the procedure. An INR >2.0, a PTT >1.5 times normal, or a platelet count <60,000/μL is a contraindication for most procedures. However, after the discontinuation or reversal of anticoagulants, administration of fresh-frozen plasma, and/or platelet transfusion, many coagulopathies can be corrected temporarily to allow for intervention.

   A history of antiplatelet drug use, uremia, or myeloproliferative disease may require measurement of the bleeding time. If the result is abnormal, consultation with a hematologist is recommended. The administration of platelets or 1-deamino-8-D-arginine vasopressin (DDAVP) may be necessary before proceeding.

6. **Which imaging modalities are used to guide interventional procedures?**
   Fluoroscopy, ultrasound (US), computed tomography (CT), and magnetic resonance (MR) imaging can be used to guide interventions. On abdominal imaging services in diagnostic radiology, US and CT are used most often (Fig. 69-1).

7. **Summarize the advantages and disadvantages of US.**
   US is widely available and portable; it allows relatively easy scanning in nonorthogonal planes. The disadvantages of US are the inability to depict small, deep lesions, to define bowel anatomy, to maintain a sterile field, and to use both hands with ease to perform the actual procedure as a single operator. In general, US is often selected for superficial and large lesions.

8. **Summarize the advantages and disadvantages of CT.**
   CT provides excellent anatomic detail, allows safe needle passes into difficult locations, is more amenable to sterile technique, and permits a single operator to use both hands for performing the procedure (Fig. 69-2). The disadvantages of CT are that it is not portable; sick patients must be monitored by support personnel in the CT suite; oblique sticks can be more difficult; and needle localization can be slower than with US, although this is less problematic when CT fluoroscopy is available. CT is selected more often for deep and small abnormalities.

9. **Discuss the uses of standard fluoroscopy.**
   Radiographic fluoroscopy is not routinely required. Sometimes it is used in conjunction with US to perform biopsy or to drain large, superficial masses and fluid collections. It is used for simple tube exchanges and can be helpful with complex tube manipulations. Fluoroscopy is used for sinograms and abscessograms, although these procedures are now performed less often. Fluoroscopy is recommended by many authors during hepatic and renal cyst sclerotherapy to check for communication with the biliary tree and urinary tract, respectively.

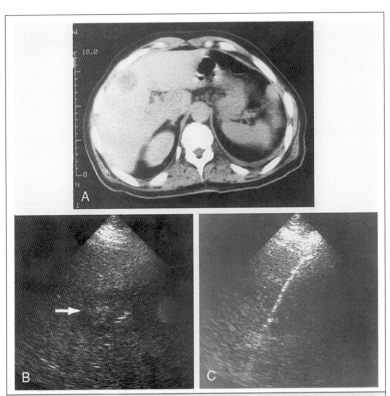

Figure 69-1. Metastatic colon cancer to the liver. *A,* Contrast-enhanced CT of the liver demonstrates a 3-cm hypodense mass. *B,* Ultrasound of the liver reveals the mass to be primarily hypoechoic *(arrow). C,* The needle tract is conspicuously demonstrated during ultrasound-guided biopsy.

0. Summarize the advantages and disadvantages of MR.

Standard and specially designed open-sided MR systems are being used selectively for interventional procedures. MR may be necessary if it is the only modality that depicts the lesion. MR can scan oblique planes. Interventions on closed-bore, high-field machines are analogous to those done with CT. Open-sided MRs allow easier access to the patient, facilitate patient monitoring, and decrease procedure time. Heat-sensitive pulse sequences, available for both standard and open-sided MRs, provide unique information during thermal ablations. Working in static and fluctuating electromagnetic fields remains the major drawback to MR-guided interventional procedures.

1. What techniques have been developed for lesion localization?

For US, CT, and MR, various trigonometric, mechanical, electronic, and computer-assisted techniques and devices have been developed for lesion localization and guidance. They are used to facilitate procedures that require oblique punctures. Although not necessary in most cases, they have the potential to facilitate the approach to small lesions and lesions in difficult locations, such as those at the dome of the liver.

KEY POINTS: CONTRAINDICATIONS TO PERCUTANEOUS FNAS AND CORE BIOPSIES

1. Written informed consent cannot be obtained

2. Patient cannot cooperate with the procedure

3. INR >2.0

4. PTT >1.5 times normal

5. Platelet count <60,000/μL

6. Prolonged bleeding time (>10 min)

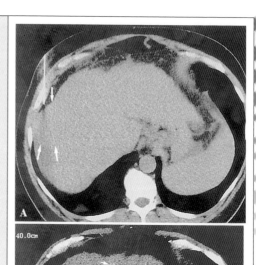

Figure 69-2. Biopsy of a hepatic mass in a 54-year-old man with end-stage alcoholic cirrhosis. *A,* Noncontrast CT performed during percutaneous biopsy of a large, solid liver lesion shows an isodense lobulation *(arrows)* of the right lobe corresponding to a tumor better demonstrated by previous dynamic CT. Two 21-G FNAs and two 18-G core biopsies of the lesion confirmed hepatocellular carcinoma. CT guidance allowed a tract to be selected that avoided aerated lung; thus, a pneumothorax was avoided. *B,* After chemoembolization, the stained carcinoma is more conspicuously shown with CT *(curved arrow).* Small satellite foci are also depicted *(small, straight arrows).*

12. **Why is it prudent to begin every biopsy of a suspected neoplasm with FNA?**
    FNA allows an initial approach with a "skinny" needle; a 21-, 22-, or 23-G needle is recommended to start. It provides the operator with a test pass before a larger needle is used. If the interventionalist has inadvertently chosen an unsafe route, it is better to discover this error using a small, "skinny" needle rather than a larger needle. If a lesion turns out to be

exceptionally hypervascular (e.g., an unexpected hemangioma), this problem usually becomes obvious when the syringe fills quickly with blood during aspiration. The procedure can be terminated before severe consequences are encountered with a larger aspiration needle or cutting needle. Finally, if a cytopathologist is present during the procedure, which is strongly recommended, his or her immediate interpretation of one to three initial FNAs can be diagnostic, obviating subsequent core biopsy.

13. **Why is FNA advantageous for initial aspiration of a suspected fluid collection?**
In addition to establishing the safety of the percutaneous approach before a much larger catheter is placed (see previous text), FNA can confirm that the lesion is, in fact, a fluid collection and not a solid mass. If necessary, a small aliquot can be sent for immediate Gram stain. If the fluid is sterile, the interventionalist, in consultation with the referring physician, has the opportunity to abort the procedure to avoid the small chance of superinfecting the collection with subsequent catheter placement. If the fluid is infected on Gram stain or by visual inspection, the operator can proceed with catheter drainage. Material should be sent for cytology to avoid the pitfall of draining a cystic, necrotic, or superinfected tumor, without recognizing the nature of the underlying lesion.

14. **What two techniques can be used to drain fluid collections?**
   - With the *Seldinger technique,* a drainage catheter is placed over a guidewire after needle puncture and tract dilatation.
   - With the *trocar technique,* the fluid collection is punctured directly with the catheter mounted on a removable sharp-tipped trocar.

15. **Which technique is used most often?**
The Seldinger technique is used most often because it starts with a smaller needle, and because catheter insertion over a guidewire is more controlled. The trocar technique is a faster, one-step procedure, but some control may be lost during catheter insertion compared with the Seldinger method. The trocar technique is usually reserved for large, superficial fluid collections or for draining a large volume of ascites.

16. **What are the major complications of percutaneous procedures?**
The major complications of percutaneous procedures are hemorrhage, infection, sepsis, solid organ injury, bowel perforation, and pneumothorax. The complication rate of "skinny" needle interventions is about 0.06–0.6%. The complication rate of catheter drainage is 3–4%. The increased risk of large-needle procedures compared with "skinny" needle procedures is the subject of some debate. However, it seems intuitive that the smallest adequate needle or catheter should be used for every procedure.

17. **How common is seeding of the needle tract during routine tumor biopsy?**
Seeding the needle tract is rare with "skinny" needle FNAs and 18-G core biopsies. A few cases of needle tract seeding have been reported for biopsy of solid, neoplastic masses of the abdomen and retroperitoneum. Although this potential complication should be discussed with the patient prior to the procedure, it should not be considered a contraindication to FNA or core biopsy.

   However, cystic lesions, like suspected cystadenomas or cystadenocarcinomas of the ovary or pancreas, should not be sampled percutaneously, even with small, "skinny" needles. This is associated with a significant risk of postprocedure needle-tract seeding and subsequent pseudomyxoma peritonei or peritoneal carcinomatosis.

   Percutaneous thermal ablation (radiofrequency, microwave, laser) of hepatocellular carcinoma and hepatic colorectal cancer metastases, which uses probes as large as 14 G, is currently associated with tumor seeding of the tract in about 2–3% of patients.

HEPATIC INTERVENTIONS

18. **What image-guided procedures are performed in the liver?**

Cross-sectional imaging is used to perform: (1) FNAs and core biopsies of primary and metastatic tumors, (2) catheter drainage of abscesses and other fluid collections, and (3) sclerotherapy of simple hepatic cysts.

19. **How is hepatic metastatic disease diagnosed?**

FNA is a simple and quick way to diagnose hepatic metastatic disease. Because of the marked difference between metastatic neoplastic cells and background hepatocytes, cytology alone is frequently diagnostic, and core biopsies are unnecessary. In difficult cases, comparison with previously obtained specimens of the primary tumor can help to establish the diagnosis.

20. **How is malignant, primary hepatic neoplasm diagnosed?**

Primary hepatic neoplasm can be diagnosed with FNA alone, depending on the tumor cytomorphology and experience of the cytopathologist. However, because many primary hepatic tumors require histologic evaluation, core biopsies are often needed (*see* Fig. 69-2). With current biopsy gun technology, 18-G cores are recommended. Core biopsy of background liver is helpful to the pathologist in cases of well-differentiated neoplasm and assists the hepatologist to choose among treatment options by detecting the presence and severity of underlying hepatocellular disease.

21. **How are pyogenic hepatic or parahepatic abscesses treated?**

At least 90% of pyogenic hepatic or parahepatic abscesses can be successfully drained percutaneously (Fig. 69-3). Almost all pyogenic abscesses can be drained with an

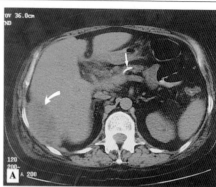

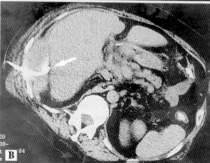

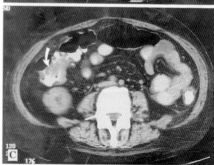

Figure 69-3. Parahepatic abscess in a 60-year-old woman, at first diagnosed with acute pancreatitis. *A,* After she failed to respond to initial management, including pancreatic duct stenting *(straight arrow),* CT revealed a fluid collection *(curved arrow)* adjacent to the liver. *B,* An 8-Fr pigtail catheter successfully drained the *Streptococcus milleri* abscess *(straight arrow). C,* A hepatic flexure mass *(curved arrow)* was suspected to be the site of origin of the parahepatic abscess.

8-Fr, self-retaining, pigtail catheter. After needle puncture, caution should be exercised during wire placement, dilatation, and catheter insertion; frequent imaging is necessary to ensure that the drainage devices have not migrated beyond the soft margin of the abscess, which can result in significant complications.

It should be noted that early (1–14 days) postprocedure CTs can result in the underestimation of the therapeutic effectiveness of percutaneous hepatic abscess drainage. Evidence for resolution of the hepatic abscess at early follow-up CT often lags behind the clinical improvement of the patient. The decision to alter patient management, or to reintervene, should not be based on the imaging alone.

Although rare, the possibility of an abscess complicating an underlying hepatic neoplasm should always be considered. Material for cytology should always be sent at the initial aspiration of a hepatic abscess. Follow-up CT scans at 3, 6, and 12 months should always be obtained to document eventual complete resolution of the lesion. Consideration should be given for FNA or core biopsy of any persistent abnormality to exclude occult hepatic tumor.

2. **Describe the treatment of simple, benign, epithelialized hepatic cysts.**
Epithelialized hepatic cysts can be drained successfully and obliterated with alcohol sclerotherapy. An 8-Fr, self-retaining, pigtail catheter can be used. After catheter placement with US or CT guidance and complete cyst aspiration, samples are sent for culture and cytology. Subsequently, water-soluble contrast is injected through the catheter under fluoroscopic guidance to ensure that there is no communication with the biliary tree. If no connection to the bile ducts is demonstrated, then 33–50% of the original cyst volume is replaced with sterile, absolute alcohol (not to exceed 100 mL). The patient is rotated into multiple positions, until the entirety of the cyst wall has been in contact with the sclerosing agent for 20–30 minutes. The entire volume of alcohol and residual cyst contents are then completely aspirated through the catheter. Patients receive prophylactic antibiotic coverage and are hospitalized for overnight drainage. The sclerosis is repeated 24 hours later. After final reaspiration, the catheter is removed.

Solitary hepatic cysts are more often successfully sclerosed than cysts in patients with polycystic liver disease. In polycystic liver disease, cysts tend to not collapse, presumably because the surrounding liver is less pliable, making cyst wall apposition and subsequent scarring of the cavity less likely (Fig. 69-4). In cases of polycystic liver disease, laparoscopic unroofing or surgical removal of multiple, symptomatic cysts is replacing alcohol sclerotherapy.

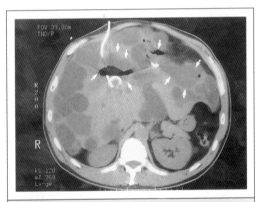

Figure 69-4. Alcohol sclerosis of hepatic cysts in a middle-aged man with polycystic liver disease who complained of abdominal distention and early satiety. Two large, dominant cysts *(small straight arrows)* have been drained with 8-Fr pigtail catheters. Despite aggressive aspiration of cyst contents and sclerotherapy with sterile absolute alcohol, neither cyst completely collapsed; air was entrained into each cyst, and wall coaptation did not occur. The patient subsequently required laparoscopic unroofing of multiple cysts for symptomatic relief.

23. **Is FNA or core biopsy safe for all hepatic lesions?**
FNA or core biopsy of some hepatic lesions is contraindicated. Carcinoid crisis characterized by profound hypotension can be precipitated by FNA of hepatic carcinoid metastases. Hepatic hemangiomas should not be intentionally needled or biopsied. Because of the ability to

characterize most hemangiomas noninvasively with cross-sectional imaging, obtaining specimens for cytology or histology is unnecessary in the management of most patients with typical hemangiomas (Fig. 69-5). Amebic abscesses do not require catheter drainage and usually respond well to medical treatment with metronidazole. In the United States, percutaneous aspiration and drainage of a suspected echinococcal lesion should not be performed; other options should be considered.

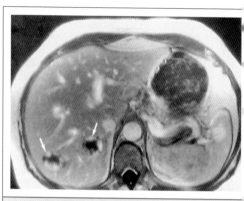

Figure 69-5. Dynamic, gadolinium-enhanced, T$_1$-weighted MR scan of the liver shows two lesions *(arrows)* with perfusion patterns characteristic of hemangiomas. Their distinctive MR features allow conservative management with surveillance imaging, obviating biopsy. Incidental note is made of a nonspecific hyperintensity in the spleen.

KEY POINTS: CONTRAINDICATED HEPATIC PERCUTANEOUS PROCEDURES ✔

1. FNA or core biopsy of suspected hemangioma

2. FNA or core biopsy of suspected carcinoid metastasis

3. Aspiration or catheter drainage of echinococcal cyst

SPLENIC INTERVENTIONS

24. **What interventions are possible in the spleen?**

Performance of percutaneous procedures in the spleen remains controversial. Some reports suggest that FNAs and catheter drainages of the spleen are possible. Although these procedures can be performed successfully, their overall risk is relatively high. Serious complications are estimated to occur in as many as 7% of cases (roughly 2–10 times more often than for other image-guided abdominal interventions). Uncontrolled hemorrhage necessitating emergency splenectomy is not uncommon. Therefore, the procedure should be clearly indicated, and its risk and benefits need to be thoroughly discussed with the patient and the referring physician. The possibility of emergency splenectomy must be emphasized. Surgical backup must be immediately available. If a percutaneous procedure is attempted, the size of the needle or catheter should be conservative. The lesion should be approached, avoiding any intervening parenchyma (Fig. 69-6). Alternatives should be considered if the abnormality is not subcapsular and is surrounded by splenic tissue.

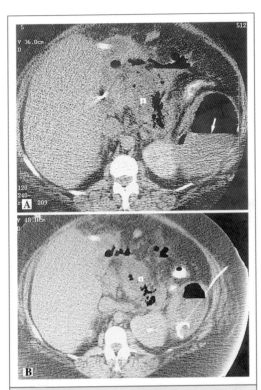

Figure 69-6. Percutaneous catheter drainage of a splenic abscess that developed after gastric bypass surgery. *A,* Diagnostic CT scan shows a large air-fluid level in the spleen *(arrow).* Although contained by the splenic capsule, the entire spleen is virtually suppurated. Note associated infected, acute pancreatic necrosis (n). *B,* An 8-Fr catheter placed into the splenic abscess drained a large volume of purulent material. No hemorrhagic complication occurred, probably because only the splenic capsule was traversed. The infected pancreatic necrosis (n) was drained separately.

PANCREATIC PROCEDURES

25. **What procedures are appropriate for solid pancreatic masses?**

Solid masses, usually suspected tumors, can be aspirated percutaneously (Fig. 69-7). Only FNAs should be performed; core biopsies should be avoided, because the use of cutting needles can result in severe pancreatitis. If a "skinny" needle is used and the lesion is solid, any organ, including the stomach, small bowel, and colon, can be traversed. Antibiotic coverage is recommended for procedures through the bowel. Major blood vessels should be avoided. The diagnosis of pancreatic adenocarcinoma can often be established by cytopathology alone; a negative result must be interpreted with caution and assumed to be a sampling error until proven otherwise. As noted previously, percutaneous biopsy of suspected cystadenomas or cystadenocarcinomas should be avoided.

26. **What procedures are used for pancreatic fluid collections?**

    Various acute and chronic pancreatic fluid collections can be aspirated and drained. Fluid collections should be defined according to the classification system adopted by the International Symposium on Acute Pancreatitis. Pancreatic-related collections can be aspirated to determine whether they are sterile or infected (Fig. 69-8). In this setting, the bowel should not be crossed with the aspiration needle, to avoid contaminating and superinfecting otherwise sterile fluid.

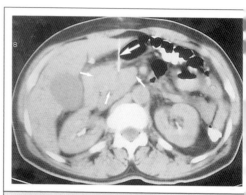

Figure 69-7. Fine-needle aspiration of pancreatic head carcinoma. CT shows mild fullness of the pancreatic uncinate process *(small, straight arrows)*. A "skinny" needle *(large, straight arrow)* passed through the liver and bowel wall without complication was used to obtain cellular material diagnostic of pancreatic adenocarcinoma.

27. **What precautions apply to percutaneous drainage of pancreatic fluid collections?**

    If endoscopic internal drainage is not possible, percutaneous drainage of most sterile and infected pancreatic collections can be undertaken if clinically indicated. The drainage of infected collections requires coverage with antibiotics. Routine techniques with 8-Fr catheters are usually adequate to treat focal pancreatic abscesses, which can be successfully drained in 7–10 days. Sterile acute or chronic pancreatic fluid collections and pseudocysts are more difficult to

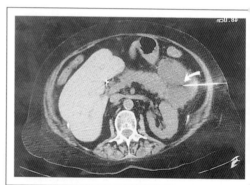

Figure 69-8. Aspiration of an acute pancreatic fluid collection associated with pancreatitis that occurred after lung transplantation. CT shows placement of a 20-G needle *(curved arrow)* into the collection. Withdrawn fluid was sterile; all cultures were negative for the growth of microorganisms.

manage and may require straight catheter drainage for 30–120 days. In these cases, concomitant endoscopic stenting of obstructing pancreatic duct pathology can facilitate catheter drainage and obviate pancreaticocutaneous fistula as a complication. Attempts at draining infected pancreatic necrosis may require aggressive treatment with multiple, large-bore, sump catheters. To prevent superinfection, percutaneous drains should be avoided in cases of sterile pancreatic necrosis.

ADRENAL BIOPSY

28. **What is the role of adrenal gland biopsy?**

    Because incidental adrenal gland adenomas can often be characterized with thin-section, dynamic CT and in-phase versus out-of-phase MR pulse sequences, fewer adrenal lesions nee a biopsy. Because of the risk of hypertensive crisis, possible pheochromocytomas should not be needled. FNA of other adrenal masses is usually sufficient for cytopathologic diagnosis. Approaching either adrenal gland can be difficult. Transhepatic access, decubitus positioning with the lesion-side down to elevate the adjacent hemidiaphragm, and angled routes may be necessary.

RENAL AND PERINEPHRIC INTERVENTIONS

29. Can a biopsy be performed on renal masses?
Given the high frequency and typical imaging features of renal cell carcinoma, most urologists are unwilling to risk the small chance of needle-tract seeding for preoperative diagnostic confirmation. In cases that are inoperable for cure, or when renal lymphoma or metastatic disease is highly suspected, FNAs are performed. Cytopathology can usually distinguish among renal cell carcinoma, lymphoma, and metastasis. In difficult cases, 18-G core biopsies can be performed. Aggressive correction of any coagulopathy is recommended because of the hypervascularity of the kidney and most renal cell carcinomas.

30. Can renal and perirenal abscesses and other fluid collections be drained percutaneously?
Renal and perirenal abscesses and other fluid collections can be drained, using routine 8-Fr catheter techniques. Gram-negative antibiotic coverage is absolutely essential to prevent urosepsis during or after the procedure. To effect a cure, a separate procedure to relieve any associated urinary tract obstruction is necessary.

31. What other intra-abdominal or retroperitoneal fluid collections can be treated percutaneously?
Most other intra-abdominal and retroperitoneal abscesses and fluid collections can be cured or palliated with routine 8-Fr catheter drainage. Pericholecystic, periappendiceal, diverticular, Crohn's-related, and postoperative abscesses can be managed percutaneously (Fig. 69-9). Percutaneous catheter drainage can allow subsequent one-stage interval

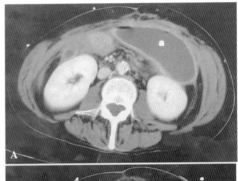
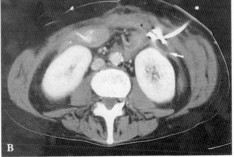

Figure 69-9. Postoperative fluid collection in a 55-year-old man who had undergone left colonic pull-up after esophagectomy for strictures. *A,* CT scan through the patient's midabdomen shows an abscess in the (a) left paracolic gutter. *B,* A 10-Fr catheter was placed into the collection, using ultrasound guidance (not shown). Follow-up CT demonstrates almost complete decompression of the abscess cavity *(straight arrow)* after short-term catheter drainage.

surgery in cases of cholecystitis, appendicitis, and diverticulitis. Most postoperative abscesses and fluid collections can be cured percutaneously, obviating the need for reoperation. Even enteric fistulas can be closed with aggressive, although sometimes prolonged, catheter drainage.

BIBLIOGRAPHY

1. Bergenfeldt M, Genell S, Lindholm K, et al: Needle-tract seeding after percutaneous fine-needle biopsy of pancreatic carcinoma. Case report. Acta Chir Scand 154:77–79, 1988.

2. Bissonnette RT, Gibney RG, Berry BR, Buckley AR: Fatal carcinoid crisis after percutaneous fine-needle biopsy of hepatic metastasis: Case report and literature review. Radiology 174:751–752, 1990.

3. Bradley EL III: A clinically based classification system for acute pancreatitis: Summary of the International Symposium on Acute Pancreatitis, Atlanta, September 11–13, 1992. Arch Surg 128:586–590, 1993.

4. Casola G, Nicolet V, van Sonnenberg E, et al: Unsuspected pheochromocytoma: Risk of blood-pressure alterations during percutaneous adrenal biopsy. Radiology 159:733–735, 1986.

5. del Pilar Fernandez M, Murphy FB: Hepatic biopsies and fluid drainages. Radiol Clin North Am 29:1311–1328, 1991.

6. Dodd GD III, Soulen MC, Kane RA, et al: Minimally invasive treatment of malignant hepatic tumors: At the threshold of a major breakthrough. Radiographics 20:9–27, 2000.

7. Freeny PC, Hauptmann E, Althaus SJ, et al: Percutaneous CT-guided catheter drainage of infected acute necrotizing pancreatitis: Techniques and results. AJR 170:969–977, 1998.

8. Gerzof SG: Triangulation: Indirect CT guidance for abscess drainage. AJR 137:1080–1081, 1981.

9. Gerzof SG, Gale ME: Computed tomography and ultrasonography for diagnosis and treatment of renal and retroperitoneal abscesses. Urol Clin North Am 9:185–193, 1982.

10. Hariri M, Slivka A, Carr-Locke DL, Banks PA: Pseudocyst drainage predisposes to infection when pancreatic necrosis is unrecognized. Am J Gastroenterol 89:1781–1784, 1994.

11. Mannucci PM, Remuzzi G, Pusineri F, et al: Deamino-8-D-arginine vasopressin shortens the bleeding time in uremia. N Engl J Med 308:8–12, 1983.

12. Price RB, Bernardino ME, Berkman WA, et al: Biopsy of the right adrenal gland by the transhepatic approach. Radiology 148:566, 1983.

13. Quinn SF, van Sonnenberg E, Casola G, et al: Interventional radiology in the spleen. Radiology 161:289–291, 1986.

14. Silverman SG, Mueller PR, Pfister RC: Hemostatic evaluation before abdominal interventions: An overview and proposal. AJR 154:233–238, 1990.

15. Soulen MC: Chemoembolization of hepatic malignancies. Semin Interv Radiol 14:305–311, 1997.

16. van Sonnenberg E, D'Agostino HB, Casola G, et al: Percutaneous abscess drainage: Current concepts. Radiology 181:617–626, 1991.

17. van Sonnenberg E, Wittich GR, Casola G, et al: Percutaneous drainage of infected and noninfected pancreatic pseudocysts: Experience in 101 cases. Radiology 170:757–776, 1981.

18. van Sonnenberg E, Wroblicka JT, D'Agostino HB, et al: Symptomatic hepatic cysts: Percutaneous drainage and sclerosis. Radiology 190:387–392, 1994.

INTERVENTIONAL RADIOLOGY: FLUOROSCOPIC AND ANGIOGRAPHIC PROCEDURES

Stephen W. Subber, MD, Paul D. Russ, MD, Dale L. McCarter, MD, and Keith M. Shonnard, MD

HEPATIC TRANSARTERIAL CHEMOEMBOLIZATION

1. **Define *hepatic transarterial chemoembolization*.**
   Hepatic transarterial chemoembolization (TACE) is a treatment for unresectable primary and secondary hepatic malignancies (Fig. 70-1). This procedure combines the intra-arterial infusion of chemotherapeutic agents with subsequent embolization of the blood vessel supplying the tumor, a combination that leads to high local drug concentrations and tumor ischemia while decreasing systemic toxicity.

2. **How safe is hepatic TACE?**
   TACE is a relatively safe therapy because liver tumors derive most of their blood supply from the hepatic artery. The unique dual blood supply to the background liver (hepatic artery and portal vein) allows safe embolization of the neoplasm's arterial blood supply, with little risk of hepatic ischemia.

3. **Why would TACE be used to treat patients with hepatic malignancy?**
   Surgical resection or transplantation are the optimal treatments for patients with hepatic malignancy. Unfortunately, many patients are not surgical candidates because of tumor extent, invasion of blood vessels, associated liver dysfunction, or distant metastases. Response to conventional treatments, such as systemic chemotherapy or radiation therapy, is also poor.

4. **How effective is TACE?**
   Response rates are encouraging for hepatocellular carcinoma as well as metastatic carcinoid and islet cell tumors but less promising for colorectal metastases. TACE has been effective in the palliation of symptoms, but increased survival rates have not been definitively shown.

BILIARY PROCEDURES

5. **Is percutaneous transhepatic biliary drainage the primary method to treat biliary obstruction?**
   The role of percutaneous transhepatic biliary drainage (PTBD) in the management of benign and malignant biliary disease has diminished significantly with the advancement of interventional endoscopy. Currently, endoscopic drainage is the primary method for biliary decompression because of its relative lack of complications and better patient tolerance compared with the transhepatic approach. However, not all endoscopic drainages are successful, and PTBD continues to play an important role in the management of biliary disease. Biliary disease is best managed by a team that includes an endoscopist, interventional radiologist, and surgeon.

6. **What are the indications for PTBD?**
   - Unsuccessful endoscopic drainage
   - Biliary obstruction at or above the level of the porta hepatis

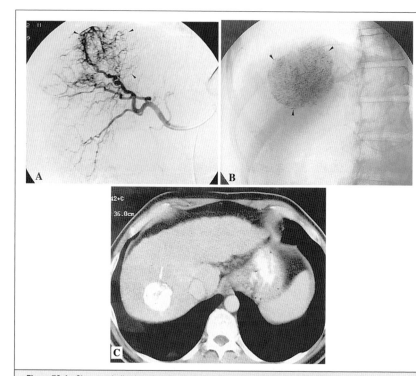

Figure 70-1. Chemoembolization of a hepatocellular carcinoma. *A,* Hepatic arteriogram demonstrates a hypervascular mass *(black arrowheads)* in the posterior segment of the right lobe. *B,* Angiographic image of the stained tumor *(black arrowheads)* after embolization with ethiodol/chemotherapeutic drug emulsion and particles. *C,* Postembolization CT scan shows persistent, dense uptake and retention of ethiodol in the lesion *(arrow).* Complete tumor staining results in tumor necrosis and, possibly, longer patient survival.

- Biliary obstruction following biliary-enteric anastomosis
- Bile duct injuries after laparoscopic cholecystectomy

The most common of these indications is failed endoscopic drainage for any reason.

KEY POINTS: INDICATIONS FOR PTBD

1. Unsuccessful endoscopic access or drainage of the biliary tree

2. Biliary obstruction in a patient with unfavorable anatomy for endoscopic retrograde cholangiopancreatography (ERCP) (e.g., surgical biliary-enteric anastomosis)

3. Hilar obstruction that involves both the right and left hepatic ducts, as can occur in cases of cholangiocarcinoma or metastatic disease

4. Multisegmental ductal obstruction (e.g., advanced primary sclerosing cholangitis [PSC])

7. **What particular problems are involved in the treatment of hilar obstruction?**
   Hilar obstruction is difficult to treat for both endoscopists and interventionalists. Usually, it is secondary to cholangiocarcinoma or metastatic disease that involves the left and right bile ducts, with frequent occlusion of intrahepatic segmental ducts. The multisegmental nature of

these obstructions makes them difficult to drain by the endoscopist; in general, drainage is better accomplished by PTBD. Bilateral drains may be required.

8. **Why is endoscopic drainage difficult in patients with biliary obstruction after biliary-enteric anastomosis?**

   The success rate for endoscopic drainage in patients with biliary obstruction after biliary-enteric anastomosis is <50% because of the technical difficulty of negotiating the endoscope through the afferent loop. PTBD may be necessary to evaluate for recurrent disease or anastomotic stricture.

9. **Describe the approach to bile duct injuries due to laparoscopic cholecystectomy.**

   Bile duct injuries due to laparoscopic cholecystectomy result from inadvertent laceration or ligation of the biliary system. PTBD is directed at relieving the obstruction or, in patients with a bile leak, diverting the bile and stenting the injury. This procedure allows healing and may be curative. Otherwise, elective surgery is performed once the patient's condition stabilizes. Endoscopic drainage can be difficult because the bile duct may be severed.

10. **Explain the advantages and disadvantages of using metallic stents for the treatment of biliary obstruction.**

    Metallic stents have supplanted plastic endoprostheses in the percutaneous treatment of malignant biliary obstructions for palliation (Fig. 70-2). Their primary advantage is the smaller-sized catheter used to deliver the stent compared with the much larger plastic endoprosthesis,

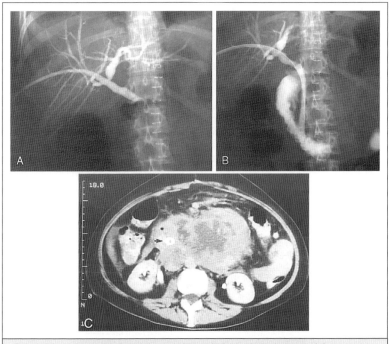

Figure 70-2. A 58-year-old woman presented with jaundice and an abdominal mass. *A,* A cholangiogram performed after percutaneous transhepatic biliary drainage shows complete obstruction of the common bile duct. *B,* After placement of a metallic stent, the common bile duct is widely patent. *C,* CT scan of the abdomen shows the large, poorly differentiated lymphoma encasing the biliary stent (*arrow*).

thus decreasing patient discomfort and liver complications. In addition, metallic stents expand to larger internal diameters (up to 12 mm or larger), affording better drainage and longer patency rates. A major disadvantage is the high cost; moreover, if they occlude because of tumor overgrowth, epithelial hyperplasia, or inspissated bile, reintervention is necessary.

11. **What are the indications for percutaneous cholecystostomy?**
Percutaneous placement of a drainage catheter into the gallbladder is a well-established technique. Its two primary indications are (1) persistent and unexplained sepsis in critically ill patients with acalculous cholecystitis and (2) acute cholecystitis in patients too ill to undergo surgery. In unstable patients, it can be performed at the bedside if necessary. Less frequent indications include temporary treatment for gallbladder perforation, drainage for distant malignant biliary obstruction, and transcholecystic biliary intervention.

GASTROINTESTINAL BLEEDING

12. **When do diagnostic angiography and percutaneous transcatheter therapy play a role in the management of gastrointestinal (GI) bleeding?**
Acute GI bleeding that is refractory to conservative management or invasive endoscopic techniques requires angiographic evaluation. For the interventional radiologist to identify the bleeding site, the following conditions must be met:
1. The patient must be actively bleeding at the time of the study.
2. The bleeding must be brisk enough to be detectable during the angiogram, usually 1.5–2.0 mL/min.
GI bleeding at lower rates is difficult to detect angiographically. Once the bleeding site is identified, transcatheter embolization is a treatment option.

13. **How important is localization of the bleeding site before angiography?**
Preangiographic localization of the GI bleeding site is extremely helpful. A visceral angiogram involves evaluation of the celiac, superior mesenteric, and inferior mesenteric arteries; selective catheterization of these vessels and the multiple angiographic projections needed when looking for a bleeding site can make this a tedious and time-consuming procedure, requiring large contrast volumes. If the preangiographic endoscopy has localized and failed to treat the bleeding, the vessel supplying this region should be studied first to shorten the procedure. If the exact site of bleeding is not known, distinguishing an upper from a lower GI source is helpful and can guide the interventionalist in choosing which vessel should be studied first. A technetium 99m-labeled red blood cell study may provide localizing information; the procedure may be repeated after 12 hours if no bleeding is demonstrated initially.

14. **What two types of transcatheter therapy are used for GI bleeding?**
Pharmacologic agents and embolic materials.

15. **Which pharmacologic agent is preferred? How is it used?**
The pharmacologic agent of choice is vasopressin (Pitressin). This pituitary hormone acts directly on the smooth muscle of arterioles and capillaries to cause vasoconstriction. The superior mesenteric, gastroduodenal, left gastric, and gastroepiploic arteries are particularly sensitive to its intra-arterial administration. After selective catheterization of the bleeding vessel, vasopressin is infused at 0.2 U/min (Fig. 70-3). A repeat arteriogram is performed after 30 minutes to assess the effectiveness of treatment, and the dose may be increased to 0.4 U/min, if necessary. With excessive vasoconstriction, the dose is reduced to 0.1 U/min. The infusion is continued for 12–24 hours, during which time the patient is monitored closely for side effects (myocardial, bowel, and extremity ischemia, water retention, hyponatremia, and cardiac arrhythmias), which may prematurely terminate the therapy. The patient is reevaluated clinically

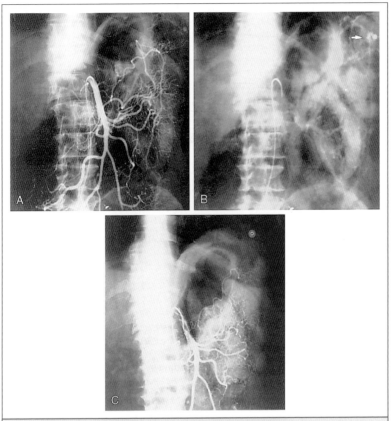

Figure 70-3. A 60-year-old man with lower GI bleeding. *A,* Diagnostic angiogram with selective injection into the superior mesenteric artery. Early arterial films show no bleeding. *B,* Later images reveal puddling of contrast in the proximal left colon consistent with a bleeding diverticulum *(arrow). C,* After a 30-minute infusion of vasopressin (0.2 U/min), the bleeding has stopped. Note the vasoconstriction of the superior mesenteric artery and its branches.

and angiographically. If the bleeding has stopped, the vasopressin is tapered slowly to normal saline with subsequent catheter removal.

16. **How is embolization of the bleeding vessel achieved?**
The catheter is selectively placed near the bleeding site for delivery of the embolic material. The embolic agents used most commonly are polyvinyl alcohol (PVA), Gelfoam, and coils. The availability of coaxial systems and microcatheters permits superselective catheterization with accurate deposition of embolic material at the bleeding site. These advances have decreased the risk of bowel infarction, making this a relatively safe procedure, even in the small bowel and colon.

TRANSJUGULAR INTRAHEPATIC PORTOSYSTEMIC SHUNT (TIPS)

17. **What is TIPS? How is it performed?**
Transjugular intrahepatic portosystemic shunt (TIPS) is a percutaneous technique that creates a shunt within the liver between the portal and hepatic veins to treat variceal bleeding or ascites,

complications of portal hypertension (Figs. 70-4 and 70-5). The procedure is performed by accessing the hepatic venous system, usually the right hepatic vein, via the right internal jugular vein. A 16-G Colapinto transjugular needle is used to puncture through the liver from the hepatic vein into the portal vein. The transhepatic tract is dilated with a balloon catheter, followed by placement of a flexible metallic stent, usually 10–12 mm in diameter.

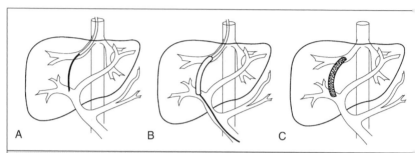

Figure 70-4. Transjugular intrahepatic portosystemic shunt procedure. *A,* After placement of a sheath in the right hepatic vein, a Colapinto needle is used to puncture through the liver to the portal vein. *B,* The liver parenchyma is dilated with a balloon catheter. *C,* A metallic stent is placed across the transhepatic tract, bridging the hepatic and portal veins.

18. **What are the benefits of a successful TIPS?**

Successful TIPS results in a reduction of the portosystemic pressure gradient (PSG) to 8–12 mmHg (bleeding from varices is rare in patients with a PSG <12 mmHg), and the stent is dilated until this goal is reached. If the PSG cannot be reduced sufficiently, parallel shunts may be necessary. Esophageal and gastric varices usually decompress once the TIPS has been placed. If the varices continue to fill at portal venography, the interventionalist may elect to embolize them.

19. **What are the indications for TIPS?**

The most important and frequent indication for TIPS is refractory variceal hemorrhage (*see* Fig. 70-5), either acute (bleeding not controlled with sclerotherapy or pharmacotherapy) or chronic (recurrent major hemorrhage, despite a course of sclerotherapy). TIPS is particularly helpful with bleeding from inaccessible intestinal or gastric varices and bleeding due to portal hypertensive gastropathy. Additional promising indications for TIPS include refractory ascites, refractory hepatic hydrothorax, and Budd-Chiari syndrome or other veno-occlusive diseases. TIPS is not indicated for the initial therapy of acute variceal bleeding, as a bridge to transplantation to reduce intraoperative morbidity, or for treatment of hepatopulmonary syndrome.

KEY POINTS: INDICATIONS FOR TIPS

1. Acute refractory variceal hemorrhage not controlled by sclerotherapy or pharmacotherapy

2. Recurrent major variceal bleeding following sclerotherapy or other treatment

3. Hemorrhage from inaccessible gastric or intestinal varices

4. Bleeding from portal hypertensive gastropathy

5. Refractory ascites or hepatic hydrothorax

6. Budd-Chiari syndrome and some other veno-occlusive conditions

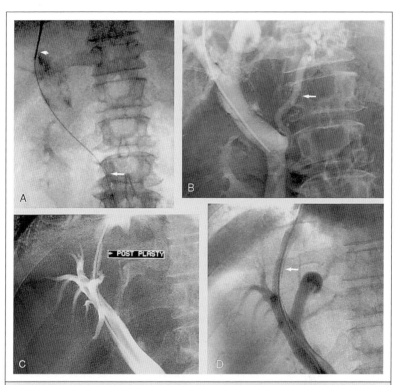

Figure 70-5. Transjugular intrahepatic portosystemic shunt in a 52-year-old woman with cryptogenic cirrhosis and refractory variceal bleeding. *A,* The portal vein has been punctured with a Colapinto needle *(arrowhead)* and a guidewire placed into the superior mesenteric vein *(arrow).* The portosystemic gradient (PSG) was 28 mmHg. *B,* Portal venogram shows a large cardiac vein and esophageal varices *(arrow). C,* After balloon dilation of the transhepatic tract, a suboptimal portosystemic shunt is shown. *D,* A metallic stent *(arrow)* has been deployed across the transhepatic tract, allowing greater luminal diameter. Postprocedural PSG was 10 mmHg.

20. **What are the contraindications to performing the TIPS procedure?**
    There are few absolute contraindications to TIPS. Because it is a portosystemic shunt, TIPS increases right-sided heart pressure and should not be performed in patients with right-heart failure. It should not be performed in patients with polycystic liver disease, in whom the risk of hemorrhage is significantly increased because the shunt tract may traverse the cysts rather than be contained by hepatic parenchyma. TIPS is also precluded if diversion of hepatic blood flow is likely to exacerbate hepatic dysfunction and severe hepatic failure. Exceptions include cases of variceal bleeding or fulminant Budd-Chiari syndrome. Relative contraindications include systemic infection, portal vein thrombosis, biliary obstruction, and severe hepatic encephalopathy.

21. **What is the technical success rate for TIPS? What are the most common causes of a failed procedure?**
    TIPS is one of the more technically challenging procedures performed by the interventional radiologist. Nonetheless, the technical success rate is >90%. Most failures are due to portal vein occlusion, when the occluded segment of portal vein cannot be catheterized from the transjugular approach.

22. **How effective is the TIPS procedure for controlling variceal hemorrhage?**
    TIPS is effective in controlling acute variceal hemorrhage. It appears to be as effective as a surgical portacaval shunt, without the added risk of hepatic injury from general anesthesia. Mid-term studies have found the rate of recurrent variceal bleeding after TIPS to be <10%. Nearly all patients with recurrent bleeding were found to have shunt abnormalities, either stenosis or occlusion. Angiographic reevaluation with shunt revision (balloon dilatation or additional stent placement) or placement of a second TIPS nearly always controls bleeding.

23. **What are the morbidity and mortality rates for TIPS?**
    TIPS is generally accepted to have lower morbidity and mortality rates than surgically created portacaval shunts. Published series show a 30-day mortality rate of 3–15%. Most deaths are in Child-Pugh class C patients. The direct procedure-related mortality rate is 2–5%. Procedure-related deaths are due to predominantly intraprocedural cardiac events or intraperitoneal hemorrhage after puncture through the liver capsule. Serious procedural complications, which occur in <10% of patients, include self-limited intraperitoneal hemorrhage, myocardial infarction, transient renal failure, hepatic arterial injury, hepatic infarction, and pulmonary edema.

24. **Describe the major short-term complications of TIPS.**
    The two main short-term complications of TIPS are shunt malfunction and hepatic encephalopathy. Acute thrombosis of the stent is infrequent but may occur immediately or shortly after the procedure. The interventionalist can treat this complication by removing or displacing the thrombus from the stent (i.e., shunt thrombectomy). Delayed shunt stenosis or occlusion usually results from pseudointimal proliferation within the stent or incomplete coverage of the parenchymal tract with the stent; treatment is shunt revision. Primary shunt patency is 70% at 1 year and 40% at 2 years. Secondary patency rates (patency after shunt revision) are >90% at 2 years.

25. **Describe the major long-term complication of TIPS. How is it treated?**
    The most significant long-term complication of TIPS is hepatic encephalopathy. New or worsened encephalopathy is seen in about 25% of patients after TIPS. Usually, it can be treated with diet and lactulose administration. Clinical variables associated with increased risk for developing post-TIPS encephalopathy include an etiology of liver disease other than alcohol, female gender, increasing age, and prior history of encephalopathy. Severe encephalopathy may require complete or partial occlusion of the shunt.

26. **How is shunt patency followed?**
    Shunt patency can be followed noninvasively by color Doppler ultrasound or venography. Protocols differ among institutions. A baseline study is obtained 24 hours after the procedure. In asymptomatic patients, routine follow-up is performed at 3 and 6 months after TIPS, then at 6-month intervals. If the patient becomes symptomatic (e.g., variceal bleeding or ascites), or if significant interval change is demonstrated by ultrasound, venography with therapeutic intervention should be performed to restore normal shunt function.

BIBLIOGRAPHY

1. Camma C, Schepis F, Orlando A, et al: Transarterial chemoembolization for unresectable hepatocellular carcinoma: Meta-analysis of randomized controlled trials. Radiology 224:47–54, 2002.

2. Chan AO, Yuen M-F, Hui C-K, et al: A prospective study regarding the complications of transcatheter intraarterial lipidol chemoembolization in patients with hepatocellular carcinoma. Cancer 94:1747–1752, 2002.

3. Gordon RL, Ring EJ: Combined radiologic and retrograde endoscopic and biliary interventions. Radiol Clin North Am 28:1289–1295, 1990.

4. Kerlan RK, LaBerge JM, Gordon RL, Ring EJ: Transjugular intrahepatic portosystemic shunts: Current status. AJR 164:1059–1066, 1995.

5. Laberge J, Ring E, Gordon R, et al: Creation of transjugular intrahepatic portosystemic shunts with the Wallstent endoprosthesis: Results in 100 patients. Radiology 187:413–420, 1993.

6. Lee BH, Choe DH, Lee JH, et al: Metallic stents in malignant biliary obstruction: Prospective long-term clinical results. AJR 168:741–745, 1997.

7. Lee K-H, Sung K-B, Lee D-Y, et al: Transcatheter arterial chemoembolization for hepatocellular carcinoma: Anatomic and hemodynamic considerations in the hepatic artery and portal vein. Radiographics 22:1077–1091, 2002.

8. Ong JP, Sands M, Younossi ZM: Transjugular intrahepatic portosystemic shunts (TIPS): A decade later. J Clin Gastroenterol 30:14–28, 2000.

9. Peck DJ, McLoughlin RF, Hughson MN, Rankin RN: Percutaneous embolization of lower gastrointestinal hemorrhage. J Vasc Interv Radiol 9:747–751, 1998.

10. Rosen RJ, Sanchez G: Angiographic diagnosis and management of gastrointestinal hemorrhage: Current concepts. Radiol Clin North Am 32:951–967, 1994.

11. Soulen MC: Chemoembolization of hepatic malignancies. Semin Interv Radiol 14:305–311, 1997.

CHAPTER 71

NONINVASIVE GASTROINTESTINAL IMAGING: ULTRASOUND, COMPUTED TOMOGRAPHY, MAGNETIC RESONANCE SCANNING

Michael G. Fox, MD, David W. Bean, Jr., MD, Steven H. Peck, MD, and Kevin M. Rak, MD

LIVER IMAGING

1. How is segmental liver anatomy defined?

Early descriptions of liver anatomy divided the organ into four lobes based on the surface configuration. Recently, the segmental anatomy has been based on the vasculature, primarily involving the hepatic veins (Fig. 71-1). The different hepatic segments are divided by intersegmental fissures, which are traversed or are in the same plane as the hepatic veins.

The main lobar fissure divides the right and left lobes of the liver and is represented by a line extending from the gallbladder recess through the inferior vena cava (IVC). In the liver, it is represented by the middle hepatic vein. The right intersegmental fissure divides the anterior and posterior segments of the right lobe of the liver and is approximated by the right hepatic vein.

The left intersegmental fissure divides the medial and lateral segments of the left lobe of the liver. It is marked on the external liver margin by the falciform ligament, and, internally, the ligamentum teres runs within it. In the liver, it is represented by the left hepatic vein. The caudate lobe is the portion of liver located between the IVC and the fissure of the ligamentum venosum.

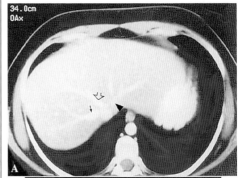
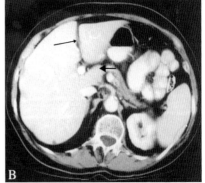

Figure 71-1. CT scans showing vascular anatomy of the liver. *A,* The right hepatic vein *(black arrow)* divides the anterior and posterior segments of the right lobe of the liver. The middle hepatic vein *(open arrow)* divides the right lobe from the left lobe. The left hepatic vein *(arrowhead)* divides the medial and lateral segments of the left lobe of the liver. *B,* The falciform ligament *(small black arrow)* divides the medial and lateral segments of the left lobe of the liver. The caudate lobe is marked by the large black arrow.

2. **What are the typical CT imaging features of liver metastases?**

On CT, most liver metastases are of low attenuation compared with the surrounding paren- chyma (Fig. 71-2); however, high attenuation metastases can be seen with pancreatic islet cell carcinoma, renal cell carcinoma, carcinoid tumor, or thyroid carcinoma.

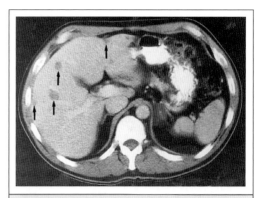

Figure 71-2. Liver metastases *(arrows)* in a patient with colon carcinoma present as hypodense lesions in the surrounding normal liver parenchyma.

3. **How does vasculature determine the detection of liver metastases on CT?**

Branches of the hepatic artery supply liver metastases, and their detection is based on the timing of the contrast bolus and the vascularity of the lesions. The liver parenchyma receives 75% of its blood flow from the portal vein and 25% from the hepatic artery. Immediately after peripheral injection of intravenous contrast, organs with only an arterial supply (e.g., spleen, kidney) enhance brightly, but the liver enhances little, because the contrast from the hepatic artery is diluted by blood from the portal vein. Only after contrast circulates through the spleen and mesentery to reach the portal vein does the dominant contrast effect occur. This takes about 60 seconds; the spleen and kidney enhance 30 seconds earlier. CT imaging is usually best performed during the portal venous contrast phase, when the contrast between the enhancing liver and low-density metastases is greatest.

The exception to this rule is imaging of hypervascular metastases. Imaging during the arterial phase, 30–40 seconds after injection, should be added to portal phase imaging. Triple-phase imaging—before contrast and 30 and 70 seconds after contrast—is helpful for evaluating metastases from renal cell, breast, thyroid, melanoma, and neuroendocrine tumors. This tech- nique should also be used for evaluating other vascular lesions, such as hepatocellular carci- noma, focal nodular hyperplasia, and hepatic adenomas.

4. **What is CT arterial portography?**

To increase liver enhancement, some medical centers place a catheter in the superior mesenteric artery for contrast injection during CT scanning. This technique, called *CT arterial portography* (CTAP), can increase the sensitivity of lesion detection to 91%. A standard contrast-enhanced CT scan has a sensitivity of 63–71%; triple-phase imaging has a sensitivity of 80%. The improved vascular contrast also improves localization of metastases to a specific subsegment. Improved localization and sensitivity are particularly helpful when partial hepatic resection is contemplated for metastases secondary to colorectal carcinoma. By detecting more lesions, needless surgery can be avoided. Other CT techniques, such as delayed contrast-enhanced CT, noncontrast-enhanced CT (NCCT), and CT scanning during contrast injection through a hepatic artery catheter, have failed to match the success of CTAP in clinical trials. About 5% of metastases contain calcification, usually from mucinous adenocarcinomas of the ovary or gastrointestinal (GI) tract. Cystic metastatic lesions can arise from tumors of the pancreas and ovary or from necrotic squamous cell carcinoma metastases.

5. **Describe the appearance of liver metastases on ultrasound (US).**
    It varies greatly. GI and more vascular tumors (e.g., islet cell, carcinoid, renal cell carcinomas) tend to produce hyperechoic metastases, but hypoechoic lesions are also common, particularly with lymphoma and cystic or necrotic metastases. Hypoechoic halos of edema surrounding hyperechoic metastases produce the common "bull's eye" appearance. The sensitivity of US for detecting metastases is about 61%; however, intraoperative US can increase the sensitivity to 96% and may be the most sensitive modality available.

6. **What is the role of magnetic resonance (MR) scanning in detection of liver metastases?**
    Studies have demonstrated increased sensitivity of dynamic gadolinium-enhanced MRI compared to single slice CT for the detection of liver metastases. In addition, MRI has a much greater sensitivity for characterizing liver lesions than CT. In general, metastases are hypointense on T_1-weighted images and hyperintense on T_2-weighted images. Exceptions occur with hemorrhagic and malignant melanoma metastases, which are hyperintense to varying degrees on T_1-weighted images. Imaging with MRI contrast agents approaches the sensitivity of CTAP for detecting metastases.

7. **What MRI contrast agents are available for use in hepatobiliary imaging?**
    The two main categories of MRI contrast agents used in hepatobiliary imaging are hepatobiliary and ferrous oxide agents. *Manganese dipyridoxyl diphosphate* (Mn-DPDP) is a hepatobiliary agent that is taken up by hepatocytes and excreted in the bile. It is convenient because it has a long (up to 10 hours) imaging window. On T_1 images, Mn-DPDP causes increased signal in the normal liver. Therefore, lesions not of hepatocellular origin do not enhance. Examples include metastases, cholangiocarcinoma, and lymphoma. However, lesions that are of hepatocellular origin (hepatocellular carcinoma [HCC], focal nodular hyperplasia [FNH], and regenerating nodules) do enhance.

    Superparamagnetic ferrous oxide agents (SPIOs) were approved by the Food and Drug Administration (FDA) for commercial use in 1997. They are used primarily to evaluate for metastases, particularly in patients with colon carcinoma. They are taken up by the reticuloendothelial system, primarily by Kupffer cells, and result in a decreased T_2 signal. Lesions that do not have reticuloendothelial elements, such as metastases and cysts, do not take up the agent and remain hyperintense on T_2. Early studies with SPIOs, such as ferumoxide, detected 27% more lesions than unenhanced MR and 40% more lesions than noncontrast CT. They can improve the detection of HCC but are limited in severe cases of cirrhosis. A limited study reported a similar detection rate of metastases with both SPIO agents and CTAP, but additional study is needed. Limitations of SPIOs include lack of effectiveness at characterizing lesions smaller than 1–2 cm and dose-related toxicity.

8. **What are the three growth patterns of HCC?**
    (1) Large solitary mass, (2) multifocal HCC with a dominant mass and satellite lesions, and (3) diffuse infiltration. In North America, underlying cirrhosis is seen in 60% and hemochromatosis in 20% of patients with HCC. HCC arising in normal livers tends to occur at a younger age (fibrolamellar HCC) and presents typically as a solitary, well-circumscribed mass.

9. **Describe the sonographic characteristics of HCC.**
    They are variable and may simulate metastatic disease. HCCs <3 cm are often hypoechoic, whereas larger lesions have mixed echogenicity. Fatty metamorphosis within the tumor may cause internal hyperechoic foci. Vascular invasion is common and suggestive of HCC, which invades portal veins more frequently than hepatic veins. Such tumor thrombus can be demonstrated with Doppler ultrasound and typically has an arterial wave form. Detecting malignant tumor thrombus is important, because it is the worst prognostic factor for tumor recurrence after surgery.

10. **How does HCC appear on CT?**

Underlying cirrhotic or hemochromatotic changes are commonly seen, and 7–10% of HCCs demonstrate calcification. Tumors are typically hypodense on noncontrast CT but may appear hyperdense in fatty livers. They are typically hypodense during portal venous phase imaging but may appear isodense. Because small HCCs may enhance much like liver parenchyma during portal phase imaging, making contour deformity and mass effect the only means of detection, arterial phase imaging should be used. Hepatic arterial phase imaging usually demonstrates a hyperdense lesion and increases detection by 10%. Central necrotic areas of low attenuation are common (Fig. 71-3). Hemoperitoneum, due to rare spontaneous rupture and vascular invasion, can be documented with CT. A hyperdense, enhancing capsule is common. CTAP increases sensitivity, especially in detecting small lesions.

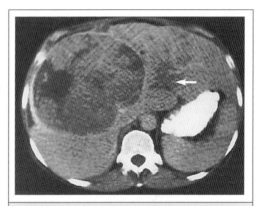

Figure 71-3. CT shows large necrotic hepatocellular carcinoma. The area of lower attenuation in the left lobe *(arrow)* is a separate focus of multifocal HCC.

11. **How does HCC appear on MRI?**

HCC is usually hypointense on T_1 images but may be isointense or hyperintense, depending on the degree of fatty change and internal fibrosis. It is usually hyperintense on T_2 images. Encapsulated HCC typically has a hypointense rim on T_1 and T_2 images. Fibrolamellar HCC appears somewhat similar to FNH. Both have a central scar with multiple fibrous septa. However, fibrolamellar HCC has a high prevalence of calcification, and the central scar is typically hypointense on T_2 images, whereas it is hyperintense in FNH. The addition of dynamic, enhanced gadolinium (Gd-DTPA) T_1 imaging increases the detection of HCC. Findings suggestive of HCC include lesion size >3 cm; increased T_2-weighted signal; intense, early gadolinium enhancement with late washout; and the presence of a "capsule."

12. **What is the most common benign neoplasm of the liver?**

Cavernous hemangiomas. Most are <5 cm in size and solitary, although they can be multiple. They are typically located in a peripheral subcapsular location, commonly in the right lobe of the liver. Blood flow within cavernous hemangiomas is usually very slow, which accounts for some of its imaging characteristics.

13. **Describe the imaging characteristics of hepatic hemangiomas.**

- US: Cavernous hemangiomas appear as well-defined hyperechoic masses. Doppler and color flow imaging show no detectable flow within the mass, but they may demonstrate a feeding vessel. Occasionally, hemangiomas have a mixed or hypoechoic appearance.
- CT: On unenhanced CT, hemangiomas are usually hypodense well-defined lesions; 20% have calcifications. They may appear isodense or hyperdense if they arise in an area of focal fatty infiltration. Triple-phase imaging may reveal a characteristic enhancement pattern, initially showing peripheral enhancement isodense to the aorta followed by slow filling of the center of the lesion. This pattern has been described as nodular or fingerlike and can take from 5–60 minutes to fill completely. Up to one fourth of lesions do not show this characteristic

pattern; they may show initial central or uniform enhancement, which may also be seen in malignant lesions.
- MRI: A typical hemangioma is well-defined and has decreased signal intensity relative to normal liver on T_1-weighted images. On T_2-weighted images, hemangiomas have increased signal compared with the liver because of their high water content. The signal is equal to or greater than the signal of bile within the gallbladder and should continue to increase with greater T_2 weighting. Using fast-scanning techniques and Gd-DTPA, a similar enhancement pattern can be seen on MRI and CT, with an accuracy approaching 95%.

14. **Outline the work-up for a suspected cavernous hemangioma.**
If a lesion has the typical US findings of a cavernous hemangioma and is <3 cm, and if the patient has normal liver function tests (LFTs and αFP) and no history of a malignancy that may metastasize to the liver, follow-up US in 3–6 months is appropriate. If the lesion is atypical on US, or if the patient has a known primary neoplasm or abnormal LFTs, further work-up is warranted. If the lesion is >2 cm, a ^{99m}Tc-tagged red blood cell (RBC) scan is the next step. This procedure is highly sensitive and specific for lesions >2 cm. If the lesion is <2 cm, the RBC scan can be attempted, but sensitivity and specificity decrease as the size of the lesion decreases. If the RBC scan is equivocal, the next study is MRI, preferably with heavily T_2-weighted and gadolinium-enhanced T_1 imaging. In this scenario, CT should be a third-line choice or used if MRI is not available.

If the initial lesion is found by CT and follows the strict criteria of a hemangioma (a well-defined, low-density lesion on unenhanced images, with peripheral enhancement followed by complete filling of the lesion), further work-up is probably not necessary. If the diagnosis needs confirmation, a tagged RBC study or ultrasound is a good choice. If the initial CT scan does not meet the strict criteria, or the patient has abnormal LFTs, a confirmatory nuclear medicine or MRI scan is appropriate. If the CT criteria are not met, it is typically due to incomplete filling of the lesion.

If these different studies do not confirm that the lesion is a cavernous hemangioma, a biopsy may be necessary for the final diagnosis.

15. **How can FNH and hepatocellular adenoma (HCA) be differentiated?**
Hepatic adenomas and FNH are more common in women, and both, particularly HCA, are associated with oral contraceptive use. FNH is benign, whereas HCA can cause morbidity and mortality because of its propensity for hemorrhage and rare malignant degeneration to HCC. If a lesion is hyperintense on T_1-weighted sequences, has a pseudocapsule, and lacks a central scar, an HCA is favored over FNH. However, in smaller lesions without hemorrhage, a biopsy may be required for differentiation.

16. **Describe the appearance of FNH on imaging modalities.**
FNH contains all of the normal liver elements in an abnormal arrangement. The characteristic feature is the central scar, containing radiating fibrous tissue with vascular and biliary elements. However, the central scar is nonspecific and may be seen with fibrolamellar HCC, hemangioma, and other lesions. On US, FNH is a well-demarcated hypoechoic to isoechoic mass, possibly demonstrating a central scar. On triple-phase CT, a central low-density scar may be seen in 20–40% of cases. The scar should be somewhat linear or branching to help distinguish it from central necrosis in a mass. On noncontrast CT, FNH is hypodense to isodense without calcification. FNH is hyperdense on arterial phase images, because it is supplied by the hepatic artery. On portal phase images, it commonly enhances much like normal liver, except for the persisting central scar, which may become hyperdense on delayed images. Thus, if no central scar is seen, FNH may be missed on CT or seen only as a deformity of the liver contour. On MR, FNH is hypointense to isointense on T_1 and isointense to hyperintense on T_2. The central scar is hypointense on T_1 and hyperintense on T_2 images. The lesion demonstrates diffuse early enhancement, with the exception of the central scar, which usually demonstrates delayed

enhancement due to the fibrous tissue. Because of the presence of Kupffer cells, *sulfur-colloid scintigraphy* demonstrates normal uptake in 50%, decreased uptake in 40%, and increased uptake or "hot spots" in 10%. However, HCA may also show normal sulfur colloid uptake in 20%.

17. **How does HCA appear on imaging modalities?**

Sonography typically shows a heterogeneous mass due to areas of internal hemorrhage; however, the mass may be hyperechoic because of the high lipid content. On *noncontrast CT,* a hypodense mass is typically seen; however, internal areas of higher attenuation may be present due to recent hemorrhage. Hemorrhage is a key distinguishing feature from FNH. *Contrast CT* may show centripetal enhancement similar to that in hemangiomas, though this enhancement does not persist in adenomas. On *MR,* HCA may be hyperintense on T_1 because of internal fat/glycogen, although similar findings may be seen in HCC. The lesions are commonly heterogeneous, as a result of necrosis and internal hemorrhage. HCA can demonstrate decreased signal on out-of-phase imaging due to the high lipid content.

18. **Describe the appearance of a hepatic abscess on imaging.**

- US: On ultrasound, a hepatic abscess appears as a complex fluid collection, typically with septations, an irregular wall, and debris or air within the fluid. Air is seen as a focal area of echogenicity with posterior shadowing. Abscesses can also appear as simple fluid collections similar to a cyst.
- CT: CT is the most sensitive imaging modality (95–98%). CT findings vary with the size and age of the abscess. Generally, the abscess appears as a low-density, well-defined mass and may be unilocular or multilocular and contain internal septations. It usually has a well-defined wall, with either smooth or irregular margins, that may enhance. Density values of the fluid range from 2–40 Hounsfield units (HU), depending on the protein content. The most specific sign is air bubbles within the abscess cavity, although this sign is seen in only 20% of cases.
- MRI: An abscess appears as a well-defined lesion of low signal intensity on T_1 images and bright signal intensity on T_2 images. The cavity may have homogeneous or heterogeneous signal, and septations may be seen. The capsule appears as a low-signal rim and may enhance with gadolinium.

Other causes of complex cysts, such as a focal hematoma and necrotic or hemorrhagic neoplasm, may have similar appearances.

19. **What causes fatty infiltration of the liver?**

Fatty infiltration of the liver is due to deposition of triglycerides within the hepatocytes and is associated with many disorders, including ethanol abuse, obesity, excessive steroids, hyperalimentation, diabetes, radiation or chemotherapy, and glycogen storage disease. It can cause slightly abnormal LFTs and hepatomegaly. Fatty infiltration may be diffuse or focal. Fatty infiltration or sparing occurs typically around the gallbladder fossa, in the medial segment near the falciform ligament and adjacent to the porta hepatis, because of the differing blood supply in these regions.

20. **Describe the imaging findings of fatty infiltration of the liver.**

- US: Fatty infiltration is seen as a focal or diffuse area of increased echogenicity. There is decreased visualization or nonvisualization of intrahepatic vessels, the deeper posterior por-tions of the liver, and the diaphragm posterior to the liver. US does not show any mass effect on adjacent biliary structures or blood vessels. The finding of diffusely increased echogenicity of the liver is nonspecific and can be seen in hepatitis or cirrhosis.
- CT: Fatty infiltration is seen as an area of decreased attenuation, which is easier to appreciate in the focal form with adjacent normal liver (Fig. 71-4). On noncontrast CT scan, the normal liver is usually 8 HU greater in density than the spleen, but in fatty infiltration it is less dense than the spleen by 10 HU or more. However, other lesions may appear as an area of decreased density on noncontrast CT, such as hepatomas and metastatic disease. In fatty infiltration, the

hepatic vessels stand out and may appear as if they contain contrast on an unenhanced scan. In focal fatty infiltration, the normal hepatic vessels traverse the area of decreased attenuation, a finding not seen in a malignant mass. Focal fatty infiltration tends to have linear margins and to be in a lobar distribution.

- MRI: Fat tissue typically has increased signal on T_1 images and decreased signal on T_2 images. Signal differences in focal fatty infiltration of the liver are not usually as dramatic as those seen in subcutaneous fat; in fact, the signal

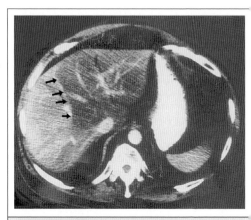

Figure 71-4. Focal fatty infiltration of the liver shown as a low-attenuation area next to normal liver *(arrows)*.

changes may be quite subtle. As with CT, it is important to see normal vessels in the area of signal abnormality and no mass effect on adjacent structures. Fat-suppression MRI scans are more sensitive than routine T_1 and T_2 scans and show fatty infiltration as areas of decreased signal intensity compared with normal liver. With chemical shift techniques, such as opposed phase imaging, fatty areas demonstrate decreased signal.

21. **Which imaging techniques are used to detect cirrhosis?**
    - US: Cirrhosis is characterized by abnormal echotexture. The hepatic parenchyma is typically hyperechoic with "coarsened" echoes, making the liver somewhat heterogeneous, and the intrahepatic vasculature is poorly defined. Unfortunately, these findings are nonspecific. Increased parenchymal echogenicity is also seen in fatty infiltration, and heterogeneity may be due to infiltrating neoplasm. Furthermore, no direct correlation exists between degree of hepatic dysfunction and sonographic appearance. More specific sonographic features of cirrhosis include nodularity of the liver surface and selective enlargement of the caudate lobe (Fig. 71-5, *A*). A caudate-to-right lobe volume ratio >0.65 is highly specific but not sensitive in diagnosing cirrhosis. In portal hypertension, the normal portal venous velocity is highly variable, but the Doppler detection of hepatofugal flow is diagnostic. Doppler also provides improved identification of portal collateral vessels, particularly the recanalized umbilical vein.
    - CT: Although early parenchymal changes may not be visible on CT, fatty infiltration (the initial manifestation of alcoholic liver disease) is well seen. The liver enlarges, and its attenuation becomes abnormally lower than that of the spleen. In later stages of cirrhosis, liver volume typically decreases. A nodular contour (due to regenerating nodules, scarring, and atrophy) may be seen, with somewhat heterogeneous enhancement. Regenerating nodules are isodense with liver and can be inferred only from contour deformity. The caudate lobe and lateral-segment left lobe are typically enlarged, and atrophy of the right lobe and medial-segment left lobe is seen. Mesenteric fat develops a higher attenuation than retroperitoneal or subcutaneous fat. CT demonstrates varices, ascites, and splenomegaly associated with portal hypertension (Fig. 71-5, *B*). Unlike sonography, CT cannot determine the direction of vascular flow, but it is superior in delineating the full extent of varices and collateral vessels.
    - MR: Early MR changes of cirrhosis include enlargement of the hilar periportal space in up to 98% of patients due to atrophy of the medial segment of the left hepatic lobe. Later findings include a caudate/right hepatic lobe ratio of >0.65. This finding has a specificity of up to 90%. An expanded gallbladder fossa sign is 98% specific for cirrhosis. MRI can help to distinguish between regenerative nodules, dysplastic nodules, and HCC. Regenerative nodules are

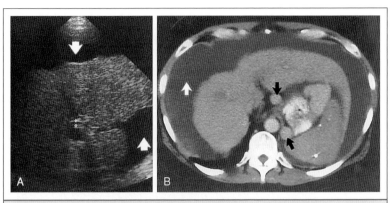

Figure 71-5. Cirrhosis. *A,* Ultrasound shows small, echogenic liver with nodular contour, compatible with cirrhosis. Low echogenicity ascites surrounds the liver *(arrows)*. *B,* CT demonstrates small liver with nodular contour and enhancing varices *(black arrows)* and extensive ascites *(white arrow)*.

variable in signal on the T_1-weighted images and usually iso to decreased in signal on the T_2-weighted sequences. Following gadolinium administration, the nodules usually demonstrate decreased T_1-weighted signal. Regenerating nodules can contain iron 25% of the time and are then known as siderotic nodules. This causes very low GRE and T_2-weighted signal. Dysplastic nodules are considered premalignant and comprise 25% of the nodules and often demonstrate increased T_1-weighted and decreased T_2-weighted signal; however, there is overlap. HCC has variable signal on both T_1- and T_2-weighted sequences but often has increased T_2 signal and demonstrates markedly increased vascularity on arterial phase imaging with portal washout. As the degree of malignancy increases, there is increased hepatic arterial flow to the nodules with decreased portal flow. A "nodule with a nodule" appearance is highly suggestive of a foci of HCC within a dysplastic nodule.

22. **What is the most sensitive examination for detecting hemochromatosis?**
MR and CT imaging rely on the increased iron content of the liver and other organs to diagnose hemochromatosis. US of the liver is normal despite iron deposition, unless underlying cirrhosis exists. Increased attenuation of the liver on CT is due to the high atomic number of iron, but it is not a specific finding; amiodarone, chemotherapy agents, gold therapy, and glycogen deposits can produce similar findings. The attenuation of the liver on noncontrast CT scans is typically >85 HU in hemochromatosis, compared with a normal attenuation of approximately 60 HU. On MR, the iron deposition causes decreased signal intensity compared with the paraspinal muscles because of paramagnetic effects. The findings are most striking on T_2 images but can be seen to a lesser extent on T_1 images. MR is more sensitive and specific than CT, and MR quantification in the future may eliminate the need for some liver biopsies.

23. **What is a normal Doppler wave form?**
The changing frequency of reflected sound waves from flowing blood allows US to calculate the velocity and direction of blood flow. A "normal" Doppler wave form is different for each artery or vein of the body. Veins have continuous low-velocity flow that frequently varies with respiration. In the portal vein, flow is hepatopetal and generally ranges from 15–25 cm/sec (Fig. 71-6, *A*). Flow velocity normally decreases during inspiration and increases during expiration. Arterial flow does not vary with respiration but varies dramatically with the cardiac cycle, showing high-velocity flow during systole and relatively high flow (i.e., low resistance) during diastole (Fig. 71-6, *B*). In fasting patients, the superior mesenteric artery has equally high systolic velocity

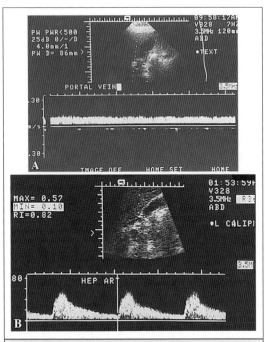

Figure 71-6. Doppler ultrasound. *A,* Normal blood flow in the portal vein. Flow registers above the baseline because it is traveling toward the ultrasound probe. *B,* Normal hepatic artery blood flow. Again, flow is toward the ultrasound probe. High-velocity flow represents systole, and lower-velocity flow represents diastole.

but minimal flow and even flow reversal during diastole (i.e., high resistance). Ingestion of a meal creates a lower resistance system by increasing the diastolic flow to the bowel with end arterial dilatation.

In both arteries and veins, color Doppler can be used to verify the presence and direction of flow. The operator determines whether blood flowing toward the transducer is blue or red, and blood flowing away from the transducer takes on the other color. Therefore, flow in arteries and veins is normally assigned a different color. Arteries also demonstrate color pulsation due to rapidly changing speed of flow.

24. **How are Doppler wave forms altered in portal vein thrombosis?**
In acute portal vein thrombosis, flow in the portal vein is markedly diminished or absent. In most instances, echogenic material is seen in the portal vein (Fig. 71-7, *A*), although in a few cases, the portal vein may appear normal. Doppler analysis yields no wave form, and with color imaging, no color is seen in the vessel. In the more chronic condition of cavernous transformation of the portal vein, the portal vein cannot be seen, but an echogenic structure in the porta hepatis represents a fibrotic remnant. The presence of multiple tubular channels in the porta hepatis with demonstrable flow by color imaging or Doppler evaluation is virtually diagnostic of cavernous transformation.

25. **Describe the effect of portal hypertension on Doppler wave forms.**
Portal hypertension can be suggested on US by a portal vein >13 mm with decreased flow velocity, although portal vein size is so variable that specific measurements are unreliable.

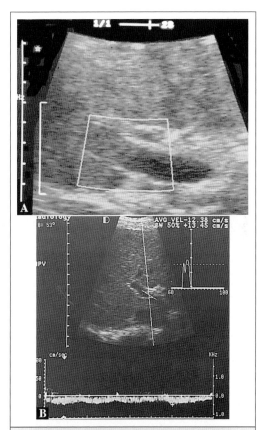

Figure 71-7. Doppler ultrasound. *A,* Echogenicity in the portal vein is due to thrombosis (inside *white square*) in a patient with HCC invading the portal vein. *B,* Hepatofugal blood flow registers below the baseline in the portal vein of a patient with known portal hypertension.

Retrograde (hepatofugal) flow in the portal vein indicates advanced disease and is a useful but late finding (Fig. 71-7, *B-C*). Detection of portosystemic collaterals aids greatly in detecting portal hypertension. The easiest collateral to detect by US is the recanalized paraumbilical vein (Fig. 71-7, *D*), which drains the left portal vein as it travels through the ligamentum teres to the abdominal wall. The coronary (left gastric) vein, another collateral vessel, originates at the portosplenic confluence and ascends to the gastroesophageal junction to feed esophageal varices. Detection of hepatofugal flow in the coronary vein is one of the best indicators of portal hypertension. Splenic varices are easily detected as tubular structures with flow in the splenic hilum. Other portosystemic collaterals include splenorenal shunts and retroperitoneal veins.

26. **How does Budd-Chiari syndrome affect Doppler wave forms?**
    Budd-Chiari syndrome refers to obstruction of hepatic venous outflow. It can occur at a number of levels, from the small hepatic venules to the inferior vena cava (IVC). Typically, the liver parenchyma is diffusely heterogeneous, but to make the diagnosis, one must observe echogenic thrombus or absent flow in one or more of the hepatic veins or the suprahepatic IVC.

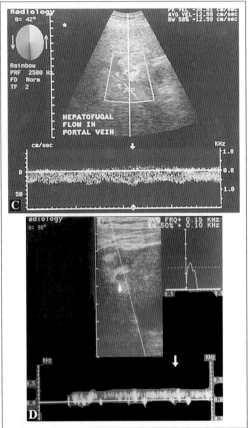

Figure 71-7. cont'd *C,* Color Doppler image registers blue (retrograde) flow in the portal vein in a patient with hypertension and hepatofugal flow. If direction of flow were normal, it would be red. (Courtesy of Patrick Meyers, RT.) *D,* Doppler-identified blood flow in the falciform ligament (in *white arrow*) is due to recanalized paraumbilical veins in a patient with portal hypertension. Note subhepatic ascites.

Twenty percent of patients have associated portal vein thrombosis, and many others have ascites.

27. **Discuss the role of US in the evaluation of transjugular intrahepatic portosystemic shunts (TIPS).**

Ultrasound is used for preprocedure evaluation and to assess shunt patency after the procedure. The preprocedure examination is obtained 24–48 hours before the TIPS. It assesses the size and parenchyma of the liver and spleen, flow characteristics of the hepatic and portal vessels, patency of the internal jugular veins, and presence or absence of varices and ascites.

A new baseline examination, documenting flow within the shunt and determining velocity measurements in the middle and at both ends of the shunt, is obtained 24–48 hours after the procedure. The flow is usually of high velocity and turbulent; however, there is a wide range of peak velocities in patent, well-functioning shunts (Fig. 71-8). A decrease in peak velocity, along

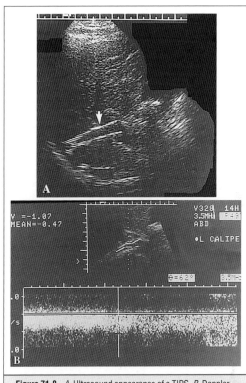

Figure 71-8. *A*, Ultrasound appearance of a TIPS. *B*, Doppler ultrasound showing flow within a patent TIPS.

with other signs of shunt failure, should prompt a portogram for further evaluation. Signs of a failing shunt include decreased velocity in the shunt, reaccumulation of ascites, reappearance or increased size of varices, and flow of blood away from the shunt. A peak shunt velocity of 50–60 cm/sec should prompt an angiographic study of the shunt to evaluate for stenosis. Routine follow-up imaging is recommended every 3 months.

BILIARY TRACT IMAGING

28. **What is the significance of gallbladder wall thickening on US?**
    A wall thickness >3 mm in a distended gallbladder is abnormal and must be explained. Abnormal wall thickness, combined with a sonographic Murphy's sign and gallstones, has a positive predictive value of >90% for acute cholecystitis, the most common cause of pathologic wall thickening. Many other conditions can cause gallbladder wall thickening. Congestive heart failure and constrictive pericarditis cause congestive hepatomegaly, which is often accompanied by a thickened, edematous gallbladder wall. Hypoalbuminemia, secondary to chronic liver dysfunction or nephrotic syndrome, results in a decrease in plasma oncotic pressure that produces generalized tissue edema, including edema of the gallbladder wall. Portal venous congestion from portal hypertension of any cause and hepatic veno-occlusive disease can produce gallbladder wall thickening. Inflammation of the gallbladder from nearby hepatitis or

AIDS-related cholangitis may produce wall thickening. Chronic cholecystitis, adenomyomatosis, primary sclerosing cholangitis, and leukemic infiltration are additional causes of wall thickening. Gallbladder carcinoma also causes wall thickening but is easily differentiated by its masslike appearance and association with adenopathy and liver metastases.

29. **Describe the radiologic work-up of suspected biliary tree obstruction.**

US is the screening examination of choice when biliary ductal disease is suspected. Normal nondilated intrahepatic ducts are 1–2 mm in diameter and are not usually visualized. The size of the common hepatic duct (CHD) is a sensitive indicator of the presence of biliary obstruction; it is more sensitive than intrahepatic ducts in assessing early or partial biliary obstruction. The normal CHD is 4–5 mm in diameter; a diameter >6 mm indicates ductal dilatation (Fig. 71-9, *A*). However, extrahepatic ductal diameter increases with age and may be increased after cholecystectomy or resolved obstruction. Thus, dilated ducts are not the equivalent of obstruction. Repeat scanning after an oral fatty meal or intravenous cholecystokinin may help to distinguish dilatation due to obstruction. A dilated CHD that fails to decrease in size or increases after this provocative test indicates obstruction. In complicated cases, Doppler examination can readily differentiate the biliary ducts from vasculature in the portal triad. With intrahepatic ductal dilatation, tubular low-echogenicity structures are seen to parallel the portal veins, producing the "too many tubes" sign.

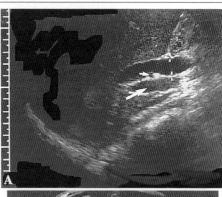

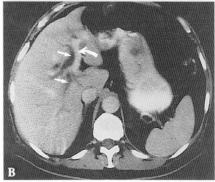

Figure 71-9. *A*, Ultrasound demonstrates a dilated common biliary duct, marked by calipers, measuring 15.7 mm in a patient with a CBD stricture. A hypoechoic portal vein *(long arrow)* and hepatic artery *(short arrow)* are seen posterior to the CBD. *B*, CT demonstrates a dilated intrahepatic biliary tree *(straight arrow)* adjacent to an enhancing portal vein *(curved arrow)* in a patient with pancreatic carcinoma.

Although US is the best screening exam for biliary disease, once disease is detected, CT is more efficacious in depicting the degree, site, and cause of obstruction. CT provides more complete delineation of the full length of the common bile duct (CBD), because bowel gas commonly obscures sonographic visualization of the distal CBD. The normal CBD is up to 6 mm, whereas a 9-mm CBD is considered dilated (Fig. 71-9, *B*).

Newer techniques allow the diagnosis of biliary ductal dilatation by MR cholangiopancreatography (MRCP). ERCP and percutaneous transhepatic cholangiography provide more detailed evaluations than US or CT but are invasive.

30. What is MRCP? What advantages does it have compared with ERCP?

MRCP is a noninvasive way to evaluate the hepatobiliary tract. MRCP can demonstrate the common bile duct in 98% of patients and can evaluate the pancreatic duct in the head, body, and tail in 97%, 97%, and 83% of patients, respectively. It can differentiate dilated from normal ducts in 95% of patients and is comparable to ERCP (and exceeds the accuracy of CT and US) in detecting choledocholithiasis. It is comparable to ERCP in detecting extrahepatic strictures, and it is 98% accurate in detecting aberrant hepatic ducts and 95% accurate in demonstrating the cystic duct.

MRCP is comparable to ERCP in diagnosing extrahepatic bile and pancreatic duct abnormalities, and it is the modality of choice for imaging patients with biliary-enteric anastomosis. It is more sensitive than ERCP in detecting pseudocysts and is potentially more accurate in evaluating biliary cystadenomas and cystadenocarcinomas.

The advantages of MRCP over ERCP are that it is noninvasive and less expensive, does not require radiation or sedation, can detect extraductal pathology, better visualizes ducts proximal to an obstruction, and visualizes the ducts in their "native" state. The drawbacks of MRCP are that it has decreased spatial resolution and difficulty with imaging nondilated, peripheral intrahepatic, or side ducts. However, the main drawback of MRCP is that it may delay therapeutic intervention in patients with a high clinical suspicion of bile duct obstruction.

31. Describe the differential imaging features seen in the common causes of biliary obstruction.

1. Biliary obstruction may be related to biliary disease (choledocholithiasis, cholangitis, cholangiocarcinoma) or extrabiliary disease (pancreatitis, periampullary carcinoma). Intrahepatic ductal dilatation with a normal CBD suggests an intrahepatic mass or abnormality. Dilatation of the pancreatic duct typically localizes the obstruction to the pancreatic or ampullary level.

2. An abrupt transition from a dilated CBD to a narrowed or obliterated duct is more characteristic of a neoplasm or stone, whereas a gradual tapering of the CBD at the pancreatic head is typical of fibrosis associated with chronic pancreatitis.

3. US is 60–70% accurate in detecting common duct stones; unlike gallbladder calculi, CBD stones do not necessarily cause acoustic shadowing. CT detection requires thin-section (3-mm) acquisition. Depending on their composition, stones may be seen as soft tissue or calcific intraluminal densities.

4. Cholangiocarcinoma should be suspected in patients with abrupt biliary obstruction but no visualized mass or stone. The primary mass is commonly difficult to identify by US or CT. Because cholangiocarcinoma often arises near or at the liver hilum (Klatskin's tumor), it commonly presents with dilated intrahepatic ducts and normal-sized extrahepatic ducts. MRCP and MR imaging with a hepatobiliary agent or gadolinium is beneficial in the diagnosis. Cholangiocarcinoma is typically low T_1, high T_2 and demonstrates progressive delayed enhancement on MRI due to the fibrous tissue in the tumor. This can be helpful in determining the area to perform a biopsy.

5. An abrupt versus tapered appearance of the CBD helps to differentiate pancreatic carcinoma from chronic pancreatitis. However, chronic pancreatitis can also present as a focal mass, and a biopsy may be required for differentiation.

PANCREATIC IMAGING

32. How can acute pancreatitis be distinguished from chronic pancreatitis on imaging?

Acute: The classic sonographic appearance of acute pancreatitis is a hypoechoic, diffusely enlarged pancreas, although focal involvement may be seen in 18% of cases. US is inferior to CT in evaluating acute pancreatitis for several reasons: (1) overlying bowel gas frequently limits complete visualization of the gland; (2) definition of extent of peripancreatic fluid collections is inferior to that of CT; and (3) US cannot diagnose pancreatic necrosis. Therefore, CT is the preferred study in patients with clinically severe pancreatitis. However, US is effective in follow-up of pseudocysts, which may be echo-free or have internal echogenicity because of hemorrhage or debris.

CT is typically performed with intravenous contrast, but if hemor-rhagic pancreatitis is suspected, noncontrast images should be first performed to detect high-attenua-tion hemorrhage. CT may be nor-mal in *mild* cases of pancreatitis, whereas with *moderate* disease the gland becomes enlarged and slightly heterogeneous, with inflammation causing peripancre-atic fat to have a higher attenuation ("dirty fat"). With *severe* disease, intraglandular intravasation of pan-creatic fluid causes intrapancreatic fluid collections, and extravasation causes peripancreatic fluid collec-tions, peripancreatic inflammation, and thickened fascial planes (Fig. 71-10, *A*). Fluid collections are most common in the anterior pararenal space and lesser sac but may have wide extension.

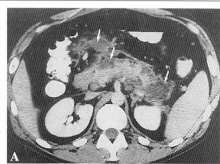
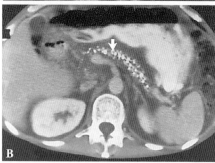

Figure 71-10. Pancreatitis. *A*, CT in acute pancreatitis demonstrates extensive peripancreatic fluid collections *(arrows)*. *B*, CT shows multiple pancreatic calcifications *(arrows)* in a patient with chronic pancreatitis.

Chronic: Sonography is 60–80% accurate in diagnosing chronic pancreatitis, and dilatation o the pancreatic duct is the most specific sonographic abnormality. Calcifications are seen as echogenic, shadowing foci within the gland. The gland may be enlarged early in the disease but atrophic or focally enlarged later. Parenchymal echogenicity is variable.

Similar findings are noted with CT. Alteration of gland size is variable, and focal enlarge-ment due to a chronic inflammatory mass may necessitate biopsy to exclude carcinoma. The pancreatic duct can be dilated (>3 mm) to the level of the papilla and may appear beaded, irregular, or smooth. Calcifications are the most reliable CT indicator of chronic pancreatitis and are seen in 50% of cases (Fig. 71-10, *B*). Pseudocysts may be seen within or adjacent to the gland.

33. **Describe the role of CT and US in assessing the complications of pancreatitis.**
   1. *Pseudocysts* evolve from fluid collections in about 30–50% of patients with acute pancreatitis. The development of a pseudocyst requires at least 4 weeks. More than half of those measuring <5 cm regress spontaneously. Pseudocysts failing to resolve or causing symptoms (pain, infection, hemorrhage, GI obstruction, or fistula) require drainage. On CT, a pseudocyst appears as an oval fluid collection with a nonepithelialized, enhancing wall. US demonstrates an anechoic fluid collection with or without internal debris surrounded by a thin wall. Gas bubbles inside a pseudocyst relate to infection or fistula formation within the bowel.

2. *Pancreatic ascites* presents as free intraperitoneal fluid with high amylase levels in about 7% of patients with acute pancreatitis. Patients tend to have severe disease with obvious additional CT abnormalities, but in rare patients, the pancreas appears normal; in such cases, percutaneous drainage of fluid and evaluation of amylase level is needed to establish the diagnosis.

3. In acute pancreatitis, CT can detect *necrosis* with a sensitivity of about 75–80%. Necrosis is defined as a lack of contrast enhancement in the expected location of pancreatic tissue, and it can develop early or late in the course of the illness. The degree of necrosis is an important prognostic factor. Patients with no CT evidence of necrosis have no mortality and a morbidity rate of only 6%. Patients with mild necrosis (<30% of the total gland) exhibit no mortality but have a rate of complications of 40%, and patients with more severe necrosis (>50%) have a morbidity rate of 75–100% and a mortality rate of 11–25%. Necrotic tissue can become secondarily infected, which is recognized on CT as gas bubbles within areas of pancreatic gland necrosis (i.e., emphysematous pancreatitis). More commonly, infected areas do not contain gas, and a culture of a percutaneous aspirate is needed to verify the diagnosis and identify the organism.

4. *Pancreatic abscesses* result from liquefactive necrosis with subsequent infection. CT shows a focal low-attenuation fluid collection with thick enhancing walls. Gas bubbles may be present. US shows a hypoechoic or even anechoic mass with a surrounding hyperechoic wall. Rates of abscess formation vary with the amount of pancreatic necrosis. Abscesses usually occur 4 weeks after the onset of acute pancreatitis. The distinction between abscess and infected necrosis can be difficult, but it is an important one because the treatment alternatives are quite different.

5. *Pseudoaneurysms,* resulting from enzymatic breakdown of the arterial wall, most commonly involve the splenic artery, followed by the gastroduodenal and pancreaticoduodenal arteries. Pseudoaneurysm rupture can cause massive hemorrhage and may occur into the retroperitoneum, peritoneal cavity, pancreatic duct, pseudocyst, or bowel, causing a GI tract bleed. CT is probably best for identifying pseudoaneurysms. High-density areas in or around a pseudoaneurysm represent either acute thrombus or hemorrhage. US with color Doppler can be just as sensitive in detecting pseudoaneurysms and their complications, provided that there is no overlying bowel gas.

6. *Splenic vein thrombosis* is detected by lack of normal enhancement in the expected region of the splenic vein on CT. Color Doppler can be used to make the same diagnosis. Thrombosis of the portal and superior mesenteric veins, although less common, is also well imaged by both modalities.

34. What are the imaging findings of pancreatic ductal adenocarcinoma?

1. *Pancreatic enlargement.* Although enlargement may be focal or diffuse, focal enlargement is more common. Diffuse enlargement is often secondary to pancreatitis caused by the neoplasm. Focal enlargement is better appreciated in the body and tail of the pancreas.

2. *Distortion of the pancreatic contour or shape.* Pancreatic cancer may also cause a focal bulge or irregularity of the organ surface. Involvement of the uncinate process of the pancreas may cause it to have a focal bulge or rounded appearance. Enlargement and contour distortion are the most frequent findings of pancreatic cancer.

3. *Difference in density or echogenicity.* On US, pancreatic cancer tends to be hypoechoic compared with normal pancreas; however, it may also appear isoechoic compared with normal pancreas. On CT, it is usually hypodense in comparison with normal pancreas; this distinction is better demonstrated with the use of intravenous contrast.

4. *Pancreatic duct dilatation* can be an important clue of a small neoplasm that may not be appreciated otherwise. It is more common when the neoplasm is located in the pancreatic head.

5. *Biliary tract dilatation.* Bile duct dilatation is more commonly seen with a neoplasm in the head of the pancreas. Isolated intrahepatic biliary ductal dilatation may be seen with pancreatic cancer that has spread to the porta hepatis.

6. *Local invasion* into the peripancreatic fat is most commonly seen, but invasion into the porta hepatis, stomach, spleen, and adjacent bowel loops may also occur.

7. *Regional lymph node enlargement.* Pancreatic cancer may spread to the nodes in the porta hepatis, para-aortic region, and region around the celiac and superior mesenteric artery axis.

8. *Liver metastasis.* The liver is a common site of metastasis for pancreatic cancer. Metastases appear as low-density lesions and may be single or multiple.

35. **Which imaging modality is best for detecting and evaluating pancreatic cancer?**
The two primary modalities to evaluate suspected pancreatic cancer are US and CT. Triple-phase CT is probably the best first-line imaging modality. CT is better at evaluating adjacent spread or nodal involvement than US, and it does not have the problem of incomplete evaluation of the body and tail of the pancreas, which occurs in up to 25% of US examinations. Overlying bowel gas can obscure these areas on US. In patients who present with biliary obstruction, both US and CT are good first-line examinations. Dynamic MR imaging with gadolinium can be performed in patients with iodine contrast allergy.

36. **What are the common cystic pancreatic neoplasms?**
Serous (microcystic) and mucinous (macrocystic) cystic neoplasms are the most common. Serous tumors are more common in women, and 82% occur in people age 60 or older. They are almost always benign and predominate in the pancreatic head. Serous tumors calcify more commonly (50%) than any other pancreatic tumors and are typified by a central stellate scar that frequently calcifies. They typically comprise numerous <2-cm cysts. On US, the mass is often hyperechoic because the multiple small cysts may not be individually resolved. The hyperechoic central stellate scar and calcifications suggest the diagnosis and may be seen on US or CT. The CT appearance is also varied; innumerable minute cysts may appear as a solid tumor, whereas multiple small but visible cysts have a honeycomb or "Swiss-cheese" appearance. Soft-tissue components enhance with contrast, and the pancreatic contour may be lobulated.

Mucinous cystic neoplasms also have a strong female predominance but tend to occur in younger patients. They have a strong predilection for the pancreatic tail (85%), calcify in 30% of cases, and must be considered malignant. They are larger lesions, averaging 12 cm, and are composed of unilocular or multilocular cysts >2 cm. US demonstrates internal septations that may be few or many, thick or thin. These septations are thicker than those in microcystic tumors, and the septations may calcify, which is better seen with CT. The tumor wall and organ of origin are better demonstrated with CT, whereas internal septations and solid excrescences are better seen by US. Differential diagnostic considerations include papillary cystic tumor, cystic islet cell tumor, cystic metastasis, pseudocysts, and abscess.

ABDOMINAL AND PELVIC IMAGING

37. **How is simple ascites distinguished from complicated ascites?**
Simple ascites is a watery transudate that is usually secondary to major organ system failure (i.e., hepatic, renal, or cardiac failure). Because it is a transudate, simple ascites has a CT density similar to water (0–20 HU). In general, as the protein content of the fluid increases, so do the Hounsfield units. By US, simple ascites is anechoic, without internal echoes or septations, and demonstrates increased through transmission. Simple ascites is "free flowing" and located in the dependent portions of the abdomen and pelvis. It is often found in Morison's pouch, paracolic gutters, and the pelvis. With large amounts of ascites, the bowel seems to float within the fluid, usually in the center of the abdomen. Simple ascites has also a sharp, smooth interface with other intra-abdominal contents (Figs. 71-11, *A–B*).

Loculated ascites is not a "simple" fluid collection, because it indicates the presence of adhesions. The adhesions may be due to benign causes (e.g., prior surgery) or an infectious or malignant process. Loculated ascites is typically located in nondependent portions of the

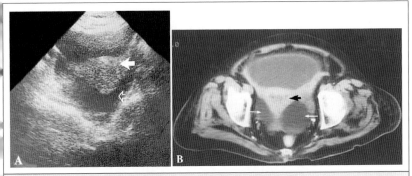

Figure 71-11. Ascites. *A,* Ultrasound and, *B,* CT scan showing simple ascites *(arrows)* in the pelvis adjacent to the uterus *(arrowhead).*

abdomen, does not move when the patient is scanned in a different position, and often displaces adjacent bowel loops.

Complex ascites is usually secondary to an infectious, hemorrhagic, or neoplastic process. The findings of complex ascites include density greater than water, internal debris or septations, air bubbles within the collection, or a thick or nodular border or capsule (Figs. 71-11, *C–D*). Usually, the density measurements must be >20 HU to be considered complex, reflecting the increased protein content. Some complex fluid collections do not have these findings and may appear simple. Often aspiration is the only way to confirm whether a collection is simple.

38. **How does one differentiate abdominal fluid from pleural fluid?**
    Both US and CT are good modalities to ascertain whether a collection is intra-abdominal or pleural. If the collection can be seen by US, it usually outlines the diaphragm, making the determination less confusing. Certain signs have been described to make this differentiation on CT:
    1. Ascites is located anterior or lateral to the diaphragmatic crus, whereas pleural fluid is located posterior or medial to the crus.
    2. Pleural effusion can extend medial to the crus and appear to touch the spine or aorta.
    3. Abdominal fluid is often contiguous with other abdominal fluid collections.
    4. Ascites has a sharp interface with intra-abdominal organs, such as the liver and spleen. Pleural fluid has a less sharp interface because the diaphragm lies between the fluid and abdominal organs.
    5. Ascitic fluid spares the bare area of the liver, which lies between the left and right coronary ligaments along the posterior border of the right lobe of the liver. These bare areas are peritoneal reflections that suspend the liver from the diaphragm; peritoneal fluid cannot pass through these ligaments to accumulate in the bare area. However, because bare area is in contact with the diaphragm, pleural fluid can accumulate behind the bare area.

39. **When is CT used to evaluate the small bowel?**
    Conventional barium examinations remain superior to CT for evaluating intraluminal and mucosal disease, but CT is far better for evaluating the intramural component of small bowel as well as the adjacent mesentery, omentum, retroperitoneum, peritoneal cavity, and viscera. Optimal evaluation requires opacification and distention with oral and intravenous contrast. With adequate distention, the thickness of the bowel wall is about 2 mm.

    Smooth and concentric thickening of the bowel wall (7–11 mm) is a typical appearance for nonmalignant disease (e.g., Crohn's, ulcerative colitis, Shönlein-Henoch purpura, intramural hemorrhage, bowel edema from portal hypertension, and ischemic, infectious, or radiation enteritis). Extraintestinal findings are an important part of the exam. For example, with Crohn's

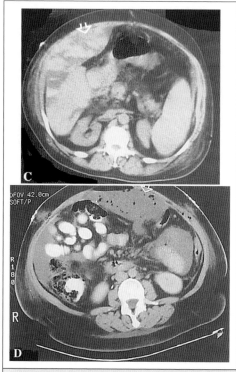

Figure 71-11. cont'd *C,* Intra-abdominal hemorrhage presenting as a complex fluid collection. *D,* Intra-abdominal abscess presenting as a complex fluid collection with multiple air bubbles.

disease, one should look for associated abscesses, fibrofatty proliferation, fistulas, and inflammation of the mesentery.

Thickening of the skin and increased density of the mesenteric and subcutaneous fat can accompany radiation enteritis, which typically involves bowel in the pelvis. Severe cases of ischemic enteritis can demonstrate portal venous gas, intramural hemorrhage, or blood elsewhere in the peritoneal cavity (Fig. 71-12).

Eccentric and irregular bowel wall thickening >2 cm is suspicious for carcinoma, especially if confined to a short segment. Lymphoma should be considered if this finding is associated with massive mesenteric or retroperitoneal adenopathy; adenocarcinoma

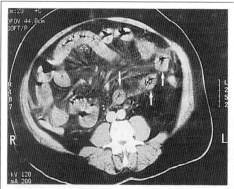

Figure 71-12. Thickening of multiple loops of small bowel due to ischemia in a patient with mesenteric infarction. Thickened loops are best seen in both longitudinal *(open arrow)* and cross-sectional *(arrows)* planes.

should be considered in the presence of associated liver lesions. Most benign small bowel tumors, such as neurofibromas and leiomyomas, are difficult to distinguish from malignant tumors. Lipomas are the exception. They are easily recognized by their low attenuation (−90 to −120 HU). Small bowel carcinoids are typically located in the right lower quadrant, characteristically contain calcification, and have a surrounding desmoplastic reaction.

Enteroenteric intussusception is easily defined by the invaginated low-density mesenteric fat situated between the higher density of the inner intussusceptum and the outer intussuscipiens. The underlying neoplasm may not be seen.

CT is also a useful tool in the evaluation of *small bowel obstruction,* especially when the diagnosis is in doubt or the patient has certain medical conditions (e.g., inflammatory bowel disease, known abdominal tumor). It can determine the cause and level of obstruction in up to 95% of cases, particularly those cases with a high-grade obstruction. CT findings can play a role in patient management by helping to separate patients requiring immediate surgery from patients who can be observed. It is also able to diagnose closed-loop obstruction and bowel strangulation.

40. How is CT used to evaluate the large bowel?

Optimal evaluation of the colon requires bowel preparation and luminal distention with rectal contrast or air to evaluate true wall thickness. Normal wall thickness of a distended colon is <3 mm. Inflammatory bowel disease, diverticulitis, appendicitis, and staging of colorectal or pelvic cancer are indications for optimal colonic distention. The addition of intravenous contrast facilitates the evaluation of the bowel wall and improves the evaluation of solid organs and vascular structures.

Diverticulitis is well suited for evaluation with CT because it is a pericolic process rather than a disease of the lumen. Acute findings include increased density in the pericolic fat, thickening of the bowel wall, and diverticula. CT is excellent for imaging complications of diverticulitis (e.g., abscess, fistula formation). It can be difficult to differentiate between perforated sigmoid carcinoma and diverticulitis with CT alone. Wall thickening that is excessive (>3 cm) or eccentric favors sigmoid carcinoma.

Circumferential wall thickening (Fig. 71-13, *A*) is a nonspecific finding in numerous conditions, including Crohn's disease, ischemic colitis, pseudomembranous colitis, radiation colitis, neutropenic colitis, and inflammatory colitis due to cytomegalovirus or *Campylobacter* infection. Benign intestinal wall thickening of an involved segment can present either as homogeneous enhancing soft-tissue density or, less commonly, as concentric rings of high and low attenuation—termed the "double halo" or target sign (Fig. 71-13, *B*). Concentric rings result from hyperemic enhancement of the mucosa and serosa (high attenuation) and submucosal edema (low attenuation).

The cause of wall thickening can sometimes be determined by location or associated findings. For example, bowel wall thickening in the region of the splenic flexure suggests ischemic disease from occlusion of the superior mesenteric artery. Thickening of the rectosigmoid colon and pelvic small bowel loops suggest radiation enteritis. Inflammation from a ruptured appendix can produce wall thickening mimicking a primary cecal process, and a severe episode of pancreatitis can cause thickening of the transverse colon, if inflammatory changes spread through the transverse mesocolon (Fig. 71-13, *C*).

Irregular, eccentric, or lobulated wall thickening is suggestive of *adenocarcinoma.* In some cases, an intraluminal polypoid mass can be seen. CT is only 50% accurate in staging the tumor by the Dukes system. However, findings of regional adenopathy, retroperitoneal adenopathy, or liver metastases help to confirm the diagnosis of carcinoma. The large tumor mass usually enhances heterogeneously secondary to regions of necrosis, and local tumor extension is usually masslike. In the absence of perforation, the surrounding pericolic fat maintains its homogeneous low attenuation in contrast to inflammatory conditions. CT is useful in evaluating anastomotic recurrence from colorectal carcinoma, which can occur in the serosa beyond the reach of the endoscope. PET (positron emission tomography) imaging is being used to stage colorectal carcinoma.

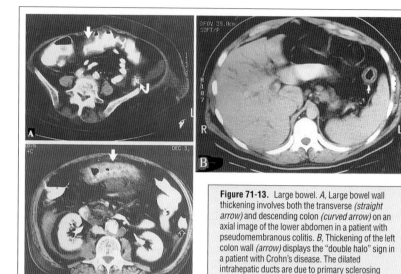

Figure 71-13. Large bowel. *A,* Large bowel wall thickening involves both the transverse *(straight arrow)* and descending colon *(curved arrow)* on an axial image of the lower abdomen in a patient with pseudomembranous colitis. *B,* Thickening of the left colon wall *(arrow)* displays the "double halo" sign in a patient with Crohn's disease. The dilated intrahepatic ducts are due to primary sclerosing cholangitis. *C,* Wall thickening of the transverse colon *(arrows)* in both longitudinal and cross-sectional planes in a patient with severe pancreatitis.

Lymphoma of the colon presents differently from adenocarcinoma. It thickens the wall to a much greater degree, often up to 4 cm. Lymphoma is rarely isolated to the colon, and additional sites of involvement should be sought.

41. **Describe the optimal radiographic work-up of diverticulitis.**

CT is generally considered the most efficacious method for the radiologic diagnosis of diverticulitis. Abdominal plain films are typically noncontributory. The barium enema depicts diverticula and may demonstrate fistulous tracts or extrinsic luminal defects related to the adjacent inflammatory process. CT is superior because it directly depicts the severity of the pericolic inflammation and the full degree of intraperitoneal or retroperitoneal extension. It is more sensitive than a barium study in detecting abscesses and fistulas.

The hallmark of acute diverticulitis on CT is increased attenuation in the pericolic fat (so-called *dirty fat;* Fig. 71-14). With greater degrees of inflammation, a soft tissue phlegmon or a fluid or, occasionally, air-containing abscess may be seen. With free perforation, air bubbles may be seen in the peritoneal cavity or retroperitoneum. Diverticula and a thickened bowel wall (>4 mm) are usually present, but these

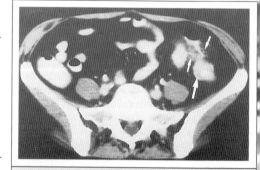

Figure 71-14. Typical CT appearance of diverticulitis, with stranding and increased density of the pericolic fat *(short arrows)* and thickening of the descending colon *(long arrow).*

findings are nonspecific and may also be seen with diverticulosis. The bowel wall thickening may, occasionally, be difficult to distinguish from that seen in colon cancer; however, an abrupt transition zone is more suggestive of tumor, and pericolic fatty inflammation suggests diverticulitis.

The assessment of the colon by CT is greatly improved with adequate colonic opacification or distention, which can be achieved with oral contrast or, if the patient has no peritoneal signs, with rectal air insufflation or water-soluble contrast per rectum.

42. What are the CT and US findings of acute appendicitis?

- US: Findings of acute appendicitis include a distended and noncompressible appendix, appendicolith, adjacent fluid collection, peritoneal fluid, and a focal mixed echogenic mass representing a phlegmon or abscess. The normal anterior-posterior dimension of the appendix is 5–6 mm; larger dimensions are considered abnormal (Fig. 71-15).
- CT: The hallmark finding is a distended (>6 mm) and thick-walled appendix. An appendicolith may be seen in one fourth of cases. Local signs of inflammation include increased density or stranding in the adjacent fat tissue, focal thickening of adjacent fascia, focal fluid collections, and adjacent phlegmon or abscess.

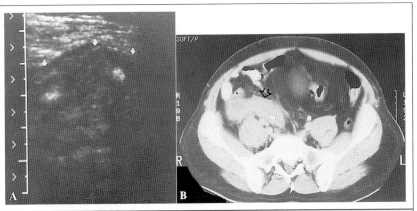

Figure 71-15. Acute appendicitis. *A,* Ultrasound shows a thickened appendix wall *(arrows)* and echogenic appendicolitis. *B,* CT shows a distal fluid-filled appendix and a calcified appendicolith.

43. Which examination is better for diagnosing acute appendicitis?

The 96% sensitivity of CT is superior to that of ultrasound (85–90%). The specificity is comparable at 90%. CT is better at showing a normal appendix and at showing the extent of adjacent inflammatory changes. The disadvantages of CT are its higher cost, use of ionizing radiation, and use of contrast material. US is highly operator-dependent but is usually a good first choice in children, pregnant women, and thin people. CT should be used for all other types of patients and is highly effective in heavier patients.

44. Discuss the role of imaging in the assessment of intra-abdominal abscess.

US: In suspected intra-abdominal abscess, US has the advantage of being performed at the patient's bedside. It is best suited for evaluation of abscesses in the pelvis and right and left upper quadrants, where the bladder, liver, and spleen, respectively, provide acoustic windows for sound transmission. However, assessment of the midabdomen is commonly impossible because of overlying bowel gas. Abscesses have a varied appearance but are commonly irregularly marginated and primarily hypoechoic, with internal areas of increased echogenicity.

CT: The entire abdomen and pelvis should be scanned after the administration of sufficient oral contrast to opacify the bowel, because fluid-filled bowel loops can easily simulate an abscess. Rectal contrast may also be helpful. The CT appearance of an abscess depends on its maturity. Initially, an abscess may appear as a soft-tissue density mass. As it matures and undergoes liquefactive necrosis, the central region develops a near-water attenuation, possibly with internal air bubbles or an air-fluid level (Fig. 71-16). Granulation tissue forming the wall of the abscess typically enhances with intravenous contrast, providing a higher attenuation rim. Mass effect with displacement of surrounding structures may be seen, and increased density in the adjacent fat is common.

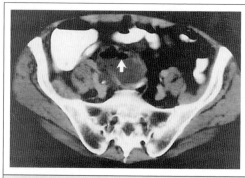

Figure 71-16. Abdominal abscess with air-fluid level *(arrow)* and internal debris.

Scintigraphy: Radionuclide imaging may be performed with gallium-67 citrate or indium-111–labeled white blood cells (WBCs). The advantage of scintigraphy is that it provides whole-body images and may detect infection in unsuspected sites. Gallium images, however, may require 48–72 hours for optimal interpretation, and normal colonic excretion of gallium may cause confusion in interpretation. Indium-labeled WBC imaging is more rapid than Ga-67, but uptake is somewhat nonspecific, and the liver and spleen are difficult to evaluate because of normal uptake in these organs.

Recommendations: CT is the first choice for detecting abscess in acutely ill patients. US can be used as the initial exam, if the abscess is suspected in the right or left upper quadrant or pelvis and in patients with suspected appendiceal abscess. Radionuclide scintigraphy can be considered the initial screening technique in patients without localizing signs and acute illness.

45. **How effective is CT colonography in screening for polyps?**
Colonography is the standard procedure for evaluating the colon because of the ability for direct visualization of the mucosa. The sensitivity for detection of lesions >1 cm is approximately 95%. The sensitivity for barium enema in detecting large adenomas is 80–90%; however, barium enemas are being performed less frequently due to the increases in colonoscopy, decreased interest in performing the procedure by radiologists, and because of the low reimbursement amounts. Using thin-section multirow detector CT, CT colonography is an effective screening test for polyps >10 mm. Sensitivities range from 73–100% for polyps >10 mm. The specificity for polyps >10 mm is reported to be >90%. However, there is a steep learning curve for the interpretation of the exams and only very well-trained and experienced radiologists should interpret the exams.

AIDS-RELATED DISORDERS

46. **What characteristic features of AIDS are seen in the biliary system?**
Gallbladder and bile duct abnormalities, including gallbladder wall thickening, sludge, cholelithiasis, bile duct dilatation, bile duct wall thickening, pericholecystic fluid, and a sonographic Murphy's sign, can be seen in as many as 20% of AIDS patients during US. The most common abnormality, *gallbladder wall thickening,* is often asymptomatic and not related to intrinsic gallbladder disease but rather to edema from hepatitis or hypoproteinemia. Gallbladder wall thickening associated with a positive Murphy's sign is suggestive of acalculous cholecystitis, either secondary to cytomegalovirus or *Cryptosporidium* infection.

AIDS-related cholangitis is usually secondary to cytomegalovirus or *Cryptosporidium* infection. US is the best noninvasive test for evaluating the extrahepatic ducts, but CT is better for evaluating the intrahepatic ducts. ERCP better displays the morphologic appearance of the entire ductal system than either modality, and the findings of dilated ducts, papillary narrowing, diffuse intrahepatic strictures, extrahepatic strictures, or any combination of these findings seen in AIDS-related cholangitis mimic those of sclerosing cholangitis, papillary stenosis, or both. Patients with papillary stenosis or isolated extrahepatic ductal involvement benefit most from sphincterotomy or common bile duct stents.

Biliary ductal dilatation can also be caused by obstruction from enlarged lymph nodes in the porta hepatis from *Kaposi's sarcoma* or *lymphoma*. Non–AIDS-related conditions, such as biliary calculi, cholangiocarcinoma, or pancreatic carcinoma, may also be a consideration. A search for these entities should be made in the appropriate clinical setting.

47. **Describe the imaging features of AIDS in the liver.**
Hepatomegaly is seen in nearly 20% of patients with AIDS. It is usually a nonspecific response to infection, hepatitis, fatty infiltration, or neoplastic infiltration from lymphoma or Kaposi's sarcoma. Approximately 10% of AIDS patients have diffusely increased liver echogenicity on US due to either *fatty infiltration* caused by malnutrition (a fatty liver has decreased attenuation on CT) or *hepatic granulomatosis* caused by *Mycobacterium avium-intracellulare, M. tuberculosis, Cryptococcus* spp., histoplasmosis, cytomegalovirus, toxoplasmosis, or a drug reaction from sulfonamides. Infection in the liver can also take the form of single or multiple liver abscesses. On US, such lesions may have increased, decreased, or mixed echogenicity, but with CT they are generally low in attenuation. Microscopic involvement of the liver may show few changes on CT and US, and a core biopsy may be the only method of diagnosis. When infection involves the liver, it is almost always secondary to disseminated disease, and one should search for associated abnormalities, such as cholangitis, adenopathy, splenomegaly, and ascites.

Kaposi's sarcoma (KS) is the most common neoplasm in AIDS; however, the diagnosis of liver involvement is rarely made antemortem. The findings are variable because the tumor is multifocal. US shows hepatomegaly and hyperechoic lesions in the parenchyma (often adjacent to the portal veins), whereas on contrast-enhanced CT, lesions are initially low in attenuation but enhance after time (4–7 min) to become either homogeneous with or more attenuated than the surrounding liver parenchyma. KS is more likely to present as adenopathy in the retroperitoneum, mesentery, or mediastinum than as lesions in the liver.

Lymphoma is more commonly extranodal in patients with AIDS than in the general population, and the liver and spleen are two of the more common extranodal sites. Both CT and US show one or more visceral lesions. With US, lesions are usually hypoechoic, whereas on CT they are generally low in attenuation. Organ involvement may be the sole manifestation, yet, normally, lymphoma is associated with bulky adenopathy of the retroperitoneum, mesentery, or mediastinum.

48. **What extrahepatic manifestations of AIDS in the GI tract can be noted by imaging?**
HIV-positive patients often demonstrate hepatosplenomegaly, and CT may show multiple, small (<5-mm) mesenteric or retroperitoneal nodes. Proctitis may be seen as a thickened rectal wall with increased attenuation of perirectal fat. Patients with clinical AIDS often demonstrate an opportunistic infection or tumor on CT or US. Enlargement of lymph nodes suggests AIDS rather than HIV disease, and focal defects in solid organs suggest either abscess or tumor infiltration.

GI tract involvement with KS is common (as is skin involvement), and submucosal nodules may be seen with barium studies anywhere in the GI tract. When the nodules become larger, they can be seen on CT, and nodular mural thickening of the gut suggests KS. Lymphadenopathy is usually absent or mild in KS, unlike lymphoma.

Lymphoma in AIDS is usually of B-cell type and aggressive, with a propensity for extranodal distribution. Lymphadenopathy is usually bulky, but an isolated node may be involved. Hepatic and splenic lesions have low attenuation on CT and are hypoechoic by US. Bowel wall thickening may be a manifestation of GI tract involvement.

Opportunistic infections are manifold: *Candida* spp., herpes simplex, or cytomegalovirus may cause esophagitis, possibly delineated with barium studies. Cytomegalovirus may involve any area of the gut, but most commonly the cecal region. CT may demonstrate thick-walled bowel with enhancing serosa and mucosa. *M. tuberculosis* may involve the ileocecal region, and wall thickening and low-density lymph nodes in the right lower quadrant are typical on CT.

M. avium-intracellulare usually involves the small bowel. Multiple nodes have central low attenuation due to liquefaction. *Cryptosporidium* infection is characterized by profuse watery small bowel contents on CT. *Pneumocystis carinii* abscesses are seen as small multifocal areas of low attenuation in the liver, spleen, pancreas, kidneys, or lymph nodes. Calcifications are common early as well as late in abscess formation.

BIBLIOGRAPHY

1. Balthazar EJ: CT of the gastrointestinal tract: Principles and interpretation. AJR 156:23–32, 1991.

2. Balthazar EJ, Freeny PC, vanSonnenberg E: Imaging and intervention in acute pancreatitis. Radiology 193:297–306, 1994.

3. Dachman AH, Yoshida H: Virtual colonoscopy: Past, present and future. Radiol Clin North Am 41:377–393, 2003.

4. Danet I, Semelka R, Braga L: MR imaging of diffuse liver disease. Radiol Clin North Am 41:67–87, 2003.

5. Ferrucci JT: Advances in abdominal MR imaging. Radiographics 18:1569–1586, 1998.

6. Foshager MC, Ferral H, Finlay DE, et al: Color Doppler sonography of transjugular intrahepatic portosystemic shunts (TIPS). AJR 163:105–111, 1994.

7. Gore RM, Levine MS, Laufer I (eds): Textbook of Gastrointestinal Radiology. Philadelphia, W.B. Saunders, 1994.

8. Ito K, Mitchell DG, Siegelman ES: Cirrhosis: MR imaging features. MR Clin North Am 10(1):75–92, 2002.

9. Lee JK , Sagel SS, Stanley RJ, et al (eds): Computed Body Tomography with MRI, 3rd ed. Philadelphia, Lippincott-Raven, 1998.

10. Low R: MR imaging of the liver using gadolinium chelates. MR Clin North Am 9(4):717–743, 2001.

11. Macari M, Bini EJ, Jacobs SL, et al: Colorectal polyps and cancers in asymptomatic average-risk patients with evaluation at CT colonography. Radiology 230(3):629–636, 2004.

12. Macari M, Bini EJ, Xue X, et al: Colorectal neoplasms: Prospective comparison of thin-section low dose multi-detector CT colonography and conventional colonoscopy for colorectal neoplasm detection. Radiology 224(2):383–392, 2002.

13. Maglinte DD, Balthazar EJ, Kelvin FM, et al: The role of radiology in the diagnosis of small-bowel obstruction. AJR 168:1171–1180, 1997.

14. Martin DR, Semelka RC: Imaging of benign and malignant focal liver lesions MR versus CT. MR Clin North Am 9(4):785–802, 2001.

15. Moss AA, Gamsu G, Genant HK: Computed Tomography of the Body with Magnetic Resonance Imaging, 2nd ed. Philadelphia, W.B. Saunders, 1992.

16. Pickardt PJ, Choi JR, Hwang I, et al: Computed tomographic virtual colonoscopy to screen for colorectal neoplasia in asymptomatic adults. N Engl J Med 349(23):2191–2200, 2003.

17. Putnam CE, Ravin CE: Textbook of Diagnostic Imaging, 2nd ed. Philadelphia, W.B. Saunders, 1994.

18. Redvanly RD, Silverstein JE: Intra-abdominal manifestations of AIDS. Radiol Clin North Am 35:1083–1125, 1997.

19. Ros PR (ed): Hepatic Imaging. Radiol Clin North Am 36:237–375, 1998.

20. Rumack CM, Wilson SR, Charboneau JW (eds): Diagnostic Ultrasound. St. Louis, Mosby-Year Book, 1991.

21. Schneiderman DJ: Hepatobiliary abnormalities of AIDS. Gastroenterol Clin North Am 17:615–630, 1988.

22. Smith FJ, Mathieson JR, Cooperberg PL: Abdominal abnormalities in AIDS: Detection at US in a large population. Radiology 192:691–695, 1994.

23. Sosna J, Morrin MM, Kruskal JB, et al: CT colonography of colorectal polyps: A metaanalysis. AJR 181(6):1593–1598, 2003.

24. Zealley IA, Skehan Stephan SJ, Rawlinson J, et al: Selection of patients for resection of hepatic metastasis: Improved detection of extrahepatic disease with FDG PET. Radiographics 21:S55–S69, 2001.

CHAPTER 72

NUCLEAR MEDICINE STUDIES

Cyrus W. Partington, MD, and Col. Mike McBiles, II, MD

1. **Outline the general advantages of nuclear medicine procedures compared with other imaging modalities.**
   - They provide functional information that is either not available by other modalities or is obtained at greater expense or patient risk.
   - High contrast (target-to-background ratio) can be achieved in many instances by nuclear medicine techniques, allowing diagnostic studies, despite poor spatial resolution.
   - Relatively noninvasive studies are the rule in nuclear medicine. They require only injection of a radioactive dose or swallowing of a substance followed by imaging.

2. **What are the disadvantages of nuclear medicine procedures compared with other radiographic studies?**
   - Spatial resolution, usually 1–2 cm, is inferior to that of other imaging modalities.
   - Imaging times can be long, sometimes up to 1 hour or more.
   - Radiation risk is obviously greater than with magnetic resonance (MR) or ultrasound (US). However, the radiation risk from most nuclear medicine studies is equal to or less than that of an average computed tomographic (CT) study. Gallium-67 and indium-111 white blood cell studies are the exceptions; they involve an average of two to four times more radiation exposure than other nuclear medicine studies. In some studies, such as gastric emptying and esophageal transit studies, radiation risk is insignificant compared with traditional imaging methods, such as fluoroscopy.
   - Availability may be limited. Specialized procedures require radiopharmaceuticals or interpretive expertise not available in all centers.

3. **What nuclear medicine tests are most helpful in gastrointestinal (GI) medicine?**
   Nuclear medicine procedures have been used in the evaluation of practically every GI problem (Table 72-1). However, improvements in and widespread use of endoscopy, manometry, pH monitoring, and traditional imaging techniques (CT, MRI, US) have limited their application to specific clinical problems.

4. **How is cholescintigraphy (hepatobiliary imaging) performed? What is a normal study?**
   The conduct of the basic cholescintigraphic study is the same for nearly all of its clinical indications (*see* question 3). The patient is injected with a technetium-99m–labeled imidodiacetic acid (IDA) derivative. Currently, commonly used compounds are diisopropyliminodiacetic (DISIDA), mebrofenin, and *hepato-IDA* (HIDA), the term used among clinicians for all of these tests. Despite their excretion by the same mechanism as bilirubin, current compounds can provide diagnostic studies at high bilirubin levels (>20 mg/dL).

   After injection, sequential images, usually 1 minute in duration, are obtained for 60 minutes or longer. Normally, the liver rapidly clears the IDA compound. On images displayed at normal intensity, blood pool activity in the heart is faint or not discernible by 5 minutes after injection. Persistent blood pool activity and poor liver uptake are indications of hepatocellular dysfunction. Right and left hepatic ducts are often seen by 10 minutes and the common bile duct and small bowel by 20 minutes. The gallbladder is usually seen at the same time but can normally be

TABLE 72-1. USES OF NUCLEAR MEDICINE PROCEDURES IN GASTROINTESTINAL DISEASES

Test/Study	Useful in Diagnosis/Evaluation
Cholescintigraphy (hepatobiliary imaging)	Acute cholecystitis
	Gallbladder dyskinesis
	Common duct obstruction
	Biliary atresia
	Sphincter of Oddi dysfunction
	Mass lesions
	Biliary leak
	Choleangiointestinal anastomosis patency
	Gastroenterostomy, afferent loop patency
Gastric emptying	Quantification of gastric motility
Esophageal motility/transit	Quantification of esophageal transit
	Evaluation/detection of reflux
	Aspiration detection
Liver/spleen scan	Hepatic mass lesions
	Accessory spleen/splenosis
Heat-damaged RBC scan	Accessory spleen/splenosis
Gallium scanning	Staging of many abdominal malignancies
	Abdominal abscess
^{131}I-MIBG, ^{111}In-pentetreotide (Octreo-scan), ^{99m}Tc-depreotide (Neotect)	Neural crest tumor staging/recurrence
^{111}In-satumomab pendetide (Oncoscint)	Colorectal/ovarian cancer staging/recurrence
^{99m}Tc-arcitumomab (CEA-scan)	Colorectal cancer staging/recurrence
In WBC scanning	Evaluation of abdominal infection/abscess
^{99m}Tc-HMPAO WBC scanning	Evaluation of sites of active inflammatory bowel disease
^{99m}Tc-RBC scanning	GI bleeding localization
	Hepatic hemangiomas
Pertechnetate scanning	Meckel's diverticulum
	Retained gastric antrum
Sulfur-colloid injections	GI bleeding localization
Peritoneovenous shunt study	Territory perfused by hepatic intra-arterial catheters
Schilling's test	Vitamin B_{12} malabsorption

MIBG = m-iodobenzylguanidine, In = indium, WBC = white blood cell, Tc = technetium, HMPAO = hexamethylpropyleneamine oxime, RBC = red blood cell, GI = gastrointestinal.

visualized for up to 1 hour, provided that the patient has not eaten within 4 hours. By 1 hour, almost all activity is in the bile ducts, gallbladder, and bowel; the liver is seen faintly or not at all.

In all of the studies listed in Table 72-1, failure to see an expected structure at 1 hour (e.g., gallbladder in acute cholecystitis, small bowel in biliary atresia) requires delayed imaging for up to 4 hours. In some cases, various manipulations, such as sincalide or morphine infusions, are performed after the initial 60-minute images, and imaging is continued for another 30–60 minutes.

5. **How should patients with acute cholecystitis be prepared? What manipulations are used to shorten the study or increase its reliability?**
Traditionally, acute cholecystitis is diagnosed on functional cholescintigraphy by noting a lack of filling of the gallbladder (usually due to a cystic duct stone) on the initial 60-minute study and on 4-hour images. Manipulations and preparations are designed to ensure that lack of gallbladder visualization is a true-positive finding or to shorten this long, sometimes tedious study. Because food is a potent and long-lasting stimulus for endogenous cholecystokinin (CCK) release and subsequent gallbladder contraction, the patient should not eat for 4 hours before the study; otherwise, a false-positive study may result. Prolonged fasting causes viscous bile formation in the normal gallbladder, which may impair its filling by the radiopharmaceutical and cause a false-positive study. Most clinics give the short-acting CCK analog sincalide, 0.01–0.04 µg/kg intravenously over 3 minutes, one-half hour before cholescintigraphy, if the patient has fasted >24 hours, receives hyperalimentation, or is severely ill.

Despite these manipulations, the gallbladder may not fill during the 60-minute cholescintigraphic study. Rather than reimage at 4 hours, morphine, 0.01 mg/kg intravenously, may be given if the gallbladder is not seen but the small bowel is seen at 60 minutes. After morphine administration, imaging is continued for 30 additional minutes. Because morphine causes sphincter of Oddi contraction, which results in increased biliary tree pressure, this manipulation overcomes functional obstruction of the cystic duct. If the gallbladder is still not seen, delayed imaging is not necessary, and acute cholecystitis is diagnosed (Fig. 72-1).

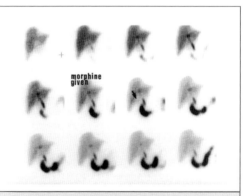

Figure 72-1. Acute cholecystitis. Hepatobiliary study with ^{99m}Tc-mebrofenin, acquired every 5 minutes after injection, shows rapid clearance and uptake by the liver, with rapid excretion into the common bile duct and small bowel. Morphine, 1 mg IV given at the 30-minute image, failed to fill the gallbladder in an additional 30 minutes of imaging. Alternatively, a 4-hour delayed image may be obtained instead of injecting morphine, but this step unnecessarily prolongs the study.

6. **If acute cholecystitis is a possibility, when should hepatobiliary scintigraphy be used?**

   Hepatobiliary scintigraphy is the most accurate imaging method to diagnose acute cholecystitis, with a sensitivity and specificity of 95%. However, it should not be used in every instance when acute cholecystitis is suspected. If, for example, the pretest clinical probability of acute cholecystitis is low (<10%), a positive study in a screening population is likely to be false. Likewise, if the pretest probability is high (>90%), a negative study is likely to be false. The same admonitions apply to CT and US, which are even less sensitive and specific.

   In the absence of obvious clinical acute cholecystitis, both US and CT are frequently the initial studies of choice, because not only the gallbladder but also adjacent structures causing the symptoms can be easily evaluated. CT is notoriously insensitive for acute cholecystitis, although the presence of inflammatory changes around the gallbladder should strongly raise this possibility. Although US is frequently the initial study of choice, only in the presence of all of the classic signs of cholecystitis (gallbladder wall thickening, gallstones, common duct dilation, and sonographic Murphy's sign) does the sensitivity of US approach cholescintigraphy. Similarly, if only a few of these US signs are present, specificity suffers.

7. **How is cholescintigraphy used to diagnose and manage biliary leak?**

   Cholescintigraphy is highly sensitive and specific for detecting biliary leak (Fig. 72-2). Because nonbile fluid collections are common after surgery, anatomic studies have a poor specificity. Because cholescintigraphy has poor spatial resolution, the exact site of the leak may not be documented; endoscopic retrograde cholangiopancreatography (ERCP) or percutaneous transhepatic cholangiography (PTC) may be necessary for anatomic definition. Cholescintigraphy can also be used noninvasively to document resolution of a bile leak.

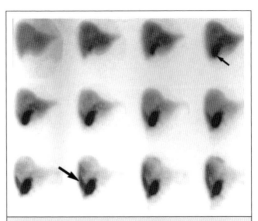

Figure 72-2. Bile leak. After percutaneous liver biopsy, the patient developed severe right upper quadrant pain. US was not helpful. Sequential 5-minute images after ^{99m}Tc-mebrofenin injection show leakage of a thin rim of bile along the inferior and lateral liver edge *(large arrow)*. Note gallbladder filling early in the study *(small arrow)* and the lack of small bowel activity, implying preferential flow of bile to the gallbladder and site of leakage.

8. **How is cholescintigraphy used in diagnosing common bile duct obstruction?**

   Ductal dilatation seen on US may be a nonspecific finding in patients with previous biliary surgery, and acute obstruction (<24–48 hours old) may not show ductal dilatation.

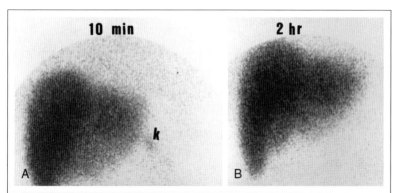

Figure 72-3. Common bile duct obstruction. After injection of the hepatobiliary agent, there is no visible activity in the intrahepatic ducts or small bowel on, *A,* 10-minute or, *B,* 2-hour images. US did not show dilated ducts, and a common duct stone was not seen, a common finding in acute common duct obstruction. Activity to left of liver (k) is the radiopharmaceutical agent excreted in the urine in an alternate pathway to biliary excretion.

Cholescintigraphy shows a lack of gallbladder and small bowel visualization and often a lack of biliary tree visualization on the 4-hour delayed images in common duct obstruction. Sensitivity and specificity are high (Fig. 72-3). Cholescintigraphy is reliable even at high bilirubin levels. It can be used to distinguish obstructive from nonobstructive jaundice.

9. **What is cholescintigraphy's role in diagnosing biliary atresia?**
   By the same rationale outlined in question 8, cholescintigraphy is sensitive and highly specific for the diagnosis of biliary atresia, if the patient is properly prepared. The major differential diagnostic possibility in neonates is severe neonatal hepatitis. US findings are insensitive. US may show ductal dilatation or gallbladder absence in biliary atresia, but dilatation is usually absent, and the gallbladder is usually present. The main scintigraphic problem is a false-positive study caused by a lack of biliary secretion in severe hepatitis. Premedication of the neonate with oral phenobarbital, 5 mg/kg/day for 5 days, stimulates bile flow and eliminates this problem. The importance of therapeutic serum levels of phenobarbital cannot be overemphasized. If radioactivity in the small bowel is seen on delayed images, biliary atresia is ruled out (Fig. 72-4).

10. **How is sphincter of Oddi dysfunction assessed by cholescintigraphy?**
    A significant number of patients continue to have pain after cholycystectomy, and sphincter of Oddi dysfunction may be the cause. Although manometry during ERCP is diagnostic, this study is invasive and not without complications. An empiric scintigraphic scoring system looking at quantitative parameters of bile movement and liver function has been developed. High correlation with biliary tree manometric findings has been demonstrated.

11. **When can cholescintigraphy help to evaluate obstruction in gastroenterostomies?**
    Afferent loops are difficult to evaluate with barium studies because the afferent loop must be filled retrograde with barium. By cholescintigraphy, afferent loop obstruction can be reliably excluded, if activity is seen in the afferent and efferent loops 1 hour after radiopharmaceutical injection. Persistent accumulation in the afferent loop with little or no efferent loop activity at 2 hours establishes the diagnosis of afferent loop obstruction.

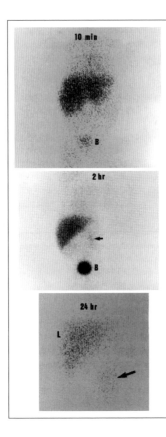

Figure 72-4. Neonatal hepatitis with suspected biliary atresia. This difficult diagnosis can be made with a hepatobiliary agent. In this case, 99mTc-mebrofenin was injected after a 5-day preparation with phenobarbital. Note the (B) continued blood pool activity in the heart on the 2-hour image and excretion into the bladder, suggesting hepatocellular dysfunction with abnormal excretion of the hepatobiliary agent into the alternate urinary pathway. At 4 hours there is a subtle focus *(arrow)* in the abdomen that may be in the bowel or radiopharmaceutical agent excreted by the alternate urinary pathway. In the 24-hour image with the bladder catheterized, ill-defined activity in the left lower quadrant *(arrow),* inferolateral to the liver (L), confirms excretion of the radiopharmaceutical agent into the bowel and rules out biliary atresia.

12. **What is gallbladder dyskinesia? How does cholescintigraphy evaluate the emptying of the gallbladder?**

A significant number of patients with normal imaging and clinical work-ups have pain referable to the gallbladder, as evidenced by relief of symptoms after cholecystectomy. The poorly understood and heterogeneous entity of gallbladder dyskinesia has been proposed as the cause of this pain. It is thought that poorly coordinated contractions between the gallbladder and cystic duct can cause pain. Gallbladder dyskinesia may be manifested by an abnormally low ejection of bile under the stimulus of cholecystokinin (sincalide).

After the gallbladder is filled during traditional cholescintigraphy, gallbladder contraction is stimulated by an infusion of sincalide, 0.01 mg/kg. The amount of gallbladder emptying over 30 minutes reflects the gallbladder ejection fraction (GBEF; normal >35–40%). This protocol has demonstrated correlation of both normal and abnormal GBEF, with surgical and medical follow-up.

13. **What is a nuclear medicine gastric emptying study?**

Both liquid and solid gastric emptying studies can be performed with nuclear medicine. Liquid studies are usually performed on infants. After the infant receives a mixture of 99mTc-sulfur colloid with milk or formula at normal feeding time, imaging is done every 15 minutes for 60 minutes, and an emptying half-time is calculated. In adults, a solid-phase emptying study is usually performed after an overnight fast by mixing 99mTc-sulfur colloid-labeled scrambled eggs with a standard meal, performing anterior and posterior imaging every 15 minutes for 90 minutes and calculating the percentage of emptying. The meal has not been standardized, and normal values depend on the meal composition. Using a 300-calorie meal of scrambled eggs, bread, and butter, solid gastric emptying is 63% at 1 hour (standard deviation of 11%).

14. **In what clinical situations is a nuclear medicine gastric emptying study useful?**
    Symptoms related to problems of abnormal gastric motility may be nonspecific, and barium studies are neither quantifiable nor physiologic. Although gastric emptying studies are semiqualitative, show less than optimal reproducibility, and are not standardized, a rough estimate of emptying in clinically important groups (such as diabetic patients and patients with partial gastrectomy) can help to explain nonspecific symptoms or suggest another etiology, if the results are clearly normal or abnormal (Fig. 72-5).

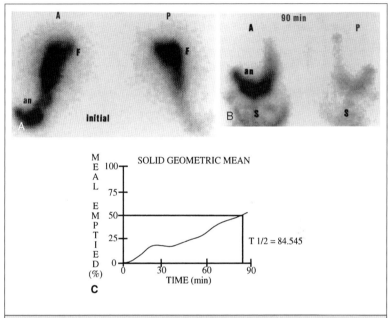

Figure 72-5. Normal gastric emptying study. *A,* Initial anterior (A) and posterior (P) images after ingestion of ^{99m}Tc-sulfur colloid-labeled scrambled eggs in beef stew show activity in the fundus (F) on posterior images and extending to the antrum (an). *B,* At 90 minutes, little radiopharmaceutical agent is left in the fundus, but a significant amount is seen in the antrum, and noticeable activity is distributed throughout the small bowel (S). *C,* At 84.5 minutes, 50% of the meal had emptied (normal = 35–60% with this type of meal).

15. **What nuclear medicine esophageal studies are available? How are they used?**
    Esophageal motility study. This study is performed by rapid sequential imaging of the esophagus during swallowing of ^{99m}Tc-colloid in water. Although it provides a precise and reproducible quantitation of esophageal function, barium studies provide usually adequate definition of the anatomic or functional problem. Esophageal motility studies are useful as an easily performed study in the noninvasive follow-up of therapy for dysmotility and achalasia.
    Esophageal reflux study. This study is performed by serial imaging of the esophagus, after the patient drinks acidified orange juice containing ^{99m}Tc-colloid and during serial inflation of an abdominal binder. Although less sensitive than 24-hour pH monitoring, the test is more sensitive than barium studies and can be used for screening study or evaluation of response to therapy.

Pulmonary aspiration studies. These studies are performed by imaging the chest after oral administration of ^{99m}Tc-colloid in water. Activity in the lungs is diagnostic of aspiration. Although sensitivity is low, it is probably higher than that of radiographic contrast studies. The test has the advantage of easy serial imaging to detect intermittent aspiration.

16. **What is the role for nuclear medicine studies in evaluating hepatic mass lesions?**
The traditional liver-spleen scan using an intravenous injection of the Kupffer cell-seeking ^{99m}Tc-sulfur has been largely replaced by US and dynamic multiphase CT and MRI. Because of superior resolution with CT and MRI, lesion blood flow characteristics are evident, and adjacent structures can be evaluated.

Virtually all neoplasms, including metastasis, focal inflammatory and infectious diseases of the liver, and vascular malformations, manifest as decreased radionuclide activity ("cold") on both liver-spleen and hepatobiliary imaging. However, *focal nodular hyperplasia* (FNH) often has a nonspecific appearance on CT, MRI, and US but appears warm (isointense with the rest of the liver) or hot on liver-spleen imaging because of the predominance of Kupffer cells. Liver-spleen scanning, therefore, has a limited role in evaluating this rare lesion. *Hepatic adenomas* are usually composed of mostly hepatocytes and appear warm or hot on hepatobiliary imaging and cold on liver-spleen imaging. This unique combination is not always seen, but its presence is diagnostic. Because focal fatty replacement does not affect Kupffer cell distribution or the kinetics of hepatobiliary scintigraphy, a normal liver-spleen strongly suggests this diagnosis (Fig. 72-6).

Most *hepatomas* avidly accumulate gallium-67; in the absence of a known gallium-67–avid primary tumor elsewhere, a gallium-avid liver lesion is highly suspicious for hepatoma.

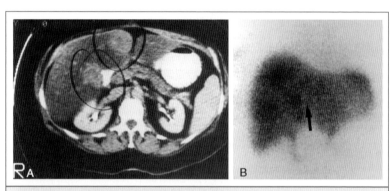

Figure 72-6. Evaluation of mass lesions. *A,* Contrast-enhanced CT scan of the liver shows diffuse fatty infiltration, with two areas of relatively normal-appearing liver *(circles)* in this patient with colon cancer treated with 5-fluorouracil. Regenerating liver nodules and metastatic disease are the diagnostic possibilities. *B,* Given the large size of these lesions and their anterior location, metastatic lesions would be readily seen as a photopenic defect on hepatobiliary imaging *(arrows)*. Because no defects are seen, the diagnosis is regenerating nodules.

Occasionally, certain kinds of metastatic lesions (see question 25) may be occult, or CT, MRI, or US may not distinguish benign or malignant nature. Radionuclide receptor or antibody imaging may be helpful.

With dynamic multiphase imaging, CT and MRI are diagnostic for *hepatic hemangioma.* Delayed imaging with single-photon emission computed tomography (SPECT), which produces three-dimensional scintigraphic images similar to CT, with ^{99m}Tc-labeled red blood cells, provides comparable sensitivity and specificity in the diagnosis of hemangiomas >2 cm (Fig. 72-7), frequently at lower cost and without contrast injection. The positive predictive value of SPECT for hemangiomata <1 cm is also high because of the high target-to-background ratio in such lesions, a result of their uniquely high proportion of blood to other tissue, at 2-hour delayed SPECT imaging. In lesions near large vessels, however, it may be difficult to differentiate the

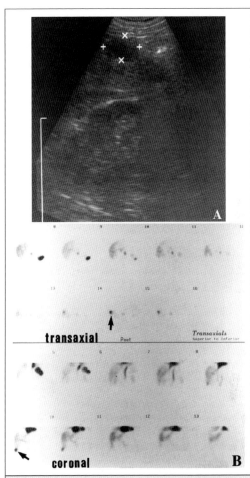

Figure 72-7. Liver hemangioma. *A,* Ultrasound shows a 3-cm hypoechoic lesion with internal echoes, consistent with hemangioma but a nonspecific finding. *B,* A ^{99m}Tc-RBC study obtained at 2 hours with SPECT shows an intense focus in the inferior right lobe of the liver on transaxial and coronal images *(arrows).*

Continued

vessel from the hemangioma, and other imaging modalities should be used. The unusual clot-filled or fibrotic lesions are not detected with high sensitivity using SPECT imaging.

17. **Describe the vitamin B$_{12}$ absorption (Schilling's) test and its use.**
    The Schilling's test measures the ability of the body to absorb and excrete vitamin B$_{12}$. Because there are many causes of vitamin B$_{12}$ malabsorption, the work-up is usually performed in stages. Each stage is designed to evaluate, in sequence, the most clinically prevalent causes of vitamin B$_{12}$ deficiency. Although some clinicians treat all B$_{12}$-deficient patients without searching for a cause, the etiology can be important because of associated or unsuspected problems that should be recognized.

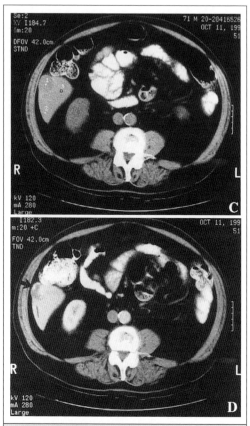

Figure 72-7. cont'd *C,* CT scan without contrast shows a lesion in this same area *(box 1). D,* CT with contrast shows centripetal, nodular filling of this lesion *(arrow),* confirming the diagnosis of hemangioma made on the ^{99m}Tc-RBC study.

It is not necessary or, in fact, desirable for the patient with severe vitamin B_{12} deficiency to abstain from vitamin B_{12} therapy before the Schilling's test. In stage 1 and all subsequent stages, nonradiolabeled vitamin B_{12}, 1 mg intramuscularly, is given to bind B_{12} receptors 2 hours after the patient takes a pill containing radioactive-cobalt-labeled vitamin B_{12}. It is extremely important that the patient not eat for 3 hours before and after taking the pill (to prevent the radiolabeled B_{12} from being bound by food) and that a 24- to 48-hour urine sample be accurately collected. Urinary creatinine and volume should be determined. Less-than-normal 24-hour urinary creatinine levels suggest inadequate collection, which artifactually decreases the amount of vitamin B_{12} excreted in the urine. The collected urine is analyzed for radioactive cobalt. Normally, >10% of the radioactive oral dose is excreted by 24 hours. If the excretion of vitamin B_{12} at 24 hours is normal, normal GI absorption is implied.

If the results of stage 1 are abnormal, the patient undergoes stage 2, which is a repeat of stage 1, except that oral intrinsic factor is given together with the radioactive B_{12} pill. Stage 3 has several variations that depend on the clinical suspicion of the etiology of B_{12} malabsorption (Fig. 72-8). A normal stage-2 excretion of vitamin B_{12} after an abnormal stage-1 excretion implies the diagnosis of pernicious anemia.

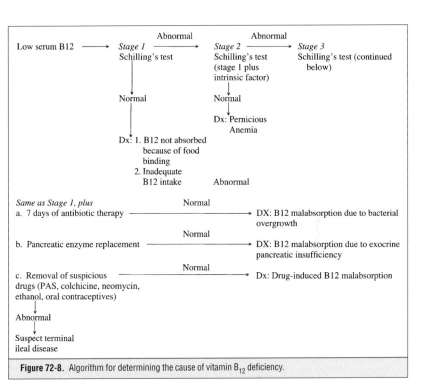

Figure 72-8. Algorithm for determining the cause of vitamin B_{12} deficiency.

18. **How can nuclear medicine procedures assist in detecting ectopic gastric tissue?**

As a source of pediatric GI bleeding, Meckel's diverticulum almost always contains gastric tissue. Because ^{99m}Tc-pertechnetate is concentrated and extracted by gastric tissue, it is an ideal agent to localize sources of GI bleeding, which can be difficult to detect with traditional contrast studies.

The study is performed by injecting pertechnetate intravenously and imaging the abdomen for 45 minutes. Typically, ectopic gastric mucosa appears at the same time as stomach tissue and does not move during imaging. The test's sensitivity is 85% for detection of bleeding Meckel's diverticula. Manipulations to increase the sensitivity of the study include pretreatment with cimetidine (to block pertechnetate excretion into the bowel lumen) and/or glucagon (to inhibit bowel motility so that ^{99m}Tc-pertechnetate is not washed away). A similar procedure for peptic ulcer disease can be performed to identify a retained gastric antrum after surgery; it has a sensitivity of 73% and specificity of 100%.

19. **Can accessory splenic tissue or splenosis be detected via nuclear medicine procedures?**

Yes. After splenectomy as treatment of idiopathic thrombocytopenia, treatment failure is associated with unremoved accessory spleen. Unrecognized splenosis may also be a cause of unexplained abdominal pain. The most sensitive imaging procedure for localization of small foci of splenic tissue is the heat-damaged ^{99m}Tc-RBC scan, because damaged red blood cells localize in splenic tissue intensely and specifically. This is the procedure of choice, especially if SPECT is used. However, the RBC-damaging process requires exquisite laboratory technique and may not be readily available in many centers. It is therefore reasonable to perform a liver-spleen scan as

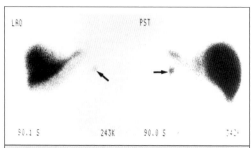

Figure 72-9. Accessory spleen in a patient after splenectomy for idiopathic thrombocytopenic purpura. The high contrast achieved with ^{99m}Tc-sulfur colloid can detect a small remnant *(arrow)* and direct surgical exploration. Left anterior oblique (LAO) and posterior (PST) images of the abdomen are shown. If ^{99m}Tc-sulfur colloid studies are negative, even higher contrast, specificity, and target-to-background ratios can be obtained by using scanning with heat-damaged RBCs, which preferentially accumulate in splenic tissue and demonstrate an almost identical scintigraphic pattern, as does ^{99m}Tc-sulfur colloid.

an initial study and, if it is positive for splenic tissue, to institute appropriate therapy (Fig. 72-9). If it is negative, a heat-damaged RBC study should be performed.

20. **What nuclear medicine studies help in the management of inflammatory bowel disease and abdominal abscesses?**
    Gallium-67 is normally excreted into the bowel, and a small amount of ^{99m}Tc-HMPAO dissociates from the WBCs and is excreted into the bowel; therefore, these agents are less useful for imaging abdominal inflammation. With gallium-67, it may be necessary to image for up to 1 week to allow bowel activity to move so that suspicious abdominal foci can be adequately characterized. This disadvantage is offset slightly by the low cost of gallium-67, despite its higher dosimetry (equal to the radiation of two to four abdominal CT scans). ^{99m}Tc-HMPAO and ^{111}In-labeled WBC studies are expensive and require special labeling expertise.

    ^{111}In-labeled WBCs, which normally accumulate in only the liver, spleen, and bone marrow, are the agent of choice in localizing abdominal infection in cases in which CT, MRI, and US are nondiagnostic. The normal WBC uptake in the liver and spleen is a minor drawback and can be overcome by dual-isotope imaging with ^{99m}Tc-colloid (liver-spleen scanning), because intrasplenic and perisplenic or liver abscess is cold on liver-spleen scanning and hot on the ^{111}In-WBC study. The necessity for delayed 24-hour imaging to maximize sensitivity is also a drawback.

    One-hour postinjection *^{99m}Tc-HMPAO WBC imaging* also correlates well with the degree of inflammation and localization of inflammatory bowel disease seen on other imaging modalities; thus, it can be used for noninvasive follow-up. This agent is preferable to ^{111}In-WBC studies because of higher sensitivity and lower radiation dosimetry.

21. **Which nuclear medicine procedures are useful in localizing lower GI bleeding?**
    The difficulty of localizing acute lower GI bleeding is well recognized. The precise nature of the bleeding lesion is frequently immaterial to patient management, because the final common therapeutic pathway often involves partial bowel resection. Even acute and rapid bleeding is intermittent and frequently not detected on angiography, or the culprit lesion is obscured by luminal blood during endoscopy. Small bowel bleeding distal to areas reachable by upper endoscopy is notoriously difficult to localize.

Two nuclear procedures have been used to localize GI bleeding sources: short-term imaging after ^{99m}Tc-colloid injection and extended imaging after ^{99m}Tc-tagged RBC injection. Despite the theoretic advantage of ^{99m}Tc-colloids in being able to detect smaller bleeds, this technique shares the limitation of angiography: short intravascular residence time (few minutes) of the contrast material. ^{99m}Tc-RBC imaging has assumed dominance because the long intravascular residence time (limited by radioactive decay) allows detection of intraluminal radioactive blood accumulation, if extended imaging is used.

The study is begun by performing an in vitro tag of RBCs with ^{99m}Tc-pertechnetate. The radiolabeled RBCs are injected, and multiple sequential computer images are obtained for 90 minutes or longer. Computer acquisition is important because sensitivity for localization is higher when the study is displayed in a sine-loop.

22. **Are nuclear medicine procedures clinically useful in localizing GI bleeding, or are simpler techniques adequate?**
   ^{99m}Tc-RBC studies are more sensitive, in general, than angiography in detecting intermittent bleeding (Fig. 72-10). Early claims that the nuclear medicine GI bleeding study should be used as a screening study prior to angiography may not be defensible. However, with rigorous technique and attention to rigid diagnostic criteria for bleeding localization, the bleeding study is helpful in many difficult cases. Knowledge of the advantages and disadvantages of each technique allows the clinician to select the most appropriate study for the specific situation.

23. **Is nuclear medicine helpful in placement of arterial perfusion catheters?**
   Yes. Occasional unrecognized systemic shunting, catheter dislodgment, and unintended perfusion of an area not suitable for highly toxic chemotherapeutic drugs hamper placement of hepatic arterial perfusion catheters. Arterial catheter injection of ^{99m}Tc-macroaggregated albumin (MAA) results in microembolization at the arteriolar level and provides an imaging map of the true area of perfusion of the catheter, especially if SPECT is used. This imaging cannot be done reliably with radiographic contrast because of its rapid dilution at the arteriolar level.

24. **How can nuclear medicine assess peritoneovenous shunt patency?**
   Increasing abdominal girth in the presence of a peritoneovenous shunt can be a diagnostic challenge because it may be due to shunt obstruction, increased ascites production, or loculation. Radiographic studies are not possible if the shunt is radiopaque; in any event, such studies require shunt cannulation. Because a one-way valve is located at the abdominal origin of the shunt, it is difficult to evaluate the shunt in a retrograde manner. Patency can be readily evaluated by injecting ^{99m}Tc-MAA intraperitoneally and imaging the chest for 30 minutes. The shunt tube may not be visualized, but trapping of the ^{99m}Tc-MAA in lung arterioles is de facto evidence of shunt patency.

25. **Can abdominal malignancies be evaluated with nuclear medicine studies?**
   Yes. Traditionally, *gallium-67,* a nonspecific tumor and infection marker, has been used to evaluate suspicious malignancy. It is not useful in staging of tumors but rather in evaluating recurrence of hepatomas and Hodgkin's and non-Hodgkin's lymphomas. Anatomic studies have difficulty separating necrosis and scar from recurrent tumor. Its utility is hampered by variable tumor avidity and by interference from GI activity caused by its excretion into the large bowel. The problem of separating GI activity from target lesion activity can be partially overcome by SPECT and serial imaging for up to 1 week to allow elimination of gallium-67 excreted into the bowel.

   Recent Food and Drug Administration (FDA) approval of ^{111}In-pentetreotide, ^{99m}Tc-depreotide, and ^{131}I-MIBG for imaging of neural crest tumors has opened new possibilities in evaluating these difficult-to-image tumors. ^{131}I-MIBG, a dopamine analog, is a particularly useful complement to CT and MRI in staging and detecting carcinoid tumors, neuroblastoma, paragangliomas, and pheochromocytomas. ^{111}In-octeotide and, possibly, ^{99m}Tc-depreotide, both of which are somatostatin analogs and therefore accumulate in tissues with somatostatin

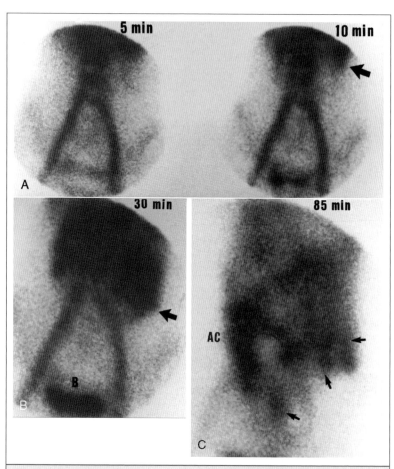

Figure 72-10. *A–C,* GI bleeding from the small bowel. After negative upper endoscopy and continued bleeding, a ^{99m}Tc-labeled RBC scan shows a focus of bleeding near the spleen *(large arrows).* Continued imaging at 85 minutes demonstrates serpiginous transit time through the small bowel *(small arrows)* toward the right lower quadrant, confirming a proximal small bowel origin. At surgery, a bleeding distal duodenal ulcer was found (B = bladder, AC = ascending colon).

receptors, are also highly sensitive and specific for a variety of neural chest tumors that express somatostatin receptors (Fig. 72-11). They frequently detect occult lesions not seen by other modalities and can lend specificity to questionable GI lesions found on MRI and CT, including gastrinoma, glucagonoma, paraganglioma, pheochromocytoma, carcinoid, and Hodgkin's and non-Hodgkin's lymphoma.

The radiolabeled antibody ^{111}In-satumomab has also been approved by the FDA and is extremely useful in evaluating colon and ovarian cancer in patients with an elevated carcinoembryonic antigen (CEA) level and an otherwise negative diagnostic evaluation; patients with known recurrent disease presumed to be isolated and amenable to surgical resection; and patients in whom the standard diagnostic work-up provides equivocal information. ^{111}In-satumomab frequently detects occult disease and significantly affects therapy in almost one fourth of these patients.

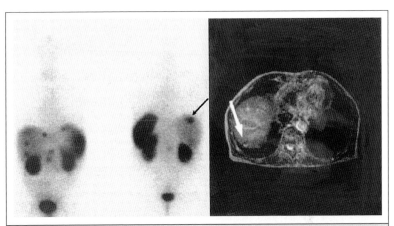

Figure 72-11. Left image shows an ^{111}In-pentetreotide scan in a patient with multiple metastases of gastrinoma to the liver. Two foci consistent with gastrinoma are seen in the pancreas. The black arrow points to one of the metastases in the dome of the liver. Note the normal homogenous distribution of the radiopharmaceutical agent in the spleen, kidneys, and bladder. The right image is a T_2-weighted transaxial MR scan at the level of the subtle metastasis in the dome of the liver *(white arrow)* seen in the nuclear medicine study.

26. **What are the advantages and drawbacks of radioactive receptor and antibody imaging?**

Many tumors express either unique antigens or high concentrations of peptide receptors. Table 72-1 lists only the radiopharmaceuticals approved by the FDA at the time of this printing; promising new agents are under development. Tumors with peptide receptors are ideally suited for radionuclide imaging with radiolabeled peptides or antibodies because of high theoretic target-to-background ratios, despite extremely low receptor or antigen concentrations. In clinical trials, these radiopharmaceuticals often have outperformed CT and MRI in both sensitivity and specificity. Nevertheless, sensitivity and specificity are frequently less than optimal (70–80%), although in certain tumor/radiopharmaceutical combinations they may be even higher. These radiopharmaceuticals may be helpful when other imaging and/or biopsy results are inconclusive, when detection of multiple lesions would affect treatment, and when a residual mass after treatment cannot be adequately characterized by CT, MRI, or US.

Several drawbacks have become evident. Radiopharmaceuticals can be expensive, and their preparation requires some expertise. The best results require state-of-the-art equipment, careful attention to imaging protocol details, and interpretive expertise not available at all imaging centers. Nonspecific accumulation of the radiopharmaceutical or its breakdown products in the liver, kidney, and bowel is a common finding and sometimes necessitates complex dual isotope subtraction techniques, multiday imaging, or bladder catheterization or bowel cleansing. Imaging times may be long, which increases the chance of motion artifacts. Some drugs may interfere with radiopharmaceutical localization. Some monoclonal antibodies derived from mouse hybrid cells may cause unwanted immune response. Careful consultation with the nuclear medicine physician is necessary for selection of the proper test, patient preparation, and statement of the clinical questions needing an answer.

BIBLIOGRAPHY

1. Arndt J, Van der Sluys, Veer A, et al: Prospective comparative study of technetium-99m-WBCs and indium-111-granulocytes for the examination of patients with inflammatory bowel disease. J Nucl Med 34:1052–1057, 1993.

2. Corman M, Galandiak S, Block G, et al: Immunoscintigraphy with ^{111}In-satumomab pendetide in patients with colorectal adenocarcinoma: Performance and impact on clinical management. Dis Colon Rectum 37:129–137, 1994.

3. Davis L, McCarroll K: Correlative imaging of the liver and hepatobiliary system. Semin Nucl Med 26:208–216, 1994.

4. Drane W: Scintigraphic techniques for hepatic imaging: Update for 2000. Radiol Clin North Am 36:309–318, 1999.

5. Fischman A, Babich J: Radiolabeled peptides: A new class of imaging agents. In Freeman L (ed): Nuclear Medicine Annual. Philadelphia, Lippincott-Raven, 1997, pp 103–131.

6. Mettler F, Guiberteau M: Essentials of Nuclear Medicine Imaging, 4th ed. Philadelphia, W.B. Saunders, 2000.

7. Pawels S, Leners N, Fiasse R, Jamar F: Localization of gastroenteropancreatic neuroendocrine tumors with indium-111-pentetreotide scintigraphy. Semin Oncol 12(Suppl 13):15–20, 1994.

8. Shapiro M: The role of the radiologist in the management of gastrointestinal bleeding. Gastroenterol Clin North Am 23:123–181, 1994.

9. Sodee D, Velchik M, Noto R, et al: Gastrointestinal system. In Early P, Sodee D (eds): Principles and Practice of Nuclear Medicine. St. Louis, Mosby, 1995, pp 476–579.

10. Sostre S, Kalloo A, Spiegler E, et al: A noninvasive test of sphincter of Oddi dysfunction in postcholecystectomy patients: The scintigraphic score. J Nucl Med 33:1216–1222, 1992.

11. Weissmann H, Gliedman M, Wilk P, et al: Evaluation of the postoperative patient with ^{99m}Tc-IDA cholescintigraphy. Semin Nucl Med 12:27–52, 1982.

12. Yap L, Wycherley AG, Morphett A, Toouli J: Acalculous biliary pain: Cholecystectomy alleviates symptoms in patients with abnormal cholescintigraphy. Gastroenterology 101:786–793, 1991.

CHAPTER 73

ENDOSCOPIC ULTRASOUND

Peter R. McNally, DO

1. **When was intraluminal gastrointestinal (GI) ultrasound first performed?**
   Wild and Reid performed the first ultrasound (rectal) in 1956. For the past decade, interest in the use of GI ultrasound (US) has been revitalized. Intraluminal ultrasound permits precise definition of the gut wall layers and examination of adjacent structures of the chest and abdomen. The proximity of the ultrasound transducer and the high scanning frequencies provide incomparable morphologic detail of the gut wall and extraintestinal anatomy.

2. **How do ultrasound waves visualize the GI tract?**
   Ultrasound pulses represent longitudinal waves that are propagated through soft tissues or fluid by motion of molecules within the conducting media. The ultrasound wavelength is the distance between two waves of compression and rarefaction. Ultrasound is defined as frequency >20,000 cycles/sec (20 Hz); most diagnostic ultrasound uses frequencies ranging from 2–20 million cycles/sec (2–20 MHz). The velocity of sound transmission through soft tissues is a constant 1540 m/sec and is independent of frequency. Transmission of ultrasound within a medium depends on the compressibility and density of the medium, two properties that tend to be inversely proportional. Because ultrasound power is diminished as it traverses tissue, the intensity of the returning echo, when related to the original echo, is expressed in negative terms.

3. **How does the frequency of the ultrasound beam influence the depth of beam penetration and image resolution?**
   For maximal resolution of ultrasound, the transmitted waves should be parallel. If the target of interest is too close or too far from the transducer, divergence of the wavelength causes distortion of the image. Hence, proper positioning of the US transducer and use of the appropriate frequency are essential to provide maximal resolution (Table 73-1).

TABLE 73-1. PROPER POSITIONING OF THE ULTRASOUND TRANSDUCER AND USE OF THE APPROPRIATE FREQUENCY		
Ultrasound Frequencies	**Penetration**	**Axial Resolution**
5 MHz	8 cm	0.8 mm
10 MHz	4 cm	0.4 mm
20 MHz	2 cm	0.2 mm

4. **What are the ultrasonographic properties of the common structures of the body?**

Water/blood	Echo poor (black)
Collagen	Echo rich (white)
Air	Reflection (reverberation echoes)
Bone	Reflection (reverberation echoes)
Muscle	Echo poor (black)

NORMAL ANATOMY

5. **What determines the thickness of the echosonographic layer visualized? What is the normal endosonographic anatomy of the intestinal wall?**
    The thickness of the intraluminal ultrasound image of the intestinal wall does not equal the total thickness of a histologic section. It has been hypothesized that the overall appearance of the ultrasound image is determined by a combination of echoes from two sources: those created at interfaces between tissue layers with different acoustic impedances and those created within the internal structures of the tissue layer. Using 5- to 12-MHz scanning frequencies, the intestinal wall has five sonographic layers (Fig. 73-1).

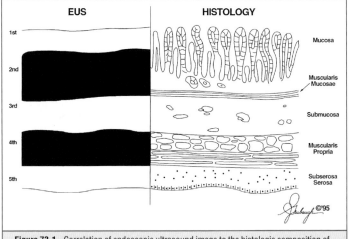

Figure 73-1. Correlation of endoscopic ultrasound image to the histologic composition of the bowel wall.

6. **What are the imaging characteristics of normal and malignant lymph nodes on endoscopic ultrasound (EUS)?**
    The high resolution of EUS imaging allows even normal lymph nodes to be visualized. Normal lymph nodes are characterized by the presence of internal echoes, a bean-like shape, and size <1 cm. Malignant lymph nodes tend to be hypoechoic, rounded, and >1 cm; they exhibit distinct margins.

7. **How are blood vessels distinguished from lymph nodes on EUS?**
    Blood vessels generally appear as anechoic, curvilinear structures that often branch. Branching and posterior wall enhancement (hyperechoic) are helpful in distinguishing paraluminal vessels from hypoechoic lymph nodes.

8. **Describe the normal EUS anatomy of the retroperitoneum. What are its major landmarks?**
    The pancreas and retroperitoneum are the most challenging and difficult areas to examine with intraluminal US. Familiarity with the gross and US anatomy is essential. The examination begins with the echoendoscope at the level of the duodenal ampulla. Antimotility agents, such as glucagon, are frequently necessary. The US examination is usually conducted with a 7.5-MHz scanning frequency. The normal paraduodenal anatomy is shown in Figure 73-2.

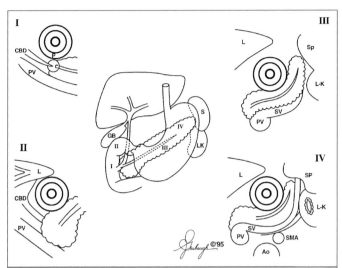

Figure 73-2. Four commonly used positions to examine the pancreas by EUS. I, Transverse section at the level of the ampulla. II, Sagittal section near the duodenal bulb. III, Transverse section of the pancreatic body through the posterior wall of the stomach. IV, Transverse section of the body and tail of the pancreas from the proximal stomach. A = ampulla, CBD = common bile duct, L-K = left kidney, PV = portal vein, SV = splenic vein, L = liver, Sp = spleen, SA = superior mesenteric artery, Ao = aorta.

The normal pancreas has a homogeneous echo pattern, usually slightly more hyperechoic than the liver. There is considerable interobserver variation in measurement of the head of the pancreas, probably due to variations in the angle of view. The remainder of the pancreas is examined from a paragastric position. In the stomach, the water-filled lumen method is used.

9. **What are the indications for EUS examination?**
   Staging of GI tumors

Esophageal carcinoma	Ampullary tumors
Gastric carcinoma	Biliary tract carcinoma
Gastric lymphoma (non-Hodgkin's lymphoma)	Colorectal carcinoma
Pancreatic lymphoma	Colorectal adenoma
Pancreatic endocrine tumors	Submucosal tumors

   Evaluation of nonneoplastic disease

Reflux esophagitis	Portal hypertension
Achalasia	Chronic pancreatitis
Gastric ulcer	Common bile duct stones
Giant gastric folds	Inflammatory bowel disease

10. **How is EUS used in the clinical evaluation of esophageal cancer?**
    Currently, EUS has no role in the diagnosis of esophageal cancer. Findings from EUS provide morphologic staging but do not supplant the need for histologic diagnosis of malignancy. EUS has not been shown to be helpful in differentiating malignant from inflammatory strictures. It is not sufficiently sensitive to use as a screening test for cancer (i.e., in Barrett's esophagus with dysplasia). Combined EUS with or without fine-needle aspiration (FNA) and computed tomographic (CT) scanning provide the most accurate method of tumor node metastasis (TNM) staging for esophageal cancer. CT should be performed first to exclude distant metastasis (M stage), followed by EUS for precise T and N staging (Table 73-2).

TABLE 73-2. TNM STAGING FOR ESOPHAGEAL CARCINOMA		
Primary Tumor (T)	**Regional Lymph Nodes (N)**	**Distant Metastasis (M)**
Tx Primary tumor cannot be assessed	Nx Regional lymph nodes cannot be assessed	Mx Presence of distant metastasis
T0 No evidence of primary tumor	N0 No regional lymph node metastasis	M0 No distant metastasis
Tis Carcinoma in situ	N1 Regional lymph node metastasis	M1 Distant metastasis
T1 Tumor invades lamina propria or submucosa		
T2 Tumor invades muscularis propria		
T3 Tumor invades the adventitia		
T4 Tumor invades adjacent structures		

11. **How can EUS findings affect clinical management of esophageal carcinoma?**
    - Direct stage-dependent treatment decisions
    - More accurate pretreatment prognosis
    - Preoperative assessment of tumor resectability

12. **What are the problematic areas for EUS in the staging of esophageal cancer?**
    - At presentation, 25–50% of esophageal cancers are so advanced that passage of the echoendoscope beyond the cancer is prohibited. Wallace et al. (2000) showed that obstructing malignant esophageal strictures can be safely dilated to permit EUS with fine-needle aspiration (FNA) in approximately 90% of such patients.
    - Accurate T_1 staging is difficult, and overstaging is common.
    - EUS features cannot accurately distinguish between malignant and inflammatory lymph nodes. Only about 25% of patients with nodal metastasis exhibit the four characteristic EUS features: round shape, size >1 cm, hypoechoic, and distinct margins. EUS-FNA of suspicious lymph nodes should be done to improve staging accuracy.
    - EUS does not accurately stage esophageal cancer after chemoradiation.

13. **Does EUS have a role in the evaluation of gastric cancer?**
    EUS has no role in the initial diagnosis of gastric cancer and should not be used as a screening tool in patients at risk for this disease. However, in patients where the suspicion of linitis plastica is not confirmed by biopsy, identification of the typical EUS pattern of this cancer contributes significantly to the correct diagnosis (Fig. 73-3). Radial sector scanning in the region of the pylorus and proximal fundus can be technically difficult. If stage-dependent treatment protocols are used, then EUS is indicated when CT shows no metastasis (M0). EUS appears to be reliable in predicting stages T1–T3, which are surgically resectable (R0).

14. **What are the problematic areas for EUS staging of gastric malignancy?**
    1. Overstaging of 20–30%, mainly in T2 lesions, is partly due to the peculiar histopathologic definition of stage T2 (infiltration into the submucosa) versus T3 (invasion of the serosa), a differentiation that cannot be made by EUS. Also, portions of the stomach are not covered by serosa.

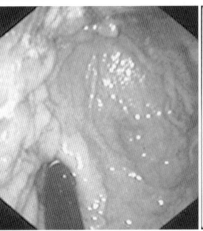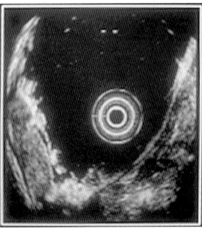

Figure 73-3. Endoscopic view of a gastric adenocarcinoma *(left)* compared with EUS findings *(right)* of a thickened tumor involving the first three echo layers, from the 7 o'clock to the 9 o'clock position. The echoendoscope is located in the center of the water-filled stomach.

2. Differentiation of gastric cancer confined to the mucosa (and therefore amenable to endoscopic treatment) from cancer involving the submucosa (with an attendant increase in the incidence of lymph node metastasis) is relatively inaccurate (60–70%). Small lesions that are flat, slightly depressed, or elevated at endoscopy and cancerous on biopsy can be assumed to be confined to the mucosa, if EUS shows no abnormality of the gastric wall in relation to the tumor. Overstaging occurs predominantly with ulcerating, early carcinomas, because EUS cannot differentiate malignancy from ulcer-related fibrosis and inflammation.

3. Distinguishing inflammatory from malignant lymph nodes requires EUS-FNA sampling.

15. **Summarize the TNM staging classification for gastric malignancy.**
    Primary tumor (T)
Tx	Primary tumor cannot be assessed
T0	No evidence of primary tumor
T1	Tumor confined to mucosa or submucosa
T2	Tumor invades muscularis propria or subserosa
T3	Tumor invades serosa without invasion into adjacent structures
T4	Tumor invades adjacent structures

    Regional lymph nodes (N)
Nx	Regional lymph nodes cannot be assessed
N0	No regional lymph node metastasis
N1	Positive perigastric lymph nodes, 3 cm from the tumor edge
N2	Positive perigastric lymph nodes, 3 cm from the tumor edge or positive lymph nodes along the gastric, common hepatic, splenic, or celiac arteries

    Distant metastasis (M)
Mx	Presence of distant metastasis
M0	No distant metastasis
M1	Distant metastasis

16. **How does staging affect treatment?**
    Resectable tumors (R0) = stages T1–T3. Chemotherapy is used for stage T4.

17. **Is EUS helpful in the evaluation of gastric lymphoma?**

Yes. Unlike gastric adenocarcinoma, gastric lymphoma has a highly characteristic pattern of horizontal extension. EUS is quite accurate in determining the T and N stages for gastric lymphoma and helps to select the most appropriate medical or surgical treatment (Fig. 73-4). Low-grade mucosa-associated lymphoid tissue (MALT) lymphoma is often associated with *Helicobacter pylori* and may regress with antibiotic eradication of the infection. When antibiotic treatment fails to reverse the malignant process, or if *H. pylori* is absent, EUS is helpful in staging and guiding treatment.

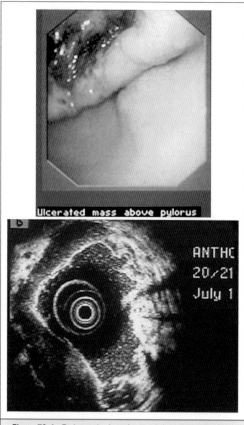

Figure 73-4. Endoscopic view of a gastric lymphoma *(top)* compared with EUS findings of a thickened hypoechoic tumor with foot-like extensions (pseudopodia) into the fourth echogenic layer at the 9 o'clock position. The echoendoscope is located in the center of the water-filled stomach *(bottom)*.

18. **How is EUS helpful in evaluating pancreatic neoplasms?**

The introduction of EUS-FNA has greatly advanced the role of EUS in the management of suspected pancreatic neoplasms. Organ-preserving pancreatic resections can be performed when tumors of low malignant potential, such as cystadenomas and neuroendocrine tumors, are diagnosed. Erickson and Garza showed that EUS-FNA is superior to CT-FNA for the diagnosis of pancreatic cancer. In their hands, EUS-FNA decreased the need for operative staging by 75%.

19. **Neuroendocrine tumors of the pancreas and peripancreas are often difficult to localize by conventional CT, ultrasound, and angiography. Does EUS examination offer any value in localizing these tumors?**

    Yes. EUS is the most accurate imaging method available for the localization of pancreatic endocrine tumors. When CT and sonographic findings are negative, EUS remains >90% accurate. However, EUS fails to detect up to 50% of extrapancreatic neuroendocrine tumors; either transabdominal ultrasound or CT remains the preferred first test. One needs considerable experience with EUS of the pancreas to achieve this accuracy rate.

20. **Describe the use of EUS in the evaluation of colon malignancy.**

    Advances in laparoscopic and endoscopic surgical techniques provide alternatives to conventional exploratory laparotomy and segmental colonic resection for patients diagnosed with early-stage colon cancer. Studies are under way to evaluate the utility of colonoscopic EUS for accurate staging and selection of patients suitable for minimal access surgery and endoscopic mucosal resection.

21. **Describe the use of EUS in the evaluation of rectal malignancy.**

    EUS is highly accurate in determining the T and N stages and superior to CT scanning. The combination of EUS and CT provides the most practical and accurate approach to staging rectal cancers, and the results of both tests should be considered in treatment planning. The surgical options are largely determined by the tumor stage: T1 is appropriate for local resection, whereas T2–T4 require radical extirpation with or without adjuvant radiation/chemotherapy. A recent comparison of endorectal surface coil magnetic resonance imaging (ERSCMRI) with EUS showed that MR and EUS tumor staging are equal, but MR is more accurate in node staging. Further studies comparing the staging accuracy of ERSCMRI and EUS with FNA are needed.

22. **Summarize the EUS characteristics of submucosal tumors.**

Aberrant pancreas	Submucosal; similar in echogenicity to the pancreas; hypoechoic ductular structure may be present
Bronchogenic carcinoma	Hypoechoic; disrupts submucosa and muscularis propria; usually irregular outer margin
Breast cancer	Metastatic; same as bronchogenic cancer
Carcinoid	Mucosal; hypoechoic (Fig. 73-5)
Fibrovascular polyp	Submucosal; mixed echogenicity (Fig. 73-6)

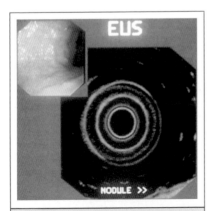

Figure 73-5. EUS finding of a mucosal hypoechoic carcinoid tumor and endoscopic findings.

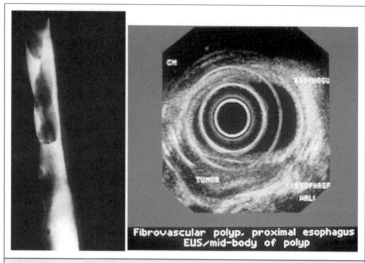

Figure 73-6. Esophageal fibrovascular polyp seen on barium swallow radiograph *(left)* and EUS findings *(right)*.

Gastric cyst	Anechoic; smooth border; submucosal
Granular cell tumors	Hypoechoic; submucosal; smooth margin
Lipoma	Hyperechoic; submucosal (Fig. 73-7)
Leiomyoma	Hypoechoic; contiguous with muscularis propria; smooth outer margin (Fig. 73-8)
Leiomyosarcoma	Hypoechoic; contiguous with muscularis propria; large lesions may have irregular outer margin; adenopathy; small lesions identical to leiomyoma
Lymphoma	Hypoechoic; may disrupt submucosa; muscularis propria and adenopathy
Pancreatic pseudocyst	Anechoic; smooth margin; compress N1 wall
Varices	Anechoic; submucosal serpentine
Vessels	Anechoic; curvilinear branching; often with through-penetration enhancement of the posterior wall

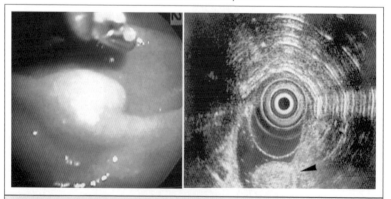

Figure 73-7. Endoscopic finding of a soft submucosal tumor *(left)* and EUS findings of a hyperechoic lipoma *(right)*.

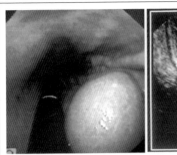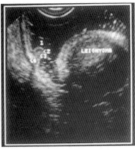

Figure 73-8. Endoscopic view of a submucosal tumor *(left)*, confirmed to be a leiomyoma, arising from the fourth hyperechoic layer *(right)*.

23. Is EUS useful in the evaluation of nonneoplastic disease?

Preliminary studies of EUS in the evaluation of reflux esophagitis, achalasia, and gastric ulcer have not shown EUS to be clinically important. EUS evaluation of enlarged gastric folds can determine the safety of large-particle biopsy devices and exclude the presence of intramural vascular structures. EUS findings contribute to the characterization of the cause of the process. Thickening of the first two layers is characteristic of inflammation, Ménétrier's disease, and lymphoma; large-particle biopsies should be safe and diagnostic. Thickening of all layers suggests lymphoma or linitis plastica. If biopsy findings are still equivocal, laparoscopy/laparotomy may be indicated.

24. How is EUS used in the evaluation of patients with portal hypertension?

EUS can demonstrate fundal varices when endoscopic results are equivocal and define the vascular patency of the splenic vein. Some authorities suggest that intramural vessel enlargement can be detected in patients with portal hypertensive gastropathy. Identification of large paraesophageal varices >5 mm by EUS is predictive of variceal hemorrhage. Others have shown that EUS can guide treatment of esophageal varices and facilitate treatment of bleeding gastric varices with injection of cyanoacrylate glue.

25. Does EUS have a role in the evaluation of recurrent idiopathic pancreatitis?

Yes. When ERCP fails to detect the anatomic cause of recurrent idiopathic pancreatitis (e.g., choledocholithiasis, microlithiasis, sphincter of Oddi dysfunction, pancreatic divism), EUS should be performed. Lui et al. (2000) showed that EUS detects stones in the gallbladder and/or common bile duct in 77% of patients with recurrent idiopathic pancreatitis and negative results with previous CT, US, or ERCP.

26. What is the stack sign? Does it have clinical significance?

The stack sign refers to a characteristic view of the bile and pancreatic ducts. The view is obtained by positioning the echoendoscope in the long scope position with the transducer in the duodenal bulb. The balloon is inflated and advanced snugly into the apex of the bulb. From this position, the bile duct (closest to the transducer) and pancreatic duct can be seen to run parallel through the pancreatic head. The absence of the stack sign may suggest pancreatic divism.

27. Describe the role of EUS in the evaluation of chronic pancreatitis.

EUS is more sensitive than CT in detection of early chronic pancreatitis. Its role in monitoring for neoplastic change in patients with hereditary or chronic alcoholic pancreatitis is under evaluation. EUS-guided celiac block appears to be superior to CT-guided block in terms of pain control and cost. EUS features of chronic pancreatitis include parenchymal and ductal abnormalities:

Parenchymal abnormalities

Hyperechoic foci (distinct 1- to 2-mm hyperechoic points)

Hyperechoic strands (hyperechoic irregular lines)

Lobularity (2- to 5-mm lobules)

Cysts (thin-walled, round, anechoic structures >2 mm in diameter within the pancreatic parenchyma)

Shadowing calcifications

Ductal abnormalities

Dilation (head >3 mm, body >2 mm, and tail >1 mm)

Irregular duct

Hyperechoic duct margins (duct wall visible as a distinct, hyperechoic structure)

Visible side branches (anechoic structures budding from the main pancreatic duct)

28. Summarize the EUS criteria for chronic pancreatitis.

Mild, chronic pancreatitis: 1–2 abnormal features

Moderate chronic pancreatitis: 3–5 abnormal features

Severe chronic pancreatitis: >5 abnormal features

29. Discuss the role of EUS in evaluating patients with common bile duct stones.

A recent study of patients with choledocholithiasis found EUS to be superior to magnetic resonance cholangiopancreatography (MRCP), but both are highly accurate (96.9% and 82.2%, respectively). However, in most hospitals, extracorporeal ultrasound will continue to be the most cost-effective first test to evaluate for choledocholithiasis. When the patient is too obese to permit diagnostic extracorporeal ultrasound, MRCP is the most accurate noninvasive test. The approximate 5% risk of pancreatitis with ERCP increases the appeal of EUS for evaluation of choledocholithiasis in high-risk patients.

WEBSITES

1. http://www.vhjoe.com

2. http://www.simbionix.com/EUS.html

BIBLIOGRAPHY

1. Ahmad NA, Kochman ML, Lewis JD, Ginsberg GG: Can EUS alone differentiate between malignant and benign cystic lesions of the pancreas? Am J Gastroenterol 96:3295–3300, 2001.

2. Ahmad NA, Lewis JD, Ginsberg GG, et al: EUS in preoperative staging of pancreatic cancer. Gastrointest Endosc 52:463–468, 2000.

3. Anderson MA, Carpenter S, Thompson NW, et al: Endoscopic ultrasound is highly accurate and directs management in patients with neuroendocrine tumors of the pancreas. Am J Gastroenterol 95:2271–2277, 2000.

4. Antillon MR, Chang KJ: Endoscopic and endosonographic guided fine-needle aspiration. Gastrointest Endosc Clin North Am 10:619–636, 2000.

5. Beseth BD, Bedford R, Isacoff WH, et al: Endoscopic ultrasound does not accurately assess pathologic stage of esophageal cancer after neoadjuvant chemoradiation. Am Surg 66:827–831, 2000.

6. Bhutani MS, Hoffman BJ, Hawes RH: Diagnosis of pancreas divism by endoscopic ultrasonography. Endoscopy 31:167–169, 1999.

7. Caletti GC, Fusaroli P, Togliani T, Roda E: Endosonography in gastric lymphoma and large gastric folds. Eur J Ultrasound 11:31–40, 2000.

8. Catalano MF, Lahoti S, Geenen JE, Hogan WJ: Prospective evaluation of endoscopic ultrasonography, endoscopic retrograde pancreatography, and secretin test in the diagnosis of chronic pancreatitis. Gastrointest Endosc 48:11–17, 1998.

9. de Ledinghen V, Lecesne R, Raymond JM, et al: Diagnosis of choledocholithiasis: EUS or magnetic resonance cholangiography? A prospective controlled study. Gastrointest Endosc 49:26–31, 1999.

10. Erickson RA, Garza AA: Impact of endoscopic ultrasound on the management and outcome of pancreatic carcinoma. Am J Gastroenterol 95:2248–2254, 2000.

11. Gress F, Schmitt C, Sherman S, et al: A prospective randomized comparison of endoscopic ultrasound- and computed tomography-guided celiac plexus block for managing chronic pancreatitis pain. Am J Gastroenterol 94:900–905, 1999.

12. Lahoti S, Catalano MF, Alcocer E, et al: Obliteration of esophageal varices using EUS-guided sclerotherapy with color Doppler. Gastrointest Endosc 51:331–333, 2000.

13. Lambert R, Caletti G, Cho E, et al: International workshop on the clinical impact of endoscopic ultrasound in gastroenterology. Endoscopy 32:549–584, 2000.

14. Lee YT, Chan FK, Ng EK, et al: EUS-guided injection of cyanoacrylate for bleeding gastric varices. Gastrointest Endosc 52:168–174, 2000.

15. Lui C, Lo C, Chan JKF, et al: EUS for detection of occult cholelithiasis in patients with idiopathic pancreatitis. Gastrointest Endosc 51:28–32, 2000.

16. Maldjian C, Smith R, Kilger A, et al: Endorectal surface coil MR imaging as a staging technique for rectal carcinoma: A comparison study to rectal endosonography. Abdom Imaging 25:75–80, 2000.

17. Marone P, Petrulio F, de Bellis M, et al: Role of endoscopic ultrasonography in the staging of rectal cancer: A retrospective study of 63 patients. J Clin Gastroenterol 30:420–424, 2000.

18. Martin SP, Ulrich CD II: Pancreatic cancer surveillance in a high-risk cohort. Is it worth the cost? Med Clin North Am 84:739–747, 2000.

19. Powis ME, Chang KJ: Endoscopic ultrasound in the clinical staging and management of pancreatic cancer: Its impact on cost of treatment. Cancer Control 7:413–420, 2000.

20. Rosch T, Dittler HK, Strobel K, et al: Endoscopic ultrasound criteria for vascular invasion in the staging of cancer of the head of the pancreas: A blind reevaluation of videotapes. Gastrointest Endosc 52:469–477, 2000.

21. Schechter NR, Yahalom J: Low-grade MALT lymphoma of the stomach: A review of treatment options. Int J Radiat Oncol Biol Phys 46:1093–1103, 2000.

22. Schwartz DA, Harewood GC, Wiersema MJ: EUS for rectal disease. Gastrointestinal Endoscopy 56:100–109, 2002.

23. Sheth S, Bedford A, Chopra S: Primary gallbladder cancer: Recognition of risk factors and role of prophylactic cholecystectomy. Am J Gastroenterol 95:1402–1410, 2000.

24. Wallace MB, Hawes EH, Sahai AV, et al: Dilation of malignant esophageal stenosis to allow EUS guided fine-needle aspiration: Safety and effect on patient management. Gastrointest Endosc 51:309–313, 2000.

CHAPTER 74

ADVANCED ENDOSCOPIC ULTRASOUND

Erik W. Springer, MD, and Mainor Antillon, MD, MBA, MPH

1. What are the major applications of advanced endoscopic ultrasound (EUS)?
- Sampling of suspected malignant lesions or lymph nodes with EUS-guided fine needle aspiration (EUS-FNA)
- EUS-guided drainage of pancreatic or peripancreatic fluid collections, such as pancreatic pseudocysts
- Celiac plexus neurolysis/block for pain control of pancreatic cancer or chronic pancreatitis

2. What are some investigational applications of advanced endoscopic ultrasound?
- EUS-guided antitumor therapy
- EUS-guided nonpapillary pancreatic and bile duct drainage.
- High-frequency ultrasound probe-assisted endomucosal resection (EMR)

3. What is the role of EUS-guided fine needle aspiration (FNA) biopsy in tissue sampling? Sampling of nodes?
EUS-FNA has been shown to aid in the diagnosis of primary lesions within or close to the gastrointestinal tract, such as rectal, esophageal, pancreatic, and lung cancers. The sensitivity and specificity are still being defined and vary with the type of lesion being evaluated. The sensitivity and specificity of EUS-FNA is higher for lesions, such as pancreatic neuroendocrine tumors and pancreatic cancer, and lower for submucosal lesions, such as gastrointestinal stromal tumors (GIST). EUS-FNA has become extremely useful in the staging of lesions within or close to the gastrointestinal tract. The main utility of EUS-FNA is in nodal staging of these lesions, allowing not only imaging of lymph nodes (Fig. 74-1) but also providing samples of these nodes.

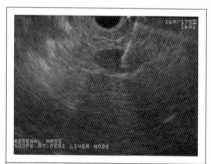

Figure 74-1. EUS-FNA of a lymph node.

4. How is EUS-FNA performed?
EUS is performed with a linear-viewing (curved linear array) scope, which provides an image along the long axis of the scope. This allows the endoscopist to visualize the exact position and action of the needle in sonographic real time. The flow and Doppler capability of this instrument allows for visualization of vascular structures that need to be avoided to perform a safe tissue sampling. The 19- to 22-G aspiration needle, with a stylet, is introduced through the scope channel and, under direct ultrasound visualization, is advanced into the area to be sampled. Once the lesion has been clearly located, the stylet is partially removed to make the needle sharp and ready for puncturing. Once the lesion has been entered, the stylet is advanced to the original position to clear any nonlesional tissue possibly adherent from the passage of the needle through the gastrointestinal tract. Suction is then applied with a syringe to the proximal end of the needle. Sometimes several

"passes" are performed to ensure that enough material is obtained. The presence of a cytologist to evaluate the sample material has been found to be very useful to ensure an adequate sample. The direct visualization of the biopsy needle, along with the resolution of endoscopic ultrasound, allows lesions to be sampled that are even smaller than 10 mm in diameter.

5. **What are the advantages of EUS-FNA over other sampling modalities?**
EUS-FNA allows definitive cytologic diagnosis of both primary and metastatic lesions and thus permits staging of the primary tumor, regional lymph nodes, and metastatic lesions (TNM system). First, the patients undergoing evaluation of a suspected gastrointestinal (GI) wall malignancy often require a EUS examination to obtain tumor (T) staging information (depth of penetration of lesion through the gastrointestinal wall) of the lesion. Nodal staging (N) with tissue acquisition can be performed in the same setting. EUS/FNA can also be useful in determining the presence of distal metastasis (M), such as to the liver. In addition, EUS-FNA allows the sampling of extremely small lesions, including pleural and ascitic fluid collections (Fig. 74-2), that cannot be obtained by other means (such as CT-guided biopsy). In general, EUS staging accuracy appears to be better than all modalities, except surgical exploration. It is also thought that EUS-guided FNA obtained through the gastrointestinal lumen is safer than percutaneous biopsy, with respect to seeding of malignant cells in the needle track.

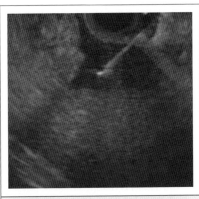

Figure 74-2. EUS-FNA of malignant ascites (not seen on CT scan).

KEY POINTS: MAJOR APPLICATIONS OF ADVANCED EUS

1. Sampling of suspected malignant lesions or lymph nodes with EUS-guided fine needle aspiration (EUS-FNA).

2. EUS-guided drainage of pancreatic or peripancreatic fluid collections, such as pancreatic pseudocysts.

3. Celiac plexus neurolysis/block for pain control of pancreatic cancer or chronic pancreatitis.

6. **What are the sensitivity and specificity of EUS-FNA for the diagnosis of malignancy?**
The sensitivity and specificity of EUS-FNA for diagnosis of malignancy depend on the type of tissue being sampled (Table 74-1).

7. **What is the role of EUS-FNA in the evaluation of mediastinal lymphadenopathy and non-small-cell lung carcinoma?**
Because the mediastinum is in close proximity to the esophagus, EUS with FNA is a useful tool for evaluation of mediastinal adenopathy secondary to any malignancy (Fig. 74-3). It is particularly useful in patients who have non-small-cell lung cancer (NSCLC). In patients with NSCLC, the most significant predictor of long-term survival is the presence of metastasis within regional bronchopulmonary or mediastinal lymph nodes. Studies have shown that 50% of

TABLE 74-1. SENSITIVITY AND SPECIFICITY OF EUS-FNA

Tissue	Sensitivity	Specificity
Pancreatic cancer	90–95%	90–100%
Mediastinal lymphadenopathy	75%	90–100%
Peri-intestinal lymphadenopathy	70–90%	93–100%
Mucosal/submucosal lesions	50–90%	80–100%

(Data from Harewood and Wiersema, 2002; Rösch T: Endoscopic ultrasonography: Imaging and beyond. Gut 52:1220–1226, 2003; Eloubeidi MA et al, 2003.)

potentially malignant lymph nodes in the mediastinum are easily visible by EUS with greater accuracy than CT. The accuracy of EUS-FNA in diagnosing metastasis to lymph nodes has been found to be 96%. In addition, the information provided by EUS-FNA has been found to change further management in the majority of the patients who have had the procedure. EUS-FNA is safer and more cost-effective than other more invasive methods of sampling, such as mediastinoscopy or thoracotomy.

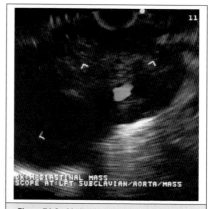

Figure 74-3. Mediastinal mass invading the left ubclavian artery.

8. **Do prophylactic antibiotics need to be used prior to EUS-FNA?**
   No. Routine use of prophylactic antibiotics prior to any EUS-FNA is not advisable. Antibiotic prophylaxis is advised prior to FNA of cystic lesions that will be sampled, especially if they are not going to be entirely drained. Use of prophylactic antibiotics prior to rectal EUS/FNA is widely practiced.

9. **What are the contraindications of EUS-FNA?**
   There are no specific absolute contraindications to EUS-FNA. Nevertheless, severe coagulopathy would be a relative contraindication to EUS-FNA. Use of prophylactic antibiotics before FNA of any cystic lesion or lower GI lesion is advisable.

10. **What are the risks of EUS-FNA?**
    The risks of EUS-FNA are thought to be extremely low, given the small diameter of the aspiration needle. In addition to the usual risks of any endoscopic procedure (bleeding, perforation, sedation risk), a 0.5% overall complication rate was reported in a multicenter trial predominantly from infectious or hemorrhagic events. EUS-FNA of the pancreas has a very small risk of acute pancreatitis, probably less than 1% (Fig. 74-4). This risk is certainly lower than other methods used to obtain tissue sampling for the diagnosis of pancreatic malignancy, such as endoscopic retrograde cholangiopancreatography (ERCP).

11. **What is the role of EUS in sampling pancreatic cystic neoplasms?**
    EUS with FNA can be used to obtain diagnosis in the case of suspected cystic neoplasms (Fig. 74-5). If a lesion in the pancreas is symptomatic or has malignant-appearing features on

EUS visualization alone, then surgical resection is indicated and FNA is not required. If the diagnosis is unclear, then FNA with cytologic evaluation can be useful. Additional analysis of aspirated fluid can also be of value, such as a mucin stain (positive in intraductal papillary mucinous tumor, mucinous cystadenoma, and mucinous cystadenocarcinoma), determination of amylase level (suggestive of a pseudocyst), and CEA level. (A high CEA level would suggest the presence of mucinous cystadenoma with malignant potential, but a normal CEA level would suggest the presence of a serous cystadenoma or pseudocyst with no malignant potential.)

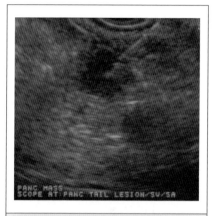

Figure 74-4. EUS-FNA of neuroendocrine tumor in the tail of the pancreas.

12. **Is there a risk of biopsy tract seeding when EUS-FNA of a suspected malignancy is sampled?**
    Yes, although the amount of risk is very low. Comparative studies have found that there is less risk of seeding with EUS-FNA when compared to percutaneous CT-guided FNA biopsy.

13. **How is EUS-guided transmural pseudocyst drainage performed?**
    Transmural EUS-guided pseudocyst drainage can be performed by a multistep or single-step procedure. The multistep procedure involves EUS localization of the pseudocyst, followed by transmural drainage using a side viewing endoscope (duodenoscope). Presence of gastric or

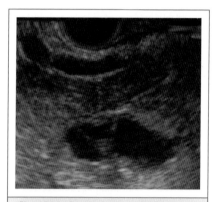

Figure 74-5. Septated cystic mass in the pancreas: biopsy positive for cystadenocarcinoma.

duodenal varices and lack of bulging of the stomach/duodenum produced by the pseudocyst are contraindications to using a duodenoscope for transmural drainage.

The single-step procedure allows the endoscopist to achieve drainage of the pseudocyst with a single linear array EUS scope. This technique allows continued EUS imaging during the whole procedure. Presence of varices or the lack of a bulge does not preclude the performance of transmural drainage with this technique.

The placement of large bore endoprostheses (10 Fr double pigtail stents) requires the use of a therapeutic EUS scope. The procedure starts with a thorough EUS examination of the pseudocyst and surrounding areas. The linear array echoendoscope with its color flow/Doppler capabilities will allow evaluation of the presence of vessels/structures that may be situated in the needle pathway. After the needle pathway is found to be safe, a 19-G FNA needle is advanced into the pseudocyst, and cyst fluid is aspirated. The resulting specimen could be sent for microbiologic and biochemical analysis to corroborate the presence of a pseudocyst and to determine the presence or absence of infection.

A 0.035-in guidewire is subsequently introduced through the needle into the pseudocyst cavity. Fluoroscopy can be used for guidance. After the guidewire is coiled into the cyst, the FNA needle is removed, leaving the guidewire in place.

A triple lumen needle knife sphincterotome is then advanced over the guidewire. Next, opening of the gut-cyst wall is performed by cutting with the sphincterotome, which is subsequently removed, leaving the guide-wire in place. Dilatation of the gut-cyst opening is performed, using a 10-mm biliary balloon dilator over the guidewire. Dilation is followed by the placement of the first 10 Fr 2- to 3-cm double pigtail stent into the cyst. The original guidewire is removed from the cyst.

Placement of the second 10 Fr 2- to 3-cm double pigtail stent is performed over the wire after recannulation of the opening next to the first stent with the sphincterotome. With the use of this technique, there is no need for nasocystic catheter drainage, even in the presence of infected pseudocysts.

Single-step EUS-guided pseudocyst drainage is illustrated in Figures 74-6 through 74-11.

14. What are the major risks of transmural EUS-guided pseudocyst drainage?

The major risk is of bleeding (significant bleeding in approximately 5% of cases). Puncture of the pseudocyst with a needle knife and subsequent balloon dilation, rather than the creation of a longitudinal incision, is thought to reduce the risk of bleeding. Perforation occurs in approximately 5% of cases. Infection can also occur after EUS-guided transmural drainage. Use of prophylactic antibiotics is advisable.

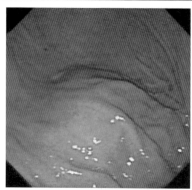

Figure 74-6. Bulge in gastric wall from pseudocyst seen endoscopically (bulge visualization is not necessary for single-step EUS-guided pseudocyst drainage).

15. What is EUS-guided antitumor therapy with radiofrequency ablation?

Radiofrequency ablation is the process of emitting high-intensity ultrasound waves to destroy targeted tissues. This could be performed with an EUS scope to specifically target small tumors. Although to date it has only been performed in a pig model, the technique could be used to ablate small neuroendocrine tumors or palliate unresectable pancreatic cancer.

16. What is the status of EUS-guided fine needle injection (FNI)?

Some preliminary studies have been performed using the injection of local immunotherapy (activated T-lymphocytes [Cytoimplant]) and modified viruses (ONYX-015) into pancreatic

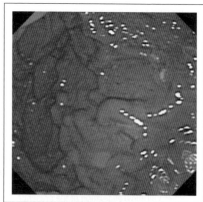

Figure 74-7. No bulge but endoscopic presence of gastric varices in a patient with pseudocyst. EUS-guided pseudocyst drainage can still be safely performed.

adenocarcinomas. Neither of these studies showed a beneficial effect but demonstrated the applicability of the concept. Further studies are currently being developed.

17. **What are the indications for EUS-guided celiac plexus block (CPB) and celiac plexus neurolysis (CPN)? What is the difference? Why do they work?**

The celiac plexus transmits pain sensations from the pancreas and most of the abdominal organs. As a result, blockage of this transmission has been found to be effective in the therapy of pain. CPB refers to the use of steroid and/or local anesthetics to temporarily inhibit celiac plexus function in patients with uncontrolled pain secondary to chronic pancreatitis. CPN refers to the use of alcohol or phenol to produce neurolysis in patients with uncontrolled pain secondary to pancreatic cancer.

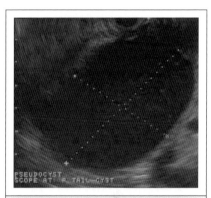

Figure 74-8. Visualization of pseudocyst with EUS.

18. **How are EUS-guided celiac plexus block and neurolysis performed?**

The celiac trunk is easily identified with EUS, because it is located in close proximity to the posterior gastric wall. Because of its close proximity, EUS fine-needle injection (FNI) can be performed. Just prior to the procedure, the patients are well hydrated with intravenous saline to reduce the risk of hypotension. Next, the EUS scope is introduced, and the celiac plexus is located by its position near the celiac trunk. A 22-G needle is advanced into the area, and bupivacaine (an anesthetic) is injected to reduce discomfort. Next, alcohol (for pancreatic cancer) or steroids (for chronic pancreatitis) is injected to the plexus.(See Fig. 74-12.)

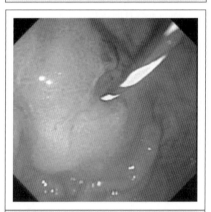

Figure 74-9. Transgastric placement of wire into cyst cavity.

19. **What is the success rate of celiac plexus neurolysis? Celiac plexus block?**

The success rates of CPN and CPB differ. CPN performed for pain from pancreatic cancer has a reported sustained response of 78% at 2 weeks with a sustained response for up to 24 weeks, independent of narcotic use or adjuvant therapy (Gunaratnam, 2001). CPB performed for pain secondary to chronic pancreatitis has a lower success rate. Although there are no randomized, controlled trials investigating

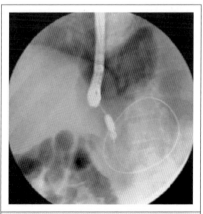

Figure 74-10. Fluoroscopic view of wire in cyst cavity and dilation of tract.

efficacy in this group, one study demonstrated a reduction in pain score and narcotic use in 50% of patients following the procedure. However, persistent pain relief was seen in only 10% of patients at 24-weeks' follow-up.

20. **What are the potential complications of celiac plexus neurolysis?**
There is a 1–2% risk of major complications. Neurologic complications include lower extremity weakness, paresthesia, or paralysis. The artery of Adamkiewicz runs along the spine between T8 and L4 and perfuses the lower two thirds of the spinal cord. Spasm or thrombosis of this artery can lead to spinal cord ischemia. In addition, direct damage to the spinal cord or somatic nerves can cause neurologic deficits. Chronic gastroparesis or diarrhea may also occur. Bleeding, infection, and inadvertent organ puncture are also recognized complications.

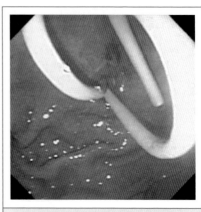

Figure 74-11. Final view of drainage stents.

KEY POINTS: MOST COMMON INDICATIONS FOR THERAPEUTIC EUS

1. Transmural drainage of pseudocysts

2. Celiac plexus block/neurolysis

3. EUS-guided placement of pancreatic and biliary stents

---

21. **Is EUS-guided cholangiography or pancreatography possible? When are they indicated?**
Yes. EUS-guided pancreatography and cholangiography can be easily achieved due to the ability of EUS to image the common bile duct (CBD) and pancreatic duct (PD). Injection of contrast into the ducts can be performed. These techniques are indicated when access to the CBD or PD cannot be achieved through ERCP techniques. EUS-guided placement of stents into the PD or biliary system has also been described.

22. **What are EUS-guided nonpapillary bile duct drainage and EUS-guided nonpapillary pancreatic duct drainage? How are they performed?**
EUS-guided transluminal drainage of the bile duct has been described. In this technique transgastric, transduodenal, or

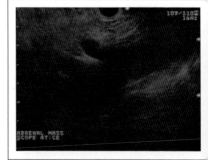

Figure 74-12. Celiac axis identified by EUS.

transjejunal access of the bile duct with stent placement can be achieved in patients whose bile duct cannot be accessed through the standard transpapillary route. This might be an issue in the case of tumor obstruction or surgically altered anatomy (Billroth II or gastrectomy with Roux-en-Y). It is essentially a modification of the technique used for transduodenal or transgastric drainage of pancreatic pseudocysts where the lumen of a dilated bile duct is accessed instead of a pseudocyst. Although it has been performed in only a few patients, it may eventually be shown to be a viable alternative to percutaneous biliary drainage.

Similarly, EUS-guided pancreatic duct drainage has been performed via a transgastric route (pancreaticogastrostomy) to alleviate pain associated with chronic pancreatitis and ductal disruption/obstruction. After identification and localization of a dilated pancreatic duct with EUS, a 19-G needle is introduced through the gastric wall, which is exchanged for a guidewire. After enlargement of this opening, a stent can be placed.

23. **What is high-frequency US probe sonography-assisted endoscopic mucosal resection (EMR)?**

A high-frequency ultrasound probe uses a frequency of 20 or 30 MHz, rather than 7.5 or 12 MHz frequencies used in a conventional EUS transducer. The probe is introduced through the working channel of a standard therapeutic endoscope. The advantage of this probe is that it can be placed directly on a lesion with direct endoscopic guidance. In addition, the higher frequency visualizes more superficially but allows more detailed evaluation of the layers of the gastrointestinal wall. This allows one to evaluate the depth of invasion of a mucosal lesion, whether in the esophagus, stomach, or colon, and determine whether it can be appropriately and safely removed by EMR, after submucosal injection. (See Figs. 74-13 and 74-14.)

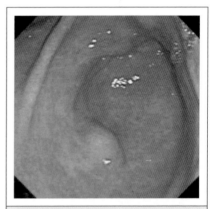

Figure 74-13. Submucosal mass seen on endoscopy.

24. **What about EUS-assisted resection of submucosal tumors?**

Traditionally, submucosal tumors have been surgically resected. The detailed evaluation of the gastrointestinal tract by high frequency EUS has changed this. High frequency EUS-assisted resection (using a high-frequency ultrasound probe) has been performed with tumors <2 cm in diameter prior to EMR. In one study, resections in 28 patients were performed with a 93% success rate. Lesions removed in this study included leiomyomas, carcinoid tumors, and lipomas of the esophagus, stomach, small bowel, colon, and rectum.

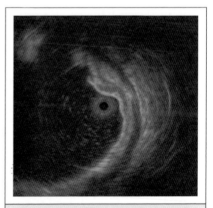

Figure 74-14. High-frequency ultrasound probe: hyperechoic lesion arising from submucosa consistent with lipoma.

BIBLIOGRAPHY

1. Antillon MR, Chang KJ: Endoscopic and endosonography guided fine-needle aspiration. Gastrointest Endosc Clin North Am 10(4):619–636, 2000.

2. Antillon MR, Shah RJ, Chen YK: Single-step endoscopic ultrasound (EUS) drainage of infected and noninfected pseudocysts using large (10-French) endoprostheses. Gastrointest Endosc 57(5):W1201, 2003.

3. Bhutani MS: Emerging indications for interventional endoscopic ultrasonography. Endoscopy 35:45–48, 2003.

4. Bhutani MS: Endoscopic ultrasonography. Endoscopy 34(11):888–895, 2002.

5. Bhutani MS: Endoscopic ultrasound guided antitumor therapy. Endoscopy 35(S1):S54–S56, 2003.

6. Burmester E, Niehaus J, Leineweber T, Huetteroth T: EUS-cholangio-drainage of the bile duct: Report of 4 cases. Gastrointest Endosc 57(2):246–251, 2003.

7. Dye CE, Waxman I: Endoscopic ultrasound. Gastroenterol Clin North Am 31:863–879, 2002.

8. Eloubeidi MA, Chen VK, Eltoum IA, et al: Endoscopic ultrasound-guided fine needle aspiration biopsy of patients with suspected pancreatic cancer: diagnostic accuracy and acute and 30-day complications. Am J Gastroenterol 98(12):2663–2668, 2003.

9. Francois E, Kahaleh M, Giovannini M, et al: EUS-guided pancreaticogastrostomy. Gastrointest Endosc 51(1):128–133, 2002.

10. Fusaroli P, Caletti G: Endoscopic ultrasonography. Endoscopy 35(2):127–135, 2003.

11. Giovannini M, Binmoeller K, Seifert H: Endoscopic ultrasound-guided cystogastrostomy. Endoscopy 35(3):239–245, 2003.

12. Gress F, Schmitt C, Sherman S, et al: Endoscopic ultrasound-guided celiac plexus block for managing abdominal pain associated with chronic pancreatitis: A single multi-center experience. Am J Gastroenterol 96(2):409–416, 2001.

13. Gress F, Schmitt C, Sherman S, et al: A prospective randomized comparison of endoscopic ultrasound- and computer tomography-guided celiac plexus block for managing chronic pancreatitis pain. Am J Gastroenterol 94(4):900–905, 1999.

14. Gunaratnam NT, Sarma AV, Norton ID, Wiersema MJ: A prospective study of EUS-guided celiac plexus neurolysis for pancreatic cancer pain. Gastrointest Endosc 54(3):316–324, 2001.

15. Harada N, Kouzu T, Arima M, et al: Endoscopic ultrasound-guided pancreatography: A case report. Endoscopy 27(8):612–615, 1995.

16. Harewood GE, Wiersema MJ: Endomography-guided FNA biopsy in the evaluation of pancreatic passes. Am J Gastroenterol 97(6):1386–1391, 2002.

17. Hawes RH: Endoscopic management of pseudocysts. Rev Gastroenterol Disord 3(3):135–141, 2003.

18. Hoffman BJ, Knapple WL, Bhutani MS, et al: Treatment of achalasia by injection of botulinum toxin under endoscopic ultrasound guidance. Gastrointest Endosc 45(1):77–79, 1997.

19. Levy MJ, Wiersema MJ: EUS-guided celiac plexus neurolysis and celiac plexus block. Gastrointest Endosc 57(7):923–930, 2003.

20. Rösch T: Endoscopic ultrasonography: Imaging and beyond. Gut 52:1220–1226, 2003.

21. Waxman I, Dye CE: Interventional endosonography. Cancer J 8(Suppl 1):S113–S123, 2003.

22. Waxman I, Saitoh Y, Raju GS, et al: High-frequency probe EUS-assisted endoscopic mucosal resection: A therapeutic strategy for submucosal tumors of the GI tract. Gastrointest Endosc 55(1):44–49, 2002.

23. Wiersema MJ, Sandusky D, Carr R, et al: Endosonography-guided cholangiopancreatography. Gastrointest Endosc 43(2):102–106, 1996.

SURGERY OF THE ESOPHAGUS

Todd A. Kellogg, MD, Brant K. Oelschlager, MD, and Carlos A. Pellegrini, MD

CHAPTER 75

GASTROESOPHAGEAL REFLUX DISEASE

1. **Define gastroesophageal reflux disease (GERD).**

   GERD is best defined as symptoms and/or esophageal mucosal injury due to the abnormal reflux of gastric contents into the esophagus. One third of the U.S. population suffers from symptoms of GERD at least once monthly, and 4–7% experience daily symptoms. Although there is a high prevalence of heartburn, not everyone with heartburn has GERD.

2. **Describe the typical and atypical symptoms of GERD.**

   The *most common complaints* in patients with GERD are heartburn, regurgitation, and, occasionally, dysphagia (more precisely, the sensation of blockage to the passage of food in the lower substernal area).

   Atypical or extraesophageal symptoms include cough, asthma, hoarseness, and noncardiac chest pain, which may manifest with or without associated heartburn and regurgitation. Atypical symptoms are the primary complaint in 20–25% of patients with GERD and are secondarily associated with heartburn and regurgitation in many more. Studies have shown nearly 50% of patients with chest pain and negative coronary angiograms, 75% with chronic hoarseness, and that up to 80% with asthma have a positive 24-hour esophageal pH test, indicating abnormal acid reflux into the esophagus. However, it is considerably more difficult to prove a cause-and-effect relationship between atypical symptoms and gastroesophageal reflux than it is for typical symptoms. Many patients with atypical symptoms benefit from antireflux surgery, but surgery is not as effective as for those patients with typical symptoms.

3. **What is Barrett's esophagus? What are the risk factors for Barrett's esophagus?**

   Barrett's esophagus is metaplasia of the normally squamous endothelium of the esophagus into columnar endothelium with intestinal metaplasia (goblet cells). It is a premalignant condition. Prospective studies have determined that the risk of developing esophageal adenocarcinoma in the presence of long-segment Barrett's esophagus is approximately 1 per 100 patient years or 1% per year. This translates into a 5–10% lifetime risk. Factors leading to Barrett's esophagus include (1) early-onset GERD, (2) abnormal lower esophageal sphincter (LES) and low amplitude of esophageal peristalsis, and (3) mixed reflux of gastric and duodenal contents into the esophagus.

4. **What factors play a primary role in altering the gastroesophageal (GE) barrier?**

   Although several factors have been identified, the two most important are hypotension of the LES and loss of the angle of His due to hiatal hernia. Either may contribute to loss of competency and thus abnormal reflux. Hypotension of the LES may take the form of transient loss of the high-pressure zone due to relaxation of the LES. Gastroesophageal reflux results from the loss of the high-pressure zone normally created by the tonic contraction of the smooth muscle fibers of the LES. Physiologic reflux or reflux in early diseases result from this transient relaxation. In severe GERD, the high-pressure zone is permanently reduced or nonexistent.

A large hiatal hernia alters the geometry of the GE junction, and the angle of His is lost. There is a close relationship between the degree of gastric distention necessary to overcome the high-pressure zone and the morphology of the gastric cardia. In patients with an intact angle of His, more gastric dilatation and higher intragastric pressure are necessary to "open" the sphincter than in patients with a hiatal hernia. This explains the association of hiatal hernia with gastroesophageal reflux. A hiatal hernia may also result in hypotension of the LES. Therefore, hiatal hernia may alter the geometry of the GE junction and also the competence of the LES. However, every patient with a hiatal hernia does not have gastroesophageal reflux, and the presence of a small, sliding hiatal hernia without gastroesophageal reflux is not an indication for medical or surgical intervention.

5. **Describe the work-up of patients with suspected GERD.**
   - *24-hour pH monitoring* provides the most direct method of assessing the presence and severity of GERD and, because it has the highest sensitivity and specificity of all available tests, has become the gold standard for the diagnosis of GERD. It is especially useful in the evaluation of patients with atypical symptoms and patients with typical symptoms but with no evidence of esophagitis on endoscopy. The test also measures the correlation between symptoms and episodes of reflux. This information can be used to predict the success of treatment.
   - *Esophageal manometry* evaluates the peristaltic function of the esophagus and the pressure and relaxation of the LES. It is not a diagnostic test but provides information about the severity of the underlying physiologic defects of the LES and esophageal body. It also determines the location of the LES for proper placement of 24-hour pH probes (i.e., 5 cm above the LES).
   - *Barium swallow* can be used to diagnose the complications of advanced GERD, including peptic strictures, but its most important role is in preoperative evaluation. The study is used to assess the size and reducibility of a hiatal hernia and the presence of esophageal shortening. It also evaluates the propulsive action of the esophagus for both liquids and solids. A large, fixed hiatal hernia or paraesophageal hernia and a short esophagus are evidence of advanced disease and may predict a long, difficult operation.
   - *Upper endoscopy* of the esophagus helps to identify the presence of esophagitis and Barrett's esophagus. It can be also used to evaluate response to treatment and to detect complications of GERD, including a peptic stricture and shortened esophagus. These findings influence therapeutic decisions. Finally, endoscopy provides valuable information about the absence of other lesions in the upper gastrointestinal (GI) tract that can produce symptoms identical to those of GERD.

6. **What is the significance of a defective LES?**
   The finding of a permanently defective LES (pressure <6 mmHg) has several implications. First, it is almost always associated with esophageal mucosal injury and predicts that symptoms will be difficult to control with medical therapy. It is a signal that surgical therapy is probably needed for consistent, long-term control. When the LES is permanently defective, the condition is irreversible, even when the associated esophagitis has healed. The worse the esophageal injury, the more likely it is that the LES is defective. Approximately 40% of patients with pH-positive GERD and no mucosal injury have a mechanically defective LES, whereas nearly 100% of patients with long-segment Barrett's esophagus have a defective LES.

7. **What is the significance of abnormal esophageal motility in patients with GERD?**
   Long-standing, severe GERD can lead to deterioration of esophageal body function. Abnormalities of esophageal body function can present as a lack of peristalsis, severely disordered peristalsis (>50% simultaneous contractions), or ineffective peristalsis (the amplitude of the contractions in one or more of the lower esophageal segments is <30 mmHg) also called *ineffective esophageal motility* (IEM). Dysphagia is generally a prominent symptom in patients with defective peristalsis. Some believe that a partial fundoplication is preferable in patients with

poor esophageal motility. We and others have demonstrated that in these patients a "floppy" or loose fundoplication does not result in an increased incidence of postoperative dysphagia and provides a superior antireflux barrier.

8. **What are the indications for an antireflux operation?**
   - Complications of GERD, including erosive esophagitis, stricture, and Barrett's esophagus
   - Dependence on proton pump inhibitors for symptom relief, even without mucosal injury
   - Atypical or respiratory symptoms that are secondary to GERD
   - Need for long-term medical therapy, particularly if escalating doses of proton pump inhibitors (PPIs) are needed to control symptoms
   - Young age of onset of disease, requiring long-term therapy

   The operation is also indicated for younger patients (below age 50) who are noncompliant with a drug regimen, or for whom medications are a financial burden, and for patients who prefer a single intervention to long-term drug treatment. Surgery may be the treatment of choice in patients who are at high risk of progression, despite medical therapy. Although this population is not well defined, risk factors that predict progressive disease and poor response to medical therapy include:
   - Nocturnal reflux on 24-hour esophageal pH study
   - Structurally deficient LES (pressure <6 mmHg)
   - Mixed reflux of gastric and duodenal juice
   - Mucosal injury at presentation

9. **What are the important technical steps of an antireflux operation?**
   Most antireflux operations are now performed using laparoscopic techniques. Five trocars are inserted in the upper abdomen to provide access to the laparoscope and instruments. The short gastric vessels are divided in the proximal part of the stomach, and the fundus of the stomach is mobilized so that it can be placed around the distal esophagus without tension. Dissection is performed to identify the right and left crura of the diaphragm. The distal esophagus is mobilized so that at least 3 cm of the distal esophagus lies without tension in the abdomen. The crura are approximated with nonabsorbable sutures, and the fundoplication is constructed around the distal esophagus. A 52-Fr bougie is placed in the esophagus to prevent a very tight fundoplication. Some surgeons anchor the wrap to the crura of the diaphragm and to the esophagus to help prevent it from slipping into the chest.

10. **List the predictors of successful antireflux surgery.**
    - Abnormal score on 24-hour esophageal pH monitoring
    - Typical symptoms of GERD (heartburn and regurgitation)
    - Symptomatic improvement in response to acid suppression therapy before surgery

    Each of these factors helps to establish that GERD is the cause of the symptoms. They have little to do with severity of the disease.

11. **What are the predictors of poor outcome after antireflux surgery?**
    Most patients with documented GERD, normal esophageal body function, and length without stricture or scarring have excellent outcomes. The presence of GI symptoms other than typical GERD symptoms predicts less than optimal results. A large hiatal hernia, stricture with persistent dysphagia, and Barrett's are characteristics of advanced GERD and may predict less than ideal results.

12. **Explain the benefits of surgical treatment of GERD.**
    Antireflux procedures performed by experienced esophageal surgeons provide several benefits that cannot be accomplished with antacid medications. A successful operation augments the LES and repairs the hiatal hernia. It prevents the reflux of both gastric and duodenal juice, thus preventing aspiration. Antireflux operations also improve esophageal body motility and speed gastric

emptying, which is often subclinically delayed in patients with GERD. Most patients (>90%) are relieved of symptoms, eat unrestricted diets, and are satisfied with the outcome of surgery.

13. **Discuss the complications of laparoscopic fundoplication.**
    Improvements in technology have led to the successful application of the laparoscopic surgical approach for the treatment of GERD over the past 10 years. A laparoscopic antireflux operation is associated with significantly reduced postoperative pain, shorter hospitalization, quicker recovery, and improved cosmesis. The overall incidence of complications after laparoscopic Nissen fundoplication is 8% (range: 2–13%). Most complications are minor and include urinary retention, postoperative gastric distention, and superficial wound infections. Mild early dysphagia is common (15–20% of patients), but the incidence of residual dysphagia after 3 months is <5%. Fewer than 1% of these patients need intervention to treat dysphagia. The incidence of serious complications is <1%, and mortality is extremely rare (<1%).

14. **Is antireflux surgery cost-effective?**
    Yes. Three cost-utility analyses from the United States and Europe have shown that the cost of open or laparoscopic surgery is less than the cost of lifelong daily therapy with PPIs. Even for men as old as ages 65–69, the cost of lifelong omeprazole (20 or 40 mg/day) exceeds the costs of either open or laparoscopic surgery. The point at which the cost of medical therapy equals the cost of surgical treatment was 4 years for open surgery and 17 months for laparoscopic fundoplication. There have been reports demonstrating an increased cost of surgical therapy compared to medical therapy, thought to be mainly related to the indiscriminate use of PPIs postoperatively. However, with the fluctuating costs of PPIs and the declining cost of laparoscopic antireflux procedures, ongoing cost-effectiveness analysis is warranted.

HIATAL HERNIAS AND PARAESOPHAGEAL HERNIAS

15. **What causes a hiatal hernia?**
    The precise cause of a hiatal hernia is unknown. Its pathogenesis is thought to involve at least two important factors: increased intra-abdominal pressure and a progressive enlargement of the diaphragmatic hiatus. The increased incidence with age suggests that these hernias are acquired.

16. **Define the three types of hernias occurring at the hiatus.**
    Type I is a sliding hiatal hernia, in which the GE junction migrates through the hiatus. *Type II* hiatal hernia is a true paraesophageal hernia (PEH), where the fundus or other organ herniates through the hiatus, while the GE junction remains in its normal anatomic position. A *type III* hiatal hernia is a combination of types I and II, where there is herniation of the GE junction and another organ (usually the stomach) into the posterior mediastinum.

17. **What are the signs and symptoms of a paraesophageal hernia?**
    Many hiatal hernias are asymptomatic and are first recognized on chest radiography. Type I is often associated with reflux but does not cause direct symptoms. PEHs can cause symptoms of postprandial pain, early satiety, abdominal bloating, and microcytic anemia, and may or may not be associated with reflux. PEHs are often the cause of unexplained anemia in the elderly with otherwise normal upper and lower endoscopy. Large PEHs can cause shortness of breath from loss of vital capacity due to impingement of hernia contents on the lung. Rarely, acute herniation occurs, causing sudden pain and symptoms of obstruction. Strangulation can cause gastric necrosis, resulting in rapid decompensation, shock, and death.

18. **How are hiatal hernias and paraesophageal hernias diagnosed and evaluated?**
    Paraesophageal hernias are often first diagnosed incidentally on chest radiography as an air-fluid level within the posterior mediastinum. Upper gastrointestinal contrast study is the gold

standard for evaluating these hernias. Upper endoscopy will verify the presence of esophagitis, gastritis, and Cameron's ulcers, or other lesions that can mimic the symptoms of a PEH. Esophageal manometry and 24-hour pH monitoring are not mandatory for diagnosis or in its work-up; it has been demonstrated that most of these patients have a defective lower esophageal sphincter, and about half have abnormal gastroesophageal reflux.

19. **What are the indications for surgical repair of paraesophageal hernias?**
A PEH repair is more complex than a typical antireflux operation and requires more technical expertise. Because of the additional risks associated with this procedure, the decision to pro- ceed with surgical repair should be carefully considered. It was once believed that all PEHs should be repaired regardless of the presence or absence of symptoms due to a high incidence of severe complications associated with nonoperative management. Recent studies and experi- ence suggest that the risk of observation is much lower than previously thought. Rattner and colleagues showed that in asymptomatic patients, elective repair would benefit only one in five patients, despite the decreased morbidity associated with the laparoscopic era. Nevertheless, it should be considered in younger, fit patients under age 60 and in those with symptoms who do not have a prohibitive operative risk.

20. **What is the operative strategy of a PEH repair?**
The steps of PEH repair are (1) return the stomach and esophagus to their normal intra-abdomi- nal positions, (2) remove the hernia sac, (3) close the hiatus, (4) anchor the stomach below the diaphragm, and (5) perform a fundoplication (according to most surgeons). This can be accom- plished either transabdominally (open/laparoscopic) or transthoracically.

ACHALASIA

21. **Define achalasia. What are the classic findings of esophageal achalasia?**
Achalasia means "failure to relax" in Greek. The disease is characterized by the triad of (1) incomplete or absent relaxation in the LES, (2) progressive loss of peristalsis in the body of the esophagus, and (3) resultant esophageal dilatation.

22. **What are the most common symptoms of achalasia?**
All patients with achalasia have a history of *dysphagia*. Many patients describe exacerbation of dysphagia when they drink cold liquids or are under emotional stress. Patients accumulate food in the esophagus until the hydrostatic pressure at the bottom of the column overcomes the resistance of the LES and pushes some food into the stomach. The sensation of dysphagia dis- appears over time in some patients as the esophagus becomes distended and food collects in the distended esophagus instead of passing into the stomach. At that stage patients may develop *heartburn* because of bacterial fermentation of retained food in the esophagus. Two thirds of patients with achalasia experience *regurgitation* and may occasionally present with aspiration pneumonia. One third to one half of patients suffer from *chest pain*. Symptoms are usually present for several years before the diagnosis is made.

23. **Describe the radiologic findings in achalasia.**
Radiologic findings depend on the stage of the disease. Nonspecific findings on chest x-ray may include mediastinal widening, presence of an air-fluid level in the mid-esophagus, absence of a gastric air bubble, and abnormal pulmonary markings due to chronic aspiration. The bar- ium upper GI study is normal in the early stages, but as the disease progresses it shows a dilated, tortuous or sigmoid esophagus with air-fluid level. When the cardia is well visualized, it has typically a narrow, tapering bird's beak appearance. This appearance may also be seen in patients with pseudoachalasia (intrinsic or extrinsic obstruction of the GE junction, usually by tumor).

24. **What is the role of endoscopy in the diagnosis of achalasia?**

    Endoscopy reveals a dilated tortuous esophagus with residual liquid or food in the lumen. Esophagitis discovered during endoscopy is usually a result of fermentation of esophageal contents in untreated cases or of gastroesophageal reflux in patients previously treated for achalasia. The LES appears puckered and does not open with air insufflation; however, unlike a stricture, it permits the passage of the endoscope with a characteristic popping sensation. Endoscopy also identifies yeast esophagitis, which can obliterate the submucosal plane due to inflammation and scarring and can contaminate the mediastinum, in case of an accidental perforation of the esophagus. Therefore, yeast esophagitis should be treated aggressively with oral antifungal agents before achalasia is treated. Endoscopy also identifies patients at a higher risk of esophageal perforation with balloon dilatation due to the presence of a hiatal hernia or an epiphrenic diverticulum.

25. **Discuss the role of esophageal manometry in the diagnosis of achalasia.**

    Manometry is the gold standard for diagnosing achalasia. There are four classic features of achalasia on manometry, but all four are *not* always present:
    - *Incomplete relaxation of the LES* is the most characteristic finding (80% of patients). Normally, the LES relaxes 100% (i.e., to the level of the gastric baseline) during swallowing. In patients with achalasia, relaxation is incomplete.
    - *Aperistalsis* of the distal (smooth-muscle) segment of the esophagus is present in all patients with achalasia. Typical peristaltic waves are of very low amplitude, and peristalsis is absent in patients with a massively distended esophagus. It may be impossible to pass the manometry catheter through the LES, even under fluoroscopy. In such patients, an esophageal body study demonstrating lack of peristalsis is sufficient documentation to proceed with treatment.
    - *Elevated LES pressure.* Most patients have elevated (>25 mmHg) LES pressure. Although LES pressure may be normal, it is usually not subnormal in untreated achalasia.
    - *Positive intraesophageal body pressure.* Normal intraesophageal pressure is subatmospheric. But, in patients with achalasia, it is positive as a result of outflow obstruction and retention of food and secretions.

26. **What is pseudoachalasia? How is it diagnosed?**

    Characteristic manometric and radiologic findings of achalasia may, occasionally, be seen in patients with distal esophageal obstruction from an infiltrating tumor. Such patients have a local tumor that may directly compress the esophagus or a remote tumor (causing paraneoplastic syndrome). Endoscopy helps to rule out the possibility of pseudoachalasia, but careful examination of the GE junction with the scope retroflexed is required to avoid missing a small cancer. However, endoscopy cannot rule out pseudoachalasia caused by a mural or extramural tumor. When this is suspected based on the history (rapid weight loss, weight loss >20 lb, or symptoms with duration <6 months), endoscopic ultrasonography and/or computerized tomography is recommended.

27. **Explain vigorous achalasia.**

    Chest pain is a common complaint in patients with a variant of the disease called *vigorous achalasia*. Such patients have high-amplitude, simultaneous esophageal contractions. They are usually younger and have chest pain as a prominent symptom. Most investigators believe that vigorous achalasia is an early form of the disease that presents in some patients. The cutoff pressure for esophageal contractions used by most experts is 40 mmHg. Patients with non-reduced pressure waves >40 mmHg are classified as having vigorous achalasia.

28. **What studies other than esophageal manometry can be used to diagnose achalasia?**

    In many patients, the esophageal manometry catheter cannot negotiate the tight LES, and some patients cannot tolerate esophageal intubations. In such patients, a radiolabeled semisolid meal has been used to assess esophageal emptying and peristalsis. This study is less specific than manometry but is noninvasive and can also be used to assess treatment response. A timed barium swallow has been suggested by de Oliveira et al. as a simple and reproducible alternative. The patient ingests 100–200 mL of low-density barium over 30–45 seconds. Three-on-one spot x-ray films are obtained at 1, 2, and 5 minutes after ingestion. The degree of emptying is estimated qualitatively by comparing the 1- and 5-minute films. The degree of emptying may also be estimated quantitatively by measuring the height and width of the barium column for both films, calculating the area for both, and determining the percentage of change in the area. Both qualitative and quantitative assessments are accurate methods of estimating esophageal emptying.

29. **What are the nonsurgical options for treatment of achalasia?**
    - *Smooth muscle relaxants,* including long-acting nitrates and calcium channel blockers, are the mainstay of medical treatment. They act by reducing the LES tone. A number of non–placebo-controlled trials, based on small patient populations, have shown satisfactory response to long-acting nitrates and calcium channel blockers. However, because these results have not been reproduced by other investigators, their use is limited to mild cases or patients unsuitable for mechanical or surgical therapies. Sildenafil (Viagra) has been shown to reduce LES pressure in patients with achalasia. Sildenafil augments the smooth muscle relaxation caused by nitric oxide. The role of this new modality in the treatment of achalasia remains to be defined.
    - *Mechanical dilation of the LES* is widely used for treatment of achalasia. The type of dilators and the technique of dilatation have improved considerably over the past four decades. Pneumatic dilatation to a diameter of at least 3 cm (>90 Fr) is recommended to achieve long-term results. Immediate complications of balloon dilatation include intramural hematoma, GI bleeding, and esophageal perforation. Most complications manifest within 6 hours after the procedure. Esophageal perforation occurs in 1–4% of cases. Factors that increase the risk of esophageal perforation include massively dilated esophagus, large hiatal hernia, and epiphrenic diverticulum. Other factors include operator aggressiveness and balloon size. The reported success rate in terms of resolution of dysphagia is 60–80%. Relief is immediate for most patients. However, long-term results show that only 60% of patients are in remission at 1 year and more than one half develop recurrent symptoms by 5 years. A second session of esophageal dilatation is equally effective in patients who respond to the first dilatation, but the chance of success in patients who did not respond to the first dilatation is <20%. The success rate of esophageal myotomy is no different in patients with prior pneumatic dilatation, but dissection and myotomy may occasionally be technically more challenging. Patients younger than age 40 have a lower success rate with esophageal dilatation. Gastroesophageal reflux after dilation has been reported in 2–30% of patients but usually responds well to medical therapy.
    - *Botulinum toxin* (Botox) injection of the LES sphincter is a newer adaptation of successful treatment of skeletal muscle disorders. Botox is a potent inhibitor of acetylcholine release from presynaptic nerve terminals. The proposed mechanism of action is reduction in cholinergic excitation. Early clinical trial results demonstrated 90% immediate clinical response. However, rapid relapse or lack of initial clinical response was noted in 45% of patients, and sustained remission at 6-month follow-up was seen in only 65%. Of those who responded, 68% remained in remission at 1 year, and the average duration of sustained response was 1.3 years. Older patients and those with vigorous achalasia had a better response than younger patients and patients with classic achalasia. Botox therapy is an option for debilitated patients who are unable to tolerate balloon dilatation or surgical myotomy.

30. **How is botulinum toxin useful in patients with an unclear presentation?**
    Botox has been used in the diagnosis and management of three groups of patients with an unclear presentation: (1) patients with symptoms consistent with achalasia but insufficient manometric criteria to make the diagnosis, (2) patients in whom factors in addition to achalasia

contribute to symptoms, and (3) patients with advanced achalasia in whom it is not clear whether sphincter-directed therapy would be of benefit before consideration of esophagectomy. The short duration of the action of Botox can be used to the advantage of such patients because little harm is done, if the injection does not help to relieve symptoms. Other advantages include minimal morbidity and ease of administration.

31. **What are the disadvantages of botulinum toxin for treatment of achalasia?**
    Preoperative use of Botox increases the technical difficulties of esophagomyotomy and thus its potential risks. Because successful dilatation disrupts the muscularis in only one area, healing and scarring are limited to that area of the esophageal wall. Botox, on the other hand, is injected at multiple sites, and injections are frequently repeated. This repeated injury may cause fibrosis of the muscularis and mucosa, eliminating the submucosal plane developed during esophageal myotomy.

32. **Describe the role of esophageal (Heller's) myotomy in the treatment of achalasia.**
    Surgical treatment of achalasia consists of a longitudinal myotomy of the distal esophagus and GE junction. Most myotomies were performed through the chest in the United States before the advent of minimally invasive surgery. The transabdominal laparoscopic approach is currenty the procedure of choice. Both laparoscopic and thoracoscopic approaches are well established and offer the benefits of minimally invasive surgery. Laparoscopic esophageal myotomy produces good long-term results in 84–94% of patients.

33. **What are the basic components of laparoscopic Heller's myotomy for achalasia?**
    Five trocars are placed in the upper abdomen in an arrangement similar to that of a laparoscopic antireflux operation. A myotomy roughly 6–8 cm in length is performed, with 3 cm below the GE junction. We have shown that an extended gastric myotomy has superior relief of dysphagia. The myotomy is carried down to the level of the mucosa. A partial fundoplication is performed after the completion of the myotomy around a 52-Fr bougie.

    There is a general consensus that a complete 360-degree wrap may cause significant obstruction at the distal end of the esophagus and lead to worsening of esophageal function in patients who already have impaired peristalsis. Therefore, most experts favor a partial fundoplication after laparoscopic Heller's myotomy. The two types—partial posterior wrap (Toupet fundoplication) and partial anterior wrap (Dor fundoplication)—are equally popular among surgeons performing a laparoscopic transabdominal myotomy. The incidence of gastroesophageal reflux after surgery for achalasia is 25–48% but with the addition of an antireflux wrap, the rate decreases to 5–20%. Most of these patients have mild-to-moderate reflux and can be easily managed medically.

34. **How do the long-term results of Heller's myotomy compare with mechanical esophageal dilatation?**
    Many retrospective studies have compared the outcome of surgery (open or minimally invasive) with balloon dilatation. Most have shown superior long-term results with surgery. Repeat pneumatic dilatations increase the effectiveness of dilatation from 66–80%, but they also increase the risk of esophageal perforation by twofold to threefold. Younger patients (below age 30) should be treated primarily with myotomy because pneumatic dilatation is <50% effective.

35. **Describe the complications of Heller's myotomy.**
    Laparoscopic Heller's myotomy is a very low-risk operation. The most common complication is perforation of the mucosa, which can be solved by immediate closure. The most feared early complication is an unrecognized esophageal perforation, but the incidence is <1%. Perforation

should be suspected in a patient with persistent fever, tachycardia, and/or left-sided pleural effusion.

Early postoperative dysphagia results usually from an incomplete myotomy. Late dysphagia results from an incomplete esophageal myotomy, an incomplete gastric myotomy, healing of the myotomy, or, more rarely, a reflux-induced peptic stricture. Incomplete myotomy responds usually to extension of the myotomy. Patients with late dysphagia are difficult to treat, especially in the presence of LES pressure <10 mmHg and when the cause of dysphagia is extremely poor esophageal body function or a peptic stricture. In these cases, pneumatic dilatation or Botox injection may be effective. Takedown of the wrap may be useful as well. When the first myotomy is complete, a second myotomy is less likely to be successful; such patients may need esophageal resection.

36. **Is there an association between achalasia and cancer of the esophagus?**
    Patients with achalasia are thought to be at increased risk for the development of squamous cell carcinoma. Tumors develop at an age 10 years younger than in the general population and carry a worse prognosis because of late diagnosis. Surveillance endoscopy is recommended every 2 years by some authors, though the incidence of cancer is still very low. The effect of treatments on the incidence of cancer is not known.

37. **Summarize the approach to patients with symptoms of achalasia.**
    Most patients with achalasia are seen by gastroenterologists and referred for surgery after failure of pneumatic dilatation or Botox injections. Every patient with suspicion of achalasia should undergo (1) esophageal manometry, (2) barium upper GI study, and (3) upper endoscopy. Patients with shorter duration of symptoms and a history of substantial weight loss (>20 lb in 6 months) should also undergo endoscopic ultrasonography to rule out the possibility of pseudoachalasia. Laparoscopic Heller's myotomy should be offered as early as possible to young patients (< age 40) with achalasia. They have a higher incidence of failure with dilatation and Botox injections, and early surgery is recommended to avoid long-term complications.

    The laparoscopic approach to esophageal myotomy provides a magnified view of the operative field and allows precise division of the muscle fibers with excellent results. Laparoscopic Heller's myotomy results in reduced postoperative pain, shorter hospitalization, and better cosmetic results. Pneumatic dilatation may be offered once or twice to patients with mild-to-moderate disease. However, superior long-term results after surgical myotomy argue strongly for surgery in any patient who is fit enough to undergo general anesthesia. Botox therapy should be reserved for patients who are unable to tolerate surgery because of significant comorbidities or whose clinical presentation is complicated and the diagnosis of achalasia is in doubt.

ESOPHAGEAL CANCER

38. **What is the incidence of esophageal cancer?**
    The incidence of esophageal cancer has risen in the past 30 years. Adenocarcinoma has become more prevalent than squamous cell carcinoma in the United States and Western European nations and now accounts for 30–50% of all esophageal cancers. Primary tumor location has shifted to the distal esophagus. The cause for the rising incidence and changing demographics is unknown.

39. **What causes esophageal cancer?**
    Risk factors have been described for squamous cell carcinoma. Tobacco and excessive alcohol consumption appear to have a synergistic effect in its pathogenesis. Diet is also a factor. Risk factors for the development of distal esophageal adenocarcinoma are less clear. The presence of Barrett's esophagus (BE) is associated with an increased risk of developing adenocarcinoma of the esophagus. A population-based case-controlled study from Sweden demonstrated that

symptomatic chronic gastroesophageal reflux is a risk factor for developing esophageal adeno-carcinoma.

40. Discuss the diagnosis and staging of esophageal cancer.

The diagnosis of esophageal cancer is made using esophagogram and esophagoscopy with tissue biopsy. Clinical staging is extremely important; stage, as defined by anatomic extent, is the best predictor of survival in esophageal carcinoma. In addition to prognosis, clinical staging directs therapy. Endoscopic ultrasound (EUS) is accurate for determining the depth of tumor invasion (T) and can be helpful in identifying regional lymph node involvement (N) with an accuracy of 80%. Computed tomography (CT) and positron emission tomography (PET) are useful for identifying distant metastatic disease (M).

41. Describe the relationship of Barrett's esophagus to esophageal cancer.

Barrett's columnar-lined esophagus is an acquired condition of the distal esophagus associated with chronic gastroesophageal reflux. The incidence of adenocarcinoma increases nearly 40-fold in patients with Barrett's esophagus. It is estimated that 5% of patients with Barrett's esophagus will eventually develop invasive cancer, and patients with histologically proven Barrett's esophagus require lifelong surveillance because of this risk. It is generally believed that disease progression occurs in an orderly fashion: Barrett's metaplasia to low-grade dysplasia to high-grade dysplasia to carcinoma. However, all steps are not observed in all patients, even if regular surveillance is performed.

42. Can Barrett's esophagus regress after antireflux therapy?

Maybe. Although there is no evidence of significant Barrett's regression with medical therapy (i.e., PPIs), there is growing evidence that Barrett's esophagus can regress after surgical antireflux procedures. In a study by DeMeester and colleagues, histopathologic regression occurred in 28 of 77 patients (36.4%) after antireflux surgery. Regression was significantly more common in short (<3 cm) than long (>3 cm) segment Barrett's esophagus; 19 of 33 (58%) and 9 of 44 (20%) patients, respectively ($p = .0016$). The majority (95%) of this regression occurred within 5 years after surgery. However, more studies need to be performed before firm conclusions can be drawn.

43. Discuss the appropriate management of patients with high-grade dysplasia (HGD).

The answer to this controversial question must take into account the morbidity and mortality of esophagectomy in context of the risk of ignoring a curable potential esophageal cancer. Extensive measures must be taken to ensure the diagnosis is correct, that is, that low-grade dysplasia or cancer is not mistaken for HGD. If surveillance is to be considered for a patient with HGD, it should be done at specialized centers experienced in endoscopic surveillance, and pathologic evaluation of these lesions is imperative to avoid missing progression to cancer. Endoscopy should be done every 3 months with intensive four quadrant biopsies taken every 1 cm. With such a protocol, cancers that do form are found at an early, curable stage, and approximately 50% of patients may avoid the morbidity of an esophagectomy. Consideration is then given to the patient's age and overall health, focusing on comorbidities that might increase operative risk. This should then be balanced with the extent of the disease to choose the appropriate therapy. A younger, healthier patient with long-segment Barrett's esophagus would be considered a more appropriate candidate for esophagectomy, whereas the older patient with comorbid disease and short-segment Barrett's esophagus may be a better candidate for ablative therapy.

44. When is neoadjuvant therapy appropriate in the treatment of patients with esophageal carcinoma?

There is no role for adjuvant therapy with curative intent, that is, adding adjuvant therapy to surgical resection does not improve the incidence of cure. The data on neoadjuvant therapy are mixed with some studies showing no statistical difference in outcomes and others demonstrating some benefit to chemoradiation followed by surgery. Most of the trials are small and lack the power to show a difference, if indeed one is present. The few prospective, randomized studies comparing neoadjuvant chemoradiation (preoperative chemotherapy and radiation followed by surgery) with surgery alone suggest possible improved local tumor control and survival for patients with stage 2 and stage 3 disease when compared with surgery alone. Walsh et al. demonstrated a survival advantage at 3 years, at which time with neoadjuvant therapy 32% of patients survived compared to 6% in the group who did not receive neoadjuvant therapy. However, more studies, particularly multi-institutional prospective studies, are needed to verify the effectiveness of neoadjuvant chemoradiation for the treatment of stage 2 and stage 3 esophageal cancer.

45. What are the surgical approaches to the patient with esophageal cancer?

Surgery is the primary treatment modality for esophageal cancer. In the United States, esophageal resection is most commonly performed, using one of the following approaches: transhiatal esophagectomy, Ivor-Lewis esophagectomy, multi-incision esophagectomy, and left thoracoabdominal esophagectomy. *Transhiatal esophagectomy* (THE) involves both a midline laparotomy and a left cervical incision. The short gastric and left gastric arteries are ligated, whereas the right gastric artery and right gastroepiploic arcade are carefully preserved. A cervical gastroesophageal anastomosis is performed through the cervical incision. The main advantage of this approach is avoidance of a thoracic anastomosis; the morbidity and mortality of a cervical leak is nearly 10-fold, less than for a thoracic leak. THE also avoids the morbidity of a thoracic incision. The *Ivor-Lewis esophagectomy* also requires two incisions, a midline laparotomy and a right posterolateral thoracotomy. En bloc resection is performed from the hiatus to the apex of the chest. Hilar, subcarinal, and periesophageal nodes can be carefully resected with the esophagus. A gastroesophageal anastomosis is performed in the right chest, and chest tubes are placed for drainage. *Multi-incision esophagectomy* is performed less often and requires three incisions: midline laparotomy, thoracotomy, and a cervical incision. A *left thoracoabdominal esophagectomy* involves one incision extended across the abdomen and posterolateral chest. Regardless of the incisional approach, the same operative procedure is performed, that is, esophagogastrectomy with regional lymph node resection. Though each approach has its proponents, THE is the most common procedure performed, with a decreased incidence of pulmonary complications, the reduced morbidity and mortality of an anastomotic leak, and no evidence that a radical lymphadenectomy benefits overall survival cited as the most compelling arguments.

46. Describe nonsurgical options for treatment of esophageal cancer.

Though, currently, surgery is the mainstay of treatment, other forms of less invasive treatment for subsets of patients is in evolution. These methods can be divided into interventions for palliation and those for cure. Nonsurgical interventions for palliation include esophageal stenting and Nd:YAG laser therapy. Precancerous lesions or superficial cancers confined to the mucosa without evidence of metastatic spread can be cured with local therapy. Appropriate candidates include patients with limited HGD and superficial adenocarcinoma associated with Barrett's esophagus. In these cases, alternative therapies, such as endoscopic mucosal resection (EMR), endoscopically applied Nd:YAG laser, KTP laser, photodynamic therapy (PDT), or argon plasma coagulation (APC), are ablative therapies that have been curative in certain cases. These approaches must still be considered investigational as definitive treatments of esophageal cancer.

47. What is the survival of patients with esophageal cancer?

The overall 5-year survival rate in patients undergoing surgery varies, depending on stage. Those patients with stage 1 disease have an excellent 5-year survival, around 80%. The 5-year survival for stage 2 disease is 35%, and for stage 3 disease is 10%. Those with stage 4 disease live rarely beyond 18 months. Unfortunately, most esophageal cancers present at later stages, when cure is not possible and palliation is the only treatment option.

WEBSITES

1. http://www.vhjoe.com

2. http://www.vhjoe.com/Volume2Issue3/2-3-3.htm

BIBLIOGRAPHY

GASTROESOPHAGEAL REFLUX DISEASE

1. Allen CJ, Anvari M: Gastro-oesophageal reflux related cough and its response to laparoscopic fundoplication. Thorax 53:963–968, 1998.

2. Andersen LI, Madsen PV, Dalgaard P, Jensen G: Validity of clinical symptoms in benign esophageal disease, assessed by questionnaire. Acta Med Scand 221:171–177, 1987.

3. Becker DJ, Sinclair J, Castell DO, Wu WC: A comparison of high and low fat meals on postprandial esophageal acid exposure. Am J Gastroenterol 84:782–786, 1989.

4. Campos GM, Peters JH, DeMeester TR, et al: The pattern of esophageal acid exposure in gastroesophageal reflux disease influences the severity of the disease. Arch Surg 134:882–887; discussion, 887–888, 1999.

5. Campos GM, Peters JH, DeMeester TR, et al: Multivariate analysis of factors predicting outcome after laparoscopic Nissen fundoplication. J Gastrointest Surg 3:292–300, 1999.

6. Castel DO: Management of gastroesophageal reflux disease. Maintenance medical therapy of gastroesophageal reflux?which drugs, how long? Dis Esophagus 7:230–233, 1994.

7. Collet D, Cadiere GB: Conversions and complications of laparoscopic treatment of gastroesophageal reflux disease. Formation for the Development of Laparoscopic Surgery for Gastroesophageal Reflux Disease Group. Am J Surg 169:622–626, 1995.

8. Costantini M, Zaninotto G, Anselmino M, et al: The role of a defective lower esophageal sphincter in the clinical outcome of treatment for gastroesophageal reflux disease. Arch Surg 131:655–659, 1996.

9. DeMeester TR, Ireland AP: Gastric pathology as an initiator and potentiator of gastroesophageal reflux disease. Dis Esophagus 10:1–8, 1997.

10. DeVault KR, Castell DO: Guidelines for the diagnosis and treatment of gastroesophageal reflux disease. Practice Parameters Committee of the American College of Gastroenterology. Arch Intern Med 155:2165–2173, 1995.

11. Fein M, Ritter MP, DeMeester TR, et al: Role of the lower esophageal sphincter and hiatal hernia in the pathogenesis of gastroesophageal reflux disease. J Gastrointest Surg 3:405–410, 1999.

12. Heudebert GR, Marks R, Wilcox CM, Centor RM: Choice of long-term strategy for the management of patients with severe esophagitis: A cost-utility analysis. Gastroenterology 112:1078–1086, 1997.

13. Hinder RA, Filipi CJ, Wetscher G, et al: Laparoscopic Nissen fundoplication is an effective treatment for gastroesophageal reflux disease. Ann Surg 220:472–481; discussion, 481–483, 1994.

14. Hunter JG, Trus TL, Branum GD, et al: A physiologic approach to laparoscopic fundoplication for gastroesophageal reflux disease. Ann Surg 223:673–685; discussion, 685–687, 1996.

15. Johnson LF, DeMeester TR: Evaluation of elevation of the head of the bed, bethanechol, and antacid form tablets on gastroesophageal reflux. Dig Dis Sci 26:673–680, 1981.

16. Katzka DA, Paoletti V, Leite L, Castell DO: Prolonged ambulatory pH monitoring in patients with persistent gastroesophageal reflux disease symptoms: Testing while on therapy identifies the need for more aggressive antireflux therapy. Am J Gastroenterol 91:2110–2113, 1996.

17. Mittal RK, McCallum RW: Characteristics and frequency of transient relaxations of the lower esophageal sphincter in patients with reflux esophagitis. Gastroenterology 95:593–599, 1988.

18. NehraD, Howell P, Williams CP, et al: Toxic bile acids in gastro-oesophageal reflux disease: Influence of gastric acidity. Gut 44:598–602, 1999.

19. Oberg S, Peters JH, DeMeester TR, et al: Endoscopic grading of the gastroesophageal valve in patients with symptoms of gastroesophageal reflux disease (GERD). Surg Endosc 13:1184–1188, 1999.

20. Oelschlager BK, Chang L, Barreca M, et al: Typical GERD symptoms and esophageal pH monitoring are not enough to diagnose pharyngeal reflux: Analysis of 518 patients. Unpublished data.

21. Oelschlager BK, Eubanks T, Oleynikov D, Pellegrini CA: Symptomatic and physiologic outcomes after operative treatment for extraesophageal reflux. Surg Endosc 16:1032–1036, 2002.

22. Peghini PL, Katz PO, Bracy NA, Castell DO: Nocturnal recovery of gastric acid secretion with twice-daily dosing of proton pump inhibitors. Am J Gastroenterol 93:763–767, 1998.

23. Peters JH: The surgical management of Barrett's esophagus. Gastroenterol Clin North Am 26:647–668, 1997.

24. So JB, Zeitels SM, Rattner DW: Outcomes of atypical symptoms attributed to gastroesophageal reflux treated by laparoscopic fundoplication. Surgery 124:28–32, 1998.

25. Viljakka M, Nevalainen J, Isolauri J: Lifetime costs of surgical versus medical treatment of severe gastro-esophageal reflux disease in Finland. Scand J Gastroenterol 32:766–772, 1997.

HIATAL HERNIA AND PARAESOPHAGEAL HERNIA

26. Hill LD: Incarcerated paraesophageal hernia: A surgical emergency. Am J Surg 126:286–291, 1973.

27. Horgan S, Eubanks TR, Jacobson G, et al: Repair of paraesophageal hernias. Am J Surg 177(5):354–358, 1999.

28. Oelschlager BK, Pellegrini CA: Paraesophageal hernias: Open, laparoscopic, or thoracic repair? Chest Surg Clin N Am 11(3):589–603, 2001.

29. Stylopoulos N, Gazelle GS, Rattner DW: Paraesophageal hernia: Operation or observation? Ann Surg 236:492–501, 2002.

ACHALASIA

30. Bortolotti MM, Lopilato C, Porrazzo C, et al: Effects of sildenafil on esophageal motility of patients with idiopathic achalasia. Gastroenterology118:253–257, 2000.

31. Hunter JG, Richardson WS: Surgical management of achalasia. Surg Clin North Am 77:993–1015, 1997.

32. Katzka DA, Castell DO: Use of botulinum toxin as a diagnostic/therapeutic trial to help clarify an indication for definitive therapy in patients with achalasia. Am J Gastroenterol 94:637–642, 1999.

33. Meijssen MA, Tilanus HW, van Blankenstein M, et al: Achalasia complicated by esophageal squamous cell carci-noma. A prospective study in 195 patients. Gut 33(2):155–158, 1992.

34. Moonka R, Patti MG, Feo CV, et al: Clinical presentation and evaluation of malignant pseudoachalasia. J Gastrointest Surg 3:456–461, 1999.

35. Moonka R, Pellegrini CA: Malignant pseudoachalasia. Surg Endosc 13:273–275, 1999.

36. Parkman HP, Reynolds JC, Ouyang A, et al: Pneumatic dilatation or esophagomyotomy treatment for idiopathic achalasia: Clinical outcomes and cost analysis. Dig Dis Sci 38:75, 1993.

37. Pasricha PJ, Rai R, Ravich WJ, et al: Botulinum toxin for achalasia: Long term outcome and predictors of response. Gastroenterology 110:1410, 1996.

38. Pellegrini C, Wetter LA, Patti M, et al: Thoracoscopic esophagomyotomy. Initial experience with a new approach for the treatment of achalasia. Ann Surg 216:291–296; discussion, 296–299, 1992.

39. Vaezi MF, Richter JE, Wilcox CM, et al: Botulinum toxin versus pneumatic dilatation in the treatment of achalasia: A randomised trial. Gut 44:231–239, 1999.

ESOPHAGEAL CANCER

40. Avidan B, Sonnenberg A, Schnell TG, et al: Hiatal hernia size, Barrett's length, and severity of acid reflux are all risk factors for esophageal adenocarcinoma. Am J Gastroenterol 97(8):1930–1936, 2002.

41. Blot WJ, McLaughlin JK: The changing epidemiology of esophageal cancer. Seminars in Oncology 26(5 Suppl 15):2–8, 1999.

42. Gusrki RR, Peters JH, Hagen JA, et al: Barrett's Esophagus can and does regress after antireflux surgery: A study of prevalence and predictive features. J Am Coll Surg 195(5):706–712, 2003.

43. Heath E, Burtness BA, Heitmiller RF, et al: Phase II evaluation of preoperative chemoradiation and postoperative adjunctive chemotherapy for for squamous cell and adenocarcinoma of the esophagus. J Clin Oncol 18:868, 2000.

44. Lagergren J, Bergstrom R, Lindgren A, et al: Symptomatic gastroesophageal reflux as a risk factor for esophageal adenocarcinoma. N Engl J Med 340(11):825–831, 1999.

45. Mabrut J, Baulieux J, Adham M, et al: Impact of anti-reflux operation on columnar-lined esophagus. J Am Coll Surg 196(1):60–67, 2003.

46. Oelschlager BK, Barreca M, Chang L, et al: Clinical and pathologic response of Barrett's esophagus to laparoscopic antireflux surgery. Ann Surg 238(4):458–464, 2003.

CHAPTER 76

SURGERY FOR PEPTIC ULCER DISEASE

Jaimie D. Nathan, MD, and Theodore N. Pappas, MD

1. **Describe the classic indications and goals for peptic ulcer surgery.**
   Since the introduction of H_2-receptor antagonists and proton pump inhibitors and the identification of *Helicobacter pylori* as an ulcerogenic cofactor, the frequency of elective operations for peptic ulcer disease (PUD) has decreased substantially. Currently, operative surgery for duodenal and gastric ulcers is generally reserved for the management of complications of PUD. The classic indications for peptic ulcer surgery are perforation, bleeding, gastric outlet obstruction, and intractability of symptoms. The main goals of surgery are (1) to treat any complications of peptic ulcer disease and (2) to eliminate the factors that contribute to ulcer occurrence. These goals should be accomplished with minimization of surgical side effects.

2. **Define *intractability* in terms of the medical treatment of PUD.**
   Intractability is defined as mucosal healing refractory to maximal medical therapy. The following three criteria define a refractory ulcer and are generally indications for operative intervention: (1) ulcer persistence after 3 months of medical therapy, (2) ulcer recurrence within 1 year, despite maintenance medical therapy, and (3) ulcer disease in which cycles of prolonged activity are interrupted by brief or absent remissions.

3. **What are the three most widely used operations for PUD?**
   1. Truncal vagotomy and drainage
   2. Truncal vagotomy and antrectomy
   3. Highly selective vagotomy (parietal cell vagotomy or proximal gastric vagotomy)

4. **What are the surgical options for reconstruction after antrectomy?**
   - The Billroth I reconstruction consists of a gastroduodenostomy in which the anastomosis is created between the gastric remnant and the duodenum (Fig. 76-1).
   - The Billroth II reconstruction consists of a gastrojejunostomy in which a side-to-side anastomosis is created between the gastric remnant and a loop of jejunum, with closure of the duodenal stump.
   - The Roux-en-Y reconstruction involves the creation of a jejunojejunostomy (forming a Y-shaped figure of small bowel) downstream from the anastomosis of the free jejunal end to the gastric remnant (gastrojejunostomy).

5. **How is the type of reconstruction determined for a given patient?**
   The decision of which type of reconstruction to perform is determined, in part, by the extent of duodenal scarring due to PUD. Severely scarred duodenum cannot be used for an anastomosis. The Billroth I reconstruction is the most physiologic anastomosis because it restores normal continuity of the gastrointestinal (GI) tract. The Billroth II reconstruction may be complicated by the afferent loop syndrome in which obstruction of the afferent limb results in accumulation of bile and pancreatic secretions, causing right upper quadrant abdominal pain that is alleviated by bilious vomiting. The Roux-en-Y reconstruction allows diversion of bile and pancreatic secretions away from the gastric outlet, thereby reducing the risk of bile reflux gastritis. It can result in a delay in gastric emptying.

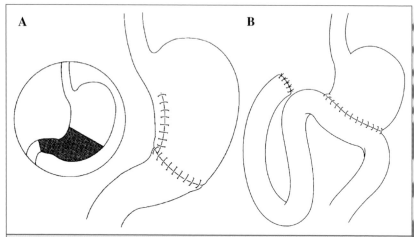

Figure 76-1. *A,* Billroth I gastroduodenostomy and, *B,* Billroth II gastrojejunostomy reconstructions following antral resection (shaded area in inset). (From Greenfield LJ: Surgery: Scientific Principles and Practice. Philadelphia, Lippincott-Raven, 1997, p 768, with permission.)

6. **Why is an outlet or "drainage" procedure added to truncal vagotomy? What are the surgical options?**

   Truncal vagotomy involves division of both anterior and posterior vagal trunks at the esophageal hiatus. This procedure results in denervation of the acid-producing mucosa of the gastric fundus as well as the pylorus and antrum, causing alteration of normal pyloric coordination and impaired gastric emptying. Thus, a procedure to eliminate function of the pyloric sphincter must be performed to allow gastric drainage. There are four primary options for an outlet procedure (Fig. 76-2):

   - *Heineke-Mikulicz pyloroplasty,* in which a longitudinal incision of the pyloric sphincter, extending into the duodenum and antrum, is closed transversely.
   - *Finney pyloroplasty,* which is used in cases of extensive duodenal scarring to create a wider gastroduodenal opening; a U-shaped incision crossing the pylorus is made, and a gastroduodenostomy is created.
   - *Jaboulay gastroduodenostomy,* which is used when severe pyloric scarring precludes safe division of the pyloric channel; a side-to-side gastroduodenostomy is created in which the incision does not cross the pyloric sphincter.
   - *Gastrojejunostomy*

7. **Describe the truncal vagotomy, selective vagotomy, and highly selective vagotomy.**

   Truncal vagotomy involves division of both anterior and posterior vagal trunks at the esophageal hiatus above the origins of the hepatic and celiac branches. Periesophageal dissection must include the distal 6–8 cm of the esophagus to ensure division of gastric vagal branches that arise from the trunks above the level of the hiatus, including the "criminal nerve of Grassi," the first and highest posterior branch supplying the fundus. Thus, truncal vagotomy results in denervation of all vagally supplied viscera. A drainage procedure, usually a pyloroplasty, must be performed with truncal vagotomy, because denervation of the pylorus results in impaired gastric emptying.

   Selective vagotomy involves division of the vagal trunks distal to the hepatic and celiac branches, thereby preserving vagal innervation to the gallbladder and celiac plexus and reducing the incidence of gallbladder dysmotility, gallstones, and diarrhea. Selective vagotomy also

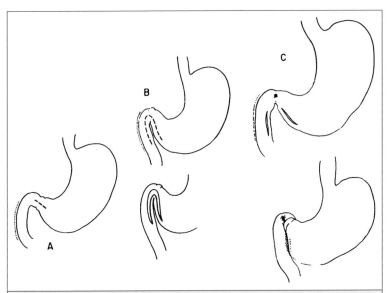

Figure 76-2. *A,* Heineke-Mikulicz pyloroplasty, *B,* Finney pyloroplasty, and, *C,* Jaboulay gastroduodenostomy are the primary options for an outlet or "drainage" procedure after truncal vagotomy. (From Zollinger RM: Atlas of Surgical Operations. New York, McGraw-Hill, 1993, p 41, with permission.)

results in complete gastric vagotomy, necessitating a drainage procedure. Selective vagotomy is not the operation of choice, because most surgeons find it needlessly complex and not superior to truncal vagotomy; therefore, it is rarely used.

Highly selective vagotomy (parietal cell vagotomy or proximal gastric vagotomy) involves selective division of the vagal fibers to the acid-producing parietal cell mass of the gastric fundus, while maintaining vagal fibers to the antrum and distal gut. The anterior and posterior neurovascular attachments are divided along the lesser curvature of the stomach, beginning approximately 7 cm from the pylorus and progressing to the gastroesophageal junction, with additional skeletalization of the distal 6–8 cm of the esophagus to ensure division of the "criminal nerve of Grassi." Innervation of the antrum and pylorus is maintained because the two terminal branches of the anterior and posterior nerves of Latarget are left intact.

8. **What are the relative indications and contraindications to highly selective vagotomy?**
Highly selective vagotomy is indicated for the treatment of intractable duodenal ulcers because, unlike truncal vagotomy, it does not require a drainage procedure. It is also the procedure of choice in the emergent treatment of bleeding or perforated duodenal ulcers in stable patients. Highly selective vagotomy is contraindicated in patients with prepyloric ulcers or with gastric outlet obstruction because they demonstrate high rates of recurrent ulceration. The ulcer recurrence rate is closely tied to the surgeon's experience with this operation.

9. **Describe the five types of gastric ulcer in terms of location, gastric acid secretory status, incidence, and complications.**
   - *Type I:* located on the gastric body, typically along the lesser curvature; associated with low-to-normal acid output; about 55% of gastric ulcers (Fig. 76-3). Bleeding is relatively uncommon.

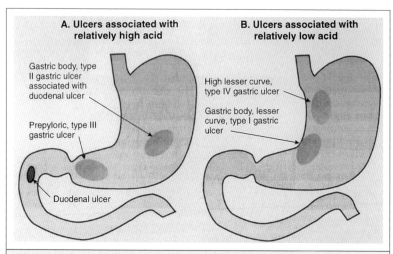

Figure 76-3. The four major types of gastric ulcers and their association with either, *A*, high acid or, *B*, low acid. (From Sabiston DC Jr: Textbook of Surgery: The Biological Basis of Modern Surgical Practice. Philadelphia, W.B. Saunders, 1997, p 854, with permission.)

- *Type II:* located on the gastric body in combination with a duodenal ulcer; typically associated with acid hypersecretion; about 20% of gastric ulcers. Bleeding, perforation, and obstruction are frequent complications.
- *Type III:* prepyloric ulcer; associated with acid hypersecretion; about 20% of gastric ulcers. Bleeding and perforation are frequent complications.
- *Type IV:* located high on the lesser curvature in proximity to the gastroesophageal junction; associated with low acid secretion; <10% of gastric ulcers. Bleeding is a frequent complication.
- *Type V:* may be located anywhere in the stomach; secondary to chronic use of aspirin or nonsteroidal anti-inflammatory drugs (NSAIDs); highly prone to bleeding and perforation.

10. **Describe the most appropriate operative procedure for each type of gastric ulcer.**

The choice of operation for gastric ulcers depends on several factors: ulcer location, acid secretory status, and presence of a coexistent duodenal ulcer. The operation of choice for *type I gastric ulcer* is antrectomy with inclusion of the ulcer in the resected specimen and reconstruction with a gastroduodenostomy (Billroth I) or, alternatively, a gastrojejunostomy (Billroth II). Although type I gastric ulcers are associated with low-to-normal acid output, most surgeons now include a truncal vagotomy, unless achlorhydria is demonstrated. Highly selective vagotomy with ulcer excision is an alternative operation, although the rate of recurrence is significantly higher.

Type II gastric ulcers are associated with high rates of acid secretion. Thus, the goal of operation is removal of the gastric mucosa at risk for ulceration (with inclusion of the gastric ulcer itself) and reduction of acid secretion. The procedure of choice is antrectomy with Billroth I reconstruction (with inclusion of the gastric ulcer in the resection) and truncal vagotomy. Truncal vagotomy with drainage procedure and excision of the ulcer is an acceptable alternative.

Patients with *type III gastric ulcers* are also acid hypersecretors. Truncal vagotomy and antrectomy (with inclusion of the ulcer) is the operation of choice and carries a recurrence rate of <2%.

Type IV gastric ulcers present a challenge, because they are located high on the lesser curvature near the gastroesophageal junction. Other factors to be considered in surgical management are size and degree of adjacent inflammation. A distal gastrectomy may be performed with extension of the resection proximally to include the lesser curvature (with the ulcer), followed by a gastroduodenal anastomosis.

Type V gastric ulcers generally heal rapidly with cessation of aspirin or NSAID and institution of an H_2-receptor antagonist or proton pump inhibitor. An intractable type V gastric ulcer should raise suspicion for underlying malignancy. Surgical intervention for benign type V gastric ulcers is reserved for the treatment of complications, such as perforation or bleeding.

11. **Describe the presentation of a patient with a perforated peptic ulcer.**
Patients usually describe a prodrome of gnawing abdominal pain in the epigastric region prior to perforation. With acute perforation, the epigastric pain becomes diffuse and is often associated with fever, tachycardia, tachypnea, and hypotension. Some patients present with GI bleeding. On examination, the patient with peptic ulcer perforation lies immobile. Bowel sounds are typically absent, and the abdomen is diffusely tender and rigid. The white blood cell count is elevated, and, in 70% of cases, free intraperitoneal air is found on upright abdominal x-rays. Although computed tomographic (CT) scan is the most sensitive radiologic test for free intraperitoneal air, it is rarely indicated because patients with perforated peptic ulcer usually present with classic signs and symptoms, and CT scanning only serves to delay operation.

12. **Why do almost all perforated gastric ulcers require operation?**
   - Perforated gastric ulcers usually fail to heal spontaneously.
   - They are associated with a risk of adenocarcinoma.
   - Gastric ulcer disease produces a hypoacidic environment with resultant bacterial overgrowth and abscess formation after perforation.

On rare occasions, patients with perforated duodenal ulcer may be managed medically, particularly if the ulcer has been perforated for longer than 24 hours, and a contrast study indicates that the perforation is contained.

13. **What are the contraindications to medical management of perforated peptic ulcer disease?**
   - Concurrent use of steroids, which makes healing unlikely.
   - Continued leak, as demonstrated by a contrast radiograph.
   - Perforation in a patient taking an H_2-receptor antagonist or a proton pump inhibitor. A definitive ulcer operation is necessary to allow ulcer healing and to reduce the risk of recurrence.

14. **What are the major risk factors for mortality in the surgical treatment of perforated PUD?**
(1) Severe comorbidities, (2) perforation present for longer than 24 hours, and (3) hemodynamic instability on presentation. Patients with one of these risk factors have a mortality rate of approximately 10%; with two risk factors, the mortality rate increases to 46%. Patients with all three risk factors have a mortality rate of nearly 100%. Thus, nonsurgical management of perforated PUD should be considered in elderly patients with any of these risk factors.

15. **What are the three major goals of operation for perforated PUD?**
(1) Repair of the perforation, which is usually performed by suturing the perforation closed and buttressing the repair with omental fat as a patch (Graham's patch, Fig. 76-4); (2) copious irrigation of the abdominal cavity; and (3) definitive ulcer operation, as necessary. A patient who has had a perforation for <24 hours and is hemodynamically stable without significant comorbidities should undergo a definitive ulcer operation if he or she has known PUD, has been receiving medical therapy for PUD, or is taking medications that increase the risk of PUD.

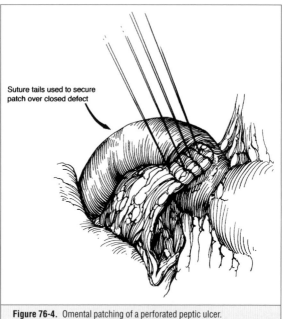

Suture tails used to secure
patch over closed defect

Figure 76-4. Omental patching of a perforated peptic ulcer.

16. **What is the preferred operation for treatment of a perforated duodenal ulcer?**
In patients who have undergone medical therapy to eradicate *H. pylori*, the classic operation for a perforated duodenal ulcer is truncal vagotomy and pyloroplasty, with incorporation of the perforation into the pyloroplasty closure. This relatively simple procedure requires a short operative time. In the ideal surgical candidate, highly selective vagotomy with patch closure of the perforation is recommended, although this procedure requires a high degree of surgical expertise. Patients who have not been treated for *H. pylori* prior to perforation should undergo repair and Graham's patch of a perforated duodenal ulcer with postoperative *H. pylori* eradication therapy, in lieu of a definitive ulcer operation.

17. **What is the preferred operation for treatment of perforated gastric ulcer?**
The major distinction between surgical management of perforated duodenal and perforated gastric ulcers is that in all cases of perforated gastric ulcers, carcinoma must be excluded. Thus, all perforated gastric ulcers must undergo biopsy or resection. One option is to perform a wedge resection as diagnostic biopsy. Controversy exists as to whether a definitive ulcer operation should be added to this procedure, but most surgeons perform an ulcer operation if the ulcer is a type II or type III variant. An alternative for perforated antral ulcers is antrectomy (with inclusion of the ulcer in the resection), to which truncal vagotomy may be added if the patient is an acid hypersecretor.

18. **Discuss the role for laparoscopy in the management of perforated PUD and the indications for conversion to an open operation.**
The surgical goals in the laparoscopic management of a perforated peptic ulcer are similar to those of open surgical management: (1) repair of the perforation, which is most easily performed in the setting of an anterior duodenal perforation, (2) copious irrigation and removal of enteric soilage, and (3) addition of a definitive ulcer operation, which depends on the skill of the surgeon and may involve either laparoscopic truncal vagotomy and pyloroplasty or a

laparoscopic highly selective vagotomy. Relative indications for conversion to an open procedure include ulcer diameter greater than 6 mm, ulcer with friable edges, posterior location of the ulcer, and inadequate localization. The presence of a perforated gastric ulcer with its suspicion for malignancy often necessitates conversion for definitive operation.

19. **In patients with GI bleeding caused by PUD, what are the predictors for rebleeding in the hospital?**
    - Hemodynamic instability
    - Hematocrit <30
    - Multiple comorbidities
    - Documented coagulopathy
    - Hematemesis
    - Inability to clear the stomach with aggressive lavage

    Findings at endoscopy help to predict which patients are at highest risk for continued bleeding or rebleeding. Active bleeding on endoscopy is a good predictor of rebleeding. A spurting artery is associated with a rebleeding rate of 70–90%; a visible nonbleeding vessel in the ulcer bed with a rebleeding rate of 40–50%; and an adherent clot with a rebleeding rate of 10–20%.

20. **What is the classic indication for operation for rebleeding after endoscopic therapy?**
    After endoscopic therapy for a bleeding peptic ulcer, patients who require further resuscitation with 6 units of blood should be strongly considered for surgical intervention. In general, the indications for surgical treatment of a bleeding peptic ulcer are: (1) hemodynamic instability as a result of massive hemorrhage, although cardiovascular stabilization must precede surgery, (2) need for multiple transfusions due to continued bleeding, and (3) failure of nonsurgical therapy to prevent rebleeding.

21. **What is the most appropriate surgical procedure for a bleeding duodenal ulcer?**
    Control of the ulcer bed is attained by performing a duodenotomy with direct ligation of the bleeding vessel or complete plication of the ulcer bed. If the ulcer has eroded into the gastroduodenal artery, bleeding may be profuse. A definitive ulcer operation is then performed, which may consist of either a truncal vagotomy and pyloroplasty or a truncal vagotomy and antrectomy. An alternative approach is to attain control of the bleeding duodenal ulcer through a pyloroplasty incision, in which case a truncal vagotomy completes the definitive ulcer operation. Evidence indicates no difference in mortality rates between local procedures (ulcer underrunning or vessel oversewing) and radical operations (partial gastrectomy). Reports suggest that the rate of rebleeding may be higher in patients treated with local procedures, but most of these studies have not been properly controlled.

22. **What are the operative options for control of a bleeding gastric ulcer?**
    Bleeding gastric ulcers require excision and biopsy to rule out malignancy. Small gastric ulcers (<2 cm) can usually be excised easily and safely, with the addition of an ulcer operation for patients who are acid hypersecretors. Large gastric ulcers, lesser curvature ulcers, bleeding ulcers associated with gastritis, and gastric ulcers that penetrate into the pancreas often require a more radical and technically demanding operation (subtotal or near-total gastrectomy) to control hemorrhage.

23. **How is gastric outlet obstruction due to PUD surgically managed?**
    Gastric outlet obstruction (GOO) can result from an acute exacerbation of PUD in the setting of chronic pyloric and duodenal scarring. Classically, patients with GOO present with nausea, emesis, early satiety, and weight loss. Although radiologic contrast studies are useful in evaluation, upper endoscopy is critical to rule out a malignant cause of the obstruction. Operative intervention is necessary in 75% of patients presenting with gastric outlet obstruction.

The two main goals of surgery are to relieve the obstruction and to perform a definitive ulcer operation. Truncal vagotomy and antrectomy with Billroth II reconstruction is performed, if the duodenal stump can be safely closed. If the stump cannot be closed, a tube duodenostomy is left in place for control of secretions until the stump closes by secondary intention. An alternative is to perform a truncal vagotomy and pyloroplasty, which often requires the Finney pyloroplasty or Jaboulay gastroduodenostomy because of severe scarring. Truncal vagotomy and gastrojejunostomy may be performed, if the severe scarring precludes an adequate drainage procedure via the duodenum.

24. **What are the long-term outcomes and risks for complications after truncal vagotomy and drainage, truncal vagotomy and antrectomy, and highly selective vagotomy?**
See Table 76-1.

TABLE 76-1. LONG-TERM OUTCOMES AND RISKS FOR COMPLICATIONS			
	Truncal Vagotomy and Drainage (%)	Truncal Vagotomy and Antrectomy (%)	Highly Selective Vagotomy (%)
Mortality rate	0.5–0.8	1.5	0.05
Recurrence rate*	12	1–2	10–15
Dumping	10	10–15	1–5
Diarrhea	25	20	1–5

*All rates are from the pre-*Helicobacter pylori* era. Currently, patients that require ulcer surgery often have difficult disease to control and probably have recurrence rates that are higher than previously published. Therefore, the numbers quoted in the table should be considered minimum recurrence rates, and certain patient subgroups, such as smokers, should be expected to have much higher recurrence rates.

25. **How should postoperative gastroparesis be managed?**
Postoperative gastroparesis typically occurs in patients who undergo surgery for gastric outlet obstruction. Such patients should receive prolonged nonoperative management. Prokinetic agents (e.g., erythromycin, metaclopramide) may be useful. The indications for reoperation are (1) early marginal ulcers refractory to medical management, (2) anatomic abnormalities of the gastric outlet, and (3) recurrent bezoar associated with weight loss.

26. **Describe the management of duodenal stump disruption ("blow-out") after truncal vagotomy, antrectomy, and Billroth II reconstruction.**
Patients presenting with low-grade right upper quadrant sepsis may be managed by percutaneous drainage of the abscess under radiologic guidance. An acute abdomen suggests free perforation with leakage of duodenal contents into the peritoneal cavity. Management requires reoperation for reclosure of the duodenal stump over a tube duodenostomy as well as an external drain around the tube. Mortality from stump blow-out approaches 10%.

27. **What are the Visick's criteria?**
The Visick's criteria are used to grade outcome after surgery for PUD:
Grade I   No symptoms
Grade II   Mild symptoms that do not affect daily life
Grade III   Moderate symptoms that affect daily life and require treatment but are not disabling

Grade IV   Recurrent ulceration or disabling symptoms

Grades I and II are considered adequate results. Most poor outcomes fall into grade III.

28. **What is the dumping syndrome? Describe its pathophysiology and treatment.**
    The dumping syndrome consists of tachycardia, diaphoresis, hypotension, and abdominal pain after meals in patients who have undergone ulcer operations, such as truncal vagotomy. Its pathophysiology is loss of receptive relaxation of the fundus in response to a gastric load. Thus, gastric pressure increases during a meal, and rapid decompression through the gastric outlet procedure causes the classic signs and symptoms. Symptoms improve typically with time and can be alleviated in some patients by separation of solids and liquids during meals. Conversion of a Billroth II reconstruction to a Billroth I or a Billroth operation to a Roux-en-Y reconstruction can improve symptoms (Fig. 76-5). Octreotide, a somatostatin analog, has also been used to alleviate symptoms.

29. **Describe the pathophysiology of bile reflux gastritis. How is it managed?**
    Bile reflux gastritis occurs when ablation of the pylorus in a gastric ulcer operation results in stasis of bile in the stomach. The diagnosis is made with the following triad of findings: (1) postprandial epigastric pain accompanied by nausea and bilious emesis, (2) evidence of bile reflux into the stomach or gastric remnant, and (3) biopsy-proven gastritis. Bile reflux gastritis can occur after truncal vagotomy and pyloroplasty or truncal vagotomy and antrectomy with Billroth reconstruction. Although up to 20% of patients who undergo these operations may have transient bile reflux gastritis postoperatively, symptoms resolve in all but 1–2%.

    Treatment of bile reflux gastritis requires revision of the pyloroplasty or the Billroth reconstruction to a Roux-en-Y gastrojejunostomy with a 50–60 cm limb (*see* Fig. 76-5). Bilious emesis resolves in nearly 100% of patients who undergo revision. The symptoms of bile reflux

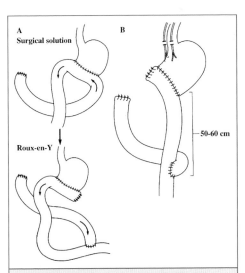

Figure 76-5. Technique for conversion of a Billroth II reconstruction to a Roux-en-Y gastrojejunostomy. After division of, *A*, the afferent limb, *B*, a jejunojejunal anastomosis is created approximately 50–60 cm distal to the original Billroth II gastrojejunostomy. (From Greenfield LJ: Surgery: Scientific Principles and Practice. Philadelphia, Lippincott-Raven, 1997, p 772, with permission.)

gastritis may be indistinguishable from those of gastroparesis. Because the Roux-en-Y gastroje-junostomy worsens the symptoms of gastroparesis, care must be taken to exclude the diagnosis of gastroparesis preoperatively.

30. **What is the presentation of Zollinger-Ellison syndrome?**
Most patients with Zollinger-Ellison syndrome present with PUD and/or diarrhea. Ulcers are typically duodenal. The diarrhea resembles steatorrhea and results from a combination of high volumes of acid and neutralization of pancreatic enzymes. In patients with Zollinger-Ellison syndrome associated with multiple endocrine neoplasia (MEN) syndrome I, signs and symptoms at presentation may be related to parathyroid or pituitary disease.

31. **How is Zollinger-Ellison syndrome diagnosed?**
A high level of suspicion is required for the diagnosis of gastrinoma. Serum gastrin should be measured in all patients undergoing peptic ulcer surgery. If the gastrin level is in the range of 1000–2000 pg/mL, gastric pH analysis demonstrating acid production confirms the diagnosis. If the gastrin level is minimally elevated, the patient should undergo gastric pH analysis and a secretin test. The secretin test is performed by comparison of basal serum gastrin level with gastrin level after the administration of secretin. Gastrinoma is suspected in patients with an increase in the serum gastrin level of 200 pg/mL after secretin administration. Normal patients have no change or a reduction in serum gastrin after secretin administration. Because achlorhydria is more common than gastrinoma, an elevation in serum gastrin is due more commonly to lack of acid as opposed to ectopic gastrin production. Therefore, measurement of acid production is essential in making the appropriate diagnosis.

32. **For which patients with Zollinger-Ellison syndrome is operative intervention indicated?**
Surgery is the treatment of choice for patients with nonmetastatic sporadic gastrinoma. In addition, patients with metastatic gastrinoma who are unable to tolerate or are refractory to medical management should be considered for operative intervention. The gastrinoma seen as part of MEN syndrome differs from sporadic gastrinomas. Sporadic gastrinomas are often solitary and located in the pancreas or duodenum, but not both, and are amenable to surgical resection and cure. Although gastrinomas seen with MEN syndrome are usually multiple, virtually always in the duodenum, and often multicentric, they are also found in the pancreas and are more difficult to cure surgically. Gastrinoma associated with hypercalcemia should suggest MEN syndrome complicated by hyperparathyroidism, and parathyroidectomy is essential for management of gastric acid hypersecretion. Elevated serum gastrin levels postoperatively after gastrinoma surgery indicate residual gastrinoma(s) that should be treated medically. Medical management is also generally indicated for patients with metastatic gastrinoma. Medical management consists of high-dose proton pump inhibitors with the goal of reducing gastric acid output to <10 mEq/hr for the hour that immediately precedes the next scheduled dose of antisecretory medication.

33. **Describe the preoperative evaluation for gastrinoma.**
CT scan with intravenous and oral contrast is routine in the preoperative evaluation for gastrinoma resection to rule out metastatic disease, and its accuracy is dependent on the size of the gastrinoma. In some cases, MRI is used because it is more sensitive than CT scan for liver metastases. Rarely, partial venous sampling for gastrin has been successful in localizing gastrinoma; however, this is an expensive and cumbersome technique with a risk of complications. The advent of somatostatin receptor scintigraphy (octreotide scan) has greatly improved the preoperative localization of gastrinomas. This study relies on the high density of somatostatin receptors on gastrinomas and uses the radiolabeled synthetic somatostatin analog, 125-iodine [^{125}I]-octreotide, to identify primary as well as metastatic gastrinomas. Recent studies have demonstrated that somatostatin receptor scintigraphy has high sensitivity and specificity for

detection of primary and metastatic gastrinomas and is now regarded as the initial imaging modality of choice for localization. Endoscopic ultrasound has recently been used to localize gastrinomas; however, it is highly operator-dependent and does not reliably identify small tumors in the duodenum. Intraoperative localization of the tumor remains the standard of care. For tumors not identified preoperatively, intraoperative ultrasound has been used successfully for gastrinoma localization. Intraoperative upper endoscopy with transillumination may also help to localize small duodenal gastrinomas. A modification of octreotide scanning is currently under evaluation as an adjunct to intraoperative localization. A handheld gamma-detecting probe is used intraoperatively to localize gastrinomas after the injection of [^{125}I]-octreotide.

34. **Where is the gastrinoma triangle? What percentage of tumors occur in this area?**

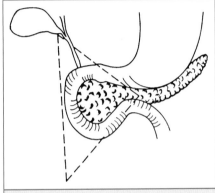

The apex of the gastrinoma triangle is at the cystic duct-common bile duct junction, and the triangle is bounded by the border of the second and third portions of the duodenum and the junction of the neck and body of the pancreas (Fig. 76-6). Approximately 60–75% of gastrinomas are found within this triangle.

35. **Describe the operative scheme for exploration, localization, and removal of gastrinoma.**

If no tumor is obvious on preoperative CT scan, and other preoperative localization studies have failed, exploration begins with exposure of the

Figure 76-6. The gastrinoma triangle.

anterior surface of the pancreas by mobilization of the transverse colon. A Kocher's maneuver is then performed to mobilize the duodenum, allowing complete bimanual palpation of the pancreas. Intraoperative ultrasound is concentrated in the gastrinoma triangle. Biopsy of lymph nodes should be performed because, occasionally, the gastrinoma is localized to a solitary node. If ultrasound of the pancreas does not reveal the tumor, duodenal gastrinoma should be suspected. A pyloroplasty incision is made, and the duodenal wall is visually inspected and manually palpated. An alternative method of localizing duodenal gastrinomas is to transilluminate the wall with intraoperative endoscopy. Gastrinomas in the duodenal wall or pancreas may be enucleated, but solitary lesions in the pancreatic tail are often treated by distal pancreatectomy.

If no lesion is found, or if the disease is found to be multicentric or metastatic, an ulcer operation may be performed as palliation. This procedure often consists of the addition of a truncal vagotomy to the pyloroplasty. Alternatively, the patient may be maintained on a proton pump inhibitor. In rare cases, a total gastrectomy may be performed for control of acid production in patients who are refractory to medical therapy or unable to tolerate the side effects of the medication.

36. **What is a giant gastric ulcer? How is it managed?**

A giant gastric ulcer is an ulcer with diameter of ≥3 cm. Typically, it is located along the lesser curvature and carries a high risk of bleeding, perforation, and obstruction. Giant gastric ulcers carry an incidence of malignancy of up to 30%, and the risk of malignancy increases with size. Because of the high risk of complications and malignancy, the treatment of choice is early surgical intervention, if the ulcer does not completely resolve with an initial course of medical therapy. Giant ulcers are treated by resection, with the addition of a truncal vagotomy for type II or type III variants.

37. **Describe the risk of gastric stump cancer after partial gastrectomy for duodenal and gastric ulcer.**

    Gastric stump carcinoma is defined as adenocarcinoma of the stomach that occurs at least 5 years after partial gastric resection for benign disease. In patients who have undergone partial distal gastrectomy for duodenal ulcer, the risk of developing stump carcinoma is low in the first 20 years postoperatively, but the relative risk rises to 2.0 after 20 years. In patients who have had a partial distal gastrectomy for gastric ulcer, the relative risk is no different than in the general population in the first 20 years but rises to 3.0 after 20 years. Multivariate analysis has indicated that the most important risk factor in the development of gastric stump cancer is the time interval since surgery. Annual screening gastroscopy and biopsy should be performed in patients who underwent gastric resection at least 15 years prior and have moderate-to-severe dysplasia on biopsy.

38. **What is the proposed mechanism for the development of stump carcinoma?**

    Postpartial gastrectomy hypochlorhydria results in bacterial overgrowth in the gastric remnant. The bacteria convert nitrates to nitrites, allowing the production of carcinogenic N-nitroso compounds. Bile reflux into the gastric remnant increases the permeability of the gastric mucosal barrier to carcinogens. A final factor believed to promote the development of stump carcinoma is the presence of gastric mucosal atrophy, which results because the trophic effects of the antrum-produced peptide gastrin are absent after antrectomy.

BIBLIOGRAPHY

1. Arai R, Barkin JS: Managing recurrent peptic ulcer bleeding: The scalpel or the scope? Am J Gastroenterol 94:3365–3367, 1999.

2. Azimuddin K, Chamberlain RS: The surgical management of pancreatic neuroendocrine tumors. Surg Clin North Am 81:511–525, 2001.

3. Benevento A, Dominioni L, Carcano G, Dionigi R: Intraoperative localization of gut endocrine tumors with radio-labeled somatostatin analogs and a gamma-detecting probe. Semin Surg Oncol 15:239–244, 1998.

4. Bulut O, Rasmussen C, Fischer A: Acute surgical treatment of complicated peptic ulcers with special reference to the elderly. World J Surg 20:574–577, 1996.

5. Chung SC, Li AK: Helicobacter pylori and peptic ulcer surgery. Br J Surg 84:1489–1490, 1997.

6. Donahue PE: Parietal cell vagotomy versus vagotomy-antrectomy: Ulcer surgery in the modern era. World J Surg 24:264–269, 2000.

7. Donahue PE: Ulcer surgery and highly selective vagotomy-Y2K. Arch Surg 134:1373–1377, 1999.

8. Dubois F: New surgical strategy for gastroduodenal ulcer: Laparoscopic approach. World J Surg 24:270–276, 2000.

9. Greene FL: Discovery of early gastric remnant carcinoma: Results of a 14-year endoscopic screening program. Surg Endosc 9:1199–1203, 1995.

10. Hansson L-E: Risk of stomach cancer in patients with peptic ulcer disease. World J Surg 24:315–320, 2000.

11. Jamieson GG: Current status of indications for surgery for peptic ulcer disease. World J Surg 24:256–258, 2000.

12. Jensen RT, Gibril F: Somatostatin receptor scintigraphy in gastrinomas. Ital J Gastroenterol Hepatol 31(Suppl):S179–S185, 1999.

13. Johnson AG: Proximal gastric vagotomy: Does it have a place in the future management of peptic ulcer? World J Surg 24:259–263, 2000.

14. Kauffman GL, Conter RL: Stress ulcer and gastric ulcer. In Greenfield LJ (ed): Surgery: Scientific Principles and Practice, 2nd ed. Philadelphia, Lippincott-Raven, 1997, pp 773–788.

15. Kleef J, Friess H, Buchler MW: How Helicobacter pylori changed the life of surgeons. Dig Surg 20:93–102, 2003.

16. Kondo K: Duodenogastric reflux and gastric stump carcinoma. Gastric Cancer 5:16–22, 2002.

17. Lagoo S, McMahon RL, Kakihara M, et al: The sixth decision regarding perforated duodenal ulcer. JSLS 6:359–368, 2002.

18. Makela JT, Kiviniemi H, Ohtonen P, Laitinen SO: Factors that predict morbidity and mortality in patients with perforated peptic ulcers. Eur J Surg 168:446–451, 2002.

19. Millat B, Fingerhut A, Borie F: Surgical treatment of complicated duodenal ulcers: Controlled trials. World J Surg 24:299–306, 2000.

20. Mulholland MW: Duodenal ulcer. In Greenfield LJ (ed): Surgery: Scientific Principles and Practice, 2nd ed. Philadelphia, Lippincott-Raven, 1997, pp 759–773.

21. Noguiera C, Silva AS, Santos JN, et al: Perforated peptic ulcer: Main factors of morbidity and mortality. World J Surg 27:782–787, 2003.

22. Ohmann C, Imhof M, Roher H-D: Trends in peptic ulcer bleeding and surgical treatment. World J Surg 24:284–293, 2000.

23. Pappas TN: The stomach and duodenum. In Sabiston DC Jr (ed): Textbook of Surgery: The Biological Basis of Modern Surgical Practice, 15th ed. Philadelphia, W.B. Saunders, 1997, pp 847–868.

24. Sabiston DC Jr: Atlas of General Surgery. Philadelphia, W.B. Saunders, 1994.

25. Simeone DM, Hassan A, Scheiman JM: Giant peptic ulcer: A surgical or medical disease? Surgery 126:474–478, 1999.

26. Svanes C: Trends in perforated peptic ulcer: Incidence, etiology, treatment, and prognosis. World J Surg 24:277–283, 2000.

27. Termanini B, Gibril F, Reynolds JC, et al: Value of somatostatin receptor scintigraphy: A prospective study in gastrinoma of its effects on clinical management. Gastroenterology 112:335–347, 1997.

28. Tersmette AC, Giardiello FM, Tytgat GNJ, Offerhaus GJA: Carcinogenesis after remote peptic ulcer surgery: The long-term prognosis of partial gastrectomy. Scand J Gastroenterol 30(Suppl):96–99, 1995.

29. Testini M, Portincasa P, Piccinni G, et al: Significant factors associated with fatal outcome in emergency open surgery for perforated peptic ulcer. World J Gastroenterol 9:2338–2340, 2003.

30. Tzu-Ming C, Stabile BE, Passaro E: Gastrinoma: Current medical and surgical therapy. Contemp Surg 29:34, 1986.

31. Von Holstein CS: Long-term prognosis after partial gastrectomy for gastroduodenal ulcer. World J Surg 24:307–314, 2000.

32. Zollinger RM: Atlas of Surgical Operations. New York, McGraw-Hill, 1993.

CHAPTER 77

SURGICAL APPROACH TO THE ACUTE ABDOMEN

Jonathan A. Schoen, MD, and Frank H. Chae, MD

1. **What are the two main goals of a surgeon consulted for an acute abdomen?**
   (1) To determine whether the patient requires surgery and, if so, (2) whether the patient has time for adequate resuscitation and diagnostic work-up before the general anesthesia.

2. **What are the critical factors in the history of present illness?**
   Age; location, character, and duration of pain; and associated problems.

3. **Which disorders are associated with specific age groups?**
   - *Neonates:* intussusception, appendicitis, Meckel's diverticulitis, mesenteric adenitis, midgut volvulus, malrotation, hypertrophic pyloric stenosis, small bowel atresia, annular pancreas
   - *Adults:* cholecystitis, gynecologic disorders, peptic ulcer disease, incarcerated hernia, ruptured spleen, renal or biliary stone, pancreatitis, small bowel obstruction
   - *Elderly patients:* diverticulitis, colon cancer, appendicitis, ruptured aneurysm, volvulus, bowel ischemia, pseudo-obstruction

4. **Summarize the significance of pain location.**
   - Right upper quadrant: biliary tract disease, liver disease, peptic ulcer disease, pulmonary disease
   - Right flank: hepatitis, pyelonephritis
   - Right lower quadrant: appendicitis (see Chapter 53), ectopic pregnancy, incarcerated hernia, rectus hematoma, torsion of ovary, Meckel's diverticulitis, Crohn's disease
   - Epigastrium: pancreatitis, peptic ulcer disease
   - Left upper quadrant: ruptured spleen, subdiaphragmatic abscess, leaking aneurysm, pulmonary disease
   - Central abdomen: bowel obstruction, mesenteric infarction, midgut volvulus
   - Left lower quadrant: diverticulitis, incarcerated hernia, torsion of ovary, perforated colon cancer.

5. **What associated problems help to pinpoint the diagnosis?**
   Past surgical and medical history. In premenopausal women, pelvic inflammatory disease and pregnancy-related problems must be screened as part of the initial assessment.

6. **What is the peritoneum, its pain innervation, and what are peritoneal signs?**
   The peritoneum is derived from mesoderm. It consists of two double-layered sheets of cells that form the visceral and the parietal peritoneal layers. These two layers have separately derived neural innervation. The visceral layer covering organs is innervated by autonomic nerves. This innervation is bilateral, and pain from these nerves is perceived as midline pain. These are slow C fibers and produce dull, crampy pain of insidious nature. The parietal layer covers the inner surfaces of the abdominal parieties and is innervated by somatic nerves of spinal origin (T7–L2). These nerves produce a sensation of pain in the local area from which it originates. These are fast transmitters and give rise to sharp and exquisite pain. Peritonitis refers to any inflammation of the peritoneal layers and can be localized, diffuse, sterile, or infected. This leads to guarding or spasm of the muscle when it is palpated. Voluntary guarding is described when the patient

can consciously eliminate the muscular response, and involuntary guarding is when the response cannot be eliminated by the patient. The latter is more foreboding. Rigidity of the muscle is when the abdominal wall is tense and boardlike and is usually associated with diffuse peritonitis.

7. **How does duration of pain help in making a diagnosis?**
Pain is sudden with a perforated ulcer or diverticulum, renal stones, and ruptured ectopic pregnancy and intermittent in bowel obstruction; it is gradual in appendicitis or pyelonephritis.

8. **Is acute abdomen ruled out by absence of fever or leukocytosis?**
No. Fever and leukocytosis are late occurrences. Elderly and immunocompromised patients are often unable to mount these responses, despite significant abdominal disease.

9. **What is the significance of bowel sounds?**
Bowel sounds are not highly reliable in surgical evaluation of the abdomen. Their absence may indicate ileus, whereas high-pitched rushes may indicate small bowel obstruction.

10. **What is the most important part of the abdominal examination?**
Palpation, which permits assessment of localized tenderness, guarding, or diffuse peritonitis. Rectal exam is also essential. A pelvic exam must be performed in all female patients with abdominal pain.

11. **What are psoas and obturator signs?**
Inflammation of the psoas muscle causes pain on hip flexion-extension, whereas inflammation of the internal obturator muscle causes pain on internal rotation and flexion of the hip. Retrocecal appendicitis or, on occasion, diverticulitis may be responsible for these signs.

12. **What is Rovsing's sign?**
Palpation of the *left* lower quadrant causes pain in the *right* lower quadrant, indicating appendicitis.

13. **What is Kehr's sign?**
Pain in the left upper quadrant radiates to the left shoulder because of diaphragmatic irritation. Kehr's sign usually indicates hematoma from splenic injury.

14. **Define *mittelschmerz*.**
Pain in the middle of the menstrual cycle from ovulation.

15. **How does urinalysis help in the assessment?**
White blood cells in the urine may indicate urinary tract infection. Hematuria may suggest ureteral stones or tumor. Glucose or ketones may reveal diabetic ketoacidosis. An inflamed appendix abutting an adjacent ureter may lead to the finding of white and/or red blood cells in the urine.

16. **What should be the first x-ray studies obtained?**
Upright chest radiograph may reveal free air under the diaphragm or suggest a pulmonary process. Free air may also be seen over the liver in a left lateral decubitus abdominal film. Air-fluid levels on the upright abdominal film may suggest bowel obstruction. Only 10% of gallstones are radiopaque, but 90% of ureteral calculi are visualized. An appendiceal fecalith may suggest appendicitis. Absence of rectal air may indicate complete bowel obstruction. Air in the biliary system indicates biliary-enteric fistula.

17. **How is ultrasound (US) used?**
US helps to evaluate the gallbladder, biliary tree, free peritoneal fluid collection, and female adnexa (to assess for ectopic pregnancy or ovarian cyst/mass). Unfortunately, US abdominal

exam is limited in the setting of obesity, bowel distention from obstruction, and poorly prepped bowel.

18. **What additional x-ray studies may help in the diagnosis?**
CT of the abdomen and pelvis with oral and intravenous contrast is useful for intra-abdominal abscess, pancreatitis, aortic aneurysm and dissection, arterial and venous occlusive disease, hepatic, splenic, retroperitoneal, and renal disorders. Upper and lower gastrointestinal (GI) series may pinpoint the level of bowel obstruction, if CT scan is inconclusive. Angiography may be needed to assess mesenteric arterial flow.

19. **If the diagnosis is in doubt, what other tests should be done?**
Surgical exploration (laparotomy) of the abdomen is the next step if CT scan cannot confirm a diagnosis, and is mandatory when the patient's condition worsens despite aggressive resuscitation.

20. **Is exploratory laparotomy justified, even if it produces no significant findings?**
Yes. Despite pain from postoperative incisions, risk of wound infection, and a small lifetime risk of bowel obstruction (<5%) from adhesions, it is still safer to undergo an exploratory laparotomy than to miss the diagnosis of developing appendicitis or bowel infarction.

21. **Discuss the role of exploratory laparoscopy.**
Laparoscopy is useful only when it provides a positive pathologic finding. If the exam is negative, the next appropriate step is conversion to laparotomy. In the setting of distended abdomen from bowel obstruction, laparoscopy is not advised; thus, its role is very limited. When the presumptive diagnosis is acute appendicitis but the appendix appears normal, it should be removed anyway to eliminate future confusion for the cause of right lower quadrant pain. Meckel's diverticulum, inflammatory bowel disease, mesenteric adenitis, and pelvic disorders may be adequately assessed via laparoscopy.

22. **In blunt trauma, CT scan of the abdomen and pelvis reveals free peritoneal fluid collections. When is observation appropriate instead of immediate surgical exploration?**
First and foremost, the patient must be hemodynamically stable, and the identified injury must be confined to the liver and spleen. Small lacerations to the liver and spleen may be managed by aggressive resuscitation. Immediate access to the operating room must be available at all times in case the patient's condition deteriorates. Evidence on CT scan that suggests biliary or bowel injury requires surgical exploration.

23. **Do all penetrating injuries to the abdomen require laparotomy?**
No. If the patient is hemodynamically stable, and the stab wound(s) or a low-velocity tangential bullet wound does not penetrate the fascia, observation and resuscitation suffice after a negative CT scan. Immediate surgery is recommended with a high index of suspicion for abdominal injury. In case of multiple trauma victims, surgical exploration may be safer than observation of a penetrating wound because adequate and frequent exams during the observation period may be impossible due to shortage of health care personnel. High-velocity bullet wounds almost always require surgery. The transmission of explosive energy on impact usually delivers severe injury to adjacent organs.

24. **Does laparoscopy have any role in trauma?**
Laparoscopy is appropriate when diaphragmatic injury is suspected or when penetration of abdominal fascia cannot be ascertained. Otherwise, its use in major trauma is not advised.

25. **When is surgery indicated for peptic ulcer disease (PUD)?**
   - *Perforation.* Closure with an omental patch (Graham's patch) is acceptable for patients without previous history of PUD and hemodynamically unstable patients. Definitive antiulcer sur-

gery is indicated for patients with a history of chronic PUD and hemodynamic stability. Resection of the ulcer crater with adequate margins should be performed for gastric ulcers. Definitive gastrectomy is performed after recovery if carcinoma is found on the specimen.

- *Obstruction.* If duodenal obstruction from ulcer is not relieved by medical therapy in 7 days, surgery should be performed. Balloon dilatation is an option in patients who are not surgical candidates.
- *Bleeding.* If more than 6 units of packed red blood cells within 24 hours are required for resuscitation, surgery should be performed.
- *Intractability.* Despite benign biopsies, if gastric ulcers do not heal after medical therapy, surgery is recommended for suspected gastric carcinoma.

26. **When is cholecystectomy optimal for acute pancreatitis, presumably due to gallbladder disease?**
Cholecystectomy should be performed before discharge from hospital after resolution of acute pancreatitis. Recurrence rates for pancreatitis may be as high as 60% within 6 months, if the source of the gallstone is not treated.

27. **How should acute pancreatitis due to biliary tract stone be managed?**
The stone should be extracted as soon as possible. Endoscopic retrograde cholangiopancreatography (ERCP) should be tried first; if it is unsuccessful, surgery is necessary.

28. **When is surgery indicated for severe acute pancreatitis?**
Patients with progressively hemorrhagic or necrotizing pancreatitis and infected debris should undergo surgery when resuscitative measures fail. CT-guided catheter drainage may be an option for well-localized pancreatic abscess. Despite aggressive surgery, mortality rates are still as high as 40%. The impact of surgery on long-term survival is still debatable.

29. **Describe treatment for a pancreatic pseudocyst.**
An asymptomatic cyst <4 cm in diameter on CT scan should be followed. Larger cysts with symptoms or infected cysts should be drained by endoscopy, CT-guided catheterization, or surgery. Patients with an isolated pancreatic cyst and no previous history of pancreatitis should undergo partial pancreatic resection for suspicion of cystadenocarcinoma.

30. **How can one diagnose small bowel ischemia due to vascular obstruction?**
Despite advances in technology, a high index of suspicion based on history and physical exam remains the best indicator. Pain out of proportion with abdominal exam, atrial fibrillation, recent cardiac surgery, and hypercoagulable state should arouse suspicion of bowel infarction. Base deficit from arterial blood gas may reflect a late and fulminant course of bowel infarction, but a normal blood gas should not delay surgery. Immediate surgical exploration, based on high index of suspicion, is not only justified but also mandatory.

31. **Describe the surgical strategy for the treatment of Crohn's disease.**
The goal is to preserve as much small bowel as possible. Only segments with complete obstruction should be excised. Partial obstruction may be repaired by stricturoplasty. Diseased appearance by itself at the time of surgery is not an indication for resection. If resection is required, grossly normal-appearing margins and not microscopically normal margins are the goal.

32. **When should surgery be offered for uncomplicated acute diverticulitis?**
After more than two recurrent episodes, although the risk of recurrence after the first episode may be as high as 30–40%. Age less than 50 is a relative, not an absolute, indication. Complications, such as perforation with diffuse peritonitis, bowel obstruction, fistula formation, or severe bleeding, require immediate surgery. Localized perforation with abscess in a nontoxic

patient can be treated by percutaneous drainage and antibiotics with colectomy planned 6–8 weeks later. This avoids the need for a colostomy in the acute setting.

33. **Should elderly patients with sigmoid or cecal volvulus undergo surgery?**
Yes. After immediate reduction with barium enema or endoscopy, the recurrence rate may be as high as 50–90%. If the patient is not in a moribund state, surgery should be offered during the same hospital stay.

34. **How should toxic megacolon in the setting of ulcerative colitis be managed?**
Aggressive resuscitation in the intensive care unit with bowel rest, broad spectrum antibiotics, intravenous corticosteroids, and frequent abdominal exams. There is some evidence that cyclosporine may be helpful as rescue therapy. Serial abdominal radiographs are usually obtained to evaluate for bowel distention, pneumatosis, or free air. If there is no improvement after 48 hours, total abdominal colectomy with ileostomy may be the only course available. Barium enema, antidiarrheal agents, and morphine should be avoided because they might intensify the colonic dilatation.

35. **How should Ogilvie's syndrome be managed?**
The vast majority of cases may be treated by colonoscopic decompression, with or without addition of prokinetic agents. Intravenous neostigmine has gained acceptance as a first-line prokinetic agent. Surgical resection should be offered when signs of ischemia or peritonitis are noted or when cecal diameter reaches 12 cm of distention. Ileostomy with mucous fistula is established after bowel resection. Decompression by tube cecostomy should be reserved for moribund patients.

36. **After ERCP, a patient develops upper abdominal and back pain. What steps should be considered?**
CT scan and/or repeat ERCP usually reveals the injury. The main focus should be the location of leak: is it the biliary-pancreatic system or the duodenum? Bile duct injury may be treated by endoscopic stent placement with percutaneous drainage of intra-abdominal collection or surgery if the injury is complex. Pancreatitis should be treated expectantly. A contained, small leak in the posterior wall of the duodenum may be treated with bowel rest and gastric decompression; however, ongoing leakage should be repaired immediately, before onset of inflammatory tissue response. Late manifestation of duodenal leak requires extensive drainage and possible duodenal exclusion. Perforation involving the ampulla of Vater usually requires surgical repair.

37. **How should esophageal perforation be managed after endoscopy? What if the patient has achalasia? Esophageal carcinoma?**
Small, contained leaks may be treated with avoidance of oral ingestion and antibiotics, although decompression with chest tubes is usually required. More extensive leaks require surgical repair. In the setting of achalasia, concomitant Heller's myotomy with fundoplication should be performed. In the presence of esophageal carcinoma, the tumor, including the area of injury, should be resected, followed by an esophagogastrostomy at the same time.

38. **How should colonic perforation be managed after colonoscopy?**
With well-prepped bowel, patients may be treated with bowel rest, antibiotics, and observation for a small perforation. Immediate laparoscopic repair is a viable, minimally invasive alternative. With extensive laceration or with signs of diffuse peritonitis, surgery is required.

39. **How should colonic perforation be managed after barium enema?**
Unlike colonoscopic injuries, colonic perforation after a barium contrast study requires immediate surgery. As much barium contaminant as possible must be removed from the peritoneal cavity to minimize the risk of chemical peritonitis. Fluid resuscitation is delivered to offset

third-space fluid shift. Diverting proximal colostomy and resection of perforated segment are usually required.

BIBLIOGRAPHY

1. Boyd WP, Nord HJ: Diagnostic laparoscopy. Endoscopy 32:153–158, 2000.

2. Chae FH, Stiegmann GV: Current laparoscopic gastrointestinal surgery. Gastrointest Endosc 47:500–511, 1998.

3. Heaton KW: Diagnosis of acute non-specific abdominal pain. Lancet 355:1644, 2000.

4. Marco CA, Schoenfeld CN, Keyl PM, et al: Abdominal pain in geriatric emergency patients: Variables associated adverse outcomes. Acad Emerg Med 5:1163–1168, 1998.

5. McKellar DP, Reiling RB, Eiseman B: Prognosis and Outcomes in Surgical Disease. St. Louis, Quality Medical Publishing, 1999.

6. Mindelzun RE, Jeffrey RB: The acute abdomen: Current CT imaging techniques. Semin Ultrasound CT MR 20(2):63–67, 1999.

7. Norton LW, Stiegmann GV, Eiseman B: Surgical Decision Making. Philadelphia, W.B. Saunders, 2000.

8. Simic O, Strathausen S, Hess W, Ostermeyer J: Incidence and prognosis of abdominal complications after cardiopulmonary bypass. Cardiovasc Surg 7:419–424, 1999.

CHAPTER 78

COLORECTAL SURGERY

Martin D. McCarter, MD

POLYPOSIS SYNDROMES AND INFLAMMATORY BOWEL DISEASE

1. Name four different types of intestinal polyps.
Neoplastic, hamartomatous, inflammatory/lymphoid, and hyperplastic.

2. What is a hamartoma?
A hamartoma is an exuberant growth of normal tissue in an abnormal amount or location. An isolated hamartomatous polyp has no malignant potential.

3. Which intestinal polyposis syndromes are associated with hamartomatous polyps?
- Peutz-Jeghers syndrome
- Juvenile polyposis (familial or generalized)
- Cronkhite-Canada syndrome (hamartomatous polyps with alopecia, cutaneous pigmentation, and toenail and fingernail atrophy)
- Intestinal ganglioneuromatosis (isolated or with von Recklinghausen's disease or multiple endocrine neoplasia type 2)
- Ruvalcaba-Myhre-Smith syndrome (polyps of colon and tongue, macrocephaly, retardation, unique facies, pigmented penile macules)
- Cowden's disease (gastrointestinal [GI] polyps with oral and cutaneous verrucous papules [tricholemmomas], associated with breast cancer, thyroid neoplasia, and ovarian cysts)

4. How is Peutz-Jeghers syndrome manifest?
This autosomal, dominant trait is often heralded by the presence of melanin spots on the lips and buccal mucosa (*see* Chapter 71, Noninvasive GI Imaging: Ultrasound, Computed Tomography, Magnetic Resonance Scanning). Hamartomas are almost always present on the small intestine and, occasionally, on the stomach and colon. Previously considered a benign process, patients with Peutz-Jeghers syndrome are at increased risk for cancer.

5. Describe the manifestation of familial adenomatous polyposis (FAP).
FAP is a mendelian-dominant, nonsex-linked disease in which >100 adenomatous polyps affect the colon and rectum. FAP is caused by mutation in the adenomatous polyposis coli (APC) gene on the long arm of chromosome 5 at the 5q21–q22 locus. The APC protein is a tumor suppressor that, when mutated, fails to bind β-catenin and allows for unregulated cellular growth. One third of patients present as the propositus case (presumed mutation) with no prior family history. The disease invariably leads to invasive colon cancer if not treated. The average age at diagnosis of colon cancer is 39 years compared with 65 years for routine colon cancer.

6. What extracolonic abnormalities are associated with FAP?
See Table 78-1.

7. What is Gardner's syndrome?
FAP plus fibromas of the skin, osteomas (typically of the mandible, maxilla, and skull), epidermoid cysts, desmoid tumors, and extra dentition.

TABLE 78-1. EXTRACOLONIC ABNORMALITIES ASSOCIATED WITH FAMILIAL ADENOMATOUS POLYPOSIS (FAP)

Benign	Malignant
Congenital hypertrophy of retinal pigment epithelium (CHRPE)	Gastric cancer
Gastric fundic gland polyps	Periampullary carcinoma
Antral adenomas	Duodenal adenocarcinoma
Duodenal adenomas	Pancreatic adenocarcinoma
Jejunoileal adenomas	Cholangiocarcinoma
Desmoid tumors	Small intestinal carcinoma
Adrenal adenomas	Ileal carcinoids
Pituitary adenomas	Adrenal adenocarcinoma
	Medulloblastoma
	Turcot's syndrome or glioblastoma
	Thyroid carcinoma
	Osteogenic sarcoma
	Hepatoblastoma

8. **How does one screen for FAP?**

   When family history is positive, children should undergo annual sigmoidoscopic surveillance beginning at ages 10–12. When polyps are identified, a full colonoscopy is recommended. Once multiple adenomas are documented, colectomy is recommended. State-of-the-art presymptomatic detection uses molecular genetic screening. Direct mutational analysis of the APC gene, restrictive fragment length polymorphism linkage analysis, or protein truncation assay can determine whether a person is affected with 95–99% certainty, if genetic material is available from affected and unaffected members of the kindred. Ophthalmoscopic exam for congenital hypertrophy of the retinal pigment epithelium (CHRPE) can detect involved patients as early as age 3 months with a 97% positive predictive value for developing FAP. CHRPE is present in 55–100% of FAP patients and is documented with wide-angle fundus photography.

KEY POINTS: CHARACTERISTICS OF POLYPOSIS SYNDROMES

- Genetic mutation

- Hundreds of intestinal polyps

- Extraintestinal manifestations

- Risk for developing cancer

9. **What is attenuated FAP?**

   Attenuated FAP is rare but should be considered when there are multiple but fewer than 100 colorectal adenomas present on colonoscopy. There is a tendency toward rectal sparing, a delay in onset of adenomatosis and bowel symptoms of 20–25 years, and a delay in onset of colorectal cancer (CRC) of 10–20 years. A more limited expression of the extracolonic features is seen, but gastric and duodenal adenomas are frequently encountered.

10. **What is Crohn's disease?**
A nonspecific inflammatory disease that may involve any portion of the GI tract; regional enteritis commonly causes abdominal pain and diarrhea. The distribution of disease in the GI tract may be discontinuous. Presenting patterns are ileocolic in about 40%, colonic Crohn's alone in 30%, small bowel involvement alone in 25%, and anorectal disease alone in 5%. Historic use of immunologic therapies (azathioprine, cyclosporin, infliximab) lends support to the recent discovery of a genetic mutation in an immune regulatory gene associated with Crohn's disease.

11. **What is ulcerative colitis?**
A nonspecific inflammatory bowel disease that involves the colon and rectum. Bloody diarrhea is the classic presenting symptom. Disease may be limited to the rectum (proctitis), left colon (proctosigmoiditis), or entire colon (pancolitis). The rectum is always involved; the disease process is one of continuous inflammation (no skip areas).

12. **How is Crohn's disease differentiated from ulcerative colitis?**
See Table 78-2.

13. **What are the surgical indications for ulcerative colitis?**
   - Intractability or failure of medical management
   - Fulminant colitis (toxic megacolon, bleeding, diarrhea)
   - Prophylaxis of carcinoma (presence of high-grade dysplasia)
   - Treatment of carcinoma

14. **Identify the extracolonic manifestations of ulcerative colitis.**
   - *Skin:* Pyoderma gangrenosum, erythema nodosum
   - *Liver:* Fatty infiltration of the liver, pericholangitis, cirrhosis
   - *Biliary:* Primary sclerosing cholangitis, bile duct carcinoma
   - *Eye:* Uveitis, episcleritis, conjunctivitis, retrobulbar neuritis
   - *Joints:* Monoarticular arthritis, ankylosing spondylitis, sacroiliitis
   - *Mouth:* Aphthous ulcers, stomatitis
   - *Renal:* Pyelonephritis, nephrolithiasis
   - *Systemic:* Amyloidosis, thromboembolic disease, hypercoagulability, vasculitis, pericarditis

15. **What are the elective surgical options for FAP and chronic ulcerative colitis?**
   - Total proctocolectomy with end (Brooke end) ileostomy
   - Total proctocolectomy with continent ileostomy reservoir (Kock's pouch)
   - Abdominal colectomy with ileorectal anastomosis
   - Near-total proctocolectomy ± rectal mucosectomy and ileal pouch-anal anastomosis (IPAA)

16. **Can one always tell the difference between Crohn's disease and ulcerative colitis?**
No. Colitis that cannot be categorized as definitely Crohn's or ulcerative colitis is called *indeterminate colitis* and may account for 5–10% of cases referred for surgical consideration. The postoperative result when IPAA is performed for indeterminate colitis has been held to be generally the same as that obtained with definite ulcerative colitis. However, a recent Mayo Clinic review notes that pouch failure is twice as common in indeterminate colitis as in ulcerative colitis (18% and 9%, respectively).

TABLE 78-2. ULCERATIVE COLITIS VERSUS CROHN'S DISEASE

	Ulcerative Colitis	Crohn's Disease
Clinical manifestation		
Bleeding per rectum	3+	1+
Diarrhea	3+	3+
Abdominal pain	1+	3+ (especially with ileal involvement)
Fever	R	2+
Palpable abdominal mass	R	2+
Internal fistula	R	4+
Intestinal obstruction (stricture or infection)	0	4+
Rectal involvement	4+	1+
Small bowel involvement	0	4+
Anal and perianal involvement	R	4+
Thumbprinting sign on barium enema	R	1+
Risk of cancer	2+	1+
Clinical course	Relapses/remissions	Slowly progressive
Gross appearance		
Thickened bowel wall	0	4+
Shortening of bowel	2+	R
Fat creeping onto serosa	0	4+
Segmental involvement	0	4+
Aphthous ulcer	0	4+
Linear ulcer	0	4+
Microscopic picture		
Depth of involvement	Mucosa and submucosa	Full thickness
Lymphoid aggregation	0	4+
Sarcoid-type granuloma	0	4+
Fissuring	0	2+
Surgical treatment		
Total proctocolectomy	Gold standard	Indicated in total large bowel involvement
Segmental resection	Infrequent	Frequent
Ileal pouch procedure	Excellent option in selected patients	Contraindicated
Recurrence after surgery	0	3+

R = rare, 0 = not found, 1+ = may be present, 2+ = common, 3+ = usual finding, 4+ = characteristic (not necessarily common).
From Nivatvongs S: The colon, rectum and anal canal. In James EC, Corry RJ, Perry JF Jr (eds): Basic Surgical Practice. Philadelphia, Hanley & Belfus, 1987, p 325.

17. **What is pouchitis? How is it treated?**

Pouchitis, one of the most frequent long-term complications of IPAA, is a nonspecific acute and/or chronic inflammation of the reservoir. Pouchitis is found in 7–44% of patients with IPAA; it presents with watery, bloody stools, urgency, frequency, abdominal pain, fever, malaise, and possible exacerbation of extraintestinal manifestations of inflammatory bowel disease. The cause is uncertain, but the risk is greater in chronic ulcerative colitis than in familial polyposis. Pouch stasis, bacterial overgrowth, colonification of ileal mucosa, ischemia, pelvic sepsis, oxygen-derived free radicals, altered immune status, and lack of mucosal trophic factors have been proposed as etiologies.

Successful treatment regimens include metronidazole and other antianaerobic antibiotics as well as steroid or 5-aminosalicylate enemas. Topical volatile fatty acids and glutamine have been used with variable success. Although half of patients with pouchitis at some time suffer a recurrence, very few develop intractable involvement requiring pouch excision.

18. **Does a defunctionalized colon develop colitis?**

Yes. Perhaps 30% of patients with a portion or the entire colon out of the fecal stream develop an inflammation difficult to distinguish from ulcerative colitis on biopsy. The diagnosis of diversion colitis is suggested when bloody mucopus is passed from the separate colorectal segment. The colon may be isolated by diverting ileostomy, end or loop colostomy, mucous fistula, or Hartmann's procedure. Short-chain fatty acids normally produced by anaerobic bacteria serve as a trophic factor for the colonocytes. The diversion colitis quickly resolves restoration of intestinal continuity; when restoration is not possible, the administration of short-chain fatty acid enemas is beneficial.

CONTROVERSIES

19. **What are the risks/benefits of performing a rectal mucosectomy?**
   - *Risks:* increased incontinence, decreased discrimination of air/liquid/formed stool, anastomotic leak.
   - *Benefits:* decreased risk of recurrent polyps or colitis.

20. **Should the IPAA be stapled or hand-sewn?**

If a mucosectomy is performed, a hand-sewn anastomosis of the pouch to the dentate line is created. If the anal transition zone mucosa is preserved, a stapled anastomosis may be performed at the top of the anorectal ring. Complication rates are nearly equivalent.

21. **Should IPAA be a one- or two-stage operation?**

The procedure has classically been two-staged, with construction of a temporary ileostomy followed at an interval by ileostomy takedown. Recent experience has shown that the morbidity of a one-stage IPAA may be less, if the patient is taking no or low-dose steroids and the operation is performed without complication. Because there is really only "one shot" at getting it right, intraoperative judgment is at a premium.

22. **What type of pouch should be used?**

Higher-volume pouches are advocated. W (quadruplicated) pouches have a greater capacity than S (triplicate) and J (two-limbed) pouches. The functional results may not be that different. Shorter efferent limbs (for S pouches) are also used to avoid outlet obstruction. The author prefers a long (15 cm) J pouch (when feasible in one stage) preserving the anal transition zone.

ANORECTAL DISEASE

23. **What are anal fissures?**
A generally painful rip or tear in the sensitive anoderm of the anal canal. Most anal fissures are located in the posterior (90%) or anterior (10%) midline of the anal canal.

24. **What disorders should be considered in patients with laterally situated anal fissures?**
Crohn's disease, ulcerative colitis, syphilis, tuberculosis, leukemia, carcinoma, and AIDS.

25. **What does anorectal manometry demonstrate in patients with an anal fissure?**
After transient relaxation, the internal sphincter shows a prolonged elevation in pressure above the normal baseline—the "overshoot" phenomenon associated with the pain/spasm cycle of fissure disease.

26. **How are acute fissures managed?**
Conservative treatment consists of stool softeners and bulk agents to avoid hard bowel movements, sitz baths to help decrease sphincter spasm, topical anesthetics, and topical steroids. Suppositories should generally be avoided because they may induce anal spasm. Topical nitroglycerin or nifedipine ointment reduces anal spasm. Injection of botulinum toxin has also been used to relax the anal sphincter.

27. **How does nitroglycerin ointment work?**
Nitroglycerin ointment breaks down into the active moiety nitric oxide, an inhibitory neurotransmitter for the internal sphincter. Thus, it allows relaxation of the muscle, relief of spasm, and, ultimately, increased blood flow and increased oxygen delivery through the microcapillaries to the area of anoderm breakdown. To avoid the common side effect of headache seen with the use of 2% nitroglycerin ointment used for angina, 0.2% strength should be used for anal fissure.

28. **What are the signs of a chronic anal fissure? What do they imply?**
A chronic anal fissure can be identified by the presence of a sentinel pile (skin tag or hemorrhoid), anal ulcer (with fibropurulent material or visible internal sphincter muscle in the base), and a hypertrophied anal papilla arising from the dentate line. A chronic anal fissure does not usually respond to conservative treatment, and surgical intervention is in order.

29. **Which surgical procedures are available for treatment of a chronic anal fissure?**
Open or closed lateral internal sphincterotomy, excision (ulcerectomy), excision and Y-V or other anoplasty, or anal dilation.

30. **What are hemorrhoids?**
Hemorrhoids are difficult to define precisely. Everyone has vascular cushions in the anal canal that contain veins (and arteries), elastic and connective tissue, and smooth muscle. Hemorrhoids are not "varicose veins of the anus"; they may play a role in fine control of anal continence. It has been suggested that the term "hemorrhoid" be reserved for symptomatic involvement of these structures.

31. **How are hemorrhoids classified?**
   - *External* hemorrhoids originate distal to the dentate line of the anus and are covered by squamous epithelium. External hemorrhoids may thrombose or become filled with clotted blood. Typically, these are painful involving the anoderm.
   - *Internal* hemorrhoids arise above (proximal to) the dentate line and are covered with transitional and columnar epithelium. First-degree hemorrhoids swell and bleed. Second-degree

hemorrhoids prolapse and spontaneously reduce. Third-degree hemorrhoids prolapse and can be manually reduced, whereas fourth-degree hemorrhoids are irreducible. Typically, these are not painful above the anoderm.

32. How are acute hemorrhoids treated?
- *Topical medicines:* anesthetics, hydrocortisone preparations, astringents (witch hazel, glycerine, magnesium sulfate).
- *Emergency hemorrhoidectomy* (ouch!) requires 2 weeks of recovery time. Circular stapling devices have been used to treat larger hemorrhoids.

33. Where in the anal canal are hemorrhoids classically found?
Left lateral, right anterior, and right posterior locations are typical. The use of clock face times as descriptions of hemorrhoids (e.g., "large bundle at 9 o'clock position") is confusing and should be avoided, because patients may be examined in lithotomy, jackknife, or decubitus positions by different examiners with resulting confusion.

34. List several minimally invasive outpatient treatments of internal hemorrhoids.
Rubber band ligation, bipolar cautery, direct current electrical therapy, infrared coagulation, sclerotherapy, and cryotherapy.

35. Who is the patron saint of hemorrhoid sufferers?
Fiachra (Irish), Fiacre (French), or Fiacrius (Latin). An Irish holy man famed for cures of such less desirable maladies, he died in France on August 30, 670 AD.

KEY POINTS: BENIGN ANORECTAL CONDITIONS

- Fissures
- Hemorrhoids
- Fistulas
- Rectal prolapse
- Perianal Paget's disease

36. How is an acute thrombosed external hemorrhoid best treated?
Excision of the clot and involved hemorrhoidal complex (as opposed to incision alone) better prevents future recurrence at the same site.

37. Explain the cause of anorectal abscesses and fistulas.
A cryptoglandular origin seems to provide the best explanation. Four to 10 anal glands enter the anal canal at the level of the crypts in the dentate line. The glands extend back into the internal sphincter two thirds of the time and into the intersphincteric space half the time. Blockage of the gland leads to an overgrowth of bacteria, with resultant pressure necrosis and abscess formation. An abscess or infection that causes an abnormal communication between two surfaces (such as the anal canal and perianal skin) creates a fistula.

38. List the various types and locations of anorectal abscesses.
Submucosal, intersphincteric, perianal (anal verge), ischiorectal (perirectal), and supralevator.

39. **What is a horseshoe abscess?**
A perirectal abscess that connects the ischiorectal fossae bilaterally through the deep postanal space posteriorly or anteriorly.

40. **What is the best treatment for an anorectal abscess?**
Prompt incision and drainage! Antibiotics play little or no role (exceptions are immunocompromised patients and patients with prosthetic heart valves or severe cellulitis), and waiting for the abscess to "point" or become fluctuant is not necessary before surgical treatment.

41. **What is Goodsall's rule?**
See Figure 78-1.

42. **What is a seton?**
A drainage device used to control and treat an anal fistulous abscess. It is inserted through a fistula tract and secured to itself, thus making a circle about some portion of the anal sphincter muscle. Typical setons are Penrose drains, silastic "vessel loops," or silk sutures.

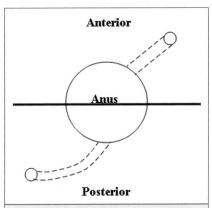

43. **Why is a seton used?**
  - To provide permanent drainage, as in perianal Crohn's disease with multiple fistulas
  - To serve as a cutting device to slowly exteriorize the fistula
  - To act as a temporizing agent while awaiting a staged fistulotomy
  - To treat primarily by sequential downsizing of the seton material until, eventually, all drains are removed

Figure 78-1. This rule helps predict the location of the internal opening of an anal fistula based on the site of its external opening. Accurately determining the "criminal crypt" of fistula origin on the dentate line is important at the time of surgical treatment, generally fistulotomy. If the anus is divided into imaginary anterior and posterior halves in the coronal plane, posterior fistulas tend to curve into the posterior midline. Anterior fistulas shorter than 3 cm tend to proceed radially to the dentate line, whereas anterior fistulas longer than 3 cm may track back to the posterior midline.

44. **What are the common indications for inserting a seton?**
  - High fistulous abscesses involving greater than one-half the length of the anal canal muscle
  - Anterior fistulas in a woman
  - Inflammatory bowel disease
  - Elderly patients or patients with multiple previous anorectal surgeries

45. **List new developments for treatment of anorectal fistulas.**
  - Fibrin sealant glues
  - Monoclonal antitumor necrosis factor antibodies for Crohn's fistulas
  - Revival of Park's fistulotomy procedure, with excision/debridement of the fistula tract, muscle repair, advancement flap coverage of the internal opening, and drainage of the external portion of the fistula tract

46. **When is anorectal suppurative disease especially dangerous?**
In the presence of neutropenia, as associated with chemotherapy, the mortality at 1 month may approach 50%. Unfortunately, surgery and even anorectal digital examination may be

contraindicated. Often bacterial infection is widespread without formation of purulence or a classic abscess.

47. **Describe perianal Paget's disease.**
Perianal (extramammary) Paget's disease is characterized by a scaly, inflamed dermis resembling eczema. Biopsy reveals typical Paget cells with round, pale, vacuolated mucin positive cytoplasm and an eccentric reticular nucleus. Often a chronic condition, underlying carcinoma must be ruled out because cancer is associated with Paget's disease.

48. **Which patient characteristics are associated with rectal prolapse?**

Chronic constipation	Deep pouch of Douglas
Neurologic disease	Patulous anus
Female gender	Diastasis of the levator ani muscles
Nulliparity	Lack of fixation of the rectum to the sacrum
Redundant rectosigmoid colon	Previous anorectal surgery

49. **What radiologic procedure may document a prolapse that cannot be reproduced in the office?**
Cine defecography may reveal an internal intussusception beginning on the anterior rectal wall several centimeters above the anal verge, which may progress to complete prolapse.

50. **What is the relationship between rectal prolapse and anal continence?**
Some degree of incontinence almost always accompanies rectal prolapse. Surgical repair may not correct incontinence problems. Abdominal approaches tend to have higher success rates for continence than perineal operations, but the results vary widely.

51. **What surgical options are available for rectal prolapse?**
In general, procedures can narrow the anal orifice (Thiersch's operation), obliterate the pouch of Douglas (Moschcowitz' procedure), restore the condition of the pelvic floor (levator plication), excise (abdominally or perineally) the excess rectosigmoid colon, and/or fixate or suspend the rectum. Combinations of these options are often used.

52. **How is rectal prolapse handled in pediatric patients?**
Most prolapses in children are mucosal prolapses alone. A bowel management program to reduce constipation and straining is used to handle prolapse. Surgical or invasive methods, such as sclerosis, encirclement, or excision, are rarely necessary.

BENIGN COLON AND SMALL BOWEL DISEASE

53. **Which type of colonic volvulus is most common?**
Sigmoid volvulus accounts for 75% of cases seen in the United States. It is far more common than cecal volvulus.

54. **List the characteristics of a typical American patient with colonic volvulus.**
Male, black, elderly, and possibly from a nursing home or mental institution.

55. **What are the findings of sigmoid volvulus on plain abdominal film and contrast enema?**
The plain film demonstrates a "bent inner tube" or "coffee bean" sign of massively dilated, air-filled sigmoid colon arising out of the pelvis. The contrast enema shows a "bird's beak" appearance as the colon narrows at the twist at the rectosigmoid junction.

56. **How is a nonstrangulated sigmoid volvulus treated?**
Rigid or flexible sigmoidoscopic or colonoscopic decompression, followed by elective sigmoid resection.

57. **Why should elective surgery be performed after a successful endoscopic detorsion and decompression of a sigmoid volvulus?**
Recurrence is the rule with sigmoid volvulus. Elective sigmoid resection of prepped and decompressed bowel can generally be accomplished with a mortality rate <5%. Emergency operation for a sigmoid volvulus involves a mortality rate of 35–80%.

58. **What is the most common cause of mechanical large bowel obstruction in Western society?**
Carcinoma far outnumbers diverticular causes and volvulus.

59. **What is Ogilvie's syndrome?**
Colonic pseudo-obstruction presents with signs, symptoms, and radiologic findings suggestive of obstruction without a mechanical source. Ogilvie's syndrome is most often seen in hospitalized patients with other underlying medical conditions found to have marked colonic air on abdominal x-ray. Treatments include managing the underlying medical issues, colonoscopic decompression, and neostigmine.

60. **What does plain x-ray study of the abdomen reveal in large bowel obstruction?**
Differential air-fluid levels (stair steps) of the small intestine or a massively dilated colon. The colon is identified by the presence of haustral folds, as compared to the *valvulae conniventes* of the small intestine. The rectum is usually gasless, although gas distal to a colonic obstruction may not have completely cleared the distal colon. A picture resembling small bowel obstruction alone may appear in a very proximal colon obstruction. Colonic pseudo-obstruction may also give a roentgenographic picture similar to true obstruction.

61. **How can one safely differentiate true from false colonic obstruction?**
A water-soluble enema contrast study reveals the presence or absence of an organic obstructing lesion. Barium should be avoided because a perforation during the study or a leak of colonic contents and barium at the time of surgery may lead to severe barium peritonitis.

62. **What is a bezoar?**
A concretion formed in the alimentary tract that may produce an obstruction. It can be caused by vegetable matter (phytobezoar), hair (trichobezoar), or a combination of hair and food (trichophytobezoar).

63. **What radiologic findings are associated with gallstone ileus?**
Air in gallbladder or biliary tree, small bowel obstruction at the level of the ileocecal valve, large bowel obstruction at the sigmoid colon, and, occasionally, a calcified mass at the previously mentioned points.

64. **What does endometriosis have to do with the alimentary system?**
Endometriosis is the presence of functioning endometrial tissue outside the uterus. When this hormonally active tissue implants on intestinal surfaces, it can cause pain, cyclical bleeding, and obstructive symptoms.

65. **What is a primary bowel obstruction?**
An intestinal obstruction without a known etiology, such as adhesions or a prior cancer diagnosis. Primary bowel obstructions will virtually always require an operation.

66. **How is postoperative ileus differentiated from postoperative small bowel obstruction?**
This distinction can be extremely difficult. Postoperative ileus generally occurs up to 1 week after operation, whereas postoperative small bowel obstruction (SBO) may last 7–30 days or longer. SBO is associated with nausea, vomiting, distention, and abdominal pain, whereas an ileus may be associated with painless failure to pass bowel movements. The radiographic picture may or may not include differential air-fluid levels in each disorder.

67. **Is treatment of postoperative SBO different from treatment of SBO remote from surgery?**
Yes. Generally, one waits out a postoperative obstruction for an indefinite period, as long as there is no evidence of strangulation or impending perforation. Approximately 80% resolve without surgery. Nasogastric suction is the mainstay of treatment for postoperative SBO, whereas "the sun never sets" on a suspected mechanical SBO remote from surgery; one generally operates as soon as the diagnosis of complete obstruction is made.

KEY POINTS: INDICATIONS FOR OPERATING ON INTESTINAL OBSTRUCTION

- Complete obstruction
- Fever
- Intractable pain
- Evidence of strangulation
- Primary obstruction

68. **What is the leading cause of SBO?**
Adhesions.

69. **Can adhesions be prevented?**
Absorbable hyaluronate and carboxymethylcellulose membranes lead to a statistically significant reduction in the number and severity of intra-abdominal adhesions, although it is unclear if it translates into a reduced future need for operative intervention.

70. **What are the pathologic findings of late radiation enteritis?**
Obliterative arteritis. Severe fibrosis is commonly accompanied by telangiectasia formation. The pelvis may be "frozen" because of incredibly dense adhesions and fibrosis.

71. **What are the general principles of managing radiation enteritis?**
Medical management options are generally exhausted before surgery is contemplated or attempted. Cholestyramine, elemental diets, and total parenteral nutrition are commonly used. Although surgery is not withheld for urgent indications (complete obstruction, perforation, abscess not amenable to percutaneous drainage, bleeding, or unresponsive fistulas), it carries significant morbidity (up to 65%) and mortality (up to 45%) rates. Enterolysis, or separating of adhesions, in radiated bowel is associated with a high rate of fistula formation. Anastomosis can be performed safely, if at least one end of bowel to be connected has not been radiated. Intestinal bypass procedures without resection may be necessary.

72. **What treatments are available for bleeding radiation proctitis?**
Topical anti-inflammatories (steroids, mesalamine enemas, or suppositories), laser ablation of telangiectasias, and application of 4% formaldehyde solutions (under controlled situations in the operating room).

BIBLIOGRAPHY

1. Bailey HR, Ott MT, Hartendorp P: Aggressive surgical management for advanced colorectal endometriosis. Dis Colon Rectum 37:747, 1994.
2. Corman ML: Colon and Rectal Surgery, 4th ed. Philadelphia, Lippincott-Raven Publishers, 1998.
3. Gordon PH, Nivatvongs S: Principles and Practice of Surgery for the Colon, Rectum and Anus. St. Louis, Quality Medical Publishing, 1999.
4. Guillem JG, Smith AJ, Puig La Calle J, Ruo L: Gastrointestinal polyposis syndromes. Curr Probl Surg 36(4):217–324, 1999.
5. Hizawa K, Iida M, Matsumoto T, et al: Neoplastic transformation arising in Peutz-Jeghers polyposis. Dis Colon Rectum 36:953, 1993.
6. Keighley MR, Williams NS: Surgery of the Anus, Rectum and Colon. London, W.B. Saunders, 1993.
7. Knudsen AL, Bisgaard ML, Bulow S: Attenuated familial adenomatous polyposis (AFAP): A review of the literature. Fam Cancer 2(1):43–55, 2003.
8. Knutson D, Greenberg G, Cronau H: Management of Crohn's disease: A practical approach. Am Fam Physician 68(4):707–714, 2003.
9. Longo WE, Vernava AM III: Prokinetic agents for lower gastrointestinal motility disorders. Dis Colon Rectum 36:696, 1993.
10. McCarter MD, Quan SH, Busam K, et al: Long-term outcome of perianal Paget's disease. Dis Colon Rectum 46(5):612–616, 2003.
11. McIntyre PB, Pemberton JH, Wolff BG, et al: Indeterminate colitis: Long-term outcome in patients after ileal pouch-anal anastomosis. Dis Colon Rectum 38:51, 1995.
12. Metcalf AM: Anal fissure. Surg Clin North Am 82(6):1291–1297, 2002.
13. Mignon M, Stettler C, Phillips SF: Pouchitis: A poorly understood entity. Dis Colon Rectum 38:100, 1995.
14. Saclarides TJ, King DG, Franklin H, et al: Formalin instillation for refractory radiation-induced hemorrhagic proctitis. Dis Colon Rectum 39:196, 1996.
15. Vrijland WW, Tseng LN, Eijkman HJ, et al: Fewer intraperitoneal adhesions with use of hyaluronic acid-carboxymethylcellulose membrane: A randomized clinical trial. Ann Surg 235(2):193–199, 2002.

CHAPTER 79

OBESITY AND SURGICAL WEIGHT LOSS

Jonathan A. Schoen, MD, and Frank H. Chae, MD

1. **What is the definition of *obesity*?**
   Excess body fat.

2. **How is body fat relative to weight usually measured?**
   By calculating the body mass index, or BMI:

$$BMI = \frac{Weight\ (kg)}{Height\ (m)^2}$$

or

$$BMI = \frac{Weight\ (lb)}{Height\ (in)^2} \times 703$$

3. **Describe the BMI classification system.**
   - <18 = underweight
   - 18–24 = healthy weight
   - 25–29 = overweight
   - 30–39 = obese
   - ≥40 = morbidly obese

4. **What are the limitations of BMI?**
   - Those with a higher proportion of fat relative to muscle: the elderly
   - Those with an unusually high proportion of muscle: bodybuilders

5. **What percentage of the U.S. adult population is considered overweight?**
   The percentage is 64%, or 127 million.

6. **What percentage of the U.S. adult population is considered obese?**
   The percentage is 31%, or 60 million adults; obesity is now considered a national epidemic.

7. **Are there health implications associated with a BMI ≥30?**
   Obesity is considered a major factor contributing to many health problems, including: diabetes mellitus, hypertension, sleep apnea and pickwickian syndrome, asthma, coronary artery disease, cardiomyopathy and cardiac failure, gastroesophageal reflux disease, degenerative joint disease, hypercholesterolemia, fatty liver, gout, urinary incontinence, gallbladder disease, psychological disorders, menstrual irregularities, and certain cancers (endometrial, colon, postmenopausal breast, and kidney).

8. **Can obesity lead to premature death?**
   Yes. Individuals who have a BMI >30 have a 50–100% increased risk of premature death from all causes compared to individuals with a BMI of 20–25.

This increased mortality is directly proportional to increasing BMI. Obesity causes 400,000 preventable deaths in the United States and is a close second to smoking as the leading cause of preventable death.

9. **What does the term *bariatric* mean?**
   Bariatric was derived in the 20th century from the Greek *barros*, meaning heavy or large. Bariatrics is weight treatment.

10. **How is obesity best treated?**
    The National Institutes of Health (NIH) consensus statement in 1991 concluded that medical therapy was ineffective for severe clinical obesity, and that surgery was indicated for this population of patients.

11. **Who qualifies for surgical weight loss procedures?**
    Those with severe clinical obesity defined as a BMI ≥40 (morbid obesity) or a BMI of 35–39 with severe, debilitating comorbidities.

12. **Define the four main categories of surgical weight loss procedures, and provide a main example of each category.**
    - *Restrictive:* adjustable gastric band
    - *Malabsorptive:* biliopancreatic diversion, with or without duodenal switch
    - *Combination restrictive/malabsorptive:* Roux-en-Y gastric bypass
    - *Other:* gastric pacing

13. **Can these operations be performed laparoscopically?**
    Yes. Not to perform these laparoscopically is now the exception.

14. **What is the most common weight loss operation performed in the United States?**
    The laparoscopic Roux-en-Y gastric bypass.

15. **Describe the operation and resulting anatomic changes.**
    1. A 15- to 30-mL gastric pouch is created by completely dividing the proximal stomach (the restrictive part).
    2. The proximal jejunum is divided 15 cm from the ligament of Treitz. The distal end of this divided proximal jejunum is measured out between 75 and 150 cm, and the roux limb is anastomosed to the gastric pouch (the malabsorptive part).
    3. The proximal end of divided jejunum (biliopancreatic limb) is anastomosed to roux limb at the previously measured length, creating the Y configuration (Fig. 79-1).

16. **What are the weight loss expectations after a Roux-en-Y gastric bypass?**
    Expressed as percentage of excess weight loss (excess weight = preoperative weight – ideal weight), the longest term data has shown is a 50% loss of excess body weight maintained after 14 years. Most current laparoscopic literature shows up to 5-year excess weight loss in the 70% range.

17. **Is this just a cosmetic operation?**
    No. Ninety to 100% of the patient's obesity-induced comorbid conditions are improved or resolved within 1 year.

18. **What are the complications of laparoscopic Roux-en-Y gastric bypass?**
    Complications can be divided into early (<30 days) and late. Early complications include mortality (0.2%), anastomotic leaks (2.1%), gastrointestinal (GI) bleeding (1.9%), pulmonary

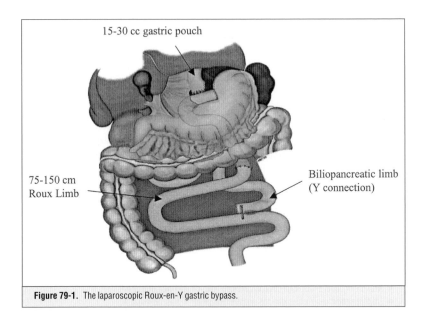

15-30 cc gastric pouch

75-150 cm
Roux Limb

Biliopancreatic limb
(Y connection)

Figure 79-1. The laparoscopic Roux-en-Y gastric bypass.

embolus (0.4%), and wound infection (3.0%). Late complications include anastomotic stenosis (4.7%), small bowel obstruction from internal hernias (2.9%), marginal ulceration (1.4%), cholelithiasis (1.4%), and vitamin/mineral deficiencies.

19. **How are anastomotic leaks handled?**
Usually at the gastrojejunostomy anastomosis and can be treated conservatively with total parenteral nutrition (TPN), NPO, and percutaneous catheter drainage, if the patient is stable. An unstable patient or a nonhealing fistula requires surgical repair.

20. **How is an anastomotic stenosis treated?**
Many surgeons purposely make the gastrojejunostomy anastomosis small (approximately 1 cm) to enhance the restrictive aspect of the operation. If this anastomosis becomes too small for the patient to tolerate, endoscopic balloon dilatation is usually successful.

21. **What is a marginal ulcer? How is it treated?**
This is an ulcer found usually on the jejunal side of the gastrojejunostomy. It is often related to local ischemia or nonsteroidal anti-inflammatory drug (NSAID) use and heals with H_2-blocker therapy.

22. **What are the vitamin/mineral deficiencies and potential long-term risks?**
Vitamin B_{12}, folate, and iron deficiency anemia can occur in up to 40% of patients without lifelong supplementation. Hypocalcemia and resulting osteoporosis can also occur without lifelong supplementation. The deficiencies are a result of bypassing most of the stomach, all of the duodenum, and the proximal jejunum.

23. **What is the most common surgical weight loss procedure in Europe?**
The laparoscopic adjustable gastric band (Lap Band).

24. **Describe the Lap Band.**

A silicone ring secured around the proximal stomach 15 mL from the gastroesophageal junction. A balloon on the inside of the ring is slowly inflated over time. The inflation port is placed in the abdominal wall subcutaneous tissue.

25. **Is weight loss similar to the Roux-en-Y gastric bypass?**

According to the European and Australian data, weight loss is slower but reaches a similar 60% excess weight loss over 5 years. The U.S. data are not as impressive, with only 38% excess weight loss. Eating habits and culture may play an important role.

26. **Why would someone choose the Lap Band over a Roux-en-Y gastric bypass?**

The Lap Band is considered reversible because there is no anatomic reconfiguration. It also avoids vitamin and mineral deficiencies. It should still be considered investigational because of absence of good long-term data on weight loss.

27. **What is a biliopancreatic diversion?**

A portion of the stomach is removed, and then the ileum is divided approximately 200–300 cm proximal to the ileocecal valve. The distal end of the divided ileum is connected to the remaining stomach or first portion of the duodenum (duodenal switch), creating a 200- to 300-cm intestinal limb for food. The proximal end of the divided ileum (the long biliopancreatic limb) is connected to the food limb 50–100 cm proximal to the ileocecal valve.

28. **How does the operation work?**

It creates a fixed amount of malabsorption, whereby all fat and most starch can be absorbed in only 50–100 cm of terminal ileum.

29. **How effective is this for weight loss?**

Long-term (up to 18 years) data show a maintained excess weight loss of approximately 75%. Although at the expense of malnutrition, biliopancreatic diversion is considered the most effective weight loss procedure.

30. **Why is there malnutrition with biliopancreatic diversion? How problematic is it?**

Protein has only 200–300 cm of ileum to be absorbed. Up to 30% of patients end up with protein-calorie malnutrition requiring hospitalization and TPN or surgical revision. A high protein/low carbohydrate diet is required to avoid inducing a state of starvation mimicking Kwashiorkor's disease.

31. **Are there other health risks associated with biliopancreatic diversion?**

Yes. Vitamin B_{12}, folate, and iron deficiency anemia are common without lifelong supplementation. Hypocalcemia and bone demineralization are common, leading to bone pain and osteoporosis if calcium and vitamin D are not administered in high doses lifelong. Patients also complain of frequent diarrhea, foul-smelling stool and flatulence, and halitosis.

32. **Why would one choose biliopancreatic diversion?**

Patients can eat as much as they want. This may be the best procedure for the binge-eater or compulsive snacker who classically fails the other weight loss procedures. The biliopancreatic diversion has also been proven to be effective for the so-called super morbidly obese (BMI ≥ 50).

33. **What is the gastric pacer?**

An electrode placed in the gastric wall, connected to a pacemaker battery placed in the abdominal wall subcutaneous tissue. Originally, this was used to stimulate gastric contractions in those with gastroparesis. However, overstimulation of the gastric muscle leads to appetite suppression by various mechanisms, as of yet not fully understood. Well-selected patients may achieve 30% excess weight loss. Food and Drug Administration trials are currently underway.

WEBSITES

1. http://www.asbs.org/

2. http://www.nhlbisupport.com/bmi/bmicalc.htm

3. http://www.obesitylaw.com

4. http://www.niddk.nih.gov/health/nutrit/pubs/statobes.htm

5. http://www.weightlosssurgeryinfo.com

BIBLIOGRAPHY

1. Belachew M, Legrand M, Vincent V, et al: Laparoscopic adjustable gastric banding. World J Surg 22:955–963, 1998.

2. Biertho L, Steffen R, Ricklin T, et al: Laparoscopic gastric bypass versus laparoscopic adjustable gastric banding: A comparative study of 1,200 cases. J Am Coll Surg 197:536–545, 2003.

3. Demaria EJ, Sugerman HJ, Meador JG, et al: High failure rate after laparoscopic adjustable silicone gastric banding for treatment of morbid obesity. Ann Surg 233:809–818, 2001.

4. Hess DS, Hess DW: Biliopancreatic diversion with a duodenal switch. Obes Surg 8:267–282, 1998.

5. Higa KD, Boone KB, Ho T, Davies OG: Laparoscopic Roux-en-Y gastric bypass for morbid obesity: technique and preliminary results of our first 400 patients. Arch Surg 135:1029–1034, 2000.

6. National Institutes of Health Consensus Conference. Gastrointestinal surgery for severe obesity. Ann Intern Med 115:956–961, 1991.

7. Podnos Y, Jimenez JC, Wilson SE, et al: Complications after laparoscopic gastric bypass: A review of 3,464 cases. Arch Surg 138:957–961, 2003.

8. Pories W, Swanson MS, MacDonald KG, et al: Who would have thought it? An operation proves to be the most effective therapy for adult-onset diabetes mellitus. Ann Surg 222:339–351, 1995.

9. Schauer PR, Ikramuddin S, Gourash W, et al: Outcomes after laparoscopic Roux-en-Y gastric bypass for morbid obesity. Ann Surg 232:515–529, 2000.

10. Scopinaro N, Adami GF, Marinari GM, et al: Biliopancreatic diversion. World J Surg 22:936–946, 1998.

11. Wittgrove AC, Clark GW: Laparoscopic gastric bypass, Roux-en-Y?500 patients: Technique and results, with 3–60 month follow-up. Obes Surg 10:233–239, 2000.

HEPATOBILIARY SURGERY

Anthony J. Canfield, MD, John D. Moffat, MD, Michael C. Hotard, MD, and F. Calvin Bigler, MD

CHAPTER 80

BILIARY DISEASE

1. **What are the clinical manifestations of acute cholecystitis?**
   Acute cholecystitis usually occurs in patients aged 40–80 years. The female-to-male ratio is 3:1. Most patients complain of severe right upper quadrant (RUQ) pain that radiates to the right scapula or midback, which is often accompanied by nausea and, occasionally, by vomiting. Physical findings include fever, RUQ tenderness, and Murphy's sign (inspiratory arrest with steady palpation of the RUQ). Presence of a mass in the RUQ implies omental inflammation or gallbladder dilation.

2. **How is acute cholecystitis diagnosed?**
   Laboratory tests demonstrate elevated white blood cell (WBC) count and, occasionally, a mild increase in bilirubin. Plain abdominal films may show radiopaque gallstones (15–20% of cases). Ultrasound (US) findings include thickened gallbladder wall with pericholecystic fluid. A hepato-biliary (HIDA) scan shows nonvisualization of the gallbladder. HIDA scan is highly accurate for the diagnosis of acute cholecystitis (sensitivity, 95–100%; specificity, 95%).

3. **Describe the treatment of acute cholecystitis.**
   Surgical intervention includes hydration, antibiotic therapy, and prompt cholecystectomy. The laparoscopic approach is preferred, but conversion to a conventional open cholecystectomy is required when the inflammation is severe. Percutaneous cholecystostomy is useful when the patient is too ill to tolerate surgery.

4. **Explain "hydrops" of the gallbladder.**
   Hydrops refers to the accumulation of clear mucus within a chronically obstructed and inflamed gallbladder. The gallbladder is often dilated and palpable on physical exam. Outlet obstruction of the cystic duct is usually caused by an impacted stone but may be due to chronic inflammation of the gallbladder neck or congenital stenosis of the cystic duct. The mucus is produced by the secretory epithelium of the gallbladder.

5. **What bacteria are commonly found within the gallbladder with acute cholecystitis?**
   Escherichia coli, Pseudomonas aeruginosa, anaerobic streptococci, *Streptococcus faecalis,* and species of *Klebsiella, Clostridium, Proteus,* and *Enterobacter.* Antibiotic coverage includes either ampicillin/sulbactam (Unasyn), piperacillin (Pipracil), or ticarcillin (Timentin).

6. **A 36-year-old woman presents with a 4-month history of postprandial RUQ pain with radiation to the right scapula, accompanied by nausea and occasional emesis. US shows no gallstones, and the white blood cell count is normal. What further work-up should be obtained?**
   Patients with "typical" symptoms of biliary colic but without demonstrable gallstones frequently have chronic inflammation of the gallbladder, known as chronic acalculous cholecystitis or

biliary dyskinesia. The diagnosis can be confirmed by CCK-HIDA scan, which determines cystic duct patency (accumulation of radionucleotide in the gallbladder) and the gallbladder's capacity to contract (referred to as *ejection fraction*). An ejection fraction <35% correlates strongly with chronic acalculous cholecystitis and predicts a 95% probability of symptomatic cure after cholecystectomy.

7. **A 53-year-old American Indian woman with RUQ pain undergoes laparoscopic cholecystectomy for a 3.1-cm gallstone. During the surgery, nodular indentation is found at the gallbladder fundus that appears to be extending into the liver bed. What should one do next?**
   This finding may represent gallbladder carcinoma. Biopsy with frozen section should be performed. When gallbladder carcinoma is identified, the surgery should be converted to an open laparotomy and intraoperative staging performed.

8. **List the major risk factors for gallbladder carcinoma.**
   - *Race:* The highest incidence of gallbladder carcinoma is seen among Native American Indians, Mexican Americans, and Native Alaskans.
   - *Gallstones:* Most gallbladder cancer (90%) is associated with cholelithiasis, and the presence of large gallstones (>2.5 cm) increases significantly the risk for cancer.
   - *"Porcelain" gallbladder:* 12–61% risk for gallbladder cancer.

9. **A 67-year-old woman with a history of intermittent RUQ pain for several years complains of nausea and bilious emesis for 2 days, with crampy midabdominal pain and bloating. She denies passing flatus. The abdomen is distended and nontender, and abdominal x-rays show distended loops of small bowel with air-fluid levels. What is the likely cause?**
   Gallstone ileus is the cause of nonstrangulated small bowel mechanical obstruction in 25% of patients older than age 65. The usual mechanism involves acute cholecystitis with adherence of the duodenum or jejunum to the gallbladder, followed by subsequent erosion of the gallstone into the duodenum or jejunum. The gallstones are usually >2.5 cm. Only 20% of stones are radiopaque and visible on plain abdominal radiographs.

10. **Describe the surgical management of gallstone ileus.**
    - Stage 1: removal of gallstone to relieve bowel obstruction and antibiotic therapy.
    - Stage 2: elective surgery to repair the cholecystoenteric fistula.

11. **Why is the two-stage approach preferred?**
    The mortality rate for simultaneous surgery of the small bowel obstruction and cholecystoenteric fistula is approximately 20%, whereas the mortality rate for the two-stage surgery is about 11%. Most cholecystoenteric fistulas close spontaneously with conservative management.

CYSTIC DISEASE OF THE LIVER

(See Chapter 35, Hepatobiliary Cystic Disease.)

12. **In a patient with atypical RUQ abdominal pain, CT reveals a hepatic cyst. Discuss the symptoms and characteristics of the cyst that warrant surgical treatment.**
    The simple cyst is the most common cystic lesion of the liver. It is often discovered by radiologic tests performed to evaluate unrelated symptoms or during surgery for unrelated reasons. Small, asymptomatic simple cysts do not require treatment. However, simple hepatic cysts >5 cm tend to enlarge slowly and become symptomatic. Symptoms may range from mild discomfort to

debilitating pain. Hepatic cysts may also become infected, obstruct the biliary tree, rupture, and even hemorrhage. Although hepatic cysts consist generally of biliary epithelium, they do not communicate with the biliary system. Internal cyst hemorrhage, decompression into the biliary tree, and cholangitis are rare complications that may warrant emergent surgical intervention.

13. **Discuss the nonsurgical treatment options for benign hepatic cysts.**
Treatment options vary widely and may be tailored to the patient's presentation and medical condition. Simple percutaneous aspiration is generally ineffective and associated with a high recurrence rate. Most centers limit this technique to a diagnostic role (i.e., to determine whether symptoms are related to the cyst). Percutaneous cyst aspiration combined with cyst sclerosis is gaining popularity because it is technically simple and minimally invasive and can be performed on an outpatient basis. Contraindications to cyst sclerosis include communication of the cyst with the biliary tree and systemic coagulopathy. Complications of the technique include hemorrhage, sepsis, bile duct injury, and biliary leak. Repeated attempts at sclerotherapy do not preclude subsequent surgical treatment.

14. **What are the goals of surgical treatment?**
Successful surgery for simple hepatic cysts requires complete excision and wide exposure of the superficial cyst wall. This technique permits free flow of cyst secretions into the peritoneal cavity and cyst decompression. Surgically applied coagulation or sclerosants can treat hepatic cysts that are inaccessible to complete excision of the cyst epithelium. Partial excision with fenestration, involving wide unroofing of the superficial cyst surface, is also effective when cysts are multilocular but communicate with each other. Advantages of surgical treatment include lowest recurrence rate and ability to repair cystobiliary communications and control hemorrhage.

15. **Discuss differences in presentation of adult polycystic liver disease and simple liver cysts.**
Adult polycystic liver disease is an inherited disorder that tends to progress slowly after late onset of symptoms. It is characterized by cystic transformation of both lobes of the liver. The most common symptoms include abdominal swelling, abdominal pain, pain with bending, and shortness of breath. Physical findings include increasing abdominal girth and enlarged nodular liver; tenderness is rare.

16. **How is adult polycystic liver disease treated?**
Treatment options are more limited. Aspiration and sclerosis are generally used to provide symptomatic relief of larger lesions. Surgical resection of larger cysts, with or without combined fenestration of multiple adjacent cysts, has been the mainstay of treatment to relieve symptoms. Postoperative treatment with H_2-receptor blockade and octreotide has been effective in reducing hepatic drainage. Hepatic resection of polycystic liver disease can be dangerous, but recent studies have shown that combined anatomic resection of the diffusely cystic portion of the liver, with fenestration of a less involved portion of the liver, produces good long-term results.

PARASITIC AND OTHER INFECTIOUS DISEASES OF THE LIVER

(See Chapter 32, Liver Abscess.)

17. **What are the important considerations in both presentation and management of hydatid diseases of the liver?**
The tapeworm, *Echinococcus granulosus*, causes hepatic hydatid disease. A long latent period is typical, and painless hepatomegaly may be the only sign of disease. Free peritoneal rupture of the cyst can cause fatal anaphylaxis. Preoperative administration of steroids and diphenhydramine and cyst injection with hypertonic saline and scolicidal agents may decrease the risk of

fatal anaphylaxis associated with operative leak of cyst contents. Recent studies have shown that complete pericystectomy is more effective at reducing recurrence and improves resolution of the hepatic defect.

18. **Describe the changes in etiology, diagnosis, and treatment of pyogenic liver abscess over the past 40 years.**
Earlier in the 20th century, pyogenic liver abscess was caused primarily by pylephlebitis due to complicated appendicitis or diverticulitis. For the past 40 years, biliary tract obstruction and cholangitis from either benign or malignant causes have become the most common causes of pyogenic liver abscess. Abdominal imaging with US, CT, and percutaneous fine needle aspiration and cholangiography have greatly improved the ability to diagnosis pyogenic abscess. Treatment options include antibiotics alone, antibiotics in combination with drainage procedures (e.g., percutaneous aspiration or indwelling catheter drainage), and surgical drainage. Recent studies have shown that percutaneous indwelling catheter drainage and antibiotic therapy are superior to surgical cyst drainage. Simple aspiration has a high recurrence rate and often requires repeated aspiration. Antibiotic treatment alone has a high mortality rate (up to 25%).

19. **A patient has been treated appropriately with broad-spectrum antibiotics and drainage for pyogenic hepatic abscess but fails to improve. What is a possible explanation? What treatment options should be entertained?**
The patient with a presumptive pyogenic liver abscess that fails indwelling catheter drainage and antibiotics should be carefully evaluated for a mixed fungal/pyogenic abscess. Fungal hepatic abscesses are recognized with increasing frequency, especially in immunocompromised patients.

20. **How does amebic abscess of the liver differ from pyogenic abscess of the liver in diagnosis and treatment?**
An amebic abscess is less likely to perforate than a pyogenic abscess. Circulating amebic antibody is detected by indirect hemagglutination test in >95% of cases and is sufficient to initiate treatment when a liver abscess is identified. Primary treatment for amebic abscess is metronidazole, 750 mg three times/day for 10 days, plus an intraluminal agent (e.g., iodoquinol) for cyst passers. Most amebic liver abscesses respond to metronidazole treatment alone. Mixed amebic/pyogenic abscesses occur in 15% of cases and should be considered when metronidazole treatment fails. Surgical treatment is rarely necessary.

BENIGN HEPATIC TUMORS (SEE CHAPTER 24, RHEUMATOLOGIC MANIFESTATIONS OF HEPATOBILIARY DISEASES)

21. **What are the most common benign hepatic tumors? Discuss briefly their distinguishing characteristics and recommended treatment.**
The increased use of US and CT to evaluate abdominal complaints has led to increased detection of coincidental, asymptomatic benign hepatic tumors, including cavernous hemangiomas, hepatic adenomas, and focal nodular hyperplasia (FNH).

22. **Describe cavernous hemangiomas.**
Cavernous hemangiomas are the most common benign liver tumor and occur more often in women than in men. They are usually small (<3 cm) and asymptomatic and can be safely followed radiographically. When mass effect produces symptoms or spontaneous rupture occurs, surgical excision is indicated. Preoperative biopsy is often complicated by hemorrhage and is not necessary.

23. **What causes hepatic adenomas? How are they treated?**

Hepatic adenomas occur generally in women of menstrual age and are associated with oral contraceptive use. Discontinuation of oral contraceptives may lead to regression of small, asymptomatic lesions within several months. Larger lesions are less likely to regress, and resection should be considered, especially when pregnancy is contemplated. Needle biopsy may be effective in distinguishing hepatic adenoma from other benign lesions and hepatocellular carcinoma. Symptoms from hepatic adenoma are due mostly to mass effect and include abdominal pain, early satiety, nausea, and vomiting. Hepatic adenomas are more likely to hemorrhage and may undergo malignant degeneration. Hepatic adenomas should be resected when they produce symptoms or when the diagnosis is uncertain.

24. **How is FNH diagnosed and treated?**

FNH affects primarily women of menstrual age but has not been associated with oral contraceptive use. Most patients (90%) with FNH are asymptomatic; work-up is usually initiated when it is difficult to distinguish the presence of malignancy or other benign tumors. Focal nodular hyperplasia has a highly characteristic intraoperative appearance: usually tan to dark brown, smaller than 5 cm, and usually located in the periphery of the liver. Specific radiologic imaging tests and needle biopsy are helpful in establishing the diagnosis. Once the diagnosis is established, FNH can be managed expectantly; it has no malignant potential. Wedge resection is the treatment of choice when the diagnosis is in doubt or significant enlargement occurs.

MALIGNANT HEPATIC TUMORS

25. **What is the only treatment of hepatocellular carcinoma (HCC) that can significantly prolong survival?**

Surgical resection. Unfortunately, the presence of cirrhosis and decreased hepatic reserve precludes significant liver resection in most patients. A limited disease-free margin of 1 cm has been shown to improve survival. Intraoperative US at the time of operative exploration is useful in detecting more extensive disease and avoids unnecessary and unhelpful resection. Some transplant centers offer liver transplantation for small (<5 cm), solitary HCC after preoperative chemotherapy.

26. **What is the differential diagnosis of obstructive jaundice?**

Benign: choledocholithiasis or biliary stricture (usually of surgical etiology)
Malignant: extrinsic, primary or metastatic pancreatic head tumor or gallbladder cancer; intrinsic, cholangiocarcinoma

27. **What is a Klatskin's tumor?**

A primary biliary or metastatic malignancy at the bifurcation of the left and right hepatic ducts. A Klatskin's tumor should be suspected when US or CT shows dilation of the right and left intrahepatic bile ducts but a small to normal-sized common bile duct and gallbladder.

28. **What clues may help to define the nature of the biliary obstruction?**

The history and physical exam often provide important clues to the diagnosis. Biliary tract pain develops as a consequence of sudden biliary distention, as seen clinically with migration of a gallstone. Insidious and slow obstruction is frequently painless; hence, painless jaundice is often of malignant etiology. Weight loss may suggest underlying malignancy, whereas fever, chills, and rigors may suggest a diagnosis of biliary infection, which is seen more commonly with gallstones. Recent biliary surgery suggests surgical misadventure or complication.

Physical exam frequently demonstrates jaundice and scleral icterus. A nontender, palpable gallbladder (Courvoisier's gallbladder) suggests distal biliary obstruction. A painful distended gallbladder is more often due to an impacted stone in the neck of the gallbladder that produces acute hydrops. Compression of the common bile duct by an inflamed Hartman's pouch or large cystic duct stone may produce a picture of obstructive jaundice known as Mirizzi's syndrome. Spiking fevers suggest a diagnosis of ascending cholangitis, which is seen more often with choledocholithiasis.

29. **What investigations should be undertaken in a jaundiced patient?**
    - *Laboratory tests:* complete blood count, liver panel, and coagulation studies.
    - *Radiology:* US is the best first test; dilation of the bile ducts implies obstruction. Important findings include gallstones and the size of the common bile duct and intrahepatic ducts. On occasion, common bile duct stones are identified on US. Intravenous cholangiography is of historic interest only. Endoscopic retrograde cholangiography is the gold standard for investigating patients with obstructive jaundice. Magnetic resonance cholangiography is a new, accurate, and noninvasive method, but its availability is limited.

30. **Can obstructive jaundice constitute a surgical emergency?**
    Yes. Jaundice, fever, and RUQ pain (Charcot's triad) suggest a diagnosis of ascending cholangitis. Untreated, the disease can progress rapidly to septic shock with the added features of hypotension and confusion (Reynold's pentad). Complete cardiovascular collapse and death may ensue without prompt intervention.

31. **Describe the treatment of ascending cholangitis.**
    Immediate institution of broad-spectrum antibiotics may abort the progression of ascending cholangitis, but biliary decompression is still necessary. It can be accomplished by endoscopic retrograde cholangiopancreatography (ERCP) with sphincterotomy and internal drainage or via either laparoscopic or open cholecystectomy.

32. **Is ERCP the gold standard for the investigation and treatment of obstructive jaundice?**
    Yes. In expert hands ERCP can determine the cause of biliary obstruction and provide internal biliary decompression in 90–95% of cases.

33. **What is postcholecystectomy syndrome?**
    Patients who continue to complain of upper abdominal discomfort suggestive of biliary tract pain after removal of the gallbladder have been labeled as suffering from the postcholecystectomy syndrome. Unrelated factors (e.g., hiatal hernia, gastroesophageal reflux disease, duodenal ulcer, colon cancer) may be the underlying cause of symptoms.

    Biliary manometry has demonstrated that some patients have high resting sphincter of Oddi (SO) pressures that may be caused by fibrosis or SO spasm. When biliary manometry identifies SO pressures >40 mmHg, sphincterotomy may relieve pain.

34. **List some uncommon causes of jaundice.**
    - *Primary sclerosing cholangitis* (PSC) is an inflammatory and fibrotic process that can involve part or all of the biliary tree. PSC is insidious and progresses to liver failure or cholangiocarcinoma. The cause is uncertain but may be related to viral infection and altered immune function. Coincident inflammatory bowel disease is seen in 80% of cases. PSC is diagnosed by MRCP or ERCP.
    - *Choledochal cysts* are relatively rare and have a five-part subclassification. They may not present until adulthood, when the patient develops recurrent bouts of cholangitis. Choledochal cysts are associated with an increased risk of bile duct cancer and should be treated with resection and reconstitution.

BIBLIOGRAPHY

1. Cameron JL (ed): Current Surgical Therapy, 6th ed. St. Louis, Mosby, 1998.

2. Caporale A, Guiliani A, Teneriello FL, et al: Surgical management of nonparasitic cysts of the liver: Report of 17 cases. Dig Surg 10:249–253, 1994.

3. Fong Y, Kemenly N, Paty P, et al: Treatment of colorectal cancer: Hepatic metastasis. Cohen Semin Surg Oncol 12:219–252, 1996.

4. Huang C-J, Pitt HA, Lipsett PA, et al: Pyogenic hepatic abscess: Changing trends over 42 years. Ann Surg 223:600–609, 1996.

5. Huguier M, Hobeika J, Houry S: Hydatid cysts of the liver: Surgical treatment. Dig Surg 12:314–317, 1995.

6. Lipsett PA, Huang C-J, Lillemoe KD, et al: Fungal hepatic abscesses: Characterization and management. J Gastrointest Surg 1:78–84, 1997.

7. Madariaga JR, Shunzaburo I, Starzl TE, et al: Hepatic resection for cystic lesions of the liver. Ann Surg 218:610–614, 1993.

8. Marcos-Alvarez A, Jenkins R, Washburn WK, et al: Multimodality treatment of hepatocellular carcinoma in a hepatobiliary specialty center. Arch Surg 131:292–298, 1996.

9. Meng X-J, Wu J-X: Perforated amebic liver abscess: Clinical analysis of 110 cases. South Med J 87:988–990, 1994.

10. Moskal TL, Charnsangavej C, Ellis LM: Workup, diagnosis, and treatment of benign hepatic tumors. Cancer Bull 47:385–391, 1995.

11. Sabiston DC Jr (ed): Textbook of Surgery, 14th ed. Philadelphia, W.B. Saunders, 1991.

12. Seeto RK, Rockey DC: Pyogenic liver abscess: Changes in etiology, management, and outcome. Medicine 75(2):99–113, 1996.

13. Soravia C, Mentha G, Giostra E, et al: Surgery for adult polycystic liver disease. Surgery 117:272–275, 1995.

14. Vauthey J-N, Maddern GJ, Blumgart LH: Adult polycystic disease of the liver. Br J Surg 78:524–527, 1991.

15. Yamanaka N, Okamoto E, Tsuyosi O, et al: A prediction scoring system to select the surgical treatment of liver cancer: Further refinement based on 10 years of use. Ann Surg 219:342–346, 1994.

CHAPTER 81

LAPAROSCOPIC SURGERY

Anthony J. LaPorta, MD, and Brian Barbick, MD

1. **You are evaluating a patient who may require surgery. During your work-up, the patient tells you that he is taking ginseng. What recommendations should you make?**

   Ginseng is a common herbal preparation taken by many people to increase energy levels and improve memory. Ginseng has been reported to cause tachycardia and hypertension. An interaction with ginseng and estrogens or warfarin has also been reported. Recently, the American Society of Anesthesiologists recommended that all herbal preparations be stopped 2–3 weeks before surgery.

2. **What is the difference between the hepatocystic triangle and the triangle of Calot?**

   To avoid major biliary tract injury, knowledge of the hepatocystic triangle and Calot's triangle is essential. Lateral inferior retraction of the gallbladder at the infundibulum (Hartmann's pouch) with cephalad retraction at the dome facilitates the identification of both. Dissection for laparoscopic cholecystectomy should start at the gallbladder neck (Hartmann's pouch) and proceed to the cystic duct, followed by dissection of the cystic artery. Excessive dissection toward the common bile duct is fraught with danger and may result in inadvertent injury to the common hepatic duct or an aberrant right hepatic artery (seen in 10% of cases). Identification of the hepatocystic triangle (cystic duct, common hepatic duct, and border of the liver) avoids injury to the common hepatic duct (Fig. 81-1).

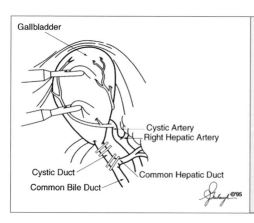

Gallbladder

Cystic Artery
Right Hepatic Artery

Cystic Duct
Common Hepatic Duct
Common Bile Duct

Figure 81-1. Calot's triangle, formed by the cystic duct, cystic artery, and common hepatic duct, is essential for dissection in laparoscopic cholecystectomy. The hepatocystic triangle is defined as the area between the cystic duct, common hepatic duct, and border of the liver.

3. **Summarize the key strategies for safe laparoscopic cholecystectomy.**
   - Dissection from the infundibulum down toward the cystic duct
   - Dissection from lateral to medial
   - Adequate inferolateral traction to open the triangle of Calot

- Dissection to develop continuity both laterally and medially from the neck of the gallbladder onto the cystic duct
- Divide no structure unless you are certain about its identity

4. **Is there any clearly defined benefit to laparoscopic appendectomy?**
No. Most studies have shown no benefit for laparoscopic appendectomy over open appendectomy in hospital length of stay, total hospital charges, operative time, recovery time or return to work, or postoperative pain. However, the false diagnosis rate for appendicitis is four times higher among women. For young women, the laparoscopic approach has a clear advantage because gynecologic disorders (ectopic pregnancy, pelvic inflammatory disease, ovarian cysts, and endometriosis) may mimic appendicitis.

5. **What is the harmonic scalpel? How does it work?**
The ultrasonic scalpel uses ultrasonic energy that causes the blade to vibrate up to 55,000 times per second. By adjusting the power level and selecting the appropriate blade, both cutting and coagulation functions are possible (Table 81-1). Vibration of the tip causes intracellular water to vaporize, allowing for the cutting function. The coagulation function allows the operator to achieve homeostasis in vessels as large as 3 mm. When the instrument contacts human tissue, high-frequency vibrations generate heat secondary to the friction created between the cells. This effectively seals the ends of the vessels by denaturing the protein and producing a sticky coagulum.

TABLE 81-1.   USES OF THE HARMONIC SCALPEL

	Straight Tip	Hook Tip
Setting 1 (55,000/sec)	Cutting	Cutting and coagulation
Setting 2	Cutting > coagulation	Coagulation
Setting 3	Coagulation	Coagulation

6. **Does laparoscopic surgery preserve immune function?**
Yes. Both human and animal studies have shown that laparoscopy preserves immune function. In contrast, open surgery causes a reduction in lymphocyte and neutrophil chemotaxis, killer cell activity, and lymphocyte and macrophage interactions as well as delayed hypersensitivity responses. After open surgery, immunosuppression persists for 6–9 days.

7. **Elder surgical statesmen are fond of saying that the incision heals from side to side and that the length of the incision does not matter. Is this true? What is the evidence for or against?**
A large portion of the recent research on immune function and surgery has been performed by Bessler and Whelan. Their series of experiments show that the immune depression is directly related to incision length. No more is the longer incision acceptable because it heals from side to side. Although adequate exposure is crucial, we must learn to perform laparoscopic surgery through smaller incisions that preserve the immune response.

8. **A 9-year-old girl presents with a 2-month history of right upper quadrant abdominal pain that most commonly occurs after eating fatty foods and resolves usually in 30 minutes. The pain radiates to the right shoulder. It is not associated with nausea or vomiting. She has no prior medical**

or surgical history. She is afebrile, and the physical exam is unremarkable. Laboratory values, including complete blood count and biliary panel, are normal. An abdominal ultrasound of the right upper quadrant demonstrates no evidence of cholelithiasis, gallbladder wall thickening, or pericholecystic fluid. What should be the next step in your evaluation?

The history is consistent with biliary colic. An initial diagnosis of cholelithiasis was not demonstrated by ultrasound. An upper gastrointestinal (GI) series or esophagogastroduodenoscopy (EGD) would demonstrate possible gastric pathology but would not evaluate the biliary system. A computed tomography (CT) scan is less sensitive than ultrasound for detection of gallstones and would not be helpful. Because the history points toward a biliary etiology, a hepatoiminodi-acetic acid (HIDA) scan should be the next step in the evaluation.

9. **The HIDA scan demonstrated rapid filling of the gallbladder and unobstructed flow into the duodenum. Cholecystikinin (CCK) is administered, and the gallbladder ejection fraction (EF) is calculated at 30%. What is the most likely diagnosis?**

Biliary dyskinesia, which is defined as the presence of symptoms of typical biliary colic without evidence of cholelithiasis and a gallbladder ejection fraction (EF) less than 35–50%. Typical symptoms of biliary colic include right upper quadrant or epigastric pain, which may radiate to the right scapula. The pain is often aggravated by eating, especially fatty foods. The cause of biliary dyskinesia is unknown.

10. **How should the patient be treated?**

Cholecystectomy is successful in 85% of patients with typical symptoms of colic and a gallbladder EF less than 35–50%. A recent study by Gollin et al. demonstrated that children with biliary dyskinesia characterized by typical biliary colic and a gallbladder EF <40% respond equally well to cholecystectomy (about 79% success rate).

11. **What percentage of patients have free intra-abdominal air on upright radiograph 24 hours after laparoscopic procedure?**

In the nonpostoperative state, the presence of subdiaphragmatic free air on upright chest radiograph is diagnostic of intra-abdominal perforation. After an open abdominal or laparoscopic procedure, the significance of free intra-abdominal air is less clear. Nonpathologic subdiaphragmatic air may be seen in 24–39% of patients after laparoscopic surgery, and in 60% of patients after open surgical procedures. The difference relates to the solubility of carbon dioxide used in laparoscopy versus the solubility of trapped room air within the abdominal cavity. Carbon dioxide is more soluble in serum than room air and is absorbed 32 times more quickly.

12. **Describe the cause and incidence of electrocautery injuries to the small bowel during laparoscopic surgery.**

Electrocautery injuries during laparoscopic surgery occur most commonly during the lysis of adhesions and dissection of Calot's triangle. The causes can be separated into two types: contact or conductive.

- *Contact injuries* occur when the electrocautery instrument directly touches the tissue. Such injuries are more likely to be recognized intraoperatively. The most common location of contact injury is the common bile duct.
- *Conductive injuries* are secondary to the conversion of electrical energy into thermal energy by passing through high-resistance tissue. Conductive injuries to the bowel are rare (0.07–0.7% of laparoscopic cholecystectomies) and usually present 2–21 days postoperatively as delayed perforations. The duodenum is the most common site of bowel injury (58%), and most are *not* recognized at the time of surgery.

13. **How do electrocautery injuries to the small bowel present?**
    Patients with bowel or bile duct cautery injuries commonly present with fever, abdominal pain, nausea, and vomiting. Common clinical findings include temperature >38°C, tachycardia, ileus, leukocytosis, and, possibly, free subdiaphragmatic air on upright chest radiograph. A recent study by Bishoff et al. (1999) demonstrated that the symptom of pain at the trocar site closest to the perforation was the most reliable clinical finding. Clinical evidence of peritonitis and sepsis after surgery requires immediate evaluation. When findings indicate visceral injury, exploration by laparoscopy or celiotomy is necessary.

14. **List the advantages and disadvantages of using carbon dioxide (CO_2) as an insufflation gas instead of other gases.**
    See Table 81-2.

TABLE 81-2. ADVANTAGES AND DISADVANTAGES OF CARBON DIOXIDE AS AN INSUFFLATION GAS	
Advantages	**Disadvantages**
CO_2 suppresses combustion and is therefore believed to be ideal for operative laparoscopy.	CO_2 is rapidly absorbed and can thus raise the arterial partial pressure of CO_2 and lower pH, with adverse potential metabolic and hemodynamic consequences in susceptible patients.
CO_2 has a high diffusion coefficient, reducing the risk of a serious gas embolism. Up to 100 mL/min of CO_2 can be injected directly into the bloodstream of animals without adverse outcome.	Insufflation of cold CO_2 (0.3°C), especially in high-flow systems or long procedures, can result in a drop in core temperature with resultant hypothermia.
CO_2 is safely absorbed and can be effectively eliminated by the lungs with moderate hyperventilation.	Tension CO_2 pneumothorax, either from occult defects in the diaphragm or in the absence of diaphragmatic injury (typically in subhiatal laparoscopic surgery), has been reported.
CO_2 is inexpensive and readily available.	CO_2 gas embolism can occur, even without direct insufflation into mesenteric veins.

15. **Which alternative gases can be used for laparoscopy?**
    Room air, oxygen, nitrous oxide, helium, and carbon dioxide have been used to create the pneumoperitoneum needed for laparoscopy, but CO_2 is the most commonly used. Research is ongoing to identify alternative gases for pneumoperitoneum. Helium shows promise in an experimental animal model of chronic obstructive pulmonary disease, in which helium compared with CO_2 pneumoperitoneum showed far less arterial CO_2 retention.

16. **What are the respiratory effects of pneumoperitoneum (planned intra-abdominal hypertension)?**
    Pneumoperitoneum alters respiratory mechanics. Intra-abdominal hypertension results in elevation of the diaphragm, decreases in functional residual capacity and total lung volume, ventila-

tion-perfusion inequalities, and atelectasis. Some patients may require increased peak inspiratory pressure to compensate for decreased respiratory compliance. No significant change occurs in arterial oxygenation in healthy patients under pneumoperitoneum, but in patients with cardiopulmonary compromise, arterial oxygen desaturation has been reported, presumably secondary to mechanical pulmonary dysfunction.

17. **What are the hemodynamic effects?**
Mean arterial blood pressure (MAP) and systemic peripheral resistance are increased (up to 35% and 160%, respectively) at operative levels of pneumoperitoneum (12–15 mmHg), presumably as a result of sympathetic vasoconstriction from hypercarbia. Cardiac index may increase 20%. As intra-abdominal pressure increases more than 20 mmHg, cardiac output falls, and abdominal venous compliance decreases, reaching a point at which effective Trendelenburg's position and higher pneumoperitoneum can combine in patients with preexisting cardiopulmonary disease to produce potential hemodynamic compromise. Portal venous blood flow is reduced by 70% when intra-abdominal pressure reaches 25 mmHg. Many workers believe that renal blood flow and therefore glomerular filtration rate also decrease with pneumoperitoneum >12–15 mmHg, although this phenomenon has not been well documented.
  In summary, intra-abdominal hypertension >15 mmHg can result in significant changes in central hemodynamics and even more pronounced changes in splanchnic circulation.

18. **What is recommended as the maximal safe pressure setting for a CO_2 insufflator?**
Based on the potential adverse cardiopulmonary effects of intra-abdominal hypertension, the maximal recommended insufflation pressure setting is 15 mmHg.

19. **A thin, 68-year-old woman with chronic obstructive pulmonary disease from 52 years of smoking undergoes laparoscopic cholecystectomy for acute cholecystitis. Because she has had a previous lower midline abdominal incision, you choose the "open" Hasson's technique for initial trocar placement and have no difficulties with access to the peritoneal cavity. You immediately insufflate with a flow rate of 10 L/min to a pneumoperitoneum of 15 mmHg and then proceed with laparoscopic cholecystectomy. Fifteen minutes into the procedure, the anesthesiologist observes that the patient's end-tidal CO_2 is elevated and plans to draw an arterial blood gas. Before the anesthesiologist can do so, the patient experiences several episodes of ventricular tachycardia and arrests. What is the pathophysiology behind these events?**
Insufflated CO_2 is directly absorbed through the peritoneum into the capillary bed and bloodstream. Typically, the partial pressure of CO_2 (PCO_2) and end-tidal CO_2 increases only slightly, but in certain circumstances the PCO_2 can rise dramatically, causing a significant drop in pH. The resulting acidemia aggravates any preexisting cardiac condition. Most patients adapt to the absorbed CO_2 by maximizing plasma and intracellular buffering systems and accelerating CO_2 transport and elimination with mild hyperventilation, but some patients have impaired CO_2 clearance mechanisms. Patients who cannot handle an acute change in PCO_2 are those with high metabolic and cellular respiratory rates (e.g., septic patients), those with large ventilatory dead space (e.g., patients with chronic obstructive pulmonary disease [COPD]), and those with poor cardiac output (e.g., patients with cardiac failure).
  During laparoscopy, special care and monitoring should be provided to prevent significant hypercarbia and acidemia. Rapid shifts in intra-abdominal pressure (with attendant PCO_2 absorption gradients) should be avoided, such as those that follow initial insufflation at a high rate with a resultant, sudden large gradient between intra-abdominal CO_2 pressure and PCO_2. Equilibrium between CO_2 pressure in blood and tissues occurs at about 20 minutes. After initial insufflation, arterial PCO_2 steadily rises for about 20 minutes then plateaus.

This septic patient with preexisting COPD was subjected to rapid CO_2 insufflation, which resulted in hypercarbia, peaking 15–20 minutes after rapid insufflation, and consequent acidemia, triggering ventricular irritability and arrest.

20. **Who introduced electrocautery? Why is the alternating cycle (AC) frequency used?**

The "Bovie" nickname for electrosurgical units in most operating rooms acknowledges the introduction in 1929 of electrocautery by William Bovie and Harvey Cushing. In most American homes, the alternating current (AC) that powers appliances and lights alternates at 60 cycles/sec. In the operating room or endoscopy suite, however, the electrosurgical unit alternates between 400,000 and 2,000,000 cycles/sec. This high-frequency electrical current is essential to avoid neuromuscular stimulation. Lower-frequency currents, such as the standard 60-cycle AC current, can cause tetany and electrocution.

21. **How do electrocautery units work? Describe the mechanisms by which the cut and coagulation modes work.**

Electrosurgery units work by producing heat at the cellular level. When the electrosurgical unit is set on *cut,* the current is "on" nearly 100% of the time, but at a lower voltage (e.g., 100 V) than during *coagulation* (e.g., 600 V), when the current is typically "on" in bursts 5–10% of the time and "off" 90% of the time. The various blends of cut and coagulation modes combine lower voltages than those used with coagulation (but higher than those used with cut) with varying percentages of time that the current is "on" for optimal effect.

- Although the precise mechanisms are not known, the *cut* mode of electrosurgery generates an uninterrupted current with movement of ions within the cell, vaporizing the cell. The release of vaporized (boiled) cell content from the disrupted cell dissipates the heat, accounting for the lack of damage to surrounding tissue.
- In the *coagulation* mode, the higher-voltage but short-duration energy "bursts" lead to cellular insult but not vaporization. The drying effect on the cells during the "off" part of the cycle (i.e., cellular desiccation) leaves an area of increased resistance to electron flow and thus allows more heat dissipation and progressive insult to deeper tissue layers. This can be explained partially by the formula $p = I^2R$, where p (power, or relative heat per unit of time) is equal to a given current (I) through a certain resistance (R). The issue is more complex than this simple formula suggests, because various body tissues have different levels of conductivity and resistance. Thus, some structures may be affected by electrosurgical energy, whereas others are spared injury.

22. **Morbid obesity, defined as >100 lb above ideal body weight, is no longer a contraindication to laparoscopic cholecystectomy. Describe the technical changes needed in morbidly obese patients.**

1. Safe access and adequate visualization of the porta hepatis structures are the major concerns for safe laparoscopic cholecystectomy in morbidly obese patients. In patients with normal body habitus, the umbilicus is typically the optimal site for the telescope trocar. In obese patients, particularly those who are taller, shifting the trocar site 1–5 inches cephalad from the umbilicus allows optimal visualization of the protal structures with a 0-degree telescope. Visualization from an umbilical port is often obscured by the visual horizon in the upper abdomen or by the heavy pannus, which the insufflation cannot sufficiently elevate.

2. Some physicians prefer to gain access to the peritoneum in obese patients by using the "closed" Verress' needle approach through the umbilicus. After insufflation they pass an extra-long trocar from the skin level at a predetermined supraumbilical approach. Preperitoneal insufflation is a common problem in obese patients because, even with mechanical elevation of the interior abdominal wall, the posterior fascia often does not become elevated. We favor an "open" Hasson's approach at a supraumbilical location.

3. Another technique to improve visualization of the porta hepatis in morbidly obese patients involves use of a 30-degree–angled telescope, which may obviate the need for a supraumbilical trocar site election. Care must be taken with placement of lateral trocars to avoid skiving the trocar to a preperitoneal position and not entering the abdominal cavity.

4. Placement of a fifth 5-mm subcostal trocar either medially or laterally may be necessary to facilitate adequate retraction and exposure. Some surgeons use a 5-mm, fan-type retractor to press down the duodenum or transverse colon. Such retractors should be used with care, particularly if they are positioned off camera.

23. **Compare the rate of conversion from laparoscopic cholecystectomy to open cholecystectomy in patients with acute versus chronic cholecystitis.**
The rate of conversion from laparoscopic cholecystectomy to open cholecystectomy is two to four times higher for acute cholecystitis than for chronic cholecystitis (typically reported at 3–5%) among experienced laparoscopic surgeons.

24. **What pathophysiologic features of acute cholecystitis increase the likelihood of technical difficulties?**
- Distended, inflamed, thick-walled gallbladder
- Intrahepatic gallbladder
- Inflammation of cystic duct and cystic artery

25. **What techniques are used to decompress the distended gallbladder?**
Decompression of the distended gallbladder with a special trocar, or even percutaneously (under direct visualization) with a central venous pressure catheter, makes it easier to grasp the gallbladder with laparoscopic forceps. It may be necessary to use traumatic/toothed forceps, but because they tend to puncture the gallbladder wall, they should be left in place to minimize bile spillage. When there is an area of bile leakage, from either the percutaneous drainage site or a tear from a traumatic grasper in the gallbladder wall, a suture or loop ligature can be used to close a small rent in the gallbladder wall. Some acutely inflamed gallbladders cannot be grasped with conventional graspers. In such cases, one solution is to use a commercial screwlike device, such as the Reddick screw, which facilitates retraction of the gallbladder.

26. **How are bile spills managed?**
Despite the best efforts by experienced surgeons, bile spill is seen in 30–50% of laparoscopic cholecystectomies. Sterile laparoscopic specimen bags are indicated to retrieve lost gallstones, to remove a friable, disrupted gallbladder, or to remove detached, necrotic tissue. Use of closed suction drains should follow the same guidelines used at open surgery.

27. **How is inflammation of the cystic duct and cystic artery managed?**
The degree of inflammation may make use of laparoscopic clip devices inadequate. In such cases, pre-tied loop ligatures can be used to control the cystic duct or cystic artery.

28. **Should we routinely use prophylactic antibiotics for laparoscopic cholecystectomy?**
Yes, for the following reasons:
- Bile spills during laparoscopic cholecystectomy occur in 30–50% of cases.
- Normal bile is often colonized with bacteria (30–40% of patients).
- Acute cholecystitis is associated with a 60% rate of bacterbilia after the first 24 hours of inflammation.

29. **Which antibiotic should be used?**

    For routine laparoscopic cholecystectomies, a first-generation cephalosporin should provide adequate prophylaxis for most common organisms, although many surgeons use a second-generation cephalosporin.

30. **At 24 hours after open upper abdominal surgery using subcostal incisions, patients show a decrease in pulmonary function tests of nearly 50%. What decreases should be expected at 24 hours after laparoscopic cholecystectomy?**

    See Table 81-3.

TABLE 81-3. POSTOPERATIVE PULMONARY FUNCTION TESTS: OPEN VERSUS LAPAROSCOPIC SURGERY		
	Percentage of Preoperative	
Measurement at 24 Hours After Surgery	**Open Surgery**	**Laparoscopic Surgery**
Forced vital capacity (FVC)	54%	73%
Forced expiratory volume at 1 sec (FEV_1)	52%	72%
Forced expiratory flow at 25–75% ($FEF_{25-75\%}$)	53%	81%

In one study, the decrease in pulmonary function measured at 24 hours after laparoscopic cholecystectomy was approximately one half of that seen with open surgery. In a related study, age-, gender-, and size-matched patients were randomized prospectively to open versus laparoscopic cholecystectomy, and pulmonary function tests were measured preoperatively and postoperatively. FVC and FEV_1 were similarly decreased but less so with laparoscopic than with open surgery. Functional residual capacity was significantly higher at 72 hours after laparoscopic than after open surgery. Respiratory function is less impaired, and recovery is improved after laparoscopic surgery compared with open surgery.

31. **What are the indications and contraindications for laparoscopic adrenalectomy? What are the advantages of laparoscopic adrenalectomy?**

    Adrenal masses can be divided into functioning, nonfunctioning, and malignant tumors. Functioning or hormonally active tumors (e.g., pheochromocytoma, aldosteronoma, androgen-producing adenoma, glucocorticoid-producing adenoma, bilateral adrenal hyperplasia) should be resected. Studies have shown that tumors as large as 10 cm can be resected laparoscopically. Nonfunctioning or hormonally inactive adrenal tumors >4 cm or tumors >3 cm that have grown on serial studies should be resected. The risk of malignancy increases with size; most adrenal cancers measure >6 cm. Laparoscopic resection of adrenocortical cancer is controversial. If the tumor is confined to the adrenal gland, laparoscopic resection may be possible. The need for clear surgical margins may necessitate conversion to an open procedure, if direct extension of tumor involves surrounding structures.

    The contraindications to laparoscopic resection of adrenal tumors are based on the surgeon's clinical judgment and laparoscopic abilities. Radiographic imaging aids the surgeon in determining laparoscopic resectability. Studies have demonstrated that laparoscopic adrenalectomy is a safe and beneficial alternative to an open procedure. Patients who undergo laparoscopic adrenalectomy have less operative blood loss, lower transfusion requirements, fewer admissions to intensive care, decreased use of pain medication, quicker return of bowel function, and decreased hospital stay. In some studies, however, operative times were significantly longer for laparoscopic surgery.

32. **Can laparoscopic cholecystectomy be performed safely in a pregnant patient?**
    Yes. Laparoscopic cholecystectomy can be performed safely in a pregnant patient, ideally in the second trimester. Indications are the same as an open operation, including repeated attacks of biliary colic, acute cholecystitis, obstructive jaundice, gallstone pancreatitis, and peritonitis. Laparoscopic cholecystectomy is associated with a decreased risk of premature contractions, though it confers no advantage or disadvantage to open operation with regards to inducing preterm labor, surgical complications, or neonatal outcomes.

33. **What are some technical considerations when performing laparoscopy on a pregnant patient?**
    Using the left lateral decubitus position, when possible, to minimize uterine compression of the IVC. Minimize reverse Trendelenburg and insufflation pressures to help reduce decreased venous return. Always use SCD or other DVT prophylaxis. Pregnant patients have increased venous stasis and increased levels of coagulation factors VII and XII, making them relatively prothrombotic.

34. **Can laparoscopic appendectomy be performed safely during pregnancy?**
    Yes. Notably, appendicitis is the most common nonobstetric surgery during pregnancy. When performed by an experienced laparoscopist, there is no difference in preterm delivery (12–16%), uterine injuries, or neonatal outcomes.

35. **Is gangrenous or perforated appendicitis a contraindication to laparoscopic appendectomy?**
    No. Though conversion rates vary between 6% and 50%, reportedly related to surgical experience, laparoscopic appendectomy is associated with a decreased wound infection rate, quicker return of bowel function, and no difference in intra-abdominal abscess rate.

36. **What are the benefits and drawbacks of laparoscopic versus open inguinal hernia repair?**
    Laparoscopic hernia repair is more expensive, technically more demanding, requires longer operative time, and is associated with increased risk of visceral and vascular injuries (especially TAP) relative to open repair. However, recurrence rates are similar between the two approaches. Additionally, laparoscopic allows the surgeon to evaluate and, possibly, repair a contralateral hernia at the time of operation. It is also noteworthy that laparoscopic repair is associated with less acute and chronic groin pain, thus allowing patients to return sooner to their normal activities.

37. **What is Mirizzi's syndrome?**
    Mirizzi's syndrome was first described in 1948 as an uncommon complication of cholelithiasis occurring in less than 1% of patients with cholelithiasis. The syndrome is characterized by gallstones impacting in the infundibulum, Hartmann's pouch, or cystic duct and thus causing direct pressure on the common hepatic duct, resulting in a stricture and jaundice.

BIBLIOGRAPHY

1. Affleck D, Handrahan D, Egger MJ, Price RR: The laparoscopic management of appendicitis and cholelithiasis during pregancy. Am J Surg 178:523–529, 1999.

2. Allendorf JD, Bessler M, Whelan RL, et al: Postoperative immune function varies inversely with the degree of surgical trauma in a murine model. Surg Endosc 11:427–430, 1997.

3. Barone J, Bears S, Chen S, et al: Outcome study of cholecystectomy during pregnancy. Am J Surg 177:232–236, 1999.

4. Berry SM, Ose KJ, Bell RH, Fink AS: Thermal injury of the posterior duodenum during laparoscopic cholecystectomy. Surg Endosc 8:197–200, 1984.

5. Bishoff JT, Allaf ME, Kirkels W, et al: Laparoscopic bowel injury: Incidence and clinical presentation. J Urol 161:887–890, 1999.

6. Brunt LM, Doherty GM, Norton JA, et al: Laparoscopic adrenalectomy compared to open adrenalectomy for benign adrenal neoplasms. J Am Coll Surg 183:1–10, 1996.

7. Cameron J: Current Surgical Therapy, 6th ed. St. Louis, Mosby, 1998.

8. Cho JM, LaPorta AJ, Clark JR, et al: Response of serum cytokines in patients undergoing laparoscopic cholecystectomy. Surg Endosc 8:1380–1384, 1994.

9. Crist DW, Gadacz TR: Complications in laparoscopic surgery. Surg Clin North Am 3:265–289, 1993.

10. Curet M: Special problems in laparoscopic surgery. Surg Clin North Am 80:1093–1111, 2000.

11. Deziel DJ, Millikan KW, Economou SG, et al: Scientific papers: Complications of laparoscopic cholecystectomy. A national survey of 4,292 hospitals and an analysis of 77,604 cases. Am J Surg 165:9–14, 1993.

12. EU Hernia Trialists Collaboration: Laparoscopic compared with open methods of groin hernia repair: Systematic review of randomized controlled trials. Br J Surg 87:860–867, 2000.

13. Farooqui MO, Bazzoli JM: Significance of radiologic evidence of free air following laparoscopy. J Reprod Med 16(3):119–125, 1976.

14. Fitzgerald SD, Andrus CH, Baudendistel DF, et al: Hypercarbia during carbon dioxide pneumoperitoneum. Am J Surg 163:186–190, 1992.

15. Fleshman JW, Nelson H, Peters WR, et al: Early results of laparoscopic surgery for colorectal cancer: Retrospective analysis of 372 patients treated by Clinical Outcomes of Surgery Therapy (COST) study group. Dis Colon Rectum 39(Suppl):S53–S58, 1996.

16. Frazee RC, Roberts JW, Okeson GC, et al: Open versus laparoscopic cholecystectomy: A comparison of operative pulmonary functions. Ann Surg 213:651–653, 1991.

17. Gollin G, Raschbaum GR, Moorthy C, Santos L: Cholecystectomy for suspected biliary dyskinesia in children with chronic abdominal pain. J Pediatr Surg 34:854–857, 1999.

18. Greene FL: The impact of laparoscopy on cancer management. Surg Endosc 14(3):217–218, 2000.

19. Hammer JH, Neilsen HJ, Moesgaard F, et al: Duration of post-operative immunosuppression assessed by repeated delayed typed hypersensitivity skin test. Eur Surg Res 24:133, 1992.

20. Jones DM, Weintraub PS: Anesthesiologists warn if you're taking herbal products, tell your doctor before surgery. ASA Publ Educ, 1999.

21. Joris JL, Noirot DP, Legrand MJ, et al: Hemodynamic changes during laparoscopic cholecystectomy. Anesth Analg 76:106–107, 1992.

22. Khalili T, Hiatt J, Savar A, et al: Perforated appendicitis is not a contraindication to laparoscopy. Am Surg 65:965–967, 1999.

23. Kumar S, Wilson R, Nixon SJ, Macintyre IM: Chronic pain after laparoscopic and open mesh repair of groin hernia. Br J Surg 89:1476–1479, 2002.

24. Lee SW, Southall JC, Gleason NR, et al: Lymphocyte proliferation in mice after full laparotomy is the same whether performed in a sealed carbon dioxide chamber or room air. Surg Endosc 14:235–238, 2000.

25. McCahill LE, Pellegrini CA, Wiggins T, Helton WS: A clinical outcome and cost analysis of laparoscopic versus open appendectomy. Am J Surg 171:533–537, 1996.

26. McLucas B, March C: Urachal sinus perforation during laparoscopy: A case report. J Reprod Med 35:573–574, 1990.

27. McVay CB, Anson BJ (eds): [Entire issue]. Surg Anat 16:622–628, 1984.

28. Miller LG: Herbal medicinals selected clinical considerations focusing on known or potential drug-herb interactions. Arch Intern Med 158(20):2200–2211, 1998.

29. Minne L, Varner D, Burnell A, et al: Laparoscopic vs. open appendectomy. Arch Surg 132:708–712, 1997.

30. Prinz RA: A comparison of laparoscopic and open adrenalectomies. Arch Surg 30:489–494, 1995.

31. Rattner DW, Ferguson C, Warshaw AL: Factors associated with successful laparoscopic cholecystectomy for acute cholecystitis. Ann Surg 217(3):233–236.

32. Reddick EJ, Olsen DO, Daniell JF, et al: Laparoscopic laser cholecystectomy [First U.S. report]. J Clin Laser Med Surg 7:38–40, 1989.

33. Reich H: Laparoscopic bowel injury. Surg Laparosc Endosc 2:74–78, 1992.

34. SAGES Committee on Standards of Practice: Guidelines for Diagnostic Laparoscopy. Santa Monica, CA, SAGES Guidelines, 1998.

35. Schauer PR, Page CP, Ghiatas AA, et al: Incidence and significance of subdiaphragmatic air following laparoscopic cholecystectomy. Am Surg 63:132–136, 1997.

36. Schirmer BD, Dix J, Edge SB, et al: Laparoscopic cholecystectomy in the obese patient. Ann Surg 216:146–152, 1992.

37. Schrenk P, Woisetschlager R, Rieger R, Wayand W: Mechanism, management, and prevention of laparoscopic bowel injuries. Gastrol Endosc 43:572–574, 1996.

38. So JB, Chiong EC, Chiong E, et al: Laparoscopic appendectomy for perforated appendicitis. World J Surg 26:1485–1488, 2002.

39. Talamini MA, Gadacz TR: Equipment and instrumentation. In Zuker KA, Bailey RW, Reddick EJ (eds): Surgical Laparoscopy Update. St. Louis, Quality Medical Publishing, 1993, pp 4–5.

40. Voyles CR, Tucker RD: Education and engineering solutions for potential problems with monopolar electrosurgery at laparoscopy. Am J Surg 164:57–62, 1992.

41. Wright D, Paterson C, Scott N, et al: Five-year follow-up of patients undergoing laparoscopic or open groin hernia repair: A randomized controlled trial. Ann Surg 235:333–337, 2002.

42. Yeh C, Jan Y, Chen M: Laparoscopic treatment for Mirizzi syndrome. Surg Endosc 17:1573–1578, 2003.

43. Yost F, Margenthaler J, Presti M, et al: Cholecystectomy is an effective treatment for biliary dyskinesia. Am J Surg 178(6):462–465, 1999.

INDEX

A

Abdomen
  abscess of, nuclear medicine studies of, 652
  acute
    AIDS/HIV infection-related, 463–464
    surgical treatment of, 463, **700–705**
    perforation of, 463–464
    radiographic evaluation of, 575–579
    traumatic injury to, 702
Abdominal cancer
  as gastroparesis cause, 113
  nuclear medicine studies of, 649–650, 651
Abdominal pain
  abdominal angina-related, 508
  acute, evaluation of, **459–464**
  AIDS/HIV infection-related, 493
  bacterial overgrowth-related, 398
  chronic pancreatitis-related, 344, 348–349
  Crohn's disease-related, 371
  duration of, 701
  hepatitis-related, 127
  intestinal ischemia-related, 504, 505
  ischemic colitis-related, 509
  location of, 700
  pancreatitis-related, 348–349
  peritonitis-related, 700–701
  post-endoscopic retrograde
    cholangiopancreatography, 704
  referred, 459, 461
  ulcerative colitis-related, 371
Abetalipoproteinemia, 252, 364
Abortion, spontaneous, maternal portal
  hypertension-related, 202
Abscess
  abdominal, nuclear medicine studies of, 652
  anorectal, 712–713
  appendiceal, 433
  diverticulitis-related, 425–426, 429
  hepatic, 214, **281–286**, 726
    amebic, 281, 283, 284, 469, 598, 726
    pyogenic, 596–597
  horseshoe, 713
  pancreatic, 358, 400
  parahepatic, 596
  renal and perirenal, 601
  retroperitoneal, 601–602
  splenic, 599
  tubo-ovarian, 425–426, 432

Acanthosis nigricans, 453
Acetaminophen, hepatotoxicity of, 223, 224
  as liver transplantation indication, 257
Acetohexamide, hepatotoxicity of, 226
Acetylcholinesterase inhibitors, 14
5-Acetylsalicylic acid products. *See also* Sulfasalazine
  as microscopic colitis treatment, 440
  as radiation colitis treatment, 441
  as ulcerative colitis treatment, 381–382, 383, 384
Achalasia, **43–50**, 677–681
  as chest pain cause, 38
  cricopharyngeal, 17, 75
  differentiated from scleroderma, 581, 582
  as esophageal cancer risk factor, 538, 681
  primary, differentiated from secondary, 582
  secondary, 45, 582
  surgical treatment of, 704
  symptoms of, 677
  vigorous, 43, 678
Achlorhydria, 85
Acid-fast bacilli, identification of, on biopsy, 304
Acid ingestion injury, esophageal, 59–60, 62
Acid suppression trial, 35
Acquired immunodeficiency syndrome (AIDS).
    See also Human immunodeficiency virus (HIV)
    infection
  gastrointestinal manifestations of, **491–499**
    abdominal pain, 493
    diarrhea, 470, 478, 494–498
    esophagitis, 32
    focal fatty liver, 219
    pancreatitis, 332
Acromegaly, 571
Actinobacter infections, 282
Actinomyces infections, 282
Acute fatty liver of pregnancy, 198–199, 200
Acute respiratory distress syndrome, pancreatitis-
    related, 336
Acyclovir, 31
Addison's disease, 483, 519, 573
Adefovir dipivoxil, as hepatitis B treatment, 133, 144,
    145, 146–147, 148
Adenocarcinoma
  esophageal, 51, 54, 69, 70–71
  gastric, 85, 86, 87, 94, 100, 657, 698
    of the gastric antrum, 107
  ovarian, 356
  pancreatic, 347, 352, 356

Adenocarcinoma (*Continued*)
  of the pancreatic head, 586, 588
  Peutz-Jeghers syndrome-related, 564
Adenoma
  adrenal, 600–601
  biliary, 214
  colonic, 401–402, 405
  colorectal, 544
  gastric, 99, 541
  hepatic, 214, 215–216, 726, 727
    drug-related, 225
  liver-cell, 306
Adenomatous polyposis coli (APC) protein, 706
Adhesions, intra-abdominal, 716
Adrenalectomy, laparoscopic, 737
  in pregnant patients, 738
Adrenal glands, biopsy of, 600–601
Adrenal insufficiency, 573
Adverse drug reactions (ADRs), in hospitalized
    patients, 227
Aeromonas infections, 465–466, 471
Aerophagia, 20, 41
African iron overload, 287
ALADIN protein, 44
Alanine aminotransferase
  alcoholic hepatitis-related increase in, 233
  assessment of, 120–121
  biliary acute pancreatitis-related increase of, 334
  congestive hepatopathy-related increase in, 241
  hepatic abscess-related increase in, 281
  hepatitis-related increase in, 127
  as liver function indicator, 119
  nonalcoholic fatty liver disease-related increase in,
    245, 248
  in pregnancy, 196, 197
    in acute fatty liver, 198
    in intrahepatic cholestasis, 197
  primary biliary cirrhosis-related increase in, 178
  veno-occlusive disease-related increase in, 240
Alanine phosphatase, hepatic abscess-related
    increase in, 281
Albendazole
  as hydatid cyst disease treatment, 315
  as microsporidiosis treatment, 498
Albumin
  ascitic fluid content of, 269, 270
  as liver function indicator, 119
Alcohol
  metabolism of, 231–232
  toxicity of, 232
Alcohol consumption, indicators of, 247
Alcohol dependency, 231
Alcohol use/abuse, adverse effects of, 231
  cirrhosis, 232, 234, 297–298, 594
  drug hepatotoxicity-potentiating effects, 223
  esophageal cancer, 51, 681
  esophageal injury, 59
  fatty liver, 219, 232, 233
  gastritis, 79, 81

Alcohol use/abuse, adverse effects of (*Continued*)
  as hepatitis cause, 232–234, 247, 298–299, 560
  hypoglycemia, 570–571
  liver disease, **231–235**
  pancreatic cancer, 353
  pancreatitis, 331, 338, 342, 562
  steatohepatitis, 247
Aldehyde dehydrogenase, 232
Alendronate sodium (Fosamax), 19
  as esophageal injury cause, 58
Alkali ingestion injury, esophageal, 59, 60, 61, 64
Alkaline, hepatitis-related increase in, 128
Alkaline phosphatase, 214
  chronic pancreatitis-related increase in, 344
  liver disease-related increase in, 121
Allergies
  differentiated from eosinophilic gastroenteritis,
    389
  as eosinophilic gastroenteritis cause, 389,
    394–395
  as hepatitis cause, 223–224
Allgrove's syndrome, 44
Allopurinol, hepatotoxicity of, 224, 225
Alopecia, necrolytic migratory erythema-related, 565
Alosetron, 536
Alpha heavy-chain disease, 366
Alveolitis, fibrosing, 153
Amebiasis, 469
  vaccine against, 285
Amebic abscess, hepatic, 469, 598, 736
Ameboma, 469
American College of Gastroenterology, 51, 52
American Society of Gastrointestinal Endoscopy, 46
5-Aminosalicylic acid, as Crohn's disease treatment,
    374, 376
Amiodarone
  hepatotoxicity of, 224, 227, 249, 252
  interaction with tacrolimus and cyclosporine,
    261
Amoxicillin
  as *Helicobacter pylori* infection treatment, 81, 95
  hepatotoxicity of, 224, 228
Amoxicillin-clavulanic acid, 272, 569
Amphotericin B, as candidal esophagitis
    treatment, 30
Ampicillin, hepatotoxicity of, 224
Amylase
  ascitic fluid content of, 269
  pancreatic cancer-related increase in, 354
  pancreatic panniculitis syndrome-related increase
    in, 557–558
  pancreatitis-related increase in, 333, 461
Amyloidosis
  as gastroparesis cause, 113
  as intestinal pseudo-obstruction cause, 112
  as thickened gastric folds cause, 100
  ulcerative colitis-related, 708
Anabolic steroids, hepatotoxicity of, 224, 225, 227
Anal fissures, 711, 712

Anastomosis
  biliary-enteric, 603–604, 605
  ileal pouch-anal, 386, 708, 710
Anemia
  bacterial overgrowth-related, 398
  hemolytic, Coombs' positive, 153
  iron-deficiency, 108, 410, 454–455, 516
  pernicious, 82, 100, 153, 352–353, 542, 567
Anesthetic agents, hepatotoxicity of, 229
Aneurysms
  hepatitis B polyarteritis nodosa-related, 207, 208
  intracranial saccular ("berry"), 312
Angina, abdominal, 506, 508–509
Angiodysplasia, 455
Angiography
  coronary, 34
  magnetic resonance, for abdominal angina
    evaluation, 506
  mesenteric, 507
Angioma, spider, 196, 215, 234, 559–560
Angiomatosis, retinal, 359
Angioplasty, for abdominal angina management, 508
Angiosarcoma, 214, 225
Anisakiasis, gastric, 100
Anismus, 415
Ankylosing spondylitis, 380–381, 552
Anorectal disease, 711–714
Anorectal dysfunction, as diabetic diarrhea cause,
  569
Anorectal dyssynergia, 415
Anorexia
  Addison's disease-related, 573
  hepatitis-related, 127
  hypercalcemia-related, 571
Anorexia nervosa, 522–524
  as gastroparesis cause, 113
Antacids
  effect on esophageal sphincter pressures, 21
  as gastroesophageal reflux disease treatment,
    23, 24
Anti-arrhythmic medications, as esophageal injury
  cause, 57
Antiarthritic medications, hepatotoxicity of, 225
Antibiotic prophylaxis, in laparoscopic
  cholecystectomy patients, 736–737
Antibiotic resistance, in diarrhea-causative bacteria,
  471
Antibiotics. See also names of specific antibiotics
  as bacterial overgrowth treatment, 399, 400
  as caustic ingestion injury treatment, 66
  as diarrhea cause, 487
  effect on Helicobacter pylori test results, 92–93
  as esophageal injury cause, 57
  as fungal esophagitis cause, 29
  as gastric MALT lymphoma treatment, 87
  hepatotoxicity of, 224, 225, 228, 262
  as pancreatitis cause, 331
  as pseudomembranous colitis cause, 435,
    436, 437

Antibodies, radiolabeled, 651
Antibody tests, 124
Anticardiolipin antibodies, 208
Anticholinergic
  as irritable bowel syndrome treatment, 535
  as nausea and vomiting treatment, 520, 521
Anticoagulants, ulcerative colitis-exacerbating effects
  of, 386
Antiemetics, 520–521
Antihistamines, as nausea and vomiting treatment,
  520, 521
Antihypertensive medications
  as diarrhea cause, 487
  as esophageal injury cause, 57
Anti-inflammatory medications
  as diarrhea cause, 487
  as esophageal injury cause, 57–58
  ulcerative colitis-exacerbating effects of, 386
Anti-mitochondrial antibody (AMA), 123, 124, 152,
  156, 159, 172
Antimotility agents, contraindication in dysentery,
  471–472
Antineutrophil cytoplasmic antibody (p-ANCA), 380
Antinuclear antibody (ANA), 123, 124, 151, 153,
  155–156, 157, 158, 208
Antioxidants, as alcoholic hepatitis treatment, 233
Antiparietal antibodies, 567
Antireflux surgery, 23, 25, 27, 675–676
  Barrett's esophagus regression after, 682
Antiretroviral therapy, highly-active (HAART), 494,
  497, 498
Antisaccharomyces antibody (ASCA), 380
Antisialoglycoprotein receptor antibody, 123
Antismooth muscle antibody (ASMA), 123, 124, 208,
  210, 212
Antispasmodic agents, as irritable bowel syndrome
  treatment, 535
Antithyroid antibodies, 208
α_1-Antitrypsin
  deficiency of, 136, 152, 291–292, 306
    diagnostic tests for, 122, 123
  function of, 122
Antiviral therapy, 132
  for hepatitis B, **143–150**
Antrectomy, 690, 694
Anus. See also Anorectal disease
  fissures of, 711, 712
  foreign bodies in, 529
APACHE-II score, for pancreatitis prognosis, 335
Appendectomy
  laparoscopic, 433, 731, 738
  during pregnancy, 433–434, 738
    contraindicated, 462
Appendicitis, **431–434**
  acute, 431, 434, 462
  atypical forms of, 462
  gangrenous, 738
  perforated, 432, 738
  during pregnancy, 461

Appendix
abscess of, 433
anatomy and function of, 431
carcinoid tumors of, 433, 573
diseases of, **431–434**
Argon plasma therapy, for esophageal cancer, 54
Arrhythmias, gastric, 113, 114
Arteriography, mesenteric, 507
Arteritis, obliterative, 716
Arthralgia, Whipple's disease-related, 363
Arthritis. *See also* Rheumatoid arthritis
celiac disease-related, 557
colitic, 380–381
drug therapy for, hepatotoxicity of, 225
enteropathic, 547–552
hemochromatosis-related, 211, 212, 213
primary biliary cirrhosis-related, 210
reactive, 552–555
Reiter's syndrome-related, 473
spinal, 548–549
Whipple's disease-related, 556
Ascaris, as pancreatitis cause, 332
Ascites, **268–280**
alcoholic liver disease-related, 234
autoimmune hepatitis-related, 166–167
cirrhotic, 178, 269–270, 271, 272–273, 274–275, 277
congestive hepatopathy-related, 241
pancreatic, 340, 348
primary sclerosing cholangitis-related, 178
refractory, 276
subserosal/serosal inflammation-related, 392
transjugular intrahepatic portosystemic shunt treatment of, 607–608, 610
Ascitic fluid
diagnostic tests of, 268–269, 272–273
infection of, 270, 272–273
Aspartate aminotransferase
alcoholic hepatitis-related increase of, 233
autoimmune hepatitis-related increase of, 164, 167, 168, 172
congestive hepatopathy-related increase of, 241
hepatic abscess-related increase of, 281
hepatitis-related increase of, 127
as liver function indicator, 119
nonalcoholic fatty liver disease-related increase of, 248
in pregnant patients, 196, 197, 198
primary biliary cirrhosis-related increase of, 178
primary sclerosing cholangitis-related increase of, 178
veno-occlusive disease-related increase of, 240
Aspergillosis, as esophagitis cause, 31
Aspiration
fine-needle, 594–595
of fluid collections, 591, 595, 596
of hepatic abscesses, 283–284

Aspirin
as esophageal cancer prophylaxis, 54
as esophageal injury cause, 58
as gastric ulcer cause, 690, 691
as gastrointestinal hemorrhage cause, 443, 444
hepatotoxicity of, 223, 224, 225
ulcerative colitis-exacerbating effects of, 386
Asterixis, 234
Asthma
carcinoid syndrome-related, 573
gastroesophageal reflux disease-related, 27, 673
Atresia
biliary, 311, 641, 642
esophageal, 76
Atrophy, intestinal villous, 153
Autoantibodies
hepatitis-associated, 151, 152, 153, 155–156, 157–160, 161
hepatitis C-related autoimmune disorders-associated, 208
primary biliary cirrhosis-associated, 177, 179, 211
primary sclerosing cholangitis-associated, 179
Autoimmune disorders
autoimmune hepatitis-related, 209
hepatic, 124
primary biliary cirrhosis as, 177
Autoimmune markers, 123–124
Autoimmune polyendocrinopathy-candidiasis-ectodermal dystrophy (APECED), 163
Azathioprine, 259, 260
as autoimmune hepatitis therapy, 166, 171, 172
as Crohn's disease treatment, 374, 375
fetal effects of, 203
hepatotoxicity of, 262
as microscopic colitis treatment, 440
use in pregnant patients, 385

B
Bacillary peliosis hepatis (BPH), 498–499
Bacillus cereus infections, 472
Bacitracin, as pseudomembranous colitis treatment, 438
Back pain, post-endoscopic retrograde cholangiopancreatography, 704
Bacterascites, 270, 273–274
Bacteremia, 467
Bacterial infections. *See also specific bacteria*
as gastritis cause, 79
as pancreatitis cause, 332
as pyogenic hepatic abscess cause, 281, 282–283
Bacterial overgrowth, **397–400**
diagnosis of, 365–366
as diarrhea cause, 484
in diabetic patients, 569
scleroderma-related, 364
Bacteroides infections, 282, 337, 397, 427
Bad breath, Zenker's diverticulum-related, 75
Balanitis, circinate, 553
Balantidium coli infections, 469

Balloon dilation, of the lower esophageal sphincter, 47–48
Balsalazide, 383
Bannayan-Ruvalcaba-Riley syndrome, 408
Bariatrics, 719
Bariatric surgery, 516, 571, 719–722
Barium, as contrast media, 579
Barium enema/studies
    for AIDS-related esophagitis evaluation, 491
    air contrast, 410
    barium swallow, 580–582
        for oropharyngeal dysphagia evaluation, 14
    for colon cancer screening, 585
    as colonic perforation cause, 704–705
    defecography, 584–585
    double-contrast, 585
    esophagraphy, of congenital esophageal
        stenosis, 76
    for gastroesophageal reflux disease evaluation,
        674
    single-contrast, 585
Bartonella henselae, 498–499
Basiliximab, 260
Bayes' theorem, 483–484
bDNA (deoxyribonucleic acid) assay, 130
Belching, as chest pain cause, 41
Bentiromide test, 345
Beriberi, 513
Bernstein test, 38–39
Beta blockers, 446–447
    gastric emptying effects of, 113
Beta-carotene, anticarcinogenicity of, 404
Bethanechol, 24, 115, 416
Bezoars, 694, 715
Bile acids
    deficiency of, 485
    malabsorption of, as diarrhea cause, 487–488, 569
Bile ducts
    common
        cancer of, 282
        in Mirizzi's syndrome, 728
        obstruction of, 587, 588
        stones in. *See* Choledocholithiasis
    congenital cysts of, 310–312
    endoscopic retrograde cholangiopancreatography-
        related injury to, 704
    endoscopic ultrasound-guided nonpapillary
        drainage of, 670–671
    endosonographic evaluation of, 661
    histopathology of, 302–303
    laparoscopic cholecystectomy-related injury to,
        604, 605
    obstruction of, 727–728. *See also* Bile duct stones
        cholescintigraphy of, 640–641
        diagnosis and treatment of, 348
        hepatic biopsy findings in, 302
        by location, 587–588
        metallic stent treatment of, 605–606
        pancreatic cancer-related, 354

Bile ducts (*Continued*)
        pancreatitis-related, 347, 348
        percutaneous transhepatic biliary drainage of,
        603–605
Bile duct stones. *See also* Choledolithiasis
    imaging of, 320–321
    as pancreatitis cause, 703
    removal of, 320
Biliary leaks
    cholescintigraphy of, 640
    laparoscopic cholecystectomy-related, 736
    post-liver transplantation, 262
Biliary sludge, 317–318, 319, 320, 321
Biliary tract
    in primary biliary cirrhosis, 180
    in primary sclerosing cholangitis, 179–180
Biliary tract disease, 723–724
    as abdominal pain cause, 462
    as hepatic abscess cause, 282, 284
Biliary tract pain, 727. *See also* Colic, biliary
Biliopancreatic diversion, 721
Bilirubin, 318–319
    assessment of, 121–122
    in cholestasis, 301
    in chronic pancreatitis, 344
    conjugated, 121–122
    in hepatitis, 127, 128
    in pancreatic cancer, 354
    unconjugated, 121
Billroth I and II gastroduodenostomies, 687, 688,
    690, 694
    conversion to Roux-en-Y reconstruction, 695
Biofeedback, as fecal incontinence treatment, 419,
    420
Biopsy
    adrenal, 600–601
    core, 591, 594, 596
        contraindications to, 597–598
    esophageal, 51–52
        of esophageal ulcers, 492
    fine-needle aspiration, 591, 594–595
        adrenal, 601
        contraindications to, 597–598
        endoscopic ultrasound-guided, 664–667
        of hepatic masses, 219–220
        pancreatic, 599, 600
        splenic, 598
    hepatic
        in acute fatty liver of pregnancy, 198
        in α-$_1$ antitrypsin deficiency, 306
        in autoimmune hepatitis, 169
        in bile duct obstruction, 302
        in bone marrow transplant recipients, 308
        in cholestasis, 301
        in cirrhosis, 297
        in fatty liver, 249, 250, 252
        in hemochromatosis, 122, 123
        in hepatitis, 134, 299, 301
        in hereditary hemochromatosis, 289–290

Biopsy (*Continued*)
  histopathologic findings in, 296, 297
  in liver cancer, 306, 594, 596
  in primary biliary cirrhosis, 180, 303
  in primary sclerosing cholangitis, 180
  prior to hepatitis therapy, 137, 144
  in steatohepatitis, 298–299
  in Wilson's disease, 123, 305
  image-guided, 591, 664–667
  renal, 601
  of tumors, needle tract seeding during, 595
  ultrasound-guided fine-needle aspiration, 664–667
Biotin, toxicity of, 514
Biotin deficiency, 514
Bismuth, as *Helicobacter pylori* infection treatment,
  81, 95
Bismuth-containing compounds, effect on
  Helicobacter pylori test results, 92–93
Bismuth subsalicylate, as microscopic colitis
  treatment, 487
Bisphosphonates, as gastritis cause, 79
Blastomycosis, 31
Blood alcohol levels (BALs), 232
Blood flow
  hepatic, 236–238
  intestinal, 500–502
Blood vessels, in intestinal circulation and
  microcirculation, 500–502
Blunt trauma, abdominal, peritoneal fluid collections
  associated with, 702
Body-cell mass, 511
Body mass index (BMI), 515, 718
  in obesity, 571
Boerhaave's syndrome, 520
Bone disease, metabolic
  post-liver transplantation, 265
  primary biliary cirrhosis-related, 181
  primary sclerosing cholangitis-related, 181
Bone marrow transplantation, 308
Botulinum toxin (Botox)
  as achalasia treatment, 48–49, 679–680, 681
  as dysphagia treatment, 17
Botulism, immunoprophylaxis against, 189
Bougienage, esophageal, 66, 73, 74, 76
Bouveret's syndrome, 319
Bovie, William, 735
Bowel. *See* Intestines
Bowel sounds, 701
BRAT diet, 473
Bravo capsule, 23
Breast cancer, 564, 565, 571
  endosonographic evaluation of, 659
  metastatic, 216
Breastfeeding, 203, 204
Breath tests, radiolabeled, for bacterial overgrowth
  diagnosis, 399
Bromfenac, hepatotoxicity of, 225
Bromosulfophthalein test, 119
Brucellosis, 304

Budd-Chiari syndrome, 200–201, 238–240, 608, 609
Budesonide, 174, 374
Bulimia nervosa, 522–523, 524
Burns, esophageal, caustic ingestion-related, 59–67
Butyrophenone, 520

C

Caffeine test, 119
CAGE questionnaire, for alcohol abuse
  diagnosis, 231
Calcineurin inhibitors, 204
Calcium, toxicity or deficiency of, 514
Calcium channel blockers
  as achalasia treatment, 46
  gastric emptying effects of, 113
Calcium pyrophosphate disease, 211
Caliciviruses, 473
Calories, "hidden" sources of, 512
Calot's triangle, 730
Cameron's erosions, 456
Campylobacter infections
  in AIDS/HIV patients, 470, 494, 495, 496, 498
  as diarrhea cause, 466–467
  as dysentery cause, 465, 471
  as enterocolitis cause, 494, 495
  as immunoproliferative small intestinal disease
    cause, 366
  as reactive arthritis cause, 552, 553–554
  as Reiter's syndrome cause, 473–474
  as traveler's diarrhea cause, 472
Cancer. *See also specific types of cancer*
  endoscopic screening and surveillance of,
    538–545
Candidas (caspofungin), 30
Candidiasis, 337
  AIDS/HIV-related, 30, 491, 492, 498
  esophageal, 29–31, 77, 491
  as esophagitis cause, 31
  fluconazole-resistant, 30
  imidazole-resistant, 30–31
CA19-9
  as liver cancer marker, 215, 353–354
  as pancreatic cancer marker, 353–354
Captopril, hepatotoxicity of, 224, 227
Caput medusae, 234
Carbamazepine
  hepatotoxicity of, 224
  interaction with tacrolimus and cyclosporine, 261
Carbon dioxide, as insufflation gas, 733, 734–735
Carcinoembryonic antigen (CEA), as colorectal cancer
  marker, 404
Carcinoid crisis, 597
Carcinoid syndrome, 572–573, 574
Carcinoid tumors, 484
  appendiceal, 433
  endosonographic evaluation of, 659
  gastric, 85, 88, 107
  metastatic, 597, 598
Cardiospasm, 43

Cardiovascular medications
  as esophageal injury cause, 57
  hepatotoxicity of, 227
Caroli's disease, 311
Caroli's syndrome, 311–312
Carotenoderma, 559
Catheters, arterial perfusion, placement of, 649
Caustic ingestion injury, 59–67
  as esophageal cancer cause, 540
Cefotaxime, 272, 273
Ceftriaxone, as gallbladder sludge cause, 317
Celecoxib (Celebrex), hepatotoxicity of, 225
Celiac disease, 362–363, 563
  autoimmune hepatitis associated with, 153
  diagnosis of, 389, 485
  as diarrhea cause, 484, 485
    in diabetic patients, 569
  fatty liver associated with, 252
  hepatitis associated with, 159
  macroamylasemia associated with, 333
  rheumatic manifestations of, 556, 557
  serologic diagnostic test panel for, 362
Celiac plexus neurolysis/block, 348–349, 354
  endoscopic ultrasound-guided, 665, 669–670
Cephalosporins, 737
  as diabetic diarrhea treatment, 569
  as pseudomembranous colitis cause, 435
Cerebral palsy, 20
Ceruloplasmin, in Wilson's disease, 123, 136, 196,
    293–294, 305
Cesarean section, 197
Chagas' disease, 32–33
Charcot's triad, 432, 728
Cheilitis, angular, 73
Chemoembolization, hepatic transarterial (TACE),
    219, 603, 604
Chemotherapy
  as diarrhea cause, 487
  hepatotoxicity of, 224
Chest pain
  of cardiac origin, 34
  esophageal causes of, **34–42**
  unexplained, psychological component of, 41
Chest-wall pain syndromes, 34
Child-Pugh scores, 277
Children
  caustic ingestion injuries in, 59, 61
  esophageal rings in, 74
  fatty liver disease in, 248, 250, 251
  Helicobacter pylori infections in, 90
  Ménétrièr's disease in, 105
  rectal prolapse treatment in, 714
Child-Turcotte-Pugh (CTP) score, 254, 259
Chlamydia infections, 470
Chlamydia trachomatis infections, 494
Chloramphenicol, hepatotoxicity of, 228
Chloroquine, hepatotoxicity of, 249
Chlorpromazine, 522
  hepatotoxicity of, 225

Chlorpropamide, hepatotoxicity of, 226
Chlorzoxazone, hepatotoxicity of, 226
Cholangiocarcinoma, 214, 218, 220, 311, 312, 381,
    727
Cholangiography
  endoscopic retrograde, 728
  magnetic resonance, 180
  retrograde, 179
Cholangiopancreatography, 311, 585–589
  endoscopic retrograde (ERCP), 303, 311, 326,
      345–346, 353, 704
    of AIDS-related cholangiopathy, 492–493
    of bile duct stones, 320, 321, 703
    of biliary acute pancreatitis, 338
    of biliary obstruction, 604
    of obstructive jaundice, 728
    of pancreatic pseudocysts, 357
    as pancreatitis cause, 326–327, 329
  magnetic resonance, 662
    of bile duct disease, 311
    of bile duct obstruction, 348
    of bile duct stones, 320, 321, 662
    of chronic pancreatitis, 346–347
    of pancreas divisum, 332
    of sphincter of Oddi dysfunction, 325–326
Cholangiopathy, AIDS-related, 492–493
Cholangitis
  ascending, 728
  autoimmune, 172, 182, 299
    differentiated from autoimmune hepatitis, 152
  bacterial
    postoperative, 185
    primary biliary cirrhosis-related, 178
    primary sclerosing cholangitis-related,
        181–182, 183–184
  chronic nonsuppurative destructive, 180
  fibrous obliterative, 180
  gallbladder sludge-related, 318
  hepatic cyst-related, 725
  primary sclerosing, **177–187**, 299, 301, 311,
      380–381, 728
    autoimmune hepatitis-associated, 172
    differentiated from autoimmune hepatitis, 152
    overlap syndrome of, 182
    small duct, 182
Cholecystectomy, 321–322
  as acute pancreatitis treatment, 703
  as bile reflux gastritis cause, 83
  as biliary acute pancreatitis treatment, 338
  as diarrhea cause, 486
  laparoscopic, 319–320, 320, 730–731, 732,
      734–735
    antibiotic prophylaxis in, 736–737
    bile spills in, 736
    conversion to open cholecystectomy, 736
    in morbidly obese patients, 735–736
    in pregnant patients, 738
  as sphincter of Oddi dysfunction cause, 325,
      327

Cholecystitis, 319
  acute, 432, 463, 638, 639, 723
    acalculous, 322
    laparoscopic cholecystectomy treatment of, 736
  chronic
    acalculous, 723–724
    laparoscopic cholecystectomy treatment of, 736
  gallbladder sludge-related, 318
Cholecystokinin, 732
  use in pancreatic exocrine function measurement, 344
Cholecystolithiasis. See Gallstones
Cholecystostomy, percutaneous, 723
  indications for, 606
Choledochocele, 310, 311
Choledochoduodenostomy, 185
Choledochojejunostomy, 185
Choledocholithiasis, 662, 727, 728. See also Gallstones
  as cholestasis cause, 182
  ultrasonographic detection of, 320–321
Cholelithiasis
  in alcohol-related pancreatitis patients, 338
  pancreatitis-associated, 331
Cholera, 472–473
Cholescintigraphy, 637, 638, 639–642
Cholestasis, 299, 305
  autoimmune hepatitis-related, 172
  drug-related, 222, 224
  intrahepatic, of pregnancy, 196, 197, 200
  liver biopsy findings in, 301
  post-liver transplantation, 262
Cholestatic liver injury, 119, 120
Cholestyramine, 183, 197, 488, 489, 569, 573
Chromium, deficiency or toxicity of, 514
Chronic obstructive pulmonary disease, 734–735
Churg-Strauss syndrome, 390
Chymotrypsin, fecal content of, in pancreatitis, 345
Cidofovir, 32, 496
Cimetidine, 24
  hepatotoxicity of, 224
Ciprofloxacin, 184, 272
Cirrhosis, 214
  alcoholic, 232, 234
    hepatic biopsy in, 594
    hepatic histopathology in, 297–298
  ascites associated with, 269–270, 271, 272–273, 274–275, 276, 277
  autoimmune hepatitis-related, 151, 166–167, 168–169, 170
  drug-related, 225
  gastrointestinal hemorrhage associated with, 445, 446
  hepatic histopathology of, 296–297
  hepatitis B-related, 148
  hepatitis C-related, 140–141
  as hepatocellular carcinoma cause, 217, 219, 220
  hydrothorax associated with, 269–270
  micronodular, 297

Cirrhosis (Continued)
  nonalcoholic fatty liver disease-related, 252
  during pregnancy, 202
  primary biliary, **177–187**
    antibodies/autoantibodies associated with, 124, 172, 177, 211
    autoimmune diseases associated with, 172, 210, 212
    autoimmune hepatitis associated with, 172
    differentiated from autoimmune hepatitis, 152
    Helicobacter-related, 90
    hepatic histopathology in, 302–303
    musculoskeletal manifestations of, 210–211
    overlap syndrome of, 182
    staging of, 302, 303
  spontaneous bacterial peritonitis associated with, 271, 272–273
Cisapride, 24, 115, 416
  effect on esophageal sphincter pressures, 21
Cisplatin, hepatotoxicity of, 224
Clarithromycin, 81
  interaction with tacrolimus and cyclosporine, 261
Clindamycin
  as pseudomembranous colitis cause, 435
  as pyogenic liver abscess treatment, 285
Clofibrate, as nonalcoholic fatty liver disease treatment, 251
Clonidine, 488, 489, 569
Clonorchis sinensis, as pancreatitis cause, 332
Clostridia, 397
Clostridium botulinum infections, 112
Clostridium difficile infections
  as colitis cause, 435–438, 470, 478, 494
  as diarrhea cause, 465–466, 478
  as dysentery cause, 471, 494
  as pseudomembranous colitis cause, 435–438
Clostridium infections, 282, 427, 723
Cobalamin deficiency, 398
Cocaine, hepatotoxicity of, 229
Codeine, as diarrhea treatment, 488, 489
Colchicine, 184, 233
Colectomy, 544
  of dysplasia-associated lesion or mass (DALM), 384–385
Colic, biliary, 317, 318, 319, 723–724, 731–732
Colitis
  Clostridium difficile-related, 478, 494
  Crohn's. See Crohn's disease
  cytomegalovirus-related, 470, 495–496, 497
  in defunctionalized colon, 710
  diarrhea associated with, 368
  indeterminate, 379
  ischemic, 465, 474–475, 509–510
  microscopic, 438–440, 487, 550, 552
    collagenous, 438, 439, 440, 550, 552
    lymphocytic, 438, 439, 440
  pseudomembranous, 435–438, 470
  radiation-induced, 440–441
  ulcerative, 178, 185, **379–387,** 561

Colitis (*Continued*)
  adenomatous colonic polyps associated with, 410, 544
  arthritis associated with, 547, 548, 551
  as colorectal cancer risk factor, 543
  definition of, 379, 708
  differentiated from bacterial dysentery, 474
  differentiated from Crohn's disease, 369, 370–371, 379, 474, 708–709
  drug-related exacerbation of, 386
  extraintestinal manifestations of, 380–381
  as hepatic abscess cause, 282
  hepatic complications of, 381
  severe, 383–384
  surgical management of, 386
  surveillance of, 384, 385
  universal, 380
Colon
  barium enema examination of, 585
    as perforation cause, 704–705
  carcinoid tumors of, 573
  foreign bodies in, 529
  redundant sigmoid, 432
Colon cancer. *See* Colorectal cancer
Colonic marker studies, for constipation, 414
Colonography, computed tomographic, 411
Colonoscopy
  colonic polyp removal during, 401–402
  for colorectal cancer screening, 405, 411
    versus barium enema, 584
  correlation with fecal occult blood test results, 454, 455
  for intestinal ischemia evaluation, 507
  for microscopic colitis evaluation, 438–439
  for pseudomembranous colitis evaluation, 436
  surveillance, 384, 542, 543, 544
  "virtual," for colorectal cancer screening, 411
Colorectal cancer, **401–412**
  acromegaly associated with, 571
  arthritis associated with, 557
  Crohn's disease-related, 544
  endoscopic screening and surveillance of, 542–544
  endosonographic evaluation of, 659
  Gardner's syndrome-related, 564
  genetic factors in, 401, 405–409
  hereditary nonpolyposis, 401, 405–406, 407, 408–409, 543
  metastatic, 216
    imaging of, 593
  prevention of, 410, 411
  resection of, 404, 543
  risk factors for, 404, 543, 544
  screening for, 405, 410, 411
    barium enema *versus* colonoscopy, 584
    endoscopic, 542–544
  staging of, 402, 403
  ulcerative colitis-related, 385, 543
Colorectal surgery, **706–717**

Colostomy, 420
Common bile duct cancer, 282
Complementary and alternative medicines (CAMs). *See also* Herbal remedies
  hepatotoxicity and drug interactions of, 227
Computed tomography (CT)
  for abdominal pain evaluation, 461
  for appendicitis evaluation, 433
  for biliary colic evaluation, 732
  of caustic ingestion injury, 66
  of diverticulitis, 424, 425–426
  of esophageal cancer, 52
  of hemochromatosis, 289
  for interventional procedure guidance, 592, 593
  for intestinal ischemia evaluation, 506
  of liver abscess, 283
  of nonalcoholic fatty liver disease, 249
  for pancreatitis diagnosis, 333, 345
  of simple hepatic cysts, 313
  of small bowel obstruction, 584
  triphasic, of hepatic masses, 215
Computed Tomography Severity Index, for pancreatitis prognosis, 336
Conjunctivitis, 473, 553
Constipation, 413–417
  effect of dietary fiber on, 534
  hypercalcemia-related, 571
  idiopathic slow transit, 112
  irritable bowel disease-related, 532, 535, 536
Contraception. *See also* Oral contraceptives
  for liver disease patients, 201
  use during and after ribavirin therapy, 140
Contractures, Dupuytren's, 234
Contrast media, 579–580
Contrast studies
  of diverticulitis, 424, 426
  of sigmoid volvulus, 714
Copper
  deficiency or toxicity of, 514
  hepatic concentration of, in Wilson's disease, 123, 152, 293–294, 305
Coronary artery disease, 34
  differentiated from gastroesophageal reflux disease, 21, 22
Corticosteroids
  as alcoholic hepatitis treatment, 233
  as autoimmune hepatitis treatment, 166–171, 172
  as caustic ingestion treatment, 65–66
  as diverticulitis cause, 425
  as eosinophilic gastroenteritis treatment, 365
  fetal effects of, 203
  hepatotoxicity of, 224
  as reactive arthritis treatment, 555
  use in liver transplantation patients, 260
Costochondritis, 34
Cough, gastroesophageal reflux disease-related, 20, 26
Councilman bodies, 297, 300
Courvoisier's sign, 352

Cowden's disease, 408, 564–565, 706
CREST syndrome, 177, 178, 212
Cricopharyngeal "bar," 75
"Criminal nerve of Grassi," in vagotomy, 689
Crohn's disease, 100, **368–378,** 561
   appendectomy in, 433
   arthritis associated with, 547, 548, 551
   as colorectal cancer risk factor, 544
   definition of, 708
   diarrhea associated with, 365, 368
   differentiated from
      bacterial dysentery, 474
      ulcerative colitis, 369, 370–371, 379, 474,
         708–709
   diseases which mimic, 369–370
   extraintestinal manifestations of, 373
   gallbladder disease associated with, 317
   genetic factors in, 372
   as hepatic abscess cause, 282
   histopathology of, 369, 370
   ileal resection in, as diarrhea cause, 365
   primary sclerosing cholangitis-related, 178
   as small bowel cancer risk factor, 373
   stricturing-type, 375
   "string sign" of, 369, 370
   surgical treatment of, 703
   surveillance schedule in, 544
Crohn's Disease Activity Index (CDAI), 368–369
Cromoglycate sodium, 394
Cronkhite-Canada syndrome, 706
Cryoglobulinemia
   autoimmune hepatitis-related, 153
   hepatitis C-related, 208, 209
   mixed, 208
Cryoglobulins, 209
Cryptococcosis, 31, 363
Cryptosporidiosis, 469, 470, 497, 498
Cullen's sign, 561
Cushing, Harvey, 735
Cyclizine (Marezine), 520
Cyclooxygenase-2 (COX-2) inhibitors, 445, 447, 541
   as esophageal cancer prophylaxis, 54
   as gastritis cause, 82
   as gastritis treatment, 81
Cyclospora, 469
Cyclosporine, 259, 260
   as autoimmune hepatitis treatment, 174
   drug interactions of, 261
   fetal effects of, 203
   neurotoxicity of, 260
Cystadenocarcinoma, 214, 599, 703
Cystadenoma, 599
   biliary, 214
   serous, 356, 358, 359
Cystic fibrosis, chronic pancreatitis associated
     with, 343
Cysts
   choledochal, 728
   duplication, 105

Cysts (*Continued*)
   epidermoid, 564
   gastric, 660
   hepatic, 214, 219–220, 312–313, 595, 724–725
     alcohol sclerosis of, 597
     simple/solitary, 313
   hepatobiliary, **310–316**
   hydatid (echinococcal), 311, 312, 313–315, 598,
     725–726
   ovarian, 461–462
   pancreatic, **356–360**
     endoscopic ultrasound-guided biopsy of, 666–667
   submucosal gastric, 105
Cytochrome P-450 systems, 223, 234, 261
   in proton pump inhibitor metabolism, 27
Cytology, of ascitic fluid, 269
Cytomegalovirus infections, 177, 304
   as acute abdomen cause, 463
   in AIDS patients, 492, 493, 495–496, 497
   as colitis cause, 470
   as Crohn's disease mimic, 369
   esophageal, 29
     as esophagitis cause, 31
   post-liver transplantation, 261, 262, 263
Cytotoxic T lymphocyte antigen, as autoimmune
     hepatitis treatment, 175

D

Daclizumab, 260
Danazol, hepatotoxicity of, 227
Dane particle, 129
Defecation, normal mechanism of, 413
Defecography, 414, 415, 419, 584–585
   cine, 714
Deflazacort, as autoimmune hepatitis treatment, 174
Dermatitis herpetiformis, 153, 557, 562, 563
Dermatologic manifestations, of gastrointestinal
     disease, **559–566**
Dermatomyositis, 390
Desmopressin, 446
Dexamethasone, 66
Diabetes mellitus
   chronic pancreatitis-related, 344
   diarrhea associated with, 567, 569
   excessive glycemic control in, 569
   focal fatty liver associated with, 219
   gallbladder disease associated with, 317
   gastrointestinal disorders associated with, 567
   gastroparesis associated with, 111, 113, 115, 116,
     567, 568
   insulin-dependent, 153
   liver transplantation-related, 264
   as nonalcoholic fatty liver disease risk factor, 247,
     248–249
   as pancreatic cancer risk factor, 352
*Diagnostic and Statistical Manual of Mental Disorders
     (DSM)*
   eating disorders diagnostic criteria of, 523, 524
   alcohol-related diseases diagnostic criteria of, 231

Diarrhea
  abdominal angina-related, 508
  acute, **465–475**
  in AIDS/HIV-infected patients, 469, 470, 478,
      494–498
  bile acid, 487–488
  bloody, 469, 470, 474
  carcinoid syndrome-related, 573
  chronic, **476–490**
    differentiated from irritable bowel syndrome,
      486
  classification of, 477–478
  Crohn's disease-related, 365, 368
  diabetes mellitus-related, 567, 569
  drug-induced, 470
  erythema nodosum-related, 560
  fatty, 479, 484–485
  hospital-acquired, 470
  iatrogenic, 486, 487
  immunoproliferative small intestinal disease-
      related, 366
  inflammatory, 479, 485, 486
  in institutionalized patients, 478
  intestinal ischemia-related, 505
  irritable bowel disease-related, 532
  malabsorption-related, 479, 484
  maldigestion-related, 479, 484, 485
  mechanisms of, 476, 477
  medullary thyroid cancer-related, 574
  microscopic colitis-related, 438
  osmotic, 477, 480, 481
  peptic ulcer surgical treatment-related, 694
  radiation-related, 440
  secretory, 477, 478, 480, 481–482, 484, 488
    systemic diseases associated with, 482, 483
  travelers', 472, 478
  ulcerative colitis-related, 368
  Whipple's disease-related, 363
Diastase, 122
Diazepam
  gastric emptying effects of, 113
  hepatotoxicity of, 225
Didanosine, as pancreatitis cause, 331
Dientamoeba fragilis infections, 469
Diet
  BRAT, 473
  for carcinoid syndrome treatment, 573
  for colorectal cancer prevention, 404
  for diabetic gastroparesis management, 568
  for diverticulitis management, 423
  for eosinophilic gastroenteritis management,
      394–395
  gluten-free, 563
  high-fiber, 416, 417
  oral, 511–512
  for ulcerative colitis management, 385
Dietary factors
  in esophageal cancer, 51
  in gastric cancer, 85

4,4'-Diethylamino ethyl hexestrol, hepatotoxicity of,
    224
Dieulafoy's ulcers, 444
"Difficult pylorus" sign, 45
Diffuse esophageal spasm (DES), relationship with
    achalasia, 43
Dilation, esophageal, 25
  in caustic ingestion injury patients, 67
Diltiazem
  as achalasia treatment, 46
  hepatotoxicity of, 225, 249
  interaction with tacrolimus and cyclosporine, 261
Dimenhydrinate (Dramamine), 520
Diphenhydramine, gastric emptying effects of, 113
Diphenoxylate, 488, 489, 569
Discriminant function value, 233
Dissolution therapy, for gallstones, 320, 321
Diuretics
  as cirrhosis-related ascites treatment, 275, 276
  as pancreatitis cause, 331
Diverticula
  as bacterial overgrowth cause, 397
  definition of, 422
  esophageal
    epiphrenic, 74, 75
    traction, 74, 75
    Zenker's, 15, 16, 74–75, 518, 527
  location of, 422–423
  Meckel's, 91, 432, 456, 462
Diverticulitis, **422–430**
  differentiated from appendicitis, 432
  as hepatic abscess cause, 282
  imaging of, 424, 425–426
  perforated, 426
  surgical treatment for, 703–704
  treatment of, 426–429
Diverticulosis, 423
  jejunal, 248
bDNA (deoxyribonucleic acid) assay, 130
Domperidone, 115, 568
  effect on esophageal sphincter pressure, 21
"Double duct sign," 588–589
Down syndrome, 20
Doxycycline, as esophageal injury cause, 57
Drainage
  of fluid collections, 591, 595
  of hepatic or parahepatic abscesses, 284, 596–597
  percutaneous transhepatic biliary, 603–605
Drug abuse
  as acute abdominal pain cause, 464
  hepatotoxicity of, 229
Drugs. *See also specific drugs*
  as diarrhea cause, 486, 487
  gastric emptying effects of, 113
  hepatotoxicity of, 162, **222–230**, 301–302
  as nausea and vomiting cause, 519
  as pancreatitis cause, 331
Dumping syndrome, 695
Duodenal stump disruption, 694

Duodenal ulcers, 703
  as gastrointestinal hemorrhage cause, 444, 693
  Helicobacter pylori-related, 93–94, 96
  perforated, 692
Duodenitis, 444
  eosinophilic, 394
Duodenum
  cancer of, 107
  obstruction of
    in chronic pancreatitis, 347
    ulcer-related, 703
Dyschezia, 415
Dysentery, 494
  acute bacterial, 474–475
  infectious, 465, 471–472
  seafood-related, 469
Dyskinesia
  biliary, 325, 723–724, 732
  gallbladder, 642
Dyspepsia, *Helicobacter pylori*-related, 94
Dysphagia
  achalasia-related, 44, 45, 677
  barium swallow evaluation of, 580–581
  caustic ingestion injury-related, 63
  definition of, 11
  differentiated from globus sensation (globus
    hystericus), 11
  eosinophilic esophagitis-related, 21
  esophageal cancer-related, 54
  esophageal strictures-related, 25
  esophageal web-related, 73
  gastroesophageal reflux disease-related, 16, 19,
    673, 674–675
  oropharyngeal, 12, 13–14
    differentiated from esophageal dysphagia, 13
  stroke-related, 14
  Zenker's diverticulum-related, 75
Dysphagia lusoria, 75
Dysplasia
  Barrett's esophagus-related, 70–71
  colonic, 384–385, 544
  esophageal, 539–540
    high-grade, 682
Dysplasia-associated lesion or mass (DALM),
  384–385

E

Eating disorders, 522–524
Ecchymoses, gastrointestinal hemorrhage-related,
  453
Echinococcosis, 311, 312, 313–315, 598,
  725–276
Ecstasy (3,4-methylene dioxymethamphetamine),
  hepatotoxicity of, 229
Edrophonium, 39
Elastase, fecal content of, in pancreatitis, 345
Elderly patients
  acute abdominal pain in, 462
  oropharyngeal dysphagia in, 13

Electrocautery, 735
  as small bowel injury cause, 732–733
Electrogastrography, 114
Electromyography, for fecal incontinence evaluation,
  419
Embolism, as ischemic bowel disease risk factor, 503,
  505
Embolization, as gastrointestinal hemorrhage
  treatment, 607
Empyema, spontaneous bacterial, 270–271
Enalapril, hepatotoxicity of, 227
Encephalopathy
  cirrhosis-related, 446
  hepatic, 166–167, 234, 446
  pancreatic, 336
  Wernicke's, 234
Endocarditis, intravenous drug abuse-related, 464
Endocrine disorders, **567–574**
  as diarrhea cause, 482, 483, 484
  drug therapy for, hepatotoxicity of, 226–227
Endometriosis, 715
Endoscopic procedures. *See also*
    Cholangiopancreatography, endoscopic
    retrograde
  diagnostic applications of
    achalasia evaluation, 45, 46, 678
    cancer screening and surveillance, **538–545**
    caustic ingestion evaluation, 64–65
    caustic ingestion injury evaluation, 61
    diarrhea evaluation, 466
    diverticulitis evaluation, 424
    eosinophilic esophagitis evaluation, 21
    esophageal cancer evaluation, 51–52
    gastric lymphoma evaluation, 103
    gastric polyps evaluation, 99–100
    gastroesophageal reflux disease evaluation, 674
    gastrointestinal hemorrhage evaluation, 454,
      455
    pill-induced esophageal injury evaluation, 57
    submucosal lesion evaluation, 105, 106
  as esophageal perforation cause, 704
  therapeutic applications of
    for gastroesophageal reflux disease, 25, 27
    for gastrointestinal hemorrhage, 445
    for pancreatitis-related pain, 349
Endoscopic retrograde cholangiopancreatography
    (ERCP). *See* Cholangiopancreatography,
    endoscopic retrograde
Enema
  barium. *See* Barium enema/studies
  for constipation treatment, 416
  contrast
    for diverticulitis evaluation, 424, 426
    for sigmoid volvulus evaluation, 714
  small bowel (enteroclysis), 455, 583–585
Enflurane, hepatotoxicity of, 229
Entamoeba histolytica infections, 281, 285, 465, 469,
  471, 494
Enteric fever, 467

Enteritis, radiation-related, 716

Enterobacter infections, 282, 427, 723

Enteroclysis (small bowel enema), 455, 583–585

Enterococcus infections, 337

Enterocolitis
  AIDS-related, 494
  cytomegalovirus-related, 495–496

Enteropathy
  gluten-sensitive. *See* Celiac disease
  nonsteroidal anti-inflammatory drugs-related,
    363–364
  protein-losing
    abdominal angina-related, 508
    intestinal ischemia-related, 505

Enzyme-linked immunosorbent assay (ELISA), for
  hepatitis C, 130

Eosinophilia
  gastroenteritis-related, 364–365, **388–396**
  pancreatic cancer-related, 556
  pancreatic panniculitis-related, 557–558

Eosinophilia-myalgia syndrome, 389

Eosinophilic gastroenteritis, 364–365, **388–396**

Episcleritis, 380–381

Epistaxis, hereditary hemorrhagic telangiectasia-
  related, 563

Epithelial tumors, hepatic, 214

Epstein-Barr virus infections, 304

Erythema
  necrolytic migratory, 565
  palmar, 196, 234

Erythema nodosum, 153, 380–381, 553, 560, 561

Erythromycin, 115, 521
  interaction with tacrolimus and cyclosporine,
    261

Erythromycin estolate, hepatotoxicity of, 228

Escherichia coli, gastrointestinal content of, 397

Escherichia coli infections, 282, 337, 465, 466, 468,
  471, 723

Esomeprazole, 24
  as *Helicobacter pylori* infection treatment, 95

Esomeprazole (Nexium), 28

Esophageal acid clearance time, 22

Esophageal cancer, **51–55,** 681–683
  achalasia-related, 46, 681
  adenocarcinoma, 51, 54, 69, 70–71
  arthritis associated with, 557
  caustic ingestion-related, 63
  diagnosis of, 682
  endoscopic screening and surveillance of,
    538–540, 682
  endosonographic evaluation of, 655–656
  intramural pseudodiverticulosis-related, 77
  metastatic, 216
  palliative therapies for, 54
  risk actors for, 681–682
  screening for, 51
  staging of, 52–54, 682
    endosonographic, 655, 656, 682
  surveillance for, 51–52

Esophageal cancer (*Continued*)
  treatment of, 682–683, 704
    curative therapies, 53–54

Esophageal felinization, 75

Esophageal function tests, 22

Esophageal motility
  disorders of, 36, 37, 38, 40
    as chest pain cause, 34
  ineffective, 674–675
  nuclear medicine studies of, 643–644

Esophageal rings, 56, 73–74

Esophageal sphincter
  lower (LES), 17
    in achalasia, 43, 44, 45, 46, 47–48, 678,
      679, 681
    balloon dilation of, 47–48
    competency evaluation of, 23
    defective, 674
    in gastroesophageal reflux disease, 20, 21, 674
    in hiatal hernia, 673, 674
    "hypertensive," 38
    myotomy of, 75
    pneumatic dilation of, 679, 681
  upper (UES), 17
    in Zenker's diverticulum, 74

Esophageal webs, 73

Esophagectomy, 70, 112, 683

Esophagitis, **29–33**
  acute alkali, 61
  in AIDS/HIV patients, 29, 30, 32
  bacterial, 32
  cytomegalovirus, 29, 31, 32
  eosinophilic, 21
  fungal, 30–31
    candidal, 29–31, 31, 77, 491
  as gastrointestinal hemorrhage cause, 444
  infectious, 29
  monilial, 30
  pill-induced, 21
  viral, 31–32
    herpes viruses-related, 29, 30, 31, 32

Esophagogastroduodenoscopy, 35, 58
  for biliary colic evaluation, 732

Esophagography, 682

Esophagopharyngeal reflux (EPR), 26, 27

Esophagoscopy, 682

Esophagus
  anomalies of, **73–77**
  Barrett's, 23, 26, 35, **69–72,** 673
    endoscopic surveillance of, 538–539
    as esophageal cancer risk factor, 69, 70–71,
      681, 682
    esophageal cancer surveillance of, 51–52
    gastroesophageal reflux disease associated
      with, 538–539
    screening for, 54
    short-segment, 540
    short-term, 69
  cancer of. *See* Esophageal cancer

Esophagus (*Continued*)
  caustic injury to, 540
  as chest pain cause, **34–42**
  comparison with the oropharynx, 15
  congenital stenosis of, 76
  dysmotility of, 36, 37, 38, 40
    as chest pain cause, 34
  foreign bodies in, 529
  infections of, **29–33**
  "irritable," 39–40
  "nutcracker," 37
  perforation of, 704
  pH of, ambulatory monitoring of, 35–36, 39
  physiologic narrowing of, 58–59
  pill-induced injury of, 56–59
  provocation testing of, 38–39
  "sigmoid," 45
  spasms of, 34, 37, 38
  surgery of, **673–686**
  tuberculosis of, 32
  ulcers of, AIDS-related, 492
Estrogens
  hepatotoxicity of, 249
  as pancreatitis cause, 331
Extracorporeal shock-wave lithotripsy, 320, 321

F
Factor replacement therapy, 446
Famciclovir, as hepatitis B treatment, 149
Familial adenomatous polyposis (FAP) syndrome,
    100, 107, 401, 405–406, 407, 408, 541
Famotidine, 24
Fasciitis, eosinophilic, 390
Fasting breath hydrogen test, 399
Fat, dietary
  fecal excretion of, 361
  malabsorption of, 361, 516
Fatty liver disease, nonalcoholic (NAFLD),
    245–253
Fecal chymotrypsin test, 345
Fecal elastase test, 345
Fecal impaction, 415
Fecal incontinence, 417–420, 486
  differentiated from diarrhea, 476
Fecal occult blood test (FOBT), 405, 453–454,
    542
Feces, fat excretion in, 361
FEESST (flexible endoscopic evaluation of
    swallowing with sensory testing), 11
Felinization, esophageal, 75
Ferritin
  hemochromatosis-related increase of, 122
  inherited liver disease-related increase of, 304
  nonalcoholic fatty liver disease-related increase
    of, 245
  serum levels of, 289
Fetal loss, ulcerative colitis treatment-related,
    385–386
α-Fetoprotein, 215, 219

Fever
  acute abdomen-related, 701
  of unknown origin, 304
Fiber, dietary, 416, 419, 534–535
Fibroma
  gastric, 105
  sclerotic, 564
Fibrosis, hepatic, 247, 296
  grading of, 300
  perisinusoidal, 250
Fistula
  anorectal, 712, 713
  colovaginal, 425
  colovesicular, 425, 426
  diverticulitis-related, 425, 426
  enteric, 397
  pancreatic, 340, 347, 348
  of small bowel, as diarrhea cause, 484
  tracheoesophageal, esophageal atresia
    associated with, 76
Fistulography, 590
Flexible endoscopic evaluation of swallowing
    with sensory testing (FEESST), 11
"Florid duct lesions," 180
Fluconazole, 491
  as candidal esophagitis treatment, 30
  candidal resistance to, 30
  interaction with tacrolimus and cyclosporine,
    261
Flucytosine, hepatotoxicity of, 228
Fluid collections
  aspiration or drainage of, 591, 595, 596
  intraabdominal, 601–602
  pancreatic, 600
  renal and perirenal, 601
  retroperitoneal, 601–602
Fluid resuscitation, in upper gastrointestinal
    hemorrhage patients, 444
Fluorine, deficiency or toxicity of, 514
Fluoroquinolone, 184
Fluoroscopy, gastrointestinal, 584, 592, 603–606
  video, of Barrett's esophagus, 73
Flushing, carcinoid syndrome-related, 573
Flutamide, hepatotoxicity of, 224
Folate/folic acid
  bacterial overgrowth-related increase in,
    398, 399
  deficiency of, 382, 514, 516, 720, 721
  toxicity of, 514
Food poisoning, 472
Foreign bodies, in gastrointestinal tract, **527–530**
Foscarnet, 32, 496–497
Fructose, 419
Fundoplication
  delayed gastric emptying associated
    with, 111
  with Heller's myotomy, 704
  as ineffective esophageal motility treatment,
    674–675

Fungal infections. *See also specific types of fungal infections*
  as hepatic abscess cause, 726
  as pancreatitis cause, 332
Furazolidone, 95
Fusidic acid, 438
Fusobacterium nucleatum infections, 282

G

Gallbladder
  Courvoisier's, 727
  distended, decompression of, 736
  dysmotility of, 322
  hydrops, 723, 727–728
  inflammation of, 723–724
  perforation of, 432
  polyps of, 321–322
  "porcelain," 322, 724
Gallbladder cancer, 587, 724, 727
Gallbladder disease, **317–323**
  as pancreatitis cause, 703
Gallbladder dyskinesia, 642
Gallbladder ejection fraction, 322
Gallbladder sludge, 317–318, 319, 320, 321
Gallium-67 scan, 648
Gallstone ileus, 319, 715, 724
Gallstones, 317. *See also* Cholelithiasis
  asymptomatic, 319–320
  as gallbladder cancer cause, 724
  as pancreatitis cause, 331
  during pregnancy, 317
  treatment of, 319–320
  ultrasonographic detection of, 320–321
GALT (gut-associated lymphoid tissue), 551
Gamma-glutamyl transaminases, 127, 128
Gamma-glutamyl transpeptidase, as hepatic function
    indicator, 119
  in focal liver masses, 214
  during pregnancy, 196, 197
    in acute fatty liver, 198
    in intrahepatic cholestasis, 197
Ganciclovir, 32, 496–497
Ganglioneuromatosis, intestinal, 706
Gangrene, appendicitis-related, 738
Gardner's syndrome, 107, 405, 406, 706
Gas, intestinal, 576–579
Gastrectomy
  as bile reflux gastritis cause, 83
  as diarrhea cause, 486
  distal, 691
  as gastric stump cancer risk factor, 541–542, 698
  survival rates after, 86
Gastric antral vascular ectasia (GAVE), 100, 108, 456, 457
Gastric bypass, as obesity treatment, 719–720, 721
  as gastric stasis cause, 112
  Roux-en-Y, 111, 695, 696, 719–720, 721

Gastric cancer, **85–89**
  adenocarcinoma, 85, 86, 87, 94, 100, 657, 658
  endoscopic screening and surveillance of, 541–542
  endosonographic evaluation and staging of, 656–658
  gastric polyps as risk factor for, 99, 107
  gastric stump, 86, 541–542, 698
  Helicobacter pylori-related, 82, 94
  lymphoma, 85, 94, 100, 101–102, 658
    aggressive, 88
    MALT (mucosal-associated lymphoid tumor), 87, 90, 95, 100, 102–104
    staging of, 87
  metastatic, 216
  staging of, 86, 87, 656–658
Gastric emptying and motility, 110
  effect of drugs on, 113
  nuclear medicine studies of, 638, 642–643
Gastric folds, large/thickened, 100–106
Gastric outlet
  anatomic abnormalities of, 694
  obstruction of, 693–694
Gastric pacer, 721–722
Gastric stump cancer, 86, 541–542, 698
Gastric tissue, ectopic, 647
Gastric ulcers
  benign differentiated from malignant, 583
  as gastrointestinal hemorrhage cause, 444, 693
  giant, 697
  Helicobacter pylori-related, 93
  perforated, 691, 692
  types of, 689–690
    operative procedures for, 690–691
  upper gastrointestinal series evaluation of, 583
Gastrinoma, 484, 572, 696-697. *See also* Zollinger-Ellison syndrome
  metastatic, 651
Gastrinoma triangle, 697
Gastritis, 21, **79–84**
  acute, 79, 80
  atrophic, gastroparesis associated with, 112
  autoimmune, 82
  bile reflux, 83, 695–696
  chronic, 79–80, 81, 82
    Helicobacter pylori-related, 79, 80, 81–83, 93, 94
    nonspecific, 83
  classification of, 79–80
  eosinophilic, 83–84, 100
  granulomatous, 83, 100
  immune, 567
  lymphocytic, 82–83
  stress-related, 81, 336
Gastritis cystica profunda, 100
Gastroduodenostomy
  Billroth I and II, 687, 688, 689, 694
  Jaboulay, 688, 689, 694

Gastroenteritis
acute, 467
eosinophilic, 364–365, **388–396**
rotavirus-related, 473
viral, 473
Gastroenterostomy, 641
Gastroesophageal barrier, compromise of, 21
Gastroesophageal reflux disease (GERD), **19–28,**
673–676
antireflux surgical treatment of, 675–676
atypical symptoms of, 26
barium swallow evaluation of, 580–581
Barrett's esophagus-related, 538–539
as chest pain cause, 34, 35, 38
differentiated from
achalasia, 44
eosinophilic gastroenteritis, 388
dysphagia associated with, 16
as esophageal cancer risk factor, 681–682
gastroparesis associated with, 112
globus sensation associated with, 11
Helicobacter pylori infection relationship with, 96
laryngeal symptoms of, 26
lower esophageal sphincter dilation-related, 48
medical conditions which mimic, 21, 22
as pill-induced esophageal injury risk factor, 56,
57, 58, 59
postoperative, 47
symptoms of, 673
treatment for, 23–25
Gastrointestinal disease
dermatologic manifestations of, **559–566**
rheumatologic manifestations of, **547–558**
Gastrointestinal stromal tumors (GISTs), 88,
105–106, 107
Gastrointestinal tract
bacterial overgrowth of, **397–400**
Helicobacter pylori localization in, 91
hemorrhage in. *See* Hemorrhage, gastrointestinal
Gastrojejunostomy, 688, 690, 694
Roux-en-Y, 695, 696
Gastroparesis, 20, 21, **110–117,** 519
diabetes mellitus-related, 567, 568
gastric pacing in, 521
postoperative, 694
Gastropathy, portal hypertensive, 456
GAVE (gastric antral vascular ectasia), 100, 108,
456, 457
GB-C virus, 132
Gene therapy, for autoimmune hepatitis, 175
Genetic testing, in acute fatty liver of pregnancy
patients, 199
Genitourinary cancer, metastatic, 216
Gestational age, relationship with maternal liver
disease, 200
Giardiasis, 469, 470, 495, 496
Gingivitis, 153
Ginseng, adverse effects of, 730
Glasgow criteria, for pancreatitis prognosis, 335

Glipizide, hepatotoxicity of, 226
Glisson's capsule, distention of, 241
Globus sensation (globus hystericus), 11
Glomerulonephritis, 153
membranoproliferative, 208
Glomus tumors, 105
Glossitis, Paterson-Brown-Kelly syndrome-related,
73
Glucagonoma, 484, 572
Glucagon-producing tumors, 565
Glucocorticoids, hepatotoxicity of, 249
Glu474Gln mutation, 198, 199
Glyburide, hepatotoxicity of, 226
Goiter, 564
Gold therapy, hepatotoxicity of, 225
Goodsall's rule, 713
Graft-*versus*-host disease, 308
Gram-negative bacterial infections, 271, 274
Gram-positive bacterial infections, 66
Gram stain, of ascitic fluid, 269
Granular cell tumors, 105, 660
Granulocytopenic patients, candidal esophagitis
treatment in, 30
Granuloma
Crohn's disease-related, 376
eosinophilic, 390
hepatic, 297, 303–304
drug-related, 225
Grapefruit juice, hepatotoxic drug interactions
of, 227
Graves' disease, autoimmune hepatitis-associated,
153
Grey Turner's sign, 561
Griseofulvin, hepatotoxicity of, 228
Guillain-Barré syndrome, 467
Gut-associated lymphoid tissue (GALT), 551
Gynecomastia, 234

H
HAART (highly-active antiretroviral therapy), 494,
497, 498
Halothane, hepatotoxicity of, 223, 229
Hamartoma, 564, 706
Hamartomatous polyp syndromes, 405–406, 408
Hashimoto's disease (autoimmune thyroiditis), 153,
210, 567
Head and neck cancer, dysphagia associated
with, 15
Heartburn, 19, 26, 673, 677. *See also*
Gastroesophageal reflux disease (GERD)
achalasia-related, 44
therapy for, 23
α-Heavy-chain disease, 366
Heavy metal poisoning, 483
Helicobacter bilis, 90
Helicobacter heilmannii, 90
Helicobacter hepaticus, 90
Helicobacter pullorum, 90
Helicobacter pylori, characteristics of, 90

Helicobacter pylori infections, 444, 446
  diagnosis of, 92–93
  as duodenal ulcer cause, 93–94
  as dyspepsia cause, 94
  as gastric cancer cause, 85–86, 87, 94
  as gastric polyps cause, 100
  as gastritis cause, 79, 80, 81–83, 93
  long-term consequences of, 82
  as mucosa-associated lymphoid tissue (MALT) cause, 102, 104
  as peptic ulcer cause, **90–97**
  as stomach cancer cause, 51, 541–452
  as thickened gastric folds cause, 100
Helicobacter winghamensis, 90
HELLP (hemolysis, elevated liver enzymes, low platelets) syndrome, 198, 199, 200
Hemangioblastoma, of the central nervous system, 359
Hemangioendothelioma, hepatic, 242
Hemangioma, hepatic, 219–220, 597–598, 644–645
  cavernous, 214, 215, 242, 243, 726–727
  giant, 215
Hematochromatosis, 304–305
Hematocrit
  in acute pancreatitis, 336
  in upper gastrointestinal hemorrhage, 444
Hemoccult fecal blood tests, 453
Hemochromatosis, 287–291
  arthritis associated with, 211, 212, 213
  diagnostic tests for, 122, 123
  differentiated from autoimmune hepatitis, 152
  genetics of, 211–212
  hereditary, 287, 288–289
    comparison with Wilson's disease, 294
  liver disease associated with, 213
Hemolytic uremia syndrome, 471
Hemorrhage
  gastrointestinal
    alcoholic hepatitis-related, 233
    angiographic evaluation of, 606–607
    chronic pancreatitis-related, 347
    diverticulitis-related, 422
    duodenal ulcers-related, 693
    gastric ulcers-related, 693
    gastric varices-related, 107–108
    gastrointestinal reflux disease-related, 19
    laser photocoagulation therapy for, 441
    lower, differentiated from upper
    nuclear medicine-assisted localization of, 648–649, 650
    occult or obscure, **453–458**
    peptic ulcers-related, 693, 703
    percutaneous transcatheter treatment of, 606–607
    upper, **443–448**
  intrahepatic, preeclampsia-related, 199
  pseudoaneurysm-related, 358
  variceal, 444, 445

Hemorrhage (*Continued*)
  during pregnancy, 202
  transjugular intrahepatic portosystemic shunt treatment of, 202, 607–608, 610
Hemorrhoids, 456, 711–712
  external, 711
  internal, 711–712
Hemosuccus pancreaticus, 336, 358, 400
Heparin, effect on ulcerative colitis, 386
Hepatic artery, 236, 237, 238
  thrombosis of, 242, 262
Hepatic iron index (HII), 250, 290
Hepatic veins, 236, 237
Hepatitis
  acute, differentiated from chronic hepatitis, 126
  alcoholic, 232–234, 247, 298–299, 560
  allergic, 223–224
  autoimmune, 124, **151–165,** 248, 301
    autoantibodies associated with, 151, 152, 153, 155–156, 157–160, 161
    drug-related, 162
    genetic predisposition to, 162–164
    overlap syndromes of, 182
    treatment of, **166–176**
    types of, 152–155
    variant syndromes of, 172
    viral, 161
    with viral features, 173
    in women, 223
  biochemical abnormalities in, 127–128
  chronic
    biochemical abnormalities in, 128
    cryptogenic, 172
    differentiated from acute hepatitis, 126
    grading and staging of, 300
    histopathology of, 299–300
  drug-related, 162, 222, 225
    differentiated from autoimmune hepatitis, 152
    nitrofurantoin-related, 302
  fulminant, 257–258, 299
  giant-cell, 131–132
  halothane-related, 229
  ischemic, 240–241
  neonatal, 642
  symptoms of, 127
  transmission of, 127
  viral, **126–135,** 189
    histopathology of, 299–301
    as jaundice cause, 196
    as liver cancer cause, 214
    lupoid (type I autoimmune), 209, 212
    during pregnancy, 201
    rheumatologic manifestations of, 207–209
    treatment of, 132–133
Hepatitis A, 126, 128, 189
  liver biopsy findings in, 299
  perinatal transmission of, 203
  during pregnancy, 201
  prevention of, 133–134

Hepatitis A (*Continued*)
vaccine/immunoprophylaxis against, 137,
188–191, 194
in pregnant women, 203
Hepatitis B, 126, 129, 189
antiviral therapy for, 132–133, **143–150**
chronic, 126
diagnosis of, 128
liver biopsy findings in, 299
perinatal transmission of, 203–204
polyarteritis nodosa associated with, 207–208
post-liver transplantation, 149
during pregnancy, 201
rheumatologic manifestations of, 207–208
vaccine/immunoprophylaxis against, 128–129,
134, 137, 188–189, 191–194
in neonates, 204
Hepatitis B anticore antibody (HBcAb), 129
Hepatitis B core antibody-immunoglobulin M
(HBcAb-IgM), 143
Hepatitis B surface antibody (HBsAb), 128–129
Hepatitis B surface antigen (HBsAg), 128, 129,
143, 144
Hepatitis B virus-DNA polymerase chain reaction
assay, 143
Hepatitis C, 126, 189
antiviral therapy for, 133, **136–142**
chronic, 127
as cirrhosis cause, 140–141
diagnostic tests for, 130–131
differentiated from autoimmune hepatitis, 152
differentiated from liver transplant rejection,
261–262
fatty liver associated with, 252
genotype testing for, 137
human immunodeficiency virus (HIV)
infection-associated, 141
liver biopsy findings in, 299
liver transplantation treatment for, 258
perinatal
diagnosis of, 204–205
transmission of, 204
during pregnancy, 201
prevention of, 134
recurrent, after liver transplantation, 261–263,
265–266
rheumatologic manifestations of, 207,
208–209
Hepatitis D, 126, 189
chronic, 126
diagnosis of, 131
perinatal transmission of, 204
treatment of, 133
Hepatitis E, 126, 189, 194
diagnosis of, 131
pregnancy-related exacerbation of, 200
Hepatitis G, perinatal transmission of, 204
Hepatitis vaccines, **188–195**
Hepatitis viruses, types of, 126

Hepatobiliary diseases
cystic, **310–316**
dermatologic manifestations of, 559, 560
rheumatologic manifestations of, **207–213**
Hepatobiliary scans, 637, 638, 639–642, 723
Hepatobiliary surgery, **723–729**
Hepatocellular carcinoma, 214, 216–217, 727
autoimmune hepatitis-related, 170
chemoembolization of, 604
cirrhosis-related, 185, 216
drug-related, 224
fibrolamellar variant of, 218
fine-needle biopsy of, 219
hepatitis C-related, 131
histopathology of, 306–307
laboratory findings in, 217
primary biliary cirrhosis-related, 185
primary sclerosing cholangitis-related, 185
screening for, 219
treatment of, 218–219
liver transplantation as, 255
tumor marker for, 215
Hepatocellular injury
differentiated from cholestatic injury, 119
liver tests for, 120
Hepatocolithiasis, 179
Hepatocystic triangle, 730
Hepatoenterostomy, 311
Hepatoiminodiacetic acid (HIDA) scan, 461, 518,
732
Hepatoma, 644
Hepatomegaly
Budd-Chiari syndrome-related, 238, 239
ischemic hepatitis-related, 240
thyrotoxicosis-related, 568
Hepatopathy, congestive, 241
Hepatorenal syndrome, 278
Herbal remedies
gastrointestinal effects of, 515
hepatoprotective effects of, 229
hepatotoxicity of, 229
Hernia
hiatal, 456, 676–677
relationship with gastroesophageal reflux,
673–674
inguinal, 738
paraesophageal, 676–677
Herpes simplex virus infections
esophageal, 29, 31
as esophagitis cause, 31
pregnancy-related exacerbation of, 200
as proctitis cause, 494
Hiccups, 521–522
High-density lipoprotein (HDL), 179
Highly-active antiretroviral therapy (HAART), 494,
497, 498
Hilar obstruction, 604–605
Hirschsprung's disease, 415
short-segment, 415

Histamine receptor antagonists, 573
Histamine$_2$-receptor antagonists, 23, 24, 29–30, 446, 691
Histiocytosis X, 390
Histoplasmosis, 31, 363, 470
HLA (human leukocyte antigens)
    in autoimmune hepatitis, 164
    in enteropathic arthritis, 548, 549, 552
    in reactive arthritis, 554, 555
Hoarseness, gastroesophageal reflux disease-related, 20, 26, 27
Hospitals, *Clostridium difficile* epidemics in, 437
Human immunodeficiency virus (HIV) infection
    abdominal pain associated with, 462
    acute abdomen associated with, 463–464
    diarrhea associated with, 469
    esophagitis associated with, 32
    hepatitis C associated with, 141
    as liver transplantation contraindication, 258
    pancreatitis associated with, 493
Hyaline, in alcoholic hepatitis, 298
Hybridization tests, 130
Hydatid (echinococcal) cyst disease, 311, 312, 313–315, 598, 725–726
Hydralazine, hepatotoxicity of, 227
Hydrops, of the gallbladder, 723, 727–728
Hydrothorax
    hepatic, 269–270, 277
    pleural, 269–270
3-Hydroxy-3-methylglutaryl coenzyme A reductase inhibitors. *See* Statins
Hydroxyzine hydrochloride, 197
Hyperamylasemia, 333
Hypercalcemia
    gastrointestinal manifestations of, 571
    as pancreatitis cause, 332, 568
Hyperemesis gravidarum, 200
Hypereosinophilic syndrome, idiopathic, 389–390
Hypergammaglobulinemia, 151
Hyperimmune globulin, recommended dose of, 191
Hyperlipidemia, 333
Hyperlipidemia
    as nonalcoholic fatty liver disease risk factor, 247, 248
    primary biliary cirrhosis-related, 179
Hyperoxaluria, 348
    short bowel syndrome-related, 366
Hyperparathyroidism
    as pancreatitis cause, 568
    Wermer syndrome-related, 572
Hyperpigmentation, Addison's disease-related, 573
Hyperplasia, focal nodular, 216, 306, 726, 727
Hypersegmentation, 422
Hypertension
    liver transplantation-related, 264
    portal
        during pregnancy, 202

Hypertension (*Continued*)
    transjugular intrahepatic portosystemic shunt treatment of, 607–608
    ultrasonographic evaluation of, 661
Hypertriglyceridemia, as pancreatitis cause, 332, 568
Hypoglycemia, 570–571
    biochemical, 569
    pathologic, 569
Hypogonadism, 234
Hypopharynx, squamous cell carcinoma of, 73
Hypotension, pancreatitis-related, 336

I

Ibuprofen, hepatotoxicity of, 224, 225
Ileal pouch-anal anastomosis, 386, 708, 710
Ileal resection, 365
    as diarrhea cause, 487–488
Ileitis, backwash, 379
Ileocecal valve, absence or incompetence of, 397
Ileocolitis, Crohn's disease-related, 368, 369
Ileostomy, 386, 584, 708
    as bacterial overgrowth cause, 397
Ileus
    gallstone, 319, 715, 724
    paralytic, 397
    postoperative, 716
Imaging, 591–595. *See also* Radiology
Imatinib, 390
Imidazole, candidal resistance to, 30–31
Imipramine, hepatotoxicity of, 224
Immune system
    effect of incisions on, 731
    effect of laparoscopic surgery on, 731
Immunocompromised patients. *See also* Acquired immunodeficiency syndrome (AIDS); Human immunodeficiency virus (HIV) infection
    esophagitis in, 32
Immunoglobulin A deficiency, 485
Immunoglobulin M, 178–179
Immunoproliferative small intestinal disease (IPSID), 366
Immunoprophylaxis
    for hepatitis A, 189–190
    for hepatitis B, 191
    for hepatitis C, 194
Immunosuppressant therapy
    for autoimmune hepatitis, 173, 174
    for Crohn's disease, 374, 375
    in liver transplantation patients, 259–261
    side effects of, 264
    as pancreatitis cause, 331
    during pregnancy, 203, 385
Immunotherapy, endoscopic ultrasound-guided, 668–669
Incisions, effect on immune function, 731
Incontinence, fecal, treatment for, 419–420
Indocyanine green test, 119
Indomethacin, as esophageal injury cause, 58

Infections. *See also specific bacterial, fungal, and viral infections*
  esophageal, **29–33**
Infectious diseases
  as gastroparesis cause, 112
  hepatic, 725–726
Inflammation, subserosal/serosal, 392–393
Inflammatory bowel disease, 474
  as colorectal cancer cause, 404, 409, 410
  as diarrhea cause, 465, 466
  as macroamylasemia cause, 333
  as macrolipasemia cause, 333
  nuclear medicine studies of, 652
  rheumatic disorders associated with, 547–552, 554
  as ulcerative colitis cause, 379
Infliximab, 386
  as alcoholic hepatitis treatment, 233
  as Crohn's disease treatment, 375
Injection therapy, endoscopic ultrasound-guided, 668–669
Insulinoma, 570, 572
Insulin resistance, 246, 247
Intensive care unit patients, "hidden" sources of calories for, 512
Interferon, as hepatitis treatment, 132, 133, 137
Interferon, phenylated, 133
Interferon-alpha, phenylated, as hepatitis C treatment, 265
Interferon alpha-2b
  as hepatitis B treatment, 144–145, 146, 147
    "prednisone priming" prior to, 147
  phenylated, 137, 138, 139, 141–142, 145
Interleukin-10, recombinant, as autoimmune hepatitis treatment, 175
Intestinal bypass arthritis-dermatitis syndrome, 557
Intestinal wall, endosonographic anatomy of, 654
Intestines. *See also* Large intestine; Small intestine
  blood circulation and microcirculation in, 500–502
  chronic pseudo-obstruction of, 112
  foreign bodies in, 529
  motility disorders of, as bacterial overgrowth cause, 397, 398
  obstruction of
    acute, 463
    computed tomographic evaluation of, 584
    differential diagnosis of, 389
    dilation associated with, 575–578
    fluoroscopic-radiographic evaluation of, 584
    malignant, 390
    pancreatic pseudocyst-related, 400
    primary, 715
    radiographic findings in, 575–576
  perforation of, 527–528
    radiographic evaluation of, 506
Intraductal papillary mucinous neoplasm (IPMN), 356, 359
Intraesophageal balloon distention (IEBD), 39
Intravenous drug abuse, as endocarditis cause, 464

Iodine, deficiency or toxicity of, 514
Iodoquinol, 469
Iritis, 153
Iron
  absorption of, 287
  deficiency of, 287, 454–455, 514, 516, 571
    as anemia cause, 108, 410, 454–455, 516
    bariatric surgery-related, 720, 721
    Paterson-Brown-Kelly syndrome-related, 73
  distribution in body, 288
    hepatic concentration, 290
    in hereditary hemochromatosis, 289–290
    quantitative measurement of, 305
  toxicity of, 514
Iron-age index, 122
Iron-overload disorders, 287
  toxic manifestations of, 288
Irritable bowel syndrome, 325, 326, **531–537**
  constipation-predominant, 415–416
  differentiated from
    chronic diarrhea, 486
    eosinophilic gastroenteritis, 388, 389
  postinfectious, 533
  as thromboembolism risk factor, 381
Ischemic bowel disease, **500–510**
  focal (short segment), 504
  nonocclusive, 504, 505, 507, 508
  nonocclusive mesenteric (NOMI), 504, 507, 508
  occlusive, 503–505
  small bowel, 703
Ischemic heart disease, *Helicobacter pylori* infection associated with, 96
Islet cell tumors, 572
Isoflurane, hepatotoxicity of, 229
Isoniazid, hepatotoxicity of, 223, 224, 225, 228
Isospora belli infections, 470
Itraconazole, interaction with tacrolimus and cyclosporine, 261

J

Jaundice, 727–728
  alcoholic hepatitis-related, 233
  bilirubin levels in, 559
  cirrhosis-related, 178
  fulminant hepatitis-related, 257
  hepatitis-related, 127, 233, 257
  Mirizzi's syndrome-related, 738
  obstructive, 727–728
  pancreatic pseudocyst-related, 400
  in pregnancy, 196, 197
  primary sclerosing cholangitis-related, 178, 182
Jejunal intubation, for bacterial overgrowth diagnosis, 399
Jejunoileal bypass, 571
  as bacterial overgrowth cause, 397
Jejunojejunostomy, Roux-en-Y, 687
Jejunostomy, 116, 568
Jenner, Edward, 188
Johne's disease, 372

Joints
   involvement in enteropathic arthritis, 547
   involvement in reactive arthritis, 553
Juvenile polyposis syndrome, 405–406, 407

K

Kaposi's sarcoma, 100, 463–464, 492
Kayser-Fleischer rings, 123, 293
Kehr's sign, 701
Kennedy, John F., 573
Keratoconjunctivitis sicca. *See* Sjögren's syndrome
Keratoderma blennorrhagicum, 553
Ketoconazole
   hepatotoxicity of, 228
   interaction with tacrolimus and cyclosporine, 261
Ketoprofen, hepatotoxicity of, 224
Ketotifen, 394
Killian's dehiscence, 74
Klatskin's tumor, 218, 587, 727
Klebsiella infections, 282, 337, 427, 723
Kock's pouch, 708
Korsakoff's syndrome, 234
Kupffer cells, 304, 305
   in hereditary hemochromatosis, 288, 289–290
Kwashiorkor, 511
Kyphosis, 20

L

Lactase deficiency, 473
Lactose, 419
Lactose intolerance, 385
Lactulose-hydrogen breath test, 365–366
Lamivudine, as hepatitis B treatment, 144, 145, 146, 147–148
Lansoprazole
   as gastroesophageal reflux disease treatment, 24
   as *Helicobacter pylori* infection treatment, 95
Laparoscopic adjustable gastric band (Lap Band), 720–721
Laparoscopic surgery, **730–740**
   for acute abdomen evaluation, 702
   adrenalectomy, 737
   appendectomy, 433, 731
   for intestinal ischemia evaluation, 507
   for morbid obesity treatment, 719–721
   for perforated peptic ulcer treatment, 692–693
Laparotomy
   of acute abdomen, 702
   of appendicitis, 462
Lap Band (laparoscopic adjustable gastric band), 720–721
Large intestine. *See also* Anus; Colon
   obstruction of, 463, 715
Laser therapy, for esophageal cancer, 54, 683
Lavage, gastric, as caustic ingestion treatment, 64
Laxatives
   abuse of, 486–487
   bulk-forming, 416
   gastric emptying effects of, 113

Lean body mass (LBM), 511
Leiomyoblastoma, 105
Leiomyoma, 105, 660, 661
Leiomyosarcoma, 85, 105, 106, 660
Leukocytes, in stool, 465–466
Leukocytosis
   acute abdomen-related, 701
   hepatic abscess-related, 281
Lichen planus, 153
Linitis plastica, 100, 102
Lipase, pancreatitis-related increase of, 333
Lipid-lowering agents, 183
   hepatotoxicity of, 227
   statins
      hepatotoxicity of, 227
      use by nonalcoholic fatty liver disease patients, 250
Lipogranuloma, 304
Lipoma, 105, 106, 107, 660
Liposarcoma, gastric, 105
Lithotripsy, extracorporeal shock-wave, 320, 321
Liver
   abscess of, 214, **281–286,** 726
      amebic, 281, 283, 284
      aspiration of, 283–284
      drainage of, 284
      pyogenic, 281, 282, 283–285, 285
   alcohol metabolism in, 231–232
   enlarged. *See* Hepatomegaly
   fatty
      alcoholic, 219, 232, 233
      focal, 219
      histopathology of, 297–299
      of pregnancy, 198–199, 200
   histopathology of, **296–309**
      in autoimmune hepatitis, 151
      in bile duct disorders, 302–303
      in cholestasis, 301
      in drug injury, 301
      in fatty changes and steatohepatitis, 297–299
      in granulomatous inflammation, 303–304
      in inherited liver disease, 304–306
      microanatomy and injury patterns of, 296–297
      in neoplasms, 306–307
      in nonalcoholic fatty liver disease, 250–251
      in transplant recipients, 307–308
      in viral hepatitis, 299–301
   image-guided procedures in, 595–598
   iron content of, 304–305
      in hemochromatosis, 289–290
   mass lesions of
      benign tumors, 214–216, 644–645, 726–727
      focal, **214–221**
      nuclear medicine studies of, 644–645
   "nutmeg," 241
   vascular anatomy of, 236–237
   in Wilson's disease, 293

Liver-associated enzymes, 119. *See also* Alanine
aminotransferase; Aspartate aminotransferase;
Gamma glutamyl transpeptidase
Liver cancer, 727. *See also* Hepatocellular carcinoma
biopsy findings in, 594, 595
drug-related, 224–225
histopathology of, 306–307
markers for, 215
metastatic, 216
most common types of, 216–217
Liver disease, 209–213
abnormal iron studies in, 289
alcoholic, **231–235**
autoimmune, 124
bacterial infection prophylaxis in, 274
chronic, liver transplantation treatment for, 256
congenital/metabolic, liver transplantation
treatment for, 256
contraception in, 201
cystic, 724–725
drug-induced, **222–230**
hemochromatosis-related, 213
infectious, 725–726
inheritable forms of, **287–295**, 304–306
metabolic, 123
parasitic, 725–726
polycystic, 312–313
differentiated from simple hepatic cysts, 725
vascular, **236–244**
Liver failure
acute, liver transplantation treatment for, 256
drug-related, 257
fulminant, 257
Liver function, during pregnancy, 196
Liver function tests, 119, **119–125**
in liver transplant recipients, 307–308
Liver-kidney microsomal antibody type-1 (LKM-1),
123, 124
Liver/spleen scans, 644–645, 647–648
Liver transplantation, **254–267**, 307–308
as alcoholic liver disease treatment, 234
autoimmune hepatitis after, 172
as autoimmune hepatitis treatment, 167, 171–172
as bile duct cyst disease treatment, 311
as Budd-Chiari syndrome treatment, 240
as cirrhosis-related ascites treatment, 277
complications of, 262–263
contraindications to, 258–259
graft rejection in, 261–264, 307
as hepatic artery thrombosis cause, 242
hepatitis B after, 148
as hepatitis B-related cirrhosis treatment, 148
as hepatitis C-related cirrhosis treatment, 140–141
as hepatocellular carcinoma treatment, 218, 255
as hepatorenal syndrome treatment, 278
immunosuppressant therapy following, 259–261
side effects of, 264
living donor, 255–256
as nonalcoholic fatty liver disease treatment, 252

Liver transplantation (*Continued*)
pregnancy after, 202–203
as primary biliary cirrhosis treatment, 185–186
as primary sclerosing cholangitis treatment,
185–186
repeat, 264, 266
Liver tumors, benign, 214–216, 644–645, 726–727
Long chain 3-hydroxyacyl-CoA-dehydrogenase
(LCHAD) deficiency, 198, 199
Loperamide (Imodium), 471–472, 488, 489, 569, 573
Low back pain, differentiated from spinal arthritis,
548
Low density lipoprotein (LDL), 179
Lung cancer
endosonographic evaluation of, 659
metastatic, 216
non-small cell, ultrasound-guided fine needle
aspiration of, 665–666
small-cell, achalasia symptoms in, 45
Lycopene, as dermatosis cause, 559
Lye ingestion injury, 60–62
Lymphadenopathy, mediastinal, ultrasound-guided
fine needle aspiration of, 665–666
Lymphangiectasia, 364
Lymph nodes
endosonographic anatomy of, 654
ultrasound-guided fine-needle aspiration of, 664,
665
Lymphogranuloma venereum, 494
Lymphoma
B-cell, *Helicobacter pylori*-related, 82
celiac disease-associated, 362
endosonographic evaluation of, 660
gastric, 85, 94, 100, 101–102, 658
aggressive, 88
MALT (mucosal-associated lymphoid tumor),
87, 90, 95, 100, 102–104
staging of, 87
human immunodeficiency virus (HIV)-related,
463–464
primary hepatic, 214
Lymphoproliferative disorders, post-transplant, 264

M
Macroamylasemia, 333
Macroglobulinemia, 363
Macrolides, as gastritis cause, 79
Macrolipasemia, 333
Madelung's lipomatosis, 252
Magnesium
deficiency of, 514
toxicity of, 514
Magnetic resonance angiography, of focal liver
masses, 219
Magnetic resonance imaging (MRI)
of dysphagia lusoria, 75
of focal liver masses, 219
of hemochromatosis, 289
for hepatic iron content assessment, 122

Magnetic resonance imaging (MRI) (*Continued*)
  of hepatic masses, 215
  for interventional procedure guidance, 592, 593
  of liver abscess, 283
  of nonalcoholic fatty liver disease, 249
  of pancreatitis, 345
  of simple hepatic cysts, 313
Malabsorption, 361–362
  bacterial overgrowth-related, 398, 399
  as diarrhea cause, 479, 484
  of fat, 361
  immunoproliferative small intestinal disease-related, 366
Maldigestion, as diarrhea cause, 479, 484, 485
Mallory's bodies, 233, 250, 297
Mallory-Weiss tears, 444, 520
Malnutrition
  biliopancreatic diversion-related, 721
  definition of, 511
  focal fatty liver associated with, 219
MALT (mucosal-associated lymphoid tumor), 87, 90, 95, 100, 102–104
Manganese, deficiency or toxicity of, 514
Manometry
  for achalasia diagnosis, 45
  anorectal, 414, 418–419
  esophageal, 23, 674, 678–679
  of sphincter of Oddi, 326–327, 328
Marasmus, 511
Mastocytosis, 100, 484
Mauriac's syndrome, 252
McBurney's point, 431
Measles vaccine, 189
Meckel's diverticulum, 91, 432, 456, 462
Meclizine (Antivert), 520
Mefenamic acid, 364
Megacolon, toxic, 382, 384, 437, 474, 704
Megarectum, 415
MELD (Model for Endstage Liver Disease) score, 254, 255, 258, 277
Melena, 563
Ménétrièr's disease, 79, 80, 83, 100, 104–105
Menstruation, 385
6-Mercaptopurine (6-MP)
  as autoimmune hepatitis treatment, 174
  as Crohn's disease treatment, 374, 375
  use during pregnancy, 385
Mesalamine, 382, 385, 440
Mesenchymal tumors, hepatic, 214
Mesenteric circulation, 500–501
Mesenteric vascular disease, ischemic, 502–508
Mesenteric vein, occlusion or thrombosis of, 259, 504
Mestinon, 14
Metabolic disorders
  of bone
    post-liver transplantation, 265
    primary biliary cirrhosis-related, 181
    primary sclerosing cholangitis-related, 181

Metabolic disorders (*Continued*)
  hepatic, 123
  nausea and vomiting associated with, 519
Metastases
  gastric, 85
  hepatic, 214, 216
Metformin
  as diabetic diarrhea cause, 569
  as nonalcoholic fatty liver disease treatment, 251
Methimazole, hepatotoxicity of, 227
Methotrexate
  hepatotoxicity of, 224, 225–226, 252
  as microscopic colitis treatment, 440
  as reactive arthritis treatment, 555
Methoxyflurane, hepatotoxicity of, 229
Methylcellulose, 416
Methyldopa, hepatotoxicity of, 224, 228
Metoclopramide, 24, 115, 416, 520, 521, 522
  effect on esophageal sphincter pressures, 21
  effect on gastric emptying, 113
Metronidazole
  as amebiasis treatment, 285, 469, 598, 726
  as diabetic diarrhea treatment, 569
  as *Helicobacter pylori* infection treatment, 81, 95
  as pseudomembranous colitis treatment, 436, 438
Metropolitan Life Tables, 511
Microsatellite instability, 409
Microsporidiosis, 497–498
Migrating motor complex, 110
Milk thistle, 229
Milroy's disease, 364
Milwaukee Classification, 327–328
Mineral oil, hepatotoxicity of, 225
Minerals, deficiencies and toxicities of, 513–514
Mirizzi's syndrome, 322, 728, 738
Mitral valve prolapse, 312
Mittelschmerz, 432, 701
Molybdenum, deficiency or toxicity of, 514
Monoclonal antibodies, radiolabeled, 651
Monoethylglycinexylidide test, 119
Montelukast, 394
Morphine, as diarrhea treatment, 488, 489
Motility disorders, as bacterial overgrowth cause, 397, 398
Mucinous cystic neoplasms, 359
Mucosal-associated lymphoid tumor (MALT), 87, 90, 95, 100, 102–104
Mucosal resection
  high-frequency ultrasound probe-assisted endoscopic, 671
  rectal, 710
Müllerian duct, anomalies of, 210
Multichannel intraluminal impedance (MII), 22, 39
Multiple endocrine neoplasia (MEN) syndromes, 483, 570, 572, 706
Multiple hamartoma syndrome, 564–565
Münchhausen syndrome, 487
Münchhausen syndrome by proxy (Polle's syndrome), 487

Murphy's sign, 723
Muscle relaxants, effect on sphincter of Oddi
    manometry, 326
Myasthenia gravis, 14, 153
Mycobacterium avium-complex infections, 492, 498
Mycobacterium avium-intracellulare infections, 32,
    363, 470
Mycobacterium paratuberculosis infections, 372
Mycobacterium tuberculosis, identification of, on
    biopsy, 304
Mycobacterium tuberculosis infections, 32, 470
    as Crohn's disease mimic, 369
Mycophenolate, 174, 259, 260
MYH-associated polyposis (AMP), 409
Mycosis, 422
Myositis, focal, 153
Myotomy
    as achalasia treatment, 47, 48
    cricopharyngeal, 15, 16, 17, 75
    esophageal (Heller's)
        as achalasia treatment, 679, 680–681
        with fundoplication, 704

N
Naproxen, hepatotoxicity of, 224
Narcotics
    effect on sphincter of Oddi manometry, 326
    as pancreatitis-related pain treatment, 348
Nasogastric intubation
    in caustic ingestion injury patients, 67
    in upper gastrointestinal hemorrhage patients, 444
Natalizumab, 386
Nausea, 518–521
    Addison's disease-related, 573
    differential diagnosis of, 114
    gastroparesis-related, 111, 115, 116
    hepatitis-related, 127
    hypercalcemia-related, 571
Necrosis
    fat, 561–562
    pancreatic, 336–338
Needle biopsy. *See* Biopsy, fine-needle aspiration
Neonatal iron overload, 287
Nephrolithiasis
    chronic pancreatitis-related, 348
    Crohn's disease-related, 373
Neuroendocrine tumors, as diarrhea cause, 482, 483,
    484
Neurofibroma, 105
Neurologic disorders, as gastroparesis cause, 113
Neuropathy, peripheral, 153
Neutropenia, 153
Niacin. *See* Vitamin B$_3$
Nifedipine
    as achalasia treatment, 46
    hepatotoxicity of, 227, 249
    as hiccups treatment, 522
Nitrates, as achalasia treatment, 46
Nitrofurantoin, hepatotoxicity of, 224, 225, 228, 302

Nitroglycerin ointment, 711
Nocardiosis, 304
Nodules, Sister Mary Joseph's, 565
Nonocclusive mesenteric ischemia (NOMI), 504,
    507, 508
Nonsteroidal anti-inflammatory drugs
    adverse effects of
        diarrhea, 487
        diverticulitis, 425
        enteropathy, 363–364
        esophageal injury, 56, 58
        gastric injury, 58
        gastric ulcer, 94, 95, 690, 691
        gastritis, 79, 80–81, 82
        gastrointestinal hemorrhage, 443, 444–445, 447
        microscopic colitis, 439, 440
        pancreatitis, 331
        pill-induced esophageal injury, 56
    as enteropathic arthritis treatment, 551
    as esophageal cancer prophylaxis, 54
    as gastritis treatment, 81
    as reactive arthritis treatment, 555
Norfloxacin, 274
Norwalk-like viruses, 473
Nuclear medicine studies, **637–652**
    cholescintigraphy, 637, 638, 639–642
    of esophageal motility, 643–644
    of gastric emptying, 638, 642–643
    radiopharmaceuticals in, 651
Nucleic acid assays, for hepatitis C, 131
Nucleoside analogs, hepatotoxicity of, 252
Nutritional assessment and therapy, **511–517**
    for acute pancreatitis patients, 338
Nutritional status, definition of, 511
Nutritional support, in Crohn's disease patients, 377

O
Obesity, 515–516, **718–722**
    corticosteroids-related, 168
    definition of, 515, 718
    as esophageal adenocarcinoma risk factor, 69
    as gallstones risk factor, 318
    as gastroparesis risk factor, 113
    morbid, surgical treatment for, 515–516, 571,
        719–722, 735–736
    as nonalcoholic fatty liver disease risk factor, 247,
        248–249, 251
Obstructive sleep apnea, gastroesophageal reflux
    disease associated with, 26
Obturator sign, 431, 701
Octreotide
    as bacterial overgrowth therapy, 399
    as chronic diarrhea treatment, 488, 489
    as diabetic diarrhea treatment, 569
    as dumping syndrome treatment, 695
    gallbladder disease associated with, 318
    as gastrointestinal hemorrhage treatment, 446
    as short bowel syndrome treatment, 512
    use in scleroderma patients, 364, 521

Odynophagia, 520
  definition of, 19
  gastrointestinal reflux disease-related, 19
  infectious esophagitis-related, 29
Ogilvie's syndrome, 704, 715
OKT3, 260
  toxicity of, 263, 264
Olestra, 361
Omeprazole (Prilosec), 24, 28, 95
Ondansetron, 520, 521
Opiates/opioids
  contraindication in ulcerative colitis, 386
  as diarrhea treatment, 488, 489
Oral contraceptives
  focal nodular hyperplasia-exacerbating effects
      of, 216
  as gallbladder disease cause, 318
  as hepatic adenoma cause, 215–216
  hepatotoxicity of, 224, 225, 227
  as recurrent Crohn's disease cause, 372–373
Oral diets, 511–512
Oral rehydration solution, 473
Organ donation, 255
Oropharynx, comparison with the esophagus, 15
Osler, William, 34
Osler-Weber-Rendu disease, 453, 455
Osmotic gap, fecal, 479, 481
Osteoma, 564
Osteomalacia, 210, 558
  bacterial overgrowth-related, 398
  celiac disease-related, 557
  hemochromatosis-related, 213
  primary biliary cirrhosis-related, 210
Osteopenia, post-liver transplantation, 265
Osteoporosis
  corticosteroids-related, 168
  gastric bypass-related, 720
  hemochromatosis-related, 213
  inflammatory bowel disease-related, 552
  liver transplantation-related, 264
  primary biliary cirrhosis-related, 210
Ovarian cancer
  adenocarcinoma, 356
  appendectomy in, 434
Overweight, 718
Oxacillin, hepatotoxicity of, 225
Oxyphenisatin, hepatotoxicity of, 224

P
Paget's disease, perianal, 712, 714
PAIN mnemonic, for inflammatory bowel
    disease-related arthritis, 548
Palliative care, for pancreatic cancer patients,
    354
Palpation, abdominal, 701
Pancreas
  aberrant, 105, 106, 659
  abscess of, 358
  cysts of, **356–360**

Pancreas (*Continued*)
    endoscopic ultrasound-guided biopsy of,
        666–667
  endocrine tumors of, 572–574
  endosonographic anatomy of, 654–655
  percutaneous procedures in, 599–600
  pseudocysts of, 311, 339–340, 347, 356–357
    complications of, 339–340
    drainage of, 339
    endoscopic ultrasound-guided biopsy of, 665,
        668–669, 670
    endosonographic evaluation of, 660
    treatment of, 703
Pancreas cancer, **352–355**
  adenocarcinoma, 347, 352, 356
    of the pancreatic head, 586, 588, 589
  cystic, 356
  "double-duct sign" of, 353
  endoscopic ultrasound-guided biopsy of, 666–667
  endosonographic evaluation of, 658–659
  fine-needle aspiration of, 599, 600
  as hepatic abscess cause, 282
  imaging of, 353
  intraductal papillary-mucinous, 352
  as jaundice cause, 727
  metastatic, 216, 356
  Schmidt's triad of, 555
Pancreas divisum, 332, 589, 590
Pancreas-kidney transplantation, 116
Pancreatic duct
  endoscopic ultrasound-guided drainage of,
      670–671
  obstruction of, 589, 590
  prophylactic stenting of, 329
Pancreatic enzymes
  in chronic pancreatitis, 344
  as pancreatitis treatment, 348
Pancreatic exocrine deficiency, 485, 569
Pancreatic head, cancer of, 586, 588, 589
Pancreatic insufficiency, 361–362, 558
Pancreaticobiliary junction, anomalous, 311, 312
Pancreatic rest, 105, 107
Pancreatitis
  acute, **331–341**
    acute fluid collections associated with, 339, 356
    biliary, 334
    hypercalcemia-related, 332
    hypertriglyceridemia-related, 332
    metabolic causes of, 568
    NO IDEA mnemonic for, 331
    nutritional support in, 338, 512, 515
    pancreatic pseudocyst-related, 356–357
    prognostic scoring systems for, 334–335
    surgical treatment of, 703
  alcoholic, 331, 338, 342, 562
  autoimmune, 343
  chronic, **342–351**, 589
    endosonographic evaluation of, 662
    idiopathic, 343–344

Pancreatitis (*Continued*)
    obstructive, 343
        sphincter of Oddi manometry-related, 326
    core biopsy-related, 599
    cutaneous manifestations of, 561–562
    differentiated from pancreatic head cancer, 586,
        588, 589
    endoscopic retrograde cholangiopancreatography-
        related, 326–327, 329
    endosonographic evaluation of, 661–62, 662
    eosinophilic gastroenteritis-related, 393
    exocrine function measurement in, 344–345
    gallbladder sludge-related, 318
    grading of, 346
    hereditary, 342–343, 353
    in HIV-infected patients, 493
    hypercalcemia-related, 571
    idiopathic recurrent, 661
    interstitial, 334
    in lung transplant recipients, 600
    necrotizing, 334
    radiographic evaluation of, 506
    tropical, 343
Pancreatography, endoscopic retrograde, 332
Pancreolauryl test, 345
Panhypopituitarism, 483
Panniculitis, 560
    hemorrhagic, 561
    pancreatic, 557–558
Pantoprazole, 24, 95
Pantothenic acid, 514
Paracentesis, 273–274
    diagnostic, 268–269
    large-volume, 276
Parasites, detection in stool, 469–470
Parasitic infections
    as AIDS-related diarrhea cause, 497–498
    diagnosis of, 388
    as eosinophilic gastroenteritis cause, 388, 389,
        394
    as gastrointestinal hemorrhage cause, 454–455
    hepatic, 725–726
Parathyroid gland, in Wermer syndrome, 572
Parenteral nutrition, 512
Parkinson's disease, dysphagia associated with,
    16, 17
Partial thromboplastin time (PTT), assessment
    prior to percutaneous procedures, 592
Paterson-Brown-Kelly syndrome, 73
Pathergy, 561
PCR (polymerase chain reaction) assays, 130,
    131
Pellagra, 513
Pelvic inflammatory disease, 432
Penetrating trauma, abdominal, 702
Penicillin, hepatotoxicity of, 225, 228
Pentamidine, as pancreatitis cause, 331
Pentoxifylline, as alcoholic hepatitis treatment,
    233

Peptic ulcers, 432
    as gastric outlet obstruction cause, 693–694
    as gastroesophageal reflux disease mimic, 21
    as gastrointestinal hemorrhage cause, 693, 703
    as gastroparesis cause, 111
    Helicobacter pylori-related, **90–97**
    hypercalcemia-related, 571
    medical treatment for, intractability in, 687
    perforated, 691, 692, 702–703
    rebleeding in, 693
    surgical treatment of, **687–699**, 702–703
        antrectomy, 687, 694
Peptide receptors, radioactive, 651
Peptide-secreting tumors, 483–484
Pepto-Bismol. *See* Bismuth subsalicylate
Peptostreptococcus infections, 282
Percutaneous procedures
    complications of, 595
    contraindicated, 597–598
    image-guided, 591–595
    pancreatic, 599–600
    renal and perinephric, 601–602
    splenic, 598–599
Percutaneous transhepatic biliary drainage, 603–605
Perhexiline maleate, hepatotoxicity of, 224
Pericarditis, 153, 365
Periodic acid-Schiff-diastase stain, 292
Peritoneal signs, 700–701
Peritoneum, 700–701
Peritonitis, 700–701
    diverticulitis-related, 426
    eosinophilic, 392
    spontaneous bacterial, 269, 271–274
        differentiated from secondary peritonitis, 271
Peutz-Jeghers syndrome, 107, 405–406, 407, 453,
    563–564, 706
Peyer's patches, 551
Phenobarbital
    hepatotoxicity of, 227
    interaction with tacrolimus and cyclosporine, 261
    as intrahepatic cholestasis of pregnancy treatment,
        197
Phenothiazines, 520
Phenylbutazone, hepatotoxicity of, 224, 225
Phenytoin
    hepatotoxicity of, 223–224, 225, 227
    interaction with tacrolimus and cyclosporine, 261
Pheochromocytoma, 483, 484, 574, 601
Phlebotomy
    as hemochromatic arthropathy treatment, 213
    as hereditary hemochromatosis treatment, 290
pH monitoring, esophageal, 22, 23, 35–36, 39
Phosphorus, toxicity of, 514
Phosphorus deficiency, 514
Photocoagulation, as gastrointestinal hemorrhage
    treatment, 441
Phototherapy
    for esophageal cancer, 53, 54
    for pruritus, 183

Phytobezoars, 116, 715
Pill-induced injury, esophageal, 56–59
Piroxicam, hepatotoxicity of, 225
Plesiomonas infections, 465, 471
Pleural effusions
    pancreatic, 348
    pancreatitis-related, 336
Pleuritis, 153
Pneumatic dilation, of the lower esophageal
        sphincter, 48
Pneumatosis intestinalis, 506, 576–577, 578
Pneumobilia, 506
Pneumocolon, peroral, 584
Pneumocystis carinii pneumonia, 265, 383
Pneumonia
    Pneumocystis carinii, 265, 383
    presenting as acute abdomen, 576
Pneumoperitoneum, 733–735
Poliomyelitis, childhood, as dysphagia cause, 14
Polle's syndrome, 487
Polyarteritis nodosa, 207–208, 390, 464
Polyarthritis-dermatitis syndrome, 207
Polycystic liver disease, 312–313
    differentiated from simple hepatic cysts, 725
Polyenylphosphatidylcholine, as alcoholic hepatitis
        treatment, 233
Polyethylene glycol (PEG) interferon, 133, 137–138,
        139, 141–142, 145
Polymerase chain reaction (PCR) assay, 129, 130,
        143
Polymorphonuclear neutrophil count, in spontaneous
        bacterial peritonitis, 273
Polymyositis, 390
Polypectomy, 106–107
Polyposis, 706–710
    familial, 107
        adenomatous, 107, 706–708
    juvenile, 706
Polyps
    cholesterol, 321
    colonic, 384, 401–402, 405, 542, 543
        adenomatous, 544
    Cowden's disease-related, 564–565
    esophageal fibrovascular, 659, 660
    of gallbladder wall, 321–322
    Gardner's syndrome-related, 564
    gastric, 98–100, 106–107, 541
    intestinal, 706–710
        types of, 706
    Peutz-Jeghers syndrome-related, 564
Porphyria, variegated, 562
Porphyria cutanea tarda, 208
Portal vein, 236, 237, 238
    gas in, 432
    thrombosis of, 242, 259, 262
Positron emission tomography (PET), of focal liver
        masses, 219
Postcholecystectomy syndrome, 325, 728
Postpolio syndrome, 14

Potassium deficiency, 520
Pouchitis, 386, 550, 552, 710
Prednisone
    as autoimmune hepatitis treatment, 166, 167,
        170–171, 172
    as caustic ingestion treatment, 65
    use in liver transplant recipients, 259, 260
Preeclampsia, 198, 199
Pregnancy
    abdominal pain during, 461–462
    appendectomy during, 433–434
    ectopic, 432
        as abdominal pain cause, 461–462
    gallstone formation during, 317
    heartburn during, 19
    hepatitis during, 200, 201
    laparoscopic cholecystectomy during, 738
    in liver transplant recipients, 202–203
    pancreatitis during, 331
    ruptured tubal, 462
    ulcerative colitis treatment during, 385
Probiotic therapy
    for bacterial overgrowth, 400
    for ulcerative colitis, 386
Procainamide, hepatotoxicity of, 227
Proctitis, 382–383, 470
    herpes simplex virus-related, 494
    radiation-related, 441, 717
Proctocolectomy, 185, 543, 708
Proctography, evacuation, 584–585
Proctosigmoiditis, 380, 382–383
Proglottids, 313
Prokinetic agents, 24, 416, 568
    as bacterial overgrowth treatment, 399
    as chronic constipation treatment, 416
    as gastroesophageal reflux disease treatment, 24
    as gastroparesis treatment, 115, 568
Prolactinoma, 572
Promethazine (Phenergan), 520
Propofol, as "hidden" source of calories, 512
Propylthiouracil
    as alcoholic hepatitis treatment, 233
    hepatotoxicity of, 227
Protein
    ascitic fluid content of, 269
    dietary, effect on esophageal sphincter pressures,
        21
Protein deficiency, 511
Proteus infections, 282, 337, 427, 723
Prothrombin time (PT), 119
    assessment prior to percutaneous procedures, 592
Proton pump inhibitors, 23, 29–30, 691
    as Barrett's esophagus treatment, 70
    effect on *Helicobacter pylori* test results, 92–93
    empiric trials of, 27
    gastric polyp-promoting effects of, 100
    as gastritis treatment, 81
    as gastroesophageal reflux disease treatment,
        23, 24

Proton pump inhibitors (*Continued*)
  as *Helicobacter pylori* infection treatment, 79, 80, 81–82, 95
  metabolism of, 27
Provocation testing, esophageal, 38–39
Pruritus, 183, 197, 560, 562
Pseudoachalasia, 45, 46, 678
Pseudoaneurysms, pancreatic, 347
  as hemorrhage cause, 358
  pancreatic pseudocyst-related, 400
  pancreatitis-related, 336
Pseudocysts, pancreatic, 311, 339–340, 347, 356–357
  complications of, 339–340
  drainage of, 339
  endoscopic ultrasound-guided biopsy of, 665, 668–669, 670
  endosonographic evaluation of, 660
  treatment for, 703
Pseudodiverticulosis, intramural, 77
Pseudomonas aeruginosa infections, 426, 427, 723
Pseudomonas infections, 282, 337
Pseudo-obstruction
  colonic, 715
  intestinal, 397, 519
Pseudopapillary-solid epithelial neoplasm (PSEN), 356
Pseudoxanthoma elasticum, 563
Psoas sign, 431, 701
Pudendal nerve terminal motor assessment (PNTML), 419
Pulmonary aspiration studies, 644
Pulmonary function tests, postoperative, 737
Purpura, idiopathic thrombocytopenic, 153
Pylephlebitis, radiographic evaluation of, 506
Pyloroplasty, 692–693
  as bile reflux gastritis cause, 83
  Finney, 688, 689, 694
  Heineke-Mikulicz, 688, 689
Pyoderma gangrenosum, 153, 380–381, 548, 561, 708
Pyridoxine. *See* Vitamin B$_6$
Pyrimethamine-sulfadoxine, hepatotoxicity of, 228

Q
Q fever, 304
Quinidine
  as gastroesophageal reflux disease cause, 19
  as esophageal injury cause, 57
  hepatotoxicity of, 224, 225, 227
Quinine, hepatotoxicity of, 225
Quinolones, 95, 274, 569

R
Rabeprazole, 24, 95
Rabies immunoglobulin, 189
Racecadotril (acetorphan), 489

Radiation therapy, adverse effects of
  colitis, 440–441
  diarrhea, 486
  enteritis, 716
  gastroparesis, 112
  proctitis, 441, 717
Radiofrequency ablation, of hepatocellular carcinoma, 218
Radiology
  abdominal, 575–579
  interventional, **591–602**
    fluoroscopic and angiographic procedures, **603–611**
    hepatic interventions, 596–598
    image-guided interventions, 591–595
    pancreatic interventions, 599–600
    renal and perinephric interventions, 601–602
    splenic interventions, 598–599
Radiopharmaceuticals, 651
Ranitidine, 24
  hepatotoxicity of, 224
Ranson's Criteria, for pancreatitis prognosis, 334
Rapamycin, as autoimmune hepatitis treatment, 174
Raynaud's disease, 210
Rectal cancer, endosonographic evaluation of, 659
Rectal prolapse, 712, 714
Rectocele, 415, 585
Rectum, carcinoid tumors of, 573
Red blood cell transfusions, as iron overload cause, 287
Regurgitation
  differentiated from vomiting, 518
  gastroesophageal reflux disease-related, 19, 20
  Zenker's diverticulum-related, 75
Reiter's syndrome, 473–474, 553
Renal cancer, metastatic, 216
Renal cell carcinoma, 359
Renal failure, pancreatitis-related, 336
Renal masses, biopsies of, 601
Reperfusion injury, 508
Respiratory orphan (REO) virus, 177
Retinopathy, Purtscher's, 337
Retroperitoneum, endosonographic anatomy of, 654–655
Revascularization, as abdominal angina treatment, 508–509
Reynold's pentad, 728
Rheumatoid arthritis, 153, 210, 552
  comparison with
    hemochromatic arthropathy, 212
    primary biliary cirrhosis-related arthritis, 210
Rheumatoid factor, 208
Rheumatologic disorders
  gastrointestinal disease-related, **547–558**
    enteropathic arthritis, 547–552, 554
    reactive arthritis, 552–555
    Whipple's disease, 555–557
  gastroparesis associated with, 112
  hepatobiliary disease-related, **207–213**

Ribavirin, 133, 137, 265
  in combination with interferon therapy, 139
    nonresponse to, 141–142
    side effects of, 139–140
Riboflavin. *See* Vitamin B$_2$
Rickets, 513
Rifabutin, as *Helicobacter pylori* infection treatment, 95
Rifampin, 183
  hepatotoxicity of, 228
  interaction with tacrolimus and cyclosporine, 261
Right lower quadrant pain, 431
Rings, esophageal, 56, 73–74
Rituximab, 209
Rome Committee, 531
Rosiglitazone, hepatotoxicity of, 226
Rotavirus, as gastroenteritis cause, 473
Roux-en-Y gastric bypass, 111, 695, 696, 719–720, 721
Roux-en-Y reconstruction, after antrectomy, 687
Roux stasis syndrome, 111
Rovsing's sign, 431, 701
Rumack-Matthew nomogram, 223
Rumination, 525
Ruvalcaba-Myhre-Smith syndrome, 706

S
Saccharomyces boulardii, as bacterial overgrowth therapy, 400
Sacroiliitis, 549, 550, 551, 554, 556
Saliva production, in gastroesophageal reflux disease, 20
Salmonella infections
  in AIDS patients, 470, 495, 496, 498
  as diarrhea cause, 471
  as dysentery cause, 465, 471
  as proctitis cause, 494
  as reactive arthritis cause, 552, 553, 555
  as Reiter's syndrome cause, 473, 553
  as traveler's diarrhea cause, 472
Salmonella species, classification of, 467
Sandifer's syndrome, 20
Sarcoidosis, 100
Sarcoma
  Kaposi's, 100, 463–464, 492
  uterine, 211
Scalpels, harmonic, 731
Schatzki's ring, 73, 74
Schilling's test, 366, 638, 645–647
Schistosomiasis, 469
Schmidt's triad, 555
Schwannoma, 105
Scintigraphy
  esophageal, 23
  gastric, 114
  hepatoiminodiacetic acid (HIDA), 461, 518, 732
Scleroderma, 210, 212, 390
  differentiated from achalasia, 581, 582
  as esophageal clearance defect cause, 20

Scleroderma (*Continued*)
  as gastroparesis cause, 113
  intestinal motility in, 399
  as small bowel dysfunction cause, 364
Scopolamine, 520, 521
Scurvy, 513
Secretin test, 344, 485
Secrets, Top 100, **1–9**
Seldinger technique, 595
Selective intestinal decontamination (SID), 274
Selective serotonin reuptake inhibitors, 535
Selenium, deficiency or toxicity of, 514
Sentinel fold, 100
SEN-V virus, 132
Serositis, pancreatic panniculitis syndrome-related, 557–558
Serotonin, in irritable bowel syndrome, 535–536
Serotonin agonists, 416
  as chronic constipation cause, 416
  as irritable bowel syndrome treatment, 535, 536
Serratia infections, 282
Serum-ascites albumin gradient (SAAG), 270
Setons, 713
Shigella infections
  as AIDS-related enterocolitis cause, 494
  as diarrhea cause, 465–466, 467, 471, 472, 473
  in AIDS patients, 495, 496, 498
  as reactive arthritis cause, 552, 553–554, 555
  as Reiter's syndrome cause, 553–554
Short bowel syndrome, 248, 366, 512
Shunts
  peritoneovenous, 277
  patency assessment of, 649
  right-to-left, 336
  transjugular intrahepatic portosystemic (TIPS), 184, 239, 277, 607–610
Sigmoidoscopy
  for colorectal cancer screening, 405
  flexible, 474–475
  for intestinal ischemia evaluation, 507
Sildenafil (Viagra), as achalasia treatment, 47, 679
Sipple's syndrome, 483
Sirolimus, 260
Sister Mary Joseph's nodule, 565
Sitzmarks, 414
Sjögren-like syndrome, 208
Sjögren's syndrome, 20, 153, 177, 178, 210, 212
Skin cancer, post-liver transplantation, 264
Skin pigmentation, in hereditary hemochromatosis patients, 289
Skin tags, perianal, Crohn's disease-related, 368
Sleep, swallowing during, 20
Small bowel enema (enteroclysis), 455, 583–585
Small bowel follow-through (SBFT) examination, 583–584, 585
Small intestine. *See also* Duodenum; Duodenal ulcers
  bacterial overgrowth of, 397–398
  cancer/tumors of
    Crohn's disease-related, 373

Small intestine (*Continued*)
    endoscopic screening and surveillance of,
        541–542
    carcinoid tumors of, 573
    dysmotility of, 519–520
    electrocautery-related injury to, 732–733
    ischemia of, 703
    obstruction of, 716
        differentiated from postoperative ileus, 716
        mechanical, 576, 577
        nausea and vomiting associated with, 519
        radiographic evaluation of, 506
Smoking
    as Crohn's disease cause, 371–373
    drug-induced hepatotoxicity-potentiating effect of,
        227
    as esophageal cancer cause, 51, 681
    negative correlation with ulcerative colitis, 379
    as pancreatic cancer cause, 352
Smooth muscle relaxants, as achalasia treatment,
    679
Sodium restriction, as cirrhosis-related ascites
    treatment, 275, 276
Soluble liver antigen (SLA), 123, 124
Somatostatin, as pancreatitis-related pain treatment,
    348
Somatostatin analogs, 573
Somatostatinoma, 484, 572
Sorbitol, 419, 569
Spastic pelvic floor syndrome, 415
Sphincter of Oddi
    anatomy of, 324
    dysfunction of, 44, **324–330**
        cholescintigraphic diagnosis of, 641
Sphincterotomy, 328, 329, 415, 711
    endoscopic, 320, 349
Spinal cord injury, gallbladder disease associated
    with, 317
Spine, arthritis of, 548–549, 550, 552, 554
Splanchnic circulation, 501
Splanchnicectomy, chemical, 354
Spleen
    abscess of, 599
    percutaneous interventions in, 598–599
Splenectomy, 108
Splenic tissue, accessory, 647–648
Splenic vein, thrombosis of, 107, 347
Splenosis, 647–648
Spondylitis, 549, 551, 554, 556
    ankylosing, 380–381, 552
Sprue
    celiac. *See* Celiac disease
    tropical, 365
Squamous cell carcinoma
    cutaneous, 264
    esophageal, 51, 54, 74–75, 681
    hypopharyngeal, 73
Stack sign, 661
Staphylococcus aureus infections, 472

Staphylococcus infections, 282, 337
Statins
    hepatotoxicity of, 227
    use by nonalcoholic fatty liver disease patients,
        250
Steatohepatitis, 250
    alcoholic, 247
    nonalcoholic (NASH), 245, 298–299
        differentiated from autoimmune hepatitis, 152
Steatorrhea, 344, 365
    abdominal angina-related, 508
    bacterial overgrowth-related, 398
    intestinal ischemia-related, 505
Steatosis, 232, 233, 245, 248
Stenting
    for abdominal angina management, 508
Stents
    esophageal, 54, 66
    metallic, as biliary obstruction treatment, 605–606
    palliative
        in pancreatic cancer, 354
Steroids
    anabolic, hepatotoxicity of, 224, 225
    as Crohn's disease treatment, 374
    as microscopic colitis treatment, 440
Stomach
    carcinoid tumors of, 572
    electric pacesetter in, 110
    foreign bodies in, 529
    gastroparesis of, **110–117**
    large/thickened folds in, 100–106
    polyps of, 98–100, 541
    submucosal masses in, 105–106
    "watermelon," 108, 456, 457
Stomach cancer. *See* Gastric cancer
Stomatitis, aphthous, 548
Stool, leukocytes in, 465–466
Stool tests
    for fat malabsorption, 361
    fecal occult blood test (FOBT), 405, 453–454
    for *Helicobacter pylori* infections, 92
    for leukocyte content, 466
    for parasite detection, 469–470
Streptococcus bovis infections, 410
Streptococcus faecalis infections, 723
Streptococcus infections, 282, 337
Streptococcus milleri abscess, 596
Stress
    as gastritis cause, 81
    as gastroparesis cause, 113
    as irritable bowel syndrome cause, 533, 534
    as ulcerative colitis cause, 385
Strictures
    bacterial, 181–182
    biliary, 178, 179–180, 184, 262, 588, 727
    bowel, radiation-related, 441
    diverticular, 425
    esophageal, 25, 56, 59, 60–61, 63, 65, 77
Stroke, as oropharyngeal dysphagia cause, 14

Stromal tumors, gastrointestinal (GISTs), 85, 105–106, 107
Submucosal tumors
endoscopic ultrasound-assisted resection of, 671–672
endosonographic evaluation of, 659–661
Sucralfate, 24
Sulfa drugs, hepatotoxicity of, 262
Sulfasalazine, 381–382, 383
as enteropathic arthritis treatment, 551, 552
as microscopic colitis treatment, 440
as reactive arthritis treatment, 555
side effects of, 382, 386
Sulfonamides, hepatotoxicity of, 224, 225, 228
Sulfonylureas, hepatotoxicity of, 226
Sulindac, hepatotoxicity of, 224, 225
Suplatest tosilate, 394
Surgery
in the acute abdomen, **700–705**
colorectal, **706–717**
esophageal, **673–686**
gastric, as gastroparesis cause, 112, 113
hepatobiliary, **723–729**
for peptic ulcer disease, **687–699**
Swallowing
disorders of, **11-18**. *See also* Dysphagia
in gastroesophageal reflux disease, 20
sensory cues in, 11
Swallowing studies, 580–582
Swallowing therapy, 16
Synovitis, 153
Syphilis, 100
Systemic lupus erythematosus, 153, 464
comparison with type I autoimmune hepatitis, 209

T

TACE (hepatic transarterial chemoembolization), 219, 603, 604
Tachygastria, 113
Tacrolimus, 259, 260
as autoimmune hepatitis treatment, 174
drug interactions of, 261
fetal effects of, 203
hepatotoxicity of, 262
neurotoxicity of, 260
Tamoxifen, hepatotoxicity of, 224, 227, 249, 252
Tapeworms, 725–726
Target sign, 336
T-cell vaccination, as autoimmune hepatitis treatment, 175
Technetium-99m studies, 637, 638, 639, 642, 643–644, 645–646, 647, 648–649–650
Tegaserod, 25, 115, 416, 536
Telangiectasia
facial or oral, 453
hereditary hemorrhagic, 563
Tenofovir, 145
Tensilon, 14

Tetracyclines, 19, 81
as diabetic diarrhea treatment, 569
as esophageal injury cause, 57, 58
hepatotoxicity of, 223, 224, 228
Theophylline, 40–41
Thiamine. *See* Vitamin B$_1$
Thiazolidinediones
hepatotoxicity of, 226
as nonalcoholic fatty liver disease treatment, 251
Thiourea derivatives, hepatotoxicity of, 227
Thoracocentesis, for pleural hydrothorax diagnosis, 269–270
Thoracotomy, as pill-induced esophageal injury risk factor, 56
Thorium oxide (Thorotrast), hepatotoxicity of, 224, 225
Thromboembolism, irritable bowel disease-related, 381
Thrombosis, as ischemic bowel disease risk factor, 503, 504, 505
Thyroid cancer, 571
medullary, 483, 484, 574
Thyroid disease, Cowden's syndrome-related, 564–565
Thyroiditis, 552
autoimmune (Hashimoto's disease), 153, 210, 567
Thyrotoxicosis, 567–568
Ticrynafen, hepatotoxicity of, 227
Tietze's syndrome, 34
Tissue transglutaminase, 362
Tolazamide, hepatotoxicity of, 226
Tolbutamide, hepatotoxicity of, 225, 226
Top 100 Secrets, **1–9**
Total iron-binding capacity (TIBC), 122, 289, 304
Total parenteral nutrition (TPN)
in caustic ingestion injury patients, 67
in Crohn's disease patients, 377
gallbladder disease associated with, 318
Toxic oil syndrome, 224
Transaminases, 120, 124. *See also* Alanine aminotransferase; Aspartate aminotransferase
Transferrin
as nonalcoholic fatty liver disease marker, 245
serum levels of, 289
Transjugular intrahepatic portosystemic shunt (TIPS), 184, 202, 239, 277, 607–610
Trauma
abdominal, 702
as pancreatitis cause, 332
Trazodone, hepatotoxicity of, 224
Trichilemmoma, 564
Trichobezoar, 715
Trichophytobezoar, 715
Trimethoprim/sulfamethoxazole, 265, 274, 427, 471
hepatotoxicity of, 224
Triple-A syndrome, 44
Troglitazone, hepatotoxicity of, 226
Tropheryma whippelii, as Whipple's disease cause, 363

Trophozoites, 469–470
Trousseau's sign, 565
Trypanosoma cruzi infections, 32, 112
Trypsinogen, in chronic pancreatitis, 345
L-Tryptophan, as eosinophilia-myalgia syndrome
    cause, 389
TT virus, 132
Tuberculosis, esophageal, 32
Tularemia, 304
Tumor seeding, 667
Tylosis, 540
Typhoid fever, 467

U

Ulcers. *See also* Duodenal ulcers; Gastric ulcers;
    Peptic ulcers
    antral, eosinophilic gastritis-related, 83–84
    aphthous, Crohn's disease-related, 369, 371, 376
    Dieulafoy's, 456
    esophageal, 31
        AIDS-related, 492
        idiopathic, 32
    marginal, 720
    visible vessels of, 446
Ultrasonography
    for abdominal pain evaluation, 461, 462
    for acute abdomen evaluation, 701–702
    for appendicitis evaluation, 433, 462
    of biliary sludge, 318
    of diverticulitis, 424, 426
    Doppler, for intestinal ischemia evaluation,
        506–507
    endoscopic, **653–663**
        advanced, **664–672**
        with bile duct or pancreatic duct drainage,
            670–671
        for cancer diagnosis, 665–667
        with celiac plexus neurolysis/block, 665,
            669–670
        of cystic pancreatic lesions, 359–360
        of distal common bile duct obstruction, 348
        of esophageal cancer, 52
        for fecal incontinence evaluation, 419
        with fine-needle aspiration biopsies, 664–667
        of focal liver masses, 219
        for gastric cancer staging, 86
        of gastric wall bands, 100, 101
        indications for, 655
        intraluminal, 653
        of normal anatomy, 654–655
        with pancreatic fluid/pseudocyst drainage, 665,
            667–668, 670
        for pancreatitis diagnosis, 346
        for pseudo-achalasia evaluation, 46
        technical aspects of, 653
    of hepatic abscess, 283
    of hepatic masses, 215
    for interventional procedure guidance, 592, 593
    for jaundice evaluation, 728

Ultrasonography (*Continued*)
    of nonalcoholic fatty liver disease, 249
    for pancreatic cancer evaluation, 353
    of simple hepatic cysts, 313
    transabdominal
        for gallbladder disease evaluation, 320–321
        for pancreatitis evaluation, 345
Upper gastrointestinal (GI) series, 583
    for biliary colic evaluation, 732
Urea breath test, 92–93
Urethritis, Reiter's syndrome-related, 473
Urinalysis, for acute abdomen diagnosis, 701
Ursodeoxycholic acid, 172, 174, 182, 184–186, 197,
    381
Urticaria, 153
Uveitis, 380–381, 553
    acute anterior, 548

V

Vaccines, 96, 188
    hepatitis, **188–195**
Vaginitis, diverticulitis-related, 425
Vagotomy
    as diarrhea cause, 486
    as gastric atony cause, 111
    highly selective, 689, 692–693, 694
    selective, 688–689
    truncal, 687, 688, 690, 692–693, 694, 697
Valentino's sign, 432
Valganciclovir, 496
Valproic acid, hepatotoxicity of, 223, 224
Valvulae conniventes, 715
Vancomycin, as pseudomembranous colitis
    treatment, 436, 438
Varices
    endosonographic evaluation of, 660
    esophageal, 170, 196, 348, 560
    gastric, 100, 107–108, 336, 347, 348
    hemorrhagic, 107–108, 444, 445
        during pregnancy, 202
        transjugular intrahepatic portosystemic shunt
            treatment for, 202, 607–608, 610
Vascular disease, hepatic, **236–244**
Vascular medications, as esophageal injury cause, 57
Vasculitis
    lupus, 464
    polyarteritis nodosa-like, 208
    systemic syndromes of, 390
Vasoactive intestinal polypeptide-secreting tumors
    (VIPoma), 484, 572
Vasopressin (Pitressin), 606–607
Veno-occlusive disease, 240, 308
Ventricular tachycardia, carbon dioxide insufflation-
    related, 734–735
Verapamil
    as achalasia treatment, 46
    hepatotoxicity of, 227
    interaction with tacrolimus and cyclosporine,
        261

Verner-Morrison syndrome, 484
Very-low density lipoprotein (VLDL), 179
Vestibular disorders, nausea and vomiting
    associated with, 519
Viagra (sildenafil), as achalasia treatment, 679
Vibrio cholerae, 466, 472
Vibrio parahaemolyticus, 469
Vinyl chloride, hepatotoxicity of, 224, 225
VIPoma (vasoactive intestinal polypeptide-secreting
    tumor), 484, 572
Viral infections. *See also specific viruses*
    as gastritis cause, 79
    as pancreatitis cause, 332
Visceral hypersensitivity, 39–40
Visceral pain, 459
Visible vessels, 446
Visick's criteria, for peptic ulcer surgical outcome,
    694–695
Vitamin(s)
    deficiencies of, 513–514
      bacterial overgrowth-related, 398
      bariatric surgery-related, 720, 721
      of fat-soluble vitamins, 348, 516
      gastric bypass-related, 720
    toxicity of, 513–514
Vitamin A
    deficiency of, 183, 348, 513
    toxicity of, 513
Vitamin B$_1$
    deficiency of, 513, 571
    toxicity of, 513
Vitamin B$_2$
    deficiency of, 513
    toxicity of, 513
Vitamin B$_3$, toxicity of, 227
Vitamin B$_6$
    deficiency of, 513
    toxicity of, 513
Vitamin B$_{12}$
    deficiency of, 85, 514, 516, 571
      bacterial overgrowth-related, 398, 399
      bariatric surgery-related, 720, 721
    malabsorption of, 348, 364
      Schilling's test for, 638, 645–647
    toxicity of, 514
Vitamin C
    anticarcinogenicity of, 404
    deficiency of, 513
    toxicity of, 513
Vitamin D
    deficiency of, 181, 348, 513
    malabsorption of, 558
    toxicity of, 513
Vitamin E
    anticarcinogenicity of, 404
    deficiency of, 181, 183, 348, 513
    as nonalcoholic fatty liver disease treatment,
      251
    toxicity of, 513

Vitamin K
    deficiency of, 181, 183, 348, 513
      bacterial overgrowth-related, 398
    effect on prothrombin time, 119
    as intrahepatic cholestasis of pregnancy treatment,
      197
    toxicity of, 513
Vitiligo, 153
Vocal cord injuries, 20
Volume expanders, 276
Volvulus
    cecal, 714
      in elderly patients, 704
    radiographic evaluation of, 506
    sigmoid, 714–715
      in elderly patients, 704
Vomiting, 518–521
    Addison's disease-related, 573
    differential diagnosis of, 114
    differentiated from regurgitation, 518
    eating disorders-related, 524
    gastroparesis-related, 111, 115, 116
    hepatitis-related, 127
    hypercalcemia-related, 571
    psychogenic, 520
von Hippel-Lindau disease, 359
von Recklinghausen's disease, 706

W
Water, difficulty in swallowing of, 11, 16
Waterbrash, 19
Weber-Christian disease, 248, 252
Webs, esophageal, 73
Weight, desirable, 511
Weight loss
    achalasia-related, 44, 46
    Addison's disease-related, 573
    bacterial overgrowth-related, 398, 399
    chronic pancreatitis-related, 344
    Crohn's disease-related, 368
    as gastroesophageal reflux disease treatment, 23
    as nonalcoholic fatty liver disease treatment, 251
    rapid, as gallstone risk factor, 318
    surgical procedures for, 516, 571, 719–722
Werner's syndrome, 483, 572
Wernicke-Korsakoff syndrome, 513
Whipple, George Hoyt, 555
Whipple's disease, 112, 354, 363, 555–556
Whipple's triad, 570
White blood cell count, of ascitic fluid, 269
Willis, Thomas, 47
Wilson's disease, 123, 292–294, 305
    ceruloplasmin concentration in, 123, 136, 196,
      293–294, 305
    copper concentration in, 152, 305
    diagnosis of, 123
    fatty liver associated with, 252
    hepatitis C-associated, 136
    during pregnancy, 201, 202

X

Xerostomia, 16
X-rays
    abdominal
        for abdominal pain evaluation, 461
        for acute abdomen evaluation, 701, 702
        of large bowel obstruction, 715
    chest
        for achalasia evaluation, 677
        for liver abscess evaluation, 283
    of diverticulitis, 424
D-Xylose test, 361–362

Y

Yersinia infections, 369, 432, 465–466, 468, 471, 473–474, 485, 552–554, 555

Z

Zalcitabine, 492
Zenker's diverticulum, 15, 16, 74–75, 518, 527
Zidovudine, hepatotoxicity of, 224
Zinc, deficiency or toxicity of, 514
Zollinger-Ellison syndrome, 94, 100, 484, 572, 696
Zonula occludens toxin (ZOT), 472